G N R S

Geriatric Nursing Review Syllabus

A Core Curriculum in Advanced Practice
Geriatric Nursing

3rd Edition

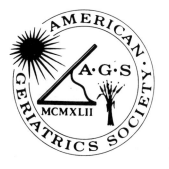

As new research and clinical experience broaden our knowledge of medicine, changes in treatment and drug therapy are required. This publication is intended only to facilitate the free flow of information of interest to the medical community involved in the care of older persons.

No responsibility is assumed by the editors or the American Geriatrics Society, as the Publisher, for any injury and/or damage to persons or property, as a matter of product liability, negligence, warranty, or otherwise, arising out of the use or application of any methods, products, instructions, or ideas contained herein. No guarantee, endorsement, or warranty of any kind, express or implied (including specifically no warranty of merchantability or of fitness for a particular purpose) is given by the Society in connection with any information contained herein. Independent verification of any diagnosis, treatment, or drug use or dosage should be obtained. No test or procedure should be performed unless, in the judgment of an independent qualified physician, it is justified in light of the risk involved.

Inclusion in this publication of product information does not constitute a guarantee, warranty, or endorsement by the American Geriatrics Society (the Publisher) of the quality, value, safety, effectiveness, or usefulness of any such product or of any claim made about such product by its manufacturer or an author.

The Chief Editors were Ellen Flaherty, PhD, RN, GNP-BC, and Barbara Resnick, PhD, CRNP, FAANP, FAAN; Editors were Carolyn Auerhahn, EdD, ANP, GNP-BC, FAANP, Marie Boltz, PhD, CRNP, Elizabeth Capezuti, PhD, RN, FAAN, and Elizabeth Galik, PhD, CRNP; Consulting Editor on Pharmacotherapy was Judith L. Beizer, PharmD, CGP, FASCP; Medical Writer was Susan E. Aiello, DVM, ELS; Indexer was L. Pilar Wyman; and Managing Editor was Andrea N. Sherman, MS.

Many thanks to Fry Communications for assistance with the production work including typesetting, graphic design, and printing. With more than 60 years in the information industry, Fry offers printing and ancillary services to publishers and other content providers.

Citation: Flaherty E, Resnick B, eds. *Geriatric Nursing Review Syllabus: A Core Curriculum in Advanced Practice Geriatric Nursing*. 3rd edition. New York: American Geriatrics Society; 2011.

Geriatric Nursing Review Syllabus: A Core Curriculum in Advanced Practice Geriatric Nursing. 3rd edition. Cataloging in publication data is available from the Library of Congress.

Library of Congress Control Number: 2011900981

ISBN Number: 978-1-886775-55-8

Printed in the United States of America

10 9 8 7 6 5 4 3 2 1

TABLE OF CONTENTS

SYNDROMES

GNRS3 EDITORIAL BOARD

ORIGINAL *GRS7* EDITORIAL BOARD AND AUTHORS

CO-EDITORS

James T. Pacala, MD, MS, AGSF

Gail M. Sullivan, MD, MPH, AGSF

SYLLABUS EDITORS
James T. Pacala, MD, MS, AGSF
Colleen Christmas, MD
G. Paul Eleazer, MD, AGSF
Anne Fabiny, MD
Melinda S. Lantz, MD
Annette Medina-Walpole MD, AGSF

SPECIAL ADVISORS
Samuel C. Durso, MD, MBA, AGSF
Michelle Eslami, MD

QUESTION EDITORS
Gail M. Sullivan, MD, MPH, AGSF
John D. Gazewood, MD, MSPH
C. Bree Johnston, MD, MPH
Gary J. Kennedy, MD

CONSULTING EDITOR FOR PHARMACOTHERAPY
Judith L. Beizer, PharmD, CGP, FASCP

CONSULTING EDITOR FOR ETHNOGERIATRICS
Carmel Bitondo Dyer, MD, AGSF

AUTHORS OF ORIGINAL *GRS7* CHAPTERS

CURRENT ISSUES IN AGING
Demography — Jennifer L. Wolff, PhD
Biology — Neal S. Fedarko, PhD
Psychosocial Issues — Kenneth W. Hepburn, PhD
Legal and Ethical Issues — Margaret A. Drickamer, MD
Financing, Coverage and Costs of Health Care — Chad Boult, MD, MPH, MBA
Richard G. Stefanacci, DO, MGH, MBA, AGSF, CMD

APPROACH TO PATIENT
Assessment — Thomas M. Gill, MD
Cultural Aspects of Care — Reva N. Adler, MD, MPH, FRCPC
Physical Activity — David M. Buchner, MD, MPH
Prevention — Mara A. Schonberg, MD, MPH
Pharmacotherapy — Todd P. Semla, MS, PharmD, BCPS, FCCP, AGSF
Complementary and Alternative Medicine — Marc R. Blackman, MD
Julie C. Chapman, PsyD
Mistreatment of Older Adults — Terry Fulmer, PhD, RN, FAAN, AGSF
Perioperative Care — Colleen Christmas, MD
James T. Pacala, MD, MS, AGSF
Palliative Care — Stacie T. Pinderhughes, MD
R. Sean Morrison, MD
Persistent Pain — Jennifer M. Kapo, MD

CARE SYSTEMS

Hospital Care

Rehabilitation
Nursing-Home Care

Community-Based Care

Outpatient Care Systems

William L. Lyons, MD
C. Seth Landefeld, MD
Cynthia J. Brown, MD, MSPH
Suzanne M. Gillespie, MD, RD
Paul R. Katz, MD
Robert McCann, MD, AGSF
G. Paul Eleazer, MD, FACP, AGSF
Steven R. Counsell, MD, AGSF

SYNDROMES

Frailty
Visual Impairment

Hearing Impairment
Dizziness
Syncope
Malnutrition

Eating and Feeding Problems
Urinary Incontinence
Gait Impairment
Falls

Osteoporosis

Dementia

Behavior Problems in Dementia

Delirium
Sleep Problems
Pressure Ulcers and Wound Care

Linda P. Fried, MD, MPH, AGSF
JoAnn Giaconi, MD
David Sarraf, MD
Anne L. Coleman, MD, PhD
Priscilla F. Bade, MD
Aman Nanda, MD
David Bush, MD
Gordon L. Jensen, MD, PhD
James Powers, MD
Paige E. Miller, MD
Colleen Christmas, MD
Catherine E. DuBeau, MD
Neil Alexander, MD
Sarah D. Berry, MD, MPH
Douglas P. Kiel, MD, MPH
Pamela Taxel, MD
Leen Bakkali, MD
Cynthia Barton, RN, MSN
Kristine Yaffe, MD
Melinda S. Lantz, MD
Ali Khanmohamadi, MD
Pui Yin Wong, MD
Edward R. Marcantonio, MD, SM
Cathy A. Alessi, MD, AGSF
Courtney H. Lyder, ND, GNP, FAAN

PSYCHIATRY

Depression and Other Mood Disorders
Anxiety Disorders

Psychotic Disorders
Personality and Somatoform Disorders
Addictions
Mental Retardation and Developmental Disabilities

Gary J. Kennedy, MD
Judith Neugroschl, MD
Amanda Itzkoff, MD
Susan W. Lehmann, MD
Marc E. Agronin, MD
David W. Oslin, MD
Mark H. Fleisher, MD

DISEASES AND DISORDERS

Dermatologic Diseases and Disorders

Oral Diseases and Disorders
Respiratory Diseases and Disorders

Cardiovascular Diseases and Disorders
Heart Failure
Hypertension
Gastrointestinal Diseases and Disorders

Sumaira Z. Aasi, MD
Jaehyuk Choi, MD, PhD
Kenneth Shay, DDS, MS
Margaret Pisani, MD
E. Wesley Ely, MD, MPH
Michael W. Rich, MD, AGSF
Michael W. Rich, MD, AGSF
Mark A. Supiano, MD, AGSF
George Triadafilopoulos, MD
Richard Sims, MD

Kidney Diseases and Disorders	Sanjeevkumar R. Patel, MD, MS
	Jocelyn E. Wiggins, MA, BM, BCh, MRCP
Gynecologic Diseases and Disorders	G. Willy Davila, MD
	Maria L. Diaz, MD
Prostate Disease	Lisa J. Granville, MD, AGSF
Disorders of Sexual Function	Angela Gentili, MD
	Thomas Mulligan, MD, AGSF
Musculoskeletal Diseases and Disorders	Shari M. Ling, MD
Back and Neck Pain	Leo M. Cooney, Jr, MD
Diseases and Disorders of the Foot	Alfred J. Phillips, DPM, FACFAS
	Douglas A. Albreski, DPM
Neurologic Diseases and Disorders	R. Charles Callison, MD
	Harold P. Adams, Jr., MD
Infectious Diseases	Kevin P. High, MD, MS, FACP
Endocrine and Metabolic Disorders	David A. Gruenewald, MD
	Anne M. Kenny, MD
	Alvin M. Matsumoto, MD
Diabetes Mellitus	Caroline S. Blaum, MD, MS
Hematologic Diseases and Disorders	Gurkamal S. Chatta, MD
Oncology	William B. Ershler, MD
	Dan L. Longo, MD

CONTRIBUTING QUESTION AUTHORS

Tara Aghaloo, DDS, MD, PhD
Douglas A. Albreski, DPM
Kathryn A. Atchison, DDS, MPH
R. Morgan Bain, MD
Rachelle Bernacki, MD, MS
Peter A. Boling, MD, AGSF
Rebecca Boxer, MD
Kenneth Brummel-Smith, MD, AGSF
Susan Charette, MD
Carl I. Cohen, MD
Leo M. Cooney, Jr., MD
Ann R. Datunashvili, MD
Michelle Eslami, MD
Helen M. Fernandez, MD
Mark H. Fleisher, MD
Gordana Gataric, MD
Angela Gentili, MD
Shelly L. Gray, PharmD, MS
Blaine S. Greenwald, MD
William R. Hazzard, MD, AGSF
Kevin P. High, MD, MS, FACP
Lyn M. Holley, PhD
Sam J. Holley, PhD
Michael S. Irwig, MD, FACE
Gail Ishiyama, MD
Jerry C. Johnson, MD, AGSF
Theodore M. Johnson II, MD, MPH
Bree Johnston, MD, MPH
Fran E. Kaiser, MD, AGSF, FGSA
Catherine McVearry Kelso, MD
Anne Kenny, MD
Mary B. King, MD
Steve Koenig, MD
George A. Kuchel, MD, FRCP, AGSF

Larry W. Lawhorne, MD
Eric Lenze, MD
Michael C. Lindberg, MD, FACP
Shari M. Ling, MD
Joanne Lynn, MD, MA, MS, AGSF
Bill Lyons, MD
Victoria Maizes, MD
Mathew S. Maurer, MD
Ellen M. McMahon, MD
Lynn McNicoll, MD
Daniel Ari Mendelson, MS, MD, FACP
Diana V. Messadi, DDS, MMSc, DMSc
Karin Ouchida, MD
Joseph G. Ouslander, MD, AGSF
Arash Naeim, MD, PhD
James T. Pacala, MD, MS, AGSF
Joe W. Ramsdell, MD
M. Carrington Reid, MD, PhD
Julie Robison, PhD
Mitchell H. Rosner, MD
Amy E. Sanders, MD
Alessandra Scalmati, MD
Gary J. Schiller, MD
Janice B. Schwartz, MD
Pushpendra Sharma, MD
David H. Stern, MD
Gwen K. Sterns, MD
Dennis H. Sullivan, MD, AGSF
Joe Verghese, MD, MS
Katie Ward, MD
Barbara E. Weinstein, PhD
Phyllis C. Zee, MD, PhD
Richard A. Zweig, PhD
Steven Zweig, MD, MSPH

ACKNOWLEDGMENTS

As the chief editors, it is our great pleasure to acknowledge the many people who have made the *Geriatric Nursing Review Syllabus: A Core Curriculum in Advanced Practice Geriatric Nursing, 3rd Edition (GNRS3)* possible. We express our gratitude to our Co-Editors: Carolyn Auerhahn, EdD, ANP, GNP-BC, FAANP; Marie Boltz, PhD, CRNP; Elizabeth Capezuti, PhD, RN, FAAN; and Elizabeth Galik, PhD, CRNP. All of them devoted long hours to the development of this program. We are thankful for the assistance from our Consulting Editor Judith L. Beizer, PharmD, CGP, FASCP. We especially thank the contributing *GRS7* authors of chapters and questions for lending us their expertise to this publication.

We thank Andrea Sherman, MS, GRS Managing Editor, for her guidance, organization, and coordination overseeing the administrative, editorial, and distribution aspects of the program. Thanks also to Susan E. Aiello, DVM, ELS, our medical writer, and to L. Pilar Wyman for her comprehensive index.

We wish to express our appreciation for the support of the AGS Board of Directors and AGS staff members Jennie Chin Hansen, RN, MS, FAAN, Chief Executive Officer; Nancy Lundebjerg, MPA, Deputy Executive Vice President; Elvy Ickowicz, MPH, Assistant Deputy Executive Vice President; Linda Saunders, MSW, Senior Director, Professional Education and Special Projects; and Dennise McAlpin, Manager, Professional Education and Special Projects.

Finally, we thank our patients, who continually inform, inspire, challenge, and sustain us.

Ellen Flaherty, PhD, RN, GNP-BC
Barbara Resnick, PhD, CRNP, FAANP, FAAN
GNRS3 Editors-in-Chief

PREFACE

The American Geriatrics Society (AGS), with almost 6,000 members, works to improve the health, independence, and quality of life of all older adults. The AGS is committed to increasing the number of healthcare professionals employing the principles of geriatrics by supporting the expansion of geriatric education in nursing and all applicable health professions. The AGS recognizes the critically important role that nurses play as members of the team providing care to older adults. In 2003, the AGS created the *Geriatrics Nursing Review Syllabus (GNRS)* for advanced practice nurses, and it has since served as the premier up-to-date geriatric resource supporting both clinicians and students. Over the years, geriatrics nursing faculty across the United States have used the *GNRS* as the core syllabus for the courses taught to advanced practice nurses focused on geriatrics and gerontology. They recognize that the syllabus provides up-to-date evidence-based information that helps nurses to deliver high quality care to older adults.

We are releasing the third edition of the *Syllabus* as advance practice nursing education enters a new era that will require all nurse practitioners who focus on caring for adults to have expertise in caring for older and frailer adults. The *GNRS*, given its focus on the complexities of caring for those with multiple co-morbidities, can help to support the nursing profession's efforts to ensure that the entire nursing workforce is prepared to care for the increasing numbers of older adults.

Ellen Flaherty, PhD, RN, GNP-BC
Barbara Resnick, PhD, CRNP, FAANP, FAAN
GNRS3 Editors-in-Chief
Jennie Chin Hansen, RN, MS, FAAN
Chief Executive Officer, American Geriatrics Society

INTRODUCTION

The *Geriatric Nursing Review Syllabus, 3rd edition (GNRS3)* is modified from the *Geriatrics Review Syllabus, 7th edition (GRS7)* and contains 62 chapters and references that allow the interested reader to pursue topics in greater depth, 120 case-oriented, multiple-choice questions and is accompanied by an answer sheet and the repeated questions with answers and supporting critiques to aid learner self-assessment.

The Syllabus is divided into six sections—Principles of Aging, Approach to the Patient, Care Systems, Syndromes, Psychiatry, and Diseases and Disorders. *GNRS3* particularly highlights developments in geriatric medicine since publication of the second edition. When discussing specific drugs, the authors and editors verified that the information provided was up to date at the time of publication. Any mention of uses not specifically approved by the U.S. Food and Drug Administration (so called "off-label" uses) are tagged as OL.

New Features

New features in the third edition include added emphases on evidence-based medicine and on quality assessment and improvement. Authors were encouraged to include strength-of-evidence (SOE) ratings for key diagnostic, prognostic, and therapeutic information. Authors and editors also have endeavored to present measures of association (between risk factors or therapies and conditions) in terms of absolute risk as well as relative risk. The Assessing Care of Vulnerable Elders-3 (ACOVE-3) quality indicators have been appended to applicable chapters in *GNRS3*. The 392 ACOVE-3 indicators, published in 2007 in the *Journal of the American Geriatrics Society*, can be used by practitioners to measure and improve the quality of care they provide to older adults. Please see the inside cover for further explanation of the SOE rating system and of the ACOVE-3 indicators.

Multiple Choice Questions

The questions are designed to complement material in the Syllabus chapters. The questions draw on the entire knowledge base of geriatric medicine, rather than just material from the Syllabus text. We recommend that participants prepare for answering these questions by first reading through the Syllabus chapters. Material addressed in the questions that is not discussed in the chapters is discussed in the critiques. The questions have been developed independently of any specialty board and will not be a part of any secure board certification examination.

We hope the *GNRS3* will meet our goal of enhancing participants' knowledge base and practice patterns when caring for older adults by providing a self-study tool that is current, concise, scholarly, and clinically relevant. We encourage your comments and suggestions, as the AGS continually strives to better serve its members and the older adults they treat.

Learning Objectives

The learning objectives for this activity have been designed to address participant knowledge, competence, performance, and patient outcomes. At the conclusion of this program, participants should be able to:

- Describe the general principles of aging and the biomedical and psychosocial issues of aging (knowledge);

- Discuss legal and ethical issues related to geriatric medicine (knowledge/competence);

- Evaluate the financing of health care for older adults (knowledge/competence);

- Identify the basic principles of geriatric medicine, including assessment, geriatric pharmacotherapy, prevention, exercise, palliative care, rehabilitation, and sensory deficits (knowledge/competence);

- Use state-of-the-art approaches to geriatric care while providing care in hospital, office-practice, nursing-home, and home-care settings (performance);

- Diagnose and manage geriatric syndromes, including dementia, delirium, urinary incontinence, malnutrition, osteoporosis, falls, pressure ulcers, sleep disorders, pain, dysphagia, and dizziness (performance);

- Apply relevant information from the fields of internal medicine, neurology, psychiatry, dermatology, and gynecology to the care of older patients (performance);

- Adjust patient care in the light of evidence-based data regarding the particular risks and needs of ethnic, racial, and sexual patient groups (patient outcomes);

- Use quality indicators to assess and improve the care of older adults in their own practices (performance/patient outcomes); and

- Employ evidence-based data to increase the effectiveness of teaching geriatrics to all health professionals (performance).

Additional American Geriatrics Society Resources

Geriatrics Review Syllabus, 7th edition (GRS7) is available as a 3-volume set of books and in CD-ROM format. The *Syllabus* offers 62 chapters on the diseases and disorders of older adults with references that allow the interested reader to pursue topics in greater depth. It also provides 290 case-oriented, multiple-choice questions that can be used for self-assessment and also to earn continuing education credits. Finally, it provides supporting critiques and references to aid learner self-assessment.

The *GRS7* self-assessment program provides participants with the option of applying for 85 Continuing Medical Education (CME) credits through the American Medical Association, American Academy of Family Physicians, and American Osteopathic Association. Additionally, the American Board of Internal Medicine (ABIM) has approved the *GRS7* CD-ROM program for 110 lifelong learning points for ABIM diplomates who are enrolled in the Maintenance of Certification (MOC) program.

Geriatrics at Your Fingertips, published annually, provides practical, up-to-date information for clinicians in a pocket-sized format.

Doorway Thoughts: Cross-Cultural Health Care for Older Adults is a three-volume series that helps the health practitioner to understand host best to care for an increasingly multi-cultural patient population.

GRS Teaching Slides are available as a subscription through the AGS Web site (http://teachingslides. americangeriatrics.org). The slide presentations in Microsoft® Power Point® are based on each of the *GRS* chapters and suitable for faculty, fellows, residents, and students. Each presentation is designed for approximately a 1-hour seminar and may be used as a stand-alone lecture or as a complement to one's own personal teaching materials.

GRS7 Audio Companion includes 30-minute audio discussions on 62 topics based on the GRS7 content with chapter authors and experts in the field. Continuing education credits can be obtained by successfully completing 124 multiple-choice questions derived from the audio content. The program offers 35 *AMA PRA Category 1 Credits*™ or 35 AAFP Prescribed Credits. Available at: http://grsaudio.com.

These and other publications, including resources and clinical practice guidelines, are available at **www.americangeriatrics.org.**

PROGRAM INFORMATION

CONGRUITY OF CONTENT BETWEEN SYLLABUS AND QUESTIONS

Because the Syllabus chapters and the questions with critiques are written by different authors, questions may not always correlate directly with the Syllabus. In the event that a question's content is not addressed in the correlating chapter, its answer is fully supported in the question critique.

REVIEW QUESTIONS

The *GNRS3* review questions are provided as learning aides but not as practice items for the Geriatric Nurse Practitioner Examination for the American Nurses Credentialing Center or the American Academy of Nurse Practitioners.

SELF-ASSESSMENT PROGRAM

For self-assessment testing, answer sheets are available for download at: http://www.americangeriatrics. org/publications/gnrs3.

USER EVALUATION

The AGS would appreciate participants' comments about the *GNRS3* program through the User Survey located at: http://www.americangeriatrics.org/ publications/gnrs3. Comments and suggestions will be taken into consideration by those planning the next edition.

UPDATES AND ERRATA

Important updates, such as medication alerts, will be posted as necessary on the AGS Web site: http://www.americangeriatrics.org/publications/gnrs3.

Please report any errata to: info.amger@american geriatrics.org, Attention: GNRS Managing Editor. Identified errata will be posted on the AGS Web site: http://www.americangeriatrics.org/publications/gnrs3.

AHRQ	Agency for Healthcare Research and Quality
ACE	angiotensin-converting enzyme
AIDS	acquired immune deficiency syndrome
ALT	alanine aminotransferase
AST	aspartate aminotransferase
BUN	blood urea nitrogen
cAMP	cyclic adenosine monophosphate
cGMP	cyclic guanosine monophosphate
CBC	complete blood count
CDC	Centers for Disease Control and Prevention
CMS	Centers for Medicare & Medicaid Services
CNS	central nervous system
COPD	chronic obstructive pulmonary disease
CT	computed tomography
ECG	electrocardiogram
FDA	Food and Drug Administration
GABA	γ-aminobutyric acid; GABAergic
GnRH	gonadotropin-releasing hormone
hCG	human chorionic gonadotropin
HIV	human immunodeficiency virus
IGF-1	insulin-like growth factor
INR	international normalized ratio
IQ	intelligence quotient
mo	month(s)
MRI	magnetic resonance imaging
NSAID	nonsteroidal anti-inflammatory drug
OTC	over-the-counter
RBC	red blood cell
SSRI	selective serotonin-reuptake inhibitor
WBC	white blood cell
yr	year(s)

Drug Prescribing

d	day(s)
h	hour(s)
IM	intramuscular
IV	intravenous
OL	off-label, ie, not approved by FDA for this use (note: used as superscript)
po	per os (orally)
prn	as needed
SC	subcutaneous
wk	week(s)

Measures of Effect

AR	absolute risk
ARI	absolute risk increase
ARR	absolute risk reduction
NNH	number needed to harm
NNT	number needed to treat
RR	relative risk
RRI	relative risk increase
RRR	relative risk reduction

CHAPTER 1—DEMOGRAPHY

KEY POINTS

- The composition of the older United States' population is far from static. The large and growing numbers of aging baby boomers are becoming more racially and ethnically diverse. With increasing longevity, greater numbers of older adults are surviving to the oldest ages.

- Relative to their predecessors, older Americans today are generally more educated, better off financially (although racial and ethnic minority populations lag behind white Americans), increasingly live alone or in alternative residential settings, and are less functionally impaired.

- The population of older adults is characterized by heterogeneity across measures of health status, functioning, and socioeconomic position.

- Among older adults, heart disease, cancer, and stroke remain the leading causes of death, while other age-related conditions such as Alzheimer's disease are becoming more common.

GLOBAL AGING TRENDS

As a result of declining fertility and mortality rates, the world today is experiencing pervasive and unprecedented population aging. According to the United Nations, the proportion of older adults ($\geq$60 yr old) comprised 8% of the worldwide population in 1950 but will represent 21% of the global population by 2050, by which time they will exceed the number of young for the first time in history. The pace of aging varies by region and age group, and is much faster in developing countries and among the oldest-old age groups. The rate of growth in the numbers of older adults between 2006 and 2030 is projected to increase by 140% among developing countries, as compared with growth of approximately 50% in more developed countries. Given the pace of population aging, developing countries will have less time to prepare for consequences associated with demographic change in their age structure. For example, older adults' workforce participation rates tend to be higher among less developed countries, where pension systems are less established. Individuals $\geq$80 yr old currently comprise the fastest growing age group in the world, increasing at a rate of 3.8% per year.

DEMOGRAPHY OF AGING IN THE UNITED STATES

In 2000, about one in eight Americans living in the United States was $\geq$65 yr old, but in light of declining birth rates and increases in longevity, older adults are anticipated to comprise one of every five Americans by 2030. This major demographic shift has prompted numerous concerns regarding U.S. social and health policy in recent years. Not only will the sheer number of older adults increase dramatically, but the composition and characteristics of the older population will also change. Although clinicians primarily attend to the needs of individual patients, some of the attributes that an older patient brings to the patient-clinician relationship are a function of the cohort to which he or she belongs. Aging baby boomers (the generation born between 1946 and 1964) will influence the health and social service systems of the United States, although the exact nature of this impact remains unclear.

During the 20th century, the U.S. population <65 yr old tripled, while the group $\geq$65 yr old increased by a factor of more than 11, growing from 3.1 million in 1900 to 36.8 million in 2005. This group is anticipated to more than double again by the middle of the next century, to 82 million people, with most of this growth occurring between 2010 and 2030. The United States is not unique in its growing numbers of older people. At present it is surpassed by many other developed countries, including Italy, Japan, Germany, Sweden, and the United Kingdom, where the proportion of people $\geq$60 yr old already comprise 20% or more of the overall population.

Older adults are not evenly distributed across geographic regions of the United States. Half of people $\geq$65 yr old live in nine states, led by California, Florida, New York, and Texas. Older adults disproportionately live in urban or suburban areas; just one in every five live in nonmetropolitan areas. While the older U.S. population is predominantly white, it is becoming increasingly diverse. Minority populations comprised approximately 18% of the adults $\geq$65 yr old in 2004 but are expected to represent 39% by 2050. While the older black American population is anticipated to increase by 50% during this period, the older Asian American and Hispanic American populations are anticipated to triple. The number of older Hispanic Americans is projected to exceed that of older blacks by 2050.

Table 1.1—Years of Life Expectancy at Birth and at Ages 65 and 85 by Gender and Race, 2004

	All Races			White			Black		
	Both sexes	Male	Female	Both sexes	Male	Female	Both sexes	Male	Female
At birth	77.8	75.2	80.4	78.3	75.7	80.8	73.1	69.5	76.3
Age 65	18.7	17.1	20.0	18.7	17.2	20.0	17.1	15.2	18.6
Age 85	6.8	6.1	7.2	6.8	6.0	7.1	7.1	6.3	7.5

SOURCE: Data from *National Vital Statistics System*. December 2007;56(9):3. Available at http://www.cdc.gov/nchs/ (accessed Jan 2011).

Life Expectancy

In the United States, the average life expectancy is currently highest for white women, followed by that for black women and white men, who have nearly identical life expectancies, and that of black men (Table 1.1). Women who survive to age 65 can, on average, expect to live to age 85, and those surviving to age 85 can expect to live to age 92. Up to age 85, the life expectancy of white American men and women exceeds that of their black counterparts. At age 85, these racial differences in life expectancy largely disappear. There is disagreement about whether these findings reflect errors in documenting age (for older black Americans) or are a true cross-over in mortality rates. The exact number of centenarians in the United States is difficult to gauge, but their numbers are growing and expected to exceed 800,000 by 2050.

Socioeconomic Status and Employment

Improvements in the Social Security system and the adoption of Medicare have had an important impact on the economic well-being of older adults in the United States. In the early 1960s, 35% of people ≥65 yr old had incomes below the federal poverty level, and only 70% received Social Security pensions. By the early 1970s, over 90% of older people received Social Security retirement benefits, and 97% were covered by Medicare. Today, the percentage of older people with incomes below the poverty line is about 10%. Another 6.6% are classified as "near poor," ie, with an income between the poverty level and 125% of this level. For impoverished seniors (generally having an income well below the poverty line), Medicaid plays a key role in filling in the gaps in Medicare by covering nursing-home and other long-term care services, other healthcare services not covered by Medicare, as well as paying for Medicare premiums and cost-sharing. Currently, there are approximately 7.5 million older adults enrolled in both Medicare and Medicaid (ie, "dual eligibles").

Although the overall economic position of older people in the United States has improved significantly over the past three decades, these gains have not been shared by all. Poverty rates among older people are higher among black Americans (23%); Hispanic Americans (20%); people ≥85 yr old (13%); and those living in rural areas (12%), principal cities (13%), in the South (12%), or alone (19%). Rates in some groups of older adults are much higher—nearly half (46%) of older Hispanic American women and more than one-third (37%) of older black women living alone are poor, for example.

While labor force participation of older adults declined throughout most of the past century, this trend has reversed during the last 20 yr, and growth in employment among older adults is expected to continue. In 2005, an estimated 5.3 million older adults were either working or actively seeking work, representing approximately one in five older men and one in ten older women. Labor force participation is influenced by a variety of factors relating to both economic necessity (eg, declines in defined benefit pension plans, the increase in the full retirement age for Social Security benefits, the high costs of health insurance), as well as personal choice. Higher levels of education and improvements in health have afforded greater numbers of older adults the opportunity to continue to work.

Education and Literacy

One of the most dramatic changes in the older U.S. population of the future will be in levels of educational attainment. Between 1965 and 2004, the percentage of individuals ≥65 yr old who completed high school increased from 24% to 73%, and the percentage with a bachelor's degree or more increased from 5% to 19%. Education is closely related to lifetime economic status, and many studies have shown that individuals with more education generally enjoy better health and lower rates of disability than those with low levels of educational attainment. Despite gains in education, education and literacy levels of older adults lag far behind those of working-age adults; older adults are also approximately one-half as likely to possess a personal computer and make use of the Internet. According to the 2003 National Assessment of Adult Literacy, older adults on average have lower levels of health literacy, defined as "...the capacity to obtain, process, and understand basic health information and services needed to make appropriate health decisions," than working-age adults. Given the greater

Table 1.2—Marital Status and Living Arrangements of Community-Dwelling Older Americans by Age, 2006 (individuals as a percentage of column total)

	All (%)			Male (%)			Female (%)		
	65–74	75–84	85+	65–74	75–84	85+	65–74	75–84	85+
Marital Status									
Married	65.6	51.3	32.0	76.7	72.2	60.6	56.1	36.8	17.6
Widowed	17.5	38.0	61.1	7.3	17.6	32.4	26.3	52.3	75.5
Other	16.9	10.7	6.9	16.1	10.3	7.0	17.6	10.9	6.9
Living arrangements									
Lives alone	23.2	35.4	46.9	16.9	21.2	28.8	28.5	45.3	56.0
With spouse	63.9	49.4	29.4	75.1	70.3	57.8	54.3	34.9	15.1
With relatives	10.0	12.9	21.7	6.5	6.9	12.4	14.4	17.8	27.2
With nonrelatives	3.0	2.3	1.9	1.6	1.6	1.1	2.7	2.0	1.7

SOURCE: Data from *Current Population Survey*, 2006; Table A.1.

Table 1.3—Perceived Health of Older Adults by Age and Race/Ethnicity, 2006

	White, non-Hispanic (%)			Black, non-Hispanic (%)			Hispanic (%)		
	65–74	75–84	85+	65–74	75–84	85+	65–74	75–84	85+
Excellent/very good	46.1	38.4	32.5	25.2	23.7	*	33.4	21.1	*
Good	34.5	37.5	36.4	38.9	35.3	30.9	36.7	38.3	*
Fair/poor	19.4	24.2	31.1	35.8	41.1	50.7	29.9	40.6	45.7

*Cell sizes too small for reliable estimates

SOURCE: Data from *National Health Interview Survey*, NCHS Vital and Health Statistics, 2007; Series 10 (235). Table 21.

availability of health and medical information via the Internet and mainstream media (eg, direct-to-consumer advertising) as well as the introduction of the voluntary Medicare Part D drug benefit, the relevance of health literacy is arguably more important today than ever before.

The Older Foreign-Born Population

In 2003, there were 3.3 million foreign-born people ≥65 yr old in the United States. More than one-third (34%) of older foreign-born people originated in Europe, another 33% from Latin America, 25% from Asia, and 8% from other parts of the world. Older foreign-born people are increasingly likely to originate from Latin America or Asia, as compared with Europe. Older foreign-born people are more likely than their native counterparts to live in family households and to live in poverty; they tend to be concentrated in western states.

Marital Status and Living Arrangements

Among Americans living in the United States who are 65–74 yr old, two-thirds are married and living with their spouse, approximately twice the proportion of older adults ≥85 yr old (Table 1.2). Not surprisingly, given older women's greater life expectancy, older men are far more likely to be married than are older women. Conversely, widowhood is much more common among older women; 52% of women 75–84 yr old and 76% of women ≥85 yr old are widows, compared with 17.6% of men 75–84 yr old and 32.4% of men ≥85 yr old.

Trends in Health, Functioning, and Mortality

The burden of disease and disability is greater for older people than working-age adults and children. In fact, the vast majority of older adults have one or more chronic conditions. In 2006, the most common self-reported conditions included hypertension (53%), arthritic symptoms (50%), heart disease (31%), cancer (21%), and diabetes (18%) (Figure 1.1). There is great heterogeneity in health status among older adults. Data on self-assessed health, which have been shown to correlate highly with mortality and risk of functional decline, illustrate this. Among white non-Hispanic Americans 65–74 yr old, 46% regarded their health as "excellent" or "very good," 35% indicated their health to be "good," and 19% reported their health to be "fair" or "poor" (Table 1.3). As might be expected, the percentages who viewed their health as only fair or poor increased with age. The proportion of older adults who reported their health to be "fair" or "poor" was higher in all age groups among black and Hispanic Americans than white Americans. Physical functioning is closely associated with both chronic disease and age. For example, approximately 70% of adults 65–74 yr old and 56% of adults 75–84 yr old reported no difficulty with ADLs or IADLs, compared with just one-third of individuals ≥85 yr old (Figure 1.2). Older women exhibit a higher percentage of limitations in functioning at all ages than older men.

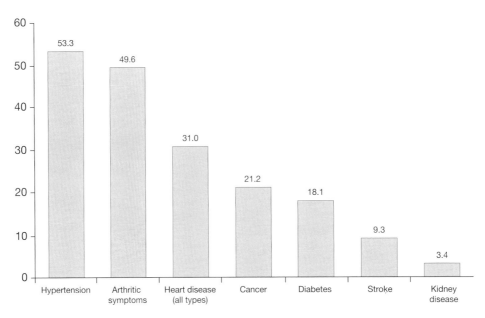

Figure 1.1—Prevalence of selected self-reported chronic conditions among adults ≥65 yr old, all races

SOURCE: Data from Data Warehouse on Trends in Health and Aging: Health Status and Chronic Conditions, from the *National Health Interview Survey*. Estimates for 2005–2006.

Deaths of older people comprise nearly 75% of all deaths in the United States. About one-fourth of all deaths occur at age 85 or older, and given broader demographic trends, this proportion is expected to grow. For many decades, heart disease, cancer, and stroke have been the leading causes of death among people ≥65 yr old, accounting for 6 of 10 deaths (Table 1.4). Causes of death vary by race, ethnicity, and gender, however. Diabetes mellitus was the fourth leading cause of death among older Hispanic and black Americans, while ranking seventh among older white Americans. Alzheimer's disease ranks fifth among all causes of death. Some causes of death usually associated with younger people also are of concern in the older population. In the United States, the death rate from motor vehicle accidents is twice as high in older men than in older women, both overall and within racial and ethnic groups. The highest suicide rates among older people are for white men aged ≥85 yr old (48.4 per 100,000, compared with 3.6 per 100,000 for older white women of comparable age).

Trends in Disability

Disability dynamics have been an area of active research, in part due to the salience of disability to public programs such as Medicare and Medicaid. Increases in life expectancy have led to debate over whether additional years of life gained will be achieved free of disability, or whether these incremental years of life gained will be spent with functional disability. Studies of active life expectancy, which use mortality and disability estimates to project disability-free years, suggest an advantage for people with more education. Because of their greater total life expectancy, older women experience both greater active life expectancy and more years of disability than do older men. It has been suggested that if there is a limit to increases in life expectancy, increases in disability-free years could produce a *compression of morbidity*, with the period of disability before death gradually compressed as active life expectancy (or disability-free years) increases.

Several longitudinal studies of older adults indicate aggregate declines in disability have occurred over the course of the last 20 yr, although the magnitude of decline across types of disability and subgroups of older Americans is more controversial. For example, estimates from the National Long Term Care Survey find that the proportion of chronically disabled or institutionalized older adults declined from 25% to 20% between 1984 and 1999. However, most of this decline was attributed to lower rates of IADL disability (shifting from 6% to 3%); ADL disability rates were more stable (from 13% to 12%) during this time period. While the trend toward a decline in IADL disability and general stability in ADL disability has been substantiated by a number of national surveys, variability in sampling strategy and measurement of disability challenge definitive conclusions regarding the magnitude of such findings. For example, the extent to which questions explicitly assess respondents' use of assistive devices (eg, remote devices, canes, walkers) or the built environment (eg, growth in residential settings that have adopted universal design) may influence disability estimates.

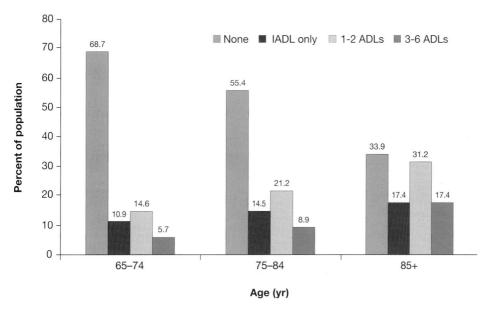

Figure 1.2—Self-reported functional limitations of community-dwelling Medicare beneficiaries by age group, 2006
SOURCE: Data from Medicare Beneficiary Survey, 2006.

Table 1.4—Leading Causes of Death and Numbers of Deaths, for Adults Aged 65 and Older, 2004

Rank	Cause of Death	Number of Deaths	% of Deaths
	All causes	1,755,669	100
1	Cardiac diseases	533,302	30.4
2	Malignant neoplasms	385,847	22.0
3	Cerebrovascular diseases	130,538	7.4
4	Chronic lower respiratory disease	105,197	6.0
5	Alzheimer's disease	65,313	3.7
6	Diabetes mellitus	53,956	3.1
7	Influenza and pneumonia	52,760	3.0
8	Nephritis, nephrotic syndrome, and nephrosis	35,105	2.0
9	Accidents (unintentional injuries)	35,020	2.0
10	Septicemia	25,644	1.5

SOURCE: *National Vital Statistics Reports* 2007:56(5) (Table 1). Available at http://www.cdc.gov/nchs/data/nvsr/nvsr56/nvsr56_05.pdf (accessed Jan 2011).

Whether the benefits of greater literacy and increased longevity have been universally experienced by all subgroups of older Americans in terms of improved functioning is less clear. Recent studies substantiate the existence of disparities in disability across racial and ethnic subgroups and by education, and suggest that such disparities are growing. For example, between 1996 and 2006, the proportion of older adults without functional limitations or disability was relatively stable among white non-Hispanic Americans, increased among black non-Hispanic Americans, but decreased among Hispanic Americans (Figure 1.3). A parallel trend is observed with regard to trends of severe disability. Between 1996 and 2006, the proportion of older adults with three or more ADL limitations was relatively stable for both white non-Hispanic and black non-Hispanic adults, but increased among Hispanic Americans (Figure 1.4). The reasons for such disparities are multifaceted, reflecting a lifetime of behavior and experience, environmental exposure, and access to and use of medical care.

Disability Accommodation

Individuals may use a variety of approaches to compensate for a physical disability, including assistive technology, personal care, environmental modifications, or a change in residential setting. Use of assistive technology is widespread among disabled older adults, with mobility-related devices, such as canes and walkers, being used most commonly. In 1999, about 26% of chronically disabled older adults were estimated to rely on assistive technology alone, an additional 58% were estimated to rely on both assistive technology and personal care, and just 16% of chronically disabled older adults relied exclusively on personal care. Individuals who rely on personal care alone tend to be most highly disabled and often possess both physical and cognitive impairment. The vast majority of older adults who receive personal care rely on help from a family member or a friend ("family caregiver"); less than 1 in 10 receives help from a paid caregiver. Family caregivers for chronically disabled older adults are predominantly spouses or adult children who live either with one another or in close proximity. While family caregivers commonly assist with household and personal care task assistance, they are also frequently involved in providing or coordinating older adults' medical care. For ex-

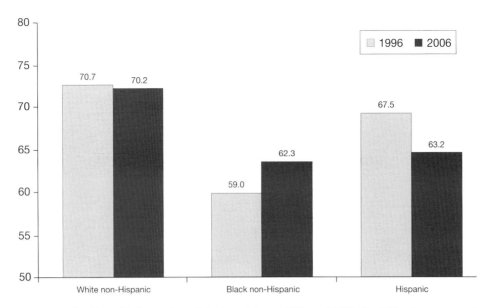

Figure 1.3—Community-dwelling Medicare beneficiaries without ADL or IADL disability by race and ethnicity, 1996 and 2006

SOURCE: Data from Medicare Beneficiary Survey, 1996 and 2006.

ample, family caregivers commonly assist with wound care, medication management, and coordination of care between clinicians or across settings of care; approximately 2 in 5 older adults are routinely accompanied to clinician office visits by a family member or friend.

Assisted-Living Facilities

Assisted-living facilities are a rapidly growing residential setting in the United States. This type of facility provides greater supervision and assistance than is typically available in a private home, while allowing more autonomy and freedom than traditional nursing-home facilities. Approximately 800,000 people were estimated to be living in 33,000 assisted-living facilities in the United States in 2002. A typical assisted-living resident is a woman between 75 and 85 yr old who is mobile but needs assistance with ADLs. Residents move to assisted-living residences from a variety of settings. More than half move from their own private apartment or residence, with the remainder being about equally distributed from other assisted-living residences, hospitals, nursing homes, or other private residence, such as an adult child's home. The average length of residency is 2 yr.

Nursing Facilities

Over the course of the past 20 yr, nursing facilities have increasingly developed skilled nursing capabilities to provide postacute care to individuals transitioning out of the acute hospital setting. How-

ever, nursing facilities continue to play an important role as a provider of long-term care to a particularly vulnerable segment of the population, caring for older adults with cognitive and/or physical impairment, and with considerable ongoing medical needs. Not surprisingly, nursing-home use rates vary considerably by age group. According to the 2004 National Nursing Home Survey, <1% of adults 65–74 yr old were living in a nursing home, compared with approximately 4% of adults 75–84 yr old and 14% of adults ≥85 yr old. There were approximately 1.3 million nursing-home residents ≥65 yr old in 2004 (3.6%), a significant decline from 4.2% in 1985. The trend of declining nursing-home use is likely a result of both improvements in older adults' health and functioning, as well as increases in system-wide community supports and the growth of alternative residential arrangements, such as assisted-living facilities and continuing-care retirement communities. Regardless, the net effect is that the nursing-home population has become older and more disabled. For example, the proportion of residents ≥85 yr old increased from 35% to 47% between 1977 and 1999. Between 1985 and 2004, the proportion of nursing-home residents needing help with five or six ADLs increased from 50% to 65%.

Future Issues

The older U.S. population is among the most heterogeneous subgroups, encompassing the entire spectrum of health and functioning, from the bedridden Alzheimer's patient to the marathon runner. One of the important unresolved questions is whether gains

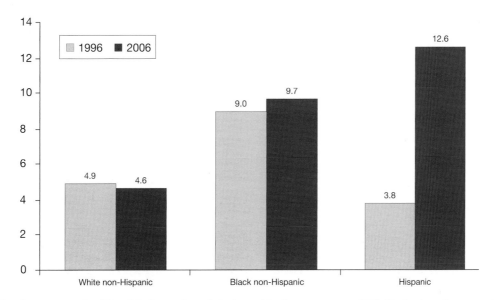

Figure 1.4—Community-dwelling Medicare beneficiaries with three or more ADL limitations by race and ethnicity, 1996 and 2006

SOURCE: Data from Medicare Beneficiary Survey, 1996 and 2006.

in longevity after age 65 are accompanied by gains or declines in years of disability-free life. It is unlikely that one answer will fit this large and diverse group. There are many questions in other areas as well. Will the increasing numbers of better-educated, longer-lived older adults contribute to the larger society, and in what ways? Will the sheer numbers of older people strain to the breaking point the medical care system and public programs that finance health care and retirement, as some analysts fear? Or will improvements in health behavior, medical breakthroughs, and financial prosperity diminish these threats? Under any scenario, chronic illness will remain a constant in the lives of many older people. Clinicians treating this population face the challenge not only of treating

chronically ill adults but also of assisting all older people in preventing or at least delaying the onset of chronic disease.

REFERENCES

■ Administration on Aging, U.S. Department of Health and Human Services. *A Profile of Older Americans: 2009*. Available at: http://www.aoa.gov/AoAroot/Aging_Statistics/Profile/index.aspx

■ Federal Interagency Forum on Aging-Related Statistics. *Older Americans 2008: Key Indicators of Well-Being*. Washington, DC: U.S. Government Printing Office; May 2006. Available at: http://www.agingstats.gov/agingstatsdotnet/main_site/default.aspx

CHAPTER 2—BIOLOGY

KEY POINTS

- Aging is a loss of homeostasis, or a breakdown in maintenance of specific molecular structures and pathways; this breakdown is the inevitable consequence of the evolved anatomic and physiologic design of an organism.

- Evolutionary theories of aging (mutation accumulation, antagonistic pleiotropic, and disposable soma theories) address the "why" of aging.

- Physiologic theories of aging (genetic, mitochondrial DNA, error catastrophe, free radical, protein modification, rate of living, immune, epigenetic, and stem/progenitor cell theories) address the "how" of aging.

- The many theories of aging are not necessarily competing or mutually exclusive; rather, the theories reflect our current understanding of the individual multiple maintenance and homeostasis mechanisms that allow us to live as long as we do.

- Some of the molecular and cellular changes that occur with aging are unique to the specific cellular and tissue context of the organ, while others occur across a number of organ systems with a common effect on functional capacity.

Aging's most visible imprints on our bodies are loss of hair and pigmentation of hair; diminished height and muscle and bone mass; and increasingly wrinkled, thinned skin. These progressive and accelerating changes have a biologic basis in altered molecular and cellular structure and function. The biology of aging includes studying the evolutionary aspects, molecular mechanisms, and organ system changes of aging. Individuals are extremely heterogeneous in the onset of the aging process, the rate at which it progresses, and the extent to which it progresses. Thus, biologic age, based on an individual's functional capacity (and not chronologic age), is the metric for the biology of aging. Functional capacity is a direct measure of the ability of cells, tissues, and organ systems to function properly and optimally and is influenced by both genes and environment. Within this context, aging is defined as the progressive decline and deterioration of functional properties at the cellular, tissue, and organ level that lead to a loss of homeostasis, decreased ability to adapt to internal or external stimuli, and increased vulnerability to disease and mortality.

INTRODUCTION

The biology of aging includes the study of the "why" of aging (evolutionary theories), the "how" of aging (physiologic theories), and the "what and where" of aging (the molecular, cellular, and organ system changes associated with increasing age). Inherent in these multiple approaches to investigating aging is the definition of what aging is. For some gerontologists, aging is a normal physiologic outcome, part of the process of being and persistence through time, manifested by simple wear and tear. For others, aging is a pathologic outcome that results from the complex cumulative interplay of multiple diseases brought about by genetic mutations, environment, and time. Underlying these two perspectives is the question of whether the goal of understanding the biology of aging is adding years to life (life extension) or life to years (improving quality of remaining years).

Aging is characterized by progressive changes in cells, tissues, and organs of the body that lead inexorably to death. These changes—the physiologic events of aging—are the consequences of the inability to maintain cells, tissues, and organ systems indefinitely. That is, aging is a necessary counterpart to and by-product of the body's maintenance systems. Aging is due to the eventual breakdown of maintenance processes—an inevitable consequence of the evolved anatomic and physiologic design of the organism.

THEORIES OF AGING

Evolutionary theories of aging explain historical and evolutionary aspects of aging, addressing why aging exists in living things, how aging evolved as a process, whether there was selective pressure for aging to occur, and whether aging can be considered a positive or negative selection factor impacting the organism's fitness. Physiologic theories explain structural and functional age changes in present-day organisms. These theories concentrate on genetic programs (specific genes), molecules and their chemical reactions (free radicals, glucose, and glycation), activities of cell organelles (mitochondria), and whole-body homeostatic systems (immune, endocrine). Programmed theories hold that aging occurs because of intrinsic timing mechanisms and signals. Stochastic theories hold that aging occurs by accidental chance events. Mixed theories hold that aging occurs because programmed genetic signals make an organism more susceptible to accidental events. The genetic theories of aging emphasize nuclear gene mutations or damage, mitochondrial DNA mutations or damage, or programmed "aging" genes. Altered molecule theories emphasize damaged and abnormal proteins, cross-linkage, glycation, waste accumulation, and general molecular wear and tear. Free radical theories emphasize free radical formation and free radical defense mechanisms. Cell organelle theories emphasize specific cellular components such as mitochondria or telomeres.

Evolutionary Theories of Aging

Evolution deals with the impact of natural selection (selective pressure) on the reproductive fitness of a species. In the 19th century, August Weismann proposed a theory of programmed death, in which aging was adaptive—a specific mechanism designed by natural selection to eliminate the old and free up resources for the reproductively fit young. There are currently three main evolutionary theories of aging: mutation accumulation theory, antagonistic pleiotropy theory, and disposable soma theory.

Mutation Accumulation Theory

Mutation accumulation theory proposes that aging is a nonadaptive trait, a by-product and inevitable result of the declining force of natural selection with age. Because no selective pressure is brought to bear on organisms expressing a mutation at older post-eproductive ages (which has minimal effects on fitness), these late-acting genes accumulate over time. The detrimental effects from these late-acting genes are "aging."

Antagonistic Pleiotropy Theory

The antagonistic pleiotropic theory proposed that aging is an adaptive trait, and genes that can influence several traits (ie, have pleiotropic effects) are selected for and affect individual fitness in opposite (ie, antagonistic) ways. Pleiotropic genes have beneficial effects on early fitness components in the young but harmful effects on late fitness components, and yet are nevertheless favored by natural selection. There is thus an evolutionary trade-off between reproductive capacity and longevity.

Disposable Soma Theory

Disposable soma theory proposes that the body's allocation of metabolic resources between growth, reproduction, and somatic maintenance is sufficient to keep the body (soma) in good condition but less sufficient than would be required for indefinite survival. Aging is the cumulative damage done to the relatively more vulnerable soma cells.

Physiologic Theories of Aging

Physiologic theories address how we age. A great deal of information on changes during aging at the organ system, cellular, molecular, and genetic levels has been gathered over the past few decades.

Target Theory of Genetic Damage

Underlying the genetic theories of aging is the idea that aging is heavily influenced or caused by genes. The genome is the repository for all genetic material, and the integrity of this information is essential for reproductive fitness and survival. DNA is subject to a number of insults, including spontaneous chemical changes, environmental damage by ionizing radiation such as UV light, aflatoxin, and alkylating agents that methylate DNA. Mechanisms of repair depend on the efficiency of many enzymes that depend on information in the DNA. Thus, the target theory of genetic damage states that genes and chromosomes are susceptible to inactivating hits from radiation or other damaging agents and that cumulative hits give rise to an aging phenotype.

Mitochondrial DNA Theory

Mitochondrial DNA (mtDNA) is not protected by proteins (eg, histones, chromatin) as nuclear DNA is, and mtDNA is attached to the inner mitochondrial membrane, where most free radicals are produced. Thus, mtDNA damage occurs 10–20 times faster than nuclear DNA damage. In addition, mtDNA cannot repair itself, and damaged mitochondria replicate faster than undamaged mitochondria, which gives rise to expansion of aberrant mitochondria. As a consequence, genes encoded for by the mitochondria are more likely to lose their integrity over time. The damaged mtDNA has more deleterious effects than does damage to nuclear DNA, because each cell uses almost all its mtDNA genes and only approximately 7% of its nuclear DNA. Thus, nearly any adverse change in mtDNA will have adverse effects on mitochondrial function. These effects include less energy production, more free-radical formation, reduced control of other cell processes, and accumulation of damaged harmful molecules, leading to aging and certain age-related diseases. The mitochondrial DNA theory of aging is closely allied with the free radical theory of aging (see below).

Protein Error Theory

This theory holds that damage is not to genes themselves but to RNA and proteins (that read the genes and carry out their instructions). The damaged molecules spread, increasing the number of mistakes and loss of molecular function causing biologic changes that are seen as "aging." The protein error theory ("error catastrophe") holds that errors in subsets of proteins involved in transfer of information from DNA to protein (RNA polymerase, aminoacyl tRNA synthetase, ribosomal proteins, etc) are normally below a threshold, so a steady state exists with random perturbations. Critical errors can destabilize the machinery for protein synthesis, causing an irreversible increase in the error level and accelerating loss of function.

Protein error theory predicts that treatments that induce errors in proteins will accelerate aging, that senescent cells should contain abnormal protein molecules, that the accuracy of synthesis should be lower in old cells/organisms, and that mutations that reduce accuracy of synthesis should accelerate aging. These predictions have been tested experimentally, and this theory has equivocal support.

Free Radical Theory

The most widely accepted theory among the physiologic theories is the free radical theory. Free radicals (including superoxide, hydrogen peroxide, and hydroxyl ions) are chemical species that have an unpaired electron in an outer orbital and are extremely reactive and unstable. Free radicals are produced in mitochondria, in oxidative enzymes in the endoplasmic reticulum, in peroxisomes (fatty-acid breakdown generates hydrogen peroxide), and by phagocytes. Free radicals are normally policed by enzymes that inactivate them (superoxide dismutase, catalase, glutathione peroxidase), antioxidants that neutralize them (α-tocopherol, ascorbic acid, uric acid), sulfhydryl-containing compounds (cysteine, glutathione, bilirubin, ubiquinol, and carnosine), and β-carotene.

Positive correlations have been observed between metabolic rate and free radical production, age and rate of free radical formation, and age and amount of free radical damage. Negative correlations have been observed between longevity and free radical production, and age and free radical defenses. Free radicals cause DNA base adducts, lipid peroxidation (which preferentially affects long-lived cells such as neurons), lipofuscin (the oxidized lipid "age pigment") generation, and protein oxidation. Free radicals can act as causative agents in other physiologic theories of aging, including DNA damage, mitochondrial DNA, protein error, and protein modification theory.

Protein Modification Theory

This group of theories posits that the structures of proteins are altered with increasing age. These protein modifications include abnormal posttranslational modifications, deamidation of asparagines and glutamine, nonenzymatic protein glycation (between lysine residues of proteins and sugars), cross-linking of lysine residues, racemization of L-amino acids, phosphorylation, sulfation and methylation, and ADP ribosylation. Cross-links reduce movement of molecules for chemical reactions, normal turnover of proteins, transport of materials through the body, and movement of body parts. Surveillance and removal of

aberrantly modified and structured proteins is done by chaperonins, proteases, and proteasomes. Examples of age-related increases in modified proteins include collagen cross-links in skin and bone, neurofibrillary tangles and plaque formation in the brain, and advanced glycation end products in multiple organ systems.

Rate of Living Theory

This theory holds that organisms possess a finite amount of some vital substance and when this substance has been consumed, aging and death occurs. A number of limiting substances have been proposed, including the number of breaths and heartbeats as well as oxygen metabolism. Aging is determined by the rate of metabolism because aerobic metabolism causes damage, primarily through the production of oxygen-free radicals. The rate of living theory predicts that the higher the rate of metabolism, the faster the rate of aging and the shorter the life span.

Epigenetic Theory

Most cells in the human body are somatic cells. A major mechanism maintaining these cells' appropriate, differentiated phenotype is epigenetic, dependent on DNA-protein interactions, DNA methylation, and histone acetylation. The epigenetic theory posits that phenotypic drift arising from inappropriate epigenetic modifications leads to altered gene expression and cellular function and the aging phenotype. Hypermethylation in a gene's promoter region is associated with transcriptional silencing, whereas hypomethylation results in increased expression. In general, DNA methylation increases with age, but within a tissue there can be variation. The degree of hypermethylation depends on multiple factors, including age, diet, and exposure to environmental agents/insults (eg, carcinogens, epimutagens, toxins). Chronic inflammation is also associated with increased methylation. Epigenetically modified (methylated) cells exhibit inappropriate gene expression, with, for example, genes involved in tumor suppression or defense against free radicals being silenced. Epigenetic silencing of repressive transcription factors may contribute to differentiated cells switching to a senescent phenotype.

Endocrine Theory

With increasing age, the synthesis and secretion of a number of hormones change. In addition, cell receptors on target organs can change in terms of number and functional signal transduction. The circadian cycles of certain hormones also become irregular. The endocrine theory of aging posits that the occurrence of changes in hormone levels and signaling are a major cause of loss of homeostasis. This theory views aging as mainly a multiple hormone deficiency syndrome. For example, excessive stimulation of insulin/insulin growth factor leads to faster cell reproduction, larger cell size and body size, and a depletion of physiologic reserves. While slightly increased glucocorticoid levels keep the body's adaptive mechanisms at peak performance and prevent damage from excess inflammatory or immune responses, prolonged increased glucocorticoid exposure promotes the death of neurons. When reproductive hormone levels decrease, loss of gene repression or detrimental gene signals occurs (bone loss and sarcopenia being two end points of this pathway).

Immune Theory

Relatively slow-growing organisms must confront infection by rapidly growing pathogens or parasites, and the immune system has evolved to do this. The decline in the immune response during aging is well documented. There is a progressive quantitative and qualitative loss in ability to produce antibodies, a decline in T-lymphocyte function, atrophy of the thymus with age, and a decline in the diversity of memory cells. Homeostasis of the immune systems is maintained by innate or nonspecific mechanisms such as humoral mechanisms (complement) and cellular mechanisms (macrophage, neutrophils, natural killer cells), as well as by the specific, acquired immune response involving humoral mechanisms (antibodies) and cellular mechanisms (T and B lymphocytes). Deleterious events (mutations, chromosomal abnormalities, or epigenetic changes) have a more severe consequence for immune cells and their function and a lesser effect on other tissue or organs. The increase in circulating pro-inflammatory cytokines seen in older individuals is consistent with such immune dysregulation.

Stem Cell/Progenitor Cell Theory

Homeostasis is maintained by a continuous supply of progenitor cells that replenish depleted reserves. Adult stem cells in the brain, bone marrow, and circulation aid in this. Examples include satellite cells that contribute to muscle mass and repair of muscle tissue, and osteoprogenitor cells that replenish osteoblasts and form bone. Over time, precursor cells become depleted either by phenotypic drift or perhaps by injury, illness, or environmental challenge. Normally, adult bone marrow stem cells can produce cells in the osteoblastic, myoblastic, or adipocytic lines. Aging is associated with osteopenia, sarcopenia, and an increase in fat content in bone marrow and muscle. These age-related changes may arise from a shift in the pathway commitment of bone marrow stem cells (away from bone and muscle cells) toward the adipocytic cell line.

THE BIOLOGY OF AGING

These changes represent either biologic processes common to everyone or common disease states. The many theories of aging should not be viewed as competing or mutually exclusive. Rather, the theories reflect our current understanding of the individual maintenance pathways and homeostatic mechanisms that allow us to live as long as we do. The theories provide the framework for translating the "what" and "where" of aging from molecules to systems biology. Aging nerves, muscle, skin, hair, cartilage and bone, vasculature, and other organs exhibit changes at the molecular and cellular level. Some molecular changes with aging are shared between tissue types and organ systems, while others are unique. For example, in skin, bone, and cartilage, increases in cross-links (both enzymatic and nonenzymatic) alter compressibility and resiliency, and decreases in structural components (eg, proteoglycans and glycosaminoglycans) alter tissue hydration and function. In contrast, changes in the immune system (eg, diminished ability of dendritic cells to present antigen) are unique to the specific cell type, organ system, and function. A brief overview of significant age-related changes in the major organ systems follows. Not all of these are directly age-related but may occur in age-related disease states (see Table 2.1).

Nerves

With increasing age, both the number and functioning of sensory neurons decline. Age-related changes in somatic motor functioning include changes in somatic cell number, action potentials, and transmission rates. The number of somatic motor neurons decreases, reducing the number of cells that can be stimulated, decreasing the maximal strength of contraction that muscles can produce. The speed of action potentials in their axons decreases slightly, such that impulses arrive over an increasingly long period and contractions of muscle cells are spread out over a longer period; the slower transmission results in further delay in starting a motion. Neurons remaining in the brain have less fluid and stiffer cell membranes, internal membranes that become irregular in structure and accumulate lipofuscin, and tangled neurofibrils. The ability of neurons to grow branches of both axons and dendrites decreases, reducing fine motor control. Changes in motor neuron cell membranes, myelin, or blood vessels within the nerves reduce blood flow in nerves, decreasing the supply of nutrients and the elimination of wastes, which contribute to the slower action potentials and spreading of muscle cell contraction. The slower contraction, lower peak strength of contraction, and slower relaxation reduce maximal muscle strength when performing quick movements.

Table 2.1—Physiologic Changes of Aging

Body System	Change	Consequences
Nervous	↓ Number of neurons ↓ Action potential speed ↓ Axon/dendrite branches	↓ Muscle innervation ↓ Fine motor control
Muscle	Fibers shrink ↓ Type II (fast twitch) fibers ↑ Lipofuscin and fat deposits	Tissue atrophies ↓ Tone and contractility ↓ Strength
Skin	↓ Thickness ↑ Collagen cross-links	Loss of elasticity
Skeletal	↓ Bone density Joints become stiffer, less flexible	Movement slows and may become limited

Cardiovascular
  Heart
 	
  Vasculature
	
	↑ Left ventricular wall thickness
	↑ Lipofuscin and fat deposits
	↑ Stiffness
	↓ Responsiveness to agents
		
		Stressed heart is less able to respond

Pulmonary	↓ Elastin fibers ↑ Collagen cross-links ↓ Elastic recoil of the lung ↑ Residual volume ↓ Vital capacity, forced expiratory volume, and forced vital capacity	↓ Effort dependent and independent respiration (quiet and forced breathing) ↓ Exercise tolerance and pulmonary reserve
Eyes	↑ Lipid infiltrates/deposits ↑ Thickening of the lens ↓ Pupil diameter	↓ Transparency of the cornea Difficulty in focusing on near objects ↓ Accommodation and dark adaptation
Ears	↑ Thickening of tympanic membrane ↓ Elasticity and efficiency of ossicular articulation ↑ Organ atrophy ↓ Cochlear neurons	↑ Conductive deafness (low-frequency range) ↑ Sensorineural hearing loss (high-frequency sounds)
Digestive	↑ Dysphagia ↑ Achlorhydria Altered intestinal absorption ↑ Lipofuscin and fat deposition in pancreas ↑ Mucosal cell atrophy	 ↓ Iron absorption ↓ B_{12} and calcium absorption ↑ Incidence of diverticulum, transit time, and constipation
Urinary	↓ Kidney size, weight, and number of functional glomeruli ↓ Number and length of functional renal tubules ↓ Glomerular filtration rate ↓ Renal blood flow	↓ Ability to resorb glucose ↓ Concentrating ability of kidney
Immune	↓ Primary and secondary response ↑ Autoimmune antibodies increase ↓ T-cell function, fewer naive and more memory T cells Atrophy of thymus	↓Immune functioning ↓ Response to new pathogens ↓ T lymphocytes, natural killer cells, cytokines needed for growth and maturation of B cells
Endocrine	↑ Atrophy of certain glands (eg, pituitary, thyroid, thymus) ↓ Growth hormone, dehydroepiandrosterone, testosterone, estrogen ↑ Parathyroid hormone, atrial natriuretic peptide, norepinephrine, baseline cortisol, erythropoietin	Changes in target organ response, organ system homeostasis, response to stress, functional capacity

Muscle

Lean body mass decreases, caused in part by loss of muscle tissue (atrophy). The rate and extent of muscle changes seem to be genetically determined. Muscle changes often begin in the 20s in men and in the 40s in women. Lipofuscin (the oxidized lipid "age pigment") and fat are deposited in muscle tissue. The muscle fibers shrink. Muscle tissue is replaced more slowly, and lost muscle tissue may be replaced with a tough fibrous tissue. This is most noticeable in the hands, which may appear thin and bony. Changes in muscle tissue, combined with normal aging changes in the nervous system, lead to reduced muscle tone and contractility. Muscles can become rigid with age and can lose tone even if exercised regularly, leading to changes in strength and endurance.

Skin

Cellular changes in the skin include a thinner epidermis with a reduced mitotic rate in epidermal basal cells, shortened and attenuated rete ridges, reduced epidermal appendages, and fewer fibroblasts and capillaries in the dermis. Melanocytes in both exposed and unexposed skin decrease with age, while those remaining become larger but produce less melanin. At the molecular level, the dermal thickness decreases as the collagen content per unit area of the skin decreases. Loss of skin elasticity (caused by increased collagen cross-links and decreased elastin) leads to skin sagging and wrinkling. Hair follicles atrophy, and hair density and color decrease uniformly in both men and women. Hair turns gray because melanocytes are lost at the base of the hair follicles. Eyebrows, ear, and nasal hair coarsen and get longer, especially in men. Linear nail growth slows and nail thickness increases development of longitudinal ridges. Nails become brittle, dull, opaque, and yellowish.

Bone

Bone mass or density is lost, especially in women after menopause, and bones become more brittle and can break more easily. Height decreases, primarily caused by shortening of the trunk and spine as the intervertebral discs gradually lose fluid and become thinner, and vertebrae lose some of their mineral content, making each bone thinner. The spinal column becomes curved and compressed. The foot arches become less pronounced, contributing to slight loss of height. The long bones of the arms and legs, although more brittle because of mineral losses, do not change length, making the arms and legs look longer in relation to the shortened trunk. The joints become stiffer and less flexible. Fluid in the joints may decrease, and the cartilage may begin to rub together and erode. Minerals may deposit in some joints. Hip and knee joints may begin to lose structure due to degenerative changes. The finger joints lose cartilage, and the bones thicken slightly. Inflammation, pain, stiffness, and deformity can result from breakdown of the joint structures. The posture can become progressively stooped, and the knees and hips more flexed. The neck may become tilted. The shoulders may narrow while the pelvis may become wider. Movement slows and may become limited. The gait becomes slower and shorter. Walking may become unsteady, with less arm swing.

Cardiovascular System

Macroscopically, the heart increases in size and weight. The increasing thickness of the left ventricular wall is thought to be a compensatory mechanism in the face of increased afterload. Four components contribute to this increased afterload: increased aortic diameter, decreased central arterial compliance, premature timing of the reflected wave (in systole rather than diastole), and increased peripheral resistance. The size of the left ventricular cavity does not change, although the left atrium dilates. The thickened myocardium is due to not only myocyte hypertrophy but also collagen deposition due to decreased turnover. These changes, in addition to lipofuscin deposits, fatty infiltration, and fibrosis, result in ventricular stiffness. The endocardium undergoes diffuse thickening, and valves may become thickened and calcified. Fibrosis, myocyte hypertrophy, and calcium deposition can impact the rest of the conduction system, which may manifest as prolongation in the PR and QRS intervals on electrocardiography and right bundle-branch block.

Pacemaker cells are lost at a rate of 10% per decade and can result in sinus arrest or tachy-brady syndrome. Despite these changes of normative aging, resting cardiac function remains unchanged throughout life in the absence of disease. Resting heart rate, left ventricular ejection fraction, cardiac output, cardiac index, and stroke index do not change with age. Heart rate variability is diminished and hypertrophy, especially in older women, may actually result in an increased (hyperdynamic) resting ejection fraction. The heart is less responsive to β-adrenergic stimulation and thus does not speed up as much when stimulated by exercise as in a stress test. With physical or mental stress, the inotropic (contraction) and lusotropic (relaxation) response to adrenaline are also diminished in older compared with younger hearts despite higher levels of circulating catecholamines in the former; maximal oxygen consumption, an objective measure of exercise, declines with advancing age due to declines in maximal heart rate, maximal cardiac output, and muscle extraction of oxygen from the blood. All of these changes accompany advancing age, but occur at different rates in individuals. These changes may also be magnified by the impact of atherosclerosis and hypertension, the risk of which both increase with age.

The arteries become dilated, and the vessels increase in length, become more rigid, and lose their sensitivity to receptor-mediated agents. Macroscopically, the intima and basement membrane progressively thicken, while endothelial cells become irregular in size and shape. Smooth muscle cells and blood-derived macrophages infiltrate, followed by increased matrix synthesis (ie, intimal sclerosis). In the media, internal elastic lamina becomes thinner and straighter, and elastin fibers fragment and are replaced by collagen, causing decreased elasticity; calcification increases, and lipids accumulate intra- and extracellularly.

Pulmonary System

The costal cartilages undergo calcification, there is kyphosis, and the compliance of chest wall decreases. The bronchial mucous glands increase. Elastin fibers in the parenchymal framework decrease with increasing cross-linkage between these fibers, which decreases elastic recoil of the lungs. Decreased recoil can lead to reduced intrathoracic negative pressure and airway collapse. Collagen levels also decrease. Alveolar duct volume increases at the expense of the alveolus (ductectasia). The surface area of the lung decreases, residual volume increases by 20 mL/yr, vital capacity decreases, and forced expiratory volume and forced vital capacity decrease by 30% by 80 yr of age. Effort-independent respiration (ie, quiet breathing) decreases due to decreased elastic recoil and airway collapse in the lower lung zones. Effort-dependent respiration (ie, forced breathing) decreases with decreasing respiratory musculature. All the above factors can contribute to decreased arterial partial pressure of oxygen, exercise tolerance, and pulmonary reserve.

Eyes

Loss of periorbital fat produces sunken eyes and laxity of eyelids, leading to senile entropion (in which the lower lid curls in and the eyelashes irritate the cornea) and ectropion (in which the eyelids fall away from the orbit, resulting in excessive tear production and poor siphoning). Both entropion and ectropion increase susceptibility to conjunctivitis. Transparency of the cornea decreases as lipid infiltrates/deposits (ie, arcus senilis) accumulate. The anterior chamber becomes progressively shallower because of the thickening of the lens. Pupil diameter decreases progressively. Increasing fibrosis of the iris reduces accommodation and slows dark adaption. The eye needs double the illumination every 13 yr to maintain recognition in subdued light. The lens increases in size and becomes more rigid because of the constant formation of new central epithelial cells at the front of the lens. Consequences of these changes include presbyopia (ie, difficulty in focusing especially on near objects due to lens rigidity), reduced concentration of soluble proteins with an increase in insoluble complexes, general decline in transparency with an increase in yellow pigment filtering out blue light, reduced metabolic activity, and increased cataract formation (due to a progressive increase in the annular layers of the lens and a compression of central components that become hard and opaque).

In the retina, rods constantly produce pigment membranes, but with age less phagocytosis of the pigment membranes leads to buckling and kinking of rods. Cones show a major deterioration of membranes with age, and a decline in numbers that is particu-

larly marked after age 40. Pigment epithelial cells are captive macrophages that die off throughout life. They phagocytose 250,000 membranes per day, thus becoming full of debris that they try to extrude through Bruch's membrane, forming yellow or white plaques (termed drusen) that are visible through an ophthalmoscope. Macrophages migrate in and break up Bruch's membrane, allowing blood vessels to invade, which can lead to senile macular degeneration and visual impairment. The lens, cornea, and macula contain yellow pigment that filters out damaging blue light. These pigment levels increase with age, possibly as an innate protection against environmental damage.

Ears

In the external ear, the pinna continues to grow, and ear wax accumulates and hardens. In the middle ear, the tympanic membrane thickens with a loss of both elasticity and efficiency of ossicular articulation. These changes may lead to conductive deafness, which affects predominately low-frequency sounds. In the inner ear, a gradual bilaterally symmetrical sensorineural hearing loss (ie, presbycusis) predominately affects high-frequency sounds. The multiple forms of presbycusis include sensory (atrophy of the hair cells in the organ of Corti), neural (loss of cochlear neurons in the basal part of the spiral ganglion), metabolic (patchy atrophy of the stria vascularis over the middle and apical regions of the cochlea, restricting blood supply to the neurosensory receptors), and mechanical (changes in the motion mechanics of the cochlear duct such as that caused by increasing stiffness of the basilar membrane). The auditory canal narrows progressively.

Digestive System

The tongue develops varicosities, and decreased saliva production predisposes the mouth to oral infections. An increase in nonperistaltic spontaneous contractions of the esophagus produces difficulty in swallowing (ie, dysphagia). In presbyesophagus, normal swallowing is not often followed by the primary peristaltic wave, nonpropulsive contractions increase relaxation, and the lower esophageal sphincter is uncoordinated. Clinically, diverticulae and herniation are common in older adults. In the stomach, the incidence of atrophic gastritis increases (16% of the population >70 yr old), showing atrophy of the mucosa and muscularis mucosae, and inflammation and loss of gastric glands. The incidence of achlorhydria increases; pepsin activity decreases while plasma gastrin levels increase. Gastric emptying is delayed after fatty meals (not seen with carbohydrate meals).

The proximal jejunal villi become broader and shorter. Cell production in jejunal crypts decreases, incidence of diverticula increases, and chronic intestinal ischemia due to atheroma in supply vessels also increases. Intestinal fat absorption is delayed and reduced because of delayed gastric emptying and decreased lipase production. Vitamin B_{12} absorption and calcium absorption decrease; iron absorption also decreases in the presence of achlorhydria. In the pancreas, there is duct hyperplasia, increased cyst formation, deposition of lipofuscin granules in acinar cells, and increased fatty deposition. In the large intestine, mucosa cells atrophy. There is cellular infiltration of the lamina propria and mucosa and hypertrophy of the muscularis mucosae. Atrophy of other muscle layers leads to an increase in connective tissue, development of diverticula, transit time, and constipation.

Urinary System

Kidney size and weight decrease. The number of functional glomeruli decreases, and the number of abnormal and sclerotic glomeruli increases. The number of functional renal tubules decreases, and these tubules decrease in length. These changes lead to an increase in tubular diverticula and an increase in tubular basement membrane thickness; impaired permeability decreases the ability to resorb glucose. The glomerular filtration rate (GFR) declines. Renal blood flow falls as a consequence of altered vascular pattern, atherosclerotic changes, altered arteriole-glomerular flow, and focal ischemic lesions. Filtration fraction (GFR/renal plasma flow) increases; therefore, renal plasma flow must decline relatively more than GFR. The concentrating ability of the kidney declines. Acid-base and water balance, and regulation of electrolyte concentrations remain normal, but the system is unable to maintain homeostatic conditions under times of stress. In the bladder, there is edema, lymphocyte infiltration, trabeculae and diverticula, prolapse, and urethral mucosal atrophy.

Immune System

The general effects of aging on the immune system include a variable but gradual average decline in immune functioning. The immune system requires more stimulus and more time to become activated, produces less primary and secondary responses, and loses memory cells faster. Autoimmune antibodies also increase. T-cell function decreases gradually, and fewer naive and more memory T cells reduce the ability to mount an immune response when new exposures to pathogens occur. B-cell function decreases gradually, as does the response by naive B cells to newly introduced antigens. Aging B cells also increase production of abnormal antibodies. Atrophy

of the thymus reduces function and production of T lymphocytes, proliferation of natural killer cells, and production of cytokines needed for growth and maturation of B cells. Loss of self-renewal capacity by hematopoietic stem cells contributes to immune-cell dysfunction.

Endocrine System

Age-related changes in the endocrine system vary with the individual gland and can involve changes in hormone levels, in receptor numbers on target cells, or in signal-transducing pathways. The pituitary gland exhibits minimal changes. Growth hormone exhibits a variable but average decline in pulsatile secretion pattern, contributing to a decrease in size of structures and in lean body mass to fat ratio. Prolactin also decreases nocturnal pulsatile secretion. In the pineal gland, a reduced diurnal melatonin rhythm can contribute to altered sleep patterns and a deficit in free-radical defenses. Norepinephrine secretion increases, and an altered responsiveness contributes to age-associated changes in systemic vasoconstriction and decreased cardiac function. Epinephrine levels and metabolism do not change.

The thyroid gland atrophies with increased fibrosis and nodule formation. T_4 production declines with very old age, but blood concentrations of thyroxine are normal because the clearance rate of T_4 decreases. There is an evolving debate over whether thyrotropin levels do not change with normal aging, or whether levels associated with hypothyroidism in older adults reflect a change in the set point of this hormone. Total serum calcitonin levels decrease, although bioactive calcitonin levels remain unchanged. The parathyroid glands show increased fat deposition but no atrophy. In women >40 yr old, parathyroid hormone levels increase and its metabolism decreases, associated with decreased 1,25(OH)D serum concentrations and changes in bone mineral homeostasis.

The adrenal glands do not atrophy but show an increase in fibrous tissue. A moderate decrease in aldosterone secretion can contribute to orthostatic hypotension. Cortisol secretions also decrease, although the steady-state levels of circulating cortisol stay the same. Adrenocorticotropic hormone (ACTH) secretion (unstimulated and stimulated), cortisol secretion, and circadian rhythms remain unchanged, although negative feedback is delayed after a stressor, resulting in a delayed restoration of ACTH and cortisol to unstimulated levels. The adrenals also produce androgens and estrogens, although the adrenal contribution is usually masked by the testes and ovaries. However, after menopause, androgen secretion and masculinization arise from the adrenals. There are minimal changes in the pancreas, and an age-related decline in insulin signaling occurs at the target cell level, where decreased receptors and cellular glucose transporters contribute to reduced sensitivity. In the heart, atrial natriuretic peptide (ANP) levels increase, renal responsiveness to ANP decreases, and the hypotensive response to infused ANP increases. The thymus atrophies with age, and thymosin levels decrease as does immune function, contributing to an age-related increase in risk of infection and cancer.

In the kidneys, the response of antidiuretic hormone to osmotic stimuli increases, and the response of vasopressin to volume change decreases. Erythropoietin secretion increases in both the mid-aged and old as its metabolic clearance rate also increases. Circulating renin levels decrease as a consequence of decreased renin synthesis and impaired renin release. In the gonads, dehydro-epiandrosterone (DHEA) and its more abundant sulfated form, DHEA-S, decrease, as do pregnenolone levels. Testosterone exhibits an average decrease in level and diurnal rhythm, which contributes to changes in skin, hair, muscle, and bone. In women, a large decrease in estrogen and progesterone is associated with altered skin, increased low-density lipoprotein levels, and decreased bone mineral. Leptin levels (produced by adipose tissue) decrease in women >70 yr old, concomitant with decreases in body fat. Leptin levels increase in older men despite decreasing body fat because of an age-associated decrease in testosterone levels. A number of hormones exhibit an altered two-hormone synchrony. For example, older men secrete luteinizing hormone (LH) and testosterone more irregularly and jointly more asynchronously. Other hormone pairs that exhibit age-related asynchronous secretion include insulin and growth hormone, ACTH and cortisol, LH and prolactin, and LH and follicle-stimulating hormone.

SYSTEMS BIOLOGY AND AGING

The changes that occur with aging contribute to systems-wide dysregulation and loss of maintenance. For example, the physiologic parameter of body temperature maintenance can be used to explore systems-wide aging effects. With increased age, biologic changes to structures (loss of fat and thinning of skin, loss of sweat glands, decreased number of blood vessels and blood flow to skin surface, decreased muscle mass) have discrete molecular correlates and contribute to decrements in the functional capacity to maintain body temperature. Also, with increased age, biologic changes to negative feedback pathways (eg, nervous system changes such as fewer nerve cells that monitor/sense temperature and weakly functioning remaining nerve cells) also impinge on thermal regulation. Thus, aging is associated with a decreased detection and response to thermal variance.

Similarly, malnutrition in older adults can be viewed through the contributions of age-related changes in specific organ systems. In addition to the well-known age-related changes in the digestive system that affect nutrition (eg, decreased absorption of vitamins A, D, and K, and zinc in the small intestines, decreased vitamin D production by skin and activation by kidneys causing reduced calcium), other organ systems contribute to altered nutrition. Aging in the nervous system leads to a decreased sense of smell; altered flavor preferences lead to an altered diet. Decreased sensory function and coordination, muscle weakness, changes in cartilage and in bone mobility and stability can make it more difficult to obtain, prepare, and eat nutritionally adequate food. In the circulatory system, thicker blood vessels reduce blood flow through the digestive system, causing reduced digestion and absorption of various nutrients. In the respiratory system, decreased compliance and capacity can also lead to difficulty in obtaining, preparing, and eating a proper diet.

Thus, the biologic changes that occur with aging act across multiple systems and create expanding perturbations to homeostasis and functional capacity. The challenge for the clinician is to provide care to an ever-increasing older patient population in the context of numerous subtle and not-so-subtle primary aging-related physiologic changes, along with increasing comorbid medical conditions, frailty and other geriatric conditions, and disability.

REFERENCES

■ Holliday R. *Aging: The Paradox of Life: Why We Age.* 1st ed. New York, NY: Springer; 2007.

■ Hunt KJ, Walsh BM, Voegeli D, et al. Inflammation in aging part 2: implications for the health of older people and recommendations for nursing practice. *Biol Res Nurs.* 2010;11(3):253–260.

CHAPTER 3—PSYCHOSOCIAL ISSUES

KEY POINTS

- Older adults face many psychosocial issues. Stressors can be modified or mediated by factors both internal and external to the individual. Positive modification of the stressors can improve outcomes.

- Stressors such as caregiving, loss and grief, and changes in social status and social roles, including movement out of the workforce, are more common in the lives of older adults. Successful adaptation to stressors can improve health outcomes; unsuccessful adaptation can lead to health declines.

- Implementing healthy behaviors can be beneficial, regardless of age.

- Social networks and positive interpersonal relationships can significantly moderate age-related stressors and lead to improved health.

Appreciating the role and scope of psychosocial aspects of aging improves clinicians' ability to address and treat factors that have important bearing on the overall well-being of older adults. Health events have broad ramifications. When they are viewed within a framework that includes both the stressors and the means to ameliorate the impact of stress, other factors besides the treatment of the disease itself can be seen to need clinical attention.

Stressors are any demands that induce a physiologic, behavioral, or emotional response; often, such demands are perceived as threats. Unchecked stressors can lead to negative outcomes directly related to the situation, as well as to more indirect negative outcomes across the spectrum of physical and mental health, economic welfare, and family life. Given the range of demands posed by stressors, it is evident that they can greatly affect a person's physical and mental health, including every aspect of his or her well-being. The person's ability to function in the world may be reduced, as well as the enthusiasm the person brings to and the pleasure he or she experiences from social interaction. The use the person makes of financial, health, and social service resources may also be strongly affected.

STRENGTH-OF-EVIDENCE (SOE) RATING DEFINITIONS

A = consistent and good quality patient-oriented evidence
B = somewhat inconsistent or limited quality patient-oriented evidence
C = very inconsistent or very limited patient-oriented evidence, disease-oriented evidence, and/or consensus from professional organizations
D = unstudied common practice or opinion

See inside front cover for detailed information regarding the SOE classification.

For a framework for considering the complex interaction of physical and psychosocial factors shaping the outcomes of stressors confronting older adults, see Figure 3.1. This chapter briefly discusses common psychosocial threats faced by older adults, but it is principally focused on immutable and mutable factors that bear on the direct and indirect outcomes of stress situations, all with an eye to offering the clinician important tools for treatment as well as targets for therapeutic intervention. The chapter highlights findings from social science research that indicate ways in which unchangeable facts about a person's life (eg, gender) contribute to the outcome of stress situations—and to a person's ability to respond to them. In particular, the chapter discusses mediators and moderators, factors that can serve to filter, although not entirely protect against, the impact of stress through different mechanisms. Mediators involve the older adult's perceptions of and responses to the stress situation. Moderators—which may be constituents of an older adult's environment or behaviors in which the individual engages—can be thought of as acting on the stressor itself to lessen its intensity or buffer its effect; they also affect an individual's ability to respond to the stressor. Assisting older adults to see and work toward health outcomes that impact the quality of their life is an appropriate and effective clinical strategy for helping them to confront declines in physical health and the issues of mortality.

STRESSORS

Older adults face a great number and variety of stressors that are produced by a broad range of events and conditions. The stressors may be chronic, or they may have a sudden, dramatic onset. They may be based in diseases or be of a more social nature. A chronic stressor may be health related (eg, the pain and mobility limitation of arthritis) or physiologic (particularly with regard to disrupted or inadequate sleep), or it may be psychologic (eg, the prolonged worry over a chronically ill spouse). An acute stressor might also be physical or psychologic (eg, learning of a newly diagnosed medical condition or experiencing the unexpected death of a close friend). Other stress demands include changes in social identity because of role changes at work as a person ages, role loss in retirement, or the function-driven need to move to a more supportive living arrangement. Losses in physical ability and reserve may place demands on an individual, not only because he or she perceives them as threats or increased physical demands, but also because of their accompanying psychologic compo-

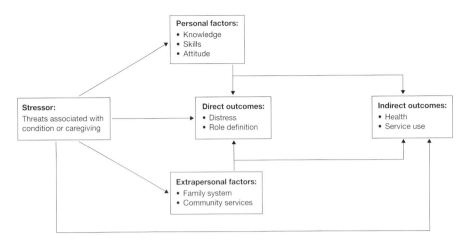

Figure 3.1—Stress Theory Model

nent, the perception that he or she may have less ability to respond to other demands. Always in the background for older adults are the various risk factors for incident or recurrent morbidity and mortality.

Some risk factors—particularly those involving behaviors over which the person (with some encouragement, teaching, and counseling) might exert control—can be modified. Other risk factors, such as gender and race, cannot be modified and produce accumulated assaults that can amplify other stressors. The increasing incidence of diseases with age means that the number and frequency of stressors are likely to increase with age.

Caregiving

Caregiving is nearly endemic; more than 46 million Americans provide informal health and social care for family members of all ages. Gender is an important factor; more than 70% of all caregivers are women. Many older adults are caregivers for a family member. Chronic diseases affect a large proportion of older adults, and much of the care they receive is provided by family members, especially spouses. The burden of caregiving for dementing disorders like Alzheimer's disease is formidable. Dementia caregivers spend many hours each day in caregiving activities, and they do so for many years (20% are caregivers for >5 yr). Such caregiving exacts a heavy toll. Caregivers are at twice the risk as their noncaregiving peers of adverse physical and mental health outcomes and more than twice as likely to be taking psychotropic medications (SOE=A). Social isolation, family disharmony, and economic hardships are common sequelae of caregiving; because, as discussed below, social networks and social interaction are important buffers against stress, their deterioration adds further to the impact of caregiving. Race and ethnicity play important roles both in establishing the pattern of family caregiving (solo caregiving is more the norm among whites than in other groups in which family caregiv-

ing is more prevalent) and the physical and mental health responses to caregiving (eg, it appears that black caregivers demonstrate less serious adverse events than do whites).

It is important to delineate and consider the roles that people assume when providing care for an acutely or chronically ill family member. Family caregivers play a number of "clinical" functions: becoming "expert" in the particular condition with which they are dealing; managing, assisting with, and monitoring prescribed therapeutic regimens (including medications); functioning as liaison with primary and specialist providers (both to report on status and to advocate for further attention); providing emotional support to the person dealing with the disease; and, often surreptitiously, initiating treatments and home remedies. In redesigning environments to accommodate for any illness-produced losses, securing or inventing devices to compensate for functional losses, and assisting with rehabilitative regimens, family caregivers assume physical and occupational therapy roles. And in serving as the point of contact for the health and social service resources that are brought to bear to address the demands of living with or recovering from an illness, family caregivers become case managers.

Caregivers need training, information, and support; they also need a positive alliance with the person's healthcare providers. They cannot be expected to be able to assume or to be effective in their various roles just because they have a relational bond with their family member. Acknowledgement of the role, provision of information about the disease, guidance and instruction regarding the work the caregiver needs to be able to do, and referral to appropriate professionals and/or health educators are all essential. Caregivers should be regularly observed for signs of the known effects of caregiving. Appropriate referrals—for direct help for themselves, for help in the home, and for respite—are all important.

Caregiving also can have positive benefits for the caregiver: relationships can be strengthened, and caregivers can experience a sense of satisfaction for a job well done and an obligation fulfilled. Such rewards can be pointed out and affirmed. Attention to family dynamics may also be useful in identifying issues contributing to stressors that can be modified. A number of intervention programs (eg, those providing education, counseling, and cognitive-behavioral therapy) have proved effective in ameliorating the stress associated with caregiving. There is some evidence that religious involvement buffers the stress of caregiving (SOE=B). Disease-specific support activities offer only modest relief but may be the conduit for more focused help.

Loss and Grief

Being widowed, especially for women, is a common occurrence in old age, as are deaths in extended families and larger social networks. More than 1.5 million spouses will be widowed annually by 2030. In 2000, 8.3% of those between 65 and 74 yr old were widowed; 22.7% of those older than 75 were widowed. Other losses, such as sensory and functional losses imposed by the onset of chronic or acute illnesses, also produce grief. Such losses are generally understood to be among the major negative life events, and they place a substantial demand on a person. For most, the intense experience of grief lasts 6–12 mo, generally a time of withdrawal and depression. After about a year, a more accepting period ensues, during which a reemergence into a social milieu occurs, or a less affecting form of more permanent memorialization of the lost person is established. Acknowledgment and monitoring of the grieving process and active treatment of the depression associated with loss can help in avoiding prolongation of this process. See also "Depression and Other Mood Disorders," p 295.

Role Loss and Acquisition

People typically encounter a large number of role shifts in aging. They leave work and social roles that may have provided economic rewards as well as status. For example, the number of Social Security beneficiaries ≥65 yr old rose from 32.9 million in 2001 (a year in which 2 million Americans turned 65) to 34.5 million in 2006 (a 4.7% increase). This appears to be just the leading edge of a trend. From 1996 to 2006, while the total U.S. workforce was growing by 13.1%, there was a 59.4% increase in workers ≥55 yr old (an additional 46.7% increase in this cohort is expected to occur from 2006 to 2016); of note, a 68.7% increase was seen in female workers in this age group in the 1996–2006 period. The average age of retirement has been declining steadily,

dropping to slightly under 62 yr of age in 1995–2000 (down more than 5 yr since 1950–1955). Within relationships, roles may change, and wage-earning spouses, after retirement, may find themselves spending much more time with each other. Grandparenthood and great-grandparenthood bring both new demands and opportunities. Functional losses can place older adults in help-seeking rather than help-providing roles or, as noted above, another's losses may place one in a caregiving role. These role changes can be stressful and negatively affect mental or physical health. Programs to enhance older workers' sense of self-efficacy and retirement planning can help make these positive experiences. The clinician's assessment of an older adult's role loss and acquisition may suggest the need for interventions.

Social Status

Three factors are consistently associated in the United States with a broad range of negative psychosocial and physical outcomes: being nonwhite, female, and poor or poorly educated (usually a surrogate for being poor). They should serve as warnings for clinicians, because the presence of one or more of these factors can add to the person's stress load. They can also affect the kinds of coping mechanisms the person has available. Lack of disposable income, for example, may exclude the use of some formal services or involvement in community activities that charge a fee.

Race has a direct bearing on health stresses and longevity in old age. A 65-yr-old black American man can expect to live nearly 2 yr less than a 65-yr-old white American man (a pattern mirrored among black American and white American women). Ethnic or cultural background and community context can substantially affect a person's outlook on a situation, the kinds of moderating activities he or she deems acceptable, and the importance he or she places on various outcomes. Older adults may understand disease through frameworks specific to other cultures, and treatment may need to include or rely principally on culturally centered options. A concept such as autonomy, which has become so central in issues of patient choice and advance directives, has a different weight and value in cultures in which choice belongs more to the community as a whole (as with some Native American groups) or to a community or family leader (eg, in Hmong societies). Choices like hospice care may be viewed in some cultures as tantamount to wishing for and bringing about the death of the person. A procedure like autopsy can strongly violate cultural or religious beliefs. The clinician is advised to proceed attentively in cross-cultural situations. See also "Cultural Aspects of Care," p 49.

MEDIATORS

Mediators shape a person's responses to stress. They are the internal and external resources the person can use to assess and interpret the stress, to assess his or her own capacities for addressing it, and to formulate a coping response to it. Many key mediators are modifiable through psychosocial intervention. Instruction and information can affect the person's understanding of a situation. Various forms of psycho-education have been shown to be effective in enhancing an older adult's sense of mastery within a stress situation and in increasing his or her awareness and use of formal services. Family counseling and therapy can strengthen the involvement of older adults with their social network.

Self-Efficacy Beliefs

A number of constructs have been studied that relate to a person's sense of his or her own ability to manage situations. The concept of self-efficacy is comparable to concepts such as mastery, internal locus of control, resilience, and competence; although it is singled out here, self-efficacy resembles these in representing a key personal quality to be considered when dealing with an older adult facing any stress situation. Self-efficacy is an important consideration for the mental and physical health of older adults for two reasons:

First, there is a relationship between strong or positive self-efficacy and a number of important health and mental health outcomes (Table 3.1) (SOE=B). A large number of longitudinal studies—most notably the MacArthur study of "successful" or healthy aging—have produced a coherent set of conclusions about self-efficacy. The way a person approaches a situation—whether it be a specific threat (eg, the onset of an acute condition) or a more pervasive one (eg, change of life roles or decline in physical performance)—affects the eventual outcome. Of particular note is the broad range of effects of strong self-efficacy beliefs, which influence physical and mental health as well as overall function (Table 3.1). In addition, self-efficacy seems to contribute to a person's ability to be actively engaged in life, an important moderating factor.

The second reason self-efficacy is important is that it can change. It can be weakened by repeated assaults and poor outcome, but it can also be strengthened. Among the strategies effective for strengthening self-efficacy are the following:

- performance accomplishment (seeing oneself succeed in a series of increasingly difficult tasks)
- vicarious learning and social modeling (seeing others like oneself succeed in a targeted area)

Table 3.1—Physical and Mental Health Impacts of Self-Efficacy Beliefs

Strong self-efficacy beliefs
- Buffer the effects of stress exposure on physical and mental health
- Contribute to overall physical performance, independently of ability
- Help maintain good function
- Slow functional decline among those with poor physical performance
- Contribute to good choice making, good performance, and persistence of effort (especially in women)
- Contribute to increased productivity

Weak self-efficacy beliefs
- Are associated with declines in functional status, especially in those with decreased physical performance

- encouragement (being persuaded to undertake a targeted activity)
- reinforcement (experiencing pleasure from success)

A number of training programs aimed at improving specific performance (eg, reducing the fear of falling or increasing adherence to an exercise regimen after a heart attack) have succeeded by working to strengthen participants' self-efficacy beliefs in the targeted area. Strong self-efficacy beliefs appear to be better predictors of performance than measures of physical ability. In falls prevention studies, for example, those with strong self-efficacy beliefs related to falling were found to show reduced fear of falling, despite low objective measures for risk of falling. Self-efficacy appears to play an important role in coping and overall well-being in older adults. Clinicians should assess the older adult's sense of his or her own competence and intervene, when possible, to strengthen it.

Coping Strategies

A number of theorists have studied the manner in which older adults meet and address the accumulated challenges of aging. Cultivating an emotional response to a stressor can mediate its effect and result in a better outcome. Thus, invoking confidence and optimism in the face of bad news helps a person to meet the challenge and strengthens the likelihood of a positive outcome. One strategy older adults can use consists of selection, optimization, and compensation. In this strategy, as people age, they begin to hone down the number and kinds of things in which they engage in on the basis of what they believe they do well, selecting activities in which they are more likely to succeed. They also reframe the way they judge their own performance, looking, for example, at people their own age or older for a source of comparison. They do the selected things more, and they derive optimal credit for doing them. As losses continue and performance diminishes, people use compensatory strategies that allow them to put their remaining performance abilities in the best light possible. A person known for preparing elaborate dinners might, for example, choose a simpler main course (selection) that he or she does well and has prepared many times (optimization) and surround it with numerous but very simple courses and side dishes as a way of favorably setting it off (compensation). Other coping strategies (eg, assimilation, accommodation, immunization, or resilience) also build essentially on the notion of reframing the self or one's performance to provide positive reinforcement and to reinforce self-esteem. Clinicians should attempt to learn how their patients typically form successful responses to challenges and help them to address new challenges in these same terms.

Social Involvement

Like people at all ages, older adults are faced with developmental tasks and challenges. In Erikson's theory of staged development, the task of old age is integration—putting the pieces together in a way that both celebrates and continues to act on the learning and accomplishments of life. In this conception, and consistent with many other findings, involvement (sometimes termed *productivity*) plays an important role. Becoming more involved, actively seeking out ways to contribute to and participate in the broader world, even engaging in paid work are all mediators that can lead to better outcomes. Taking part and making a contribution—through volunteering, productive (sometimes paid) labor, active family roles (especially child care), and participation in group activities—are all associated with older adults' continued well-being.

In terms of the framework of factors affecting health outcomes, social involvement can be understood as a positive, problem-focused coping response, a way of filtering the effects of a stressor by strengthening the connection of the person to the community (affirming the person's value in the community). Older theories of normal aging saw disengagement—the systematic withdrawal of ties to the social world—as normative. In current thinking, however, such disengagement is not encouraged and might even be considered an abnormal behavior. At the very least, there is an association between lack of social involvement and affective disorders such as depression.

MODERATORS

Moderators are components of a person's life or behaviors in which the person engages that act to

Table 3.2—Physical and Mental Health Impacts of Robust Social Networks*

- Reduced mortality risks
- Better physical health outcomes
- Better mental health outcomes
- Reduced risk of ADL disability or decline
- Increased likelihood of ADL recovery
- Buffered impact of major negative life events
- Promotion of strong self-efficacy beliefs
- Assistance that does not preclude self-care but that can increase risk of new or recurrent ADL disability (especially in men)

*SOE=A

affect the demands of the various stressors he or she faces. Moderators may be in place before the onset of a stressor, or they might be developed in response to it. A person who has a long history of exercise already has a good base of conditioning to deal with an emergent condition affecting mobility (eg, arthritis). Alternatively, making a decision to begin to exercise, to control diet or alcohol consumption, to seek help to improve sleep, or to cease smoking is a possible—and healthy—response to stressors ranging from the onset of illness to a realization that one has slowed down. These healthy behaviors directly moderate the effect of the threat or demand and contribute to better physical and mental health outcomes. Having a strong social network and calling on it in a time of crisis (rather than withdrawing) can help moderate age-related demands (eg, the loss of a loved one).

Three major activities moderate stress or demand and appear to contribute to healthy aging: social involvement, spiritual or religious activity, and engaging in healthy behaviors. Older adults' activities in these areas should be assessed regularly and encouraged, as appropriate.

Social Networks

The older adult's social network is a critical resource for overall well-being, and social isolation is a powerful risk factor for broad declines and mortality. The effect of a social network on an older adult's overall well-being has been extensively studied, with conclusive results (Table 3.2) (SOE=B). The literature points to the importance of quality over quantity but does not discount the latter. The closeness of social relationships is most important; thus, a well-functioning marital or familial relationship—a relationship that provides a person with a confidante—offers the kinds of support and protection suggested in Table 3.2. Dysfunctional close relationships—those characterized by negative and conflict-filled interactions—appear to work in the contrary direction. The size of an older adult's social network appears to work in both directions. Although having a larger social network offers the opportunity for greater involvement and contribution, it also presents the likelihood of experiencing a greater number of losses within the network (because of death or increased disability).

A robust social network both mediates and moderates age-related stresses. Social networks provide emotional and instrumental help in times of crisis. Families help older adults, for example, cope with the death of a spouse or close friend, but they also provide direct and indirect help when more functional losses occur. The social network can provide a person under stress with a context within which to envision and frame responses to various demands. Social networks seem to exert a positive effect on older adults by strengthening their self-efficacy beliefs (the person feels valued within the social network, and this contributes to a sense of self-worth). It also provides opportunities for taking action to address demands (eg, calling on family for specific functional assistance, spending more time with children after the death of a spouse, increasing time spent with friends after retirement).

Provision of such help is positive and contributes to recovery, unless it sends the wrong message. Too much instrumental assistance provided to older adults (particularly men) by the social network can contribute to continued disability. Rather than being encouraged to work toward restored function, a person may receive too much help or not be encouraged to engage in self-care and may, therefore, accept a modifiable condition as permanent. Thus, although assistance from the social network should be encouraged, it should be done with attention to promoting maximal function by the person receiving the help.

Spiritual or Religious Involvement

There is a developing but as yet incomplete understanding of the role of religion and spirituality in the lives of older adults and of the effect of the presence or absence of these involvements on health and well-being. Studies consistently demonstrate that religion plays a more important part in the lives of the current cohort of older adults than in the lives of younger persons. More than 50% of older adults report frequent attendance at religious events (with little variation by gender or race), and this has been a lifelong practice—rather than a late-life development (SOE=A).

A number of studies have demonstrated positive associations between religiousness, typically measured as regular attendance in organized religious activities, and a variety of markers of health (eg, blood pressure) and mental health (eg, depression). There is evidence that regular attendance at religious services is associated with a lower composite measure of allostatic load among older women (but not men) (SOE=B). The literature suggests that religious participation may be beneficial, in part, because it promotes social interaction; however, one study suggests evidence that the effect is independent of social interaction. However, a number of studies have found that the beneficial effects of religious participation are not universal, and there is a suggestion that it may be most beneficial for those with the least social resources, eg, women and minorities (SOE=B).

One benefit of this growing body of literature is an increasing clarity of the distinction between the two elements. While religion and spirituality are in no way mutually exclusive, neither do they necessarily overlap. In particular, the literature emphasizes the individualized quality of spirituality, portraying it in terms of practices through which a person seeks to establish or strengthen a link with a higher power or truth. In studies that have focused more on spirituality, findings generally indicate that such practices (eg, meditation or daily spiritual experiences) also are associated with better health and mental health outcomes (SOE=B). One study characterized the distinction between religion and spirituality as having positive associations for well-being related, in the case of religiosity, to positive social linkages and a sense of community service and, in the case of spirituality, to a sense of personal growth.

Overall, issues of religiosity and spirituality can provide clinicians with another dimension for assessing older adults. Ascertaining whether an older adult is engaged in a religious community or with religious practice and/or is involved in spiritual practices can provide insights about strengths that can be called on or areas in which resources are lacking.

Healthy Behaviors

Implementing positive behaviors (eg, exercising; controlling intake of food, tobacco, and alcohol; improving sleep; and participating in active relaxation or stress-reduction techniques) has positive effects on overall well-being, regardless of age when the behaviors are begun. Although these are physical behaviors, they often rely on and benefit from strong psychosocial mediators, particularly self-efficacy and social networks. Clinicians should use these mediators when proposing that older adults begin or strengthen healthy behaviors. It can help to invoke a person's understanding of benefits and appreciation of his or her own proven ability to make changes, while at the same time offering suggestions about how the targeted behavior might contribute to a strong social network (eg, "you could walk every day with your daughter," "you and your husband could take the healthy cooking class together").

REFERENCES

- Fry PS, Debats DL. Self-efficacy beliefs as predictors of loneliness and psychological distress in older adults. *Int J Aging Human Dev.* 2002;55(3):233–269.

- Pinquart M, Sorensen S. Associations of stressors and uplifts of caregiving with caregiver burden and depressive mood: a meta-analysis. *J Gerontol B Psychol Sci Soc Sci.* 2003;58(2):P112–P128.

- Sullivan MT. The Modified Caregiver Strain Index (CSI). *Try This: Best Practices in Nursing Care to Older Adults.* 2007;(14). Available at http://consultgerirn.org/uploads/File/trythis/try_this_14.pdf

- Wink P, Dillon M. Religiousness, spirituality and psychosocial functioning in late adulthood: findings from a longitudinal study. *Psychol Aging.* 2003:18(4):916–924.

CHAPTER 4—LEGAL AND ETHICAL ISSUES

KEY POINTS

- Four guiding ethical principles of American medical practice are respect for autonomy, nonmaleficence, beneficence, and justice.

- Decisional capacity is situation specific and changes over time. A consent-assent model is often useful for decision making for individuals with different degrees of incapacity.

- Substituted judgment is the process of constructing what a person would have wanted. Beneficence is the weighing of benefits and burdens of an intervention for that individual.

- Patients and their surrogates have the right to refuse treatment whether that treatment is already in place or has not yet been started.

- Respect for the patient's autonomy may come in conflict with our duty to keep an incapacitated patient safe, and with the safety of others and the public health.

INTRODUCTION TO MEDICAL ETHICS

Normative ethics is the inquiry into the standards of what we see as right or wrong action. It focuses on the question "What *ought* I do?" Medical ethics is based on a utilitarian ethical structure; that is, it is not based on deontologic overarching moral imperatives, as a religious ethic would be. Rather, it seeks the answer to the *ought* question through the principles that are applied in the context of the clinical situation. The goal of medical ethical deliberation is to maximize good consequences and minimize bad consequences (beneficence). These principles are tied to values and perspectives that are unique to each culture and that may also differ depending on whether one is addressing a specific case (situational ethics) or public policy.

The four guiding principles of American medical ethics most often cited are respect for autonomy, nonmaleficence, beneficence, and justice. How each of these principles guides the practice of medicine today is different from even 50 yr ago. These principles and their application also differ widely within various subcultures within the wider American culture.

The primacy of individual autonomy is a foundation of American culture, from the early pioneers to modern medical practice. Respect for individuals' autonomy should include respect for their right to subjugate their individualism to family, culture, or religion. In many cultures, family structure dictates who will be the decision maker for individuals within that family, and that person is deferred to even when the individual involved has the cognitive ability to make his or her own decisions. However, it is unethical to defer decision making to an adult child of an older patient who is capable of making decisions for himself or herself if that is not the cultural practice of the patient and family, or not the patient's wish.

Nonmaleficence is, in essence, the Hippocratic oath of "do no harm." Definitions or perceptions of harm differ widely between cultures and between individuals within cultures. The most frequently cited medical conflict between mainstream culture and subculture perspectives is blood transfusions for a Jehovah's Witness. For a Jehovah's Witness, blood transfusion may be thought to cause more harm than good, even if the outcome of not having the transfusion might be death. Understanding the values of subcultures within our society may help give us clues to the spectrum of values that underlie an individual's perspective on harm. Similarly, what constitutes beneficence, doing more good than harm, is largely determined by culture as well as by each individual. See "Cultural Aspects of Care," p 49.

Finally, the concept of justice in the context of health care in our society remains ambiguous. There is not a recognized right to health care in the United States. The distribution of healthcare benefits and the use of healthcare technologies continue to be uneven and reflect biases regarding gender, age, race, and ethnic origin. Researchers have frequently excluded older adults in their study populations, and the lack of knowledge on the relative effectiveness of interventions when they are used for older adults can lead to the under- or overuse of interventions in this age group. Furthermore, assumptions that equate age with chronic illness and comorbidity can deny beneficial treatment to healthy older adults. Patients from groups that have long been denied many of the benefits of our society, especially our healthcare dollars, may be more reluctant than more historically privileged patients to step back from aggressive treatments because of a perception of continued prejudice.

It is important to keep these differences in mind when considering the following discussions of ethical decision making and its application to individual patients. The discussions that follow are, in a true utilitarian sense, guiding principles, not moral imperatives.

DECISIONAL CAPACITY

Because of the nature of diseases affecting older adults, clinicians are often called on to assess a person's decision-making capacity and to use other sources of decisional authority when that capacity is impaired. Although the focus of much of the literature has been on clinicians' assessments of patients' capacity to make medical decisions, clinicians are also asked to render opinions on patients' ability to make decisions about other matters, such as managing money, writing a will, continuing to drive, possessing firearms, and even the everyday decisions involved in ADLs. A clinician may evaluate a patient's capacity to make decisions, but *competence* and *incompetence* are legal terms, and they imply that a court has taken action.

Assessment of Decisional Capacity

Assessing the patient's ability to understand the consequences of a decision is the overarching principle used in making a judgment of decisional capacity. To make a medical decision, the patient must be able to understand basic information about his or her condition, the probable progression and

outcomes of the disease, and the effects of various potential interventions. This requires the ability to understand the disease process; the proposed therapy and alternative therapies; the advantages, adverse events, and complications of each therapy; and the possible course of the disease without intervention. The patient also needs to be able to understand the broad consequences of accepting, deferring, or rejecting a proposed intervention. Admittedly, even clinicians cannot predict the full implications of complex medical decisions, because they can rarely know all the consequences of an intervention or the precise natural history of an illness in any individual. The patient should be allowed to make decisions that are based on his or her beliefs and values. Therefore, it is often most helpful for the clinician to explore a patient's hopes and fears and to help the patient clarify his or her goals so that the treatment options offered are compatible with these goals.

Cultural differences between clinicians and patients who are members of different ethnic groups can make assessing decision-making capacity an even more difficult task. Capacity assessment involves abstract concepts not easily translated into another language. It also involves interpreting value judgments on the basis of what is considered reasonable; this may differ according to culture. Because of this, it is important to ascertain the need for an interpreter. In emergency situations, this may have to be a family member or a staff member, but it is always preferable to offer the services of a professional interpreter. Issues of privacy arise when using a family member or a member of a small ethnic community who may have other connections with the patient. Family members may filter or modify what is being said out of embarrassment, lack of familiarity with medical terminology, or other motivations (conscious or unconscious). Patients may be unwilling to share sensitive information. In all such situations, confidentiality is lost. A professional interpreter can often accurately translate the nuances of language as well as act as a cultural broker when explanations need to be made. On the other hand, clinicians must avoid making assumptions based solely on ethnic background and evaluate each patient as an individual.

The capacity to make a living will is similar to that of being able to make treatment decisions, although it is somewhat more complicated because the patient is being asked to think in the abstract with a "what if?" frame of reference. The ability to choose a healthcare proxy (see below) is much less complex, and even fairly impaired patients are often able to choose someone to make decisions for them.

The requirements are even less stringent for testamentary competence (the ability to make a last

---

STRENGTH-OF-EVIDENCE (SOE) RATING DEFINITIONS

A = consistent and good quality patient-oriented evidence
B = somewhat inconsistent or limited quality patient-oriented evidence
C = very inconsistent or very limited patient-oriented evidence, disease-oriented evidence, and/or consensus from professional organizations
D = unstudied common practice or opinion

See inside front cover for detailed information regarding the SOE classification.

will and testament). In general, a person's ability to decide how he or she wishes to dispose of belongings after death is felt to be preserved even when the person is severely cognitively incapacitated in other ways. As long as the person can identify the individuals involved, is not delusional or in other ways so psychiatrically ill that their judgment is impaired (eg, paranoia), and is capable of understanding the consequence of signing the will, he or she is considered to have testamentary competence.

For a summary of the elements of decisional capacity in each of these four areas, see Table 4.1.

Standardized Tests of Decisional Capacity

Traditional tests of cognitive function have some, but limited, use in determining decisional capacity. An overall score on the Folstein Mini–Mental State Examination (MMSE) of ≤10 indicates such diminished cognitive ability that it is unlikely that the person retains decisional capacity. Some deficits uncovered by the use of the MMSE may be relevant (eg, immediate memory, attention, word finding, understanding simple verbal or written instructions, and ability to express simple ideas in writing); others are not (eg, calculation and visuospatial relationships). As we come to appreciate the influence of frontal lobe dysfunction on a patient's capacity to function, especially to perform complex IADLs, we are also coming to appreciate the influence that the cognitive domains of executive function have on decisional capacity. Executive functions include problem solving, planning (including appreciating consequences of an action), initiation, capacity to monitor one's own behavior, and inhibition of inappropriate behaviors. The Executive Interview 25-item examination of executive function correlates well with subjective measures of decisional capacity. Observation of the patient while completing tasks on the examination may reveal poor insight, impulsivity, the intrusion of irrelevant material, poor self-monitoring, and impaired ability to form and follow through on a plan. Clinicians can make similar observations by observing a patient draw a clock.

Specific tests of decisional capacity have been developed, but most deal in hypothetical situations, thereby requiring a greater degree of abstraction than does real-time decision making. The MacArthur Competency Assessment Tool for Treatment tests the person's ability to make a specific decision and has the advantage of dealing with decisions that are currently facing the individual, but it has not found a practical niche. Tools for the assessment of executive functioning or structured interviewing can be helpful for determining decision-making capacity, but there is no substitute for critical observation of the process itself.

Table 4.1—Elements of Decisional Capacity

Medical decisions
- Ability to understand relevant information
- Ability to understand consequences of the decision
- Ability to communicate a decision

Decisions of self-care
- Ability to care for oneself
- Ability to accept needed help to keep oneself safe

Finances
- Ability to manage bill payment
- Ability to appropriately calculate and monitor funds

Last will and testament
- Ability to remember estate plans
- Ability to express logic behind choices

Table 4.2—Hierarchy of Decision-Making Strategies

Patient's current wishes
- If the patient has decisional capacity, this **always** takes precedence

Substituted judgment
- Done by the surrogate decision maker only when the patient is not fully capable of making the decision
- Based on the patient's prior values and wishes
- Advance directive is used as guide
- Patient input is used when possible, even if the patient is not fully capable of making the decision

Beneficence
- Done by the surrogate decision maker when the patient lacks decisional capacity and evidence does not exist for substituted judgment
- Weighing of benefits and burdens as based on the patient's present indications of pleasures and burdens
- Input from caregivers is very important

Principles Governing Decision Making for Patients Who Lack Decisional Capacity

The hierarchy of decision-making strategies for those making the decisions for incapacitated patients is as follows: 1) respect their last capable indication of their wishes, 2) use substituted judgment, and 3) determine their best interests (ie, an analysis of benefits versus burden). Table 4.2 summarizes the hierarchy.

The last competent indication of wishes is most relevant in cases when patients are able to foresee that they will become incapacitated and can know what decisions may need to be made. Patients entering the terminal phase of an illness who know that at some point they will become confused or unconscious can give clear advance directives (also called *advance care plans* in some contexts) stating their preferences for care. As long as the circumstances remain substantially as predicted, other individuals should not be allowed to reverse these decisions.

Substituted judgment is the process of constructing what the person would have wanted if he or she had been able to foresee the circumstances and give directions for care. In theory, those who know the person best and understand what his or her fears, pleasures, values, and goals were (ie, what the patient's rationale for a decision would have been) can provide substituted judgment. This is usually, but not always, the next of kin. A patient can appoint someone to hold durable power of attorney for health affairs (designating that person as what is also referred to as a *healthcare agent* or *proxy*). The patient should choose the person who can best represent him or her. Any such surrogate makes decisions only if the patient has become incapable of making decisions. The person granted durable power of attorney takes precedence over the next of kin.

The best-interest standard, or the principle of beneficence, means making medical decisions for an incapacitated patient on the basis of the benefits and burdens an intervention poses for that patient. When there is no expressed wish by the patient and no one to offer substituted judgment, then the surrogate decision maker must weigh the benefits and the burdens of treatment for that patient to make a decision. Such analysis is best done by someone who is knowledgeable about what gives that patient pleasure; what causes agitation, fear, pain, or discomfort; and how the patient reacts to a change in setting, use of restraints, and similar matters.

Conservatorships and Living Wills

In the absence of next of kin or durable power of attorney for a patient lacking decisional capacity, the court may appoint a conservator (called a *guardian* in some states). There are usually two types of conservatorship: conservator of finance and conservator of person. Incompetence in matters of finance is usually determined either by the demonstrated incapacity of the patient to manage financial matters (eg, unpaid bills, uncashed checks) or through specific testing by either an occupational therapist or a neuropsychologist. A conservator of person is required when patients have demonstrated that either they can no longer make personal decisions (such as medical decisions), or they are both unable to care for themselves to the point that they endanger themselves through neglect or risk of injury and they cannot understand and accept the need for help.

Living wills are advance directives that attempt to demonstrate what decisions a person would make under certain circumstances. Most living wills address a couple of hypothetical clinical situations (eg, vegetative state, terminal illness) and four possible treatment options (cardiopulmonary resuscitation, respirator therapy, artificial food and hydration, and

dialysis). A living will has limited use because of its vagueness and because it cannot be generalized to the decisions that most commonly need to be made. Some living wills offer a detailed set of hypothetical case scenarios and treatment decisions, but these can be difficult for patients to understand and may not add information about the patient's rationale for decisions. Also, an individual's reaction to a hypothetical event may differ from how he or she will deal with reality. Nonetheless, a living will can be used as evidence of preferences when one is trying to construct how a patient who lacks decisional capacity might have felt about an intervention.

The Role of the Incapacitated Patient in Decision Making

Even when patients are not capable of making complex decisions, they can still participate in decision making about issues of lesser complexity. A task assessment of decision-making ability around a specific issue is always appropriate. A patient with little cognitive ability can still give some indication when something causes discomfort or displeasure or when something brings pleasure. The surrogate decision maker must consider these expressions when analyzing the benefits and burdens of an intervention. This consideration of the patient's indications of preference is supported by case law.

The perceived relative burden of an intervention can vary from one person to the next because of differences in mental status and ability to cope with change or disability. A demented patient who is accustomed to one environment will have a much harder time adjusting to hospitalization and may need restraints to undergo something as simple as intravenous antibiotic therapy. The relative benefit of this therapy should be weighed against the burden of hospitalization for such a patient. In less incapacitated patients, an assent-consent model of decision making may be appropriate. Performing certain interventions is nearly impossible without the cooperation of the patient. For instance, if a conservator has consented to a cataract operation but the patient refuses to cooperate, it is doubtful that the procedure can be performed. In this case, the conservator may consent, but the patient must assent to be treated. In other situations, patients may be able to understand the consequences of their decision well enough to give consent, but because of memory impairment or frontal lobe dysfunction or other cognitive deficit, the clinician may wish to have the family assent as well.

Temporary Loss of Decisional Capacity

Patients can temporarily lose the ability to make decisions during acute confusional states, acute psychotic episodes, periods of unconsciousness from anesthesia or illness, or during an acute CNS event. Although the patients may be expected to regain this ability over time, the rules described above still apply. Decisions that the patient has made before becoming temporarily incapacitated should be respected. A patient may reverse his or her do-not-resuscitate status while undergoing anesthesia with the understanding that it can be reinstated after the procedure. However, a patient who has stated that they would never agree to resuscitation should not have this reversed by a family member during a temporary confusional state due to a concurrent illness.

When using either substituted judgment or the best-interest standard in surrogate decision making for a patient with a transient loss of decisional capacity, the decision maker should err on the side of more aggressive intervention if there are situations when the patient's wishes are not known or the circumstances are substantively different from what the patient had anticipated.

Informed Consent for Research

The new emphasis on the quality of consent obtained for participants in research must extend to the vulnerable populations of older adults. Still, it is imperative that researchers study dementia and related problems so that the care of these patients can be improved. The two most vulnerable populations are patients with cognitive impairment, by virtue of their inability to understand the study or their role in it, and institutionalized patients, who may feel coerced to consent. Research involving vulnerable populations needs to be particularly well designed and focused on issues of importance to that population and have a potential to benefit the individuals involved.

For guidelines developed by the American Geriatrics Society for informed consent for research on cognitively impaired older adults, see Table 4.3.

DECISIONS NEAR THE END OF LIFE

Although the issues discussed in this section focus on the period near the end of life, the decision-making process and ethical principles described are the same for all medical decisions. All patients make decisions, consciously or subconsciously, concerning treatment of minor conditions, adherence with medical regimens, and related issues by weighing competing values and needs. When a person is faced with a terminal illness or a chronic, disabling, or progressive disease, decision making becomes more acute and focused. Patients, families, and clinicians must attempt to balance benefits and burdens when making many healthcare decisions. This difficult task is

Table 4.3—American Geriatrics Society Guidelines for Research on Cognitively Impaired Older Adults

- The research must be justified on scientific, clinical, and ethical grounds but can be focused on conditions other than dementia itself.
- The capacity to give consent should be assessed for each individual for each research protocol because decision-making capacity is task specific, and some cognitively impaired individuals will be able to give consent.
- Advance consent to participate in research given before the loss of decisional capacity should, in general, be respected.
- The traditional surrogates for decision making can be used to obtain consent.
- Research protocols that involve more than minimal risk or that do not have a likelihood of direct benefit for the subjects should be offered only to individuals who are able to consent or who have an advance directive consenting to participate in research. Exceptions might be made for exceptionally promising treatments, but this should be reviewed at a national level.
- Surrogates can refuse participation or withdraw the individual from participation if the surrogate determines that the research protocol is not what the individual intended to consent to or is not in the individual's best interest, even if there is advance consent.
- Only in very unusual circumstances would the refusal to participate of even an incapacitated individual be overridden.

SOURCE: Data from AGS Ethics Committee. Informed consent for research on human subjects with dementia. *J Am Geriatr Soc.* 1998;46(10):1308–1310.

further complicated by the fact that only probabilities of the benefits and burdens can be known, not certainties.

For more information on end-of-life decision making and care, see "Cultural Aspects of Care," p 49; and "Palliative Care," p 102.

Forgoing and Discontinuing Interventions

A patient's right to refuse unwanted treatment was confirmed by the Supreme Court of the United States in the 1991 case of *Cruzan v. Director, Department of Health of Missouri.* This refusal can occur before the intervention has been started or after it is in place. There is no ethical or legal distinction made between these two situations, often referred to in the more dramatic terms of *withholding* or *withdrawing* therapies. For example, in the case of uremia, a patient with kidney failure can refuse to begin dialysis, thus increasing the risk of death from uremia. Alternatively, a patient can try dialysis for a period of time, even years, and then choose to stop this treatment and die from uremia. This same principle holds for discontinuing ventilatory support for a patient who will die from his or her underlying respiratory disease whether ventilatory support is never started or if it is discontinued. The act of extubating a patient with the expectation that he or she will die is difficult for many clinicians because of the proximity of the act performed by the clinician and the death of the patient, but the decision is informed by the same ethical principles as is the decision to discontinue dialysis or to decline other medical interventions.

Clinicians and families often feel uncomfortable when a patient declines tube feeding and intravenous fluids. Case law, as well as the *Cruzan* case, characterizes these methods of delivering food and fluid as medical interventions; therefore, they are subject to the same ethical right of refusal that applies to any other medical intervention. Many people worry that the terminally ill patient will suffer without these interventions, but accumulated experience in hospice care has shown that it is usually easier to make someone comfortable without them: intravenous and nasogastric administration of food and fluid can cause discomfort through decreased gastric emptying and gastric distention, the need to replace intravenous lines or nasogastric tubes, and fluid overload as membranes become more permeable. These interventions can dampen or eliminate some of the physiologic comfort measures that occur, such as the release of endorphins.

Interventions That Can Hasten Death

Palliative care, defined here as interventions that are given to relieve discomfort or suffering without intent to cure, can at times have the unintended effect of hastening death. We have come to accept that there may be two effects of such a treatment: one (intended) effect of palliation, and the other possible (unintended) effect of hastening death. This is sometimes referred to as *the rule of double effect*. The intention of the application of the medical intervention is not to hasten death, but to palliate symptoms. Aggressive pain management, when respiratory depression is foreseeable but not intended, is generally seen as an ethical practice. Furthermore, most evidence shows that gradually increasing narcotic dosage does not hasten death. The rule of double effect has been extended by some to cover the use of terminal sedation (without hydration) in cases in which any level of consciousness will constitute continued suffering, as is frequently the case in death from head and neck cancer, for example. See "Palliative Care," p 102.

Physician-assisted suicide and euthanasia occur when an intervention is made with the clear intention of ending the patient's life. The underlying motivation of patients who wish to hasten death varies. In population-based surveys, people commonly cite fear of pain and other suffering (such as shortness of breath, anorexia, nausea, constipation, insomnia, and anxiety) as the reason for considering physician-assisted suicide. Fear of being dependent or a burden to others is mentioned at least as often. Other motivating factors that clinicians mention are depression, problems with personal relationships, spiritual issues, grief, and sleep disorders.

In the United States, unlike in some other countries that have addressed this issue, only physician-assisted suicide (and not euthanasia) has been legalized or is being considered for legalization. Because suicide is an act committed by the person who will suffer the consequences, it is felt that such a death is more clearly voluntary than a death that results from another person's administration of a lethal intervention. Although the Supreme Court has ruled that there is not a constitutional right to physician-assisted suicide, it did not rule that it is unconstitutional, either. Each state has been left to make its own laws in this regard. Some states have yet to act; many have made physician-assisted suicide explicitly illegal. Oregon has had legalized physician-assisted suicide since 1997. Experience there has shown that relatively few terminally ill patients request physician assistance with suicide. In the first 3 yr after physician-assisted suicide was legalized, 91 patients of 90,000 who died in Oregon requested it, yielding a rate of 1 per 1,000 deaths. Prominent motivating factors were loss of autonomy and determination to control the way in which one dies. The state of Washington has also legalized physician-assisted death, but no information is yet available on its application there.

The Continuum of End-of-Life Decisions Based on Goals

Decisions near the end of life are not all-or-nothing choices. The absence or presence of do-not-resuscitate orders (more accurately referred to as do-not-attempt-resuscitation orders) is often misinterpreted as instruction to the clinician either to do everything to maintain life or to stop all forms of medical treatment, including palliative measures. This dichotomy is false.

Other medical interventions for seriously ill patients with similar prognoses can have very different outcomes. For example, a patient with New York Heart Association Class IV or American Heart Association Stage D heart failure from a cardiomyopathy may ask not to receive cardiopulmonary resuscitation but might choose to accept placement of an automatic implantable cardiac defibrillator or be given a "dobutamine holiday." A patient who is dying of lung cancer might weigh the relative burdens and benefits of antibiotic treatment for pneumonia before deciding whether to treat an infection. The benefits and burdens of enteral feeding are highly influenced by the condition being treated. Most studies that have been done on the utility of enteral feeding for patients who aspirate have grouped all patients with feeding tubes together, which may not be appropriate. Many variables should be considered, for example:

- Patient 1 has had surgery for a localized pharyngeal cancer followed by radiation. The procedure has left the patient freely aspirating, making it difficult for him to take sufficient calories by mouth. The patient's overall prognosis is still uncertain.

- Patient 2 has Parkinson's disease and still functions well. His pharyngeal muscle coordination is slow, and he recurrently chokes on his food, especially thin liquids.

- Patient 3 has end-stage Alzheimer's disease. Although she has evidence of aspiration on a swallowing examination and has had two documented pneumonias that are probably related to aspiration, she is comfortable when she eats. One of her few remaining discernible pleasures is eating.

The balance between benefits and burdens is very different for each of these patients. Enteral feeding may or may not prolong their lives, and restrictions on eating could have a different meaning for each. The recommendations by clinicians for each patient or patient's surrogate might include everything from placing a feeding tube to avoiding oral intake to oral intake as tolerated for pleasure, using antipyretic medications for fevers caused by the aspiration and allowing nature to take its course. Before a choice is made, the patient or family must first clarify their priorities. The clinician can then decide how different approaches can best meet these goals. See "Eating and Feeding Problems," p 203.

Treatment Decisions in the Extended-Care Setting

Until policymakers and clinicians paid attention to the resuscitation status of patients in nursing homes, residents were assumed not to be candidates for attempted resuscitation; it was rarely, if ever, attempted. Studies that have looked at the outcomes of attempted resuscitation of patients in long-term care facilities show that it is used infrequently and associated with low long-term survival (SOE=A). However, the number of patients in long-term care settings for short-term recuperation and rehabilitation has grown, which may change the statistics concerning the utility of attempted resuscitation of nursing-home patients.

Staff perceptions of the utility of resuscitation efforts differ by profession. Nursing staff strongly prefer to limit interventions in this setting, especially for older patients and those with cognitive impairments (SOE=C). On the other hand, clinicians tend to overestimate the benefit of interventions for these patients (SOE=C). Patient participation in the process is variable. Federal legislation requires the systematic inquiry into advance directives for all patients in institutions receiving federal funds. With the advent of this more systematic approach to discussions about treatment status, nursing homes have transferred fewer patients to acute-care settings, and yet patient and family satisfaction has not declined.

Some regulatory agencies have encouraged enteral feeding of patients in nursing homes to prevent nutritional deficits in patients who may not be getting enough nourishment by eating. Although the motives for enacting these regulations were compassionate, the usefulness of enteral feeding, especially for patients with advanced dementia, is questionable. Also, it is not ethical to use enteral feedings for a patient capable of taking oral sustenance but who may not be getting enough nutrition because a facility fails to provide patients with the help they need in eating. See "Malnutrition," p 195.

SPECIAL ETHICAL ISSUES IN DEMENTIA

Although most of the topics discussed above involve the ethics of caring for cognitively impaired persons, some areas of particular concern for this population merit further discussion.

Truth Telling

The ethics of truth telling has evolved considerably through the last half of the 20th century in mainstream American culture, breaking with the longstanding tradition of paternalism in medicine that advocated withholding bad news from patients to do no harm. In many other cultures, telling bad news is still not felt to be appropriate. In the United States, however, telling a patient that he or she has a dementing illness may be the last area of controversy about truth telling. Increasingly in the United States, both professional and lay people agree that patients with dementia should be given a chance to understand what is happening to them. The opportunity for the older adult with early dementia to prepare legal documents (powers of attorney, a will, advance directives), to address personal issues, and to make plans is important. As therapies become available and research advances, patients with dementia should be informed of their options and given the opportunity to voice their preferences, even though they may no longer be fully capable of giving informed consent.

Autonomy

Ensuring personal safety and avoiding harm to others are important concerns in caring for patients with dementia. Because of the very nature of the disease process and its effect on recent memory, insight, and judgment, patients may not perceive how they have changed; they may not be able to recognize when their problem interferes with their ability to make decisions. Some patients with cognitive impairment may not understand the consequences of their actions and may have difficulty planning because of frontal lobe dysfunction. This puts them at risk of behaviors that can endanger themselves or others, including unsafe driving, the continued possession of firearms, wandering, and socially inappropriate behaviors. Their care needs can exceed what their caregivers can provide, and they may be unable to understand the rationale for having help at home, day care, or nursing-home care. The clinician plays a crucial role in being able to objectively recognize when this has happened and to help the family or others take the necessary steps to protect the patient and others.

Clinicians face complex ethical problems when caring for older adults who endanger themselves and others by driving. The conflicting interests are powerful: respect for the patient's autonomy, duty to protect the patient from harm, duty to protect others from predictable danger, and respect for patient-doctor confidentiality. Educating the patient and family members is often the key to developing a practical solution. Legal requirements regarding clinician reporting of unsafe older drivers vary from state to state. In some states, clinicians are required to report patients who may be unsafe; in other states they are permitted to do so; and in a few states, reporting may be considered a violation of patient-clinician confidentiality. See also the older driver in Assessment, p 47.

Another area of controversy is the use of physical and chemical restraints. The use of physical restraints in the long-term care setting has become closely regulated and monitored. Studies have shown that using physical restraints has little, if any, value in preventing injuries from falls (SOE=B). Less restrictive alternatives are usually available. Clinicians and patients' surrogates must consider several factors in deciding whether to use restraints. If the patient is engaging in activities that might harm other residents or staff, and when intervention is ineffective or the patient's surrogate refuses it, then the institution's responsibility to protect others may require that it send the patient elsewhere. In medical settings, restraints are often used to protect medical devices. Because of the dire physical, cognitive, and psychologic consequences of restraints, it is incumbent on clinicians to assess the necessity of such devices and to find the least restrictive way of protecting those that are deemed absolutely necessary. The use of sitters and other interventions to keep the patient safe, as well as the prevention and treatment of delirium, allow the patient to be treated with dignity and respect his or her autonomy as much as possible.

Definition of Personhood and Advance Directives

Adults with intact decisional capacity not only have the right to make their own decisions but also always have the right to change their minds. If their last competent statements were made close to an event that rendered them incapable of decision making, the likelihood is low that their rationale for the decision or that their goals, fears, and pleasures had changed significantly. If life experiences do mold their thinking, or if new interventions or approaches to problems occur, they can alter their directive to fit with these changes. A person with a progressive cognitive disorder can change substantially over time. What brings pleasure and what causes fear or pain can change substantially from year to year; almost certainly a patient's perceptions change greatly as the disease progresses. The demented person is unable to comprehend the future and slowly becomes more and more disconnected from the past. In some ways, the patient with advancing dementia becomes suspended in time: he or she loses his or her connection to previous and future selves, the essence of what many define as personhood. A demented person is connected to the decisions and perceptions of a previous self who he or she may not even remember. The decisions made by this prior "self" can inform current decision making, even though that person did not know what he or she would need or want at this time. Therefore, conflict can arise between the previous directives made by that person and what is best for the demented patient in the here-and-now (ie, what gives the patient pleasure and what may disturb him or her).

Sexuality and the Cognitively Impaired Individual

Expressions of sexuality and sexual desire do not end with aging or disappear with cognitive impairment. Certain aspects of cognitive impairment, specifically the disinhibition sometimes seen in frontal lobe dysfunction, can increase individuals' expression of their sexuality. Medications, particularly hormonal therapies and anti-Parkinson's medications can also increase expressions of sexuality and sexual desire.

Although patients with cognitive impairment should not be denied pleasure through sexual gratification, there are ethical concerns regarding their sexual activity that need to be addressed. As certain cognitive areas become affected by disease, the individual may no longer recognize social boundaries and engage in lewd behavior toward others or in public autoerotic acts. Beyond the fact that such behavior is disturbing to others, it is behavior that the person would likely have been mortified by before the onset of dementia. Such behaviors need to be forestalled, but all such pleasures should not be forbidden or punished. The person should be allowed some privacy if this is possible. Families may be uncomfortable with this because it may not be consistent with their image of their parent (rightly or wrongly). Institutions are often uncomfortable with expressions of sexuality because staff may find it offensive and be concerned that families will be upset.

Cognitively impaired individuals can be vulnerable to unwanted and unpleasurable sexual activity as well. This can be everything from sexual abuse by a cognitively intact family member or caregiver to incidental sexual contact by another demented individual. Cognitively impaired individuals may perceive sexual abuse when none was intended, eg, they may not have the ability to understand why someone would be undressing them when having a bath or a physical examination. Demented individuals may engage in sexual activity that is pleasurable but under a misapprehension as to who they are with or where they are. Protecting vulnerable individuals from harm obviously depends on how one defines harm but is still a fundamental responsibility of social institutions and caregivers.

ACOVE-3* QUALITY INDICATORS PERTAINING TO LEGAL AND ETHICAL ISSUES

Advance care planning documented

- All vulnerable older adults should have in their outpatient chart the patient's surrogate decision maker and documentation of a discussion to identify or search for a surrogate decision maker.

Advance directive continuity

- If a vulnerable older adult has an advance directive in the outpatient, inpatient, or nursing-home medical record, or the patient ports the existence of an advance directive in an interview, and the patient receives care in a second venue, then the advance directive should be present in the medical record at the second venue, or documentation should acknowledge its existence and its contents.
- If a vulnerable older adult is admitted to the hospital or nursing home, then within 48 hours of admission, the medical record should contain the patient's surrogate decision maker or documentation of a discussion to identify or search for a surrogate decision maker.

Care preference documentation of the hospitalized vulnerable older adult

- If a vulnerable older adult with severe dementia is admitted to the hospital and survives 48 hours, then within 48 hours of admission, the medical record should document that the patient's preferences for care have been considered or an attempt was made to identify them.
- If a vulnerable older adult is admitted to the intensive care unit and survives 48 hours, then within 48 hours of intensive care unit admission, the medical record should document that the patient's preferences for care have been considered or an attempt was made to identify them.

Mechanical ventilation preference

- If a hospitalized vulnerable older adult requires mechanical ventilation for more than 48 hours, then within 48 hours of the initiation of mechanical ventilation, the medical record should document the goals of care and the patient's preference for mechanical ventilation or why this information is unavailable.

Life-sustaining treatment decisions

- If a vulnerable older adult with decision-making capacity has orders in the hospital or nursing home to withhold or withdraw a life-sustaining treatment (eg, do-not-resuscitate order), then the medical record should document patient participation in the decision or why the patient did not participate.

Follow treatment preferences

- If a vulnerable older adult has documented treatment preferences to withhold or withdraw life-sustaining treatment (eg, do-not-resuscitate order, no tube feeding, no hospital transfer), then these treatment preferences should be followed.

Gastrostomy tube placement

- If a vulnerable older adult with dementia has a gastrostomy or jejunum tube placed, then before placement, the medical record should document one of the following:
  ◦ Patient preferences concerning tube feeding
  ◦ If patient is decisionally incapacitated and a surrogate decision maker is available, discussion of patient preferences or best interests
  ◦ If patient is decisionally incapacitated and a surrogate decision maker is not available, use of a formal decision mechanism

End-of-life care preferences and management

- If a vulnerable older adult dies an expected death with metastatic cancer, oxygen-dependent pulmonary disease, New York Heart Association (NYHA) Class III–IV congestive heart failure, end-stage liver disease, end-stage (Stage IV) renal disease, or dementia, then the chart should document the following within the 6 mo before death:
  ◦ Pain and other symptoms
  ◦ Spiritual and existential concerns
  ◦ Caregiver burdens and need for practical assistance
  ◦ Advance care planning

- If a vulnerable older adult dies an expected death with metastatic cancer, oxygen-dependent pulmonary disease, NYHA Class III–IV congestive heart failure, end-stage liver disease, end-stage (Stage IV) renal disease, or dementia, then the chart should document one of the following within the 6 mo before death:
  - Discussion of the medical condition and goals for treatment with a designated surrogate
  - Patient's preference for not involving a designated surrogate in discussions
  - Note that a surrogate decision maker is unavailable

Related quality indicators for Legal and Ethical Issues

End-of-life care (see "Palliative Care," p 102)

Assessing Care of Vulnerable Elders – 3ʳᵈ Set. See inside front cover for explanation.

REFERENCES

- Appelbaum PS. Assessment of patients' competence to consent to treatment. *N Engl J Med.* 2007;357:1834–1840.

- Kapp MB. Medical mistakes and older patients: admitting errors and improving care. *J Am Geriatr Soc.* 2001;49(10):1361–1365.

- Powers BA. *Nursing Home Ethics: Everyday Issues Affecting Residents with Dementia.* NY: Springer Publishing Company; 2006.

- Snyder CH. Dementia and driving: autonomy versus safety. *J Am Acad Nurse Pract.* 2005;17(10):393–402.

CHAPTER 5—FINANCING, COVERAGE, AND COSTS OF HEALTH CARE

KEY POINTS

- Medicare Part A covers hospital, skilled nursing home, home-health, and hospice services. Medicare Part B covers physicians, nurse practitioners, social workers, psychologists, therapists, laboratory tests, and durable medical equipment. Medicare Part D covers some of the cost of prescription medications. Medicare Part C provides the benefits offered under Medicare Parts A, B, and D through Medicare Advantage plans, which are managed care plans.

- Medigap supplemental insurance plans are available that cover Medicare Part A and Part B deductibles and co-insurance costs, as well as preventive care and other health-related goods and services.

- The Medicare Personal Plan Finder (http://www.medicare.gov) has search tools that can assist patients in selecting a Medicare Advantage (MA) plan or a medigap plan and in comparing nursing-home facilities and home-health care agencies.

- Medicaid is a joint federal and state program that provides supplemental health insurance (including long-term custodial care in nursing homes) to people of all ages who have low incomes and limited savings.

- While the details of health care reform will be defined over the next several years, the movement toward coordination of care and delivery systems that operate in an efficient and effective manner has already begun to take shape. Systems such as accountable care organizations and medical homes are likely to play a major role in care delivery.

In 1965, the U.S. government passed legislation designed to improve access to acute health care for people who are old, disabled, or poor. During the decades that followed, the resulting Medicare and Medicaid programs expanded, evolved, and spawned thousands of supplemental commercial insurance plans. Today, a complex and often confusing array of personal payments, public programs, and private insurance plans (Figure 5.1) pays for and thereby determines much of the health care that older Americans receive.

MEDICARE

Medicare is a federal insurance program run by the Centers for Medicare and Medicaid Services (CMS), which pays health professionals and organizations to provide acute health care for Americans who are ≥65 yr old, disabled, or suffering from end-stage renal disease. As originally enacted, Medicare comprises two separate fee-for-service (FFS) plans (Part A and Part B), each of which pays predetermined amounts for specified health-related goods and services that are needed by its beneficiaries. More than 80% of older Americans are covered by both plans.

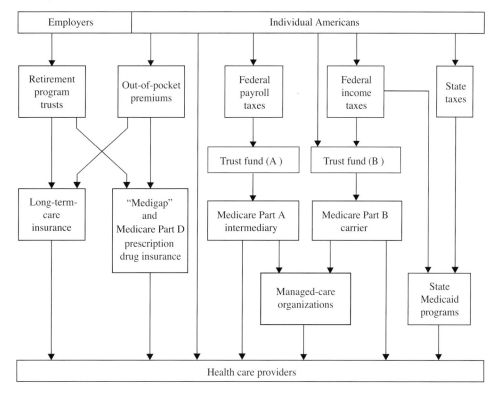

Figure 5.1—The Flow of Funds for the Health Care of Older Americans

Parts A and B

Medicare Part A uses regional insurance companies ("intermediaries") to pay hospitals, nursing homes, home-care agencies, and hospice programs for the Medicare-covered services they provide. Older Americans (and their spouses) who have had Medicare taxes deducted from their paychecks for at least 10 yr are entitled to coverage through Part A without paying premiums. Others may be able to purchase Part A coverage (for up to $461/mo in 2010, depending on how long they had Medicare taxes deducted from their paychecks).

Medicare Part B uses other regional insurance companies ("carriers") to pay physicians, nurse practitioners, social workers, psychologists, rehabilitation therapists, home-care agencies, ambulances, outpatient facilities, laboratory and imaging facilities, and suppliers of durable medical equipment for the Medicare-covered goods and services they provide. At age 65, older adults become eligible for Part B coverage if they are entitled to Part A coverage or if they are citizens or permanent residents of the United States. To obtain this coverage, eligible older adults must enroll in Part B and pay premiums ($96–$354/mo in 2010, depending on income), usually by agreeing to have them deducted from their monthly Social Security checks.

Providers must choose among three options for participating in the FFS Medicare program: participation, nonparticipation, and private contracting. For each Medicare-covered service provided, a participating provider submits a claim to the Part B carrier, accepts Medicare's fee for the service (80% of its preestablished "allowed" amount), and bills the patient or the patient's secondary insurer for no more than a 20% co-insurance payment. Providers electing nonparticipation status can bill patients directly for up to 15% more than 95% of Medicare's allowed amounts. The patients pay the providers and then submit their requests to Medicare for partial reimbursement (ie, for 80% of 95% of the allowed amounts). For services not covered by Medicare, the provider may bill the patient, if the patient agrees in advance in writing.

Neither Part A nor Part B of the Medicare program covers periodic health maintenance physical examinations, outpatient medications, dental care, hearing aids, eyeglasses, foot care, orthopedic shoes, cosmetic surgery, care in foreign countries, or custodial long-term care at home or in nursing homes. Part B covers some preventive services (Table 5.1).

Beneficiaries pay out-of-pocket for the following (rates are for 2010):

- monthly premiums for Part B (standard premium is $96 but can be as high as $354 depending on income)

- annual deductible for Part B ($155)

- the deductible for Part A ($1,100 per benefit period, ie, the first 60 days after an admission)

Table 5.1—Health Insurance Coverage for Older Americans (all dollar amounts from 2010)

Covers the cost of:	Fee-for-Service Medicare		Supplemental Coverage			Medicare Advantage Insurance[b] (Part C)
	Part A	Part B	Medicaid[a]	Part D	Medigap Insurance	
Hospitals	100%[c]	—	$1100	—	$550–1100	100%
Postacute care in skilled-nursing facility	100%[d]	—	—	—	—	100%
Hospice	100%[e]	—	—	—	—	—
Home care ("medically necessary")	100%	100%	—	—	—	100%
Durable medical equipment	80%[f]	80%[f]	20%	—	20%	100%
Diagnostic laboratory tests	—	100%	—	—	—	100%
Diagnostic imaging tests	—	80%	20%	—	20%	100%
Physicians, nurse practitioners	—	80%	20%	—	20%	100%
Outpatient PT, OT, ST	—	80%	20%	—	20%	100%
Outpatient services, supplies	—	80%	20%	—	20%	100%
Emergency care	—	80%	20%	—	20%	100%
Ambulance services	—	80%	20%	—	20%	100%
Preventive services	—	[g]	20%	—	20%	[g, h]
Outpatient mental health care	—	50%	50%	—	50%	100%
Custodial care in nursing home	—	—	100%	—	—	—
Hearing, vision services	—	—	[i]	—	[i]	[i]
Outpatient medications	—	—	[i]	75%[j]	[i]	[i]
Additional costs to patient:						
Deductibles	$1,100[k]	$155[l]	—	$310	[i]	[i]
Monthly premiums	—	$96–$354	—	$32[m]	[i]	[i]

NOTE: PT = physical therapy; OT = occupational therapy; ST = speech therapy

[a] Under the Balanced Budget Act of 1997, state Medicaid programs were given the option whether or not to pay deductibles and co-insurance costs.

[b] Some Medicare Advantage plans require members to pay deductibles and co-payments.

[c] After the beneficiary or secondary insurer pays the Part A deductible

[d] For the first 20 days of care in skilled-nursing facility after a hospital stay of at least 3 days

[e] Patient makes co-payments of $5.00 per outpatient prescription and 5% of cost of respite care.

[f] When patient is receiving Medicare-covered home care

[g] 100% of allowed cost of fecal occult blood test, Pap smear interpretation, prostate-specific antigen test, blood tests for diabetes and cardiovascular disease, and influenza and pneumococcal vaccinations; 80% of allowed cost of mammograms and clinical examination of breast and pelvis (no deductible applies); after the annual Part B deductible has been paid, 80% of allowed cost of a general physical examination at age 65, glaucoma screening, sigmoidoscopy or colonoscopy or barium enema, digital rectal examination (men), measurement of bone mass, hepatitis B vaccination, and diabetic education and equipment (coverage subject to change by health reform legislation)

[h] Some Medicare Advantage plans cover additional preventive services.

[i] Benefits and costs vary widely among medigap insurance plans, state Medicaid plans, prescription drug plans, and Medicare Advantage plans.

[j] Starting in 2011, the coverage gap ("doughnut" hole) will gradually be closed over the next 10 yr. In 2011, beneficiaries will pay 50% of the cost of brand name medications and 93% of the cost of generic medications while in the coverage gap.

[k] Per benefit period (first 60 days after hospital admission)

[l] Annually

[m] Base premium for 2010; premiums vary by plan.

- co-insurance payments (usually 20%) for goods and services for which Medicare or other insurance pays only a portion
- the full cost of those goods and services that are not covered by Medicare or other insurance

Part C

As an alternative to traditional FFS Parts A and B, Medicare beneficiaries can instead elect to enroll in a Medicare managed care plan, an option known as Part C or Medicare Advantage (MA). MA plans, operated by private insurers, hold contracts with CMS specifying that, for each Medicare beneficiary they enroll, they will provide at least the standard Medicare benefits in return for fixed monthly capitation payments. To attract enrollees, most MA plans also cover additional benefits and charge low or no premiums, deductibles, and co-payments. The plans achieve cost savings by managing their enrollees' use of services within their networks of providers, with whom they negotiate price discounts in return for patient volume. Each January, MA plans have the option of changing their premiums, benefits, and provider networks—or of discontinuing their plans altogether.

There are several types of MA plans:

- Medicare Health Maintenance Organizations (HMOs)—insurance companies that accept capitation payments from CMS and provide or purchase Medicare-covered health services

- Preferred provider organizations (PPOs)—alliances of providers that accept capitation payments and deliver Medicare-covered health services to their enrolled patients

- Provider-sponsored organizations (PSOs)—partnerships of physician groups and hospitals that accept capitation payments and deliver Medicare-covered health services to their enrolled patients

- Private FFS plans—plans that may charge beneficiaries a premium, pay providers more liberally than the original Medicare FFS program does, and allow physicians to charge their patients co-payments of up to 15%

- Special needs plans—plans designed for patients with certain chronic diseases or other special needs

- Medical savings accounts (MSAs)—accounts into which Medicare beneficiaries can make tax-deductible contributions and out of which they can withdraw funds to purchase routine health-related goods (including medications) and services (including long-term care insurance) from any Medicare provider. Linked to the MSA is a catastrophic insurance policy that limits the individual beneficiary's out-of-pocket expenses for health care to $6,000/yr.

Each November, beneficiaries covered by Medicare Part A and Part B have the option of joining any MA plan operating in their area; they cannot be denied enrollment because of any health problems except end-stage renal disease. Enrollees must continue to pay their monthly Medicare Part B premiums to Medicare, plus any additional premium that the MA plan charges to cover additional services, and they must obtain their healthcare services from the plan's provider network. They have the option of leaving the plan at any time and returning to the FFS Medicare program.

Part D

In 2003, Congress enacted a Medicare reform bill that included an option (Medicare Part D) for beneficiaries to purchase insurance coverage for outpatient prescription medications. The Part D option is open to all Medicare beneficiaries, whether enrolled in traditional FFS or MA. Part D benefits can be purchased as stand-alone policies or as sponsored by MA plans. For most Medicare beneficiaries, there is a dizzying array of plans from which to choose, with premiums, deductibles, co-payments, and formularies differing from plan to plan. CMS has set up a Medicare Prescription Drug Plan Finder (http://www.medicare.gov/MPDPF/Public/Include/DataSection/Questions/MPDPFIntro.asp), where enrollees can enter their location and medications to compare Part D options available to them.

Part D coverage policies as set by law are also confusing to many beneficiaries, because different levels of coverage apply to cumulative yearly prescription drug expenditures. Many plans have a relatively small deductible; the maximal allowable deductible by law in 2011 is $310. After the deductible is paid, Part D plans usually cover 75% of the ensuing drug costs up to a specified amount ($2,840 in 2011). Starting in 2011, the coverage gap ("doughnut" hole) will gradually be closed over the next 10 yr. In 2011, beneficiaries will pay 50% of the cost of brand name medications and 93% of the cost of generic medications while in the coverage gap.

Medigap and Medicaid

Medigap supplemental plans fill some of the holes in the insurance coverage provided by Medicare Part A and Part B. Private insurance companies offer FFS medigap plans of 12 types (A through L), classified according to the benefits they offer. For new Medicare beneficiaries at age 65, the premiums for A-level (basic) plans across the United States vary considerably. These policies cover a person's Part A and Part B co-insurance costs, eg, 20% of Medicare's allowed fees for durable medical equipment and primary provider services. (In Minnesota, Wisconsin, and Massachusetts, A-level medigap policies are required by law to cover more than just the costs of Medicare co-insurance.) B-level plans cover Part A and Part B co-insurance, plus the Part A deductible. Each successive level of medigap policy provides additional benefits and costs more. J-level plans cover co-insurance, deductibles, care in foreign countries, and preventive services. Less expensive medigap coverage can be obtained by purchasing plans that require the insured to pay high deductibles (F- and J-level plans only) or plans that cover the services of only selected providers and hospitals ("Medicare SELECT" policies). Medigap policies do not cover long-term care, dental care, eyeglasses, hearing aids, or private-duty nursing. They also do not cover out-of-pocket costs for MA plans.

Within 6 mo of their initial enrollment in Medicare Part B, beneficiaries are entitled to purchase any medigap policy on the market at advertised prices. After this open enrollment period, medigap insurers can refuse to insure individual beneficiaries or charge them higher premiums because of their past or present health problems.

Medicaid is a joint federal and state program that provides health insurance to people of all ages who have low incomes and limited savings. The exact criteria for Medicaid eligibility and the benefit packages provided by Medicaid programs vary considerably from state to state. Most programs pay Medicare Part B premiums, and some pay Medicare deductibles and co-insurance costs. Most important, Medicaid pays for long-term custodial care in nursing homes for those who qualify. Several states have begun offering fixed capitation payments to managed-care organizations that are willing to provide Medicaid and Medicare benefits to residents who are "dually eligible" (for Medicaid and Medicare).

Extensive information about all the options is available to consumers at each state's medical assistance office, at 1-800-MEDICARE (1-800-633-4227) or 1-877-486-2048 for hearing impaired TTY users, and at the Medicare Personal Plan Finder (http://www.medicare.gov/ [accessed Jan 2011]).

FINANCING OF CARE AT DIFFERENT SITES

This section describes, through the eyes of both patients and providers, how the various programs influence the day-to-day care of older adults. It illustrates their effects during a year in the life of Mrs. Rose Murat, an imaginary 79-yr-old retired schoolteacher who lives with her 83-yr-old husband in a small, older home. Mrs. Murat has hypertension, coronary artery disease, and mild heart failure, for which she takes hydrochlorothiazide, metoprolol, lisinopril, and nitroglycerin. She is covered by traditional Medicare Parts A and B. Mrs. Murat has also purchased a Part D drug plan, for which she pays annual premiums ($383), deductibles ($310), and co-insurance (25% of her remaining medication expenses = $298). As a result, her total out-of-pocket medication costs were reduced 34% from $1,500 to $991 per year (from $125 to $83 per month). For the primary advantages and disadvantages of each of Mrs. Murat's coverage options, see Table 5.2.

Outpatient Care

Mrs. Murat sees her primary provider quarterly for monitoring of her chronic conditions.

Fee for Service

Under the Medicare FFS system, providers obtain the fairest possible reimbursement by understanding and following CMS's payment system, which is based on evaluation and management (E&M) codes (Table 5.3).

For each Medicare-covered service provided, the provider submits to the regional Medicare carrier the appropriate E&M code and the international classification of disease (ICD) code that indicates the diagnosis for which the service was provided. Entries in the medical record, which are subject to audit, must document that the data collection and medical decision-making aspects of the service conform to standards established for the E&M code submitted. By providing and documenting services efficiently, providers can maximize their FFS reimbursements within the (tight) limits imposed by the Medicare fee schedules.

At the end of her quarterly office visit, Mrs. Murat asks for advice on joining a managed care organization that has been marketing an MA plan in her county. She is impressed by the MA plan's offer of free eyeglasses, hearing aids, and preventive check-ups, all of which she has purchased out-of-pocket in the past. Her options are as follows: staying with traditional FFS Medicare as her only coverage, keeping FFS Medicare and applying for either Medicaid or supplemental (medigap) coverage, or exchanging her FFS Medicare coverage for membership in the MA plan (Table 5.2). Depending on the Murats' income, savings, and state of residence, they may also qualify for a Medicare assistance program that pays for some combination of their Medicare premiums, deductibles, and co-insurance costs. Some older Americans may have additional health insurance options through the federal Department of Veterans Affairs or through their (or their spouses') present or previous employer or union.

Managed Care

Mrs. Murat's primary care provider, knowledgeable about her health and prognosis, can help her to choose the plan(s) that will cover the goods and services that she needs, both now and in the future. If she can obtain what she is likely to need from the MA plan's network of providers, joining the plan might be her best option, because it will likely cover eyeglasses, hearing aids, and preventive services, and she can avoid paying the usual Medicare deductibles and co-insurance. Data about the quality of care and the satisfaction of other enrollees in all the local MA plans are available at the Medicare Personal Plan Finder.

If Mrs. Murat needs health care that is not available from the MA plan's network, or if she is reluctant to change providers, retaining the flexibility

Table 5.2—Advantages and Disadvantages of Four Types of Health Insurance

Type of Insurance	Primary Advantages	Primary Disadvantages
Fee-for-Service Medicare (Parts A, B, and D)	Traditional Medicare benefits, choice of any provider that participates in the Medicare program, partial coverage for prescription medications	Cost of co-insurance, deductibles, noncovered goods and services (eg, eyeglasses, hearing aids)
Medicaid	Coverage of co-insurance, deductibles, and some benefits[a] not covered by Medicare	Choice of providers restricted to a single network in some states
Medigap insurance	Coverage of co-insurance, deductibles, and some benefits[b] not covered by Medicare	Out-of-pocket monthly premiums may be expensive, depending on the coverage provided by the policy purchased
Medicare Advantage plan (ie, Part C)	Traditional Medicare benefits plus coverage of additional goods and services[b]	Choice of providers restricted to a network; potential for changes in premiums, co-payments, deductibles, benefits, and providers at the discretion of the plan

[a] Benefits vary from state to state.

[b] Benefits vary from plan to plan.

Table 5.3—Fee-for-Service Reimbursement by Medicare, 2009

E&M Service	E&M Code	"Allowed" Amount ($)[a]	% Covered	CMS Payment ($)[b]
Comprehensive office visit, new patient	99205	180	× 0.80 =	144
Detailed office visit, established patient	99213	62	× 0.80 =	50
Detailed office visit (mental health problem), established patient	99213	62	× 0.50 =	31
Comprehensive office consult	99245	228	× 0.80 =	182
Comprehensive inpatient consultation[c]	99255	198	× 0.80 =	158
Complex hospital admission	99223	176	× 0.80 =	141
Complex hospital follow-up visit	99233	93	× 0.80 =	74
Comprehensive nursing facility initial assessment	99305	109	× 0.80 =	87
Detailed nursing facility follow-up visit	99308	60	× 0.80 =	48
Comprehensive initial home visit	99345	197	× 0.80 =	158
Detailed follow-up home visit	99349	114	× 0.80 =	91
Home-health certification	G0180	61	× 0.80 =	49
Home health care supervision	G0181	108	× 0.80 =	86

NOTE: E&M = evaluation and management

[a] For physicians who participate in Medicare; amounts vary by location (see http://www.cms.hhs.gov/PfsLookup for local rates and annual updates).

[b] For eligible services provided by nurse practitioners, payment is 85% of the amount shown.

[c] Hospital or nursing-facility consultation.

of her traditional FFS Medicare coverage (which covers her use of any provider that participates in the Medicare program) might be a better choice, especially if she also qualifies for Medicaid or buys a medigap policy. Information from Medicare's information line or from the Medicare Personal Plan Finder would help her compare the prices and coverage of the medigap policies available in her area.

The primary care provider's recommendations to Mrs. Murat are likely to be influenced by the characteristics of the different plans she is considering. For instance, if the primary care provider is not in the MA plan's service network, he or she would likely point out to Mrs. Murat that her enrollment in the MA plan would require her to select a new

primary care provider. If the primary care provider is in the MA plan's network, Mrs. Murat's enrollment might change (ie, probably reduce) the payment for her care. The payments would depend on the type of plan involved (Table 5.4). If it is a group or independent practice association model, the MA plan may pay providers "discounted FFS," ie, possibly less than Medicare Part B would pay for each service. Or it may pay primary providers a fixed capitation amount each month to cover specified services. If these services are limited to primary ambulatory care, the capitation amount will be relatively small. Plans may choose to reward primary care providers with bonus payments for efficient and effective use of resources for the patients for whom they are respon-

Table 5.4—How Medicare Advantage Plans Pay Healthcare Providers

	Staff Model	Group Model	Independent Practice Association Model
		Type of Medicare Advantage Plan	
Providers	Employees	One large group practice	Many small independent practices
Method of payments	Salary	Fee-for-service or capitation[a]	Fee-for-service or capitation[a]

[a] The services covered by the capitation payments range from "primary care only" in some plans to "medications and all acute care" in others.

sible. If the covered services also include specialty and inpatient care, the capitation amounts will be considerably larger, and the provider will have incentives to use these services judiciously because he or she will have to pay for them, at least in part.

Regardless of the payment mechanism, the crucial question is whether the amount of payment suffices to support high-quality care. For example, if capitation rates are below the aggregate cost of the services they are intended to cover, the provider will feel pressure to take on more patients and to limit the amount of service that each patient receives. Similarly, if FFS amounts are too small, the provider will feel pressure to schedule more visits and procedures and to reduce the time devoted to each patient. Each provider should, therefore, monitor carefully and continually the many changing elements in the practice environment (eg, payment schedules, covered services, expenses, patients' and families' expectations, population demographics) to help determine the numbers and types of services that are appropriate for each older patient.

Inpatient Care

Four months later, Mrs. Murat awakes dysarthric and unable to feel her left hand. Her face is asymmetric, and her left arm and left leg are weak. Her husband calls 911; the ambulance rushes her to the nearest emergency department, where the physician on duty diagnoses a right hemispheric stroke and admits her to the hospital.

Fee for Service

If Mrs. Murat had retained traditional Medicare as her only health insurance, she would have to pay Medicare's required deductibles (in 2010, $155 per year under Part B for the ambulance and the emergency medical care, plus $1,100 under Part A for the hospital admission) and co-insurance amounts (20% of Medicare's allowed charges by physicians and the ambulance service). She would also have to pay any ambulance charges in excess of Medicare's approved fee. If she had supplemented her Medicare coverage, her Medicaid or private medigap coverage would cover some of these deductibles and co-insurance payments, and she would not be transferred to another hospital for insurance reasons.

The hospital would submit its claim for emergency and inpatient care, which would be based on the diagnosis-related group (DRG) of her discharge diagnosis, to Medicare's Part A regional intermediary insurance company. The involved physicians and the ambulance service would submit their E&M coded claims to Medicare's Part B regional insurance carrier. The intermediary and the carrier would pay their shares of these costs and, if Mrs. Murat had supplemental coverage, they would forward requests for payment of the balances to the state Medicaid program or to Mrs. Murat's medigap insurance company. Ultimately, CMS would reimburse the intermediary from the Medicare Part A Trust Fund and the carrier from the Medicare Part B Trust Fund.

Managed Care

If Mrs. Murat had joined the MA plan, the MA plan would pay for the ambulance, emergency, and physician services; in most cases, it would pay the hospital a prenegotiated lump sum or a per diem fee to cover all of her inpatient care. The amount of this lump sum would be determined by the DRG of her discharge diagnosis, in this case, stroke. If the admitting hospital had no contract with her MA plan, Mrs. Murat would probably be transferred to a hospital in the plan's provider network as soon as she was medically stable. Depending on the MA plan's benefit package, she might be responsible for co-payments and deductibles for some of these services.

Postacute Rehabilitation

After 4 days of stabilization, evaluation, and rehabilitation, Mrs. Murat is deemed stable enough for discharge from the acute-care hospital. She has improved somewhat, but she is still mildly hemiparetic and dysarthric, and she is apathetic and easily fatigued. Because her days in the hospital are fewer than the average number of hospital days associated with the DRG of her discharge diagnosis (ie, 5.9 days) and because her discharge diagnosis is one of those listed in Table 5.5, CMS regards her "early" discharge as a "transfer." This permits CMS to reduce the amount it pays the hospital for her care. The consulting neurologist advises her and her husband that her progress during the next few weeks will

Table 5.5—Primary Diagnoses for Which "Early" Discharges from Hospitals Are Regarded as "Transfers" to Postacute Care

Primary Diagnosis	DRG Number	Hospital Days, National Average
Degenerative nervous system disorders	12	8.1
Specific cerebrovascular disorders, except transient ischemic attack	14	5.9
Seizure and headache with complications and comorbidities	24	5.0
Seizure and headache without complications and comorbidities	25	3.2
COPD	88	5.1
Simple pneumonia and pleurisy with complications and comorbidities	89	6.0
Simple pneumonia and pleurisy without complications and comorbidities	90	4.1
Amputation for circulatory system disorders, except arm and toe	113	12.3
Circulatory disorders with acute myocardial infarction and major complications, discharged alive	121	6.4
Circulatory disorders with acute myocardial infarction without major complications, discharged alive	122	3.7
Heart failure and shock	127	5.3
Peripheral vascular disorders with complications and comorbidities	130	5.7
Peripheral vascular disorders without complications and comorbidities	131	4.2
Major joint and limb reattachment procedures for leg	209	5.1
Hip and femur procedures except major joint with complications and comorbidities	210	6.8
Hip and femur procedures except major joint without complications and comorbidities	211	4.9
Fractures of hip and pelvis	236	5.2
Pathologic fractures and musculoskeletal and connective tissue malignancy	239	6.3
Cellulitis with complications and comorbidities	277	5.7
Cellulitis without complications and comorbidities	278	4.3
Diabetes mellitus	294	4.6
Nutritional and miscellaneous metabolic disorders with complications and comorbidities	296	5.2
Nutritional and miscellaneous metabolic disorders without complications and comorbidities	297	3.4
Kidney and urinary tract infections with complications and comorbidities	320	5.3
Kidney and urinary tract infections without complications and comorbidities	321	3.8
RBC disorders	395	4.4
Organic disturbances and mental retardation	429	10.0
Extensive operating room procedure unrelated to principal diagnosis	468	13.0
Tracheostomy for face, mouth, and neck diagnoses	483	39.6

NOTE: DRG = diagnosis-related group

determine her potential for functional recovery. Mr. Murat asks the neurologist to recommend a rehabilitation facility for his wife.

Fee for Service

If Mrs. Murat could participate in rehabilitative therapy, Medicare Part A would pay for 20 days of postacute rehabilitation, in either a rehabilitation facility or a transitional (postacute) care unit of a nursing home. On Mrs. Murat's admission to either type of postacute care unit, rehabilitation professionals would evaluate her functional status, establish a plan for her care, and certify her as needing one of 26 levels of intensity of care according to the resource utilization group system (RUGS). Her RUGS category would determine the daily rate that Medicare Part A would pay the facility for the first 2 wk of her

care as long as she was demonstrating progress in rehabilitation. After 2 wk, a nurse would reevaluate her status, update her plan of care, and adjust her RUGS category, thereby adjusting Medicare's payments to the facility for the next 2 wk. Under this prospective payment system, the facility would be responsible not only for Mrs. Murat's nursing, rehabilitative, and social services but also for the costs of her medications, laboratory tests, and visits to an emergency department not resulting in admission to the hospital.

Using nursing-home rates, Medicare Part B would pay 80% of the allowed charges for the postacute medical care provided by Mrs. Murat's provider. Any postacute care related to an inpatient surgical procedure would be the responsibility of the surgeon, who would receive a "global fee" to cover the surgery and all postoperative surgical care. The Murats would need to satisfy Medicare Part B's $155 annual deductible and then make 20% co-insurance payments for the provider's care. Their out-of-pocket expenses would be reduced or eliminated by any Medicare supplements in effect, such as Medicaid, medigap, or long-term care coverage.

Managed Care

If Mrs. Murat had joined the MA plan, her insurance coverage would include postacute rehabilitative care, probably at a nursing home in the MA plan's provider network rather than at a rehabilitation facility. Some nursing homes concentrate such high-acuity patients in transitional (or postacute) care units and provide them with coordinated rehabilitative (physical, occupational, and speech), social, and nursing services. Most homes, lacking such units, offer only custodial care supplemented by rehabilitative services as needed. The MA plan would also cover the physician's postacute services, but the Murats may be responsible for a deductible and co-payments.

More than 3 million Americans have long-term care insurance policies, but these policies pay for <2% of all nursing-home care. The high premiums for these policies, combined with consumers' uncertainty about needing long-term care in the future and their doubts about the policies' ability to cover the costs of long-term care in the future, have limited the growth of the long-term care insurance sector. Many middle-aged Americans believe they will retain good health and independence into old age; they appear to be relying on a combination of good fortune, social insurance (ie, Medicaid), and their personal assets to see them through their later years. Those who are interested in long-term care insurance can obtain information by reading *Choosing Long-Term Care: A Guide for People with Medicare* (CMS Publication No. 02223) or *A Shopper's Guide to Long-Term Care Insurance* (available from state insurance departments or the National Association of Insurance Commissioners, 2301 McGee St, Suite 800, Kansas City, MO 64108-3600).

Home-Health Care

During the first 10 days of rehabilitative therapy, Mrs. Murat regains her ability to speak, and her left arm becomes stronger. During the next 8 days, however, she makes few additional gains. After 18 days, she is still unable to walk, cook, bathe, or dress herself without help. Her lack of continued progress toward functional independence will probably make her ineligible for coverage of additional rehabilitative services in either the MA plan or the FFS Medicare program. The Murats will have to pay for any future physical therapy or occupational therapy on their own.

To obtain long-term care for Mrs. Murat's functional deficits, the Murats will need to choose between a home-health agency and a custodial nursing home. If Mrs. Murat returns home, neither the FFS Medicare program nor the MA plan will be likely to pay for a home-health aide unless she is homebound and requires the services of a registered nurse or rehabilitation therapist. Local community agencies, however, may be able to offer assistance. The Murats' choice of a home-health agency could be informed by comparisons of their local agencies' recent clinical performance, available at Home Health Compare (http://www.medicare.gov/HHcompare/home.asp).

Fee for Service

In the FFS environment, if Mrs. Murat were homebound and dependent on skilled professional services, then traditional Medicare Part A would pay any Medicare-certified home-health agency a fixed fee to provide her with the services and equipment necessary to treat her primary diagnosis. Medicare Part B would pay her primary care provider 80% of the allowed charges for house calls, office visits, and care plan oversight services. In addition, Medicare Part B would pay her provider for home-health certifications and recertifications. The Murats would be responsible for the Part B annual deductible ($155) and the 20% co-insurance payments, unless they had supplemental coverage through Medicaid, a medigap policy, or a long-term care policy. See also "Community-Based Care," p 150.

Managed Care

If Mrs. Murat's condition made her homebound and dependent on skilled professional services, her MA plan probably would pay a home-health agency a fixed fee to provide her with the services and equipment necessary to treat her primary diagnosis. The MA plan would also provide her with the services of a primary care provider.

Program for All-inclusive Care of the Elderly

If a healthcare organization in the area had contracted with CMS and the state Medicaid agency to create a Program for All-inclusive Care of the Elderly (PACE), it could provide community-based long-term care for "dually eligibles" (people eligible for both Medicare and Medicaid) whose disabilities qualified them for custodial care in a nursing home. (See also "Community-Based Care," p 150.) If she were eligible for Medicaid and she enrolled in PACE, Mrs. Murat would attend an adult day healthcare center several days each week and receive comprehensive outpatient, inpatient, acute, and long-term care from a salaried interdisciplinary team composed of a physician, a nurse practitioner or physician assistant, a nurse, a social worker, rehabilitation therapists, and other members of the PACE staff.

Nursing-Home Care

Three months after Mrs. Murat returns home, Mr. Murat, now 84 yr old, suffers a myocardial infarction and is no longer able to care for his wife at home. Their daughter logs on to Nursing Home Compare (http://www.medicare.gov/NHcompare/home.asp) to shop for a nursing home. After comparing the local facilities' nurse-to-resident ratios, results of recent quality-of-care inspections, and rates of pressure ulcers and behavior problems, she arranges for her mother to enter a high-quality nursing home in her neighborhood, at least until Mr. Murat recovers.

Fee for Service

The FFS Medicare program would pay 80% of the allowed charges submitted by Mrs. Murat's provider for visits to the nursing home. The Murats would be responsible for the Medicare Part B annual deductible ($155) and the 20% co-insurance payments. Medicare would not cover any of the nursing home's per diem charges.

Managed Care

If Mrs. Murat had joined the MA plan, one of the MA plan's clinicians would provide her primary care in the nursing home. Unless she was covered by Medicaid or a long-term care policy, however, she and her husband would be responsible for the nursing home's per diem charges for room, board, and other basic services (about $200/day). After "spending down" their savings at this rate, the Murats might become sufficiently impoverished to qualify, if they had not qualified previously, for Medicaid coverage. If the Murats owned their house, some states would put a lien on it to recover some of its payments to the nursing home when the house was eventually sold.

Hospice Care

After residing in the nursing home for 6 mo, Mrs. Murat suffers a massive stroke that leaves her physiologically stable but in a persistent vegetative state. Her husband reports that she had always said she would not want to go on living in such a condition if there were little hope of recovery. Mrs. Murat is unable to swallow thin liquids, and her husband says she would not want to be fed through any sort of tube. Her physician says that, with oral feeding, she is likely to live for several weeks. Her husband agrees to enroll Mrs. Murat in a hospice program with the understanding that she will receive palliative care without life-prolonging interventions.

Enrollment in hospice would require the traditional FFS Medicare program (Part A) to pay a Medicare-certified hospice program a daily fee that would cover all care for the terminal diagnosis, including home care, medications, equipment, respite, counseling, and social services even if Mrs. Murat had enrolled in (and remained in) the MA plan.

If she had remained in the FFS Medicare program, Part B would pay her primary care provider 80% of the allowed charges for home or office visits and care-plan oversight services. Mr. Murat would be responsible for the 20% co-insurance and small co-payments for outpatient prescription medications, as well as for respite care.

CHANGES IN THE FEDERAL FINANCING OF HEALTH CARE

The complex and evolving combinations of coverage and programs create difficult choices for older Americans and powerful incentives for their healthcare providers. The U.S. Congress and CMS continue to revise the Medicare program.

The Balanced Budget Act of 1997 (BBA 97)

BBA 97 required CMS to adjust capitation amounts according to enrollees' risk of requiring expensive health care. This results in higher capitation payments for high-risk enrollees and lower payments for low-risk enrollees. This risk-adjustment method is based on the diagnoses associated with beneficiaries' health care during a recent 12-mo period. If a hospital or outpatient provider designates as a reason for providing a healthcare service a diagnosis included in CMS's list of "selected significant disease" groups, CMS increases the amount of its capitation payment for that beneficiary during the following year. For example, if a beneficiary received care for heart failure during the 12 mo from July 2008 to June 2009, CMS would adjust its capitation payments for the beneficiary during 2010 to provide the extra funds typically needed to care for people who have heart failure. To make this risk-adjustment system cost-neutral, CMS offsets the diagnosis-related increases in capitation payments by reducing its capitation payments for beneficiaries who have not received care for diagnoses in the selected significant disease groups during this 12-mo period.

BBA 97 provisions for improving the quality of health care for older Americans include the following:

■ the Quality Improvement System for Managed Care (QISMC)

■ the Healthcare Employers' Data Information System (HEDIS), which requires MA plans to monitor and report to CMS their rates of compliance with selected processes and outcomes of health care (eg, mammography and immunization against influenza)

- the Medicare Health Outcomes Survey, which requires MA plans to contract with third parties to survey a sample of their members and report information to CMS about their health status, functional ability, and satisfaction with their recent health care

CMS summarizes the information generated by all three systems and makes it available at the Medicare Personal Plan Finder to help older Americans make informed choices about Medicare's FFS program and its various managed care options.

Balanced Budget Revision Act of 1999

Within the first 18 mo of the enactment of BBA 97, the quality of health care for older Americans began to erode, and the decreases in the payments to providers proved to be steeper than projected. For example, Medicare payments for home-health care decreased by 45% between 1997 and 1999. In response, Congress passed the Balanced Budget Revision Act at the end of 1999. This legislation restored some of the budget cuts made 2 yr earlier, including $4.5 billion to MA plans.

Medicare Modernization Act of 2003

The Medicare Prescription Drug Improvement and Modernization Act of 2003 required dramatic changes in the nature and scope of the Medicare program, including the following:

- The creation of the Medicare Part D program covering prescription medications
- Subsidies for employers who continue to provide their retirees with insurance that covers prescription medications
- Elimination of coverage for prescription medications by Medicaid
- Competition between traditional FFS Medicare and MA plans
- Higher premiums for Medicare Part B to be paid by beneficiaries with higher incomes
- Expanded coverage for preventive services
- Increased reimbursement rates to providers and hospitals in rural areas

The Future of Medicare and Medicaid

CMS is now (in 2010) conducting dozens of demonstration projects designed to improve the quality and outcomes of care for beneficiaries with chronic conditions. In most of these demonstrations, CMS is paying provider and managed-care contractors capitated monthly fees for providing case-management or disease-management services to beneficiaries with specified chronic conditions, such as heart failure, diabetes mellitus, or other "special needs." Many of these demonstrations are based on the principle of "pay for performance," which stipulates that CMS will pay the capitation fees only to the extent that the contractor attains pre-agreed standards of performance, eg, performing certain diagnostic tests, reducing Medicare's overall FFS payments, and satisfying beneficiaries with the services they provide.

Another Pay-for-Performance program is the Physician Quality Reporting Initiative (PQRI). Physicians and other healthcare providers who report data about the quality of their care when they submit their bills to their Medicare carriers may earn bonuses of up to 1.5% of their total Medicare payments. CMS also sends them personal reports comparing their PQRI data to that of peers nationwide. In 2008, there were 118 quality measures that could be reported, but some are specific to certain specialties. Additional information is available at http://www.cms.hhs.gov/PQRI (accessed Jan 2011).

The aging of the baby-boom generation, technology-driven increases in healthcare spending, and a decline in the number of workers per Medicare beneficiary will contribute to serious financial challenges for the Medicare program in the years ahead. Similarly, imminent sharp increases in the number of older Americans with serious disabilities will soon surpass states' ability to pay for their long-term care. To meet these challenges, the nation needs visionary leaders, committed professionals, and rapid major changes in its systems for providing and paying for health care.

In December 2009 the Patient Protection and Affordable Care Act (H.R. 3590) was signed into law. Several organizations such as the Gerontological Society of America (see http://www.geron.org/HCR provisions.pdf; accessed Jan 2011) and the Kaiser Family Foundation (see http://www.kff.org/health reform/8023.cfm; accessed Jan 2011) have distributed guidelines regarding how this comprehensive healthcare reform bill may affect older adults.

REFERENCES

- Centers for Medicare and Medicaid Services, Department of Health and Human Services. Medicare Physician Guide: A Resource for Residents, Practicing Physicians, and Other Health Care Professionals. Available at http://www.cms.hhs.gov/MLNProducts/downloads/physicianguide.pdf

- Kaiser Family Foundation. *Talking about Medicare: Your Guide to Understanding the Program, 2009.* Available at http://www.kff.org/medicare/7067./med_prescription.cfm

- Sullivan-Marx EM. Lessons learned from advanced practice nursing payment. *Policy Polit Nurs Pract.* 2008;9(2):121–126.

CHAPTER 6—ASSESSMENT

KEY POINTS

- Geriatric assessment is a multifaceted approach to the care of older adults with the goal of promoting wellness and independent function.

- Assessment of function includes the physical, cognitive, psychologic, and social domains.

- Time-efficient, valid tools are available for use in a variety of settings to evaluate the status of older adults in all these domains.

- Time tends to be a less important element than the skills of the clinician in successful communication with older adults.

Geriatric assessment is a multifaceted approach to the care of older adults with the goal of promoting wellness and independent function. Function is defined broadly to encompass the physical, cognitive, psychologic, and social domains. The scope of the assessment of any individual domain depends on the goals of care, the site of care, the patient's level of frailty, time constraints, and the availability of a multidisciplinary team. The essential aspects of geriatric assessment should be performed routinely in all sites of care, including the ambulatory setting, the emergency department, the hospital, the nursing home, and the home. Whenever possible, assessments should be performance based. An informant, ideally a caregiver or family member who lives with the patient, is often required to provide or to verify pertinent historical information about the older adult's day-to-day functioning.

Try This, a publication of the Hartford Institute for Geriatric Nursing, is a series of geriatric assessment tools. Each of the more than 40 *Try This* issues contains the tools and a description of their use. Each can be downloaded from the ConsultGeriRN.com Web site. Examples of topics include The Geriatric Depression Scale, Predicting Pressure Ulcer Risk, the Geriatric Oral Health Assessment Index, and Decision Making and Dementia.

STRENGTH-OF-EVIDENCE (SOE) RATING DEFINITIONS

A = consistent and good quality patient-oriented evidence
B = somewhat inconsistent or limited quality patient-oriented evidence
C = very inconsistent or very limited patient-oriented evidence, disease-oriented evidence, and/or consensus from professional organizations
D = unstudied common practice or opinion

See inside front cover for detailed information regarding the SOE classification.

THE ROUTINE OFFICE VISIT

Incorporating geriatric assessment into routine office practice requires use of efficient strategies. One such strategy entails rapid screening of targeted areas (Table 6.1), followed by comprehensive assessment in areas of concern. Many of the initial screens can be completed by trained office staff; some can be completed by the patients themselves while seated in the waiting area or at home before the visit. The use of a "rolling" assessment, which targets at least one area for screening during each office visit, should be considered. Finally, in the absence of specific target symptoms, parts of the routine examination, such as auscultation of the chest and palpation of the abdomen, can be replaced by aspects of geriatric assessment, such as observation of gait, balance, and transfers. Office-based screening for common geriatric conditions, however, has not been shown to improve patient outcomes (SOE=A).

PATIENT-CLINICIAN COMMUNICATION

Because of the demands of a busy clinical practice, the time available for office visits is often constrained. Time tends to be less important, however, than the skills of the clinician in successful communication with older adults. For several simple strategies that can be used to enhance communication, see Table 6.2. See also the table on communication in "Hearing Impairment," p 181. To accommodate the high prevalence of sensory deficits among older adults, particular attention should be given to the environment of the examination room. The use of simple, inexpensive amplification devices with lightweight earphones can be especially effective, even for severely hearing-impaired adults. During the course of the interview, the clinician should go beyond the customary clinical inquiries by asking open-ended questions such as, "What would you like me to do for you?" Finding out what the patient wants can be a prime mechanism for solving potential problems, generating trust, and improving mutual satisfaction in the patient-clinician relationship.

Effective communication can be compromised by low health literacy—the diminished ability to obtain, process, and understand basic health information and services needed to make appropriate health decisions. Increasing evidence suggests that low health literacy, which has been documented in about one of every four community-living older adults, has deleterious effects on health and survival, due at least in part to deficiencies in self-management skills, poor adher-

Table 6.1—Rapid Screening Followed by Assessment and Management in Key Domains

Domain	Rapid Screen	Assessment and Management
Functional status	Answers "Yes" to one or more of the following: Because of a health or physical problem, do you need help to: • shop? • do light housework? • walk across a room? • take a bath or shower? • manage the household finances?	Assess all other ADLs listed in Table 6.3. Evaluate cognitive function and mobility using performance-based tests. Assess social support. Consider use of adaptive equipment.
Mobility	"Timed Up and Go" test: unable to complete in <20 sec	Treat underlying musculoskeletal or neurologic disorder. Refer to physical therapy.
Nutrition	Answers "Yes" to "Have you lost more than 10 lbs over the past 6 mo without trying to do so?" (or BMI <20 kg/m²)	See "Malnutrition," p 195.
Vision	If unable to read a newspaper headline and sentence while wearing corrective lenses, test each eye with Snellen chart; unable to read greater than 20/40	See "Visual Impairment," p 167.
Hearing	Acknowledges hearing loss when questioned or unable to perceive a letter/number combination whispered at a distance of 2 feet	See "Hearing Impairment," p 197.
Cognitive function	3-item recall: unable to remember all 3 items after 1 min	Administer Folstein Mini–Mental State Examination.
Depression	Answers "Yes" to either of the following: In the past month, have you been bothered by: • feeling down, depressed, or hopeless? • having little interest or pleasure in doing things?	Administer 15-item Geriatric Depression Scale or 2- or 9-item Patient Health Questionnaire (see "Depression and Other Mood Disorders," p 295).

Table 6.2—Effective Strategies to Enhance Communication

- Use a well-lit room and avoid backlighting.
- Minimize extraneous noise and interruptions.
- Introduce yourself to establish a friendly relationship.
- Face the patient directly, sitting at eye level.
- Address the patient, using his or her last name.
- Speak slowly.
- Inquire about hearing deficits; raise the volume and lower the tone of your voice accordingly.
- If necessary, write questions in large print.
- Allow sufficient time for the patient to answer.
- Touch the patient gently on the hand, arm, or shoulder during the conversation.
- Provide patient education materials that are appropriate for individuals with low health literacy.

ence, and inadequate use of preventive services (SOE=A). Helpful information on low health literacy, including risk assessment and strategies to enhance communication, is available at http://www.reynolds.med.arizona.edu/EduProducts (accessed Jan 2011).

PHYSICAL ASSESSMENT

The importance of a complete, appropriately detailed physical examination cannot be overstated. Many older adults cannot see well enough to report signs of disease, or have cognitive impairment that prevents them from being able to accurately report symptoms. The clinician cannot assume that "no news is good news" in the care of older adults.

Functional Status

Functional status refers to the person's ability to perform tasks that are required for living. These tasks, usually referred to as activities of daily living (ADLs), are listed in Table 6.3. When assessing function, ask whether the patient is independent or requires the help of another person to complete the tasks. Bathing is typically the basic ADL with the highest prevalence of disability, and disability in bathing is often the reason why older adults receive home aide services. To identify patients with "preclinical" disability, ie, those who do not yet require personal assistance but who are at risk of becoming disabled, ask about perceived difficulty with the tasks and whether the patient has changed the way he or she completes the task because of a health-related problem or condition. Assess the use of any assistive devices, such as a cane or walker, as well as duration and circumstances of use.

Outside of a rehabilitation setting, performance-based testing of most of the self-care and instrumental ADLs is not practical. Hence, performance-based testing of functional status focuses primarily on mobility, including transfers, gait, and balance. Ask

Table 6.3—Activities of Daily Living

Self-care

Bathing	Toileting
Dressing	Grooming
Transferring from bed to chair	Feeding oneself

Instrumental

Using the telephone	Doing laundry
Preparing meals	Doing housework
Managing household finances	Shopping
Taking medications	Managing transportation

Mobility

Walking from room to room
Climbing a flight of stairs
Walking outside one's home

---

the patient to stand from the seated position in a hard-backed chair while keeping his or her arms folded. Inability to complete this task suggests leg (hip flexor/extensor and knee flexor/extensor) weakness and is highly predictive of future disability. Once the patient is standing, observe him or her walking back and forth over a short distance, ideally with the usual walking aid. Abnormalities of gait include path deviation; diminished step height or length, or both; trips, slips, or near falls; and difficulty with turning. The tasks of rising from the chair, walking 10 feet (3 meters), turning around and returning to the chair, turning, and then sitting back down in the chair make up the "Timed Up and Go" test. Individuals who can complete this sequence of maneuvers in <10 sec have intact mobility; those who take ≥20 sec require further evaluation.

An alternative assessment strategy is to measure gait speed as a predictor of future disability. A gait speed of 0.80 meters/sec allows for independent community ambulation; a speed of 0.60 meters/sec allows for community activity without use of a wheelchair. These norms indicate that patients who can walk 50 feet in an office hallway in ≤20 sec should be able to walk independently in normal activities. See "Gait Impairment," p 218.

Balance can be tested progressively by asking the patient to stand first with his or her feet side by side, then in semitandem position, and finally in tandem position. Difficulty with balance in these positions predicts an increased risk of falling. Although standardized instruments, such as the Tinetti Performance-Oriented Mobility Assessment, can be used to quantify impairments in gait and balance, a qualitative assessment is usually sufficient to make recommendations about the need for an assistive device, such as a cane or walker. When assessing gait and balance, particularly in older women, clinicians should observe for the use of proper footwear, ie, flat, hard-soled shoes.

Finally, clinicians can often glean useful functional information by observing older adults as they complete simple tasks such as undressing or dressing, picking up a pen and writing a sentence, touching the back of the head with both hands, and climbing up and down from an examination table.

Nutrition

Poor nutrition in older adults can reflect concurrent medical illness, depression, dementia, inability to shop or cook, inability to feed oneself, or financial hardship. Aside from visual inspection for signs of malnutrition, older adults should have their weight and height measured routinely. A low body mass index (ie, kg/m^2 <20) or an unintentional weight loss of >10 pounds in 6 mo suggests poor nutrition and requires further evaluation. See "Malnutrition," p 195.

Vision and Hearing

Although visual impairment from cataracts, glaucoma, macular degeneration, and abnormalities of accommodation usually worsens with age, older adults are often unaware of their visual deficits. Asking about difficulty with driving, watching television, or reading may uncover a problem with vision. As a brief performance-based screen, an older adult can be asked to read (using corrective lenses, if applicable) a short passage from a newspaper or magazine. Significant visual impairment can be confirmed through the use of a Snellen chart or Jaeger card; the inability to read greater than 20/40 is the standard criterion. See "Visual Impairment," p 167.

The high prevalence of hearing loss among older adults and its association with depression, dissatisfaction with life, and withdrawal from social activities make it an important target for assessment. Hearing loss is usually bilateral and in the high-frequency range. In the absence of cerumen impaction, older adults who acknowledge hearing loss when questioned should be referred directly for formal audiometric testing. If hearing loss is denied, further screening with the whisper-voice test is indicated. Inability to perceive a letter/number combination whispered at a distance of 2 feet is considered abnormal and warrants a discussion about referral for formal audiometric testing. See "Hearing Impairment," p 176.

COGNITIVE ASSESSMENT

The prevalence of cognitive decline doubles every 5 yr after the age of 65 and approaches 40%–50% at age 90. Most patients with dementia do not complain of memory loss or volunteer symptoms of cognitive impairment unless specifically questioned. Older adults with cognitive impairment, even in the absence of dementia, are at increased risk of accidents, delirium, medical nonadherence, and disability.

Therefore, an important feature of every assessment of an older adult, especially those ≥75 yr old, is a brief cognitive screen (SOE=C).

Because short-term memory loss is typically the first sign of dementia, the best single screening question is recall of three words after 1 min. Anything other than perfect recall should lead to further testing. An alternative strategy adds orientation to day of the week, month, and year to the three memory items. A cut-off of three or more errors has a sensitivity and specificity of nearly 90% for a diagnosis of dementia. The most commonly used instrument for formal testing of cognition is the Folstein Mini–Mental State Examination (MMSE), which assesses orientation, registration and recall, attention and calculation, language, and visual-spatial skills. Although scores on the MMSE need to be interpreted in the context of educational attainment, race, and age, scores <24 generally warrant further evaluation for possible dementia.

An often overlooked area of cognition, which is essential for proper goal-directed behaviors, is executive function. The clock-drawing test is valuable because it assesses executive control and visual-spatial skills, two domains of cognition that are not tested or incompletely tested by the MMSE. In the clock-drawing test, the patient is asked to draw the face of a clock and to place the hands correctly to indicate 2:50 or 11:10. The clock-drawing test is combined with the three-item recall in the Mini-Cog Assessment Instrument for Dementia, a validated screening test that takes about 3 min to administer. The Mini-Cog has an advantage over the MMSE of being relatively uninfluenced by level of education or language differences.

Another useful question to assess executive function is asking the patient to name as many four-legged animals as possible in 1 min. Fewer than 8 to 10 animals or repetition of the same animals is abnormal and suggests the need for further evaluation. See "Dementia," p 245.

PSYCHOLOGIC ASSESSMENT

Although the prevalence of major depressive disorder among community-dwelling older adults is only about 1%–2%, a large number of older adults suffer from significant symptoms of depression below the severity threshold of major depression as defined by the *Diagnostic and Statistical Manual of Mental Disorders, 4th Edition, Text Revision*. These subthreshold depressive symptoms, which often include somatic complaints such as poor sleep and fatigue, increase the risk of physical disability and slower recovery after an acute disabling event (SOE=A). They are also associated with a significant increase in the cost of

medical services, even after accounting for the severity of chronic medical illness (SOE=A). Hence, clinicians should have a high index of suspicion for depressive symptoms and a low threshold for treatment. The best single question to ask is, "Do you often feel sad or depressed?" An affirmative response warrants further evaluation of other depressive symptoms, perhaps through the use of a standardized instrument such as the 15-item Geriatric Depression Scale. The PHQ-2 is a very short, validated instrument for depression screening as well. See "Depression and Other Mood Disorders," p 295.

Anxiety and worries are also important symptoms in older adults and are often a manifestation of an underlying depressive disorder. Finally, because older adults are particularly likely to experience the loss of a loved one, special efforts should be made to recognize and manage the consequences of bereavement. See "Depression and Other Mood Disorders," p 295.

SOCIAL ASSESSMENT

A social assessment consists of several elements, including ethnic, spiritual, and cultural background; the availability of a personal support system; the need for a caregiver, his or her role, and presence of caregiver burden; the safety of the home environment; the patient's economic well-being; the possibility of mistreatment of the older adult; and the individual's advance directives. Although a comprehensive social assessment may not be feasible in a busy office practice, clinicians caring for older adults should be mindful of these aspects of an older adult's life. Clinicians can uncover important clues to unmet needs by inquiring about the availability of help in case of an emergency. For frail older adults, particularly those who lack social support, referral to a visiting nurse or physical therapist may be helpful in assessing home safety and level of personal risk. See "Psychosocial Issues," p 17; "Cultural Aspects of Care," p 49; and "Mistreatment of Older Adults," p 87.

QUALITY OF LIFE

During the past decade, *quality of life* has been embraced as a convenient "catch phrase" to denote important patient outcomes other than death and traditional physiologic measures of morbidity. Although a gold standard does not exist, most instruments designed to measure quality of life include various aspects of physical, cognitive, psychologic, and social function. Perhaps the most commonly used instrument is the Short Form-36 Health Survey (SF-36), which includes 36 items organized into eight domains: physical function, role limitations due to physical health, role limitations due to emotional health, bodily pain, social functioning, mental health, vitality, and general health perceptions. The SF-36 has been tested extensively among community-living adults and hospitalized patients, but it may not be suitable for use among the oldest-old group, especially those who are frail, because of floor effects and insensitivity to clinically important changes in health status.

When assessing quality of life, clinicians should ask about patient preferences regarding medical care and goals of care. Goals can be multiple, diverse, and sometimes conflicting. Older adults exhibit striking heterogeneity with respect to physiologic function, health status, belief systems, cultural and ethnic backgrounds, values, and personal preferences. The successful management of chronic conditions, such as diabetes mellitus, arthritis, and heart failure, requires that patients, families, and clinicians work collaboratively to define the specific problems, to elicit personal preferences, and to establish the goals of care. Patients' cultural and ethnic heritages have an important role in their understanding of their illness, its meaning in their lives, and their response to it. It is crucial, therefore, for the cliniciian to have an appreciation of that heritage and the role it plays in the patient's understanding of health and illness. (See "Cultural Aspects of Care," p 49.) Treatment plans that include patient preferences enhance adherence and increase satisfaction, and they have the potential to improve patient outcomes.

ASSESSING THE OLDER DRIVER

Evaluating the older driver is a difficult challenge. The automobile is the most important—and often the only—source of transportation for older adults. Yet a variety of age-related changes, chronic conditions, and medications place the older adult at risk of automobile accidents. Although the absolute number of crashes involving older drivers is low, the number of crashes per mile driven and the likelihood of serious injury or death are higher than for any age group other than those aged 16–24 yr.

The vast majority of older adults make prudent adjustments in their driving behaviors by avoiding rush hour or congested thoroughfares or by not driving at night or during adverse weather conditions. Nonetheless, impaired older adults who continue to drive are a hazard not only to themselves but also to other drivers, passengers, and pedestrians. Pertinent risk factors for automobile accidents include poor visual acuity (less than 20/40) and contrast sensitivity; dementia, particularly deficits in visual-spatial skills and visual attention; impaired neck and trunk rotation; and poor motor coordination and speed of movement. Alcohol and medications that adversely affect alertness, such as narcotics, benzodiazepines, antihistamines, antidepressants, antipsychotics, sedatives, and muscle relaxants, can impair driving skills and increase crash risk. Hence, caution is warranted when starting or adjusting the dosage of these medications, and patients should be warned about potential adverse events on driving safety.

Any report of an accident or moving violation should trigger an assessment of an older adult's driving ability. Safety concerns should be discussed honestly with the older driver, and ideally with a spouse or other family member as well, particularly when the older driver lacks insight into his or her driving limitations. Alternative modes of transportation should be considered. Recommendations to stop driving, however, should not be proffered lightly, because driving cessation can lead to a decreased activity level and increased depressive symptoms. Referral for a formal driving evaluation by a skilled occupational therapist may be helpful in confirming unsafe driving behaviors, or perhaps in suggesting interventions such as adaptive equipment to correct for specific physical disabilities. In the interest of public safety, clinicians should know their state's law on reporting impaired drivers. In most states, clinicians are encouraged, and in some states mandated, to report their concerns to the licensing agency. (See also driving in "Legal and Ethical Issues," p 30.) An excellent reference for clinicians caring for older drivers is *The Physician's Guide to Assessing and Counseling Older Drivers*. Developed by the American Medical Association in cooperation with the National Highway Traffic Safety Administration, it is available free of charge at http://www.ama-assn.org/ama/pub/category/10791.html (accessed Jan 2011).

ACUTE FUNCTIONAL DECLINE

An acute decline in functional status is usually precipitated by an illness or injury. Most new disability episodes are attributable to illnesses or injuries leading to hospitalization. The most severe forms of disability commonly arise from a relatively small number of acute conditions, including hip fracture, stroke, heart failure, and pneumonia. The adverse functional consequences of hospitalization reflect not only the disabling effects of these and other serious conditions but also the hazards of immobility and hospital-acquired complications. Up to 20% of new disability episodes are attributable to less serious illnesses or injuries that lead to restriction of activity but not to hospitalization. These restrictions are usually caused by several concurrent health-related problems, although a fall or injury is most likely to result in disability. Among older adults who are physically frail, about a third of new disability episodes occur insidiously, ie, in the absence of a discernable illness or injury. These episodes may be attributable to relatively subtle perturbations in physiologic status or to the loss of compensatory strategies among highly vulnerable older adults with relatively little reserve capacity. Contrary to conventional wisdom, most older adults who become newly disabled recover independent function within 6 mo. However, these individuals are at high risk of subsequent disability.

COMPREHENSIVE GERIATRIC ASSESSMENT

See "Hospital Care," p 119 and "Outpatient Care Systems," p 157.

ACOVE-3* QUALITY INDICATORS PERTAINING TO ASSESSMENT

Cognitive and functional screening and assessment

- If a vulnerable older adult is new to a primary care practice or inpatient service, then there should be a documented assessment of cognitive ability and functional status.
- All vulnerable older adults should be evaluated annually for changes in memory and function.

Screening and assessment of common geriatric conditions

- All vulnerable older adults should have documentation of the presence or absence of urinary incontinence during the initial evaluation.
- All vulnerable older adults should have documentation of the presence or absence of urinary incontinence every 2 yr.
- All vulnerable older adults should have documentation that they were asked annually about the occurrence of recent falls.
- If a vulnerable older adult reports a history of two or more falls (or one fall with injury) in the previous year, then there should be documentation of a basic fall history (circumstances, medications, chronic conditions, mobility, alcohol intake) within 3 mo of the report (or within 4 weeks of the report if the most recent fall occurred in the previous 4 weeks).
- If a vulnerable older adult has involuntary weight loss of ≥10% body weight in ≤1 yr, then weight loss (or a related disorder) should be documented in the medical record as recognition of undernutrition as a potential problem.
- If a vulnerable older adult presents for an initial evaluation, then a quantitative and qualitative assessment for persistent pain should be documented. (If cognitively impaired, a standardized pain scale, behavioral assessment, or proxy report of pain should be used.)
- If a vulnerable older adult has symptomatic osteoarthritis of the knee or hip, then functional status should be assessed when new to a primary care or musculoskeletal disease practice and annually.
- All vulnerable older adults should be screened for persistent pain annually.

Driving

- If a vulnerable older adult has newly diagnosed dementia, then one of the following should occur (consistent with state law):
  ○ Patient advised not to drive a motor vehicle
  ○ Referral to the Department of Motor Vehicles to test driving ability
  ○ Referred to a driver's safety course that includes assessment of driving ability

Related quality indicators for Assessment

- There are numerous additional ACOVE-3 indicators pertaining to assessment scattered through this syllabus, particularly in the following chapters: "Visual Impairment," 167; "Hearing Impairment," 176; "Malnutrition," 195 ; "Eating and Feeding Problems," 203; "Urinary Incontinence," 207; "Falls," 224; "Osteoporosis," 234; "Dementia," 245; "Sleep Problems," 272; "Pressure Ulcers and Wound Care," 283; "Depression and Other Mood Disorders," 295; and "Musculoskeletal Diseases and Disorders," 437.

*Assessing Care of Vulnerable Elders – 3ʳᵈ Set. See inside front cover for explanation.

REFERENCES

- Cigolle CT, Langa KM, Kabeto MU, et al. Geriatric conditions and disability: the Health and Retirement Study. *Ann Intern Med.* 2007;147(3):156–164.

- Fulmer T, Wallace M. Fulmer SPICES: An Overall Assessment Tool for Older Adults. *Try This: Best Practices in Nursing Care to Older Adults.* 2007;(1). Available at http://consultgerirn.org/uploads/File/trythis/try_this_1.pdf

- Graf C. The Lawton Instrumental Activities of Daily Living (IADL) Scale. *Try This: Best Practices in Nursing Care to Older Adults.* 2007;(23). Available at http://consultgerirn.org/uploads/File/trythis/try_this_23.pdf

- Graf C. The Hospital Admission Risk Profile (HARP) *Try This:*

- *Best Practices in Nursing Care to Older Adults.* 2008;(24). Available at http://consultgerirn.org/uploads/File/trythis/try_this_24.pdf

- Hall K, Chyun DA. General Screening Recommendations for Chronic Disease and Risk Factors in Older Adults. *Try This: Best Practices in Nursing Care to Older Adults.* 2010;(27). Available at http://consultgerirn.org/uploads/File/trythis/try_this_27.pdf

- Hardy SE, Gill TM. Factors associated with recovery of independence among newly disabled older persons. *Arch Intern Med.* 2005;165(1):106–112.

- Shelkey M, Wallace M. Katz Index of Independence in Activities of Daily Living (ADL). *Try This: Best Practices in Nursing Care to Older Adults.* 2007;(2). Available at http://consultgerirn.org/uploads/File/trythis/try_this_2.pdf

CHAPTER 7—CULTURAL ASPECTS OF CARE

KEY POINTS

- The capable clinician incorporates into geriatrics practice a nuanced understanding of the role that culture and religious beliefs play in promoting the health of older adults.

- The astute clinician remains alert to the differences among individual patients from a given culture or religious tradition and guards against stereotyping on the basis of ethnic, cultural, or religious affiliation.

- Communication and clinical care are enhanced when the patient and healthcare provider make an effort to negotiate a common understanding of causation, diagnosis, and treatment, while maintaining respect for the beliefs and constructs of both individuals.

As the cultural and religious diversity of older Americans continues to grow, it is increasingly important for clinicians to develop an approach to working with older adults from a broad range of cultural and religious groups. The purpose of this chapter is to assist clinicians in developing and improving their skills during cross-cultural and interfaith patient encounters. Readers are also referred to the *Doorway Thoughts* series, published by the American Geriatrics Society (see the references). Other chapters in the *Doorway Thoughts* series demonstrate how the general approaches outlined here in each topic relate to working with patients from a variety of cultural or religious groups. It is very important to keep in mind when using the *Doorway Thoughts* series that, although the information offered in each chapter is accurate *in general*, the beliefs, traditions, customs, and preferences of individuals in all cultural and religious groups vary widely. The astute clinician never assumes that any person's cultural or religious background will dictate his or her health choices or behavior. The capable clinician remains alert to the differences among individual patients and families from a given culture or religious tradition, and on guard against stereotyping older adults on the basis of their cultural or religious affiliation.

STRENGTH-OF-EVIDENCE (SOE) RATING DEFINITIONS
A = consistent and good quality patient-oriented evidence
B = somewhat inconsistent or limited quality patient-oriented evidence
C = very inconsistent or very limited patient-oriented evidence, disease-oriented evidence, and/or consensus from professional organizations
D = unstudied common practice or opinion

See inside front cover for detailed information regarding the SOE classification.

DOORWAY THOUGHTS IN CROSS-CULTURAL HEALTH CARE

The key concepts discussed in this chapter are "doorway thoughts"—factors that the astute practitioner reflects on before walking through the doorway of any examining, consultation, or hospital room. These factors can shape intercultural and interfaith healthcare encounters and relationships for good or for ill. Cultural, spiritual, and historical facts and issues relating to the members of an entire minority group can be in play in any cross-cultural or interfaith encounter or relationship. The practitioner should be sensitive to the possibility that they may affect their relationships with individual patients and families and may also affect patients' willingness or ability to understand, accept, and adhere to prescribed regimens.

The quality of any encounter between a clinician and a patient from different religious or cultural backgrounds depends on the clinician's skill and sensitivity. Questions about the individual patient's attitudes and beliefs should be worked naturally and carefully into the clinical interview. The clinician must remember that no culture or religious tradition is monolithic; attitudes and beliefs vary widely from one individual to another within a single group. Prior familiarity with a patient's background will not suffice, for it is inaccurate to assume that a person's outlook is inflexibly determined by his or her cultural or religious heritage. The concepts presented here are intended to serve as guidelines in formulating appropriate questions, and not as a rigid list of attributes or clinical scenarios.

PREFERRED TERMS FOR CULTURAL OR RELIGIOUS IDENTITY

The terms referring to specific cultural, ethnic, or religious groups can change over time, and individuals in any one group do not always agree on the terminology that is appropriate. It is important to learn the term that the individual patient prefers for his or her cultural or religious identity, and to use that terminology in conversation with the patient, as well as in his or her health records.

FORMALITY

Attitudes regarding the appropriate degree of formality in a healthcare encounter differ widely among cultural groups. Learning a new patient's preferences with regard to formality and allowing those preferences to shape the relationship is always advisable. Initially, a more formal approach is likely to be appropriate.

Addressing the Patient

The patient's correct title (eg, Dr., Reverend, Mr., Mrs., Ms., Miss) and his or her surname should be used unless and until he or she requests a more casual form of address. Another important issue is to determine the correct pronunciation of the person's name, as well as the appropriate ordering of names; for those from a variety of countries, an individual's family name is given first, followed by their given name.

Addressing the Healthcare Provider

It is also important to learn how the patient would prefer to address the clinician and to allow his or her preference to prevail. For example, in some cultures, trust in the physician depends on his or her assuming an authoritative role, and informality would undermine the patient's trust. This is an aspect of the clinical relationship in which the clinician's personal preferences may be relinquished.

LANGUAGE AND LITERACY

- What language does this individual feel most comfortable speaking? Will a medical interpreter be needed?

- Does this patient read and write English? Another primary language? If so, which one(s)?

- If the patient is not literate, does he or she have access to someone who can assist at home with written instructions?

It is worthwhile to consider these questions early in the healthcare relationship to determine whether interpretation services are needed and to make certain that communication with the patient is effective. Even those who speak English fluently may wish to discuss complicated issues in their native language. It is the clinician's responsibility to explain medical terms and to ask the patient for explanations of any cultural or foreign terms that are unfamiliar.

RESPECTFUL NONVERBAL COMMUNICATION

Body position and motion is interpreted differently from one cultural group to another. Specific hand gestures, facial expression, physical contact, and eye contact can hold different meanings in different cultures. The clinician should watch for particular body language cues that appear to be significant and that might be linked to cultural norms that are

important to the patient, in an effort to cultivate sensitivity to the conditions that facilitate and improve communication.

Conservative body language is advisable early in a relationship with a patient or when in doubt about a patient's background or preferences; assume a calm demeanor and avoid expressive extremes (eg, very vigorous handshakes, a loud and hearty voice, many hand gestures, an impassive facial expression, avoidance of eye contact, standing at a distance). The clinician should remain alert for signals that the patient is comfortable or uncomfortable. Directly asking the patient questions about body language may also help. Making negative judgments about a patient that are rooted in unconscious cultural assumptions about the meaning of his or her gestures, facial expressions, or body language should be avoided.

The distance from others that individuals find comfortable varies, depending in part on their cultural background. The clinician should determine what distance seems to be the most comfortable for each patient and, whenever practicable, allow the patient's preference to establish the optimal distance during the encounter.

HISTORY OF TRAUMATIC EXPERIENCES

Is the patient a refugee or survivor of violence or genocide? Are family members missing or dead? Have patients or family members been tortured? Such experiences could negatively affect the healthcare encounter without the clinician's knowledge unless relevant questions are included among standard questions about the patient's history.

Clinicians should remember that in some historical periods and jurisdictions, healthcare providers have participated in torture and genocide. For example, during World War II, Nazi medical personnel were responsible in concentration camps for selecting individuals for gassing, supervising the gassing process, and administering lethal injections to inmates in "hospitals." The methods and tools of torture used have sometimes resembled legitimate clinical procedures and tools. Patients who have survived such experiences may not feel safe in medical or governmental settings, and contact with all clinicians may invoke feelings of vulnerability, fear, panic, or anger. Great sensitivity is necessary in providing health care for these individuals.

ISSUES OF IMMIGRATION

Immigration Status

Some individuals may be living in North America without the protection of appropriate immigration documents. Clinicians may wish to assure each patient that information given within the medical encounter will be kept in the strictest confidence.

History of Immigration or Migration

The history of the movements of a large portion of a religious or cultural group can affect the attitudes and behavior of an individual in that group even when he or she has not immigrated to North America from another country. In addition, understanding an individual's specific migration history often provides insight into the key life transitions informing his or her outlook. Knowing how a person came to live in North America can be important. The time and effort the clinician invests in learning more about a cultural or religious group's history and current situation can be repaid not only in a better relationship with the individual patient but also in an enhanced appreciation of the factors affecting clinical relationships with other patients from that group.

ACCULTURATION

Acculturation is a process in which members of one cultural group adopt the beliefs and behaviors of another group. Acculturation of a group may be evidenced by changes in language preference, adoption of common attitudes and values, evolution of religious practices, or gradual loss of separate ethnic identification. Although acculturation typically occurs when a minority group adopts the habits and language patterns of a dominant group, acculturation may also be reciprocal between groups.

It is essential to keep principles of acculturation in mind during any cross-cultural or interfaith health encounter. Beginning by determining how long a person has lived in North America and whether he or she was born here is helpful. However, remember that the degree to which the person is acculturated to North American customs and attitudes is the consequence of many factors and not just of the number of years since he or she immigrated. Older adults who follow the traditions of their cultural or religious group may have been born outside of the United States, may be recent arrivals to the continent, or may even be lifelong North American residents.

A patient's level of cultural or spiritual shifting can impact not only his or her health behavior but also preferences in end-of-life planning and decision making. Acculturation can also be an issue dividing family members, and a person's resistance to or ease of acculturation may be a matter of pride or shame and guilt. Developing sensitivity about the issues of acculturation for one's older minority patients is a key element in effective cross-cultural health care. Asking patients directly about their adherence to cultural and spiritual traditions can be useful.

TRADITION AND HEALTH BELIEFS

People from a variety of cultural groups may not conceive of illness in North American terms. Some may have highly developed concepts of the causes of health and disease that are incompatible with the concepts that form the foundations of North American medicine. Some other paradigms of wellness and illness include beliefs that illnesses have spiritual causation or are the result of imbalance among bodily humors, or that they are caused by a person's actions in past lives, to name but a few.

Patients may be making unexamined assumptions that are based on traditional beliefs, and these can cause confusion or create misunderstanding. The more the clinician knows about specific cultural and religious traditions, the more he or she can promote effective clinical communication.

In addition, patients holding traditional beliefs may be using alternative remedies (eg, rituals, herbal preparations) that they do not mention, and questions about such practices should be included among other questions about the patient's history. It is unrealistic to expect that a patient will simply "adapt" to North American approaches to health and health care, just as it is impractical to expect the clinician to accept a new conception of wellness and disease. Clinical communication and efficacy will be enhanced when patients and healthcare providers make an effort to negotiate a common understanding of causation, diagnosis, and treatment for a specific health problem, while maintaining respect for the beliefs and constructs of both individuals.

UNSPOKEN CHALLENGES

Are there any issues that are critical to the success of the healthcare encounter that are present but may go unspoken? Clinicians should remain alert for the possibility that such issues may be present. Examples include the following:

- lack of trust in healthcare providers and the healthcare system
- fear of medical research and experimentation
- fear of medications or their adverse events
- unfamiliarity or discomfort with the Western biomedical belief system

Some patients may not feel comfortable in customary North American healthcare settings for a variety of reasons. Explanations for the discomfort, distrust, or uneasiness can include lack of familiarity with Western practices, dissatisfying previous encounters with the healthcare system, or the belief that insensitivity or discrimination is inevitable for anyone in the cultural or religious group. Such feelings may result from having been stereotyped or treated insensitively or even unfairly by clinicians in the past.

Sensitive exploration of these issues with patients is often both worthwhile and necessary. In general, sensitivity to the possibility that such issues are in play is advised in all patient encounters.

THE INTERFACE BETWEEN CULTURE AND RELIGION

In some cultural groups, the large majority of individuals share one religious heritage; in others, there is a great deal of religious and spiritual diversity. As a result, the relative impact of religion and culture on health behavior and decision making for older adults may be subtle and complex, warranting respectful exploration on the part of the astute clinician.

Several studies have documented that most patients either prefer or would accept clinicians asking them about their spiritual beliefs and what impact such beliefs might have on their world view, health behavior, and health decision making (SOE=A). Questions regarding religion and spirituality should be incorporated sensitively and early in the patient-provider relationship, and reexplored when significant health problems arise.

APPROACHES TO DECISION MAKING

Western bioethics emphasizes individual autonomy in all health decisions, but for many other cultures, decision making is family or community centered. Autonomy principles allow competent individuals to involve others in their health decisions or to cede those rights to a proxy decision maker. The clinician should ask patients if they prefer to make their own health decisions or if they would prefer to involve or defer to others in the decision-making process. Some may wish to assign the decision-making authority wholly to another individual or a group. In some cultures, the definition of family may include fictive kin. In families in which the degree of acculturation of the generations differs, the older adult may defer to or depend on younger relatives, even though the tradition might suggest that the reverse would occur.

Many studies have documented the impact of religious and spiritual beliefs on preferences regarding end-of-life practices and decision making. Some religious traditions characterize health outcomes as divinely willed and emphasize acceptance in the face of adversity. Other traditions stress the religious obligation for individuals to save or extend life at almost any cost.

Establishing an understanding of each patient's decision-making construct and preferences early in the clinical relationship will, in most instances, promote better communication and avoid the difficulties inherent in trying to address the issues at a time of crisis. When the patient's and clinician's cultural or religious backgrounds differ, careful exploration of the issues is all the more important because the clinician cannot proceed if he or she and the patient are not starting from common assumptions.

ATTITUDES REGARDING DISCLOSURE AND CONSENT

Cultural attitudes toward truth telling and disclosure of terminal diagnoses vary widely. In some cultures, it is commonly believed that patients should not be informed of a terminal diagnosis, because this may be injurious to health or hasten death. Obtaining informed consent from patients with this belief may prove difficult. There is no consensus in bioethics concerning the rigorous application of full clinical disclosure in every situation. However, it is generally agreed that incorporating a patient's beliefs concerning disclosure and truth telling into clinical planning whenever possible is desirable. Some patients may prefer not to know if they are terminally ill and ask that family members or other caregivers receive all diagnostic information and make all treatment decisions. It is advisable to explore each patient's preferences regarding disclosure of serious clinical findings early in the clinical relationship and to reconfirm these wishes at intervals. See also "Legal and Ethical Issues," p 23.

GENDER ISSUES

Culture and religion intertwine in describing traditions and structures with regard to gender roles. Societies seemingly based on the same patriarchal or matriarchal model may vary widely in their expressions of the model. A person's gender influences the sorts of experiences he or she has had, not only within the family but also in the community and healthcare system. Another level of complexity may be added to healthcare encounters when an older adult's group struggles with conflicting traditional and contemporary views on gender roles. Cultural norms for men and women can influence their health behavior, and such norms for the genders vary widely from one culture to another. Gender-based norms may also affect how patients choose a healthcare provider and make health decisions, as well as how they form their preferences for disclosure and consent.

The clinician is strongly advised to explore each patient's attitudes regarding the interplay among gender, choice of healthcare provider, autonomy, and personal decision making early in the patient-provider relationship, to confirm his or her preferences at intervals, and to follow the individual patient's wishes whenever possible.

CARE INTENSITY AT THE END OF LIFE

Cultural, religious, and spiritual beliefs are an important influence in a person's formation of his or her attitudes toward supportable quality of life, approach to suffering, and beliefs about medical feeding, life-prolonging treatments, and palliative care. Some cultures and religious traditions value a direct struggle for life in the face of death, and both patients and families expect an intensive approach to treatment. Others avoid personal confrontation of death and dying and prefer to leave such decisions to the clinician. Still others take a direct approach to death and dying but reject too aggressive an approach.

Research has shown that physicians and patients from shared cultural and religious backgrounds have similar values in these areas (SOE=B); the implications of such findings for clinicians and patients from differing backgrounds are obviously important. Both clinicians and patients bring their own attitudes and beliefs to any clinical encounter. Clinicians should be aware of their personal views, cultural values, and religious beliefs when discussing end-of-life plans with patients, and respect patients' beliefs and preferences even when they are different from their own.

In negotiating end-of-life decisions with a patient whose background is different from his or her own, the clinician must listen especially carefully to the patient's goals and concerns and exert every effort to avoid making assumptions that do not apply. For example, the assumption that "no one would want to live in that condition" or that "everyone would want treatment in this situation" is likely to be faulty. To ensure that end-of-life plans and decisions reflect an individual's rights and wishes, the clinician must strive to understand the older adult's overall approach to life and death and, as far as possible, provide care that is consistent with that approach.

ATTITUDES TOWARD ADVANCE DIRECTIVES

The use of advance directives and healthcare proxies has become more common over the past 25 yr, but research indicates that the use of written directives may be more common among older adults in the dominant North American culture than among older adults in minority cultural groups (SOE=A). In cross-cultural situations, when discussing attitudes and beliefs regarding written directives with a patient, clinicians should be sensitive to the possibility that some minority older adults will prefer to use alternatives (eg, verbal directives or directives dictated to family members or others), while others will need to avoid any such discussion so as to observe proscriptions against talking about death. In view of the fact that preferences for care intensity may also differ according to cultural and religious backgrounds, patients should also be given the opportunity to indicate the interventions they *do* want as well as those they do not want in any written or verbal directive used.

APPROACHES: THE ETHNICS MNEMONIC

The ETHNICS mnemonic, as described by Kobylarz et al (2002), is a tool to facilitate effective health interviews and care planning in cross-cultural settings. Rather than serving as a prescribed outline of questions to ask, the ETHNICS mnemonic provides a framework in which to ascertain a wide variety of information and to negotiate effective therapeutic next steps, all within a routine 15-min clinical session.

ETHNICS stands for the following:

Explanation: Asking patients to describe what they think is happening to them in their own words.

Treatments: Inquiring as to which treatments patients have used for their health problem(s) before the interview. The astute clinician will inquire about both biomedical interventions as well as any complementary and alternative treatments patients may have used.

Healers: Respectfully inquiring about other healers involved in a patient's care. Many patients will seek treatment from alternative practitioners or traditional healers, as well as from conventional healthcare providers, and incorporating this information into the healthcare encounter is important to overall care planning and efficacy.

Negotiate: Negotiating with each patient and/or his or her designated caregiver(s) as to which treatments the patient will accept and participate in is a part of every healthcare encounter with an older adult.

Intervene: Putting together a care plan that is acceptable from the perspectives of both the provider and the patient. This still frequently incorporates a blending of "scientific" explanations of wellness and disease, as well as each individual patient's concepts of their health status and acceptable approaches to addressing concerns.

Collaborate: Focusing on building a trustful and resilient relationship with each older patient is one of the goals of every healthcare encounter. Incorporating formal and informal caregivers into a broader team alliance is also critical to the success of health care for all older adults.

Spirituality: Inquiring respectfully about patients' spiritual beliefs, and how these might impact on their healthcare preferences and behavior, particularly at the end of life.

There is no gold standard definition of cultural competence. Most definitions emphasize a careful coordination of individual behavior, organizational policy, and system design to facilitate mutually respectful and effective cross-cultural and interfaith interactions.

Cultural competence combines attitudes, knowledge base, acquired skills, and behavior. It is an approach, not a technique. Cultural competence is not a form of "political correctness." Ideally, it is a nuanced understanding of the determining role that culture plays in all of our lives and of the impact culture has on every healthcare encounter, for both the clinician and the patient.

Clinicians are encouraged to view each cross-cultural and interfaith encounter as an opportunity to learn more, not only about the individual patient and his or her culture or religion, but also about themselves. It is recommended that clinicians continually learn more about the impact of cultural and religious beliefs on healthcare decisions. Additionally, clinicians are urged to work with the entire interdisciplinary healthcare team, including administrators, to promote cultural competence in the healthcare organizations in which they practice.

ACOVE-3* QUALITY INDICATORS PERTAINING TO CULTURAL ASPECTS OF CARE

Interpreter
- If a vulnerable older adult is deaf or does not speak English, then an interpreter or translated materials should be used to facilitate communication

*Assessing Care of Vulnerable Elders – 3ʳᵈ Set. See inside front cover for explanation.

REFERENCES

- American Geriatrics Society, Ethnogeriatrics Committee. *Doorway Thoughts: Cross-Cultural Health Care for Older Adults.* Volumes 1–3. Boston, MA: Jones and Bartlett; 2004, 2006, 2008.
- Kobylarz FA, Heath JM, Like RC. The ETHNIC(S) mnemonic: a clinical tool for ethnogeriatric education. *J Am Geriatr Soc.* 2002;50(9):1582–1589.
- Kwak J, Haley WE. Current research findings on end-of-life decision making among racially or ethnically diverse groups. *Gerontologist.* 2005;45(5):634–641.
- Wilson-Stronks AL. The role of nursing in meeting the healthcare needs of diverse populations. *J Nurs Care Qual.* 2008;23(4):289–291.

CHAPTER 8 – PHYSICAL ACTIVITY

KEY POINTS

- Regular physical activity provides numerous and substantial health benefits for older adults.

- The health benefits of physical activity accrue independently of risk factors. Greater amounts of physical activity have greater health benefits.

- To obtain substantial health benefits of physical activity, older adults are commonly recommended to do at least 150 minutes of moderate-intensity aerobic activity each week. If they cannot do this amount of activity, they should do the amount that is possible according to their abilities, so as to avoid inactivity. Doing at least 30 minutes of moderate-intensity aerobic activity on ≥5 days each week is an appropriate way for older adults to be active.

- Older adults should also engage in muscle-strengthening activity on ≥2 days each week.

- Older adults at risk of falls should do balance training.

- Promoting physical activity is one of the most important and effective preventive and therapeutic interventions in older adults.

- Counseling by a healthcare provider is an important way of promoting physical activity in clinical settings. Referral of patients to community resources, particularly evidence-based programs, is also important.

Physical activity can be defined broadly as movement of the body produced by skeletal muscles that expends energy. However, in public health, "physical activity" usually refers to *health-enhancing physical activity*. Health-enhancing physical activity generally involves the large muscle groups of the body and significant energy expenditure. Movement that expends small amounts of energy, sometimes called *baseline activity*, includes light-intensity activity such as standing and walking slowly. People who do only baseline activity are considered inactive. In this chapter, the term "physical activity" is used to refer to health-enhancing physical activity. The term "exercise" is used to refer to the subset of physical activity that involves a structured program to improve physical fitness.

BENEFITS OF PHYSICAL ACTIVITY

Preventive Health Benefits

Regular physical activity in adults and older adults improves cardiorespiratory and muscular fitness (SOE=A). It reduces the risk of many diseases, including coronary heart disease, stroke, hypertension, some lipid disorders, type 2 diabetes, colon cancer, breast cancer, osteoporosis, and depression (SOE=A). It also reduces the risk of unhealthy weight gain and assists in weight loss (SOE=A). In older adults, physical activity reduces the risk of falls (SOE=A) and sarcopenia, and regularly active older adults have a lower risk of hip fracture (SOE=B). The evidence that physical activity reduces the risk of cognitive impairment is growing and substantial (SOE=B). There is some evidence that physical activity can reduce the risk of lung cancer, endometrial cancer, osteoarthritis, sleep problems, and anxiety disorders (SOE=B).

Consistent with its broad physiologic effects, regular physical activity decreases both cardiovascular and noncardiovascular mortality in older adults. This benefit is large. The risk of premature mortality is estimated to be 40% less in adults who are active ≥7 hours each week than in those who are active for <0.5 hours each week (SOE=B). While this estimate is based on cohort studies that determined amounts of physical activity from questionnaires, one study of older adults determined level of physical activity objectively using doubly labeled water. In this study, adults in the highest tertile of energy expenditure per day had a 67% lower mortality rate than adults in the lowest tertile of energy expenditure (SOE=B).

In general, greater amounts of physical activity have greater health benefits, although the relationship between the amount of physical activity and the amount of benefit appears nonlinear for many health conditions. That is, the absolute increase in benefit is greatest at low levels of activity, and less at high levels of activity. The "dose-response" relationship varies by disease in a manner that is incompletely understood. Risk of cardiovascular disease decreases with amount of aerobic activity over a wide range of dose. Blood pressure shows little dose-response effect, with most of the effect of physical activity on blood pressure occurring at low to medium levels of activity.

The health benefits of physical activity accrue independently of risk factors. For example, sedentary smokers experience health benefits of increasing physical activity even if they continue to smoke. The health benefits of physical activity are also generally independent of body weight: overweight and obese adults obtain benefits from physical activity even if it does not promote weight loss.

Strong, consistent observational evidence indicates that regularly active older adults are at reduced risk of moderate or severe functional limitations and role limitations (SOE=B). One review estimated that moderate amounts of aerobic physical activity reduced risk of functional decline by 30%. There appears to be a dose-response relationship, with greater amounts of physical activity producing more benefit.

Therapeutic Benefits

Physical activity is commonly recommended in clinical practice guidelines as therapy for specific conditions. Clinical practice guidelines identify a substantial therapeutic role for physical activity in coronary heart disease, peripheral vascular disease, hypertension, type 2 diabetes, osteoarthritis, osteoporosis, some lipid disorders, obesity, claudication, and COPD. Physical activity also has a role in the management of depression, anxiety disorders, pain, heart failure, syncope, sleep disorders, stroke, dementia, back pain, and constipation, and in prevention of venous thromboembolism.

In a systematic review, there was moderate evidence from controlled trials that physical activity has a beneficial effect on functional limitations in older adults with existing mild, moderate, or severe limitations (SOE=B). Evidence that physical activity improves role limitations (eg, measures of ADLs) was only limited. Most evidence was from studies that prescribed periods of 30–90 minutes of exercise, on 3 to 5 days per week, in which most of the time was devoted to aerobic and muscle-strengthening activities.

Economic Benefits

Regularly active adults are consistently reported to have lower medical expenditures than sedentary adults (SOE=B). In one study comparing older adults

---

STRENGTH-OF-EVIDENCE (SOE) RATING DEFINITIONS

A = consistent and good quality patient-oriented evidence
B = somewhat inconsistent or limited quality patient-oriented evidence
C = very inconsistent or very limited patient-oriented evidence, disease-oriented evidence, and/or consensus from professional organizations
D = unstudied common practice or opinion

See inside front cover for detailed information regarding the SOE classification.

Table 8.1–Recommended Types and Amounts of Physical Activity

Type of Exercise	Frequency/Duration	Examples of Activities	Examples of Targeted Conditions
Aerobic	≥150 minutes of moderate-intensity activity each week, spread throughout the week, *or* ≥75 minutes of vigorous-intensity activity each week, spread throughout the week	Walking, running, swimming, bicycling	Many conditions, including cardiovascular disease, cancer, diabetes, and depression
Muscle strengthening	≥2 days each week	Resistance training (eg, using weight machines)	Falls, frailty
Flexibility	As necessary to maintain adequate flexibility	Stretching	Osteoarthritis
Balance training	≥3 days/wk	Backward walking, heel-to-toe walking, Tai Chi exercise	Falls, osteoporosis

who remained sedentary to older adults who became active ≥3 days each week, medical expenditures of the active group were lower by about $2,200 per year. In one managed-care plan that offered a physical activity benefit consisting of paying per-visit costs for Medicare-eligible enrollees who participated in an exercise program called EnhanceFitness, participants adjusted total costs were $1,186 lower per year than those of nonparticipants by year two.

RECOMMENDED AMOUNTS OF PHYSICAL ACTIVITY

A public health recommendation for ≥20 min of vigorous aerobic activity on ≥3 days per week was developed in the 1980s. In 1995, the CDC and the American College of Sports Medicine (ACSM) developed a moderate-intensity recommendation: "Every US adult should accumulate 30 minutes or more of moderate-intensity physical activity on most, preferably all, days of the week." In 2007, the ACSM and the American Heart Association (AHA) updated the 1995 recommendation by issuing separate recommendations for adults and for older adults. In 2008, the U.S. Department of Health and Human Services issued the first national guidelines for physical activity, the *2008 Physical Activity Guidelines for Americans* (see Table 8.1).

Aerobic Activity

An older adult can achieve recommended levels of aerobic activity by doing either moderate-intensity aerobic physical activity for at least 150 minutes each week, or vigorous intensity activity for at least 75 minutes each week. Doing a combination of moderate- and vigorous-intensity activity is also acceptable. Aerobic activity should be spread throughout the week, preferably on 3 or more days per week. Doing at least 30 minutes of aerobic activity on 5 or more days each week remains an appropriate way for older adults to obtain the health benefits of activity.

Several comments help clarify this recommendation. First, episodes of moderate-intensity activity of ≥10 minutes count toward meeting the recommendation. Second, the recommendation does not refer to just leisure activity or exercise. Occupational activity (eg, carpentry), domestic activity (eg, mowing the grass), and transportation activity (eg, walking to the store) all count toward meeting recommendations. Third, participation in physical activity above the minimum recommended levels results in greater health benefits. Some physical activity is clearly preferable to none for those who are unable to meet these targets. Older adults should be strongly encouraged to avoid an inactive lifestyle, even if they do not (or cannot) obtain recommended amounts of activity. Finally, as indicated earlier, the recommended activity is in addition to routine (baseline) activity of light-intensity or of short duration (<10 minutes).

In these guidelines, older adults should use the relative intensity of the activity to guide the level of effort. That is, the intensity of activity is relative to a person's level of aerobic fitness (or capacity). In exercise physiology, relative intensity is expressed as a percent of a person's aerobic capacity (VO_2max) reserve, or as a percent of a person's measured or estimated maximal heart rate, or as a percent of heart rate reserve. The large variation in fitness levels among older adults means that for more fit older adults, a brisk walk is moderate-intensity; for less fit adults, a slow walk is moderate-intensity.

The most difficult part of explaining the recommendation to patients is describing how to judge intensity. To help explain intensity, both the ACSM/AHA recommendation and the HHS 2008 guidelines described the range of relative intensity using a scale from 0 to 10, in which sitting is 0 and all-out effort is 10. With this scale, moderate-intensity activity is a 5 or 6 and produces noticeable increases in heart rate and breathing. On the same scale, vigorous-intensity activity is a 7 or 8 and produces large increases in heart rate and breathing. The "talk test" can be used to help judge relative intensity. During moderate-intensity activity, a person should be able to talk without pauses but not sing. During vigorous activity, a person cannot say more than a few words without pausing for breath. Older adults should monitor their subjective perception of effort. However, the ACSM/AHA recommendation notes that older adults vary in their ability to match a certain level of effort (eg, a "5" on a 0 to 10 scale). A period of supervised exercise can help a person learn how to monitor level of effort. If maximal heart rate is known from an exercise test, then heart rate reserve can be used to set a range of intensity. Typically, 40%–59% of heart rate reserve is moderate intensity, and 60%–84% is vigorous intensity. When maximal heart rate is not known, equations can be used to predict maximal heart rate. However, the standard deviation of maximal heart rate at a given older age is large (in the range of 15 beats per minute), and the usefulness of setting a heart rate range (eg, for moderate-intensity aerobic activity) for a specific person based on these equations alone is limited.

Muscle-Strengthening Activity

ACSM/AHA recommendations and the HHS 2008 guidelines state that older adults should perform muscle-strengthening activities of the major muscle groups on ≥ 2 days each week. The major muscle groups are usually regarded to be the arms, shoulder, legs, hip, back, chest, and abdomen. A typical routine for older adults involves 2 or 3 nonconsecutive days each week. For adults who chose resistance training (eg, weight machines), one set of 8 to 10 different exercises is sufficient, with 10 to 15 repetitions per set. There is some evidence that two or three sets are more effective than one. Moderate-intensity or high-intensity training is recommended, in which level of effort of moderate intensity is 5 or 6 on a 0 to 10 scale (0=no movement and 10=maximal effort). High-intensity is 7 or 8 on the same scale.

Flexibility Activity

Flexibility activity is recommended for older adults as a means of maintaining the flexibility needed for regular physical activity and daily life. Flexibility is an important aspect of fitness, and flexibility activities like stretching are effective in increasing flexibility. Unlike aerobic activity and muscle-strengthening activity, flexibility activity by itself has no known health benefits. Evidence that flexibility training prevents injury is insufficient.

Balance Training

Balance training is recommended for older adults at risk of falls, including adults with frequent falls or mobility problems. Examples of balance exercises include backward walking, heel-to-toe walking, and standing using a narrow base of support. With balance training, exercises can be graduated in difficulty. For example, a tandem walk is easiest when holding on to a table and becomes progressively more difficult with arms in any positions, arms close to the body, and arms close to the body while holding a weight.

The optimal types and amounts of balance training are unclear. Several effective interventions to prevent falls included balance training on ≥ 3 days per week. Hence, it is preferable that older adults do standardized balance exercises from a program demonstrated to reduce falls. There is moderate evidence that Tai Chi exercise is effective in fall prevention, although the optimal amount and forms of Tai Chi are unclear (SOE=B).

Management of Body Weight

The *2005 Dietary Guidelines for Americans* included recommendations about physical activity and management of body weight. These guidelines recommended 60 minutes of moderate- to vigorous-intensity aerobic activity on most days of the week to help manage body weight and prevent gradual, unhealthy body weight gain in adulthood. For sustaining weight loss in adulthood, the guidelines recommended at least 60–90 minutes of daily moderate-intensity physical activity.

However, the Physical Activity Guidelines Advisory Committee concluded that the amount of physical activity needed for weight maintenance over the long term is unclear. Further, a great deal of variability exists among individuals in the amount of activity needed for weight control. It is a major challenge, if not impossible, for some older adults to obtain 60–90 minutes of physical activity in a day. Further, when dietary intake is not controlled, changes in weight due to increases in physical activity are unpredictable. A reasonable approach for physical activity and weight management in older adults is to follow the HHS 2008 guidelines. Overweight and obese older adults should first achieve minimal recommended levels of physical activity (150 minutes of moderate-intensity aerobic activity per week). If a healthy weight is not achieved with this level of activity, then caloric intake should be controlled, physical activity increased gradually, and body weight monitored. Physical activity can be increased to the point that is individually effective in controlling weight. If an older adult is not capable of sufficiently high amounts of activity, then additional dietary restriction is necessary.

When older adults lose weight, they lose not only fat mass but also muscle mass and bone mass. Because physical activity, particularly muscle-strengthening activity, acts to preserve bone and muscle mass, older adults should not attempt to lose weight by diet alone.

Screening

For older adults, especially older adults with chronic conditions, the ACSM/AHA recommends they develop an activity plan in consultation with their primary care provider. The activity plan should integrate public health preventive recommendations (summarized above), with any therapeutic use of physical activity recommended, eg, by clinical practice guidelines. Older adults should understand if, and how, chronic conditions limit the amounts and types of activity they can do.

This recommendation changes screening guidelines. Rather than advise older adults to consult a healthcare provider before starting to increase physical activity, ACSM/AHA recommends that healthcare provider consultation about physical activity should occur regardless of whether an adult currently plans to increase physical activity. One quality of care measure for older adults ascertains whether older adults discuss physical activity with a healthcare provider at least once a year. At the time of a consultation about physical activity, the clinician should ensure that the patient does not have any undiagnosed symptoms and is up-to-date on preventive care, and that medical conditions are stable. Further, the clinician should assess if and how the patient should limit his or her activity because of chronic conditions.

Thus, "screening" older adults can be used to match them to an activity plan appropriate for their abilities. Most, if not all, studies of exercise in people with disabilities have assessed potential participants to ensure the exercise intervention is appropriate. These study populations have included adults with osteoarthritis, lower limb loss, cerebral palsy, multiple sclerosis, muscular dystrophy, Parkinson's disease, spinal cord injury, stroke, traumatic brain injury, dementia, intellectual disability, and mental illness. A review concluded that the benefits of physical activity for such people with disabilities clearly outweigh the risks.

It is appropriate for providers of exercise programs to ask new participants (who are not referred after an examination by a healthcare provider) to complete a symptom checklist. People with undiagnosed symptoms should seek medical care before starting an exercise program.

The Physical Activity Guidelines Advisory Committee concluded, after a systematic review of the literature, that "the protective value of a medical consultation for persons with or without chronic diseases who are interested in increasing their physical activity level is not established." The U.S. Preventive Services Task Force does not recommend any type of routine preexercise screening of healthy asymptomatic adults. Specifically, for adults at increased risk of coronary heart disease, the Task Force finds insufficient evidence for routine screening with resting ECG, exercise treadmill test, or electron-beam CT scanning for coronary calcium. For adults at low risk of heart disease, the Task Force recommends against screening with these tests.

PROMOTION OF PHYSICAL ACTIVITY IN OLDER ADULTS

The public health approach to promotion of physical activity is based on a socioecologic model. This involves action at all levels of society: individual, interpersonal, organizational, community, and public policy. To illustrate the logic of the model, consider that counseling an older adult to walk regularly (individual level intervention) is more effective if the person lives in a neighborhood with good access to parks and other safe places to walk (a community level intervention). A referral to an exercise program (an individual level intervention) is more likely to succeed if the costs of the exercise program are subsidized by a health plan (organizational level intervention). Physical activity promotion in clinical settings occurs in this broader context. The Task Force on Community Preventive Services has identified eight evidence-based community approaches for promoting physical activity (http://www.thecommunity guide.org).

Clinical Settings

Clinical settings need a system for routinely assessing levels of physical activity in patients, for providing patients with a recommendation about physical activity, for helping patients achieve recommended levels, and for evaluating the effectiveness of the system in promoting physical activity. An example of an evidence-based system is the Green Prescription in New Zealand. In brief, after assessing their level of physical activity, patients are given the option of requesting a prescription from a primary care provider. The provider provides a written "green" prescription, typically for walking or other home-based activity. A copy is faxed to the local sports foundation, who contacts patients and offers them assistance by telephone counseling, face-to-face counseling, or peer group support. In a randomized trial of this approach, the intervention group averaged 35–40 more minutes of physical activity each week (SOE=A).

Assessing Physical Activity

The importance of routine assessment of physical activity is emphasized by the Exercise is Medicine

Initiative of the ACSM. This initiative advocates for physical activity as a vital sign to be checked each visit. Tools have been developed to provide quick assessments of the physical activity level of older adults, such as the Rapid Assessment of Physical Activity, a 9-item questionnaire in which patients self-rate their strength, flexibility, and frequency and intensity of exercise. Both the amount of aerobic activity and the amount of muscle-strengthening activity should be assessed.

Providing an Activity Prescription

In the ACSM/AHA recommendations, the activity prescription is considered part of a broader approach of developing the physical activity plan. The plan considers individual preferences, individual abilities and fitness, chronic conditions and activity limitations, risk of falls, strategies for decreasing risk of injury, and behavioral strategies to increase adherence to the plan. Essentially, the plan provides specific guidance on how to meet physical activity guidelines. A resource for developing the plan is ACSM's *Exercise Management for Chronic Diseases and Disabilities*. This book covers issues in exercise management for some 40 different conditions. Some guidelines for developing a plan include the following:

- The plan will commonly emphasize walking, which is a popular and safe activity in older adults.

- The plan should emphasize the importance of gradually increasing physical activity over time (see below). It can be appropriate for older adults to spend weeks or months at activity levels below recommended levels.

- The less active an adult is currently and the less experience he or she has with physical activity, the more appropriate it is to recommend starting in a supervised, evidence-based program (see below).

- Providing social support for physical activity is important. Social support can be provided by classes, formal mall walking groups, telephone counseling, and informal arrangements in which people simply meet to go for a walk.

- Vigorous-intensity activity, such as running, should be recommended with caution, mainly to older adults who are accustomed to these activities, or who have sufficient fitness, experience, and knowledge and already do sufficient moderate-intensity activity to meet recommendations.

Providing Assistance in Increasing Physical Activity

In 2002, the U.S. Preventive Services Task Force concluded that the evidence is insufficient to recommend for or against behavioral counseling in primary care settings to promote physical activity. However, some clinic-based systems of promoting physical activity have been carefully studied and reported to increase physical activity, such as the "Green Prescription" system above. A reasonable conclusion is that a clinic can implement either an existing evidence-based approach, or implement and evaluate a new approach tailored to the clinical situation based on principles of behavior change and building on existing approaches. The many negative studies of physical activity counseling in clinical settings emphasize the importance of evaluating any new approaches.

Most counseling approaches are broadly consistent with the transtheoretical model, which posits that individuals move through a series of stages when changing a health-related behavior. The counseling is based on the current stage of the patient, which in the simplest form involves 3 stages. People in the *contemplation stage* have not yet decided if they wish to be physically active, and the counseling provides persuasive messages individually tailored to the person's health situation and values. People in the *preparation* (or *ready for action*) *stage* agree they should be more physically active but have not yet started to get more activity. The counseling assists the person start to become active. People in the *maintenance stage* have been regularly active for ≥6 mo, and the counseling seeks to reinforce regular physical activity. Counseling strategies commonly seek to increase patient self-efficacy for exercise.

Particularly for adults with some functional limitations, an appropriate way to provide assistance is to make a referral to an evidence-based program. Resources, such as the National Council on Aging Web site (http://www.ncoa.org), can help identify evidence-based programs that have been tested in research studies and translated into versions that work in the community. For example, Active Living Every Day, and Active Choices are two programs that were originally tested in research studies and subsequently translated into programs appropriate for community settings. A recent study demonstrated the community versions of these programs were effective in large samples of older adults who were substantially more ethnically, economically, and functionally diverse than the samples in the original research studies.

A longstanding resource for older adults from the National Institute on Aging is *Exercise: A Guide from the National Institute on Aging.* This publication is updated periodically.

Management of Risks of Physical Activity

The most important recommendation for avoiding activity-related injuries is to increase physical activity gradually over time (SOE=B). Observational evidence is strong that the risk of injury is directly related to the size of the gap between a person's usual level of activity and their new level of activity. A series of small increments in activity, each followed by a period of adaptation, is associated with lower rates of musculoskeletal injury. The safest method for increasing activity has not been established by intervention studies. For reasonably healthy adults, adding a small amount of light- to moderate-intensity activity (eg, walking 5–15 minutes per session, 2 to 3 times per week) has low risk of musculoskeletal injury and no known risk of sudden cardiac events (SOE=B).

In contrast, during vigorous-intensity activity, all individuals are at higher risk of sudden adverse cardiac events. However, regularly active adults are at much less risk than inactive adults who abruptly engage in vigorous activity.

In older adults, cardiovascular adaptation to a target level of physical activity can take as long as ≥20 wk. This suggests that activity levels should be increased once per month instead of once per week.

Other factors also affect injury risk. The risk of injury is higher with vigorous exercise, with greater amounts of exercise, and with activities that involve frequent contact (eg, soccer, basketball) or purposeful collision (eg, football). The risk of injury is less with a higher level of fitness, supervision, protective equipment such as bike helmets, and in well-designed environments. To illustrate the safety of walking, one community-based study estimated 0.2 injuries per 1,000 hours of walking for transportation. In contrast, in 1,000 hours of participation, dancing had 0.7 injuries, gardening 1.0 injuries, and running 3.6 injuries.

Master Athletes

Promoting physical activity in older adults should avoid ageism. Some older adults are capable of high levels of physical activity. Evidence is strong that high levels of physical activity provide additional health benefits over medium amounts of activity. A major issue for all athletes, including master athletes, is the prevention and management of overuse injuries. Variety (cross-training) in physical activity is recommended to reduce risk of overuse injury. While athletes may focus on one specific activity (eg, running), they should meet recommendations for both aerobic and muscle-strengthening activities. Both aerobic fitness and muscular fitness reduce risk of injury.

Older Adults with Low Fitness or Low Functional Ability

In the lifestyle interventions and independence for elders (LIFE) pilot study, a randomized trial in which older adults (70–89 yr old) with chronic diseases and reduced functional ability who were at substantial risk of mobility disability were enrolled, regular exercise improved measures of physical function without appreciably increasing risk of adverse events. This trial affirmed that older adults with functional impairments can achieve benefits from exercise (SOE=A). Similarly, an older study of resistance exercise in frail nursing-home residents demonstrated improvements in strength and function. (SOE=A).

Regardless, in such older adults with low fitness or low functional ability, it is more challenging to match abilities with types and amounts of activity. Sometimes referrals can be made to specific rehabilitation programs, such as pulmonary rehabilitation, for assessment, exercise prescription, and medically supervised exercise. Assessment by a physical therapist is generally appropriate, and the therapist can design and tailor an exercise program to the specific limitations of the patient. This assessment can also confirm a patient is capable of participating in a specific community exercise program (eg, a water exercise program designed for adults with arthritis). Given that the care of such patients often involves a geriatric team and consultants, methods should be in place to ensure the activity recommendation is communicated to all the healthcare providers.

REFERENCES

- Exercise Assessment and Screening for You: EASY Screening Tool and exercise recommendations for older adults: http://www.easyforyou.info.

- LIFE Study Investigators. Pahor M, Blair SN, Espeland M, et al. Effects of a physical activity intervention on measures of physical performance: Results of the lifestyle interventions and independence for Elders Pilot (LIFE-P) study. *J Gerontol Series A Biol Sci Med Sci.* 2006;61(11):1157−1165.

- Nelson ME, Rejeski WJ, Blair SN, et al. Physical activity and public health in older adults: recommendations from the American College of Sports Medicine and the American Heart Association. *Med Sci Sports Exerc.* 2007;39(8):1435−1445.

- Resnick B, Galik E, Gruber-Baldini AL, et al. Implementing a restorative care philosophy of care in assisted living: pilot testing of Res-Care-AL. *J Am Acad Nurse Pract.* 2009;21(2):123–133.

CHAPTER 9—PREVENTION

KEY POINTS

- It is important to consider a patient's remaining life expectancy and cognitive status when deciding which preventive health measures to offer.

- Many preventive health measures are underutilized among older adults, including immunizations (eg, flu shots, pneumococcal vaccinations), exercise counseling, depression screening, and counseling on geriatric health issues (eg, falls prevention, incontinence).

- Tools are available to help clinicians appropriately target cancer screening for those with ≥5 yr of remaining life expectancy.

- Medicare covers screening for breast, colon, prostate, and cervical cancer; for osteoporosis; and for diabetes and glaucoma for those at high risk. The flu and pneumococcal vaccinations are also covered.

Many preventive health measures are available to older adults, including *screening* tests (eg, colonoscopy), *counseling* about a healthy lifestyle (eg, exercise) and/or geriatric health issues (eg, incontinence), *immunizations* (eg, flu shot), and *chemoprophylaxis* (eg, aspirin). Ideally, older adults should receive preventive health measures from which they are most likely to benefit based on their health and remaining life expectancy. Remaining life expectancy decreases uniformly with age, but it can vary from one individual to the next according to illness burden and functional status. Predicted remaining life expectancy and cognition are important determinants to consider when offering preventive services to older adults. For example, experts generally recommend that clinicians screen older adults for breast cancer who have ≥5 yr of remaining life expectancy.

This chapter reviews the preventive health measures available to older adults and discusses which measures are appropriate based on remaining life expectancy. Table 9.1 provides an overview of all measures available and their recommended use in different populations of older adults, including robust individuals with ≥5 yr remaining life expectancy,

frail individuals with <5 yr remaining life expectancy, those with moderate dementia, and those at the end of life. The recommendations given in Table 9.1 are based on reports from geriatric expert panels, as well as on guidelines from the American Geriatrics Society (AGS) and the United States Preventive Services Task Force (USPSTF). This chapter focuses mainly on primary (ie, disease avoidance) and secondary (ie, early detection and treatment of asymptomatic disease) prevention rather than on tertiary prevention (ie, preventing functional decline from established illness). Table 9.2 shows cost-effectiveness of measures and which measures are covered under Medicare. A service that costs less than $50,000 per life-year saved is generally considered cost-effective, while those costing more than $100,000 per life-year are generally not considered cost-effective. Finally, the chapter discusses effective ways to counsel older adults about preventive health measures and tools available to target cancer screening for older adults with adequate remaining life expectancy.

Several criteria should generally be met before recommending disease screening: 1) The condition being screened for must be serious and prevalent in the population being tested. 2) The disease should have a significant asymptomatic phase that can be detected by the screening test. 3) The screening test must be safe, sensitive, and specific to limit false-positive and false-negative tests. 4) Effective treatment must be available for use early in the natural course of the disease that results in a better prognosis than treatment given after symptoms develop. 5) The costs of screening should be acceptable. 6) Ideally, the screening test should have been found effective in a randomized controlled trial (RCT). Few older adults have been included in RCTs that evaluate screening measures; therefore, recommendations are often based on indirect evidence. Clinicians are encouraged to consider the effect of preventive health measures not only on quantity of life but also on quality of life.

CANCER SCREENING TESTS

The main potential benefit of screening is reducing cancer mortality experienced by individuals whose cancer is detected early and that otherwise would have resulted in death if the cancer was not treated early. The potential harms of screening that can affect all who are screened include complications from screening tests or diagnostic evaluations after false-positive test results, false reassurance from false-negative test results, detection and treatment of

Table 9.1—Preventive Health Measures Available for Older Adults and Recommended Use

Procedure	Clinical Condition of Patient				SOE
	Robust (≥5 yr life expectancy)	*Frail (<5 yr life expectancy)*	*Moderate dementia (2–10 yr life expectancy)*	*End of life (<2 yr life expectancy)*	
Cancer Screening					
Mammography	Every 1–2 yr	Don't do	Consider	Don't do	A/C[a]
PAP smear	May stop after age 65	May stop after age 65	May stop after age 65	May stop after age 65	B
Prostate-specific antigen	Discuss pros/cons	Don't do	Don't do	Don't do	B
Colon cancer screening					A/C[b]
Fecal occult blood test	Do yearly, may stop at age 75	Don't do	Consider	Don't do	
Colonoscopy	Every 10 yr, may stop at age 75	Don't do	Don't do	Don't do	
Other Screening Tests					
DEXA screening for osteoporosis	At least once after age 65, or 60 if high risk			Consider	A
Blood glucose	Screen those with sustained blood pressures >135/80 mmHg[c]			Don't do	C
Cholesterol screening	Consider for those 65–75 yr old with additional risk factors[d]			Don't do	C
Ultrasonography for abdominal aortic aneurysm	Once for men 65–75 yr old who ever smoked			Consider	A
Thyrotropin	Every 2–5 yr	Every 2–5 yr	Every 3 yr	Consider	C
Blood pressure	Consider each visit	Consider each visit	Consider each visit	Consider each visit	A
Height	Once a year	Once a year	Don't do	Don't do	C
Weight	Each visit	Each visit	Each visit	Each visit	C
Immunizations					
Influenza	Annually	Annually	Annually	Annually	A
Pneumococcal	Once after age 65[e]	Once after age 65[e]	Once after age 65[e]	Once after age 65[e]	A
Tetanus	Booster every 10 yr	Booster every 10 yr	Booster every 10 yr	Booster every 10 yr	C
Herpes zoster	Once after age 60	Once after age 60	Once after age 60	Once after age 60	A
Healthy Lifestyle Counseling					
Smoking cessation	Every visit	Every visit	Discuss with caregiver	Don't do	A
Exercise	Annually	Annually	Consider annually	Consider	C
Alcohol misuse	Do initially, then if symptomatic	Do initially, then if symptomatic	Do initially, then if symptomatic	Do initially, then if symptomatic	A
Sexual function	Annually	Annually	Consider annually	Don't do	D
Geriatric Health Issues					
Urinary incontinence screening	Annually	Annually	Annually	Annually	C
Visual acuity testing	Consider annually	Consider annually	Consider annually	Don't do	C
Hearing impairment screening	Consider annually	Consider annually	Consider annually	Don't do	C
Cognitive impairment screening	Do if symptomatic	Do if symptomatic	Do if symptomatic	Do if symptomatic	C
Gait and balance screening	Annually	Annually	Annually	Annually	C
Depression screening	Annually	Annually	Annually	Annually	C
Falls risk assessment	Annually	Annually	Annually	Annually	C

Table 9.1—Preventive Health Measures Available for Older Adults and Recommended Use (continued)

Procedure	Clinical Condition of Patient				SOE
	Robust (≥5 yr life expectancy)	Frail (<5 yr life expectancy)	Moderate dementia (2–10 yr life expectancy)	End of life (<2 yr life expectancy)	
Advance directives completion	Complete and update as needed	Complete and update as needed	Complete and update as needed	Complete and update as needed	C
Chemoprevention					
Aspirin	See below[f]	See below[f]	See below[f]	See below[f]	A
Calcium	Recommended[g]	Recommended[g]	Recommended[g]	Recommended[g]	A
Vitamin D	Recommended[g]	Recommended[g]	Recommended[g]	Recommended[g]	A
Multivitamin	Consider	Consider	Consider	Consider	D
Hormone therapy (women)	Don't do	Don't do	Don't do	Don't do	A

SOURCE: Adapted with permission from Flaherty JH, Morley JE, Murphy DJ, et al. The development of outpatient clinical glidepaths. *J Am Geriatr Soc.* 2002;50(11):1886–1901.

[a] A for women up to age 74; C otherwise
[b] A for robust category; C otherwise
[c] Optimal screening interval is unknown, possibly every 3 yr.
[d] Examples: smoking, diabetes, hypertension
[e] If vaccinated before age 65, may vaccinate once 5 or more years later.
[f] *Men:* 45–79 yr old when benefit from myocardial infarction reduction outweighs risk of GI hemorrhage; coronary heart disease risk estimation tool: http://hp2010.nhlbihin.net/atpiii/calculator.asp (accessed Jan 2011)
   Women: 55–79 yr old when benefit from ischemic stroke reduction outweighs risk of GI hemorrhage; stroke risk estimation tool: http://www.westernstroke.org/index.php? (accessed Jan 2011)
   Men and women ≥80 yr old: insufficient data for recommendation
[g] If there are no contraindications

disease that never would have become clinically significant during a person's lifetime, and psychological distress.

Cancer screening research is subject to three main types of bias: lead time, length, and selection biases. These biases can make a test appear to be effective when it actually is not. Lead-time bias occurs when the underlying disease is not able to be affected by treatment. It results in earlier diagnosis but does not alter the time until death. Thus, the person spends more time as a patient, but the course of the disease is basically unaltered.

Length bias occurs when a test identifies clinically slowly progressive or nonprogressive disease that would never have become a symptomatic problem. Screening for prostate cancer is affected by length bias. Increased levels of prostate-specific antigen can detect cancers that may never cause the patient's death. This leads to overdiagnosis, the detection of "disease" that is of no consequence, also called pseudodisease.

Selection bias is based on the observation that people willing to be screened for cancer may not reflect the population as a whole. Volunteers may be more health conscious or have other personal habits that favorably influence prognosis. Thus, their outcome from screening may be better than what would be seen in a random population.

Controlled prospective randomized trials are the only method of documenting the value of screening while effectively eliminating these sources of bias. Study populations must be followed for many years to document the cancer cause-specific survival advantage, if any, for the screened group. However, no RCTs have been done that support screening for cervical cancer, and data that support screening individuals ≥70 yr old for colorectal or breast cancer are limited.

Breast Cancer

Because the mammography screening trials did not include women >74 yr old, it is unknown whether screening mammography results in a survival benefit for older women. The AGS recommends screening mammography every 1–2 yr for women with ≥5 yr remaining life expectancy up until age 85 and for women >85 yr with excellent health or functional status, or for patients who feel strongly that mammography will benefit them. The recommendations are based on 5-yr remaining life expectancy because cancer-specific survival did not significantly differ between the screened and unscreened groups in RCTs until at least 5 yr from enrollment. The risk of finding clinically insignificant disease increases as women age. In one retrospective cohort study, women with breast cancer and more than three comorbid conditions were estimated to be 20 times more likely to die of a cause other than breast cancer within 3 yr. To help determine who should be screened for breast cancer among the oldest populations, investigators have divided the U.S. population into 5-yr age categories and into quartiles of life expectancy and

Table 9.2—Medicare Coverage of Preventive Health Services and Summary of Cost-Effective Data Available

Measure	Medicare Coverage	Cost-Effectiveness Data*
Preventive health-care visit	Medicare will cover a one-time preventive physical examination within the first 6 mo of enrollment. The examination includes education and counseling about preventive services (eg, depression, hearing impairment, ADLs, falls risk, home safety); it should include a blood pressure measurement, height and weight, ECG, a visual acuity screen, administration of immunizations, a plan for obtaining cancer screening tests, glaucoma screening, bone mass measurements, diabetes outpatient self-management training, medical nutrition therapy for individuals with diabetes or renal disease, and diabetes screening for those at high risk.	Uncertain
Bone density	Once every 2 yr for women at clinical risk of osteoporosis and for men at high risk (eg, on prednisone, primary hyperparathyroidism, history of fracture or osteoporosis)	Bone densitometry combined with alendronate therapy for those found to have osteoporosis is highly cost-effective for women ≥65 yr old and may be cost-saving for ambulatory women ≥85 yr old. It is also cost-effective for men 80–85 yr old with no prior fracture and possibly for men ≥65 yr old with a self-reported prior clinical fracture.
Colon cancer screening	Colonoscopy every 10 yr (every 2 yr for those at high risk), sigmoidoscopy every 4 yr, FOBT every 12 mo, or barium enemas every 48 mo (24 mo for those at high risk)	The current screening strategies of FOBT, flexible sigmoidoscopy combined with FOBT, or colonoscopy are all cost-effective.
Diabetes screening	Only for those at high risk (hypertension, dyslipidemia, obesity, history of high blood glucose) or if someone has ≥2 of the following: >65 yr old, overweight, family history of diabetes, history of gestational diabetes or of a baby weighing >9 pounds	Unknown
Glaucoma screening	Covered every 12 mo for people at high risk (history of diabetes, family history of glaucoma, or black Americans who are >50 yr old)	Population screening is not cost-effective; however, targeted screening of high-risk groups may be.
Routine hearing examinations	Medicare does not cover routine hearing examinations or hearing aids; in some cases, diagnostic hearing examinations are covered.	A simple systematic screen, using an audiometric screening instrument, may be cost-effective for those 55–74 yr old.
Immunizations	Medicare currently covers flu, pneumonia, and hepatitis B vaccinations (for those at medium to high risk). All Part D plans offer partial or full coverage for the zoster vaccine.	The flu shot is cost-effective for adults ≥50 yr old. The pneumonia vaccine is cost effective for adults ≥65 yr old. A single tetanus booster at age 65 is also cost-effective.
Mammograms	Every 12 mo	Somewhat cost-effective for women <80 yr old, may be cost-effective for women ≥80 yr old at the top quartile of life expectancy.
Pap tests and pelvic exams	Every 24 mo and every 12 mo if at high risk of cervical or vaginal cancer	Cost-effective to stop between 65 and 70 yr old as long as there were three normal prior Pap smears.
Prostate cancer screening	A screening digital rectal exam and a screening prostate-specific antigen blood test are covered once every 12 mo	Uncertain
Smoking cessation	Eight face-to-face visits per year for people who are diagnosed with a smoking-related disease and those who take any of the many medications that have their effectiveness complicated by tobacco use.	Telephone quit lines and counseling are cost-effective; brief counseling by primary care physicians may also be cost-effective.
Substance abuse	Medicare covers substance abuse treatment in outpatient treatment centers.	Screening and brief behavioral counseling interventions for alcohol abuse are cost-effective.

NOTE: FOBT = fecal occult blood test

* Cost-effectiveness is the ratio of costs of a test/procedure compared with the benefits of the test/procedure. It is expressed as the cost per year of life saved or the cost per quality-adjusted-life-year saved. Less than $50,000 per life-year gained is considered cost-effective.

then examined the number needed to screen (NNS) for at least one person to benefit in each age and life expectancy category. Although no threshold NNS has been defined, the higher the NNS, the less chance a screening test will benefit a patient and the greater chance the test may cause harm. The NNS with mammography ranges from 176 for women aged 75–79 yr in the top quartile of remaining life expectancy to 1,361 for those in the lowest quartile of remaining life expectancy. As for breast self-examination (BSE) and clinical breast examinations (CBEs), two large RCTs of women of all ages found no benefit of BSE compared with no breast cancer screening, and no trials have compared CBE alone to no screening. The AGS recommends that CBEs be performed periodically and neither endorses nor discourages BSEs. Similarly, the USPSTF found insufficient evidence to recommend for or against CBEs and recommends against teaching BSEs. A Cochrane review in 2008 also recommended against BSE, concluding that BSE was associated with unnecessary biopsies without a survival benefit (SOE=B).

Colon Cancer

Several tests are considered effective for colon cancer screening among adults 50–75 yr old, including colonoscopy every 10 yr, home-based high-sensitivity fecal occult blood tests (FOBT) annually, and flexible sigmoidoscopy every 5 yr with high-sensitivity FOBTs every 3 yr. Although air-contrast barium enemas every 5 yr were previously considered for screening, this test has not been subject to screening trials, has lower sensitivity than other screening strategies, and is thus not commonly used. The likelihood that detection of adenomas and early intervention will yield a mortality benefit declines after age 75 because of the slow growth of an adenoma into invasive cancer (thought to be at least 10 yr) and competing risks of mortality. Decisions about first-time screening after age 75 need to be made in the context of patient health. Colonoscopy is the most sensitive and cost-effective screening test for colon cancer and has specificity similar to that of flexible sigmoidoscopy. Serious complications (eg, major bleeding, perforation, death) from colonoscopy occur in 25 per 10,000 procedures. The USPSTF recommends against routinely screening adults ≥75 yr old and against ever screening adults ≥85 yr old because the risks of screening outweigh the benefits. These recommendations do not apply to adults who have had previous adenomas on colonoscopy and are undergoing surveillance. "Virtual" colonoscopy, a new method using thin-section helical CT, could help reduce colorectal cancer mortality among patients who would otherwise refuse screening with other modalities. However, the

lifetime cumulative risk from radiation exposure could be significant.

Cervical Cancer

Guidelines recommend stopping cervical cancer screening for women 65–70 yr old who have been previously screened and are not otherwise at high risk of cervical cancer. These recommendations are based on evidence that shows that the incidence of high-grade cervical lesions significantly declines after middle age and that the risk of false-positive tests resulting in invasive procedures is increased. Also, older women who have undergone total hysterectomy (no cervical tissue remaining) for a benign indication are not at risk of cervical cancer and should not be screened. An older woman of any age who has never had a Pap smear should be screened with at least two Pap smears 1 yr apart. Risk factors for the development of cervical cancer (eg, new sexual partners) should be assessed on an ongoing basis and taken into consideration when deciding how often and for how long to screen older women for the development of cervical cancer.

Prostate Cancer

In 2008, the USPSTF updated recommendations for prostate cancer screening, stating that there is insufficient evidence to recommend for or against routine screening using prostate-specific antigen (PSA) testing or digital rectal examination (DRE) among men <75 yr old, and recommended against screening men ≥75 yr old. Although the PSA and DRE can effectively detect prostate cancer at early pathologic stages, there is limited and conflicting evidence that the treatments available (radical prostatectomy, radiation therapy, or hormonal therapy) reduce morbidity and/or mortality from early prostate cancer. Initial results of two RCTs of prostate cancer screening in men <75 yr old published in 2009 showed no significant improvement in prostate cancer mortality in one and a 20% mortality reduction in the other; both trials documented detection of numerous clinically insignificant tumors. The number needed to screen (NNS) to prevent one death from prostate cancer is 1,410 with 48 additional men needing to be treated for prostate cancer. Given the uncertainties surrounding prostate cancer screening, it is recommended that clinicians discuss potential benefits of PSA screening (modest reduction of morbidity and mortality from prostate cancer) and the possible harms (false-positive results, unnecessary biopsies, and possible complications of treatment) of prostate cancer screening. If there is a benefit to screening, the populations most likely to benefit are men 50–70 yr old or men >45 yr old at increased risk (black American men and men with a family history of a first-degree relative with prostate cancer). Men with remaining life expectancies of <10 yr are unlikely to benefit from screening. See "Prostate Disease," p 420, for more discussion of prostate cancer screening.

OTHER SCREENING TESTS

Thyroid Disease

Because of the low cost of screening, the increasing risk of subclinical and clinical hyperthyroidism and hypothyroidism with age, and the low risks of treatment (particularly for hypothyroidism), screening of older adults for thyroid dysfunction by measurement of serum thyrotropin is recommended by some clinical experts every 2−5 yr. However, the USPSTF states there is insufficient evidence on whether or not to recommend screening for thyroid disease among adults.

Hypertension

In the United States, hypertension is responsible for 35% of all cardiovascular events (myocardial infarction and stroke) and 49% of all episodes of heart failure. Strong indirect evidence supports screening for hypertension. Randomized trials have confirmed that treatment of isolated systolic hypertension in patients >60 yr old with pharmacologic therapy reduces the risk of stroke, coronary disease, and total mortality (SOE=A). A trial reported in 2008 found that treatment of hypertension among adults ≥80 yr old also reduced the risk of these end points. The USPSTF and geriatric consensus panels recommend screening as frequently as each visit or at least biennially.

Diabetes

No RCT of screening for diabetes has been performed, and the magnitude of benefit of initiating tight glycemic control during the preclinical phase of diabetes is unknown. In one RCT, intensive lifestyle modification in persons with prediabetes delayed progression to clinical diabetes, but it is unknown whether early treatment affects micro- or macrovascular outcomes of diabetes or decreases mortality. Individuals with hypertension do benefit from knowing whether or not they have diabetes, because blood pressure targets are lower for diabetics than for nondiabetic individuals. Therefore, the USPSTF recommends screening for type 2 diabetes in asymptomatic adults with sustained blood pressure of 135/80 mmHg (treated or untreated). The USPSTF found insufficient evidence to recommend screening for type 2 diabetes in asymptomatic adults with blood pressure of 135/80 mmHg or lower. Diabetes is diagnosed by a fasting plasma glucose of 126 mg/dL or more on two separate occasions.

Abdominal Aortic Aneurysm (AAA)

AAAs are found in 4%–8% of older men and in <2% of older women. Although AAAs may be asymptomatic for years, as many as one in three eventually rupture. In a meta-analysis, screening men aged 65–75 yr and surgical repair of those with AAAs ≥5.5 cm was associated with a significant reduction in AAA-related mortality (odds ratio 0.6 –0.7) but no significant difference in all-cause mortality. Because the prevalence of AAAs was very low among men who never smoked, and because screening and early treatment are associated with significant harms (increased number of surgeries with associated clinically significant morbidity and mortality), the USPSTF concluded that the balance between the benefits and harms of screening for AAAs was too close to make a general recommendation; however, the USPSTF does recommend screening men aged 65–75 yr who have ever smoked. No significant reduction in AAA-related mortality was found among women, and screening is not recommended.

Osteoporosis

Four of every ten white U.S. women ≥50 yr old will eventually experience a hip, spine, or wrist fracture. Over half of women ≥80 yr old have osteoporosis (T score less than or equal to –2.5). No clinical trials have evaluated the effectiveness of screening older women for osteoporosis. However, age-based screening is supported by prevalence data. The NNS to prevent one hip fracture ranges from 731 for women 65–69 yr old to 143 for women 75–79 yr old. Routine screening (ie, measurement of bone mineral density through dual x-ray absorptiometry [DEXA]) is recommended by the USPSTF for all women ≥65 yr old and for women ≥60 yr old at high risk. An appropriate interval for screening has not been determined, but Medicare will pay for bone density testing every 2 yr. There are no consensus recommendations for screening men for osteoporosis; however, screening men ≥65 yr old with a prior clinical fracture and all men ≥80 yr old has been shown to be cost-effective.

Hyperlipidemia

The National Cholesterol Education Program Expert Panel recommends that all adults ≥20 yr old obtain a fasting lipoprotein profile every 5 yr. However, few people >70 yr old have been studied in primary prevention studies. Because older adults generally are at higher risk of cardiovascular events, lipid-lowering therapy is likely to be effective as long as their remaining life expectancy is sufficient to allow the benefits of therapy to be realized (at least 5–7 yr in high-risk patients). Secondary prevention trials with statins have included many adults 65–75 yr old. In these trials, older adults showed significant risk reduction in cardiovascular events with statin therapy (SOE=A). The low-density lipoprotein goal for those at average risk is <130 mg/dL.

HEALTHY LIFESTYLE COUNSELING

Physical Activity

Physical inactivity is recognized as a risk factor for many diseases (eg, coronary artery disease, diabetes, and obesity). Increasing physical activity in sedentary older adults may reduce morbidity and mortality and improve psychological health, promote functional independence, and prevent falls. Almost all older adults can engage safely in a program of moderate physical activity (such as walking) or lifestyle modification, without special screening. Stress testing is recommended for any older adult who intends to begin a vigorous exercise program (eg, strenuous cycling, jogging). The AGS encourages clinicians to counsel patients about the importance of exercise. When counseling older adults about exercise, providers should consider patient-specific goals and barriers for exercise and expand on patients' current exercise habits. Exercise for older adults should include endurance (eg, walking, cycling), strengthening (eg, weight training), flexibility (eg, stretching), and balance training (eg, Tai Chi, dance). The exercise prescription should address the type, frequency, duration, and intensity of physical activity for each fitness component. See "Physical Activity," p 54.

Alcohol Misuse

Approximately half of the population ≥65 yr old drinks alcohol, and many may experience health risks from consuming alcohol or from the combination of alcohol use with medications; 2%–4% may have abuse or dependence. The AGS recommends that all older adults ≥65 yr old be asked annually about their alcohol use to detect abuse. Those who report alcohol use in the past year should be given the CAGE (ie, Cut down, Annoy, Guilt, Eye-opener) questionnaire or the Alcohol Use Disorders Identification Test (AUDIT), which performs better than the CAGE questionnaire, especially in women, and behavioral counseling interventions should be performed to reduce alcohol misuse. See "Addictions," p 322.

Smoking Cessation

Regular tobacco cessation counseling is recommended for all older adults who use tobacco products. Smoking cessation at any age decreases rates of COPD, many cancers, and coronary artery disease. If an older adult uses tobacco, he or she should be counseled to quit. Once he or she is ready to quit, there should be documentation of a quit date, discussion of therapies to aid cessation, and a follow-up visit within 1 mo of the quit date. See "Addictions," p 322.

Sexual Dysfunction and Sexually Transmitted Infections

Increasingly, Americans ≥50 yr old are afflicted with sexually transmitted infections (STIs) and HIV. Clinical practice guidelines recommend screening older adults who report high-risk sexual behaviors for STIs and HIV. Although the prevalence of sexual activity declines with age (73% among adults 57–64 yr old versus 26% among adults 75–85 yr old) and is significantly less common among women than men, many older adults are sexually active and about half report at least one bothersome sexual problem. The most prevalent sexual problems among women are low desire (43%), difficulty with vaginal lubrication (39%), and inability to climax (34%). Among men, the most prevalent sexual problems are erectile difficulties (37%). These problems are infrequently discussed with providers. To date, there are no guidelines around clinician counseling for sexual disorders or STIs among older adults.

GERIATRIC HEALTH ISSUES

Although there are little data examining the effectiveness of screening or counseling about geriatric health issues, expert panels generally recommend clinicians screen for these conditions annually. A Comprehensive Geriatric Assessment (CGA) is recommended for frail older adults new to a primary care practice to reduce their risk of functional decline. The elements of a CGA include assessment of medications, cognitive status, functional status, nutritional status, hearing, vision, affect, social support, gait, and balance. CGA has been associated with improvements in general well-being, life satisfaction, IADLs, and fewer clinic visits (SOE=A). See "Hospital Care," 119; and "Outpatient Care Systems," p 157.

Falls

Approximately 30% of noninstitutionalized older adults fall each year, and the annual incidence of falls approaches 50% in those >80 yr old. Extrinsic factors that contribute to falls include poor lighting, obtrusive furniture, slippery floors, loose floor coverings, and bathrooms without handrails or grab bars. A comprehensive risk assessment for falls incorporates a review of all potential intrinsic and extrinsic factors, as well as a focused physical examination. See "Falls," p 224.

Incontinence

Incontinence is estimated to affect 11%–34% of older men and 17%–55% of older women. Continence problems, which have major social and emotional consequences, are frequently treatable but are not often raised by patients as a concern. Two straightforward questions to screen for incontinence are "Do you ever lose urine when you don't want to?" and "In the past year, have you lost urine on at least 6 separate days?" See "Urinary Incontinence," p 87.

Cognitive Status

The USPSTF concluded that evidence is insufficient to recommend screening older adults for dementia. The AGS does not recommend routine screening but does recommend testing older adults with mild cognitive impairment for dementia because of their increased risk of developing the disease. Others recommend screening older adults on their initial visit, with repeated testing only if patients become symptomatic. Two of the more commonly used screening tools are the Mini–Mental State Exam (MMSE) and the Mini-Cog (clock drawing test combined with a three-item recall test). Scoring of the MMSE must be adjusted for older members of minority groups and individuals with educational levels below the eighth grade.

Depression

Studies report a 1%–2% prevalence of a major depressive disorder, 2% prevalence of dysthymia, and 13%–27% prevalence of subsyndromal depression among community-dwelling older adults. However, depression is often missed by primary care providers. The USPSTF recommends that clinicians screen adults for depression as long as they work in practice settings equipped to treat and follow patients with this disease. The PHQ-2, the Geriatric Depression Scale, and the one-question Yale Depression Screen (ie, "Do you often feel sad or depressed?") are effective screening tools. See "Depression and Other Mood Disorders," p 295.

Vision

Visual problems occur in 21%–50% of older adults. The most common causes are presbyopia, cataracts, glaucoma, diabetic retinopathy, and age-related macular degeneration. In an RCT of 4,340 people ≥75 yr old, no improvement was found in visual outcomes among those who underwent routine visual acuity testing and those who underwent examination only if they reported visual complaints. The USPSTF found insufficient evidence to recommend for or against visual acuity screening by primary care providers. Medicare covers annual glaucoma screening for those at high risk but not routine eye examinations. See "Visual Impairment," p 167.

Hearing

Hearing problems are a major cause of morbidity in older adults. Some degree of hearing loss is present in >33% of adults >65 yr old and in >50% of adults >85 yr old. While pure-tone audiometry is the gold standard for screening hearing, a whispered voice test has a positive predictive value of approximately 75%. Formal audiometry is not needed if a patient is unwilling or unable to use assisted devices. See "Hearing Impairment," p 176.

Nutrition

The weight of older adults should be obtained each visit and the height should be tested annually and a body mass index (BMI, in kg/m²) calculated. Experts recommend that obese (BMI ≥30) older adults be encouraged to lose weight because obesity is associated with poor function and greater comorbidities (eg, diabetes, sleep apnea), and one study found that BMI ≥35 was associated with increased mortality among adults 60–69 yr old. However, in a systematic review of prospective cohort studies of adults ≥65 yr old, most studies did not show an association between increased BMI and all-cause mortality, and several found an inverse relationship. On the other end of the spectrum, malnutrition and undernutrition are common yet frequently unidentified problems in the geriatric population; 15% of older outpatients are malnourished. Nutritional health screens for use in primary care are currently being evaluated. Screening evaluations include questions on meal frequency, unintentional weight loss, dental health, alcohol intake, money for food, and on the ability to shop, cook, and feed oneself. See "Malnutrition," p 195.

Mistreatment of Older Adults

Estimates of mistreatment of older adults range from 3% to 8%. Older adults who present with contusions, burns, bite marks, genital or rectal trauma, pressure ulcers, or BMI ≤17.5 with no clinical explanation should be asked about possible mistreatment or referred to social work for assessment. See "Mistreatment of Older Adults," p 87.

Safety and Preventing Injury

Older adults should be advised to check their smoke detectors and carbon monoxide detectors, and to not set their hot water heaters higher than 120°F–125°F. Those at high risk (light-skinned or history of skin cancer) should be counseled to avoid excess sun exposure and use SPF 30 sun protection when outdoors. Older adults should be encouraged to wear seat belts and to undergo regular driving tests. To date, there are no clinical guidelines for the evaluation of older drivers. Older adults are also encouraged to develop an advance directive and determine a healthcare proxy.

IMMUNIZATIONS

Several immunizations are currently recommended for older adults. An annual influenza vaccination is recommended for adults ≥65 yr old without contraindications (eg, egg allergy). In a meta-analysis of RCTs, inactivated vaccine reduced the risk of developing influenza by 58% among older adults and was associated with significant reductions in the risk of hospitalization for heart disease, cerebrovascular disease, and pneumonia, and in the risk of mortality during influenza season. Despite these benefits, many older adults, especially those of racial and ethnic minorities, do not receive the influenza vaccine. Individuals ≥65 yr old should also receive at least one pneumococcal vaccination in their lifetime. If the person was vaccinated before age 65, the vaccine should be repeated after 5 yr. In a meta-analysis of RCTs, the pneumococcal vaccine reduced the odds of pneumococcal pneumonia (OR=0.3 [0.2–0.5]). The incidence of tetanus and diphtheria (Td) has greatly declined; however, 60% of infections are in adults ≥60 yr old. Although the Td booster is recommended every 10 yr, a single booster at age 65 yr may be cost-effective. Herpes zoster vaccine is available for those ≥60 yr old. In an RCT, the vaccine reduced the incidence of herpes zoster–related disease by 61% after 3 yr.

CHEMOPROPHYLAXIS

Aspirin

In a meta-analysis of prospective RCTs, aspirin therapy (dosage range 100 mg q48h to 500 mg q24h) reduced the risk of cardiovascular events by 12% and stroke by 17% among women with no significant effect on cardiovascular mortality. Among men, aspirin therapy reduced the risk of cardiovascular events by 14% and of myocardial infarction by 32% with no significant effects on stroke or cardiovascular mortality. Aspirin therapy increased the risk of bleeding by approximately 70% in both men and women. The Women's Health Study found that aspirin reduced the risk of strokes, specifically ischemic strokes, among women but did not find that aspirin reduced women's risk of myocardial infarctions, death from cardiovascular disease, or all-cause mortality. Based on these studies, the USPSTF now recommends aspirin prophylaxis for men with a 10-yr risk of coronary heart disease of ≥4% for men aged 45−59, ≥9% for men aged 60−69, and ≥12% for men aged 70−79; and for women with 10-yr stroke risk of ≥3% for women aged 55−59, ≥8% for women aged 60−69, and ≥11% for women aged 70−79. See Table 9.1 for Web sites where providers can enter individual patient data to calculate these risks.

Calcium, Vitamin D, and Multivitamins

Calcium supplementation can prevent bone loss and mildly increase bone density (SOE=A). A meta-analysis of RCTs showed that calcium supplementation at 1,200 mg/d among postmenopausal women results in a 12% reduction in fractures of all types (SOE=A). Calcium supplements are best taken with meals and in divided doses (typically 500 mg or less at one time) to maximize absorption. However, foods should be the primary source of calcium intake. Approximately 3 cups of dairy products daily provide the 1,200-mg target. Vitamin D can prevent bone loss and mildly increase bone density. Supplementation with 700–800 units of vitamin D reduces the risk of hip and nonvertebral fractures and has been shown to reduce all-cause mortality in a meta-analysis of RCTs (RR=0.93 [0.90–0.99]). Supplementation with a multivitamin formulated at 100% recommended daily values can decrease the prevalence of suboptimal vitamin status in older adults. However, there are no RCTs demonstrating a beneficial effect of multivitamins on morbidity or mortality.

Hormone Therapy

Hormone therapy for chemoprophylaxis is not recommended because the Women's Health Initiative Trial showed that it (ie, estrogen plus progesterone) increased the risk of ischemic stroke, coronary artery disease, venous thrombosis, pulmonary embolism, decline in cognitive function, and invasive breast cancer among older women.

COUNSELING ON CANCER SCREENING AND PREVENTIVE HEALTH

Despite expert recommendations, studies have found poor targeting of cancer screening tests for older adults by life expectancy and low rates of counseling about geriatric health issues. Delivery of preventive health services to older adults is complicated for many reasons. Many preventive health services are available, and primary care providers are encouraged to deliver or at least discuss most of these services. Meanwhile, there is little reimbursement for counseling about screening tests and/or geriatric health issues, and clinic visits are often needed for caring for patients' medical conditions, which often increase as individuals age. In addition, it can be difficult for clinicians to determine remaining life expectancy, as well as uncomfortable to discuss cessation of screening.

Fortunately, tools are available to help clinicians estimate patient's remaining life expectancy and guide screening decisions. One prognostic index includes 11 questions (eg, history of diabetes, difficulty walking several blocks) that patients can answer during an office visit to help predict their risk of 5-yr mortality. In another framework, clinicians are asked to estimate whether an individual patient for his or her age is in the top quartile of health, the bottom quartile of health, or in average health, and then are referred to stratified life expectancy tables. Providers can use these tools to help determine which of their older adult patients have adequate remaining life expectancy to screen for cancer. When discussing stopping cancer screening with older adults in poor health, clinicians should discuss the limitations and risks associated with screening older adults who have multiple comorbidities and should focus on the preventive health measures that can be offered and the benefits of which are likely to be achieved in a short time frame (eg, counseling on falls prevention, immunizations).

Several studies have examined ways to improve health promotion for older adults in primary care but have found limited success. Recommendations include clinician education seminars, preventive health check lists, computer reminders, staff screensfor disease, and addressing preventive health topics at multiple visits. Greater compensation would also likely increase provider counseling about healthy lifestyle and geriatric health issues. Medicare does not pay for preventive health visits; however, it covers a "Welcome to Medicare" physical examination in which some important areas of preventive health can be addressed (Table 9.2).

ACOVE-3* QUALITY INDICATORS PERTAINING TO PREVENTION

Immunization

- If a vulnerable older adult has not received a tetanus-diphtheria booster after age 49, then he or she should receive a Td booster.
- All vulnerable older adults should be offered an annual influenza vaccination.
- All vulnerable older adults should have documentation of whether they have received a pneumococcal vaccination and, if so, at what age.
- If a vulnerable older adult has not received a pneumococcal vaccination or received it longer than 5 yr ago and before age 65, then he or she should be offered pneumococcal vaccination.

Alcohol misuse

- All vulnerable older adults should be screened for alcohol misuse within 3 mo of entering a new primary care practice.
- If a vulnerable older adult misuses alcohol, then he or she should be counseled to decrease intake or be referred to an alcohol program within 3 mo.

Tobacco

- All vulnerable older adults should be screened for tobacco use within 3 mo of entering a new primary care practice.
- If a vulnerable older adult uses tobacco, then he or she should be counseled to quit within 3 mo and annually.
- If a vulnerable older adult is ready to quit using tobacco, then there should be documentation of a quit date, discussion of therapies to aid cessation, and a follow-up visit within 1 mo of the quit date.

Exercise

- All vulnerable older adults should have an assessment of activity level (with encouragement to be active) annually.

Weight, height, and body mass index

- All non-wheelchair-bound vulnerable older adults should have their height, weight, and body mass index documented within 3 mo of the initial primary care visit.
- All vulnerable older adults should be weighed at each primary care visit, and weights documented in the medical record.

Hormone replacement therapy

- If a female vulnerable older adult is taking hormone therapy, then there should be documentation that the risks and benefits were discussed since January 2003.

Calcium and vitamin D

- All vulnerable older adults at an initial primary care visit should be counseled about intake of calcium and vitamin D and weightbearing exercises.
- All vulnerable older adults in stable health states should take 800 IU (or equivalent) of vitamin D supplementation daily.

Screening dual x-ray absorptiometry (DEXA) scan for women

- All female vulnerable older adults without a diagnosis of osteoporosis should have documentation that they were offered a DEXA scan.

Vision and hearing

- All vulnerable older adults should have a comprehensive eye examination every 2 yr.
- All vulnerable older adults should have an annual evaluation of hearing status.

Cognitive and functional screening

- If a vulnerable older adult is new to a primary care practice or inpatient service, then there should be a documented assessment of cognitive ability and functional status.
- All vulnerable older adults should be evaluated annually for changes in memory and function.

Cancer screening

- If a female vulnerable older adult is <70 yr old, then she should be offered mammographic screening for breast cancer every 2 yr.
- If a vulnerable older adult is <70 yr old, then there should be documentation that the option of colorectal cancer screening was discussed.
- If a male vulnerable older adult receives a screening prostate-specific antigen test, then the chart should document a discussion of the pros and cons of the test.
- If a female vulnerable older adult has had a total hysterectomy and has a Papanicolaou smear, then the reason for the Papanicolaou smear should be documented.

Screening for common conditions in geriatric patients

- All vulnerable older adults should have documentation that they were asked annually about the occurrence of recent falls.
- All vulnerable older adults should be screened annually for sleep problems.
- All vulnerable older adults should have documentation of a screen for depression during the initial primary care evaluation and annually.

Prevention reminders

- If a vulnerable older adult misses a required preventive care event that is recurrent with a specific periodicity, then there should be medical record documentation of a reminder that the preventive care is needed within one full interval since the missed event.

Related quality indicators for Prevention

Advance directives and preferences (see "Legal and Ethical Issues," p 23)

Screening and assessment of common geriatric conditions (see "Assessment," p 43)

Cognitive and functional evaluation (see "Dementia," p 245)

Screening for depression (see "Depression," p 295)

Screening for falls (see "Falls," p 224)

*Assessing Care of Vulnerable Elders – 3rd Set. See inside front cover for explanation.

REFERENCES

- Brassard A. Identification of patients at risk of ischemic events for long-term secondary prevention. *J Am Acad Nurse Pract.* 2009;21(12):677–689.

- Gnanadesigan N, Fung CH. Quality indicators for screening and prevention in vulnerable elders. *J Am Geriatr Soc.* 2007;55 Suppl 2:S417–423.

- Kennedy R, Cullamar K. Immunizations for Older Adults. *Try This: Best Practices in Nursing Care to Older Adults.* 2007;(21). Available at http://consultgerirn.org/uploads/File/trythis/try_this_21.pdf

- Schonberg MA, Davis RB, McCarthy EP, et al. Index to predict 5-year mortality of community-dwelling adults aged 65 and older using data from the national health interview survey. *J Gen Intern Med.* 2009;24(10):1115–1121.

- Whittemore R, Melkus G, Wagner J, et al. Translating the diabetes prevention program to primary care: a pilot study. *Nurs Res.* 2009;58(1):2–12.

CHAPTER 10—PHARMACOTHERAPY

KEY POINTS

- Risk factors associated with inappropriate prescribing and overprescribing include having more than one prescriber, poor record keeping, and using more than one pharmacy.

- Evidence suggests that underprescribing of indicated medications for older adults is a bigger problem than the prescribing of inappropriate medications.

- Cardiovascular drugs, diuretics, NSAIDs, hypoglycemics, atypical antipsychotics, and anticoagulants are the drug classes most often associated with preventable adverse drug events.

- Age-associated changes in body composition, metabolism, and pharmacodynamics make benzodiazepine use by older adults especially hazardous.

- Collaboration with pharmacists and access to up-to-date drug information can help to minimize the total number of medications and dosages prescribed for individual patients and to avoid important drug-drug and drug-disease interactions.

Adults ≥65 yr old are prescribed the highest proportion of medications in relation to their percentage of the U.S. population. Currently, approximately 13% of the U.S. population is ≥65 yr old; this age group purchases 33% of all prescription drugs. These figures are expected to increase to 25% and 50%, respectively, by the year 2040.

Drugs are the most common treatment for acute and chronic diseases. They are also used to prevent many of the diseases and disorders experienced by older adults. Successful pharmacotherapy requires the correct medication at the correct dosage, for the correct disease or condition, for the correct patient. Unfortunately, achieving these goals is not simple or easy. Many other factors come into play, including the patient's other disease states, other medications, adherence, beliefs, functional status, physiologic changes due to aging and disease, and ability to afford the medication. The basic principle of prescribing for older patients—briefly, "start low, go slow"—is

---

STRENGTH-OF-EVIDENCE (SOE) RATING DEFINITIONS

A = consistent and good quality patient-oriented evidence
B = somewhat inconsistent or limited quality patient-oriented evidence
C = very inconsistent or very limited patient-oriented evidence, disease-oriented evidence, and/or consensus from professional organizations
D = unstudied common practice or opinion

See inside front cover for detailed information regarding the SOE classification.

---

widely disseminated. However, even when this principle is adhered to, some patients will have negative outcomes from one or more of their medications.

Although the principles of pharmacotherapy have not changed significantly during the past 20 yr, drug treatment has become much more complex. More medications are available every year, some with a new pharmacologic profile or mechanism of action. In addition, many available agents have expanded indications, some of which are approved by the FDA and some of which are off-label. Additional complicating factors include frequent changes in the managed-care formulary, scientific advances in the understanding of drug-drug interactions (eg, the cytochrome P-450 system), the change of many medications from prescription to nonprescription, and the boom in an unregulated third class of medications called *nutriceuticals,* ie, nutritional supplements, alternative medicines, and herbal preparations. Finally, very little information is available about the use of nutriceuticals in older adults and acute and/or chronically ill patients on multiple medications.

AGE-ASSOCIATED CHANGES IN PHARMACOKINETICS

Pharmacokinetic studies define the time course of a drug and its metabolites throughout the body with respect to absorption, distribution, metabolism, and elimination. The effects of aging on each of these four parameters have been studied, with the resulting generalizations incorporated into the principles of prescribing for older adults.

Absorption

Aging does not affect the extent of drug absorption via the GI tract to any clinically significant degree, although the rate of absorption may be slowed. Consequently, the peak serum concentration of a drug in older patients may be lower and the time to reach it delayed, but the overall amount absorbed (*bioavailability*) does not differ in younger and older patients. Exceptions include drugs that undergo an extensive first-pass effect (eg, nitrates); they tend to have higher serum concentrations or increased bioavailability, because less drug is extracted by the liver as a consequence of decreased hepatic size and blood flow.

Factors that have a greater impact on drug absorption include the way a medication is taken, what it is taken with, and a patient's comorbid illnesses. For example, the absorption of many fluoroquinolones (eg, ciprofloxacin) is reduced when they are taken with divalent cations such as calcium, magnesium, and iron, which are found in antacids, sucralfate, dairy products, or vitamins. Enteral feedings interfere with the absorption of some drugs (eg, phenytoin). An increase in gastric pH from proton-pump inhibitors, H_2 antagonists, or antacids can increase the absorption of some drugs, such as nifedipine and amoxicillin, and decrease the absorption of other drugs, such as the imidazole antifungals, ampicillin, cyanocobalamin, and indinavir. Agents that promote or delay GI motility, such as stimulant laxatives and metoclopramide, can, in theory, affect a drug's absorption by increasing or decreasing the time spent in the segment of the GI tract necessary for dissolution or absorption. Another mechanism that can increase or decrease drug absorption is the inhibition or induction of enzymes in the GI tract (see the section on drug interactions, below).

Distribution

Distribution refers to the locations in the body a drug penetrates and the time required for the drug to reach those locations. Distribution is expressed as the volume of distribution (Vd), with units of volume (eg, liters) or volume per weight (eg, L/kg).

Age-associated changes in body composition can alter drug distribution. In older adults, drugs that are water soluble (*hydrophilic*) have a lower volume of distribution, because older adults have less body water and lean body mass. Examples include ethanol and lithium. Digoxin, which distributes and binds to skeletal muscle, has been reported to have a reduced volume of distribution in older adults because of their reduced muscle mass. Drugs that are fat soluble (*lipophilic*) have an increased volume of distribution in older adults because fat stores are greater in older than in younger people. Thus, in older adults, lipophilic drugs take longer to reach a steady-state concentration and longer to be eliminated from the body. Examples of fat-soluble drugs include diazepam, flurazepam, thiopental, and trazodone.

The extent to which a drug is bound to plasma proteins also influences its volume of distribution. Albumin, the primary plasma protein to which drugs bind, is often decreased in older adults; thus, a higher proportion of drug is unbound (free) and pharmacologically active. Drugs that bind to albumin and that have been shown to have an increased unbound fraction in older adults include ceftriaxone, diazepam, lorazepam, phenytoin, valproic acid, and warfarin. Normally, additional unbound drug is eliminated; however, age-related decreases in the organ systems of elimination can result in accumulation of unbound drug in the body. Phenytoin provides an example of the way an increase in unbound drug can lead to an unnecessary and potentially harmful dosage increase. A patient with a low serum albumin (≤ 3 g/dL) whose phenytoin dosage is increased because his or her total phenytoin concentration is subtherapeutic can develop symptoms and signs of phenytoin toxicity after the dosage increase because the concentration of free phenytoin is increased.

Metabolism

The liver is the most common site of drug metabolism, but metabolic conversion also can occur in the intestinal wall, lungs, skin, kidneys, and other organs. Aging affects the liver by decreasing hepatic blood flow as well as by decreasing hepatic size and mass. Consequently, the metabolic clearance of drugs by the liver may be reduced in older adults. Drug clearance is also reduced with aging for drugs that are subject to the phase I pathways or reactions, which include hydroxylation, oxidation, dealkylation, and reduction. Most drugs metabolized through phase I pathways can be converted to metabolites of lesser, equal, or greater pharmacologic effect than the parent compound (eg, diazepam). Drugs metabolized through the phase II pathways are converted to inactive compounds through glucuronidation, conjugation, or acetylation (eg, lorazepam). Medications subject to phase II metabolism are generally preferred for older adults, because their metabolites are not active and will not accumulate.

Age and gender differences also have been reported. For example, oxazepam is metabolized faster in older men than in older women. The reason is unknown. Nefazodone concentrations have been reported to be 50% greater in older women, but no differences were found between older men and younger persons of either sex.

In drug metabolism, factors other than aging can exaggerate or override the effects of aging. For example, hepatic congestion due to heart failure decreases the metabolism of warfarin, resulting in an increased pharmacologic response. Smoking stimulates monooxygenase enzymes and increases the clearance of theophylline, even in older adults.

Elimination

Elimination refers to a drug's final route(s) of exit from the body. For most drugs, this involves elimination by the kidney as either the parent compound or as a metabolite or metabolites. Terms used to express elimination are a drug's *half-life* and its *clearance*.

A drug's half-life is the time it takes for its plasma or serum concentration to decline by 50%, eg, from 20 μg/mL to 10 μg/mL. Half-life is usually expressed in hours. Steady state is reached when the amount of drug entering the systemic circulation is equal to the amount being eliminated. For a drug administered on a regular basis, 95% of steady state in the body is achieved after five half-lives of the drug.

Clearance is usually expressed as volume per unit of time (eg, L/h or mL/min) and represents the volume of plasma or serum from which the drug is removed (ie, cleared) per unit of time. Clearance can also be expressed as volume per weight per unit of time (L/kg/h). Half-life and clearance can also refer to metabolic elimination.

The effects of aging have been studied to a greater extent on kidney function than on liver function. Glomerular filtration declines as a consequence of a decrease in renal size and blood flow and a decrease in functioning nephrons. On average, kidney function begins to decline when people reach their mid-30s, with an average decline of 6–12 mL/min/1.73 m^2 per decade. Follow-up studies (conducted in men only) over 10–15 yr found three normally distributed groups: those whose creatinine clearance declined to the extent that it was clinically significant, those whose creatinine clearance declined to the extent that it was statistically but not clinically significant, and those whose creatinine clearance did not change. Renal tubular secretion also declines with age.

Serum creatinine is not an accurate reflection of creatinine clearance in older adults. Because of the age-related decline in lean muscle mass, production of creatinine is reduced in older adults. The decrease in glomerular filtration rate (GFR) counters the decreased production of creatinine, and serum creatinine stays within the normal range, not revealing the change in creatinine clearance.

The conservative approach in treating older adults is to calculate the appropriate dosage for renally eliminated medications as if the patient's kidney function actually has declined with aging. Measuring a patient's 24-hour creatinine clearance is the most accurate way to determine the appropriate dosage, but this is time consuming and requires an accurate 24-hour urine collection. An 8-hour urine collection time has been shown to be accurate but has not been widely accepted.

The Cockcroft-Gault equation can be used to initially estimate a patient's creatinine clearance (CrCl) (SOE=B in older adults for dosage adjustment):

$$CrCl = \frac{(140 - age) \times weight}{72 \times serum\ creatinine}$$

Weight in kg; serum creatinine in mg/100 mL; 85% less in women.

The equation is widely applied, but it has limitations. First, not all patients experience a significant age-related decline in renal function, and for them, the equation would underestimate creatinine clearance. Second, for patients whose muscle mass is reduced beyond that of normal aging, the creatinine clearance would be overestimated. This would apply to individuals whose serum creatinine is less than normal, ie, <0.7 mg/dL. It has been suggested that 1 mg/dL be substituted for a low serum creatinine. However, normalizing the serum creatinine has not been shown to be a precise estimate, and it generally underestimates the actual creatinine clearance.

Another method for estimating glomerular filtration rate (eGFR) is the Modification of Diet in Renal Disease (MDRD), which is endorsed by the National Kidney Foundation in its Kidney Disease Outcomes Quality Initiative (KDOQI) and the NIH National Kidney Disease Education Program for identifying and staging individuals with chronic kidney disease. The MDRD has not been validated in adults ≥70 yr old or in racial or ethnic groups other than white and black Americans. A patient's eGFR value is reported when it is <60 mL/min/1.73 m^2. Because of the lower precision of the MDRD equation and creatinine assay variability, the eGFR should be reported only as "≥60 mL/min/1.73 m^2" for patients with normal renal function or Stage 1 or 2 chronic kidney disease. The routine appearance of eGFR on laboratory reports has created confusion about its use to adjust medication dosages, and it is not recommended by KDOQI to adjust dosage in those with normal renal function (SOE=A).

FDA-labeled dosing is based on the Cockcroft-Gault estimated CrCl and the drug's pharmacokinetic characteristics. Substituting eGFR for estimated CrCl can result in suboptimal dosing, especially in patients with Stage 2 chronic kidney disease as their GFR approaches 60 mL/min/1.73 m^2.

In cases in which the patient's kidney function may be impaired but estimates of function are uncertain, the clinician should consider the following:

- Avoiding drugs that depend entirely on renal elimination and for which accumulation would result in toxicity (eg, imipenem).
- Obtaining an accurate measure of kidney function via an 8- or 24-hour creatinine clearance.
- Monitoring serum or plasma concentrations of the drug (eg, aminoglycosides).

AGE-ASSOCIATED CHANGES IN PHARMACODYNAMICS

The pharmacodynamic action of a drug—ie, its time course and intensity of pharmacologic effect—can change with increasing age. An excellent example of such pharmacodynamic changes in older adults has been demonstrated with the benzodiazepines. After a single dose of triazolam, older adults experience more sedation and lower performance on a psychomotor test than younger adults. These differences are attributed to pharmacokinetic changes, ie, to significantly higher plasma triazolam concentrations that are due to reduced clearance in older adults. However, a different pattern has been found for nitrazepam, an intermediate-acting benzodiazepine similar to lorazepam: the pharmacokinetics of nitrazepam were found to be no different in young and older individuals after a single 10-mg dose; yet, 12 hours and 36 hours after a 10-mg dose, older adults made significantly more mistakes on a psychomotor test than when they had taken placebo. Younger individuals did not demonstrate significant impairment at any time. In addition, even with short-term use, young older adults can experience impaired balance and posture after a single dose of a benzodiazepine.

It is uncertain whether the age-associated pharmacokinetic changes of morphine account for the increased level and prolonged duration of pain relief experienced by older adults. Morphine has a smaller volume of distribution, higher plasma concentrations, and longer clearance in older adults than in younger adults. Older adults experience pain relief at least equivalent to that experienced by younger patients at half the intramuscular dose, and the pain relief lasts longer. Thus, the dose or frequency, or both, of morphine given intramuscularly or by intravenous infusion should be lower, at least initially, in older adults who are narcotic naive.

Pharmacodynamic and pharmacokinetic changes, alone or together, generally result in an increased sensitivity to medications in older adults. In some patients, particularly those who are frail, the use of lower doses, longer intervals between doses, and longer periods between changes in dose are ways to successfully manage drug therapy and to decrease the chances of medication intolerance or toxicity. Disease- and drug-specific monitoring are also necessary to ensure a successful outcome.

OPTIMIZING PRESCRIBING

Optimizing drug therapy for older adults means achieving the balance between overprescribing and underprescribing of beneficial therapies. Overprescribing of drug therapies not only refers to the use of multiple medications but also implies a lack of appropriateness in medication selection, dosage, or use. In one survey, 40% of nursing-home residents had an order for at least one potentially inappropriate medication. Analyses of national medication use

Table 10.1 – Common Inappropriate/Overprescribed and Underprescribed Medications/Classes

Inappropriate/Overprescribed

Anti-infective agents

Anticholinergic agents

Urinary and GI antispasmodics

Antipsychotics

Benzodiazepines

Digoxin for diastolic dysfunction

Dipyridamole

H_2 receptor antagonists

Laxatives and fecal softeners

NSAIDs

Propoxyphene*

Proton-pump inhibitors

Sedating antihistamines (H_1 receptor antagonists, eg, diphenhydramine)

Tricyclic antidepressants

Vitamins and minerals

Underprescribed

ACE inhibitors for patients with diabetes and proteinuria

Angiotensin-receptor blockers

Anticoagulants

Antihypertensives and diuretics as evidenced by uncontrolled hypertension

β-blockers for patients after myocardial infarction or with heart failure

Bronchodilators

Proton-pump inhibitors or misoprostol for GI protection from NSAIDs

Statins

Vitamin D and calcium for patients with or at risk of osteoporosis

*Voluntarily withdrawn from market Nov 2010.

surveys in the ambulatory setting have consistently shown that >20% of older adults received at least one potentially inappropriate medication, with at least one potentially inappropriate medication prescribed at approximately 8% of office visits. Furthermore, nearly 4% of office visits and 10% of medical hospital admissions resulted in a prescription for one or more medications classified as "never" or "rarely appropriate" for older adults. The potential consequences of overprescribing include adverse drug events, drug-drug interactions, duplication of drug therapy, decreased quality of life, and unnecessary costs. Medications frequently deemed unnecessary based on lack of indication, lack of efficacy, or therapeutic duplication are often from the same medication classes as those considered inappropriate or overprescribed (Table 10.1). In studies in the U.S. Veterans Administration, 44% of veterans at hospital discharge and 57%–59% of outpatients had prescriptions for one or more unnecessary medications.

For factors associated with inappropriate prescribing or overprescribing, see Table 10.2. Simply limit-

Table 10.2—Factors Associated with Inappropriate Prescribing or Overprescribing

Patient Factors

Advanced age

Female gender

Lower educational level

Rural residence

Belief in using "a pill for every ill"

Multiple health problems

Use of multiple medications

Use of multiple pharmacies

System Factors

Multiple prescribers for individual patient

Poor record keeping

Failure to review a patient's medication regimen at least annually

---

Table 10.3—Risk Factors for Adverse Drug Events in Older Adults

- Age >85 yr
- Low body weight or body mass index
- Six or more concurrent chronic diagnoses
- An estimated creatinine clearance <50 mL/min
- Nine or more medications
- Twelve or more doses of medications per day
- A prior adverse drug event

---

ing the number of medications for a given patient is not always possible or desirable. For example, a patient with heart failure may be appropriately treated with three or four drugs: a diuretic, an ACE inhibitor, a β-blocker, and perhaps digoxin. If this patient has hyperlipidemia and diabetes mellitus, another two or three medications could be required. Hence, such a patient would be taking five to seven indicated medications for major medical conditions alone.

The underprescribing of medications to older adults is also of concern. Underprescribing can result from an effort to avoid overprescribing, a complex medication regimen, adverse effects, patient preferences, and medication costs. It can also result from the thinking that older adults will not benefit from medications intended as primary or secondary prevention, or from aggressive management of chronic conditions, such as hypertension and diabetes mellitus. In a VA outpatient clinic, underuse of medications was found in 64% of 125 veterans. Medications to optimally treat cardiovascular conditions (including hypertension, anticoagulants, and lipid-lowering agents), GI conditions, diabetes, osteoporosis, and COPD were commonly omitted. For other medications often cited as underprescribed in older adults, see Table 10.1.

Investigators from the Assessing Care of Vulnerable Elders (ACOVE) project developed explicit medication quality indicators divided into four categories: prescribing indicated medications; avoiding in-appropriate medications; education, continuity, and documentation; and medication monitoring. These indicators were applied to "vulnerable" older adults enrolled in two managed care organizations, and the results were reported as the percentage of eligible patients who met the indicator or "pass rate." The prescribing of indicated medications category had an overall pass rate of 50% (range 11%–94% for the 17 indicators); avoiding the prescription of inappropriate medications had an overall pass rate of 97% (range 79%–100% avoidance across the 9 indicators). The overall pass rate for education, continuity, and documentation indicators was 81% (range 10%–99% for the 8 indicators). The 9 indicators for medication monitoring had an overall pass rate of 64% (range 22%–80%). These results suggest that the prescribing of inappropriate medications is less of a problem than the underprescribing of indicated medications and the failure to monitor medications, document information about medications, maintain continuity, and educate patients.

ADVERSE DRUG EVENTS

An adverse drug event (ADE) is defined as an injury resulting from the use of a drug. Preventable ADEs are among the most serious consequences of inappropriate drug prescribing among older adults. An adverse drug reaction (ADR) is a type of ADE; it refers to harm that is directly caused by a drug at usual dosages. For a listing of risk factors for ADEs in older patients, see Table 10.3.

ADEs are estimated to be responsible for 5%–28% of acute geriatric medical admissions; the estimated annual incidence rate is 26 per 1,000 beds for hospitalized patients. It has been estimated that in the nursing home, for every dollar spent on medications, $1.33 in healthcare resources is consumed in the treatment of drug-related morbidity and mortality. A cohort study of all long-term care residents in 18 nursing homes in Massachusetts demonstrated that ADEs are common and often preventable in nursing homes. During the 28,839 resident-months of observations, 546 ADEs were identified. Overall, 51% of these adverse events were judged to have been preventable. Most of the errors occurred at the ordering and monitoring stages. In a cohort study of residents of two long-term care facilities, the overall rate of ADEs was 9.8 per 100 resident-months. Second-generation antipsychotics, anticoagulants, and diuretics were the drug classes most frequently associated with ADEs.

In the ambulatory setting, the ADE rate has been reported to be 50.1 per 1,000 person-years, and the preventable ADE rate to be 13.8 per 1,000 person-years. Cardiovascular drugs, diuretics, NSAIDs,

Table 10.4—Common Adverse Drug Events of Selected Medications

Adverse Drug Event	Medications
Cardiovascular effects	
Decreased heart rate	Cholinesterase inhibitors, β-adrenergic blockers, diltiazem, verapamil, digoxin
Hypotension	Antihypertensives, diuretics, nitrates, phosphodiesterase type 5 inhibitors, α-blockers, tricyclic antidepressants, trazodone
CNS effects	
Delirium	Anticholinergic agents, antiparkinson agents, antidepressants, opioids, glucocorticoids, benzodiazepines, antihistamines (eg, diphenhydramine)
Depression	β-Adrenergic blockers, benzodiazepines, central-acting antihypertensives
Dizziness	SSRIs, cholinesterase inhibitors
Parkinsonism	Antipsychotics, metoclopramide
Sedation	Antidepressants, antipsychotics, antihistamines (eg, diphenhydramine), opioids, anticonvulsants, benzodiazepines
Falls	Benzodiazepines, antidepressants, antipsychotics, sedative/hypnotics, anticonvulsants, opioids, diuretics, antihypertensives, anticholinergic agents, antiarrhythmics
GI effects	
Bleeding/ulceration	NSAIDs, aspirin, glucocorticoids, bisphosphonates, antiplatelet agents
Constipation	Opioids, iron- or calcium-containing antacids, calcium channel blockers, anticholinergic agents, cholestyramine
Diarrhea	Magnesium-containing antacids, SSRIs, cholinesterase inhibitors
Nausea/vomiting	Digoxin, cholinesterase inhibitors, bisphosphonates
Kidney/electrolyte effects	
Hyperkalemia	ACE inhibitors, angiotensin-receptor blockers, potassium supplements, potassium-sparing diuretics
Hypokalemia	Diuretics
Kidney impairment	NSAIDs
SIADH/hyponatremia	Carbamazepine, SSRIs, diuretics
Urinary retention	Agents with anticholinergic properties, opioids, calcium channel blockers, α-adrenergic agonists

hypoglycemics, and anticoagulants are the drug classes found to be most often associated with preventable ADEs. Again, errors occurred most often at the time of prescribing or were related to inadequate monitoring. Most ADEs (≥95%) experienced by older adults are considered to be predictable. For examples of common ADRs experienced by older adults and the medications that frequently cause them, see Table 10.4.

A common pathway for ADEs and polypharmacy has been described as the "prescribing cascade." One form of this cascade occurs when a medication results in an ADE that is mistaken as a separate diagnosis and treated with more medications, which puts the patient at risk of additional ADEs and more medications. Examples that have been studied include metoclopramide-induced parkinsonism and the subsequent prescribing of antiparkinson medications, and calcium channel blockers that result in peripheral edema and the subsequent use of diuretics.

DRUG INTERACTIONS

A drug-drug interaction (DDI) is defined as the pharmacologic or clinical response to the administration of a drug combination that differs from that anticipated from the known effects of each of the two agents when given alone. DDIs are important because they may lead to ADEs. The likelihood of DDIs increases as the number of medications a patient is taking increases. Among prescription drugs, cardiovascular and psychotropic drugs are most commonly involved in DDIs. A positive correlation exists between the number of potential DDIs and the number of adverse events experienced by hospitalized older patients. The most common adverse events are neuropsychologic (primarily delirium), arterial hypotension, and acute kidney failure. For drug combinations that are reported to result in increased risk of hospitalization for older adults, see Table 10.5. Risk factors associated with DDIs include the use of multiple medications, receiving care from several prescribing clinicians, using more than one pharmacy, and combining use of pharmacies and mail-order medications.

Drug interactions can take many forms. For example, absorption can be altered, drugs with similar or opposite pharmacologic effects can result in exaggerated or impaired effects, and drug metabolism can be inhibited or induced. Research focusing on

Table 10.5—Most Common Drug-Drug Adverse Events Identified on Hospitalization

Combination	Risk
ACE inhibitor + diuretic	Hypotension, hyperkalemia
ACE inhibitor + potassium	Hyperkalemia
Antiarrhythmic + diuretic	Electrolyte imbalance, arrhythmias
Benzodiazepine + antidepressant	Confusion, sedation, falls
Benzodiazepine + antipsychotic	Confusion, sedation, falls
Benzodiazepine + benzodiazepine	Confusion, sedation, falls
Calcium channel blocker + diuretic	Hypotension
Calcium channel blocker + nitrate	Hypotension
Digitalis + antiarrhythmic	Bradycardia, arrhythmias
Diuretic + digitalis	Arrhythmias
Diuretic + diuretic	Dehydration, electrolyte imbalance
Diuretic + nitrate	Hypotension
Nitrate + vasodilator	Hypotension

SOURCE: Data from Doucet J, Chassagne P, Trivalle C, et al. Drug-drug interactions related to hospital admissions in older adults: a prospective study of 1000 patients. *J Am Geriatr Soc.* 1996;44(8):944–948.

the cytochrome P-450 system has proposed or studied numerous DDIs (in vivo or in vitro) involving the different P-450 isozymes. The effect of aging on the cytochrome P-450 system and the clinical implications for prescribing have not been completely determined. Cross-sectional data have shown that cytochrome P-450 content declines incrementally, once in the fourth decade and again after age 70. In vitro microsomal activity of cytochrome (CYP) 3A4 is not altered by aging, but in vivo age- and gender-related reductions in drug clearance have been found for CYP3A4 substrates erythromycin, prednisolone, verapamil, alprazolam, nifedipine, and diazepam. CYP3A4 accounts for 30% of the P-450 content in the liver and is also prominent in the intestinal tract. This isozyme is involved in the metabolism of >50% of medications on the market and can be induced by drugs such as rifampin, phenytoin, and carbamazepine, and inhibited by many drugs, including the macrolide antibiotics, nefazodone, itraconazole, and ketoconazole, as well as grapefruit juice. The isozyme CYP2D6 is involved in the metabolism of 25%–30% of marketed medications and has been associated with only minimal age-related changes. CYP2D6 is involved in the metabolism of many psychotropic drugs and can be inhibited by many agents. In addition, approximately 10% of white people are deficient in CYP2D6 and have reduced ability to clear and increased sensitivity to CYP2D6 substrates. Clinically, these patients and those taking CYP2D6 inhibitors (eg, quinidine,

paroxetine, fluoxetine) cannot convert codeine and tramadol to their active metabolites and, therefore, have a reduced analgesic response to these agents.

For DDIs involving herbal preparations, see "Complementary and Alternative Medicine," p 81.

DRUG-DISEASE INTERACTIONS

Drug-disease combinations common in older adults can affect drug response and lead to adverse drug events. Obesity and ascites alter the volumes of distribution of lipophilic and hydrophilic drugs, respectively. Patients with dementia can have increased sensitivity or paradoxical reactions to drugs with CNS or anticholinergic activity. Patients with renal insufficiency or impaired hepatic function due to cirrhosis or hepatic congestion have impaired detoxification and excretion of drugs.

PRINCIPLES OF PRESCRIBING

For principles of prescribing for older adults, see Table 10.6. This basic approach applies primarily to medications that are used to treat chronic conditions for which an immediate, complete therapeutic response is not necessary. Dosage adjustment may still be needed for medications used to treat conditions requiring an immediate response (eg, when prescribing antibiotics for a patient with impaired kidney function). Medications that have been newly approved by the FDA should be used cautiously in treating older adults. Such medications are likely to be more expensive, and information about their use in older adults is often limited.

Overprescribing can be prevented by reviewing a patient's medications at each encounter. The importance of maintaining accurate records of all medications taken by the patient cannot be overemphasized. Many patients do not consider vitamins, herbal preparations, or OTC medications (eg, acetaminophen, aspirin) to be medications, so clinicians should be specific when inquiring about a patient's use of other medications.

It is best if the patient brings all medications to the review, including OTC medications, vitamins, and any herbal preparations or other types of supplements (a "brown-bag" evaluation). Examining the containers and labels and asking what each medication is for and how and when it is taken can provide insight into the patient's understanding and adherence to his or her medication regimens. Any medication for which there is no longer an indication for its continued use should be discontinued. A new complaint or worsening of an existing condition should prompt consideration of whether or not it could be drug-induced. When considering treatment for a new medical condition, nonpharmacologic approaches should always be considered first. If drug therapy is still indicated, a

Table 10.6—Principles of Prescribing for Older Adults

The basics:

- Start with a low dosage.
- Titrate the dosage upward slowly, as tolerated by the patient.
- Try not to start two medications at the same time.

Determine the following before prescribing a new medication:

- Is the medication necessary? Are there nonpharmacologic ways to treat the condition?
- What are the therapeutic end points, and how will they be assessed?
- Do the benefits outweigh the risks of the medication?
- Is one medication being used to treat the adverse events of another?
- Is there one medication that could be prescribed to treat two conditions?
- Are there potential drug-drug or drug-disease interactions?
- Will the new medication's administration times be the same as those of existing medications?
- Do the patient and caregiver understand what the medication is for, how to take it, how long to take it, when it should start to work, possible adverse events that it might cause, and what to do if such events occur?

At least annually:

- Ask the patient to bring all medications (prescription, OTC, supplements, and herbal preparations) to the office; for new patients, conduct a detailed medication history.
- For prescription medications, determine whether the label directions and dosage match those in the patient's chart; ask the patient how he or she is taking each medication.
- Ask about medication side effects.
- Note if other medications are being prescribed (by other healthcare providers) for the patient, and what the medications are and their indications.
- Look for medications with duplicate therapeutic, pharmacologic, or adverse event profiles.
- Screen for drug-drug and drug-disease interactions.
- Eliminate unnecessary medications; confer with other prescribers if necessary.
- Simplify the medication regimen; use the fewest possible number of medications and doses per day.
- Always review any changes with the patient and caregiver; provide the changes in writing.

medication that minimizes the risk of an ADE should be selected. When initiating therapy, the basic principle should be "start low and go slow." Although the FDA requires that labeling for new medications regarding dosing in older adults not be extrapolated from another patient population (eg, patients with kidney impairment), it does not require that a drug be studied explicitly in older adults. Older adults are included in phase I and II dose tolerability and pharmacokinetic and pharmacodynamic studies of many drugs, but the older adults chosen for these studies are usually healthy and free of concomitant illnesses. Much of what is known about medications and how to use them in sick older patients, particu-

larly those who are frail and >90 yr old, is learned only after a medication has been available for several years.

Finally, before prescribing a new medication or renewing a prescription, the clinician should consider the patient's life expectancy, time required to achieve therapeutic benefit, goal of treatment, and treatment targets.

NONADHERENCE

Nonadherence and underadherence to medication regimens is a huge and often unrecognized problem. It is estimated that nonadherence among older adults may be as high as 50%. Patients may be reluctant to admit that they are not taking medications or not following directions. Because there are many possible reasons for nonadherence, there is no simple screen. Predictors of nonadherence include asymptomatic disease, inadequate follow-up (missed appointments or lack of scheduling a follow-up), patient's lack of insight or perception of the value of treatment, drug side effects, drug access, and poor healthcare provider-patient communication. If nonadherence is suspected, clinicians should inquire about difficulties taking medication and adverse events; they should also ask (in a nonjudgmental manner) patients to review which medications they are taking and how they are taking them. Measuring a drug's serum concentration is one way to assess adherence, but assays are available for a small percentage of medications such as tricyclic antidepressants, lithium, and anticonvulsants. Measuring a physiologic or therapeutic response such as blood pressure, heart rate, intraocular pressure, hemoglobin A_{1c}, or a change in hormone concentration is possible for many medications to treat chronic conditions. Other measures include pill counts, refill history, and confirmation by a caregiver. All these measures have limitations, and none is foolproof. The clinician needs to consider the patient's financial, cognitive, and functional status, as well as his or her beliefs about and understanding of medications and diseases.

Prescription drug costs have increased substantially, and supplemental prescription drug benefit plans are expensive. Some plans may still leave a patient with a co-payment that he or she cannot afford or with only a fixed dollar amount for the year. Clinicians should avoid prescribing expensive new medications that have not been shown to be superior to less expensive generic alternatives.

A systematic review of interventions to improve medication compliance in older, community-living adults concluded that multifaceted, tailored interventions to individual barriers were more effective than single interventions (SOE=B). Medication reviews and counseling can be used to identify individual barriers, simplify regimens, and provide education. Telephone call reminders have demonstrated improved compliance in patients with heart failure or cognitive impairment. Reminder charts and calendars have been shown to be less effective. Technology-based interventions are increasing in number to help with medication management across all levels of care.

Combination products, ie, medications containing more than one medication, offer the advantages of decreased pill burden and increased adherence. Potential disadvantages include exposure to higher dosages than necessary, patients not recognizing that there is more than one medication in the product, and increased cost. Before starting a combination product, it needs to be determined that both medications are necessary and that the fixed doses in the product are appropriate for the patient.

Cognitive impairment can also cause nonadherence, because patients may forget to take medications or confuse them. Simplifying the regimen and involving a caregiver to oversee medication management can be helpful approaches. Medication trays also can help with organization, and they are very useful for patients who have difficulty remembering when they last took a medication.

The older adults' ability to read labels, open containers, or pour medications or even a glass of water may be impaired, so functional assessment can be useful. Some patients may need additional education or reinforcement about the purpose of a medication, especially those used to treat conditions that are usually asymptomatic, such as hypertension and diabetes mellitus. Older adults also may need reassurance regarding the safety and possible adverse events of certain medications, particularly newly prescribed medications or those associated with serious adverse events, such as warfarin.

ACOVE-3* Quality Indicators Pertaining to Pharmacotherapy

Medication list

■ All vulnerable older adults should have an up-to-date medication list readily available in the medical record that is accessible to all healthcare providers and that includes OTC medications.

Drug regimen review

■ All vulnerable older adults should have an annual drug regimen review.

Drug indication

■ If a vulnerable older adult is prescribed a drug, then the prescribed drug should have a clearly defined indication.

Patient education

■ If a vulnerable older adult is prescribed a drug, then he or she (or a caregiver) should receive appropriate education about its use.

Response to therapy

■ If a vulnerable older adult is prescribed an ongoing medication for a chronic medical condition, then there should be a documentation of response to therapy.

Medication continuity

■ If an outpatient vulnerable older adult is prescribed a new medication for a chronic disease and he or she has a follow-up visit with the prescribing clinician, then one of the following should be noted at the follow-up visit:

  ○ Medication is being taken.
  ○ Patient was asked about the medication (eg, adverse events, adherence, availability).
  ○ Medication was not started, because it was not needed or changed.

Avoid chronic or high-dose benzodiazepines

■ If a vulnerable older adult is taking a benzodiazepine (>1 mo), then there should be annual documentation of discussion of risks and attempt to taper and discontinue the benzodiazepine.

Avoid strong anticholinergics

■ No vulnerable older adults should be prescribed any medication with strong anticholinergic effects if alternatives are available.

Avoid barbiturates

■ If a vulnerable older adult does not require seizure control, then barbiturates should not be used.

Antipsychotic medication response

■ If a vulnerable older adult is started on an antipsychotic drug, then there should be documentation of an assessment of response within 1 mo.

*Assessing Care of Vulnerable Elders – 3rd Set. See inside front cover for explanation.

REFERENCES

- Bowie MW, Slattum PW. Pharmacodynamics in older adults: a review. *Am J Geriatr Pharmacother.* 2007;5(3):263–303.

- Chew ML, Mulsant BH, Pollock BG, et al. Anticholinergic activity of 107 medications commonly used by older adults. *J Am Geriatr Soc.* 2008;56(7):1333–1341.

- Farris KB, Phillips BB. Instruments assessing capacity to manage medications. *Ann Pharmacother.* 2008;42(7):1026–1036.

- Holmes HM, Hayley DC, Alexander GC, et al. Reconsidering medication appropriateness for patients late in life. *Arch Intern Med.* 2006;166(6):605–609.

CHAPTER 11—COMPLEMENTARY AND ALTERNATIVE MEDICINE

KEY POINTS

- The use of complementary and alternative medicine appears to be on the rise in all adult age groups, including the older adult population.

- When self-prayer is excluded, herbal/dietary products and chiropractic services are among the complementary and alternative medicines most frequently used by older adults. Because these practices are associated with potential risks, patients should always be queried and educated about them.

- Although widely used as a remedy for the vasomotor symptoms associated with menopause, black cohosh has not been found to significantly reduce patient- or disease-oriented symptoms in good quality clinical trials.

- Saw palmetto is commonly used to reduce the symptoms associated with benign prostatic hyperplasia. Recent evidence from clinical trials has been inconsistent with regard to efficacy.

INTRODUCTION

Complementary and alternative medicine (CAM), as currently defined by the National Center for Complementary and Alternative Medicine (NCCAM) of the National Institutes of Health, refers to "a group of diverse medical and health care systems, practices, and products that are not presently considered to be part of conventional medicine." Although some scientific evidence exists regarding certain CAM therapies, for most there are key questions that are yet to be answered through well-designed research studies—questions such as whether they are safe or effective for the diseases or medical conditions for which they are used.

NCCAM conceptualizes the diversity of CAM modalities as follows:

- Mind-body interventions, such as meditation, prayer, relaxation, and art, dance, and music therapies

- Biologically based therapies, such as herbal preparations, botanicals, and dietary supplements

- Manipulative and body-based methods, such as chiropractic, therapeutic massage, and osteopathic manipulation

- Energy therapies such as Reiki, therapeutic touch, and bioelectromagnetic-based therapies

- Whole medical systems, such as traditional Chinese medicine, Ayurvedic medicine, homeopathy, and naturopathic medicine, which incorporate many or all of the above-noted therapies.

The list of what is considered to be CAM is continually evolving, as therapies that are proved to be safe and effective become adopted into conventional health care and as new approaches to health care emerge.

The use of CAM is increasing within the U.S. adult population, particularly among middle-aged adults. The National Health Interview Survey (NHIS), a nationally representative sample of over 31,000 U.S. adults ≥18 yr old, found that 36% of those interviewed made some use of 27 different CAM modalities during the previous 12 mo. When CAM was defined to include self-prayer for health reasons, usage increased to 62%. Most CAM use is complementary, ie, in addition to conventional therapy; only a minority of CAM use serves as an alternative to conventional therapy.

Studies consistently demonstrate that, except for self-prayer, older adults use CAM less frequently than middle-aged adults, the largest group of CAM users.

Table 11.1—CAM Usage Patterns in Adults

CAM Modality	Older Adults Usage (n=5,837) Mean (%)	All Adults Usage (n=30,802) Mean (%)	Most Frequent Users (All Adults) By Ethnicity
Self-prayer	56.2	42.9	Black
Biologically based method	15.6	22.0	Asian
Mind-body	11.7	18.5	Asian
Manipulative and body-based methods	7.6	10.9	White
Alternative medical system	1.4	2.7	Asian
Energy therapy	0.3	0.7	Asian

SOURCE: Data from Grzywacz JG, Suerken CK, Neiberg RH, et al. Age, ethnicity, and use of complementary and alternative medicine in health self-management. *J Health Soc Behav.* 2007;48(1):84–98.

However, it is logical to predict that, as middle-aged adults grow older, they will continue the CAM practices begun in earlier decades of their lives.

The use of CAM by older adults is beginning to be more closely studied, in part to help design safer and more efficacious treatments specific to the needs of those >65 yr old. In one small study, 30% of adults ≥65 yr old (n=311) reported using alternative medicine, and 19% visited an alternative medicine provider. The CAM modalities used most commonly by the older adults in this study were herbal preparations and chiropractic therapies. Another small study examined the use, attitudes, and knowledge about herbal and dietary products among older adults (n=267) in Kansas City, Missouri. Fifty-six respondents (21%) reported using at least one of such products, with glucosamine, garlic, echinacea, and *Gingko biloba* cited most frequently.

CAM use can vary depending on ethnic group. An analysis of 2002 NHIS data revealed the patterns shown in Table 11.1. This analysis is noteworthy because it represents a change in consensus. A 2005 review by the Institute of Medicine found that most prior studies reported lower uses of CAM by individuals of ethnic minority groups than by whites.

The socioeconomic status and degree of acculturation may be important factors in the choice of CAM by individuals belonging to ethnic minority groups. For example, Mexican Curanderos may be the first line of health care for impoverished individuals of Mexican descent. Curanderos are community "healers" who recognize illness as resulting from natural, as well as spiritual, causes. They often use herbal remedies in the form of teas, baths, or poultices, depending on the symptoms. Native Americans may mix modern and traditional medicines, sometimes

using "white man's medicine" to treat "white man's diseases." Many clinicians may be unaware that some Western pharmaceuticals were derived from Native American herbal medicines. Traditional Native American medicine covers a broad range of interventions including ceremony, fasting, sweating, herbal and/or animal medicines, or avoidance or inclusion of specific foods. See also "Cultural Aspects of Care," p 49.

SAFETY OF CAM THERAPIES

Approximately 60% of CAM users (adults of all ages) in the United States do *not* discuss their use of CAM modalities with their healthcare providers. This statistic is of particular concern in the care of older adults because of the increased risk of adverse interactions between conventional medications and various CAM biologic agents. Moreover, aging impacts the metabolism of numerous prescriptions and OTC medications, and possibly that of many herbal preparations, botanicals, and dietary supplements. Age-related changes in hepatic and renal function contribute importantly to these phenomena, both in the absence and presence of disease.

Notwithstanding self-prayer, older adults report using herbal/dietary products and chiropractic services most frequently, both of which can pose health risks. Negative outcomes from chiropractic interventions have included stroke, transient ischemic attack, and other focal neurologic signs. Additionally, data suggest that older adults are ill-informed about the dangers associated with herbal/dietary products. In a study (N=267) of older adults in the central United States, the following percentages of respondents inaccurately believed that herbal/dietary products:

- were routinely tested by the FDA — 70%
- posed no risk to the general population — 66%
- were regulated by the FDA — 60%

However, most CAM practices have not been regulated, and licensure and certification among CAM practitioners can vary among practices and by geo-

---

STRENGTH-OF-EVIDENCE (SOE) RATING DEFINITIONS

A = consistent and good quality patient-oriented evidence

B = somewhat inconsistent or limited quality patient-oriented evidence

C = very inconsistent or very limited patient-oriented evidence, disease-oriented evidence, and/or consensus from professional organizations

D = unstudied common practice or opinion

See inside front cover for detailed information regarding the SOE classification.

Table 11.2—Safety Issues Related to Dietary Supplements Used by Older Adults

Supplement	Common Uses	Adverse Events	Interacts With:
Coenzyme Q$_{10}$	Statin-related myopathy; Parkinson's disease	Infrequent nausea, emesis, epigastric pain, headaches >300 mg/d linked to increased liver transaminase	Warfarin
Dehydroepiandrosterone (DHEA)	There is currently no evidence to support the use of DHEA in older adults for the treatment of osteoporosis, sarcopenia, or frailty, and it is not to be recommended. If a physician sees a patient who is taking it, he or she should recommend that the patient stop taking it.	Women: weight gain, voice changes, facial hair, headaches Men: prostatic hypertrophy, possible increase in hormone-sensitive tumors	Calcium channel blockers, sildenafil
Echinacea	Prevention and treatment of common cold	Allergic reactions, hepatitis, asthma, vertigo, anaphylaxis (rare)	Immunosuppressants
Gingko biloba	Treatment of Alzheimer's dementia, prevention of memory loss, intermittent claudication, macular degeneration	All rare: serious bleeding, seizures, headaches, dizziness, vertigo	Anticoagulants
Glucosamine	Osteoarthritis, rheumatoid arthritis	Nausea, diarrhea, heartburn	Hypoglycemic drugs (reduces effectiveness)
Omega-3 fatty acids	Hypertension, increased high-density lipoprotein, decreased triglycerides and low-density lipoprotein	Belching, halitosis, increased blood glucose	Antiplatelets, anticoagulants, antihypertensives
S-adenosylmethionine (SAM-e)	Depression, fibromyalgia, insomnia, osteoarthritis, rheumatoid arthritis	Nausea, vomiting, diarrhea, anxiety, restlessness	Tricyclics and SSRIs
Saw palmetto	Benign prostatic hyperplasia	All rare: constipation, diarrhea, decreased libido, headaches, hypertension, urine retention	None described
St. John's wort	Depression, anxiety	Nausea, allergic reactions, dizziness, headache, photosensitivity (rare)	Anticoagulants, antivirals, SSRIs

graphic location. There is substantial potential for adverse reactions with the use of herbal preparations and of botanical and dietary supplements in older adults (Table 11.2).

Under the Dietary Supplement Health and Education Act (DSHEA) of 1994, the FDA is not empowered to evaluate or regulate dietary supplements, and the manufacturers are not required to prove that the advertised ingredients provide the health benefits or safety they claim. Multiple studies have found that dietary supplements often contain little, none, or more of what the product labels claim, as well as contaminants or adulterants with unlisted products and prescription drugs. In November 2004, the FDA announced initiatives to monitor and evaluate ingredient quality, safety, and labeling of herbal and dietary products. However, no policy changes have followed to date.

Without the knowledge of what these products contain in their entirety, or the consequences of their use, consumers and healthcare professionals must increase communication while continued research is conducted to provide accurate evaluations. It is imperative that practitioners ask patients specifically about their use of dietary supplements and biologic products and look at the ingredients in those supplements. Older adults have consistently indicated a willingness to receive more information about CAM treatments. Thus, it is important for healthcare providers to disseminate such information.

CAM EFFICACY FOR MANAGING ILLNESS IN OLDER ADULTS

The aging of the baby-boomer generation is contributing to the already established largest group of healthcare consumers—older adults. Among the most common health challenges in older men are diseases of the musculoskeletal and connective tissues and of the circulatory and genitourinary systems. In older women, the most common health challenges are musculoskeletal, circulatory, and mental health disorders. Demographic considerations assure that the need of the expanding aging population for medical services will continue to increase, and it is logical to predict that specific interest in, and use of, CAM modalities will expand as well.

Numerous anecdotal reports or claims exist of the efficacy of diverse CAM modalities, yet there is a general lack of product and practice standardization. Although studies examining the efficacy of CAM interventions continue to accumulate, evidence remains inconclusive for most treatments.

Musculoskeletal Disorders

Osteoarthritis is one of the most common chronic diseases affecting older adults. Strong levels of evidence have been found for the use of transcutaneous electrical nerve stimulation (SOE=B), acupuncture (SOE=B), exercise (aerobic walking and quadriceps muscle strengthening for osteoarthritis in the knee and hip), and topical capsaicin (SOE=B) to treat the pain of osteoarthritis; data on the effectiveness of glucosamine and/or chondroitin are conflicting. Phytoestrogen and soy products are increasingly used to prevent or treat osteoporosis in postmenopausal women, although there is little evidence confirming their benefits (SOE=D). Dehydroepiandrosterone (DHEA), a widely used dietary supplement, is the most abundant adrenal steroid in people. Circulating DHEA levels decline progressively with age. Small-scale trials of DHEA supplementation in older adults have produced conflicting results regarding its effects on bone density, and further studies are needed to determine its use in preventing or treating osteoporosis in older adults.

Omega-3 polyunsaturated fatty acid supplementation (SOE=B) is recommended for inflammatory joint pain from rheumatoid arthritis and inflammatory bowel disease. Therapeutic massage, acupuncture, mind-body relaxation, and energy modalities are all used in the treatment of lower back pain. For a summary of considerable evidence related to these treatments, see Table 11.3. Exercise and herbal medicines are also used to treat lower back pain. Short-term improvements in pain were found for *Harpagophytum procumbens* (devil's claw) (SOE=A), *Salix alba* (white willow bark) (SOE=B), and *Capsicum frutescens* (cayenne) (SOE=B). One group of researchers has hypothesized the existence of subtypes of lower back pain, each of which may have a different pathogenesis. These authors suggest that patients can be matched to specific exercise, stabilization exercise, spinal manipulation, or traction treatment based on the location and type of symptoms.

Myopathy is a well-known adverse event of statin therapy. It is currently unknown whether decreased levels of coenzyme Q_{10} contribute to statin-related myopathy. One group of investigators has suggested that statins may interfere with the manufacture of coenzyme Q_{10} in the mitochondria, disturbing the

Table 11.3—Efficacy Related to CAM for Lower Back Pain (All Adults)

	SOE	
Treatment	Acute Lower Back Pain	Chronic Lower Back Pain
Acupuncture	A	A
	(lack of effect)	
Massage*	C	B
Neuroreflexotherapy	D	B
Spinal manipulation	B	B

*Contraindicated in areas of inflammation, infection, fracture, burn, deep-vein thrombosis, or active tumor.

SOURCE: Data from van Tulder MW, Furlan AD, Gagnier JJ. Complementary and alternative therapies for low back pain. *Best Pract Res Clin Rheumatol.* 2005;19(4):639–654.

respiratory chain and impeding energy production in skeletal muscle. Efficacy studies of coenzyme Q_{10} supplementation in the treatment of statin-related myopathy have yielded mixed results (SOE=C).

Cardiovascular Disorders

The use of stress-management techniques, such as relaxation breathing, music therapy, and meditation, may reduce blood pressure in hypertensive patients and improve sleep quality in older adults. See also "Physical Activity," p 54; "Sleep Problems," p 272; and "Hypertension," p 384.

Psychiatric Disorders

Depression is one of the most common and debilitating major public health problems, and its incidence increases with advancing age. CAM use by older adults can assist in the management of mild to moderate depression. However, adequate treatment of severe depression may involve psychotherapy and psychotropic medication to prevent further morbidity and mortality. Recent research suggests that depression is also a systemic disease and is associated with an increased incidence of sleep disorders, osteoporosis, obesity, insulin resistance, and immune dysfunction. The impact of CAM modalities on these outcomes is unclear.

The botanical known as St. John's wort has received considerable attention for its potential to treat depression (SOE=B) and remains widely used. The adverse events of St. John's wort include GI upset, fatigue, dizziness, headache, dry mouth, and photosensitivity. St. John's wort interacts with the hepatic P-450 enzyme system that induces the metabolism of many drugs, thus causing clinically significant adverse interactions and potential therapeutic failure with various antiretroviral, anticoagulant, immunosuppressant, antidepressant, and chemotherapeutic medications.

S-adenosylmethionine (SAM-e) is a naturally occurring compound that is necessary for adequate production of dopamine and serotonin in the brain. This compound is currently marketed as an antidepressant. In one study involving 195 patients, 400 mg of SAM-e daily lessened depressive symptoms (SOE=C). See also "Depression and Other Mood Disorders," p 295.

Neurologic Disorders

Some studies have investigated the use of supplements for treatment of dementia from Alzheimer's disease and vascular insufficiency. *Ginkgo biloba* extract (EGb 761) has shown some benefit in improving cognitive ability and memory impairment in Alzheimer's patients in some, but not all, studies (SOE=C). Brain tissue studies and spinal fluid abnormalities in Alzheimer's patients also offer reasonable rationale for supplementing with various antioxidants, including vitamins A, C, and E and selenium, although evidence of their effect has yet to be demonstrated in clinical trials. See also "Dementia," p 295.

Parkinson's disease patients have reduced brain levels of glutathione, an antioxidant involved in neuroprotective functions. Parkinson's patients also have deficiencies in coenzyme Q_{10}. Supplementation with these two naturally occurring substances has been shown to slow the progression of disease and reduce the severity of symptoms (SOE=C). Coenzyme Q_{10} is found in foods such as salmon, sardines, and mackerel. Acupuncture, music therapy, and physical therapy are used by Parkinson's patients to attempt to reduce disabilities and improve cognitive, emotional, and social functioning. See also "Neurologic Diseases and Disorders," p 464.

Sleep disorders are common in older adults, affecting both sleep quality and quantity. Studies suggest that abnormalities in slow-wave and rapid-eye-movement sleep may also be linked to psychologic, endocrine-metabolic, and immune system dysfunctions. Nutritional and exercise modifications are among the safest recommendations when working with older adults. Milk contains tryptophan, which is a precursor of serotonin. Having warm milk before bedtime or eating other tryptophan-containing foods such as bananas, brown rice, and turkey may be helpful in relieving depression-associated sleep difficulties. Chamomile is an herbal tea that is also known for its relaxing properties. Evidence suggests that use of valerian root (SOE=C) or melatonin (SOE=B) can also promote improved sleep quality. Aerobic exercise in the early evening has been shown to contribute to improved sleep quality. However, exercise later in the evening can be too stimulating and counteract restful sleep. Other CAM modalities for improving sleep used by older adults include aromatherapy combined with a warm bath and relaxing music. See also "Sleep Problems," p 272.

Urogynecologic Disorders

Perceptions about menopause have become more realistic in recent years with this transition becoming less frequently viewed as a pathologic process than as a natural progression in the life cycle. In addition, concerns about the safety of long-term conventional estrogen use have increased. These changes have influenced the use of alternatives, such as nutritional, nonpharmacologic supplements and exercise, for symptom management. Approximately 80% of menopausal women report using one or more CAM modalities, such as natural and plant estrogens and other herbal preparations. See also hormone therapy in "Gynecologic Diseases and Disorders," p 415.

Alternative treatments under current study consist primarily of herbal and phytoestrogen remedies. Although very popular, black cohosh has not been found to reduce patient- or disease-oriented symptoms in good quality clinical trials (SOE=A). Phytoestrogens are naturally occurring sources of estrogen found in plant foods. Isoflavones, such as daidzein, are found in soy products and have been studied as alternatives to conventional estrogen therapy. Although existing trials have not found any harmful effects of isoflavones on menopausal symptoms, the current evidence is either inconsistent or weakly positive (SOE=B). Both aerobic exercise and mind-body relaxation techniques are also helpful in decreasing irritability, restlessness, and anxiety.

Symptomatic benign prostatic hyperplasia (BPH) affects >40% of men ≥70 yr old approximately equally among racial groups. In recent decades, men in the United States have begun to self-treat this condition with saw palmetto, which has become the fifth leading medicinal herb consumed in the United States. Saw palmetto and other supplements, such as South African star grass, stinging nettle, pumpkin seed extracts, rye pollen, and African plum, have been studied but need further, more rigorous scientific investigation that meets World Health Organization BPH Consensus Conference standards. The American and European Association of Urology do *not* currently recommend plant extracts in the treatment of BPH. See also "Prostate Disease," p 420.

Diabetes

Type 2 diabetes mellitus, a major public health problem, is associated with increased incidence of obesity, hypertension, dyslipidemia, and macro- and microvascular disease. Normal aging is associated with increased insulin resistance and glucose intolerances, and increased risk of developing type 2 diabetes. In one survey, approximately 50%–60% of diabetic patients reported the use of CAM interventions, including folk remedies in ethnic populations. There is considerable interest in examining the potential benefit of using various CAM biologic agents (eg, chromium, vitamin C, other dietary antioxidants) or other modalities (eg, stress-reduction techniques) in combination with dietary modifications, exercise, and weight management. This includes attempts to develop an algorithm for clinical and research use of CAM in patients with type 2 diabetes mellitus. See also "Diabetes Mellitus," p 504.

Cancer

Approximately 30%–50% of cancer patients in one survey noted that they were using CAM interventions to manage their specific cancer. Cancer CAM therapies purportedly can be used to strengthen the body's innate immune systems as well as to manage the adverse events of conventional treatments, such as chemotherapy and radiation. One of the most important benefits for many cancer patients who use CAM modalities is the experience of feeling more empowered while dealing with the challenges of cancer. This has been substantiated by numerous studies examining various indices of health-related quality of life. The CAM therapies most frequently used are herbal preparations, exercise, and spiritual and energy modalities (eg, qi gong, therapeutic touch, Reiki, polarity, healing touch, Johrei).

Controversy remains regarding the role of diet as a possible risk factor for developing breast cancer. Of particular importance is the link between obesity and increased estrogen levels that can contribute to de novo breast cancer and recurrence after early-stage disease. High-fiber, low-fat diets with fruits, vegetables, whole grains, fish, and legumes are associated with a decreased risk of disease. Biologic agents, herbal preparations, and vitamins have all been tried by patients; however, most of these modalities have not had much scientific study. In addition, lifestyle changes to include exercise and stress management have been helpful with managing mood and energy changes associated with breast cancer.

Prostate cancer usually develops slowly in older men, and use of CAM in combination with conventional treatment has been reported to reduce associated discomforts and improve quality of life. Risk of death in this population is higher from heart disease than from prostate cancer per se. The botanical mixture known as PC-SPES, a CAM dietary supplement, was found in early small-scale trials to lead to decreases in serum prostate-specific antigen levels and pain, plus improved quality of life. However, in June 2002, several lots of PC-SPES were found to be adulterated with diethylstilbestrol, warfarin, and other undeclared prescription ingredients. As a result, PC-SPES was removed from the market. At present, exercise and healthy diet remain the safest CAM recommendations to assist with the management of adverse events and to improve quality of life in these patients. See also "Prostate Disease," p 420.

Lung cancer has been linked not only to smoking but also to excesses in dietary intake of dairy products, red meats, and saturated fats, though these associations have been questioned. In addition, preliminary research has suggested that ingestion of vitamin A by those who smoke may be harmful, whereas vitamin A intake in those who do not smoke may be beneficial. Dietary changes as well as mind-body interventions may help lung cancer patients to manage emotional distress and the adverse effects of treatment. Cancer patients using relaxation and stress-management techniques have been able to manage cravings when trying to quit smoking. These mind-body techniques are also effective in managing the emotional and physical distress associated with the adverse effects of treatment.

Currently, there are no herbal preparations or botanic supplements that appear to be useful in the prevention or management of colon cancer. A fiber-rich diet has been postulated to possibly prevent the onset of colon cancer; however, studies are inconclusive. Lutein, which is present in broccoli, carrots, oranges, and spinach, was found in one study to be beneficial for colon cancer prevention. See also "Oncology," p 521.

REFERENCES

■ Barnes PM, Bloom B, Nahin RL. Complementary and alternative medicine use among adults and children: United States, 2007. *Natl Health Stat Report.* 2009;12:1–23.

■ Cuellar NG, Rogers AE, Hisghman V. Evidenced based research of complementary and alternative medicine (CAM) for sleep in the community dwelling older adult. *Geriatr Nurs.* 2007;28(1):46–52.

■ Grzywacz JG, Suerken CK, Neiberg RH, et al. Age, ethnicity, and use of complementary and alternative medicine in health self-management. *J Health Social Behav.* 2007;48(1):84–98.

■ Marinac JS, Buchinger CL, Godfrey LA, et al. Herbal products and dietary supplements: a survey of use, attitudes, and knowledge among older adults. *J Am Osteopath Assoc.* 2007;107(1):13–23.

■ Shreffler-Grant J, Hill W, Weinert C, et al. Complementary therapy and older rural women: who uses it and who does not? *Nurs Res.* 2007;56(1):28–33.

CHAPTER 12—MISTREATMENT OF OLDER ADULTS

KEY POINTS

- Mistreatment of older adults affects almost 4% of those ≥65 yr old.

- Screening for mistreatment of older adults is important and most effective when conducted in a sensitive manner.

- Indicators of mistreatment of older adults range from dramatic (eg, bruising, fractures) to subtle (eg, withdrawn behavior, dehydration).

Mistreatment of older adults is referred to by the National Research Council in its report on elder mistreatment as "(a) intentional actions that cause harm or create a serious risk of harm (whether or not harm is intended) to a vulnerable elder by a caregiver or other person who stands in a trust relationship to the elder or (b) failure by a caregiver to satisfy the elder's basic needs or to protect the elder from harm." The authors of the American Medical Association (AMA) *Diagnostic and Treatment Guidelines on Elder Abuse and Neglect* describe mistreatment of older adults as acts of omission or commission that result in harm or threatened harm to the health or welfare of an older adult. It can manifest itself in a variety of ways, including physical or emotional abuse, intentional or unintentional neglect, financial exploitation, or abandonment, or it may be a combination of these. Research suggests that the U.S. national incidence of mistreatment of older adults is approximately 450,000 annually, with a prevalence range of 700,000 to 1.2 million older adults, accounting for approximately 4% of those ≥65 yr old. Given these estimates, routine screening for mistreatment is an appropriate part of primary care for older adults.

Research conducted in the context of a longitudinal aging cohort study sought to determine mortality related to mistreatment. In a pooled logistic regression analysis that adjusted for demographics, chronic disease, functional status, social networks, cognitive status, and depressive symptoms, the risk of death was found to remain increased for cohort members experiencing either mistreatment or self-neglect (SOE=A). To date, no intervention studies have evaluated the impact of screening on health outcomes, and such studies are needed. However, screening for

mistreatment appears warranted, given the findings of case studies and longitudinal studies that document risk factors, as well as the information in databases of adult protective services organizations across the country.

RISK FACTORS AND PREVENTION

Risk factors for mistreatment include poverty, dependency of older adults for caregiving needs, age, race, functional disability, frailty, and cognitive impairment (SOE=B). Some factors may actually be proxies for other variables. For example, lower socioeconomic status is often associated with fewer resources to meet caregiving demands.

Frail, debilitated older adults may need a level of care that at times exceeds caregiver ability. In particular, the demented person who exhibits disturbing behaviors (eg, hitting, spitting, screaming) poses immense challenges to caregivers. Caregiver stress can give way to any of the forms of mistreatment, and a careful assessment of caregiver stress can identify opportunities to prevent mistreatment. Minority older adults may be preferentially targeted for healthcare fraud by unscrupulous home care organizations and/or durable medical equipment suppliers. For factors that indicate a risk for the development of inadequate or abusive caregiving, see Table 12.1.

HISTORY

An interdisciplinary approach to assessment and care planning is optimal. Comprehensive interdisciplinary geriatric assessment (see "Hospital Care," p 119; and "Outpatient Care Systems," p 157) that includes the physical, psychosocial, and financial domains of older adults should detect potential or any alleged mistreatment.

The mistreatment history, provided by both the older adults and caregiver(s), should be conducted in private so that all individuals can speak freely and frankly. Studies suggest that the different cultures of racial and ethnic groups define abuse and neglect very differently; thus, cultural sensitivity is important. (See "Cultural Aspects of Care," p 49.) The older adult or caregiver from a different culture than the clinician's may be offended by some mistreatment screening questions; carefully worded questions can avoid alienating the older adult or caregiver, which could abolish any further opportunity to help the patient and family.

If the older adult's responses to the mistreatment questions indicate that mistreatment may be occurring, progressively focused follow-up questions are indicated. For example, the clinician might first ask, "Is there any difficult behavior in your family you

---

STRENGTH-OF-EVIDENCE (SOE) RATING DEFINITIONS
A = consistent and good quality patient-oriented evidence
B = somewhat inconsistent or limited quality patient-oriented evidence
C = very inconsistent or very limited patient-oriented evidence, disease-oriented evidence, and/or consensus from professional organizations
D = unstudied common practice or opinion

See inside front cover for detailed information regarding the SOE classification.

Table 12.1—Risk Factors for Inadequate or Abusive Caregiving

- Cognitive impairment in patient, caregiver, or both
- Dependency of the caregiver on the older patient, or vice versa
- Family conflict
- Family history of abusive behavior, alcohol or drug misuse or abuse, mental illness, or mental retardation
- Financial stress or lack of funds to meet new health demands
- Isolation of the patient or caregiver, or both
- Living arrangements inadequate for the needs of the ill person
- Stressful events in the family, such as death of a loved one or loss of employment

would like to tell me about?" If the answer is positive, the questions to follow then might be, "Has anyone tried to hurt or hit you?" "Has anyone made you do things that you did not want to do?" "Has anyone taken your things?" Obtaining such information requires sensitive clinical interviewing skills similar to those needed when asking about sexual orientation, alcoholism, or substance abuse.

Private interviews with caregivers can detect not only abusive or neglectful behavior but also signs of stress, isolation, or depression in the caregiver, in which case help for the caregiver can also be provided. Caregivers may be reluctant to discuss their own problems in the presence of the older adult who depends on their care. Because caregivers can range from registered professionals to well-intended neighbors, it is important to know and to document the level of skill the caregiver has, as well as his or her understanding of the situation. The caregiver's level of understanding is an essential factor in evaluating the underlying intention of any mistreatment of a dependent older adult. For example, a registered nurse in a nursing home is held to a different level of accountability than a frail spouse providing care in the home setting.

Identification of shortcomings in the older adult's care can be the most elusive aspect of a comprehensive assessment. The symptoms and signs of incomplete, inadequate, or neglectful caregiving can be subtle (eg, when an older adult does not do as well as expected on a given regimen) or attributable to the older adult's physical or emotional disorders (eg, weight loss in an older adult with a history of depression).

Effective assessment is that which detects mistreatment without directing undue suspicion on well-meaning caregivers or undermining a family's ability to care for an older adult with appropriate support and counseling.

For examples of symptoms and signs that indicate a particularly high level of risk of mistreatment, see Table 12.2. A number of assessment instruments have been developed to help clinicians screen for and assess mistreatment, although none has been fully validated yet, and research is ongoing.

PHYSICAL ASSESSMENT

Key signs of mistreatment are physical indicators that are incongruent with the history; examples are bruises and welts in unusual places or in various stages of healing. Bilateral bruises on the upper torso are rarely the result of falls and warrant follow-up. Other indications of possible mistreatment include frequent, unexplained, or inconsistently explained falls and injuries, multiple visits to the emergency department, delays in seeking treatment, inconsistent follow-up, or constant switching among providers. The clinician needs to search for unusual patterns or marks, such as bruises on inner arms or thighs; cigarette, rope, chain, or chemical burns; lacerations and abrasions on the face, lips, and eyes; or marks on areas of the body usually covered by clothes. Head injuries, hair loss, or hemorrhages beneath the scalp as a consequence of hair pulling are significant markers. Cachectic states can be the result of malnutrition that is a consequence of neglect. Unusual discharges, bruising, bleeding, or trauma around the genitalia or rectum raise concern of possible sexual abuse, prompting gynecologic and rectal examination.

The behavior of the older adult when in the presence of the suspected abuser may be significant. A victim of mistreatment may avoid eye contact, or dart his or her eyes continually. He or she may sit a distance away from an abusive caregiver, cringe, back off, or startle easily as if expecting to be struck. The caregiver may be nervous and fearful, or quiet and passive. The older adult may defer excessively to the caregiver, who may invariably answer for the older adult or even try to prevent a private interview with or examination of the older adult. Dubious explanations may be given to explain the older adult's injuries.

The emergency department is an important setting for assessment of mistreatment. The emergency department may see older adults in crisis, and every effort should be made not to simply treat and release patients whose situation merits further assessment. Astute emergency personnel can identify cases in which there may be serious safety problems in the caregiving situation.

PSYCHOLOGICAL ASSESSMENT

Mistreatment is not invariably or entirely physical. Psychological abuse or neglect is generally more difficult than physical abuse to detect and confirm, but it can be equally dangerous to the dependent older adult. The behavior of both the older adult and the caregiver can provide important clues about the quality of their relationship and of the care the older

Table 12.2—Screening for Mistreatment of Older Adults

Assessment Domain	Key Indicators
General	▪ Clothing: inappropriate dress, soil, or disrepair
	▪ Hygiene
	▪ Nutritional status
	▪ Skin integrity
Abuse	▪ Anxiety, nervousness, especially toward caregiver
	▪ Bruising, in various healing stages, especially bilateral or on inner arms or thighs
	▪ Fractures, especially in various healing stages
	▪ Lacerations
	▪ Repeated emergency department visits
	▪ Repeated falls
	▪ Signs of sexual abuse
	▪ Statements about abuse by the patient
Neglect	▪ Contractures
	▪ Dehydration
	▪ Depression
	▪ Diarrhea
	▪ Failure to respond to warning of obvious disease
	▪ Fecal impaction
	▪ Malnutrition
	▪ Medication under- or overuse or otherwise inappropriate use
	▪ Poor hygiene
	▪ Pressure ulcers
	▪ Repeated falls
	▪ Repeated hospital admissions
	▪ Urine burns
	▪ Statements about neglect by the patient
Exploitation	▪ Evidence of misuse of patient's assets
	▪ Inability of patient to account for money and property or to pay for essential care
	▪ Reports of demands for money or goods in exchange for caregiving or services
	▪ Unexplained loss of Social Security, pension checks
	▪ Statements about exploitation by the patient
Abandonment	▪ Evidence that patient is left alone unsafely
	▪ Evidence of sudden withdrawal of care by caregiver
	▪ Statements about abandonment by the patient

SOURCE: Data in part from Fulmer T. Elder mistreatment assessment. *Try This: Best Practices in Nursing Care to Older Adults*. 2008;15. (http://www.consultgerirn.org/)

adult is receiving. Factors that suggest a poor or deteriorating social and emotional situation are an important focus of assessment for mistreatment.

Psychological abuse includes taunting, name-calling, promoting regressive behaviors by infantilization, making painful jokes at the expense of the older adult, or other activities that are demeaning. The caregiver's style of communication can provide important clues. Impatience, irritability, and demeaning statements can indicate a pattern of verbal abuse. However, psychological neglect or mistreatment by the caregiver can also take more subtle forms. For example, not providing social or emotional stimulation, or restricting or preventing normal activities can result in total social isolation of the older adult.

The older adult's demeanor and emotional status can suggest the presence of psychological neglect or abuse. For example, ambivalence or high levels of anxiety, fearfulness, or anger toward the caregiver indicate the need for further assessment. Unexpected depression or uncharacteristic withdrawal also merits follow-up. Other high-risk behaviors include lack of adherence with treatment recommendations, frequent requests for sedating medication, or frequently canceled appointments.

Cognitive impairment, dementia, and depression are prevalent in older adults referred for evaluation for possible mistreatment. It is therefore appropriate to check any older adult presenting with cognitive impairment, dementia, or depression for symptoms and signs of neglect or mistreatment. Aggressive behaviors associated with dementia can trigger abusive responses in caregivers. See also "Behavioral Problems in Dementia," p 256.

FINANCIAL ASSESSMENT

Financial mistreatment includes unauthorized use of the older adult's funds, possessions, or property. Fiscal neglect consists of the failure to use the older adult's funds and resources to provide for his or her needs. Signs that an older adult is being mistreated financially include the following (SOE=C):

- a recent marked disparity between the older adult's living conditions or appearance and his or her assets
- a sudden inability to pay for health care or other basic needs
- an unusual interest on the part of caregivers in the older adult's assets
- the sudden acquisition of expensive possessions by a caregiver who has apparently limited financial assets
- unwillingness of a caregiver to allow access to the home of an older adult

SELF-NEGLECT

For some older adults, especially those who live in isolation or who choose to accept and endure mistreatment, self-neglect may be an issue. Successful management in such cases requires an assessment of the older adult's capacity to understand the risks and benefits of the situation, as well as the consequences of allowing the circumstances to continue. (See decisional capacity in "Legal and Ethical Issues," p 23.) These are complex situations, but the older adult's right to autonomy and self-determination must be honored. Paternalistic viewpoints regarding what the older person "should do" need to be avoided. In self-neglect cases, the clinician may need support when coming to terms with the requirement to respect the decisionally capable older adult's wishes when this involves his or her choosing to remain in an abusive or neglectful situation. (The clinical dilemma resembles that confronting clinicians who treat battered women.) Intervention contrary to the decisionally capable older adult's choice is generally inappropriate, as well as being uncomfortable for the clinician. See autonomy versus protectionism in "Legal and Ethical Issues," p 29.

THE ROLE OF THE OLDER ADULT

The relationship of the older adult with caregivers can be very complex, and dysfunctional relations between a dependent older adult and a caregiver may not be entirely the fault of the caregiver. To approach such situations with the idea that the older adult is inevitably the victim infantilizes the person and is unfair to caregivers. Situations in which older adults are mistreated fall along a spectrum from victimization to mutual abusiveness to relationships in which the older adult can be viewed as a witting cause of the mistreatment. Of course, there are cases in which the older adult and his or her caregivers are making the best of a tragic situation.

To determine the best possible approach for ameliorating if not solving a dysfunctional caregiving relationship, the clinician needs to make every effort to determine the facts in the situation, including the motives of the people involved. Consultation with social workers, psychologists, or psychiatrists can be useful. Legal reporting requirements are not limited in any way by these considerations. If an older man hits his son and the son strikes back, clinicians in most states are required to report the latter hitting.

INSTITUTIONAL MISTREATMENT

Mistreatment in the setting of home care by family or friends has been the focus of much of the discussion so far, but detecting and intervening to prevent mistreatment in the institutional setting is also important. Several factors in this setting could aggravate the problem, including poor working conditions, low salaries, inadequate staff training and supervision resulting in poor motivation, and prejudiced attitudes. Disruptive or insulting behavior by the older adult can also be a factor.

The Omnibus Budget Reconciliation Act of 1987 set a new standard for care in nursing homes. (See "Nursing-Home Care," p 142.) The clinician who is alert to the possibility of abuse and neglect in any institutional setting plays an important role in protecting vulnerable older adults. Equally important is the clinician's readiness to use the resources available through the institution itself or through state regulatory agencies to investigate and intervene when appropriate. In cases of suspected institutional mistreatment, the challenge is to balance the rights of staff members with the rights of residents. State departments of public health are usually responsible for investigating cases of abuse and neglect in nursing homes. Evidence is growing (SOE=B) regarding the phenomenon of resident-to-resident mistreatment in long-term care facilities, which warrants careful attention. In such cases, residents may assault, rob, or psychologically abuse other residents, and this will be an important area for further research.

INTERVENTION

The clinician who suspects mistreatment can use the following questions to guide intervention:

- How safe is the older adult if he or she returns to the current setting, or does he or she need to be removed to a safe environment?

- What services or resources are available locally to support the care of this older adult?

- Are there any caregivers who have health problems of their own that need attention?

- Does this situation need the expertise of others (eg, in medicine, nursing, social work), and if so, who would best serve the older adult's needs?

Successful intervention in cases of mistreatment can become complex. The factors governing the clinician's course of action include the exact nature and degree of the mistreatment, whether the patient can or will cooperate with evaluation and intervention, and whether the caregiver(s) can or will cooperate with evaluation and intervention.

Local resources in support of interventions for mistreatment vary, but information is readily available. Consultation with the social work staff of the hospital, nursing home, or local health department can be a useful early step. Each state's Adult Protective Services can provide relevant information as well as direct assistance. In addition, the AMA Web site (http://www.ama-assn.org) provides a convenient starting point in the search for information and resources, as does the National Center on Elder Abuse (http://www.ncea.aoa.gov/).

THE MEDICAL-LEGAL INTERFACE

It is important to know state laws applicable to cases of mistreatment of older adults; 46 states have a reporting mechanism for mistreatment, either through Adult Protective Services or state agencies associated with aging. Clinicians need to be familiar with the reporting mandates in their area. In some states, neglect by others must be reported, while reports of self-neglect are not required. Adult children can be charged with neglect of the older parent if a caregiving relationship can be proved and it can also be proved that care has been precipitously withdrawn without substitute services. In states where self-neglect is reportable, this is usually the largest intake category. Finally, states can mandate reports for self-neglect but may not provide any services unless the older adult agrees to accept them.

Clinicians are in a key position to assess and report suspected mistreatment of older adults, and most states require such reporting. Although clinicians are appropriately wary of acting precipitously, they should be willing to enlist the help of government agencies and the courts when mistreatment is clearly dangerous for an older adult. Penalties can be assessed against a nonreporter in some regions. Reports of mistreatment of older adults are confidential, and as is the case with reports of child abuse, the clinical reporter is protected from litigation unless it can be proved that the report was made maliciously. The home page for the National Center on Elder Abuse (cited above) provides one means for reporting information.

Especially when a case is to be reported, photographs and body charts may be required to document the findings on physical examination. Risk management personnel can provide guidance in documentation and assist the clinician when evidence suggests that there may be a need for police or court action. In any case in which the clinician is called to court to discuss his or her findings, documentation is an important part of testimony. Cases of mistreatment are often extremely complicated, and it is likely that experts in several fields will need to work with clinicians and administrators to avoid under- or over-reporting of mistreatment of older adults and to provide the best outcomes for the victims of mistreatment.

REFERENCES

■ Dong X, Simon M, Mendes de Leon C, et al. Elder self-neglect and abuse and mortality risk in a community-dwelling population. *JAMA.* 2009;302(5):517–526.

■ Fulmer T, Guadagno L, Bitondo Dyer C, et al. Progress in elder abuse screening and assessment instruments. *J Am Geriatr Soc.* 2004;52(2):297–304.

■ Fulmer T. Elder Mistreatment Assessment. *Try This: Best Practices in Nursing Care to Older Adults.* 2008;(15). Available at http://consultgerirn.org/uploads/File/trythis/try_this_15.pdf

■ Lachs M, Bachman R, Williams CS, et al. Resident-to-resident elder mistreatment and police contact in nursing homes: findings from a population-based cohort. *J Am Geriatr Soc.* 2007;55(6):840–845.

CHAPTER 13—PERIOPERATIVE CARE

KEY POINTS

- Operative therapy is an important option for many health problems affecting older adults.

- The preoperative evaluation should include an appraisal of the patient's medical conditions, functional status, and risk of cardiac and other perioperative complications, as well as recommendations for preoperative testing and therapy to minimize surgical risk.

- Risk indices and practice guidelines for common cardiac, pulmonary, and neuropsychiatric problems assist in decision making and management of older surgical patients.

- While age is a risk factor for perioperative and postoperative complications, these problems can be minimized with appropriate proactive assessment and management.

OVERVIEW OF OPERATIVE THERAPY FOR OLDER ADULTS

Surgery is a common form of treatment for older adults; currently >55% of all operative procedures are done in patients ≥65 yr old, and the proportion is expected to grow. Many of the chronic conditions that increase in prevalence with advancing age—cataracts, arthritis, vascular occlusions, and cancers—are amenable to surgery. Over half of all malignancies are seen in patients ≥65 yr old, and the primary treatment for many tumors is surgical. Advances in surgical, anesthetic, and medical care have lowered surgical risks and shifted the risk-benefit ratio to favor surgery in increasingly older patients with more complex conditions. Nevertheless, although older patients account for just over half of all surgical procedures, they suffer three-quarters of the postoperative mortality as well as a disproportionate majority of the postoperative morbidity.

Many of the changes of normal aging physiology impact the perioperative management of the older surgical patient. For example, altered body composition, and decreased kidney function, hepatic blood flow, and hepatic enzyme activity all contribute to changes in the pharmacokinetics of drugs. Cardiac and vascular stiffening complicate fluid management and optimization of intravascular volume. Both volume overload and volume depletion occur commonly and are poorly tolerated by many older adults. Stiffening of the thoracic cage and decrements in ciliary function contribute to decreases in pulmonary reserve and heightened risk of postoperative pneumonia. Because of decreased thermoregulation, the older surgical patient is at particular risk of perioperative hypothermia. Finally, by mechanisms that are not yet fully elucidated, changes in the brain that accompany aging make older individuals exquisitely susceptible to postoperative cognitive changes. The cumulative effect of multiple organ systems with limited physiologic reserve results in "homeostenosis," a condition that greatly increases the risk of iatrogenic events.

It is well recognized that the aging process is extremely variable from person to person and that within a person not all organ systems age at the same rate, producing dramatic heterogeneity even among healthy older adults. Older individuals may have several chronic conditions that can impact on perioperative care, either directly or through the medications being used to treat those conditions. The heterogeneity in physiologic aging combined with the potential for multiple comorbidities means that older patients require a more complex and individualized preoperative evaluation. They often benefit from a multidisciplinary approach to perioperative care and recovery.

PREOPERATIVE ASSESSMENT AND MANAGEMENT

Preoperative evaluations are conducted to reduce the risks of complications and death and to optimize patient outcomes. The outcome of such a consultation should not be to "clear" the patient for surgery, but rather to maximize the possibility of a good outcome from surgery. This consultation should appraise the patient's medical and functional status, assess risk of perioperative and postoperative complications, and provide recommendations for preoperative testing and/or therapy to minimize potential complications. Preoperative assessment should include evaluation of the patient's cardiovascular, respiratory, renal, metabolic, and neuropsychiatric status, as well as the patient's risk of iatrogenic problems. Usually the preoperative assessment can be accomplished with a history and physical examination alone for low-risk procedures, eg, ambulatory, breast, cataract, endoscopic, or superficial surgery (SOE=B). For patients undergoing procedures that are not low risk, or

Table 13.1—Classification of Physical Status

Class	Description
I	A healthy patient
II	A patient with mild systemic disease
III	A patient with severe systemic disease
IV	A patient with severe systemic disease that is a constant threat to life
V	A moribund patient who is not expected to survive without surgery
VI	A declared brain-dead patient whose organs are being harvested for donor purposes

NOTE: There is no additional information to help further define these categories.
SOURCE: Data from American Society of Anesthesiologists. ASA Physical Status Classification System. Available at http:/www.asahq.org/clinical/physicalstatus.htm (accessed Jan 2011).

in whom the history and physical examination have uncovered other potential risks, further assessment and testing are indicated.

Cardiovascular System

It is estimated that 25%–30% of postoperative deaths are from cardiac causes, and the rate of postoperative cardiac events is directly related to age. Cardiac risk assessment is the most fully developed and widely investigated portion of the preoperative medical assessment. Several schemes are available to help calculate cardiac risk, and decision trees have been well described to guide risk assessment and management. The American Society of Anesthesiologists classification of patient physical status relies heavily on clinical judgment and is not specific for cardiovascular morbidity and mortality (see Table 13.1). This system has been used by anesthesiologists for years and has consistently been shown to be useful in predicting postoperative outcomes. Several indices and algorithms for specifically assessing cardiac risk in noncardiac surgery have been published since the 1970s. In 2007, the American College of Cardiology and the American Heart Association (ACC/AHA) published a new algorithm for preoperative cardiac assessment (Figure 13.1). The guideline calls for consideration, in order, of the following clinical factors:

1. Urgency of surgery; if emergent, proceed to surgery if consistent with patient's overall goals (SOE=C).

2. Presence of active major cardiac risk factors, eg, unstable coronary syndromes, decompensated heart failure, significant arrhythmias, or severe valvular disease; if present, correct these conditions before reconsidering surgery (SOE=B).

3. Type of surgery; if low-risk procedure, proceed to surgery (SOE=B).

4. Patient's functional capacity; if good, proceed to surgery (SOE=B).

5. Presence of other clinical risk factors (see Figure 13.1 for definitions); if none, proceed to surgery (SOE=B).

6. Type of surgery; recommendations vary depending on number of risk factors and whether surgery is of high or intermediate risk (SOE=B).

Aside from a careful history and physical examination to determine the presence of active major cardiac risk factors and to assess functional capacity, supplemental cardiac testing or therapy should be considered in only a few specific circumstances. ECG testing is not necessary in asymptomatic patients undergoing low-risk procedures (SOE=B). An ECG can be helpful for prognostic purposes only if step 6 above is reached in the decision-making algorithm, particularly in patients with clinical risk factors undergoing high-risk (vascular) procedures (SOE=B). ECG findings suggestive of ischemia, left ventricular hypertrophy, or left bundle branch block portend a higher risk of cardiac complications and death. Measurement of left ventricular function through echocardiography, radionuclide angiography, or contrast ventriculography should be considered in patients with dyspnea of uncertain etiology, current or prior heart failure and worsening dyspnea, or cardiomyopathy; an ejection fraction <35% is associated with higher rates of postoperative heart failure (SOE=C). When newly diagnosed heart failure is determined to be the cause of unexplained dyspnea, it should be maximally treated before surgery.

Recommendations for preoperative noninvasive cardiac stress testing have been scaled back over the past few years. Stress testing should be considered in patients with clinical risk factors who are undergoing intermediate- or high-risk procedures if the results of the stress testing will change management, eg, postponement or cancellation of surgery (SOE=B). Stress testing should be particularly considered in patients with ≥3 clinical risk factors who are undergoing vascular (high-risk) surgery.

It is under comparatively rare circumstances that coronary revascularization (with coronary artery bypass graft surgery or percutaneous coronary intervention) should be performed before noncardiac surgery to decrease risk of cardiac complications. The major indications for preoperative coronary revascularization are significant left main vessel disease; 3-vessel disease with stable angina; 2-vessel disease with proximal left anterior descending stenosis, stable angina, and either left ventricular ejection fraction (LVEF) <50% or ischemia on noninvasive stress testing; acute coronary syndrome; and acute ST-segment myocardial infarction (SOE=A).

Certain medications given before or after surgery reduce cardiac and vascular complications of surgery

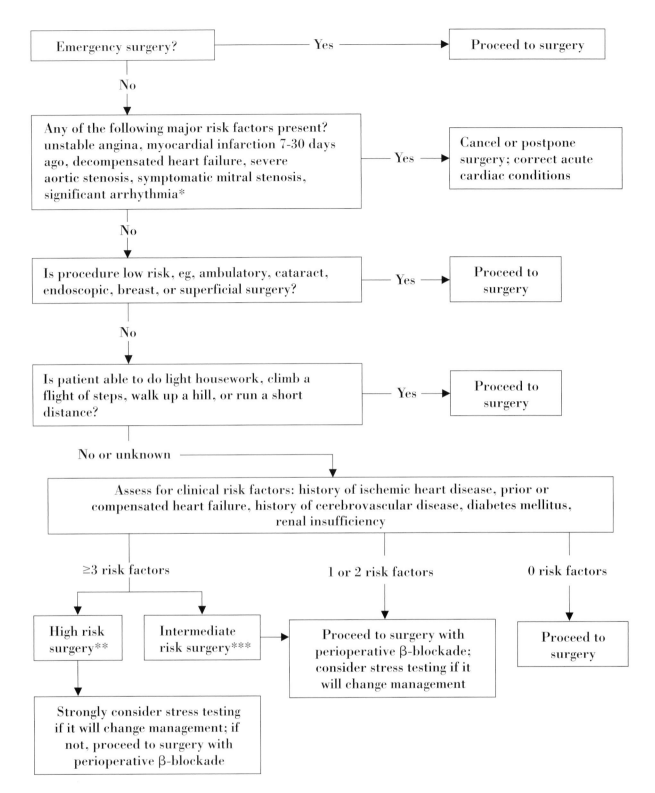

Figure 13.1—Assessing Cardiac Risk in Noncardiac Surgery

* High-grade AV block, Mobitz II AV block, third-degree AV block, symptomatic ventricular arrhythmias, supraventricular arrhythmias with resting heart rate >100 beats per minute, newly recognized ventricular tachycardia

** Open aortic or other major vascular surgery, peripheral vascular surgery

*** Intraperitoneal or intrathoracic surgery, carotid endarterectomy, endovascular abdominal aortic aneurysm repair, head and neck surgery, orthopedic surgery, prostate surgery

SOURCE: Data from Fleisher LA, Beckman JA, Brown KA, et al. ACC/AHA 2007 guidelines on perioperative cardiovascular evaluation and care for noncardiac surgery: a report of the American College of Cardiology/American Heart Association Task Force on Practice Guidelines (Writing Committee to Revise the 2002 Guidelines on Perioperative Cardiovascular Evaluation for Noncardiac Surgery). *Circulation.* 2007;116(17):e418–e499.

Table 13.2—Perioperative Medical Therapy to Reduce Cardiovascular Complications of Surgery

Medication	Target Conditions to be Prevented	Dosage	Indications[a]	SOE
β-Blocker	Myocardial infarction, ischemia, death	Long-acting agent begun days to weeks before surgery to achieve resting heart rate of 60, and continued throughout postoperative period	Continue usual dosage if already on a β-blocker	C
			Recommended in patients with one or more clinical risk factors and/or demonstrated coronary artery disease undergoing vascular (ie, high-risk) or intermediate-risk surgery	B
			Consider in patients with one clinical risk factor undergoing intermediate-risk surgery or in patients with no clinical risk factors undergoing vascular surgery	C
Statin	Myocardial infarction, ischemia, death	Uncertain timing, specific drug, and dosage; one randomized trial used atorvastatin 20 mg/d po begun an average of 30 d before surgery	Continue usual dosage if already on a statin	B
			Consider in all patients undergoing vascular surgery	B
			Consider in patients with more than one clinical risk factor undergoing intermediate-risk surgery	C
Aspirin	Coronary events, transient ischemic attack, stroke	81–325 mg/d po	For patients already on aspirin, consider not withdrawing it before surgery unless patient is undergoing tonsillectomy, prostate surgery, or intracranial surgery	B
			Begin <24 hours after coronary artery bypass surgery	A
Anticoagulant	Deep vein thrombosis, pulmonary embolus	See Table 13.3	Begin postoperatively for patients >60 yr old undergoing most types of surgery	A
Antibiotic	Infective endocarditis	Amoxicillin 2 g po 30–60 min before procedure[b]	Patients with selected cardiac conditions undergoing selected dental, respiratory tract, infected skin, or infected musculoskeletal tissue procedures[b]	C

[a] See Figure 13.1 for definitions of clinical risk factors, high-risk surgery, and intermediate-risk surgery.

[b] See Table 58.5 for alternative dosing regimens and specific indications.

SOURCE: Adapted with permission from *Geriatrics At Your Fingertips*, 12th ed. New York: American Geriatrics Society; 2010:199–200.

(Table 13.2). In general, prior antiplatelet therapy can be safely continued in patients undergoing neuraxial anesthesia, cutaneous surgery, dental procedures, diagnostic endoscopy, ophthalmologic procedures, and peripheral vascular surgery (SOE=C). For patients already on an anticoagulant, its protective benefits need to be weighed against the risk of perioperative hemorrhage. Anticoagulation therapy does not need to be withheld (as long as the INR is therapeutic) for cutaneous surgery (SOE=C), dental extractions and minor oral procedures (SOE=B), or cataract surgery (SOE=C). For other surgical procedures, cessation of warfarin, with or without bridging therapy with low molecular weight heparin (LMWH), can be based on the patient's risk factors for thromboembolism (Table 13.3). For patients receiving bridging therapy, LMWH can generally be restarted 24 hours after surgery, longer in cases of major surgery with increased risk of major bleeding. The indications for infective

endocarditis prophylaxis were dramatically reduced with the publication of new guidelines by the American Heart Association in 2007. See Table 58.4, p 487, and Table 58.5, p 488.

Respiratory System

Postoperative pulmonary complications, most commonly atelectasis and pneumonia, occur more often in older adults than in younger age groups. Pulmonary complications are predictive of increased short- and long-term mortality in older adults, and have been reported to prolong the hospital stay by an average of 1–2 wk in this age group. A comprehensive review published by the American College of Physicians (ACP) in 2005 found that age is a powerful independent risk factor for postoperative pulmonary complications (SOE=A). Other patient-associated major risk factors include COPD, ASA Class II or greater (Table

Table 13.3—Cessation of Anticoagulation Before Surgery in Older Adults[a]

Thromboembolic Risk	Patient Conditions Determining Risk	Recommendations for Cessation of Anticoagulation
Low	No VTE in past 12 mo; AF without prior TIA/stroke and 0–2 stroke risk factors; bileaflet mechanical aortic valve without AF, prior TIA/stroke, or stroke risk factors	If INR therapeutic, stop warfarin 5 days before surgery, earlier if INR is supertherapeutic or >3; bridging therapy with LMWH at prophylactic dosage is optional
Intermediate	VTE in past 3–12 mo; recurrent VTE; active malignancy; AF without prior TIA/stroke and with 3–4 stroke risk factors; bileaflet mechanical aortic valve with AF, prior TIA/stroke, or any stroke risk factors	Stop warfarin 5 days before surgery and begin LMWH 3 days before surgery at therapeutic (preferred) or prophylactic (optional) dosage; give last preoperative LMWH dose at one-half total daily dosage 24 hours before surgery
High	VTE within past 3 mo; TIA/stroke within 3 mo; rheumatic heart disease; AF with prior TIA/stroke and 3–4 stroke risk factors; mechanical mitral valve or ball/cage mechanical aortic valve	Stop warfarin 5 days before surgery and begin LMWH 3 days before surgery at therapeutic dosage; give last preoperative LMWH dose at one-half total daily dosage 24 hours before surgery

[a] SOE=C

VTE = venous thromboembolism; AF = atrial fibrillation; TIA = transient ischemic attack; INR = international normalized ratio; LMWH = low molecular weight heparin

NOTE: stroke risk factors: age ≥75 yr, hypertension, diabetes mellitus, history of heart failure

SOURCE: Data from Douketis JD, Berger PB, Dunn AS, et al. The perioperative management of antithrombotic therapy. American College of Chest Physicians Evidence-Based Clinical Practice Guidelines (8th Ed). *Chest*. 2008;133:299–339S.

13.1), heart failure, deficit in ADLs, and a serum albumin <3.5 g/dL (SOE=A). Minor patient-associated risk factors include acute confusion or delirium, alcohol use, smoking, weight loss, pulmonary findings on physical examination, and an increased BUN concentration (SOE=B). The following procedures are associated with increased pulmonary complications: emergency surgery; prolonged (>3 hour) surgery; repair of abdominal aortic aneurysm (AAA); neurosurgery; and thoracic, abdominal, head and neck, or vascular surgery (SOE=A). General anesthesia is also a risk factor (SOE=A).

In 2007, the ACP published a guideline for risk assessment and perioperative management of pulmonary complications associated with noncardiothoracic surgery. It calls for preoperative assessment of pulmonary complications by appraising the above risk factors through history, physical examination, and modest laboratory testing. Routine chest radiography is not recommended; a thoracic radiograph can be helpful for detection and management of pulmonary conditions in patients with known cardiac or pulmonary disease who are undergoing thoracic, upper abdominal, or surgery for AAA. Spirometry should be reserved for evaluating lung function in patients suspected of having undiagnosed COPD on history and physical examination, with findings such as dyspnea or wheezing.

The ACP guideline primarily recommends postoperative lung expansion therapy, which has been associated most consistently with reduced pulmonary complications of atelectasis, pneumonia, bronchitis, and severe hypoxemia (SOE=A). Lung expansion therapy can be accomplished through deep breathing exercises, incentive spirometry, and/or continuous positive airway pressure. Use of nasogastric tube for management of postoperative nausea and vomiting, inability to tolerate oral feeding, or abdominal distention can also be helpful for minimizing pulmonary complications (SOE=B). The evidence is also good for using short-acting neuromuscular blocking agents (as opposed to long-acting agents) to reduce complications (SOE=B). Less clear are the efficacies of preoperative smoking cessation, use of laparoscopic versus open procedures, epidural versus general anesthesia, and epidural analgesia.

Kidneys and Metabolism

Glomerular blood flow decreases with age. Concomitantly, there is a loss of muscle mass with age, such that an apparently normal serum creatinine can be misinterpreted as indicating normal kidney function. The glomerular filtration rate (GFR) can be estimated by calculating the creatinine clearance using the Cockcroft-Gault equation or by relying on the MDRD (Modification of Diet in Renal Disease study) method that some laboratories use to automatically calculate GFR (see the section on elimination in "Pharmacotherapy," p 72). Because many drugs administered during the perioperative period may require dosage adjustments in patients with diminished renal function, accurate estimation of GFR is important.

Also, because of decrements in the ability of the kidney to appropriately retain salt or to maximally concentrate or dilute urine in response to intravascular volume, the use of intravenous fluids needs to be monitored carefully. Volume resuscitation is best achieved with normal saline or blood (if appropriate), because half-normal saline or water are hypotonic and more readily diffuse to the extravascular tissues.

Neuropsychiatric Concerns

Delirium is a common event in the postoperative period. The type of surgery appears to be an important determinant of delirium, with incidence rates ranging from about 4%–5% in cataract or urologic procedures to 50%–60% in some series of patients with infrarenal AAA repair or hip fracture surgery. Both preoperative and intraoperative factors have been evaluated as risk factors for delirium. Preoperative factors in patients undergoing noncardiac surgery that predispose to postoperative delirium include age ≥70 yr; cognitive impairment; limited physical function; a history of alcohol abuse; abnormal serum sodium, potassium, or glucose; intrathoracic surgery; and AAA surgery. The most important intraoperative factor found to be associated with delirium is intraoperative blood loss. Patients with a postoperative hematocrit <30% have an increased risk of delirium irrespective of the presence or absence of preoperative risk factors (SOE=B). When preoperative risk factors are present, the clinician can identify patients at greatest risk of developing delirium and can be especially vigilant about correcting fluid, electrolyte, and metabolic derangements; optimizing replacement of blood loss; maintaining circadian rhythms (by promoting mobility and physical activity during the day and minimizing sleep interruptions at night); promoting adequate nutrition; and prescribing medications cautiously. See also the section on postoperative delirium in "Delirium," p 264.

Avoiding Iatrogenic Complications

Untoward effects of well-intentioned interventions are common among older hospitalized adults. Some of the more common pitfalls to be avoided include mobility restriction, excessive use of catheters, inattention to nutrition and hydration status, and inappropriate use of medications. Few disease states benefit from bed rest. It is important to maintain mobility and function as much as possible by encouraging time out of bed, promoting of physical activity, and avoiding restraints. The risks of skin breakdown, muscle atrophy, joint stiffness, and bone loss can be reduced by preserving mobility (SOE=C). Although bladder catheters can sometimes be critical in accurately measuring urine output, prolonged use of an indwelling catheter carries substantial risk of infection. Indwelling catheters can also contribute to restricted mobility and should be removed as soon as possible. Restricted diets and lack of access to water can contribute to compromise in nutrition and hydration.

Studies demonstrate that the traditional use of nothing by mouth beginning the night before surgery to reduce the risk of aspiration is not more beneficial than nothing by mouth for 6 hours except water, with the latter approach more comfortable for the patient and less likely to cause volume depletion (SOE=B). Conversely, continued administration of intravenous fluids after the patient is able to maintain hydration orally can result in volume overload and impaired oxygenation. A regular review of medication administration can avoid unnecessary drug use and inappropriate dosing.

PERIOPERATIVE AND POSTOPERATIVE MANAGEMENT OF SELECTED MEDICAL PROBLEMS

Surgery in older adults often results in destabilization of chronic, coexistent medical conditions. Additionally, because of the diminished physiologic reserve common in older adults, new medical problems can arise in the postoperative period. Some of the most common medical issues to contend with postoperatively are discussed here.

Cardiovascular Problems

The most common cardiovascular problems that arise in older adults after surgery are hypertension, rhythm disturbances, and heart failure. Postoperative hypertension should initially prompt a search for a noncardiovascular cause, such as pain or urinary retention. Next, it is important to assess volume status, review fluid administration records, and note whether antihypertensive medications were mistakenly omitted before the procedure. To treat uncontrolled essential hypertension, parenteral formulations are available in several classes of medications: β-blockers, calcium channel blockers, ACE inhibitors, and drugs that block both α- and β-adrenergic receptors. Topical agents, such as topical nitroglycerin, could also be considered useful when the patient is unable to take medications by mouth.

Cardiac rhythm disturbances are a concern because they can lead to myocardial ischemia and heart failure. Supraventricular tachycardia, commonly seen in older adults, is associated with a history of prior supraventricular dysrhythmias, asthma, heart failure, and premature atrial complexes on a preoperative ECG. This rhythm disturbance is also more common in patients who have had vascular, abdominal, or thoracic procedures. Early restoration of sinus rhythm, or at least controlling the ventricular rate, can be attempted with an infusion of adenosine, a β-blocker, or a calcium channel blocker. If the rhythm is atrial fibrillation, conversion to sinus rhythm can be at-

Table 13.4—Deep Venous Thrombosis/Pulmonary Embolism (DVT/PE) Prophylaxis in Older Surgical and Medical Inpatients

DVT/PE Risk	Surgeries or Medical Conditions	Thromboprophylactic Options
Low	Healthy and mobile patients undergoing minor surgery, including laparoscopic gynecologic procedures, transurethral or other low-risk urologic procedures, spine surgery, knee arthroscopy	Aggressive early ambulation after procedure
Moderate	Most general surgeries; major vascular procedures; thoracic surgery; open gynecologic and urologic surgery; medical or surgical patients admitted for heart failure or severe respiratory disease, or who are at bedrest with active cancer, previous DVT/PE, sepsis, active neurologic disease, or inflammatory bowel disease	LMWH, fondaparinux, or unfractionated heparin[a]
High	Total hip replacement, total knee replacement, hip fracture surgery, trauma, spinal cord injury	LMWH, fondaparinux, or warfarin[a]

LMWH = low-molecular-weight heparin

[a] For patients at high risk of bleeding, acceptable alternative is intermittent pneumatic compression and/or use of graduated compression stockings.

SOURCE: Reuben DE, Kerr KA, Pacala JT, et al. *Geriatrics At Your Fingertips*, 12th ed. New York: American Geriatrics Society; 2010:23. Reprinted with permission.

tempted with electrical cardioversion or by an infusion of amiodarone if the atrial fibrillation is poorly tolerated. Because spontaneous reversion to sinus rhythm often occurs by 6 wk after surgery, long-term use of an antidysrhythmic such as amiodarone may not be necessary. Persistent atrial fibrillation beyond 24–48 hours is associated with an increased risk of thromboembolism, and consideration should be given to anticoagulation therapy to reduce the risk of stroke (SOE=A).

Cardiac reserve is often compromised among older adults, especially those with chronic hypertension or coronary artery disease. Heart failure can develop as a result of excessive fluid administration, new cardiac ischemia, or a rhythm disturbance. It can be extremely challenging to ensure optimal ventricular filling pressures based on the clinical assessment of volume status in older adults by physical examination and standard laboratory parameters alone. Although some have recommended the use of pulmonary artery catheters in high-risk patients, studies have not shown a decreased mortality rate for this intervention, and most authorities advise against this approach (SOE=C).

Most older adults who are undergoing surgery or who are hospitalized for significant medical problems should receive prophylaxis for deep venous thrombosis and pulmonary embolism. See Table 13.4 for general guidelines regarding venous thromboembolism prophylaxis.

Kidney and Electrolyte Disorders

Impaired preoperative kidney function increases the risk of postoperative kidney failure. The impaired reserve makes the aging kidney more susceptible to the effects of even transient reductions of cardiac output or brief exposure to nephrotoxic medications.

When kidney damage has been sustained, early clinical manifestations include oliguria, isosthenuria, and an increase in serum creatinine. When impaired renal blood flow is the cause, the urine sodium will typically be <40 mEq/L and the urine-to-plasma creatinine ratio will be greater than 10:1. In contrast, if acute tubular necrosis is the mechanism of injury, the urine sediment may have granular or epithelial cell casts, and the urine sodium will be >40 mEq/L with a urine-to-plasma creatinine ratio of less than 10:1. When acute tubular necrosis is suspected, vigorous efforts should be made to preserve kidney function by withholding all potentially nephrotoxic medications and meticulously maintaining a euvolemic state. (See "Kidney Diseases and Disorders," p 404.) The indications for dialysis are no different in the perioperative period or in older adults and include hypervolemia, hyperkalemia, metabolic acidosis, or encephalopathy. Another important mechanism of postoperative kidney failure is obstructive nephropathy, especially in older men with prostatic hyperplasia. The partial outflow obstruction combined with immobility, frequent constipation, and exposure to medications with anticholinergic effects compromising detrusor function can easily precipitate acute urinary retention. In addition to oliguria and an increase in serum creatinine, the bladder is typically palpable because of distention. Treatment consists of insertion of a bladder catheter to reduce the risk of hydronephrosis and impaired kidney function. Commonly, men with prostatic hyperplasia who develop postoperative obstruction are unable to void after immediate removal of the catheter and may need α-blocking medications and continued use of the catheter for 2–4 wk until another voiding trial can be attempted (SOE=C).

Gastrointestinal Concerns

Constipation is quite common postoperatively, as a consequence of the combined effects of altered diet, immobility, and usually use of narcotics and other constipating medications. At times, ileus and obstipation can be severe and produce significant anorexia, nausea, delirium, and even vomiting. Postoperative iron therapy, commonly prescribed for anemia, is an unproven but likely contributor to postoperative constipation. Given the common co-occurrence of these risk factors for constipation in the postoperative period, a reasonable approach is to simultaneously order a laxative and a stool softener every time a narcotic is prescribed, particularly if the patient has a history of constipation or it is reasonably anticipated that mobility will be reduced for more than 1 day. Prunes or prune juice, applesauce, and bran can all also have promotility effects. For medications useful in preventing and managing constipation, see Table 49.3, p 399.

Postoperative diarrhea should raise concern for fecal impaction and antibiotic-associated or *Clostridium difficile* diarrhea in the setting of recent antibiotic use. Checking manually for fecal impaction and testing fecal specimens for leukocytes and *C difficile* toxin may be appropriate. Management must focus carefully on volume resuscitation and treating the underlying cause. Antimotility agents, while effective in reducing fecal incontinence from diarrhea, are very risky in older adults in the postoperative period and significantly increase the risk of delirium, constipation, and toxic megacolon.

Finally, nausea is not uncommon in the postoperative period, often as a result of narcotic, anesthetic, and other medications; new infection; or slowed gut motility. See the section on nausea and vomiting in "Palliative Care," p 104, for a discussion on approach to management.

Managing Common Endocrine Abnormalities

Type 2 diabetes mellitus is a common comorbid condition of many older adults undergoing surgery. Usually, given the long half-life of oral hypoglycemic agents and the nothing-by-mouth status for surgery, oral diabetes medications are withheld the day of surgery. It may be especially important to withhold metformin, given the potential additional risk of metabolic acidosis from this medication during a time of stress, although the actual risk of this complication is likely widely overestimated. To optimize glucose control, an intravenous solution containing glucose can be administered at a constant rate while blood glucose by finger stick assay is closely monitored; subcutaneous insulin should be administered as necessary to control glucose concentrations until the patient is able to resume eating. For a patient with type 2 diabetes who uses insulin, insulin should be withheld on the day of surgery and sliding-scale insulin given (SOE=C). Once the patient is able to start eating, usually half the outpatient dosage of diabetes drugs are administered the first day of oral intake, with additional sliding-scale insulin coverage as needed; full doses are resumed as the patient consumes a usual diet.

Perioperative hyperglycemia among diabetic and nondiabetic patients is associated with morbidity and mortality in medical and surgical intensive-care-unit (ICU) patients (SOE=B) and in patients undergoing coronary artery bypass grafting (SOE=C) or carotid endarterectomy (SOE=B). Maintaining glucose concentrations of <150 mg/dL with intravenous insulin in the perioperative period for patients undergoing vascular or major noncardiac surgery with planned ICU admission has reduced morbidity and mortality (SOE=B). However, maintaining tight glycemic control (≤110 mg/dL) among ICU patients has been associated with increased hypoglycemia and no reduction in mortality (SOE=B), so moderate glucose control in these patients is advised. The value of strict glycemic control in other surgical or medical inpatient populations has not been demonstrated.

Patients taking supplemental corticosteroids require special consideration during the perioperative period. Those taking prednisone at dosages >20–30 mg/d for longer than a week or with known adrenal insufficiency should be given "stress doses" of steroids after surgery (SOE=C). A single measurement of cortisol, if increased, is useful to assess the hypothalamic-pituitary axis (HPA) in patients who chronically use steroids when the function of the HPA is in question. If the cortisol level is not high, a 30-minute ACTH test may be useful. The dosage of steroids to use is debated, but some authorities advise 25 mg of hydrocortisone equivalents the day of surgery only for minor procedures, 50–75 mg of hydrocortisone equivalents daily (eg, hydrocortisone 20 mg q8h IV) for 1–2 days for moderate surgical stress, and 100–150 mg of hydrocortisone equivalents daily (eg, hydrocortisone 50 mg q8h IV beginning within 2 hours of surgery) continuing for 2–3 days after surgery and then transitioned to the usual steroid regimen for high surgical stress. Other authorities simply recommend continuing usual dosages of steroids for elective, uncomplicated surgeries, or doubling or tripling the outpatient dosage by giving hydrocortisone at dosages up to 100–150 mg/d IV for higher risk or anticipated complicated operations.

Delirium and Postoperative Cognitive Decline

Delirium is one of the most common postoperative complications, and certainly the one for which a geriatrician is most likely to be consulted. In a randomized study, a multicomponent intervention that focused on reducing sleep interruptions, minimizing medications and immobility, enhancing sensory input, and reducing dehydration reduced the rate of developing delirium by one-third over standard care for hospitalized medical patients (SOE=A). This approach, although not specifically studied in the postoperative setting, is likely to be beneficial in this phase as well (SOE=C). For the postoperative geriatric surgical patient, undertreated pain, constipation, electrolyte abnormalities, and perioperative myocardial infarction must be particularly considered.

Postoperative cognitive dysfunction, characterized by abnormalities in learning and memory, can be subtle or dramatic and is considered to be a syndrome distinct from delirium. It has been reported most commonly after cardiac surgery but is experienced by patients undergoing procedures that do not involve extracorporal circulation. Although the symptoms are often short-lived, they persist for many months in 10%–30% of patients. Efforts to define the cause of the syndrome have not yet been successful; studies have not been able to demonstrate links with hypotension, hypoxemia, or type of anesthesia. Because a better understanding of the pathophysiology is lacking, treatment efforts are supportive. See "Postoperative Delirium," p 267, for more information on postoperative delirium and postoperative cognitive dysfunction.

Pain Management

Management of postoperative pain remains a challenge, particularly in patients with dementia, delirium, or both. The key points to the evaluation and management of acute pain are quite similar to those discussed in "Persistent Pain," p 109; for a useful guide to tools used to help assess postoperative pain in cognitively impaired patients, see Table 15.2. The oldest-old and cognitively impaired patients appear to be at highest risk for undertreatment of pain, so they deserve particular attention. Undertreatment of pain, at least in nondemented individuals, appears to be a more powerful predictor for development of postoperative delirium than narcotic use (SOE=A).

Most postsurgical pain requires narcotic analgesia. Cognitively intact patients may have improved pain relief and overall lower use of narcotics if administered by patient-controlled analgesia pump (SOE=A). Individuals with less severe pain may be able to tolerate scheduled acetaminophen (not to exceed 4 g/d) with only as-needed use of narcotic analgesics, if they are able to ask for them. Patients who are unable to communicate effectively and have pain should be given standing orders for narcotic analgesics, with guidelines as to when to withhold the medications, combined with frequent assessment of medication effect. NSAIDs are best avoided in this setting because of the potential for GI bleeding, delirium, fluid retention, nephrotoxicity, and cardiovascular risks. Because narcotic analgesics can precipitate constipation, concomitant use of laxatives and stool softeners is generally advised. A small body of literature is accumulating supporting the benefits of "preemptive" analgesia to reduce anticipated pain and total doses of narcotic required to control pain postoperatively, but this has yet to be studied in older adults. For comprehensive, up-to-date information on pain medications and dosing, see http://www.geriatricsatyourfingertips.org.

Nonpharmacologic therapies, such as ice packs, heating pads, massage, and relaxation techniques, are also useful adjuncts to therapy and often underused.

Planning for Transitions

Clinicians can significantly aid older patients by anticipating and planning for transitions in care. For useful information about discharge planning and transitioning care from the hospital, see "Hospital Care," p 119.

ACOVE-3* QUALITY INDICATORS PERTAINING TO PERIOPERATIVE CARE

PREOPERATIVE CARE

Capacity to consent

■ If a vulnerable older adult is to have inpatient or outpatient elective surgery, then there should be documentation of the patient's capacity to understand the risks and benefits of the proposed procedure before the operative consent form is presented for signature.

Preoperative discussion

■ If a vulnerable older adult is to have elective major surgery, then the following should be discussed preoperatively.

  ○ Patient priorities and preferences regarding treatment options

  ○ Operative risks

  ○ Anticipated postoperative functional outcome

  ○ Advance directive and designated surrogate decision maker

Preoperative evaluation

- If a vulnerable older adult is to have elective major surgery, then a review of the respiratory system (history of smoking, baseline exercise tolerance, history of COPD or asthma) and chest auscultation should be performed preoperatively.
- If a vulnerable older adult is to have elective major surgery, then cardiovascular risk should be assessed preoperatively.

Preoperative diabetes mellitus evaluation

- If a vulnerable older adult is to have elective major surgery, then the presence or absence of diabetes mellitus should be documented preoperatively.
- If a vulnerable older adult with diabetes mellitus is to have elective major surgery, then the diabetes regimen and adequacy of diabetes control should be documented preoperatively.

Preoperative delirium assessment

- If a vulnerable older adult is to have elective major surgery, then he or she should be screened for risk factors for development of postoperative delirium within 8 wk before surgery.

Venous thrombosis prophylaxis

- If a hospitalized vulnerable older adult is at very high risk of venous thrombosis, then he or she should be on deep venous thrombosis prophylaxis (pharmacologic or sequential or intermittent compression).

PERIOPERATIVE CARE

Prevention of surgical site infection

- If a vulnerable older adult has elective major surgery, then prophylactic antibiotics should be administered within 1 hour before incision (2 hours for vancomycin or fluoroquinolone) and discontinued within 24 hours after surgery has ended.

Perioperative β-blockade

- If a vulnerable older adult with coronary artery disease has elective major surgery, then preoperative β-blockade should be considered, and if started, continued until discharge.

Anticoagulation for hip fracture

- If a vulnerable older adult has sustained a hip fracture, then an anticoagulant regimen should be started.

Anticoagulation for hip replacement

- If a vulnerable older adult is to have a total hip replacement, then an anticoagulation regimen should be started preoperatively or on the evening after surgery.

POSTOPERATIVE CARE

Mobilization

- If a vulnerable older adult who was ambulatory as an outpatient has major surgery and is not in intensive care, then ambulation should be performed by 2 days after surgery.

Diabetes mellitus control

- If a vulnerable older adult with diabetes mellitus has major surgery, then blood glucose concentration should be kept below 200 mg/dL on the day of surgery and the first 2 days after surgery (or attempts to achieve this should have been performed and documented).

Screen for postoperative delirium

- If a vulnerable older adult has major surgery, then a daily screening examination for delirium should be performed for the first 3 days after surgery.

Cognition and function at discharge

- If a vulnerable older adult has major surgery, cognition and functional status should be assessed before discharge and compared with preoperative levels.

Related quality indicators for Perioperative Care

- Follow up after hospitalization, discharge summary in outpatient chart (see "Hospital Care," p 119)

*Assessing Care of Vulnerable Elders – 3ʳᵈ Set. See inside front cover for explanation.

REFERENCES

- Douketis JD, Berger PB, Dunn AS, et al. The perioperative management of antithrombotic therapy: American College of Chest Physicians Evidence-Based Clinical Practice Guidelines (8th Edition). *Chest.* 2008;133(6 Suppl):299–339S.

- Dunn D. Preventing perioperative complications in an older adult: learn how his advancing age affects his risks so you can take steps to head off trouble. *Holistic Nursing Practice.* 2005;19(2):54–59.

- Fleisher LA, Beckman JA, Brown KA, et al. ACC/AHA 2007 guidelines on perioperative cardiovascular evaluation and care for noncardiac surgery. A report of the American College of Cardiology/American Heart Association Task Force on Practice Guidelines (Writing Committee to Revise the 2002 Guidelines on Perioperative Cardiovascular Evaluation for Noncardiac Surgery). *Circulation.* 2007;116(17):e418–e499.

- Qaseem A, Snow V, Fitterman N, et al for the Clinical Efficacy Assessment Subcommittee of the American College of Physicians. Risk assessment for and strategies to reduce perioperative pulmonary complications for patients undergoing noncardiothoracic surgery: a guideline from the American College of Physicians. *Ann Intern Med.* 2006;144(8):575–580.

- Robinson TN, Eiseman B, Wallace JI, et al. Redefining geriatric preoperative assessment using frailty, disability and co-morbidity. *Ann Surg.* 2009;250(3):449–455.

- Zarowitz BJ, Tangalos E, Lefkovitz A, et al. Thrombotic risk and immobility in residents of long-term care facilities. *J Am Med Dir Assoc.* 2010;11(3):211–221.

CHAPTER 14—PALLIATIVE CARE

KEY POINTS

- For many older adults, dying is characterized by inadequately treated physical distress; fragmented care systems; poor to absent communication among clinicians, patients, and families; and enormous strains on family caregiver and support systems.

- Geographic variations in practice patterns and services available, religious beliefs, economic status, medical differences, gender, and cognitive status all affect the experiences of dying individuals.

- Pain assessment is especially challenging in individuals with poor communication skills, and the clinician must be sensitive to nonverbal clues.

- Loss of appetite is almost a universal symptom at the end of life; often it is more distressing to loved ones than to the patient.

- The patient's self-report is the only reliable measure of dyspnea, one of the most distressing symptoms experienced by many dying individuals.

In the United States, the overwhelming majority of deaths occur among the older adult population. Older adults typically die slowly of chronic diseases, with multiple coexisting problems, progressive dependency on others, and heavy care needs that are met mostly by family members. Many of these deaths become protracted processes for patients, family members, and physicians, who must make difficult decisions about the use or discontinuation of life-prolonging treatments. Evidence is abundant that the quality of life during the dying process is often poor. For many older adults, dying is characterized by inadequately treated physical distress; fragmented care systems; poor to absent communication among physicians, patients, and families; and enormous strains on family caregiver and support systems.

Although most Americans spend most of their final months at home, in most parts of the country, their deaths actually occur in the hospital or nursing home. The experience of dying, however, varies greatly from one part of the country to another. In Portland, Oregon, for example, only 35% of adult deaths occur in hospitals, but in New York City more than 80% occur in hospitals, a difference associated in part with differences in regional hospital bed supply and the availability of community support for the dying. Social and medical differences also account for some patterns. The need for institutionalization or paid caregivers in the last months of life is much higher among poor individuals and women. Similarly, older adults suffering from cognitive impairment and dementia are much more likely than cognitively intact older adults to spend their last days in a nursing home.

OVERALL CARE NEAR DEATH

The Hospitalized Elderly Longitudinal Project (HELP) attempted to characterize the last 6 mo of life and dying in 1,266 adults ≥80 yr old. Results showed that people tend to overestimate their chances of survival near the end of life (SOE=A). Patients who died within 1 yr of enrollment had significant functional impairment in ADLs and expressed strong preferences for not being resuscitated and for comfort care (SOE=A). The number of patients reporting severe pain increased toward the end of life, with one in three reporting severe pain within 3 mo of death (SOE=A). These results highlight the need for physicians to talk with their patients early about their preferences, as well as to provide better symptom control and palliative measures at the end of life.

Part of the challenge in providing excellent end-of-life care stems from the inability to adequately predict end of life, particularly for patients with chronic diseases such as heart failure and COPD, in whom exacerbations and remissions are common and unpredictable.

ETHNOGRAPHIC DATA

Respect for life has been shown to affect decision making in some Asian cultures. For example, cardiopulmonary resuscitation as a means of doing everything possible to preserve life is viewed as an act of respect. In the Chinese culture, filial piety implies strong devotion to the dying person, and the oldest child is expected to accompany the parent through the final stage of life as an expression of filial piety. Discussions of death are thought to perhaps bring it about or bring it about sooner, so clinicians must be respectful when entering into discussion about end-of-life issues. Healthcare decisions are viewed as family decisions in Chinese culture, so it is important for clinicians to determine who should be present for delivery of bad news.

A number of studies have found that compared with white Americans, black Americans are less likely to use living wills or complete advance directives, and prefer more aggressive medical care for terminal illness (SOE=B). These preferences can conflict with hospice goals that emphasize comfort versus cure. Studies assessing attitudes and values consistent with hospice care have shown that black Americans are more likely than whites to believe that death should be avoided at all costs and to want to live as long as possible, even with terminal medical conditions. They are also less likely to want to die at home.

Studies of African Americans show that as a group, spirituality plays a dominant role in how end-of-life is experienced and interpreted (SOE=A). Data indicate that black Americans are more likely to pray for a miracle rather than accept death, to believe in the omnipotence of God, to believe that God (rather than medical treatment or the lack of it) determines death, to view the physician as God's instrument, and to believe God is able to perform a miracle (SOE=A).

Knowledge of the tendencies of diverse ethnic groups may facilitate communication between clinicians and patients and their families regarding the end of life. Often, the physician can better understand the patient's viewpoint by first asking, "Is there anything about your culture or your beliefs that would be helpful for me to know as we plan together for the future?" See also "Cultural Aspects of Care," p 49.

PALLIATIVE CARE AND HOSPICE

Palliative care is interdisciplinary care that aims to relieve suffering, improve quality of life, optimize function, and assist with decision making for patients with advanced illness and their families. It is offered simultaneously with all other appropriate medical treatment, either by the primary medical team or in conjunction with a palliative care consultant.

Hospice is the comprehensive care system for patients with limited remaining life expectancy at home or in institutional settings. Hospice as a Medicare healthcare benefit was established in 1982 by the federal government. Initially, hospice coverage was made available through an expanded Medicare benefit; now it is supported through a Medicare or Medicaid benefit, and it is also a benefit of most commercial insurance policies. The benefit is a highly regulated, fully capitated healthcare system, which is now implemented through more than 3,000 hospice services (most nonprofit) and is dedicated to providing comprehensive palliative care for patients with all types of terminal illnesses and their families. Hospice is primarily a home-care program, with access to inpatient beds for the management of acute problems. Hospice programs receive one of four daily rates for reimbursement that are based on four levels of care: home care, inpatient level of care, continuous care, and respite care. For a summary of the services hospice provides, see Table 14.1.

Access to hospice is based on two conditions:

- A licensed physician must certify that he or she believes that the patient has a remaining life expectancy of ≤6 mo if the disease runs its expected course.

- The patient or proxy must elect hospice and thereby agree that the care plan with respect to the terminal illness will be managed by the hospice program.

The patient must be recertified on a regular basis. If the physician cannot state that remaining life expectancy is still anticipated to be ≤6 mo, then the patient must be discharged from hospice. The patient can revoke the hospice benefit at any time.

STRENGTH-OF-EVIDENCE (SOE) RATING DEFINITIONS

A = consistent and good quality patient-oriented evidence
B = somewhat inconsistent or limited quality patient-oriented evidence
C = very inconsistent or very limited patient-oriented evidence, disease-oriented evidence, and/or consensus from professional organizations
D = unstudied common practice or opinion

See inside front cover for detailed information regarding the SOE classification.

Table 14.1—Hospice Services

- Care provided by an interdisciplinary team: nurse, social worker, chaplain, aides, volunteers, physical therapist, music therapist
- Case management by a hospice nurse
- Access to a hospice physician
- Medications at no cost, as long as they are related to the terminal diagnosis and are palliative, as determined by the hospice plan of care
- Tests and other treatments at no cost, as long as they are related to the terminal diagnosis and are palliative, as determined by the hospice plan of care
- Durable medical equipment
- Bereavement services for 13 mo after a death

The referring physician must certify that the prognosis for remaining life expectancy is ≤6 mo and decide whether to remain the physician of record or to transfer care of the patient to the hospice medical director. If the referring physician remains the physician of record, he or she continues to direct the care of the patient, becomes part of the hospice interdisciplinary team, must coordinate treatment decisions related to the terminal illness with the case manager (primary nurse), and may bill under Part B of Medicare or Medicaid.

See also "Financing, Coverage, and Costs of Health Care," p 32.

QUALITY INDICATORS FOR PALLIATIVE CARE

Research demonstrates that patients want to communicate with their healthcare providers about their future medical care and that many want to discuss end-of-life issues with their physicians (SOE=A). It is recommended that physicians address advance care directives, identify surrogate decision makers, and document patient preferences well before the onset of terminal illness, and update these preferences with cognitively intact patients regularly. This should include discussions about preferences for or against mechanical ventilation and other attempts at resuscitation, which have been identified by experts as important quality indicators.

Symptoms are a major cause of distress and suffering during the end stages of life. Studies show that clinicians often tend to underemphasize routine symptom assessment (SOE=C). Clinicians should seek to treat dyspnea, pain, and other distressing symptoms at the end of life.

Family and other informal caregivers risk financial as well as health consequences in caregiving. In one study of nearly 1,000 caregivers, 35% reported that their employment was affected, and significant time and money were spent on caregiving. Both patients and caregivers identify minimizing caregiver burden as a major concern.

Although no controlled trials have demonstrated that patient outcomes improve with attention given to advance care planning, symptom management, spirituality, and caregiver stress, expert opinion recommends the use of quality indicators addressing these issues in palliative and end-of-life care (SOE=D). See the ACOVE-3 quality indicators at the end of this chapter for specific examples.

PALLIATION OF SYMPTOMS

Pain

For assessing and treating pain, see "Persistent Pain," p 109, which also includes a section on pain in cognitively impaired older adults, and postoperative pain management in "Perioperative Care," p 92.

Constipation

Constipation is one of the most common and distressing symptoms seen in terminally ill patients. Opioid pain medications significantly contribute to constipation, which is exacerbated by the reduced mobility and poor fluid intake that accompanies most serious and life-threatening illnesses. Other unwanted effects of opioids generally diminish over time, but constipation usually persists, requiring ongoing bowel management as long as opioid therapy is used (SOE=D). Patients on opioids should receive prophylactic laxatives consisting of a stool softener (eg, docusate sodium) and a bowel stimulant (eg, senna, bisacodyl) unless diarrhea has already been a problem. If these measures are not effective, then an osmotic laxative (eg, sorbitol, lactulose, or polyethylene glycol) should be added. If there has been no bowel movement for ≥4 days, an enema should be considered. Patients presenting with constipation should be evaluated for bowel obstruction or fecal impaction. In cases of impaction, manual disimpaction or enemas should be used before starting laxative therapy. (See also postoperative GI problems in "Perioperative Care," p 92, especially Table 13.2.) Methylnaltrexone bromide is a newer agent approved for the treatment of opioid-induced constipation in patients with advanced illness. Methylnaltrexone antagonizes opioid binding to the peripheral mu-opioid receptors in the GI tract. It does not cross the blood brain barrier and has no effect on the central analgesic effects of opioids. It is contraindicated in known or suspected mechanical GI obstruction.

Nausea and Vomiting

The incidence of nausea and vomiting is estimated to be 40%–70% in patients with advanced cancer (SOE=B). Symptoms can be caused by disease or its treatment, so it is first important to clarify the cause of the nausea and vomiting. Emesis is mediated centrally by the chemoreceptor trigger zone in the area postrema, in the floor of the fourth ventricle. Peripherally, emesis is mediated in the gut and in the vestibular apparatus. Various receptors are involved in the mediation of emesis (eg, serotonin, dopamine, histamine, acetylcholine), and selection of an appropriate antiemetic agent should therefore seek to identify the likely cause, the pathway that is mediating symptoms, and the neurotransmitters involved (SOE=D).

Dopamine antagonists such as haloperidol[OL], metoclopramide, or droperidol act primarily on the chemoreceptor trigger zone. Serotonin antagonists such as ondansetron or granisetron act in synergy with dopaminergic antagonists in the chemoreceptor trigger zone and additionally act peripherally in the gut. Muscarinic blockers such as scopolamine or meclizine are useful for patients with disturbed vestibular function. Prokinetic agents such as metoclopramide can potentiate cholinergic activity in the GI tract and are useful if the cause is gastroparesis. Antihistamines (eg, hydroxyzine[OL], dimenhydrinate) can be useful adjunct agents when combined with either serotonergic or dopaminergic agents, although their adverse events (eg, sedation, urinary retention, delirium) can limit their use in frail older adults. It is believed that these agents act on H_1 receptors in the vestibular afferents and on the gut. Serotonin-receptor blockers, including ondansetron and granisetron, are very effective for emesis induced by radiotherapy or chemotherapy. They do not reverse nausea mediated by dopamine pathways (eg, those that are induced by opioids). Finally, corticosteroids possess intrinsic antiemetic properties and enhance the effect of other antiemetics. Corticosteroids are also useful for nausea and vomiting that is associated with increased intracranial pressure.

Diarrhea

Diarrhea affects 7%–10% of patients with cancer being admitted to hospice (SOE=C). Diarrhea is defined as the passage of more than three unformed bowel movements within a 24-hour period. The clinician should be alert to the possibility of fecal impaction that presents as watery diarrhea, particularly in immobile older adults on opioids. The treatment of impaction should begin with manual disimpaction and tap-water enemas, followed if unsuccessful by high colonic enemas. Laxatives should not be administered until the impaction is cleared because of the risk of bowel perforation. Untreated fecal impaction can be life threatening. Another common cause of diarrhea in palliative medicine is excessive laxative therapy, especially after laxative

dosages have been increased to clear an impaction; this can respond to temporarily stopping laxatives and reintroducing them at a lower dosage. Radiotherapy involving the abdomen and pelvis causes diarrhea, peaking during the second or third week of therapy. This typically responds to cholestyramine at 4–12 g q8h (SOE=C). Diarrhea caused by fat malabsorption (eg, pancreatic insufficiency or small-bowel disease) responds to pancreatic enzymes such as pancreatin (SOE=B). Diarrhea after ileal resection also responds to cholestyramine.

Anorexia and Cachexia

Loss of appetite is almost a universal symptom of patients with serious and life-threatening illness. Anorexia in those who are actively dying and who do not express a desire to eat should not be treated. Symptoms of dry mouth can be alleviated with ice chips, popsicles, moist compresses, or artificial saliva. Lemon glycerin swabs should not be used, because they irritate dry and cracked mucosa. Megestrol acetate and corticosteroids[OL] have been found to enhance appetite, cause weight gain (primarily fat), and improve quality of life in some patients with anorexia (SOE=B). However, these agents have not prolonged survival, improved function, or improved treatment tolerance of cancer therapies, and they are associated with their own adverse events (SOE=B). In general, patients should be encouraged to eat whatever is most appealing without regard to dietary restrictions.

Delirium

Delirium, agitation, and confusion are common in terminally ill older patients and are often distressing to both patients and family members. Initial efforts should be directed at identifying potentially reversible causes (eg, infection, impaction, uncontrolled pain, urinary retention, hypoxia). Antipsychotics such as haloperidol[OL] or risperidone[OL] in low dosages are effective treatments for both hypoactive and hyperactive delirium if medications are thought to be indicated either to ensure the patient's safety or because the delirium appears to be causing distress. Actively dying patients who are nonambulatory and who experience terminal delirium often appear less distressed with use of sedating antipsychotics such as chlorpromazine[OL]. Because benzodiazepines are often associated with paradoxical agitation and a worsening of the delirium in older adults, their use should be carefully considered. See also "Delirium," p 264.

Depression

Depression is under-recognized and undertreated, both in older adults and terminally ill patients. It may be underdiagnosed because of clinicians' mistaken belief that it is either a normal consequence of aging or appropriate in the context of a terminal illness. Because of underlying illness, standard vegetative symptoms described in the *Diagnostic and Statistical Manual of Mental Disorders* (insomnia, anorexia, weight change) are often not reliable indicators. Instead, clinicians should watch for change in mood, loss of interest, and suicidal ideation. Suicidal ideation should be openly discussed, including any symptoms that are contributing to the patient's suffering, which may be influencing his or her consideration of suicide. Aggressive treatment of symptoms, antidepressant therapy, cognitive-behavioral therapy, and psychiatric consultation are all appropriate initial responses. Continued discussion with the patient about the wish to hasten death often reveals a change of mind as time passes.

Standard antidepressant therapy is effective, but most agents have a delayed onset of 2–6 wk. Psychostimulants (eg, methylphenidate[OL], dextroamphetamine[OL]) are well tolerated, safe, and effective short-term treatments for medically ill depressed patients (SOE=B). Additionally, they have a rapid onset and beneficial effect on energy, mood, appetite, and mental alertness. Methylphenidate can be started at 2.5 mg in the early morning hours and given concurrently with standard antidepressants; it should be avoided in the evening hours. Finally, electroconvulsive therapy is an effective, safe method of rapidly treating depression and should be used for those who are severely depressed. The American Psychiatric Task Force Report states that electroconvulsive therapy be considered a first-line therapy when rapid response is needed (SOE=D). The presence of space-occupying CNS lesions is an important contraindication. See also "Depression and Other Mood Disorders," p 295.

Dyspnea

Dyspnea, the subjective experience of breathlessness, is one of the most distressing symptoms experienced by dying individuals. Patient self-report is the only reliable measure of dyspnea, because respiratory rates and laboratory tests often do not correlate with breathlessness. Physicians may mistakenly fear that treating dyspnea in patients close to the end of life is associated with unacceptably high risks, leading some to withhold treatment and others to prescribe inadequate dosages of medications, which will not alleviate the patient's suffering.

Because breathlessness has many causes (eg, anxiety, airway obstruction, bronchospasm, hypoxemia, pneumonia), symptomatic management should begin immediately while the underlying cause is being investigated. Like pain, dyspnea is mediated through the interaction of complex pathophysiologic processes with poorly defined psychologic factors. At a physiologic level, dyspnea results from the interplay of chemoreceptors in the respiratory tract and CNS, upper airway receptors that sense the mechanical effect of airflow or the temperature changes that accompany it, stretch receptors in chest wall skeletal muscles, irritant receptors in the airway epithelium, and C fibers located in the alveolar wall and blood vessels. The experience of dyspnea, however, depends on the modulation of these physiologic events by psychologic factors and, as a consequence, the patient's perception of dyspnea may not correlate well with objective signs such as respiratory rate, pulmonary congestion, hypoxia, or hypercarbia.

The optimal therapy for dyspnea is to treat its underlying cause. When this is not possible, one of a number of agents that have been evaluated for treatment of intractable dyspnea might be used. Oxygen is considered by many to be an important component of any regimen, although caution must be used for patients retaining carbon dioxide. Although oxygen is usually used only when oxygen saturation falls to <90%, there are some circumstances when oxygen can reduce dyspnea when this saturation value is exceeded (SOE=D). Cool air moving across the face (eg, from fans or an open window) can also treat dyspnea by stimulating the second branch of the fifth cranial nerve, which has a central inhibitory effect on the sensation of breathlessness (SOE=C).

Several centrally acting agents have been evaluated for the treatment of intractable dyspnea. Benzodiazepines may be beneficial in controlling the anxiety associated with dyspnea, but they have not improved breathlessness in randomized controlled trials involving nonanxious persons with COPD (SOE=A). The fact that respiration can be depressed after benzodiazepine administration in healthy adults suggests that these medications should be used only in breathless patients with an accompanying component of anxiety. In studies using phenothiazines and the phenothiazine antihistamine promethazine[OL], dyspnea has mildly improved (SOE=C). However, anticholinergic and sedative adverse events can limit the use of these medications in older patients.

The most widely used centrally active agents for the treatment of dyspnea are opioids. Opioids are believed to act via a number of different mechanisms, although their predominant effect appears to be a reduction in the central respiratory responsiveness to carbon dioxide, resulting in a decrease in respiratory drive. The increase in PCO_2 that often accompanies this respiratory suppression can occasionally limit this approach in management of dyspnea because of somnolence induced by the hypercarbia and by a decreased respiratory response to hypoxia. Opioids also appear to act centrally by decreasing the perception of dyspnea and peripherally on opioid receptors in the lung, perhaps by decreasing ventilatory response to, and oxygen cost of, exercise without affecting respiratory drive. In randomized controlled trials, both oral and parenteral formulations were effective (SOE=A). Anecdotal evidence supports the use of nebulized morphine for intractable dyspnea, but studies supporting this approach are lacking (SOE=D). The purported advantages of nebulized morphine include the avoidance of systemic absorption and the resulting constipation, hypotension, sedation, respiratory depression, and hypercapnia; rapid and efficient absorption because of the large surface area of the lung parenchyma; and ease of administration. However, given the lack of supporting evidence, this route of administration should be reserved for patients who experience intolerable adverse events from opioids administered by other routes.

Cough

Cough is a common symptom; its prevalence has been reported in the palliative care literature as ranging from 29% to 83%. Normal cough maintains the patency and cleanliness of the airways and thus should be treated only when distressing to the patient. Cough can be caused by the production of excessive amounts of fluids (eg, blood, mucus), inhalation of foreign material, or stimulation of irritant receptors in the airway. Additionally, patients with neuromuscular disorders may be unable to swallow saliva because of the involvement of bulbar cranial nerves, with the result that saliva causes coughing as it trickles into the larynx or trachea.

Underlying causes of cough should be investigated and treated (eg, diuretics for heart failure, antibiotics for infection, anticholinergics for aspiration of saliva resulting from motor neuron disease); how-ever, resolving the underlying cause may be impossible. Opioids can be useful in these situations.

Dextromethorphan is structurally related to opioids and has central cough-suppressant action with few sedative effects (SOE=D). Codeine and dihydrocodeine, usually in the form of elixirs, are also good first-line choices (SOE=D). Methadone syrup can also be helpful when taken as a single daily dose because of its longer duration of action (SOE=D).

Cough due to an irritated pharynx because of local infection or malignancy can be helped by nebulized anesthetics (SOE=D). Nebulized lidocaine up to four times daily has been reported, anecdotally, to offer relief.

LOUD RESPIRATION

Inability to clear secretions from the oropharynx often results in noisy or "rattling" respirations at the end of life. This occurs as secretions oscillate up and down during inspiration and expiration. Although there is no indication that this causes discomfort for patients, it often produces anxiety in family and caregivers. Best management includes preparing the family and caregivers for its occurrence and administering anticholinergic medications to reduce secretions. Because anticholinergic agents do not dry up secretions already present, it is important to educate the family to notify clinicians at the first sign of rattling. Scopalamine[OL] patches can be effective and also have a sedative effect. Hyoscyamine can also be administered by the sublingual route (0.125), or glycopyrrolate can be given subcutaneously at a dosage of 0.2 mg q8h. When pooling oral secretions are problematic, caregivers may be able to periodically remove secretions by use of a suction device; alternatively, atropine[OL] eyedrops can be given on or under the tongue.

ACOVE-3* QUALITY INDICATORS PERTAINING TO PALLIATIVE CARE

Follow treatment preferences

- If a vulnerable older adult has documented treatment preferences to withhold or withdraw life-sustaining treatment (eg, do-not-resuscitate order, no tube feeding, no hospital transfer), then these treatment preferences should be followed.

End-of-life care preferences and management

- If a vulnerable older adult dies an expected death with metastatic cancer, oxygen-dependent pulmonary disease, New York Heart Association (NYHA) Class III–IV congestive heart failure (CHF), end-stage liver disease, end-stage renal disease, or dementia, then the chart should document the following within the 6 mo before death:
  - Pain and other symptoms
  - Spiritual and existential concerns
  - Caregiver burdens and need for practical assistance
  - Advance care planning
- If a vulnerable older adult dies an expected death with metastatic cancer, oxygen-dependent pulmonary disease, NYHA Class III–IV CHF, end-stage liver disease, end-stage renal disease, or dementia, then the chart should document one of the following within the 6 mo before death:
  - Discussion of the medical condition and goals for treatment with a designated surrogate
  - Patient's preference for not involving a designated surrogate in discussions
  - Note that a surrogate decision maker is unavailable

Gastrostomy tube placement

■ If a vulnerable older adult with dementia has a gastrostomy or jejunum tube placed, then before placement, the medical record should document one of the following:

○ Patient preferences concerning tube feeding

○ If patient is decisionally incapacitated and a surrogate decision maker is available, discussion of patient preferences or best interests

○ If patient is decisionally incapacitated and a surrogate decision maker is not available, a formal decision mechanism should be used.

Dyspnea assessment

■ If a vulnerable older adult is diagnosed with lung cancer or cancer metastatic to the lungs, NYHA Class III–IV CHF, or oxygen-dependent pulmonary disease, then a self-reported assessment of dyspnea should be documented in the outpatient chart.

Treatment of dyspnea

■ If a vulnerable older adult with metastatic cancer or oxygen-dependent pulmonary disease has dyspnea refractory to nonopioid medications, then opioid medications should be offered.

Management of emergent dyspnea

■ If a vulnerable older adult is in hospice or has a preference for no hospitalization and is living with oxygen-dependent pulmonary disease, lung cancer, or NYHA Class III–IV CHF, then the medical record should document a plan for management of worsening or emergent dyspnea.

■ If a vulnerable older adult who had dyspnea in the last 7 days of life died an expected death, then the chart should document dyspnea care and follow-up.

Mechanical ventilator withdrawal

■ If a noncomatose vulnerable older adult is not expected to survive, and a mechanical ventilator is withdrawn or withheld, then the chart should document whether the patient has dyspnea, and the patient should receive (or have orders available for) an infusion of an opioid, benzodiazepine, or barbiturate infusion.

Management of emergent pain

■ If a vulnerable older adult with end-stage metastatic cancer is treated with opioids for pain, then the medical record should document a plan for management of worsening or emergent pain.

■ If a vulnerable older adult who was conscious during the last 7 days of life died an expected death, then the medical record should contain documentation about presence or absence of pain during the last 7 days of life.

Management of emergent obstruction

■ If a vulnerable older adult with end-stage metastatic cancer has obstructive GI symptoms, then the medical record should document a plan for management of worsening or emergent nausea and vomiting.

Caregiver stress

■ If a vulnerable older adult is a caregiver for a spouse, significant other, or dependent who is terminally ill or has very limited function, then the vulnerable older adult should be assessed for caregiver financial, physical, and emotional stress.

Bereavement

■ If a vulnerable older adult's spouse or significant other dies, then the vulnerable older adult should be assessed for depression or thoughts of suicidality within 6 mo.

Related quality indicators for Palliative Care

■ Decision-making, care preferences at the end of life (see "Legal and Ethical Issues," p 23)

■ Treatment of persistent pain (see "Persistent Pain," p 109)

*Assessing Care of Vulnerable Elders – 3ʳᵈ Set. See inside front cover for explanation.

REFERENCES

■ Lorenz KA, Lynn J, Dy SM, et al. Evidence for improving palliative care at the end of life: a systematic review. *Ann Intern Med.* 2008;148(2):147–159.

■ Mahler A. The clinical nurse specialist role in developing a geropalliative model of care. *Clin Nurse Spec.* 2010;24(1):18–23.

■ Morrison RS, Meier DE. Clinical Practice. Palliative care. *N Engl J Med.* 2004;350(25):2582–2590.

■ Phillips RS, Hamel MB, Covinsky KE, et al. Findings from SUPPORT and HELP: Study to Understand Prognoses and Preferences for Outcomes and Risks of Treatment; Hospitalized Elderly Longitudinal Project. *J Am Geriatr Soc.* 2000;48(Suppl 5):S1–S233.

CHAPTER 15—PERSISTENT PAIN

KEY POINTS

- Pain requires a thorough assessment to determine its source, severity, and impact on the functioning and well-being of the patient.

- Multiple pain scales are available to help quantify the severity of pain. The selection of a pain scale is based on the cognitive and communication abilities of the patient.

- A stepped approach to the treatment of pain is advised; local therapies and nonpharmacologic approaches, such as heat, cold, or massage, should be considered to reduce or eliminate the systemic therapies that have greater risk of toxicity. However, systemic analgesics should not be withheld if needed in the treatment of older adults.

- Tolerance generally develops to the respiratory depression, fatigue, and sedation effects of opioid analgesics but not to the constipating effect.

Pain, defined as an unpleasant sensory and emotional experience, is common in older adults ≥65 yr old. Studies have revealed that 25%–50% of community-dwelling older adults and 45%–80% of nursing-home residents have substantial pain. Pain is also believed to be commonly undertreated. This is due to several factors: some older adults tend to minimize or not report their symptoms, and others are unable to report their pain because of language or cognitive impairments. Also, clinicians may inadequately assess pain or undertreat it with ineffective therapies because more effective therapies can result in intolerable adverse effects.

This chapter describes the evaluation and treatment of persistent pain. In contrast to acute pain, persistent pain is pain that lasts 3–6 mo or longer after the original injury has healed, pain that is associated with a chronic medical condition, or pain that recurs at intervals of a month to years.

Persistent pain is complex, involving an amalgamation of physical, social, and psychologic factors. Untreated, it can result in difficulty performing ADLs, cognitive dysfunction, depression, anxiety, social isolation, appetite impairment, and sleep disorders. In addition, patients with chronic pain accrue greater healthcare costs than patients who are pain-free.

ASSESSMENT

A major barrier to effective pain treatment is inadequate assessment. A thorough assessment is necessary to formulate a plan to successfully treat persistent pain. This assessment should include an examination of physical, emotional, and social function, recognizing the considerable impact that each of these domains has on the experience of pain and suffering and the impact of persistent pain on each of these domains on well-being. Because there are no blood tests or imaging modalities to measure pain objectively, clinicians must rely on the patient's or caregiver's description of the pain and on the findings of a thorough physical examination. The goal of the assessment is to identify the source of the pain so that it can be treated with the most effective, targeted, and specific treatment known. Assessment is complicated by several factors, including under-reporting of symptoms by many older adults, the existence of multiple medical comorbidities exacerbating the pain and impairing patient function, and the increased prevalence of cognitive impairment as people age.

Initial evaluation begins with a complete history of the pain, including inquiry about the character of the pain and its course of onset, duration, and location. Patients should be asked what relieves and exacerbates their pain. The patient's functional status needs to be carefully evaluated to determine his or her ability to perform ADLs and IADLs to help determine the effect pain may be having on function. The patient's cognitive state, participation in social activities, mood, and quality of life are all components of a complete evaluation.

Pain intensity can be quantified using pain intensity scales. Three commonly used, validated scales are the Numeric Rating Scale, the Faces Pain Scale, and the Verbal Descriptor Scale. These scales are referred to as unidimensional because they ask the patient to rate the intensity of a single characteristic of the symptom, in this case the intensity of the pain. The patient is asked to rate his or her pain by assigning a numerical value (with 0 indicating no pain and 10 representing the worst pain imaginable), a verbal description ("no pain" to "pain as bad as it could be"), or a facial expression corresponding to the pain. The choice of scale depends on the presence of a particular language or sensory impairment. For example, if the patient does not speak English well, the faces scale may be the best choice because it

---

STRENGTH-OF-EVIDENCE (SOE) RATING DEFINITIONS

A = consistent and good quality patient-oriented evidence
B = somewhat inconsistent or limited quality patient-oriented evidence
C = very inconsistent or very limited patient-oriented evidence, disease-oriented evidence, and/or consensus from professional organizations
D = unstudied common practice or opinion

See inside front cover for detailed information regarding the SOE classification.

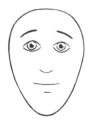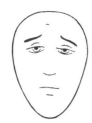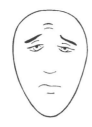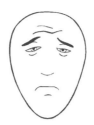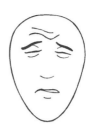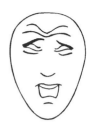

Figure 15.1—Faces Pain Scale–Revised (FPS-R)

Instruct the patient to identify which face best represents the pain he or she is feeling at that moment. Explain, "These faces show how much pain a person is feeling inside. On one end, the face is happy because the person is feeling no pain (point to the left most face). On the other end, the person is in the most pain anyone can imagine (point to the right most face). In between (point to each face from left to right), the faces show more and more pain. Point to the face that best shows the pain you are feeling now." Each face has been assigned a numerical score (0, 2, 4, 6, 8, 10). Record the score that corresponds to the face selected.

SOURCE: Hicks CL, von Baeyer CL, Spafford P, et al. The Faces Pain Scale–Revised: Toward a common metric in pediatric pain measurement. *Pain.* 2001;93:173–183. Bieri D, Reeve R, Champion GD, et al. The Faces Pain Scale for the self-assessment of the severity of pain experienced by children: Development, initial validation and preliminary investigation for ratio scale properties. *Pain.* 1990;41:139–150.

This figure has been reproduced with permission of the International Association for the Study of Pain® (IASP®). The figure may not be reproduced for any other purpose without permission.

relies on pictures rather than on words or numbers (Figure 15.1). The same scale should be used at follow-up examinations to evaluate how the pain has changed since the initial assessment. Scales such as the McGill Pain Questionnaire and the Pain Disability Scale measure pain in a variety of domains, including the intensity, location, and affect. Although lengthy, scales measuring multiple domains can provide a wealth of information about the patient's unique experience of pain.

Before the physical examination, the patient can be asked to describe the location of the pain using a drawing of a human figure, called a pain map. The patient can indicate the locations on the figure that corresponds to their own pain. Pain maps can enhance patient-clinician communication. If the patient's pain pattern is erratic and diffuse or does not conform to an anatomic distribution, referral to a mental health specialist may be appropriate to evaluate for affective disorder contributing to the discomfort.

The physical examination should include a careful examination of the reported site of the pain and any part of the body that may be a source of referred pain. The initial evaluation should include a complete musculoskeletal examination, recognizing the common findings of musculoskeletal disorders such as fibromyalgia, osteoarthritis, and myofascial pain as either the primary source of pain or an exacerbating process. Accurate diagnosis of these disorders is a critical part of formulating the correct therapeutic plan (see treatment, below). Fibromyalgia may be under-recognized in older adults. It is typically characterized by multiple tender points, sleep disturbance, fatigue, generalized pain (often with a strong axial component), and morning stiffness. Myofascial

pain is present in the vast majority of patients with persistent pain and is diagnosed by the presence of taut bands of muscles and trigger points (ie, pain that may radiate distally when firm pressure is applied to a muscle, as opposed to tender points, in which radiation of pain is absent).

Pain syndromes can be divided into at least three types: nociceptive, neuropathic, and mixed or unspecified. Nociceptive pain describes pain due to the activation of nociceptive sensory receptors by noxious stimuli resulting from inflammation, swelling, and injury to tissues. It can be defined further as either somatic or visceral pain. Somatic pain is well localized in skin, soft tissue, and bone. It is commonly described as throbbing, aching, and stabbing. Visceral pain, due to cardiac, GI, and lung injury, is not well localized and difficult to describe. Patients describe visceral pain as crampy, tearing, dull, and aching. Nociceptive pain is often adequately treated with common analgesics.

Neuropathic pain derives from the irritation of components of the central or peripheral nervous system. Patients typically report burning, numbness with "pins and needles" sensations, and shooting pains. Common causes of neuropathic pain include diabetic neuropathy and post-herpetic neuralgia, while central pain after stroke and phantom limb pain experienced after amputation are less common but often severe. Confusion between neuropathic pain and myofascial pain is possible, because patients may describe both as "burning." Careful physical examination will help to differentiate these disorders (ie, taut bands and trigger points with myofascial pain and allodynia or hyperalgesia with either disorder), although both may be present in the same patient. Neuropathic pain responds unpredictably to opioid analgesia; it may respond well to nonopioid therapies such as anticonvulsants, tricyclic antidepressants, and antiarrhythmic medications.

Mixed or unspecified pain is described as having characteristics of both nociceptive pain and neuropathic pain. An example of a mixed pain syndrome is chronic headaches of unknown causes. Older adults often have mixed pain syndromes. Lower back pain, for example, is often a combination of spinal malalignment, myofascial pathology, and neurologic impingement. Treating these patients with trials of different medications or with combinations of medicines may be necessary.

ASSESSING AND TREATING PAIN IN COGNITIVELY IMPAIRED ADULTS

While they are able to speak, patients with mild to moderate dementia are often able to self-report pain and localize it. Patients with severe cognitive impairment who are unable to verbally express pain pose a challenge to the clinicians who care for them. Not only are they unable to describe their pain and request analgesia, but clinicians may be hesitant to administer pain medications, fearing that pharmacologic treatment will worsen the patients' mental status. Clinicians must rely on observing the patient for possible pain-related behaviors as well as on noting observations reported by the patient's caregivers. For common pain behaviors in cognitively impaired older adults, see Table 15.2. Validated scales such as the Hurley Discomfort Scale and the Checklist of Nonverbal Pain Indicators have been developed; however, these require trained evaluators to complete properly. Experts suggest providing empiric analgesic therapy during procedures and conditions known to be painful. Trials of analgesia should also be considered for patients exhibiting potentially pain-related behaviors.

TREATMENT

Fundamental Approaches to Pain Treatment

Nonpharmacologic Therapy

A comprehensive review of nonpharmacologic therapies for persistent pain is beyond the scope of this chapter; however, specific therapies are worth mentioning. Many of the strategies mentioned below are appropriate suggestions for all patients' treatment plans, and highlight the importance of an interdisciplinary approach to pain treatment.

Table 15.1—Common Pain Behaviors in Cognitively Impaired Older Adults

Behavior	Examples
Facial expressions	Slight frown; sad, frightened face
	Grimacing, wrinkled forehead, closed or tightened eyes
	Any distorted expression
	Rapid blinking
Verbalizations, vocalizations	Sighing, moaning, groaning, grunting, chanting, calling out
	Noisy breathing
	Asking for help
	Verbal abusiveness
Body movements	Rigid or tense body posture, guarding
	Fidgeting
	Increased pacing, rocking
	Restricted movement
	Gait or mobility changes
Changes in interpersonal interactions	Aggressive, combative, resists care
	Decreased social interactions
	Socially inappropriate, disruptive
	Withdrawn
Changes in activity patterns or routines	Refusing food, appetite change
	Increase in rest periods
	Change in sleep or rest pattern
	Sudden cessation of common routines
	Increased wandering
Mental status changes	Crying or tears
	Increased confusion
	Irritability or distress

NOTE: Some patients demonstrate little or no specific behavior associated with severe pain.
SOURCE: American Geriatrics Society Panel on Persistent Pain in Older Persons. The management of persistent pain in older persons. *J Am Geriatr Soc.* 2002;50(6 Suppl):S211. Reprinted with permission.

Patient education and involvement in treatment decisions are an important part of all treatment plans for persistent pain. Patients should be taught how to take medications properly and how to use assessment instruments. Data also suggest that providing partner-guided pain management training to caregivers can lead to decreased discomfort and increased psychologic and social function experienced by older adults (SOE=B).

Psychologic interventions and cognitive-behavioral therapy (CBT) are also important tools for treatment of persistent pain (SOE=B). Recognizing the common overlap of depression, anxiety, and other mood disturbances should prompt early consultation with mental health professionals. In CBT, patients are asked to track their pain and record the thoughts that are associated with the pain experience to identify maladaptive coping strategies. By conscientiously replacing these maladaptive strategies with positive coping strategies, patients can increase control over pain and self-efficacy, leading to decreased perception of pain. CBT can be particularly useful in helping patients learn to cope with the stresses of persistent pain. When possible, family members and caregivers should be included in the therapy.

✓Regular physical activity has been shown to decrease pain scores, improve mood, boost functional status, and stabilize gait (SOE=A). Referral to the Arthritis Foundation or to community resources such as the YMCA for exercise classes can be considered for many patients. Frail older adults may require closely monitored rehabilitation services. For patients with advanced illness who are bed-bound, regular repositioning and gentle massage are key interventions. The goals should include improvements in flexibility, strength, endurance, and function, with reduced pain and improved quality of life.

✓Referral to a pain clinic that is geared toward an interdisciplinary team approach to treatment may be useful for patients with complex pain or who are poorly responsive to first-line treatments. Data support the use of many physical therapies such as massage therapy, acupuncture, heat/cold therapy, and transcutaneous electrical nerve stimulation (TENS) units (SOE=B). Interdisciplinary team members may also incorporate other cognitive techniques into the treatment plan such as hypnosis, aromatherapy, biofeedback, music and pet therapy, and systematic desensitization. Finally, some patients may require referral for intensive therapies such as radiation therapy for bone metastases or palliative surgery for bowel obstruction. Suboptimal treatment response should not be viewed as a permanent state, but as an opportunity for input from specialists who have additional expertise in treating these difficult problems.

See also "Complementary and Alternative Medicine," p 81.

Pharmacologic Therapy

For selected analgesics, with their starting dosages and common adverse events, see Table 15.3.

Pharmacologic therapy for patients with persistent pain should be viewed not only as an end, but as a means to promote improved function and enhance adherence with rehabilitation efforts. When starting pharmacologic therapy in older adults, the risks and benefits of the treatment should be considered and balanced carefully. If appropriate, nonsystemic therapies should be tried first. For example, patients that primarily have knee pain might respond to intra-articular corticosteroid injections, avoiding the need for systemic analgesics. However, convincing data supporting the use of intra-articular injections for knee pain are lacking. Patients with myofascial pain often respond to local treatments such as massage, gentle stretching exercises, ultrasound, and trigger-point injections (SOE=B). Topical preparations

Table 15.2—Systemic Pharmacotherapy for Persistent Pain Management

Medication	Starting Dosage*	Usual Effective Dosage (Maximal Dosage)	Titration	Comments
NONOPIOIDS				
Acetaminophen (Tylenol)	325 mg q4h to 500 mg q6h	2–4 g/d (4 g/d)	After 4–6 doses	Reduce maximal dosage 50%–75% in patients with hepatic insufficiency or history of alcohol abuse.
Anticonvulsants				
Carbamazepine[OL] (Tegretol)	100 mg/d	800–1,200 mg/d (2,400 mg/d)	After 3–5 days	Monitor liver enzymes, CBC, BUN/creatinine, electrolytes, and carbamazepine levels. Approved only for trigeminal neuralgia and glossopharyngeal neuralgia; not approved for any other types of pain. Multiple drug interactions.
Clonazepam[OL] (Klonopin)	0.25–0.5 mg hs	0.05–0.2 mg/kg/d (20 mg)	After 3–5 days	Monitor sedation, memory, CBC.
Gabapentin[OL] (Neurontin)	100 mg hs	300–900 mg q8h (3,600 mg)	After 1–2 days	Monitor sedation, ataxia, edema. Approved for post-herpetic neuralgia; not approved for any other types of pain.
Pregabalin (Lyrica)	50 mg hs	300 mg/d	After 7 days	Monitor sedation, ataxia, edema.
Antidepressants				
Tricyclic antidepressants:** desipramine[OL] (Norpramin), nortriptyline[OL] (Aventyl, Pamelor)	10 mg hs	25–100 mg hs (variable, but older adults rarely tolerate doses >75–100 mg)	After 3–5 days	Significant risk of adverse events in older adults; anticholinergic effects

Medication	Starting Dosage*	Usual Effective Dosage (Maximal Dosage)	Titration	Comments
Duloxetine (Cymbalta)	20 mg/d	60 mg/d	After 7 days	Monitor blood pressure, dizziness, cognitive effects and memory; multiple drug–drug interactions.
Venlafaxine (Effexor)	37.5 mg/d	75−225 mg/d (225 mg/d)	After 4−7 days	Associated with dose-related increases in blood pressure and heart rate
Milnacipran (Savella)	12.5 mg/d	50 mg q12h (variable)	See package insert for titration recommendations; discontinuation requires tapering.	Reduce dosage by 50% with CrCl <30 mL/min. Common reactions include nausea, constipation, hot flashes, hyperhidrosis, palpitations, dry mouth, hypertension. Contraindicated with MAOIs and narrow-angle glaucoma.
Mexiletine[OL] (Mexitil)	150 mg q12h	150 mg q6−8h (variable)	After 3–5 days	Avoid use in patients with conduction block, bradyarrhythmia; monitor ECG at baseline and after dose stabilization.
NSAIDs				Use with caution in older adults, if at all.
Celecoxib (Celebrex)	100 mg/d	100−400 mg/d		Higher dosages associated with higher incidence of GI, cardiovascular adverse events. Patients with indications for cardioprotection require aspirin supplement; therefore, older adults still require concurrent gastroprotection.
Naproxen sodium	OTC: 220 mg q12h Rx: 250 mg q6−8h	OTC: 440−660 mg/day (660 mg/d) Rx: 250–500 mg q8–12h (1,000 mg/d)		Several studies implicate this agent as having less cardiovascular toxicity.
Ibuprofen	OTC: 200 mg q8h Rx: 400 mg	400−800 mg q6−8h (3,200 mg/d)		FDA indicates concurrent use with aspirin inhibits aspirin's antiplatelet effect, but the true clinical import of this remains to be elucidated, and it remains unclear whether this is unique to ibuprofen or true with other NSAIDs.
Diclofenac sodium	50 mg q12h or 75 mg extended release daily	100−150 mg/d (150 mg/d)		May be associated with higher cardiovascular risk than other traditional NSAIDs owing to its relative cyclooxygenase-2 inhibitor selectivity.
Nabumetone (Relafen)	1 g/d	1−2 g/d (2g/d)		Relatively long half-life and minimal antiplatelet effect (>5 days).
Ketorolac				Not recommended. High potential for GI and renal toxicity; inappropriate for long-term use.
Salsalate (eg, Disalcid, Mono-Gesic, Salflex)	500–750 mg q12h	1,500–3,000 mg/d (3,000 mg/d)	After 4–6 doses	In frail patients or those with diminished hepatic or renal function, checking salicylate levels during dosage titration and after steady state is reached may be important.

OPIOIDS

Medication	Starting Dosage*	Usual Effective Dosage (Maximal Dosage)	Titration	Comments
Hydrocodone (eg, Lorcet, Lortab, Vicodin, Vicoprofen)	2.5–5 mg q4–6h	5–10 mg (see comments)	After 3–4 doses	Useful for acute recurrent, episodic, or breakthrough pain; daily dose limited by fixed-dose combinations with acetaminophen or NSAIDs. NSAIDS should be used with caution in older adults, if at all.

Table 15.2—Systemic Pharmacotherapy for Persistent Pain Management (continued)

Medication	Starting Dosage*	Usual Effective Dosage (Maximal Dosage)	Titration	Comments
Hydromorphone (Dilaudid, Hydrostat)	1–2 mg q3–4h	variable (variable)	After 3–4 doses	For breakthrough pain or around-the-clock dosing
Morphine, immediate release (eg, MSIR, Roxanol)	2.5–10 mg q4h	variable (variable)	After 1–2 doses	Oral liquid concentrate or tablet recommended for breakthrough pain.
Morphine, sustained release (eg, MSContin, Kadian)	15 mg q8–24h (see dosing guidelines in package insert for each specific formulation)	variable (variable)	After 3–5 days	Usually started after initial dose determined by effects of immediate-release opioid; toxic metabolites of morphine can limit usefulness in patients with renal insufficiency or when high-dose therapy is required; continuous-release formulations may require more frequent dosing if pain returns regularly at end of dose. Significant interactions with food and alcohol.
Oxycodone, immediate release (OxyIR, Percocet, Percodan, Tylox, Combunox)	2.5–5 mg q4–6h	5–10 mg (see comments)	After 3–4 doses	Useful for acute recurrent, episodic, or breakthrough pain; daily dose limited by fixed-dose combinations with acetaminophen or NSAIDs. NSAIDs should be used with caution in older adults, if at all. The specific oxycodone preparation being prescribed should be indicated to avoid toxicity from multiple analgesics.
Oxycodone, sustained release (OxyContin)	10 mg q12h	variable (variable)	After 3–5 days	Usually started after initial dose determined by effects of immediate-release opioid. Though intended for 12-hour dosing, some individuals may need shorter (every 8 hours) or longer (daily) dosing.
Tapentadol (Nucynta)	50–100 mg q4–6h prn	50–100 mg q4–6h prn (600 mg/d)		Avoid use of serotonergic agents (SSRIs, SNRIs, tricyclic antidepressants).
Tramadol (Ultram)	12.5–25 mg q4–6h	50–100 mg (300 mg/d)	After 4–6 doses	Mixed opioid and central neurotransmitter mechanism of action; monitor for opioid adverse events, including drowsiness, constipation, and nausea. Exert caution when used with another serotonergic drug, and observe for symptoms of serotonergic syndrome. Lowers seizure threshold.
Transdermal fentanyl (Duragesic)	12–25 mcg/h patch q72h	variable (variable)	After 2–3 patch changes	Usually started after initial dose determined by effects of immediate-release opioid; currently available lowest dose patch (25 mcg/h) recommended for patients who require <60 mg/24-hour oral morphine equivalents; peak effects of first dose takes 18–24 hours. Duration of effect is usually 3 days, but may range from 48 to 96 hours. May take 2 to 3 patch changes before steady state blood levels are reached.

NOTE: DEA = U.S. Drug Enforcement Agency; hs = at bedtime; NA = not applicable; CrCl = creatinine clearance; MAOI = monoamine oxidase inhibitor

* Oral dosing unless otherwise specified.

** Amitriptyline is not recommended.

SOURCE: Adapted with permission from American Geriatrics Society Panel on the Pharmacologic Management of Persistent Pain in Older Persons. Pharmacological management of persistent pain in older persons. *J Am Geriatr Soc.* 2009;57(8):1331–1346.

such as capsaicin or ketamine gel[OL] or lidocaine patches might be effective as primary or adjunctive therapy for treating neuropathic or myofascial pain syndromes (SOE=C). If these local therapies are ineffective and a decision is made to begin systemic therapy, older adults need to be monitored closely to ensure that the treatment is effective and to minimize adverse effects. Choice of initial dose and rate of titition depends on the individual patient's physiology, which varies considerably in older adults. In general, it is prudent to start opioid therapy at the lowest dosage possible and to titrate slowly. That said, medications should not be withheld from patients who are in a pain crisis. Rather, these patients need to be monitored closely to ensure that the dosage can be safely and adequately increased.

Acetaminophen provides adequate analgesia for many mild to moderate pain syndromes, particularly musculoskeletal pain from osteoarthritis, and is recommended as first-line therapy for persistent pain. No more than 4 g of acetaminophen every 24 hours should be administered to patients with normal hepatic and renal function, given the risk of hepatotoxicity at higher doses. Patients at risk of liver dysfunction, particularly those who have a history of heavy alcohol intake, should be treated cautiously; in these patients, the dosage should be decreased by 50%, or acetaminophen should be avoided. Acetaminophen is commonly contained in many OTC and prescription products; therefore, knowledge of all medications that a patient is taking is critical to avoiding acetaminophen toxicity. NSAIDs tend to be more effective than acetaminophen in chronic inflammatory pain but pose significantly higher threats to older adults so must be used judiciously if they are considered at all, and only after acetaminophen has been tried and only in highly select individuals. Significant adverse events, including renal dysfunction, GI bleeding, platelet dysfunction, fluid retention, precipitation of heart failure, and precipitation of delirium, limit their use in the treatment of chronic pain in older adults. The FDA has issued a particular caution against using ibuprofen with aspirin, owing to an interaction that blocks the antiplatelet effect of the aspirin. COX-2 inhibitors were developed to decrease the risk of GI bleeding by acting on a more selective receptor, but the risk of renal complications, including hypertension, remains the same as with other NSAIDs, and the degree to which longer-term GI toxicity is reduced is not clear. Several studies have confirmed high cardiovascular risks associated with COX-2 inhibitors, which is now believed to be a class effect. Although one is currently still on the market, the COX-2s should be considered with caution—if at all—in older adults. Misoprostol, a prostaglandin analogue, or a proton-pump inhibitor can be used to reduce the risk of NSAID-induced GI bleeding, but this does not reduce the risks of renal disease, hypertension, fluid retention, or delirium. Alternatively, nonacetylated salicylates such as salsalate and trisalicylate may have less renal toxicity and antiplatelet activity than other NSAIDs and therefore

may be preferable in older adults, although evidence supporting this theory is sparse. Topical NSAIDs appear to be safe and effective in the short term, but longer-term studies are lacking.

Moderate to severe pain or pain that requires chronic treatment often requires opioid medications for sufficient relief, though evidence elucidating their role in persistent noncancer pain is not well established. In general, continuous pain should be treated with 24-hour pain medications in long-acting or sustained-release formulations after opioid requirements have been estimated by an initial trial of a short-acting agent. Fast-onset medications with short half-lives may be added to cover breakthrough pain. A typical patient requires approximately 5%–15% the total daily dose offered every 2 hours orally for breakthrough pain. In general, different opioids provide similar analgesic efficacy. Cost and route of delivery can help guide the choice of medication.

Opioids are metabolized by the liver and excreted by the kidney. In kidney failure, the active metabolites of morphine, including morphine-6-glucuronide and morphine-3-glucuronide, can accumulate, increasing the risk of prolonged sedation and possible neurotoxicity. The dosing intervals should be increased and the dosage decreased to reduce this risk. Hydromorphone has fewer adverse events in patients with renal failure, and is therefore many experts' first choice for this population (SOE=C). In addition, some experts and limited data suggest that oxycodone is safer in patients with kidney failure because its metabolism results in fewer active metabolites, but this remains controversial (SOE=C).

Barriers to Using Opioids in Older Adults

Older adults may have concerns about tolerance and addiction that keep them from accepting adequate treatment for their pain. They may fear that taking opioid therapy for their current level of pain will result in the medication losing its effectiveness in the future when pain becomes more severe. Fear of addiction is a major obstacle to prescribing medications for older adults. A frank discussion of these concerns may help to alleviate these fears.

Physical dependence is an expected change in a patient's physiology that occurs while a patient is receiving chronic, continual opioid medications. If opioids are discontinued suddenly, patients who are physically dependent experience a withdrawal syndrome that may include restlessness, tachycardia, hypertension, fever, tremors, and lacrimation. Symptoms of withdrawal can be avoided by tapering opioids carefully over days to weeks. *Tolerance* refers to a change in physiology resulting in the need to increase opioid medicines over time to achieve adequate analgesic effect. Experts note that tolerance to analgesia, as opposed to tolerance to sedation and respiratory depression, develops slowly in stable disease. If medicines must be titrated rapidly to reduce pain, the cause of the pain should be evaluated, including searching for new pathologies and exacerbation of known sources of pain, as well as consideration of nonphysical factors. Of note, there is limited cross-tolerance between different opioids. Therefore, when switching a patient from one opioid to another (eg, morphine to oxycodone), the clinician should reduce the dosage to 50%–65% of the equivalent dosage.

Psychologic *dependence*, or true *addiction*, refers to a psychiatric state defined by compulsive drug seeking and drug using with disregard for adverse social, physical, and economic consequences. It is very rare for patients who have chronic pain to become addicted to opioids, but opioid abuse can become a problem in certain individuals and the potential for abuse should be carefully discussed particularly in those with a prior history of addiction. Although opioid abuse is less common in older adults, clinicians should carefully monitor for misuse of this medication. Addiction must be distinguished from *pseudoaddiction*, which refers to a patient with significant unrelieved pain who adopts behaviors similar to those of truly addicted patients while seeking relief from suffering but generally with less prominent disregard for adverse social, physical, and economic consequences.

Adverse Events of Opioids

Respiratory depression is the most serious potential adverse effect associated with opioid use, but tolerance to this effect develops quickly. Older adults and individuals with a history of lung dysfunction are at particular risk when opioid dosages are increased too rapidly or when another sedative is taken concomitantly. Naloxone, an opioid-receptor antagonist, can reverse opioid-induced respiratory depression; however, when given to a patient who has been treated chronically with opioids, it can precipitate a pain crisis and acute withdrawal symptoms. Experts suggest withholding naloxone unless the patient's respiratory rate decreases to <8 breaths per minute or the oxygen saturation drops to <90%. When it is needed, naloxone should be titrated carefully, using the lowest dosage possible.

The most common adverse event of opioid treatment is constipation, and unfortunately, tolerance to this toxicity does not occur. Opioid-induced constipation is due to multiple mechanisms, including dehydration, decreased GI tract secretions, and decreased motility of the GI tract. Although tolerance develops fairly rapidly to other adverse events of opioids, such as respiratory depression and sedation, constipation usually complicates opioid use for the duration of treatment. Therefore, education regarding the probable need for long-term laxative treatment is recommended for all patients when opioid therapy is started. Many experts recommend starting therapy with a stimulant laxative (such as bisacodyl or senna); however, these should be avoided in any patient with signs or symptoms of bowel obstruction. Bulking agents such as fiber and psyllium should be avoided in patients who are inactive and who have poor oral fluid intake because of the risk of causing fecal impaction and obstruction. All patients should be encouraged to exercise, as they are able, and to stay well hydrated. For patients who develop opioid-induced constipation despite laxative therapy, treatment with methylnaltrexone, a mu-opioid-receptor antagonist, may relieve constipation without precipitating withdrawal symptoms or pain crisis (SOE=B).

Nausea and vomiting are common adverse events of opioids. They have a direct effect on the *chemoreceptor trigger zone*, the part of the brain associated with the sensation of vomiting. Other common causes of nausea and vomiting in patients taking opioids include gastroparesis, constipation, and metabolic disorders such as renal and hepatic failure. Although the nausea and vomiting usually resolve spontaneously after the first few doses, some patients experience chronic nausea. After evaluation for reversible causes of nausea such as constipation, some patients benefit from changing to an alternative opioid (SOE=D). Others may need to be treated with chronic antiemetics, accepting the high prevalence of adverse events in older adults treated with these medications, including drowsiness, delirium, and anticholinergic effects.

Older adults can experience sedation, fatigue, and mild cognitive impairment with opioid treatment. These symptoms are common during dosage adjustment. Patients commonly overcome the fatigue and sedation over days to weeks as they become tolerant to the medication. They need to be warned of the risks of increased falls and asked not to drive or operate heavy equipment when the medication is started. A small subset of patients treated with opioids experience incessant fatigue that limits their function significantly. A limited course of a stimulant such as low-dose methylphenidate could reasonably be tried in this situation (SOE=D). Rotation to a different opioid is an alternative strategy used to alleviate opioid-induced fatigue.

Nonopioid Medication to Treat Persistent Pain

Nonopioid or adjuvant medications can be used as the sole agent or in combination with opioids. These medications can be particularly useful in treating patients with neuropathic pain or mixed pain syndromes.

Tricyclic antidepressants (TCAs) are the most extensively studied medications for neuropathic pain, though none of the TCAs has been approved for the treatment of pain. Their efficacy in the treatment of post-herpetic neuralgia and diabetic neuropathy has been shown in numerous placebo-controlled studies (SOE=A). However, they are associated with significant anticholinergic adverse events in older adults, including constipation, urinary retention, dry mouth, cognitive impairment, tachycardia, and blurred vision. Of note, desipramine[OL] and nortriptyline[OL] may have fewer adverse events than amitriptyline[OL].

Clinical depression in patients with persistent pain requires treatment to achieve optimal analgesia and quality of life. Other classes of antidepressants (eg, SSRIs) have generally been less studied than TCAs as analgesics, but older adults typically tolerate these agents better than TCAs when they are used in antidepressant doses. Duloxetine, an inhibitor of norepinephrine and serotonin uptake, is approved both as an antidepressant and for the treatment of pain from diabetic neuropathy and may offer a more favorable adverse-event profile than the TCAs.

Anticonvulsant medications such as carbamazepine, gabapentin, pregabalin, and clonazepam[OL] are commonly used as treatments for neuropathic pain. Gabapentin and pregabalin have demonstrated clinical efficacy in the treatment of post-herpetic neuralgia, and have fewer adverse events than TCAs, although their cost is substantially more. The main adverse events of gabapentin and pregabalin are sedation and dizziness, which frequently limit dosage increases.

Corticosteroids are useful adjuvants to treat pain associated with swelling, inflammation, and tissue infiltration, as well as neuropathic pain (SOE=C). In addition to their analgesic properties, they also can increase appetite and improve energy, although weight gained is predominantly fluid and fat rather than muscle. Adverse events seen with short-term use of steroids include psychosis, fluid retention, hair loss, loss of skin integrity, hyperglycemia, and immunosuppression. Corticosteroid use should be limited to clearly inflammatory conditions and metastatic bone pain, and even then used with caution. Intravenous bisphosphonates can substantially reduce pain from malignant bone metastases (SOE=B).

Tramadol has combined mechanisms binding opioid receptors and inhibiting reuptake of norepinephrine and serotonin. It can lower the seizure threshold and is therefore not recommended for patients who have a history of seizures or are taking other medications that could lower the seizure threshold. Caution should also be exercised in patients taking other medications that have serotonergic properties to avoid serotonin syndrome (ie, myoclonus, agitation, abdominal cramping, hyperpyrexia, hypertension, and potentially death).

Medications to Avoid in Older Adults

Several medications should not be administered to older adults. Propoxyphene is an older opioid medication used to treat mild to moderate pain. However, research and clinical experience has shown that it can accumulate in older adults and cause ataxia and dizziness as well as tremulousness and seizures. It has also never been shown to be a more effective analgesic than placebo (SOE=B). In November 2010, the manufacturers of the brand propoxyphene products (Darvon and Darvocet), in conjunction with the FDA, agreed to withdraw both products from the U.S. market. The FDA requested that all generic manufacturers of propoxyphene also voluntarily withdraw their products from the market. This action was due to the results of a study demonstrating an increased risk of potentially serious and fatal cardiac rhythm abnormalities with propoxyphene. Meperidine is metabolized to normeperidine, which has no analgesic properties but can accumulate in patients with decreased kidney function and cause tremulousness, myoclonus, and seizures. Neither of these medications is recommended for use in older adults.

Mixed agonist-antagonists such as nalbuphine and butorphanol also have the potential to cause restlessness and tremulousness and therefore should be avoided in older adults. As noted above, owing to their toxicities, NSAIDs and COX-2 inhibitors should rarely, if ever, be used in older adults with persistent pain.

ACOVE-3* QUALITY INDICATORS PERTAINING TO PERSISTENT PAIN

Screening for persistent pain

- If a vulnerable older adult presents for an initial evaluation, then a quantitative and qualitative assessment for persistent pain should be documented. (If cognitively impaired, a standardized pain scale, behavioral assessment, or proxy report of pain should be used.)
- All vulnerable older adults should be screened for persistent pain annually.

Ask about pain at cancer visits

- If a vulnerable older adult presents for a cancer-related clinician visit, including visits for chemotherapy or radiation, then pain should be assessed.

Treat severe pain

- If an outpatient vulnerable older adult with cancer presents with severe pain (score >5 on a 0–10 scale or similar quantifiable measurement), then pain treatment should be adjusted.
- If a hospitalized vulnerable older adult has a new complaint of moderate to severe pain, then the medical record should indicate that an intervention and follow-up assessment of the pain occurred within 4 hours.

Education for persistent pain

- If a vulnerable older adult is new to a primary care practice and has persistent pain, then there should be documentation of patient education within 6 mo that explains the likely cause of symptoms and how to use medication or other therapies.

Preventing constipation with opioids

- If a vulnerable older adult with persistent pain is treated with opioids, then one of the following should be prescribed or noted.
  - Fecal softener or laxative
  - Increased fiber, fecal-softening foods
  - Documentation of the potential for constipation or why bowel treatment is not needed

Reassessing pain control with opioids

- If a vulnerable older adult is started on new opioid therapy for persistent pain, then efficacy and adverse events should be assessed within 1 mo.

Avoid propoxyphene

- If a vulnerable older adult requires a new analgesic, then he or she should not be prescribed propoxyphene (*note*: voluntarily withdrawn from market in November 2010).

Avoid meperidine

- If a vulnerable older adult requires analgesia, then meperidine should not be prescribed.

Limit ketorolac

- If a vulnerable older adult receives ketorolac, then it should not be prescribed for >5 days.

Limit muscle relaxants

- If a vulnerable older adult receives prescription pharmacotherapy for back or neck pain, then cyclobenzaprine, methocarbamol, carisoprodol, chlorzoxazone, orphenadrine, tizanidine, or metaxalone should not be prescribed for >1 week.

Acetaminophen

- If a vulnerable older adult is prescribed chronic high-dose acetaminophen (≥3 g/d) or a vulnerable older adult with liver disease is prescribed chronic acetaminophen, then he or she should be advised of the risk of liver toxicity.

NSAIDs and aspirin

- If a vulnerable older adult is prescribed an NSAID (nonselective or selective), then GI bleeding risks should be discussed and documented.
- If a vulnerable older adult is prescribed daily aspirin (including low-dose, ≤325 mg/d), then GI bleeding risks should be discussed and documented.
- If a vulnerable older adult with a risk factor for GI bleeding (aged ≥75 yr old, peptic ulcer disease, history of GI bleeding, warfarin use, chronic glucocorticoid use) is treated with a nonselective NSAID, then he or she should be treated concomitantly with misoprostol or a proton-pump inhibitor.
- If a vulnerable older adult with two or more risk factors for GI bleeding (age ≥75 yr old, peptic ulcer disease, history of GI bleeding, warfarin use, chronic glucocorticoid use) is treated with daily aspirin, then he or she should be treated concomitantly with misoprostol or a proton-pump inhibitor.

Related quality indicators for Persistent Pain

- Pain assessment of dying patient, management of emergent pain (see "Palliative Care," p 102)
- Risks and prophylaxis of NSAIDs and aspirin, management of osteoarthritis (see "Musculoskeletal Diseases and Disorders," p 437)

*Assessing Care of Vulnerable Elders – 3rd Set. See inside front cover for explanation.

REFERENCES

■ American Geriatrics Society Panel on the Pharmacologic Management of Persistent Pain in Older Persons. Pharmacological management of persistent pain in older persons. *J Am Geriatr Soc.* 2009;57(8):1331–1346.

■ Barkin RL, Barkin SJ, Barkin DS. Perception, assessment, treatment, and management of pain in the elderly. *Clin Geriatr Med.* 2005;21(3):465–490.

■ Flaherty E. Pain Assessment for Older Adults. *Try This: Best Practices in Nursing Care to Older Adults.* 2007;(7). Available at http://consultgerirn.org/uploads/File/trythis/try_this_7.pdf

■ Herr K. Pain in the older adult: an imperative across all health care settings. *Pain Manag Nurs.* 2010;11(2 Suppl):S1–10.

■ Horgas A. Assessing Pain in Older Adults with Dementia. *Try This: Best Practices in Nursing Care to Older Adults.* 2007;(D2). Available at http://consultgerirn.org/uploads/File/trythis/try_this_d2.pdfpain/

CHAPTER 16—HOSPITAL CARE

KEY POINTS

■ Adults ≥65 yr old make up 13% of the population and account for 36% of acute-care hospital admissions and nearly 50% of hospital expenditures for all adults.

■ Older hospitalized adults should be routinely assessed for a limited number of common geriatric problems regardless of the admission diagnosis.

■ Specific system changes in providing care to hospitalized older adults have resulted in improved patient outcomes.

■ The "peridischarge" period after transition from the hospital is a time of increased risk of injury. Careful attention to the process of discharge planning can reduce the probability of unnecessary emergency department care and readmission to the hospital.

Older adults are at disproportionate risk of becoming seriously ill and requiring hospital care, whether it is in an emergency department, on a medical or surgical ward, or in a critical-care unit. Adults ≥65 yr old, who make up only 13% of the U.S. population, account for 36% of acute-care hospital admissions and nearly 50% of hospital expenditures for adults.

Hospital use rates vary as much as 3-fold for Medicare beneficiaries with the same illnesses across different regions of the United States. There is no evidence that these differences in practice patterns are explained by differences in disease rates or severity. Hospital use and the use of hospital resources is much lower among those enrolled in capitated insurance plans than among those enrolled in fee-for-service plans; this difference in resource use has not been systematically linked to differences in patient outcomes.

During hospitalization, older adults tend to receive less costly care than do younger patients. In the Study to Understand Prognoses and Preferences for Outcomes and Risks of Treatments (SUPPORT), for example, seriously ill patients in their 80s received fewer invasive procedures and less resource-intensive, less costly hospital care than similar younger patients received (SOE=A). This preferential allocation of hospital services to younger patients was not based on differences in patients' severity of illness or general preferences for life-extending care and is consistent with evidence regarding outpatient care. Differences in the aggressiveness of care have not been shown to explain differences between older and younger patients in survival or other outcomes. The best guides to assessment and management in the care of any older hospitalized patient are the clinical circumstances and the patient's preferences irrespective of the patient's age.

Preferences among seriously ill older adults for life-sustaining treatments vary widely. On the basis of SUPPORT findings, it has been recognized that even though fewer older patients prefer aggressive care than do younger patients, many older patients want cardiopulmonary resuscitation and care that is focused on life extension. Moreover, patients' families and clinicians commonly underestimate older patients' desires for aggressive care (SOE=A). Thus, in providing care for acutely ill older adults, it is essential to determine individual preferences for the site of care and to define with the patient the goals of care.

In a study of vulnerable older adults hospitalized on the medical service of an academic medical center, the quality of care provided was examined by measuring adherence to ACOVE-3 quality indicators. Adherence to indicators was significantly greater for general medical care (such as for heart failure or diabetes) than for geriatric conditions (such as delirium or pressure sores) (SOE=A). This finding is probably not peculiar to the single hospital studied. This chapter is intended to assist providers in the acute setting to adhere to effective geriatric care processes, regardless of the general medical problems of their patients.

ASSESSING AND MANAGING HOSPITALIZED OLDER PATIENTS

Many of the serious illnesses disproportionately experienced by older adults require hospital care for optimal management. The benefits of hospitalization can be remarkable: correcting serious physiologic derangements, repairing vascular obstructions and broken bones, using highly technical biomedical advances in the treatment of life-threatening illnesses. However, while in the hospital, older adults also commonly experience deteriorating functional status, adverse events of medication, or delirium. A systematic approach to assessing and managing older hospitalized adults offers the best chance of reducing the risk and consequences of these common problems.

An initial comprehensive assessment of hospitalized older patients includes an evaluation of function at the level of the organ system, the whole person, and the person's environment. This assessment can identify needs for which targeted interventions can improve function or reduce risk of adverse outcomes. This approach complements the traditional medical assessment by highlighting problems that are common in hospitalized older patients, and it is similar in concept to comprehensive geriatric assessment conducted in other settings. See "Assessment," p 43; and "Outpatient Care Systems," p 157.

For 10 hazards and opportunities that are commonly overlooked in older hospitalized patients, see Table 16.1. These problems have been selected based on their importance relative to other clinical issues, the quality of relevant evidence, and their specificity to older adults. Other important problems (eg, prevention of deep-vein thrombosis, the effects of alcohol or tobacco use, pain management, and advance directives) are not specific to older adults, and some problems specific to older adults (eg, age-related decline in renal function) are widely recognized. (See also "Legal and Ethical Issues," p 23; "Perioperative Care," p 92; "Palliative Care," p 102; "Addictions," p 322; and "Kidney Diseases and Disorders," p 404.) For suggestions on when assessment of these common geriatric problems can be incorporated into the routine of a hospital admission history and physical examination, see Table 16.2.

Two types of evidence suggest that these interventions are a good use of clinician time. First, for each problem, evidence supporting the proposed intervention is compelling, either because the efficacy of the intervention is well established (eg, anticoagulation to prevent stroke associated with atrial fibrillation), or because the associated problem is common, often overlooked, and can be improved with a safe and inexpensive intervention. Second, systematic approaches to the evaluation and management of acutely ill older adults can improve patient outcomes and reduce hospital costs.

Functional Impairments

Once hospitalized, older patients are at high risk of loss of independence and institutionalization. Among hospitalized medical patients ≥70 yr old, approximately 10% decline during hospitalization in their ability to perform basic ADLs of self-care, another 10% are discharged without recovering their baseline prehospitalization abilities, and 15% of those admitted from home are discharged to a nursing home (SOE=A). Loss of personal independence is often hastened by the combined effects of the acute illness that led to hospitalization and underlying chronic illnesses and impairments. In addition, many older patients lose their "bounce"—their ability to adapt and maintain the homeostasis of their physiologic, psychologic, and social systems in the face of acute insults to these systems both by illness and by hospitalization itself. Functional decline during hospitalization and lack of recovery to baseline function have been independently associated with increasing age, lower preadmission function in IADLs, and several admission characteristics, including cognitive impairment, symptoms of depression, and malnutrition (SOE=B). Optimal care of hospitalized older patients requires the hospital team both to manage acute illness and to simultaneously intervene to promote or maintain independent functioning. The geriatric clinician plays an important role in educating patients and families regarding the harmful effects of activity limitation and the need to engage in function-promoting activity to avoid functional decline.

The ability to perform ADLs and IADLs is necessary for older adults to live independently, and functional dependence is associated with worse quality-of-life outcomes, shortened survival, and increased resource use. The older adult's ability to perform ADLs and IADLs, determined at the time of admission, can serve as a useful baseline. If functional dependence is found, the causes can be explored (eg, dependence in IADLs is often associated with dementia), and strategies to maintain and improve functional ability can be started (eg, physical and occupational therapy). These strategies may be

Table 16.1—Common Hazards and Opportunities to Address During an Older Adult's Hospital Stay

Problem	Possible Interventions
Functional impairments	Physical therapy, occupational therapy, assess social environment
Immobility and falls	Avoid restraints, encourage ambulation in hospital, physical therapy
Sensory impairment	Eyeglasses, hearing aids; remove cerumen impaction
Depression	Pharmacotherapy, cognitive therapy, or both
Cognitive impairment	Evaluate for dementia or delirium, assess social environment
Suboptimal pharmacotherapy	Modify prescriptions
Atrial fibrillation	Rate control plus anticoagulation or conversion to sinus rhythm
Nutrition	Supplement water, calories, protein; assess social environment and medical factors that contribute to poor oral intake
Mistreatment and social support	Involve family and social services early in discharge planning
Immunization status	Vaccinate against influenza, pneumococcus, tetanus

Table 16.2—Systematic Assessment of Older Adults on Hospital Admission

Step	Assessments
Past medical history	▪ Ask about vaccination history
Medications review	▪ Assess indications for each medication, appropriateness of dosing, potential interactions ▪ Determine patient's or caregiver's method for assuring adherence (eg, pill boxes)
Social history	▪ Ask about help needed (and who provides) for ADLs and IADLs ▪ Ask about social support ▪ Ask if patient feels free and safe
Review of systems	▪ Ask about weight loss in preceding 6 mo ▪ Ask about dietary change ▪ Ask about anorexia, nausea, vomiting, diarrhea ▪ Ask about problems with memory or confusion ▪ Ask about falls or difficulty walking ▪ Ask about difficulties with vision or hearing
Physical examination	▪ Take pulse (confirm arrhythmias with ECG) ▪ Assess for loss of subcutaneous fat, muscle wasting, edema, ascites, prevalent pressure ulcer ▪ Screen for cognitive function ▪ Assess vision and hearing ▪ Use of depression screen

best implemented effectively for many patients by ward staff without consultation or referral. Social work consultation and early involvement of family or other caregivers is often necessary to plan postdischarge care for those older adults who are functionally dependent. See also "Psychosocial Issues," p 311; and "Rehabilitation," p 130.

Immobility and Falls

Walking facilitates the performance of virtually all ADLs and IADLs. The ability to walk briskly and the habit of regularly walking 1 mile or more daily are associated with prolonged survival (SOE=B). Immobility during hospitalization, however, leads rapidly to deconditioning and subsequent difficulty walking. The major risk of walking for deconditioned hospital patients is falling, which can lead to serious injury. Falls and fall-related injuries in hospitalized patients are associated with cognitive impairment; new medications and multiple medications; environmental fac-

tors in the hospital; abnormalities of gait, balance, and leg strength; multiple chronic medical conditions; and depression. At this point an individualized plan to promote physical function (engagement in self-care and physical activity) is important to maximize functional capability.

It is essential to assess the patient's gait, balance, leg strength, ability to get up from bed, cognition, and mood during the initial physical examination. At this point an individualized plan to promote physical function (engagement in self-care and physical activity) is important to maximize functional capability. Individuals able to walk independently should be encouraged to do so frequently during hospitalization. Those able to walk but unable to do so safely and independently can receive assistance from hospital staff while walking several times daily. Formal physical therapy can yield additional benefits. The initial physical examination is also a good time to assess a patient's risk of falling by inquiring about a history of falls and by careful musculoskeletal and neurologic examinations. Interventions that reduce falls in other settings can also prevent falls in the hospital. Prudent preventive strategies include avoiding restraints and tethers, providing walking assistance for those who walk with difficulty, and providing physical therapy for those with weakness or gait abnormalities. If significant soft-tissue and bony abnormalities of the feet are found, a referral for podiatric care is appropriate. See "Physical Activity," p 54; "Rehabilitation," p 130; "Gait Impairment," p 218; "Falls," p 224; and "Diseases and Disorders of the Foot," p 456.

Sensory Impairment

Most hospitalized older adults have impaired vision or hearing, and these sensory impairments are risk factors for falls, incontinence, delirium, and functional dependence. Although most visual and hearing impairments are readily corrected by eyeglasses or hearing aids, these appliances are often forgotten or inaccessible in the hospital.

Hospitalized older adults can be screened for sensory impairment by routinely asking if they have difficulty with seeing or hearing and whether they use eyeglasses or hearing aids. Physical examination including a test of visual acuity (eg, with a pocket card of the Jaeger eye test) and the whisper test of hearing, in which a short, easily answered question is whispered in each ear, is the next appropriate step in evaluation. For people with visual or hearing impairments, it is important to provide the appropriate assistive devices (eyeglasses or hearing aids brought from home), and staff may need to be instructed in the use of appliances to communicate more effectively. See "Hearing Impairment," p 176; and "Visual Impairment," p 167.

Depression

Depressive symptoms in hospitalized older adults are common, prognostically important, and potentially ameliorable. Major or minor depression occurs in roughly one-third of hospitalized patients ≥65 yr old but is often undiagnosed. The presence of depressive symptoms is associated with increased risk of dependence in ADLs, nursing-home placement, and shortened long-term survival, even after controlling for baseline function and the severity of acute and chronic illness.

It is important to consider depression in all hospitalized older patients. Simply asking patients whether they feel down, depressed, or hopeless, or whether they have lost interest or pleasure in doing things, is a good place to start. A positive response to any one of these questions is likely sensitive to the diagnosis of depression (based on evidence from outpatients) and can be followed up by a formal assessment for an affective disorder.

Detection is the first and most important step in the management of depression. Psychotherapeutic interventions (environmental, behavioral, cognitive, and family) are safe and often effective in the initial management of patients with suspected depression. Beginning pharmacotherapy during hospitalization for a medical or surgical condition may not be necessary, but follow-up shortly after discharge is critical. If pharmacotherapy is started, SSRIs are often preferred because approximately 50% of older hospitalized patients have a contraindication to tricyclic antidepressants. See "Depression and Other Mood Disorders," p 295.

Cognitive Impairment

Delirium is present in 10%–15% of hospitalized older adults on admission, and it develops in up to 30% during the course of hospitalization on a generalized medical ward (SOE=A). Delirium arising during the course of hospitalization is a predictor of prolonged hospital stay. Delirium is also associated with increased rates of in-hospital death and nursing-home placement. Patients who develop delirium can experience a worsening of a chronic cognitive impairment. Symptoms of delirium commonly persist for months after hospital discharge. Roughly one-third of cases of delirium can be prevented by appropriately managing six risk factors for delirium: cognitive impairment, sleep deprivation, immobility, visual impairment, hearing impairment, and dehydration (SOE=A). The diagnosis of delirium should be considered when any of the following is observed: fluctuation in mental status or behavior, inattention, disorganized thinking, and altered consciousness. The Confusion Assessment Method is a screening tool that incorporates all four of these features, with a positive screen consisting of both of the first two features plus one or both of the latter two. Prudent measures to prevent or ameliorate delirium include avoiding medications associated with delirium whenever possible; treating infection and fever; detecting and correcting metabolic abnormalities; frequently orienting patients with cognitive or sensory impairment; and avoiding excessive bed rest, room changes, and restraints. (See "Delirium," p 264.) Prevention is the best strategy; while the benefits of interventions to prevent delirium are well established (SOE=A), interventions for treating established delirium have not demonstrated improved outcomes (SOE=B).

Underlying cognitive impairment consistent with dementia is present on admission in 20%–40% of hospitalized older adults, and it commonly goes undetected. Preexisting cognitive impairment is a risk factor for delirium, falls, use of restraints, and nonadherence with therapy. There is also intrinsic value in identifying previously undiagnosed dementia so that appropriate evaluation and management strategies can be implemented after discharge. The medical history obtained from demented patients should be corroborated by family and caregivers. Cognitive function can be assessed by use of an established test of cognitive function, such as the Mini–Mental State Examination or the Mini-Cog test. When dementia is a possibility, it is important to exclude reversible causes and to identify those patients for whom further evaluations and interventions are warranted. See "Dementia," p 245.

Suboptimal Pharmacotherapy

Older hospitalized patients are prescribed more medications than younger ones. Moreover, hospitalization is a period of rapid turnover in medications for older patients. In one study, 40% of medications prescribed before admission were discontinued during hospitalization, and 45% of medications prescribed at discharge were started during hospitalization. Although older patients are at increased risk of inappropriate drug therapy, adverse drug events, and drug-drug interactions, they can also be undertreated when effective therapies are not used or are used in inadequate dosages. In one study, 88% of older hospitalized patients had at least one clinically significant problem related to prescribing, and 22% had at least one potentially serious and life-threatening problem (SOE=B). Consultation by clinical pharmacists can improve appropriate prescribing and improve the older patient's adherence to prescribed therapy (SOE=A).

A hospital admission is an ideal time to completely review a patient's medication regimen, discontinuing those medications that are unnecessary or have low therapeutic value (eg, sedative hypnotics) and ensuring that medical conditions are maximally treated. During hospitalization and at discharge, a medication review is useful to identify prescribing errors in six common categories: inappropriate choice of therapy, incorrect dosage, incorrect schedule, drug-drug interactions, therapeutic duplication, and allergy. Review of medications should include both prescription and nonprescription medications. See "Pharmacotherapy," p 72.

Nutrition

Serious deficiencies of macronutrients and micronutrients are common in hospitalized older patients. Key macronutrients are protein, calories, salt, water, and fiber. On admission, severe protein-calorie malnutrition is present in approximately 15% of adults ≥70 yr old, and moderate malnutrition is present in another 25%. Moreover, 25% of older patients suffer further nutritional depletion during hospitalization. Even after controlling for underlying acute illness, its

severity, and comorbid illnesses, malnutrition is associated with increased risk of death, dependence, and institutionalization.

In addition, deficiencies of vitamins and electrolytes can develop with protein-calorie malnutrition; vitamin D deficiency is especially common among older hospitalized patients. In one large hospital, nearly two-thirds of patients ≥65 yr old were found to be vitamin D deficient; vitamin D deficiency was nearly as common in patients without a risk factor for vitamin D deficiency and in those taking multivitamins as in other patients (SOE=B). See "Malnutrition," p ; "Osteoporosis," p 234; and "Endocrine and Metabolic Disorders," p 491.

One review examined the evidence from randomized controlled trials of the benefits of oral nutritional supplements for older adults at risk of malnutrition. (Of the almost 2,500 participants included in the review, 22% were from studies of hospitalized patients.) Nutritional supplementation was associated with reduced mortality and shortened length of hospital stay, although the reviewers called for additional research to substantiate these findings because most of the studies included in the analysis were of poor quality (SOE=B). Beyond considering supplements, clinicians should assess malnourished older hospitalized patients for remediable factors such as difficulty chewing, dysphagia, or insufficient time or physical ability to eat. See "Eating and Feeding Problems," p 203.

The maintenance of water and electrolyte balance requires special attention in older adults during and after fluid administration because of their decreased ability to achieve and maintain homeostasis. Initial efforts can be directed toward achieving euvolemia and correcting electrolyte abnormalities. Subsequent efforts to maintain fluid and electrolyte balance are based on estimates of daily metabolic requirements.

Mistreatment and Social Support

Hospitalization of older adults is sometimes precipitated by mistreatment, which includes physical or psychologic abuse, neglect, self-neglect, exploitation, and abandonment. Mistreatment of older adults was not recognized in the medical literature until 1975; it is now estimated to affect 700,000 to 1.2 million Americans annually. Most older adults referred to protective services because of physical abuse have been seen in hospital emergency departments, and many emergency visits lead to hospitalization.

Universal screening for mistreatment has been recommended (SOE=C) and can be implemented by asking each older adult, "Do you feel safe returning to where you live?" Further questions can explore the living situation and specific settings or aspects of mistreatment. It is important to consider the diagnosis of mistreatment when there are physical or psychologic stigmata, such as unexplained injury, dehydration, malnutrition, social withdrawal, or recalcitrant depression or anxiety. When mistreatment is suspected, most states require that Adult Protective Services or the equivalent state agency be contacted. See "Mistreatment of Older Adults," p 87.

Immunization Status

Adults ≥65 yr old should be assessed at the time of admission to the hospital for their vaccination status and updated accordingly. See also "Prevention," p 69.

DAILY ROUNDS OF OLDER PATIENTS

A systematic approach should be used on daily rounds to ensure that essential geriatric issues are not overshadowed by disease-specific or technologic concerns. For patients who are expected to recover their mobility, the progress toward that goal should be assessed. Time out of bed (eg, in a chair for meals) should be encouraged, as should ambulation and toileting (with assistance, if needed). Skin should be carefully examined for the development of pressure ulcers. When pressure ulcers are identified, in addition to therapies to treat the wound, increased mobility or frequent repositioning with appropriate padding should be prescribed. Similarly, progress on ADL recovery should be tracked, and nursing encouraged to coach patients toward functional independence.

The fraction of meals consumed is valuable information for hospitalized older adults. The intake of paltry amounts of food can suggest inadequate recovery or undetected illness. These patients may benefit from a review of the medication list because many medications disturb appetite. Another contributor to poor oral intake in the hospital is constipation. Elimination records should be reviewed regularly, and patients who have not moved their bowels in more than a couple of days may benefit from a stimulant (eg, senna) or osmotic (eg, sorbitol) laxative or from a suppository, in addition to ensuring adequate fluid and fiber intake and mobility.

Older patients commonly have difficulty sleeping in the hospital. This is not a trivial matter, because sleep deprivation is a risk factor for development of delirium. Sleep deprivation is best managed nonpharmacologically, because sedative-hypnotics can precipitate or prolong confusional states. Strategies to promote sleep include moving older adults away from noisy roommates or nursing stations; minimizing sleep interruption (eg, to take vital signs); encouraging daytime physical activity and discouraging naps; and using warm milk, herbal tea, or soft music at bedtime.

Patients accustomed to hypnotic use in the outpatient setting may require them in the hospital as well. (For prescription medications used to treat insomnia in older adults, see Table 35.4 p 281.) Patients who use a continuous positive airway pressure device at home will also need orders written for hospital use.

The daily physical examination during rounds should include identifying the devices attached to, or inserted in, each patient. Many of these devices can injure patients if used inappropriately, and a daily assessment of risks and benefits is wise. Central venous catheters, for example, allow for convenient blood draws and delivery of medications and parenteral nutrition, but they are also associated with infection, restricted mobility, deep venous thrombosis, and air embolism. Indwelling bladder catheters carry a risk of urinary tract infection and delirium, and should be reserved for three situations: 1) when accurate and timely measurement of urine output is essential and cannot otherwise be measured, 2) when urinary retention would otherwise result, or 3) when an incontinent patient's urinary leakage may contaminate a healing wound.

Restraints constitute a hazard to both safety and personal dignity. Their use should be restricted to situations in which confused patients might otherwise attempt to discontinue life-sustaining devices (eg, endotracheal tubes). "Sitters" or bedside companions are far better for monitoring and assuring the safety of confused patients.

SYSTEMS OF CARE FOR OLDER HOSPITALIZED PATIENTS

Nurses Improving Care for Health System Elders (NICHE)

NICHE is the only national nursing program designed to address the specialized needs of older patients. A program of the Hartford Institute for Geriatric Nursing at New York University College of Nursing (NYUCN), NICHE comprises a national network of hospitals and their affiliate healthcare organizations. The program provides initial and ongoing resources to assist hospitals to develop and strengthen both the individual nurse's geriatric expertise, as well as a hospital's capacity to develop, use, and evaluate best practice for older adults.

The core components of NICHE include self-evaluation tools for the hospital, a series of geriatric educational resources for staff, clinical protocols, quality improvement resources, and management tools. The Geriatric Institutional Assessment Profile (GIAP) is an instrument that helps NICHE-participating hospitals identify organizational attributes of the hospital relevant to geriatric care, including gaps in knowledge about geriatric care, attitudes and perceptions that influence how staff work with older patients, and specific practice issues and concerns. These results, as well as unit-based clinical outcomes, are benchmarked against other NICHE hospitals and used to measure organizational readiness as well as effectiveness in implementing NICHE.

The Geriatric Resource Nurse (GRN) Model is the foundation of the NICHE program (Fulmer, et al., 2002). It is based on the belief that primary nurses know the most about the daily patterns and needs of the older adults in their units. After receiving specialized education in nursing care of older adults, the GRN receives ongoing mentorship and clinical support from an advanced practice nurse. A geriatric advanced practice nurse works closely with the GRNs through clinical rounds and learning activities such as journal clubs. GRNs carry a usual caseload of patients serving as the unit's resource on geriatric best practices. GRNs are also involved in quality and research initiatives as well as the education of other staff regarding geriatric care.

Hospitals have reported improved clinical outcomes, enhanced nurse knowledge and perceptions of quality, increased compliance with protocol application, and decreased length of stay after implementing the NICHE GRN model. For additional information about the NICHE program and the GRN model, see www.nicheprogram.org.

Geriatric Evaluation and Management (GEM) Units

GEM units for older adults who have stabilized during an acute hospitalization were developed and pioneered in Veterans Affairs medical centers. These units incorporate comprehensive geriatric assessment (including screening for geriatric syndromes and assessment for and treatment of functional, cognitive, affective, and nutritional problems) with interdisciplinary team-based care. In a multicenter randomized trial, ADL function and physical performance improved for veterans assigned to GEM units relative to those who received usual hospital care (SOE=A). Some measures of health-related quality of life were also superior for patients treated on GEM units. These units did not affect mortality and were cost-neutral after consideration of costs of both initial hospitalization and care after discharge. For more information on GEM, see "Outpatient Care Systems," p 157.

Acute Care for Elders (ACE) Units

The ACE unit has been adapted in many acute-care hospitals where acutely ill older patients are admitted

to an ACE unit. ACE programs adopt a proactive, "prehabilitative" approach, comprising four components:

- a prepared environment to promote mobility and orientation (eg, carpeting, raised toilet seats, low beds, clocks, calendars, and pictures to promote orientation)
- patient-centered care with nursing-initiated protocols for independent self-care, nutrition, sleep hygiene, skin care, mood, and cognition
- planning to go home, with early social work intervention to mobilize family and other resources at home
- medical care review to promote optimal prescribing

In a randomized trial involving 651 medical patients $\geq$70 yr old in a university teaching hospital, ACE was associated with greater independence in ADLs at discharge, less frequent discharge to a nursing home, and somewhat shorter and less expensive hospitalization (SOE=A). In a second randomized trial involving 1,531 community-dwelling adults $\geq$70 yr old in a community hospital, ACE was associated with substantial differences in the satisfaction of patients, family members, physicians, and nurses but with only modest differences in ADL function (SOE=A).

The Hospital Elder Life Program (HELP)

The Hospital Elder Life Program (HELP) involves a multicomponent intervention to prevent delirium in hospitalized older patients. The intervention consists of protocols to manage 6 risk factors for delirium: cognitive impairment, sleep deprivation, immobility, visual impairment, hearing impairment, and dehydration. Older patients receiving this intervention are not segregated on a special hospital ward or unit. The program makes extensive use of hospital volunteers. In one prospective controlled study, the incidence of delirium was reduced by one-third, from 15.0% to 9.9% (SOE=A). Severity and duration of delirium episodes appeared not to be affected by HELP. The intervention was also associated with significantly improved cognitive function among patients with cognitive impairment at admission and a reduced rate of use of sleep medications among all patients. Among the other risk factors, there were trends toward improvement in immobility, visual impairment, and hearing impairment.

INTENSIVE CARE OF THE CRITICALLY ILL

Adults >65 yr old account for 42%−52% of the

intensive care unit (ICU) admissions and for almost 60% of total ICU days in the United States. Research is ongoing in an attempt to better understand which older patients are most likely to benefit from ICU care.

Patients with acute lung injury or acute respiratory distress syndrome appear to have a higher mortality with advancing age. Interestingly, in three separate studies of more than 1,500 patients, older patients recovered from their pulmonary physiologic abnormalities at a rate equal to that of their younger counterparts after acute lung injury; however, they required nearly twice as long to be successfully liberated from the ventilator and discharged from the ICU (SOE=A). Often, comorbid conditions contribute to these patients' deaths despite the apparent correction of the physiologic disturbances induced by their acute lung injury. Sedative and analgesic medications must be used judiciously; and delirium, heart failure, hypothyroidism, electrolyte disturbances, oropharyngeal dysfunction, and aspiration should be considered in patients with difficulty weaning from the ventilator. For many older adults who succumb to an acute illness, cognitive decline is the main threat to their ability to recover their former functional abilities. Determinants of this cognitive decline are poorly understood.

Establishing goals of care in older critically ill patients is of paramount importance. In caring for critically ill patients, it may become apparent to the patient, family, and clinician that further intervention would not likely be of substantial benefit, depending on the individual patient's goals, values, and hopes. Defining *futility* is often difficult. The American Medical Association recommends a standardized "fair process" rather than a strict definition of futility. As much as possible, physicians should base futility decisions on factors such as clinical efficacy of treatment, likelihood of mortality, and subsequent quality-of-life considerations rather than on chronologic age alone.

In an analysis of 6,303 ICU-related deaths, 26% of these deaths were of patients receiving full ICU care, including failed cardiopulmonary resuscitation; 24% received full ICU care without cardiopulmonary resuscitation; 14% had life support withheld; and 36% (the single largest group) had life support actively withdrawn. The limitation of life support before death is a common practice in teaching ICUs across the country. In another study of 851 patients on a mechanical ventilator, 63% were successfully liberated, 17% died while on the ventilator, and 20% had mechanical ventilation withdrawn. The top four reasons given for withdrawal of the ventilator were 1) physicians' perception that the patient did not want life support, 2) physicians' prediction that ICU survival was <10%, 3) physicians' prediction that future cognitive function would be severely impaired, and 4) the ongoing need for an inotrope or vasopressor. Given the well-described inability of physicians to accurately prognosticate beyond hours of impending death, important decisions regarding use of technology in older critically ill patients should be made with humility and through incorporating the patient's goals of care and the importance they and their families place on maintaining functional and cognitive status.

ALTERNATIVES TO HOSPITAL CARE

It is often assumed that older adults would prefer to be treated for acute illness at home rather than in the hospital whenever possible. The safety and feasibility of this approach for acutely ill older adults who would usually be hospitalized has been demonstrated. This approach, sometimes called the *home hospital*, requires intensive resources for medical and nursing care at home that are not yet widely available.

Older adults' preferences for care at home rather than in the hospital vary widely. In a study of community-dwelling older adults, virtually all preferred care in the site that would provide the higher probability of survival. When home care and hospital care provide equivalent probabilities of survival, roughly half preferred care in each site, with those preferring home care more likely to be white, better educated, living with a spouse, deeply religious, and dependent in two or more ADLs. The major difference perceived by older adults between home care and hospital care was feeling safer in the hospital than at home.

A few studies suggest that hospital-at-home care can provide safe, economical, and efficacious care for some older adults with selected medical conditions, eg, heart failure, community-acquired pneumonia, cellulitis, COPD (SOE=A).

TRANSITIONS FROM HOSPITAL CARE

Age is a strong predictor of use of hospital services, and older adults have a higher risk of death during hospitalization and higher rates of iatrogenic complications, are more likely to be admitted through an emergency department, and have longer lengths of stay than their younger counterparts. Further, older adults have more frequent transitions in location of healthcare services provided to them after hospital discharge.

Almost one-fourth of hospitalized patients ≥65 yr old are discharged to another institution. Although labor-intensive, meticulous discharge planning can maximize the probability that patients maintain the clinical and functional benefits achieved by hospitalization, and probably reduces the risk of early readmission as well as the use of emergency services. Discharge planning ideally begins at hospital admission, with the establishment of measurable, function-related goals to attain by discharge, and a projection of medical, nursing, rehabilitative, and functional support required by the patient at the time of discharge. Four indicators of high-quality transitional care (resulting in fewer readmissions) are accurate and timely transfer of information to the next set of providers, preparation of the patient and family for the move, support for self-management of medical conditions, and empowerment of the patient to assert his or her own preferences (SOE=A).

The choice of discharge destination reflects a match between the needs of a given patient and the services available at each setting. The array of possible settings includes home with family support, home with home-health care, custodial care (such as assisted living or "nursing home"), skilled-nursing facilities, acute rehabilitation hospitals, long-term acute care, or inpatient hospice. Home-health care works well for patients requiring only intermittent skilled services (nursing, physical therapy, or speech therapy), and patients with one of these needs may also receive assistance from occupational therapy, medical social work, or home health aides. Medicare requires that patients receiving home-health care be homebound. Patients appropriate for skilled-nursing facilities (according to Medicare) must also have a need for a skilled service, such as a requirement for intravenous therapy, artificial nutrition and hydration, complex wound care, ostomy care, or rehabilitation. Medicare covers all or part of skilled-nursing care for up to 100 days after a qualifying hospital stay, but coverage stops earlier if a patient's treatment goals are met or if the patient "plateaus" and no longer demonstrates improvement. Patients with substantial rehabilitation needs (more than just physical therapy, occupational therapy, or speech therapy) and considerable rehabilitation potential may be appropriate for transfer to an acute rehabilitation unit, but many older patients are deemed ineligible because of an inability to participate in 3 hours per day of intense therapy. Long-term acute care, also known as "chronic hospitalization," is appropriate for the rare hospital patient who requires prolonged, hospital-level care. Long-term acute-care facilities provide care for patients requiring long-term mechanical ventilation, multiple intravenous medications, parenteral nutrition, or complex wound care, along with a need for frequent physician monitoring.

A critical activity near the time of hospital discharge is the preparation of the discharge medication list. This list should include an indication for each medication, stop dates (eg, for antibiotics) or tapering schedules (eg, for systemic corticosteroids) as appropriate, and clear behavioral triggers for as-needed psychiatric medications. Medications added during the hospital stay (such as analgesics or laxatives with as-needed orders) can be tapered away and discontinued at this time. Finally, the discharge regimen should be formally reconciled with the preadmission regimen. Reconciliation results in clear documentation of which medications on the discharge list are new (relative to the preadmission regimen), which of the preadmission medications have been stopped, and which dosages of continued medications have been changed.

The following items should be communicated to patients (or their caregivers) who are being discharged directly home: follow-up appointments, warning symptoms or signs to watch for with instructions on whom to contact, clinical disciplines (eg, nursing, physical therapy) contracted for provision in the home, and the reconciled medication list. Patients being discharged to other care venues should be oriented with respect to the nature of the new institution, the identity of a new medical provider if known, and the expected frequency of provider visits. Tools are available to assist patients and caregivers with assessing care preferences, clarifying discharge instructions, reconciling medication inaccuracies, and facilitating communication across care sites at discharge (eg, see http://www.caretransitions.org). If the provider at the receiving institution differs from the hospital clinician, then clear and prompt communication is essential. Some items of information (critical but pending study results, nuances of goals of care or family dynamics) call for direct communication between sending and receiving clinicians. Otherwise, a brief and prompt discharge summary containing the following will suffice: summary of hospital course with care provided and results of important tests; a list of problems and diagnoses; baseline physical functional status; baseline cognitive status; physical and cognitive status at discharge; reconciled medication list; allergies; tests results still outstanding; follow-up appointments; and information related to goals, preferences, and advance directives.

ACOVE-3* Quality Indicators Pertaining to Hospital Care

Venous thrombosis prophylaxis

■ If a hospitalized vulnerable older adult is at very high risk of venous thrombosis, then he or she should be on deep venous thrombosis prophylaxis (pharmacologic or sequential or intermittent compression).

Endocarditis prophylaxis

■ If a vulnerable older adult has moderate to high risk of endocarditis, and a high-risk procedure is planned, then endocarditis prophylaxis should be given.

Central venous catheter infection precautions

■ If a hospitalized vulnerable older adult has a new temporary central venous catheter placed, then the medical record should document that maximal barrier precautions were used.

■ If a hospitalized vulnerable older adult has a temporary central venous catheter placed, then there should be daily documentation of examination of line site for signs of infection and continued need for the central line.

Indwelling bladder catheter

■ If a hospitalized vulnerable older adult has an indwelling bladder catheter placed, then the indication or continued need for the catheter should be documented at least every 3 days until its removal.

Delirium evaluation

■ If a hospitalized vulnerable older adult has a suspected or definite diagnosis of delirium, acute confusional state, or reduced level of consciousness, then there should be a documented attempt to attribute the altered mental state to a potential etiology.

Mobilization

■ If a vulnerable older adult who is ambulatory as an outpatient is hospitalized for longer than 48 hours and is not receiving intensive or palliative care, then there should be a plan to increase mobility within 48 hours of admission.

Inpatient fall evaluation

■ If a vulnerable older adult falls during hospitalization, then the following should be documented within 24 hours:

　◦ Presence or absence of prodromal symptoms

　◦ Review of medications or drugs potentially contributing to the fall

Aspiration precautions

■ If a hospitalized vulnerable older adult is tube fed, then there should be documentation of a plan to reduce risk of aspiration.

■ If a vulnerable older adult is mechanically ventilated, then the medical record should document a plan to reduce the risk of ventilator-associated pneumonia.

Discharge assessment

■ If a vulnerable older adult is discharged from the hospital, then the hospital record should contain an assessment of level of independence, need for home health services, and patient and caregiver readiness for discharge time and location.

Discharge summary

■ If a vulnerable older adult is discharged from a hospital to home or nursing home, then there should be a discharge summary in the outpatient or nursing home medical record.

■ If a vulnerable older adult is discharged from a nursing home to home, then there should be a discharge summary in the outpatient medical record.

Communication with continuity clinician

■ If a vulnerable older adult is treated at an emergency department or admitted to a hospital, then there should be documentation (during the emergency department visit or within the first 2 days after admission) of communication with a continuity clinician, of an attempt to reach a continuity clinician, or that there is no continuity clinician.

Posthospitalization follow-up

■ If a vulnerable older adult is discharged from a hospital to home and survives ≥6 wk after discharge, then a clinician visit or telephone contact should be documented within 6 wk of discharge and the medical record should document acknowledgment of the recent hospitalization.

Posthospitalization medications

■ If a vulnerable older adult is discharged from a hospital to home and received a new chronic disease medication or a change in medication before discharge, then the outpatient medical record should document the medication change within 6 wk of discharge.

■ If a vulnerable older adult is discharged from a hospital to home with a new medication that requires a serum medication level to be checked, then the medical record should document the medication level, that the medication was stopped, or that the level was not needed.

Posthospitalization tests

■ If a vulnerable older adult is discharged from a hospital to home or a nursing home and the transfer form or discharge summary indicates that a test result is pending, then the outpatient or nursing home medical record should include the test result within 6 wk of hospital discharge or indicate that the result was followed up elsewhere or why the result cannot be obtained.

Posthospitalization appointments

■ If a vulnerable older adult is discharged from a hospital to home or a nursing home and the hospital medical record specifies a follow-up appointment for a clinician visit or a treatment (eg, physical therapy or radiation oncology), then the medical record should document that the visit or treatment took place, was postponed, or was not needed.

Related quality indicators for hospital care

■ See the following chapters: "Palliative Care," p 102; "Perioperative Care," p 92; "Eating and Feeding Problems," p 203 ; "Urinary Incontinence," p 207; "Dementia," p 245; "Cardiovascular Diseases and Disorders," p 359; "Heart Failure," p 376; "Neurologic Diseases and Disorders," p 464; and "Oncology," p 521.

*****Assessing Care of Vulnerable Elders – 3rd Set. See inside front cover for explanation.**

REFERENCES

■ Arora VM, Johnson M, Olson J, et al. Using Assessing Care of Vulnerable Elders Quality Indicators to measure quality of hospital care for vulnerable elders. *J Am Geriatr Soc.* 2007;55:1705–1711.

■ Bixby MB, Naylor MD. The Transitional Care Model (TCM): Hospital Discharge Screening Criteria for High Risk Older Adults. *Try This: Best Practices in Nursing Care to Older Adults.* 2009;(26). Available at: http://consultgerirn.org/uploads/File/trythis/try_this_26.pdf

■ Boltz M, Capezuti E, Bowar-Ferres S, et al. Changes in the Geriatric Care Environment Associated with NICHE. *Geriatr Nurs.* 2008;29(3):176–185.

■ Coleman EA, Parry C, Chalmers S, et al. The Care Transitions Intervention: results of a randomized controlled trial. *Arch Intern Med.* 2006;166(17):1822–1828.

■ de Rooj SE, Abu-Hanna A, Levi M, et al. Factors that predict outcome of intensive care treatment in very elderly patients: a review. *Crit Care.* 2005;9:R307–314.

■ Frazier-Rios D. and Zembrzuski C. Communication Difficulties: Assessment and Interventions in Hospitalized Older Adults with Dementia. *Try This: Best Practices in Nursing Care to Older Adults.* 2007;(D7). Available at: http://consultgerirn.org/uploads/File/trythis/try_this_d7.pdf

■ Fulmer T, Mezey M, Bottrell M, et al. Nurses Improving Care for Healthsystem Elders (NICHE): nursing outcomes and benchmarks for evidence-based practice. *Geriatr Nurs.* 2002;23(3):121–127.

■ Mezey M, Maslow K. Recognition of Dementia in Hospitalized Older Adults. *Try This: Best Practices in Nursing Care to Older Adults.* 2007;(D5). Available at: http://consultgerirn.org/uploads/File/trythis/try_this_d5.pdf

■ Naylor ND, Feldman PH, Keating S. Translating research into practice: transitional care for older adults. *J Eval Clin Pract.* 2009;15(6):1164–1170.

■ Resnick B, Galik E, Enders H, et al. Pilot Testing of Function Focused Care-Acute Care Intervention. *J Nurs Care Quality.* 2010: Aug 4.

■ Silverstein N. Wandering in Hospitalized Older Adults. *Try This: Best Practices in Nursing Care to Older Adults.* 2007;(D6). Available at: http://consultgerirn.org/uploads/File/trythis/try_this_d6.pdf

CHAPTER 17—REHABILITATION

KEY POINTS

- The World Health Organization conceptual model of functioning and disability provides a useful framework for geriatric rehabilitation by taking into account the complex interactions of body functions and structures, health conditions, individual activities and participation in life situations, and environmental and personal factors.

- As rehabilitation treatments require active patient participation and long-term self-management, the patient and family are core members of the rehabilitation team.

- Factors that influence recovery after a hip fracture include prior mobility and functional status, comorbid conditions, cognitive status, and social support.

- Optimal rehabilitation outcomes depend on comprehensive assessment of the patient, coordinated interdisciplinary team management, multifaceted interventions, and access to appropriate and high-quality care.

OVERVIEW

Rehabilitation is a critical component of geriatric health care due to the high incidence of disabling conditions in the older adult population. Although these conditions drastically influence quality of life, they often improve with treatment. Chronic disease almost always underlies disability in older adults; for example, stroke occurs most often in people with other vascular diseases, and hip fractures occur most often in people with osteoporosis and gait disorders. Disability also worsens in progressive chronic diseases (such as osteoarthritis, Parkinson's disease, or amyotrophic lateral sclerosis) or in the context of deconditioning from inactivity during acute illness. To provide the best functional recovery possible, those providing geriatric rehabilitation must do the following:

STRENGTH-OF-EVIDENCE (SOE) RATING DEFINITIONS

A = consistent and good quality patient-oriented evidence

B = somewhat inconsistent or limited quality patient-oriented evidence

C = very inconsistent or very limited patient-oriented evidence, disease-oriented evidence, and/or consensus from professional organizations

D = unstudied common practice or opinion

See inside front cover for detailed information regarding the SOE classification.

- use systematic approaches to assess the causes of disability
- be familiar with the advantages and disadvantages of all potential sites of care
- understand the role of multidisciplinary teams and care plans
- adapt care to comorbidities and disabilities
- be familiar with the basic requirements for rehabilitation of common geriatric conditions

CONCEPTUAL MODEL FOR GERIATRIC REHABILITATION

Geriatric rehabilitation services can be organized around a conceptual model of disability for assessing the status and needs of the patient, matching treatments with specific conditions, and evaluating rehabilitation outcomes. The World Health Organization (WHO) *International Classification of Functioning, Disability, and Health* (ICF) provides a useful framework. For an ICF guide and a discussion of the ICF model of disability, see the WHO Web site (www3.who.int/icf/beginners/bg.pdf [accessed Jan 2011]). The ICF has two main domains: "Health Condition" and "Contextual Factors." Disability and functioning are viewed as outcomes of interactions between health conditions (diseases, disorders, injuries) and contextual factors, which range from a person's most immediate environment, like furniture in the room, to the more general environment, such as access to public transportation. Personal factors include a person's age, race, gender, educational background, personality, fitness, and lifestyle.

In the WHO model, interventions can be designed to modify a person's impairments, limitations in activities, and restrictions in participation. For example, a treatment plan can be developed to improve a person's strength (impairment level), but the significance of this intervention is a result of its effect on his or her physical mobility (activity) and ultimately his or her ability to return to social or physical roles (participation). The effects of gains in strength and physical mobility on participation can be modified by the person's motivation or social support. For example, if patients improve in strength and balance but their family and friends continue to "do everything for them" and do not encourage independent function, they may remain dependent. The physical environment is another powerful modifier. Even the person who achieves improved function cannot return to prior work or household roles if physical barriers to access in the community are not

Table 17.1—Rehabilitation Sites of Care and Level of Care Requirements

Rehabilitation Sites	Level of Care Requirements	Expected Intensity of Services	Payment Source
Inpatient			
Freestanding rehabilitation hospital	▪ 24-hour availability of a physician with training or experience in rehabilitation ▪ 24-hour nursing care ▪ Relatively intense level of rehabilitation services ▪ Interdisciplinary team to deliver program ▪ Coordinated program of care as evidenced by team conferences at least every 2 weeks ▪ Reasonable expectation of improvement	A multidisciplinary team approach is required and in most cases, this calls for 3 hours of therapy at least 5 days/week; this can include physical, occupational, or speech therapy in any combination.	Medicare Part A ▪ Days 1–20: full coverage ▪ Days 21–100: partial coverage but co-payment ▪ >100 days: no coverage
Medicare skilled-nursing facility	▪ Physician supervision, with access 24 hours/day on emergency basis ▪ 24-hour nursing care ▪ Less intense therapy needs ▪ Interdisciplinary team coordination usually not available ▪ Maintenance of function without progress can be goal of care	Daily therapy (5 days/week) for up to 1 hour/day, as tolerated by patient; ADL assistance and/or skilled-nursing care	Medicare Part A ▪ Days 1–20: full coverage ▪ Days 21–100: partial coverage but co-payment ▪ >100 days: no coverage
Outpatient			
Home health	▪ Physician certifies need every 60 days ▪ Skilled need requires including either intermittent skilled nursing, physical, occupational, or speech therapy	Intermittent nursing or therapy provided; can be no more than 7 days/week or 8 hours/day; patient must have support system to meet needs of living at home	Medicare Part A
Clinic (hospital-based or independent)	▪ Physician orders rehabilitation services to include physical, occupational, or speech therapy and reviews plan periodically ▪ Reasonable expectation of improvement with treatment	Intermittent physical, occupational, or speech therapy provided; patient must be able to get to therapy visits.	Medicare Part B There are caps on coverage, but these can be waived if medically necessary.

SOURCE: http://www.medicare.org (accessed Jan 2011)

removed or adapted by such means as ramps or modified bathrooms. In summary, the interaction of disease and disability is particularly complex in older adults. The ICF model is useful for structuring their comprehensive rehabilitation care.

SITES OF REHABILITATION CARE

Rehabilitation services are available through Medicare Part A on a time-limited basis. These services are offered in both inpatient and community-based sites. Inpatient care may be provided in rehabilitation centers (freestanding hospitals or units attached to acute hospitals) or nursing facilities (Medicare skilled-nursing facilities). To receive Medicare coverage for an inpatient rehabilitation stay in either type of facility, a patient must have a hospital stay of at least 3 consecutive days for a related illness or injury. Outpatient rehabilitation services can be provided in hospital-based or independent clinics, in day hospital settings, or in the home. The patient's eligibility, the particular services provided, and costs vary across sites of care. The balance of advantages and disadvantages for the individual patient are important factors for the clinician to consider in recommending a site for rehabilitation care. For a summary of the sites of rehabilitation, Medicare requirements and payment sources, and the expected intensity of the rehabilitation services, see Table 17.1.

Sites of Care: Coverage and Services

Medicare Part A covers inpatient rehabilitation for patients who have complex needs requiring a multidisciplinary team approach. In most cases, this calls for 3 hours of rehabilitation services per day. A Medicare-certified inpatient rehabilitation hospital program must demonstrate that at least a certain percentage of patients have at least 1 of 13 conditions: rheumatoid arthritis, severe advanced osteoarthritis involving 3 or more joints, amputations, brain injury, burns, congenital deformities, fractures of hip or femur, bilateral joint replacements, major multiple trauma, neurologic disorders (eg, multiple sclerosis, Parkinson's, Guillain-Barré syndrome, polyneuropathy, and others), spinal cord injury, stroke, and systemic vasculitis. Patients must have close medical supervision by a physician with spe-

Table 17.2—Functional Status and Disease-Specific Assessment Instruments

Instrument	Purpose/Description
Functional Independence Measure (www.tbims.org/combi/FIM)	▪ Measures independent performance in self-care, transfers, locomotion, sphincter control, social cognition, and communication. ▪ An 18-item ordinal scale with scores ranging from 0 (total assist) to 7 (complete independence); the possible total score ranges from 18 (the lowest) to 126 (highest), obtained by adding points for each item.
Barthel ADL Index (www.strokecenter.org/trials/scales/barthel.pdf)	▪ Used to establish degree of independence with regard to ADLs. ▪ A 10-item ordinal scale; scores vary depending on the item in question. Bathing and grooming are scored either 0 (dependent/needs help) or 5 (independent); scores for feeding, dressing, bowels, bladder, toilet use, and stairs range from 0 (dependent/unable) to 10 (independent); scores for transfers and mobility on level surfaces range for 0 (unable) to 15 (independent); the possible total score ranges for 0 (the lowest) to 100 (the highest), obtained by adding points for each item.
Stroke Impact Scale (http://www2.kumc.edu/coa/SIS/SIS_pg2.htm)	▪ An 8-domain, 59-item scale that measures the aspects of stroke recovery important to patients and caregivers, as well as stroke experts. ▪ Includes measures of physical domain such as strength, mobility, ADLs, and hand function, as well as the domains of memory, emotion, communication, and social participation.
Harris Hip Questionnaire (http://exper.ural.ru/trauma/harris_e.phtml)	▪ Asks questions regarding pain and function, including ambulation distance, presence of a limp, ability with tasks such as public transportation or stairs, and need for an assistive device. ▪ Hip deformity and range of hip motion are also included.

NOTE: Above Web sites accessed Jan 2011

cialized training or experience in rehabilitation, have 24-hour rehabilitation nursing care, and be managed by an interdisciplinary team of skilled nurses and therapists. Medicare prospective reimbursement is now based on case-mix groups using the Functional Independence Measure (Table 17.2).

The Medicare-approved skilled-nursing facility must provide 24-hour nursing care. Dietary, pharmaceutical, dental, and medical social services are also available. Physicians must supervise patient care and can visit the patient infrequently, but they must be available 24 hours per day on an emergency basis. Therapy services are available, but multidisciplinary coordination may not occur. In this setting, maintenance of function without progress may be the goal of care.

Medicare provides home-health benefits to patients who require nursing care or therapy services on an intermittent or part-time basis, defined as <7 days per week or <8 hours per day for all required services. Patients must also be homebound, defined as requiring considerable effort to leave home. Patients can leave home for medical treatments or for short, infrequent nonmedical reasons, including attendance at religious services. Home-health services must be prescribed and recertified every 60 days by a physician. There is no prior hospitalization requirement or limit on the number of visits a person may receive. Medicare provides care in 60-day episodes. Home-health services provide skilled nursing and home-health aides, therapy services, medical social services, and supplies. Home-health aide services require concomitant skilled-nursing or therapy visits.

The escalating expenditures for Medicare's postacute care benefits from $2.5 billion in 1986 to more than $30 billion in 1996 led to the Balanced Budget Act (BBA) of 1997, which mandated prospective payment systems rather than fee-for-service reimbursement. In skilled-nursing facilities, the BBA mandated the implementation of a per diem prospective payment system covering all costs (routine, ancillary, and capital) related to the services provided to the patients under Part A of the Medicare program. Per diem payments for each admission are case-mix adjusted by the use of a resident classification system (RUG III) that is based on data from patient assessments (the MDS 2) and relative weights developed from staff time data. Home-healthcare reimbursement is also under a prospective payment system. Payment rates are based on relevant data from patient assessments conducted by clinicians using the Outcome and Assessment Information Set (OASIS). The OASIS was originally developed to assess quality of care in home health. The OASIS is lengthy, encompassing sociodemographic, environmental, support system, health status, and functional status attributes; it is required for reimbursement by Medicare for home-health services. For each 60-day episode of care, national payment rates vary, depending on the intensity of care required. Home-health agencies receive less than the full 60-day episode rate if they provide only a minimal number of visits to beneficiaries.

Sites of Care and Outcomes

The effect of site of care on rehabilitation outcomes is not well established. A study of outcomes among patients with stroke and hip fracture examined rates of discharge to home and recovery of function that were based on use of inpatient or nursing rehabilitation services. When controlling for case-mix differ-

Table 17.3—Roles of Core Healthcare Providers on Rehabilitation Team

Provider	Primary Role on Rehabilitation Team
Nursing	Provides patient and family education Evaluates self-care skills Evaluates family and home factors
Physical therapist	Assesses joint range of motion and muscle strength Assesses gait and mobility Provides appropriate assistive devices Instructs in exercise training to increase range of motion, strength, endurance, balance, coordination, and gait Treats with physical modalities (heat, cold, ultrasound, massage, electrical stimulation)
Occupational therapist	Evaluates self-care skills and other ADLs Provides home assessment Provides self-care skills training; makes recommendations and provides training in use of assistive technology Fabricates splints and treats upper-extremity deficits
Speech therapist	Assesses all aspects of communication Assesses swallowing disorders Treats communication deficits Recommends changes in diet and positioning to treat dysphagia
Social worker	Evaluates family and home-care factors Assesses psychosocial factors Provides counseling
Dietician	Assesses nutritional status Recommends dietary changes to maximize nutrition
Prosthetist	Makes and fits prosthetic limbs
Physician, nurse practitioner	Certifies rehabilitation need (physician only) Supervises patient treatment Treats medical comorbidities

ences, the researchers found that stroke but not hip fracture patients were more likely to be discharged home and to recover ADLs if treated in an inpatient rehabilitation setting (SOE=B). In another cohort study, patients admitted for hip fracture to inpatient facilities had better 12-week functional outcomes than did patients undergoing rehabilitation at skilled-nursing facilities (SOE=B). This type of observational study is vulnerable to bias, despite adjusting the analyses, because the prognosis for recovery may influence discharge site; patients with a poor prognosis are more likely to go to the nursing home, while those with a better prognosis go to inpatient or home-health settings. Nevertheless, site of care may be an important factor in recovery.

Each site of care has advantages and disadvantages from the patient's perspective. Inpatient care is the most intense but may not be endurable for frail older patients, because it usually requires 3 hours per day of active (and fatiguing) therapy. Skilled nursing offers 24-hour care for those who cannot care for themselves or do not have a full-time caregiver. Outpatient services have clear advantages and disadvantages. Patients often prefer to return to their own homes but may not have the care support they need. Participation in day hospitals or outpatient clinics requires transportation, which can be costly and time consuming.

In summary, clinicians should be familiar with the services provided in a wide range of rehabilitation settings and with the advantages and disadvantages of each. The clinician is responsible for recommending the best match between patient needs and program services. However, under certain insurance plans, decisions about location of services can be heavily influenced by costs. More systematic evaluation of rehabilitation outcomes that is based on the structures and processes of care offered by various settings is essential for more rational use of rehabilitation programs. CMS is currently monitoring the quality of patient care using information from patient assessments.

TEAMS AND ROLES

An interdisciplinary team is often required to meet the complex rehabilitation needs of older adults. Coordinating this care is the function of the interdisciplinary care team; team members must be able to define roles, share tasks, and communicate within and outside the team. Team building and improving team function are important issues for geriatric rehabilitation service providers. All health professionals who work with older adults should have a basic understanding of the roles and functions of various team members (Table 17.3). The multidisciplinary team often includes nursing, physical therapy, occupational therapy, speech therapy, social work services, nutrition services, prosthetics, and geriatric medicine.

The patient and family are core members of the rehabilitation team; their expectations and preferences must be integrated into the care plan. Rehabilitation, unlike many other interventions, requires active patient participation. If the patient is the leader in decision making, he or she gains a sense of control and responsibility. Patient self-management is now an essential part of the effective management of chronic disease. Chronic disease self-management incorporates self-monitoring, knowledge about disease, and personal control over prevention and management practices.

The primary goal of multidisciplinary team management is to ensure that patients receive comprehensive assessments and interventions for the disabling illness and associated comorbid conditions, as well as for the specific impairments and environmental factors that can affect activities and participation. The team must establish common goals and a cohesive treatment plan.

IMPACT OF COMORBID CONDITIONS

In older patients, comorbid diseases and conditions can interrupt or delay treatment and often require the care plan to be modified. Many of the illnesses that can interfere with rehabilitation of older adults are predictable and potentially preventable. A systematic approach to assessment, prevention, and management of comorbid conditions can improve the patient's chance of receiving maximal benefit from rehabilitation services.

Older adults with reduced mobility are at high risk of skin breakdown, which can interfere with recovery and require extensive treatment. Immobility or altered weight bearing can precipitate pressure ulcers that heal poorly. Clinicians should monitor pressure and weight-bearing areas and be prepared to modify footwear, wheelchairs, and bedding as needed. (See also "Pressure Ulcers and Wound Care," p 283.) Because thromboembolic events are also common with reduced mobility, their prevention should be a routine part of care. Length of time for prophylaxis and medication recommendations vary depending on the medical condition.

Incontinence is prevalent among older adults; causes include detrusor overactivity, obstruction, neurogenic bladder, immobility, and cognitive deficits. Indwelling catheters increase the risk of infection and are rarely appropriate in the nonacute setting. A structured approach to the assessment and treatment of bladder problems should be a basic component of any rehabilitation service. See also "Urinary Incontinence," p 207.

The risk of pneumonia is increased by inactivity and disordered swallowing, as well as by underlying lung disease. The prevention of aspiration pneumonia involves difficult tradeoffs. Awareness of aspiration has been markedly increased by routine radiologic screening, but the clinical relevance of modest aspiration detected radiologically is unknown. Conservative measures such as changing food consistency with liquid thickeners and cohesive food substances and elevating head position while eating can help alleviate the problem. Sometimes aspiration risk is addressed by discontinuing all oral feeding and placing an enteral feeding tube. This approach eliminates the fundamental human pleasure of eating and may not be successful, because oral secretions or refluxed gastric contents can still be aspirated. (See also "Eating and Feeding Problems," p 203.) Bleeding in the upper GI tract can occur during rehabilitation as a consequence of stress or medications and may not be preceded by typical symptoms. See also "Gastrointestinal Diseases and Disorders," p 391.

Anemia is common in older adults and has been associated with adverse outcomes, including functional impairment, decreased muscle strength, and poorer quality of life. Studies are ongoing to examine the effect of erythropoietin on exercise tolerance. See also "Hematologic Diseases and Disorders," p 513.

Mental functioning is critical for rehabilitation, which requires the ability to follow commands and to learn. Because older adults who have been acutely ill are at increased risk of delirium, clinicians should assess mental status and screen for easily reversible causes in their older rehabilitation patients. (See also "Delirium," p 264.) Depression is endemic in newly disabled individuals and can manifest as low motivation; formal screens for depression and early intervention are essential. (See also "Depression and Other Mood Disorders," p 295.) Seizures can develop after stroke, and spasticity can develop during stroke recovery. Interventions for spasticity such as physical therapy or muscle relaxants have offered only modest benefit (SOE=B). Some trials of botulinum toxin have suggested promising results, but others have had no effect (SOE=B). See also stroke in "Neurologic Diseases and Disorders," p 464.

Certain comorbid conditions common in older adults, including diabetes mellitus, heart disease, peripheral vascular disease, musculoskeletal disorders, sensory impairments, and dementia, require ongoing adaptations in rehabilitation. Activity level is a powerful factor in glucose metabolism; diabetic patients are therefore likely to experience changes in glucose levels and medication requirements during rehabilitation. Increased caloric intake during recovery can also affect medication needs. Therapy personnel should know how to assess diabetic control, use a glucometer, and intervene for hypoglycemia. (See also "Diabetes Mellitus," p 504.) Most abnormal gaits increase the energy requirements of walking; an abnormal gait in a patient with coronary artery disease can cause coronary symptoms to worsen. Patients with poor cardiac output may have extreme exercise limitations. Medication adjustments for heart diseases may be necessary but can cause adverse events of their own, such as orthostatic hypotension. Patients with one vascular disease often have others; peripheral vascular disease is common, often associated with insensitive or painful feet and high risk of skin breakdown. Treatment of painful peripheral neuropathy can foster increased activity and avoid pressure ulcers. Musculoskeletal status should be monitored to avoid overuse syndromes involving increased demand on vulnerable joints. For those with vision or hearing impairment, corrections must be provided and teaching approaches adapted accordingly. In patients with dementia, rehabilitation progress is still possible, but carryover may be decreased and the need for supervision and cueing may be increased.

REHABILITATION APPROACHES AND INTERVENTIONS

The primary goals of rehabilitation treatment are restitution of function, compensation for and adaptation to functional losses, and prevention of secondary complications. Ultimately, rehabilitation should maximize the person's potential for participation in social, leisure, or work roles. Many strategies can be used to achieve these goals. Restitution of physical function usually depends on therapeutic exercises to improve flexibility, strength, motor control, and cardiovascular endurance. Exercise has been shown to improve strength, endurance, and balance in well-defined populations of disabled older adults (SOE=A). (See also "Physical Activity," p 54.) In stroke, speech and language therapy can be used to treat aphasia. Cognitive rehabilitation might improve alertness and attention. However, research evidence is insufficient to demonstrate that speech and language therapy, or cognitive rehabilitation, improve functional deficits.

Massage, heat, cold, and ultrasound are used to decrease pain and muscle spasm. These and other pain management strategies can contribute to increased function and tolerance for further rehabilitation. There is little research evidence supporting objective benefits from these therapies, but patients commonly report symptomatic relief. See also "Persistent Pain," p 109.

Equipment for mobility, dressing and bathroom assistance, orthotic and prosthetic devices, and splints all can augment or replace the function of impaired body parts and thereby reduce limitations in activities and participation. For example, an ankle orthosis can prevent foot drop and improve safety and speed of walking. A wheelchair can provide mobility for community activities.

Repeated practice of task-specific activities such as bed mobility, transfers, and walking can improve functional mobility. Arm function improves with specific functional training activities, such as grasps, reaches, and fine manipulations. Balance training may improve balance and reduce the risk of falls. Older adults can benefit from retraining in IADLs such as cooking, managing finances, or driving a car.

Contextual factors, both environmental and personal, should be addressed to minimize restrictions on a person's activities and participation. For example, motivation can be addressed by collaborative goal setting, patient and family education, detection and management of depression, and use of support groups. Environmental modifications, such as grab bars and raised toilet seats in the bathroom or curb cutouts on public streets, can promote independent functioning.

To maintain function and enhance health status after rehabilitation, patients and families should assume responsibility for long-term self-management. Rehabilitation goals include a program to prevent worsening disability, including reintegration into social programs such as senior center programs, and health and wellness programs.

COMPREHENSIVE ASSESSMENT

Comprehensive assessment of rehabilitation patients is necessary for appropriate clinical management and for the evaluation of outcomes. The treatment plan should be guided by the results of the initial assessment. The primary components of any assessment include patient demographics, social support, place of residence before illness, medical comorbidities, severity of current illness, and the patient's prior functional status. The rehabilitation stay is an ideal time for medication review and reconciliation, as patients transition from the hospital to the rehabilitation setting and ultimately to the community.

Impairments such as deficits in range of motion and flexibility, strength, sensory functions, balance, cognition, and depression should always be assessed. In conditions such as stroke, swallowing and language function should be evaluated. The patient's functional status is assessed with standardized measures of ADLs (eg, the Barthel ADL Index [Table 17.2]) and measures of IADLs. The patient's participation or quality of life is assessed with generic measures like the SF-36 Health Survey (available at http://www.sf-36.org [accessed Jan 2011]) or disease-specific measures like the Stroke Impact Scale or the Harris Hip Questionnaire (Table 17.2).

STROKE

Stroke is a major cause of mortality and morbidity in the United States, particularly among people ≥55 yr old. Acute stroke occurs in >700,000 people each year, and 80% or more are likely to survive, many with residual neurologic difficulties. Stroke-related deficits are severe in approximately one-third of the survivors. Many patients with mild and moderate stroke become independent in ADLs, but other more complex dimensions of health status may still be affected. As stroke survival continues to increase, the need for comprehensive stroke rehabilitation will rise. Rehabilitation programs must address a broad range of stroke-related disabilities, including those in basic ADLs and IADLs, and participation and integration into health and wellness programs.

Goals of Rehabilitation

The overall goals of rehabilitation for older stroke patients include regaining function, compensating for or adaptating to functional losses, and preventing secondary complications. Specific objectives include the following:

- preventing or recognizing and managing comorbid illness and medical complications
- assessing each patient comprehensively, using standardized assessments
- matching the patient's needs to the program capabilities
- training the patient to maximize independence in ADLs and IADLs
- facilitating the patient's and family's psychosocial coping and adaptation
- preventing recurrent stroke and other vascular conditions such as myocardial infarction
- assisting the patient in reintegrating into the community

Rehabilitation for older adults with stroke is complex because of the variability of causes, symptoms, severity, and recovery. Stroke patients present with varying symptoms, depending on the site and size of the brain lesions. The most common type of neurologic deficit is hemiparesis, but other deficits can include sensory impairment, aphasia, dysarthria, cognitive impairment, motor incoordination, hemianopsia, visual-perceptual deficits, depression, dysphagia, and bowel and bladder incontinence. The degree of initial recovery and the time needed to reach maximal recovery is affected by the number of deficits. For example, individuals who have hemiparesis, hemianopsia, and sensory deficits are

less likely to ambulate independently and require longer to regain skills than do those with only hemiparesis.

Stroke patients usually experience some degree of recovery. This recovery is most dramatic in the first 30 days but may continue more gradually for months. In the Framingham study, improvement in motor function and self-care slowed 3 mo after stroke but continued at a reduced pace throughout the first year. Language and visual-spatial function was recovered over 12 mo, but cognitive function improved during only the first 3 mo.

Approach to Management

Guidelines for rehabilitation after stroke have been updated by a team sponsored by the Department of Veterans Affairs and the Department of Defense (available at http://www.healthquality.va.gov/Management_of_Stroke_Rehabilitation.asp [accessed Jan 2011]). The guidelines offer algorithms for initial assessment and rehabilitation referral, followed by management in inpatient or community settings. The guidelines emphasize that clinical outcomes are better when patients with acute stroke are treated in a setting that provides coordinated, multidisciplinary stroke-related evaluation and services (SOE=A). Studies have confirmed that adherence to guidelines promotes better outcomes. Coordinated care reduces 1-yr mortality, improves functional independence, and increases satisfaction with care (SOE=A). Benefits are not restricted to any particular subgroup of patients. Stroke severity should be systematically assessed, using the NIH Stroke Scale (www.strokecenter.org/trials/scales/nihss.html [accessed Jan 2011]).

In general, therapy should be started early, but later supplementary interventions can also be beneficial. There are several philosophical approaches to physical rehabilitation after strokes that are based on neurophysiologic, motor learning, or orthopedic principles. In a Cochrane review, a mixed approach was significantly more effective than no treatment or placebo (sham treatment) control for improving functional independence (standardized mean difference 0.94, 95% confidence intervals 0.08 to 1.80). There is no convincing evidence that any one specific technique is superior to another.

Newer therapeutic interventions for regaining motor function are in development. Constraint-induced movement therapy (CIMT) discourages the use of the unaffected extremity and encourages active use of the hemiparetic extremity, with a goal of improved motor recovery. Results in patients with chronic stroke impairment suggest potential gains beyond usual therapy. In a large randomized clinical trial of constraint-induced therapy, CIMT produced statistically significant and clinically relevant improvements in arm motor function that persisted for at least 1 yr (SOE=A). Treadmill walking with partial body weight support using a harness connected to an overhead system can improve gait velocity, balance, and motor recovery. Speech and language therapy are often provided for stroke patients with aphasia. However, there is no universally accepted treatment. Although a Cochrane report states that the evidence does not support a finding of either clear effect or lack of effect, the Veterans Affairs guidelines support "good" evidence for follow-up evaluation and treatment by the speech language professional for long-term residual communication difficulties. The guidelines also support "good" evidence for cognitive retraining for attention or visual-spatial perceptual deficits and compensatory training for short-term memory deficits. The same guidelines find "good" evidence for medication treatment for depression and emotional lability. Spasticity can develop gradually after stroke and can inhibit function and interfere with hygiene. Most interventions, including surgery and medications like baclofen, have been disappointing.

The patient who has had a stroke is at high risk of recurrence: up to 7%–10% annually. The rehabilitation phase is an appropriate time to ensure that assessment and treatment for stroke prevention has occurred. Assessments for significant carotid stenosis and for atrial fibrillation should be completed. Indications for carotid endarterectomy and anticoagulation with warfarin should be reviewed. Antiplatelet medications such as aspirin alone or in combination with dipyridamole or clopidogrel should be considered in many patients. Treatment with ACE inhibitors[OL] and statins[OL] has also demonstrated reduced risk of stroke. Other risk factors to be targeted for preventing stroke recurrence include hypertension and smoking (SOE=A).

In summary, the evidence for specific interventions for stroke rehabilitation is weak. The collective benefits of well-organized multidisciplinary care, including secondary prevention, are well established. See also cerebrovascular diseases in "Neurologic Diseases and Disorders," p 464.

HIP FRACTURE

Epidemiology and Surgical Care

Each year in the United States, about 300,000 people fracture a hip. The risk of fracture is higher in women, in nursing-home residents, and in people with dementia. Mortality is about 5% during the initial hospitalization but nears 25% in the year after fracture. About 75% of survivors recover to their prior level of function, but their overall mobility is more limited; up to half still require an assistive device. About half of patients will have an initial decline requiring transient long-term care, and about 25% will still be in long-term care 1 yr later.

For medically stable patients, surgical repair is recommended 24–72 hours after fracture. This early repair has been associated with a reduction in 1-yr mortality, as well as with a lower incidence of complications such as pressure ulcers and delirium. For medically unstable patients, delaying surgery is warranted to allow sufficient improvement to tolerate the procedure. The surgical approach is determined by the location of the fracture, the presence or absence of displacement, and the prefracture mobility. One-third of hip fractures occur at the femoral neck, and the other two-thirds are intertrochanteric, occurring lateral to the femoral neck. Prefracture mobility is used as a guide to determine the goal of surgical treatment and to allow the risks and benefits of each surgical procedure to be considered.

Femoral neck fractures without any displacement can be surgically corrected with simple screws. However, femoral neck fractures with any degree of displacement are at increased risk of nonunion or avascular necrosis and therefore are usually treated with a prosthetic femoral head (hemiarthroplasty). Patients with significant underlying bony acetabular disease and a displaced femoral neck fracture may benefit from complete hip arthroplasty. Patients are usually allowed to bear weight immediately after repair of a femoral neck fracture, regardless of type of surgical procedure.

For intertrochanteric fractures, the treatment of choice is open reduction and internal fixation with a compression screw or similar device. Provided there is little or no displacement, immediate weight bearing is usually allowed. However, displaced or comminuted intertrochanteric fractures commonly remain unstable, even after surgical fixation. Therefore, full weight bearing is often not allowed for up to 6 wk or until the stability of the fracture is assured. Factors that influence recovery should be assessed, including prior mobility and functional status, comorbid conditions, cognitive status, social support, type of injury, and repair and pain status. Mobility performance can be systematically assessed with numerous instruments, including the Harris Hip Questionnaire, which was developed specifically for hip fracture.

Rehabilitation After Hip Fracture

Rehabilitation after hip fracture includes pain management, mobilization, and prevention of complications, such as delirium and thromboembolic events. The most important factors influencing recovery appear to be how soon mobilization is started and how frequently therapy is provided. Delay in mobilization is often driven by surgical recommendation, with proper healing of the fracture taking precedence over mobility. Partial weight bearing is difficult for many older adults to achieve. Prolonged inactivity is clearly associated with poorer functional outcomes, and early weight bearing is associated with low rates of surgical failure (SOE=A). Accelerated rehabilitation with rapid mobilization, coordinated planning, early discharge, and community follow-up has been associated with a 17% reduction in costs and no detriment to rates of recovery (SOE=B). Intensity of service clearly affects outcome, as those who receive physical therapy more than once a day during initial rehabilitation are more likely to be discharged directly to home than those who receive physical therapy once a day or less (SOE=A).

Prevention of Recurrence

Older adults who have had a hip fracture often have other comorbidities, such as osteoporosis and balance problems, that place them at risk of further fractures. Efforts to diagnose and treat osteoporosis, improve balance, and reduce injury risk are a key part of treatment planning during rehabilitation. (See also "Osteoporosis," p 234.) Hip protectors have been extensively studied, with mostly negative results. See hip protectors in "Falls," p 230.

TOTAL HIP AND KNEE ARTHROPLASTY

Natural History

In the United States, joint arthroplasty is the most common elective surgical procedure performed; approximately 400,000 are done annually. The primary indications for joint replacement are progressive pain and limitation of mobility despite conservative care. The most common diagnosis associated with the need for joint replacement is osteoarthrosis, followed by rheumatoid arthritis. The long-term results of joint replacement have generally been excellent and include significant pain relief and improved function. Continued success rates in the 90% range are seen 10–15 yr after joint replacement. The most common reason for failure of the hip or knee replacement is loosening of the implant. Joint infection is another major concern; infection affects 0.2%–1.1% of total hip and 1%–2% of total knee replacements. Deep infections often necessitate removal of the implant and long-term antibiotics until there is no sign of infection, followed by ultimate replacement with a new implant. See also "Infectious Diseases," p 230.

Assessment

Plain radiographs are the usual method for determining the severity of joint damage at both the hip and knee. Loss of cartilage is shown by joint-space narrowing, and often osteophyte formation is also present (Figure 54.1).

Management

Anticoagulation to prevent thromboembolism and good pain control are the major goals during the immediate postoperative period for both hip and knee arthroplasty. (See also "Perioperative Care," p 230.) Patients who have undergone a major orthopedic procedure such as total hip or knee arthroplasty are at particularly high risk of both symptomatic and asymptomatic venous thromboembolism. Current guidelines for prevention of venous thromboembolism recommend against the use of aspirin alone for any patient (SOE=A). For patients after total hip arthroplasty, extended prophylaxis with either low-molecular-weight heparin or a vitamin K antagonist (INR range 2–3) is recommended for up to 28–35 days after surgery (SOE=A). Pain control in the initial postoperative period is often achieved with opioids administered orally, intravenously, or by patient-controlled analgesia pumps. For both hip and knee arthroplasty, early mobilization is the standard of care, and weight bearing often begins on the second postoperative day. Patients at low risk can often be discharged from the acute care hospital within 5 days. For those at high risk, defined as being >70 yr old or having two or more comorbid conditions, early inpatient rehabilitation improves functional outcomes and decreases total length of stay (SOE=B). Age alone should not be used as a criterion for eligibility for joint replacement—excellent results can be achieved even in patients >80 yr old who are in good health with stable chronic conditions.

To decrease the risk of dislocation after total hip arthroplasty, patients are taught to avoid motions such as deep squats and crossing their legs. To prevent excessive hip flexion, a raised toilet seat is recommended for the first few months after surgery. Rehabilitation focuses on strengthening especially the abductors, which are weakened by the surgical approach, as well as on progressive range-of-motion and gait training. Minimally invasive surgery using an incision <10 cm long can lead to quicker recovery and return to function. This technique is currently being evaluated.

After total knee replacement, recovery of range of motion is the key to return of function and is often aided by the use of a continuous passive-motion machine (CPM). Based on a systematic review, early postoperative CPM decreased the need for postoperative manipulation and, combined with physical therapy, increased active range of motion and shortened length of stay. Surgeons have also applied the concept of minimal incisions to the total knee replacement surgery and with significantly more success. This surgery, in experienced hands, decreases blood loss and length of stay (SOE=A). Postoperative swelling is common and interferes with regaining motion. However, thigh-high compression stockings, the CPM, and possibly cryotherapy can be used to manage swelling.

AMPUTATION

Epidemiology

Approximately 75,000 people undergo leg amputation each year in the United States. Most of these people have systemic vascular disease, with or without diabetes mellitus. Those with diabetes often have other end-organ disease, such as blindness, end-stage renal disease, and peripheral neuropathy. Mortality in this group approaches 50% at 2 yr and 70% at 5 yr. For up to one-fifth of patients, amputation of the other leg is needed within the first 2 yr after the initial amputation. Most dysvascular amputees have such a burden of comorbid disease that the prosthesis is largely used for limited mobility, such as transfers and ambulation within the home.

Assessment

Key factors to assess include the patient's prior functional status, stability of comorbid conditions, cognition, and arm use, as well as the condition of the stump and the other leg. Successful prosthetic ambulation is associated with independent prior ambulation, ability to bear weight on the contralateral leg, stable medical status, and ability to follow directions. Blindness and end-stage renal disease do not necessarily preclude rehabilitation. A systematic approach to monitoring amputee status has been incorporated into an instrument, the Prosthetic Profile of the Amputee (http://www.csp.org.uk/director/effectivepractice/outcomemeasures/database.cfm [accessed Jan 2011]).

Rehabilitation for Amputation

Rehabilitation starts in the preoperative stage, when the patient begins with strength and flexibility exercises and is educated about the recovery process. Amputation surgery generally aims to preserve the knee, because the energy requirement for walking is much lower for the below-the-knee amputee than for the above-the-knee amputee. This decision must be weighed against risks of poor wound healing with more distal amputation.

Postoperative rehabilitation includes efforts at early mobilization, prevention of contractures, wound healing, and shaping of the stump. Poor wound healing delays rehabilitation in about 25% of cases. Prostheses vary in weight, socket type, style of foot, and suspensions. The older amputee benefits from a prosthesis that is lightweight, stable, and easy to use. Prosthetic rehabilitation involves progressive ambulation, teaching about prosthesis and stump care, and monitoring for stump injury.

Last, phantom limb pain is common after amputation, with an estimated incidence of 60%–80%, and pain management influences progress with rehabilitation. Treatment remains difficult, and clear evidence-based guidelines are lacking. Because tricyclic antidepressants[OL] and sodium channel blockers such as carbamazepine[OL] are generally effective for neuropathic pain, they are often used for phantom pain despite the lack of well-controlled trials (SOE=B). A number of other medication regimens, using such agents as opioids[OL] and anesthetic blocks[OL], have also had success in small trials. Two trials using memantine showed no benefit in the treatment of phantom limb pain.

MOBILITY AIDS, ORTHOTICS, ADAPTIVE METHODS, AND ENVIRONMENTAL MODIFICATIONS

Assistive devices, orthotics, adaptive methods, and environmental modifications are effective for older adults with disabilities. It is important to identify the underlying causes of disability before prescribing a device or modification, because medical or surgical treatment for individual diseases and impairments may be more effective or may enhance the usefulness of these approaches.

Mobility Aids

Canes typically support 15%–20% of the body weight and are used in the hand contralateral to the affected knee or hip. A straight cane has a single tip, while a quad cane has four tips. As the number of tips increases, the degree of support also increases, but the cane becomes heavier and more awkward to use. The handle of the cane may be curved or have a pistol grip; the pistol grip offers more support. Canes can be made of a variety of materials, but most are made of wood or lightweight aluminum. The length of the cane is important for stability. Some canes are adjustable, but wooden canes must be cut to size. One of two methods can be used to evaluate the proper cane length: measuring the distance from the distal wrist crease to the ground when the patient is standing erect, and measuring the distance from the greater trochanter to the ground.

Crutches, axillary or forearm, are usually used to provide bilateral support. Axillary crutches are seldom recommended for older adults because greater arm strength and coordination are required for use. In addition, there is a risk of brachial plexus injury if the crutches are used incorrectly. Forearm crutches are more functional because a cuff secures the crutch on the patient's arm, allowing use of the hand to manipulate objects. A single crutch can be used instead of a cane if additional unilateral support is needed.

A walker is prescribed when a cane does not offer sufficient stability. A walker can completely support one leg but cannot support full body weight. Walker types include pick-up and wheeled walkers. Walkers should be adjusted so that the user maintains an erect posture and is not required to lean forward to reach the walker. The pick-up walker is lifted and moved forward by the user, who then advances before lifting the walker again; the result is a slow, staggering gait. It requires strength to repeatedly pick up the walker and cognitive ability to learn the necessary coordination. A wheeled walker allows for a smoother, coordinated, and faster gait and takes advantage of compensated gait patterns. It is more likely to be correctly used by those with cognitive impairment. The most commonly used type is the two-wheeled walker, which brakes automatically with increased downward pressure. A "rollator" is a four-wheeled walker with hand brakes, which can be locked when the patient is transferring. This type also has a platform seat for resting, and a basket for carrying objects. Because of the use of the hand brakes, the rollator requires greater skill. It is preferred for outdoor use because the wheels are larger and move easier over sidewalks and slightly rough terrain (Figure 17.1).

Patients who cannot safely use or are unable to ambulate with an assistive device require a wheelchair. A wheelchair must be fitted according to the patient's body build, weight, disability, and prognosis. Incorrect fit can result in poor posture, joint deformity, reduced mobility, pressure ulcers, circulatory compromise, and discomfort. For the older patient with only one functional arm, the wheelchair can be lowered to allow for foot propulsion. Patients with leg amputations may have the wheels set posteriorly to compensate for a change in the center of gravity. Motorized wheelchairs can be used by mentally alert individuals with bilateral arm weakness or severe cardiopulmonary disease who lack the endurance to push a wheelchair. Motorized scooters offer less trunk support than motorized wheelchairs but are more acceptable to some people. Motorized scooters and wheelchairs increase patients' mobility but increase their risk of deconditioning, as they might otherwise push a wheelchair or ambulate. The use of a wheelchair commonly requires home modifications, including ramps and widened doorways. Cars may need to be adapted with lifts.

Orthotics, Adaptive Methods, and Environmental Modifications

Orthotics are exoskeletons designed to assist, resist, align, and stimulate function. Orthotics are named by the use of letters for each joint that the device involves in its structure. Thus, an AFO is an ankle and foot orthotic device used to support weak calf or pretibial muscles (eg, for a stroke patient with leg weakness).

Adaptations to facilitate dressing may be necessary for patients with problems such as frequent soiling or diminished flexibility, coordination, and endurance. Clothing that is easy to clean, tops that fit easily over the head or fasten in the front and allow for freedom of movement are helpful. Hook-and-loop tape is usually easier to use than buttons and can be sewn on to replace buttons and zippers. When buttons are necessary, if they are sewn on with elastic thread, the need to manipulate them can be eliminated. Putting on shoes and socks is particularly difficult for older adults with decreased agility. Longer, looser socks (eg, tubular socks) are easier to put on. For patients who find that reaching the feet to put on shoes is a problem, a long-handled shoehorn may be useful. Elastic shoelaces eliminate the need for tying and untying.

Environmental modifications can have a major impact on the older adult's ability to function independently or with minimal assistance at home. A variety of assistive devices, such as reachers, special utensils, and adapted telephones, can reduce the difficulty of performing daily tasks and have a significant impact on a person's quality of life.

The bathroom is a common place for falls. Any older adult with impaired balance or leg weakness should have bars installed near the toilet and tub or shower. Raised toilet seats and bathtub benches are available to assist those with leg weakness. These are also useful for older adults with arthritis of the hips or knees because they reduce biomechanical stress on the joint. Long-handled bath brushes, hand-held shower heads, and "soap on a rope" can be helpful for older adults with arm weakness or other impairment.

Figure 17.1.—Commonly Prescribed Mobility Aids

Canes: straight and quad
- Provide unilateral support
- Assist with balance
- Reduce weight bearing on opposite leg
- Small- and large-based quad canes available

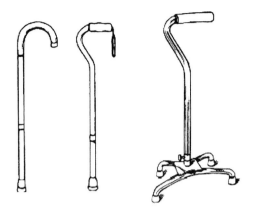

Walker: stationary "pick-up"
- Provides bilateral support
- Must be lifted and advanced, requiring strength and coordination
- Very stable and allows non-weight-bearing movement

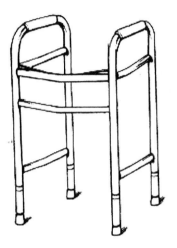

Walkers: rolling or rollator
- Less stable than stationary walker, but easier to advance
- Allows for smoother, faster gait
- Rollator requires more coordination (because of brakes)
- Rollator good for outside walking because of large wheels

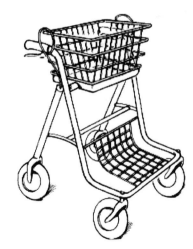

REFERENCES

■ Lin JT, Lane JM. Rehabilitation of the older adult with an osteoporosis-related fracture. *Clin Geriatr Med.* 2006;22(2):435–447.

■ Perret DM, Rim J, Cristian A. A geriatrician's guide to the use of the physical modalities in the treatment of pain and dysfunction. *Clin Geriatr Med.* 2006;22(2):331–354.

CHAPTER 18—NURSING-HOME CARE

KEY POINTS

■ Currently there are 15,850 nursing homes with 1.7 million beds, 1.3 million residents, and 2.5 million discharges each year.

■ The Omnibus Budget Reconciliation Act of 1987 requires a periodic comprehensive assessment of all nursing-home residents, sets minimum staffing requirements, and fosters residents' rights by limiting the use of restraints and psychoactive medications.

■ The care of nursing-home residents has become more complex over the past several years, commensurate with an increasing level of medical acuity in an environment constrained by lack of resources.

THE NURSING-HOME POPULATION

Currently 1.3 million Americans >65 yr old live in nursing homes. Relatively speaking, this is a small portion of the 36 million Americans in that age group. The typical nursing-home resident is a white, unmarried woman >85 yr old with limited social supports and usually widowed (60%). Most people admitted to nursing homes are older adults, with average age at admission of 79 yr. Only 9% of nursing-home residents are <65 yr old. The percentage of black residents in U.S. nursing homes has increased in recent years (9%), approaching national population norms. In fact, black Americans 65–74 yr old are more likely than white Americans to be admitted to a nursing home. Nonetheless, other nonwhite populations, such as Hispanic Americans, Asian Americans, and Native Americans, are under-represented in nursing homes despite even higher disability rates in these groups. Older adults with developmental disabilities constitute another unique population that is requiring increasing nursing-home care as their older parent-caregivers are lost. These individuals often require specialized care that many nursing homes have difficulty providing. See also "Mental Retardation," p 329.

Today's population of older adults in the nursing home is sicker than the nursing-home population of even 5 yr ago. Over two-thirds of long-stay residents in skilled-nursing facilities have multiple medical conditions. At admission, 3.9% of nursing-facility residents have pressure sores. Nearly 40% of older adults in the nursing home are diagnosed with heart failure or ischemic heart disease. Diabetes and stroke are reported in 22% and 26% of new nursing-home admissions, respectively. COPD, hypertension, arthritis, and hip fractures are also prevalent health conditions among nursing-home residents.

Although approximately 25% of older adults residing in nursing homes are diagnosed with dementia, experts estimate that 50%–70% of nursing-home residents meet the diagnostic criteria for dementia, making dementia the most commonly occurring condition in nursing homes. Depression is diagnosed in 20%–25% of residents. In 39% of nursing-home residents >65 yr old, both medical and psychiatric conditions have been diagnosed, reflecting a 60% increase in prevalence of comorbid physical and mental diagnoses in this population, when compared with 1999 data. Additionally, behavioral issues, such as verbal and social inappropriateness, wandering, and resistance to care, are observed in one-third of nursing-home residents. The prevalence of cognitive impairments is reflected in the fact that 81% of nursing-home residents are impaired in their ability to make daily decisions and two-thirds have orientation difficulties or memory problems, or both.

Functional disability is also prevalent in today's nursing-home residents. More than half of long-stay nursing-home residents require supervision or hands-on assistance from another person in five ADLs (ie, eating, dressing, bathing, transferring, and toileting). Cumulative disability is high, with about 75% of nursing-home residents requiring assistance in three or more ADLs. Assistance with bathing and dressing is needed by three-fourths of residents. Many residents require a mechanically altered diet consistency, and 52% of residents are totally dependent for eating. Difficulty with bladder and or bowel control is reported in nearly 60% of newly admitted and 40% of long-stay nursing-home residents >65 yr old. Only

Table 18.1—Selected Demographic and Functional Characteristics of Adults ≥65 yr old Living in Nursing Homes, 2004

	Older Adult Nursing-Home Population (%)		
	Recently Admitted Resident (<30 days)	Long-Stay Resident (≥90 days)	Permanent Resident (≥1 yr)
Total percent	9.9%	80.6%	56.4%
Age (yr)			
65–74	15.3	12.6	12.2
75–84	43.4	34.1	32.4
≥85	41.2	53.4	55.4
Gender			
Male	33.7	23.9	22.3
Female	66.3	76.1	77.7
Marital status[a]			
Married	28.7	19.4	18.1
Widowed	53.1	60.1	59.9
Never married	4.9	7.0	7.8
Single	3.4	4.2	4.3
Divorced/separated	6.6	8.1	8.8
Walking ability[a]			
Walks without hands-on help	17.3	27.7	27.5
Walks with hands-on help	49.8	30.9	28.2
Does not walk	32.9	41.4	44.3
Number of ADLs for which hands-on help is provided[a]			
0	10.2	5.5	5.1
1	4.7	8.9	8.9
2	4.9	7.0	6.8
3	6.3	7.7	7.3
4	46.6	36.7	35.5
5	27.2	34.2	36.3
Difficulty with bowel or bladder control[b]			
Yes	58.9	38.1	35.9
No	41.1	61.9	64.1

[a] Categories do not add up to 100% because of missing information.

[b] Includes individuals with ostomy, indwelling catheter, or other device, as well as those who were incontinent.

SOURCE: Data from Kasper J, O'Malley M. Changes in Characteristics, Needs, and Payment for Care of Elderly Nursing Home Residents: 1999 to 2004. Washington, DC: Kaiser Family Foundation; 2007. Available at www.kff.org/medicaid/7663.cfm (accessed Jan 2011).

59% of older long-stay residents are ambulatory, and few (18%) walk independent of assistance or supervision. Hearing and visual impairments are found in 36% and 39% of residents, respectively. Communication problems are noted in 60% of residents, with 44% having difficulty with both being understood and understanding others. For selected demographic and functional characteristics of older adults who live in nursing homes, see Table 18.1.

NURSING-HOME AVAILABILITY

According to CMS, there are currently 15,850 nursing homes in the United States with 1.7 million beds and 2.5 million discharges (ie, to home, hospital, or secondary to death). Of these facilities, 66.5% are proprietary (ie, for profit), with voluntary nonprofit (27.4%) and government nursing homes (6.1%) accounting for the remainder. The average nursing home operates 107 beds, and a minority (6%) has >200 beds. A little more than half of all nursing homes (56%) are part of a chain. Most admissions to nursing facilities come from acute hospitals, followed by private residences and other nursing homes. Not surprisingly, assisted-living facilities are becoming a greater source of older adults admitted to nursing facilities, accounting for 8.6% of total admissions.

By age 65, a person's lifetime risk of nursing-home admission is high, estimated at 46%. The risk of nursing-home admission rises steeply with age. While 7.4% of those ≥75 yr old reside in nursing homes, this figure approaches 16% for those ≥85 yr old. Barring breakthroughs in the treatment of dementia, the number of people ≥65 yr old using nursing homes will double by the year 2030. Interestingly, the occupancy rates in nursing homes nationally have declined over the past several years and now stand at 85%. This decline has generally been

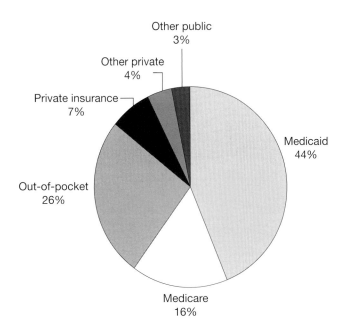

Figure 18.1—Spending for nursing-home care (2005); total spending $121.9 billion

attributed to the availability of other long-term care options, such as assisted living, but there are likely other causal social and financial variables that have yet to be identified. The availability and use of home-care services for Medicare-eligible patients have not been found to consistently reduce nursing-home admissions.

Postacute care is increasingly being offered in nursing-home settings, a response to the higher care needs of older adults in conjunction with shorter hospital stays and the presence of a Medicare payment stream. Although the types of postacute services and programs vary significantly from one locale to another (eg, dialysis, orthopedic, ventilator, postoperative, rehabilitative, wound care), they remain distinct from the standard nursing-home services by integrating the features of acute medical, long-term care nursing, and rehabilitative settings. The challenge in postacute care is that of accommodating patients with varying degrees of disease severity, functional dependence, and comorbidities. Some limited studies suggest that, for selected patient populations, postacute care in the nursing home has outcomes equal to or better than postacute care in acute hospitals. Definitions as to what constitutes postacute care, however, vary widely, as do regulatory standards, which makes comparison studies difficult. See also "Rehabilitation," p 130.

On any given day, short-stay residents, whose length of stay is <30 days after admission, comprise approximately 10% of the nursing-home population. Residents with a length of stay between 30 and 90 days comprise 9.5% of the nursing-home population. Long-stay residents, whose length of stay is ≥90 days

after admission, account for 80% of the nursing-home population >65 yr old. Among all nursing-home residents, 10% have a length of stay >3 yr. Historically, the rate of discharge of residents with length of stay <3 mo has doubled, increasing from 46 per 100 beds in 1977 to 92 per 100 beds in 1999. In contrast, the rate of discharge of those with lengths of stay >3 mo has not changed significantly. This increase in the number of residents with short length of stay coincides with increased Medicare funding of postacute care in nursing homes. Many short-stay residents are admitted for rehabilitation, and some enter nursing homes for terminal care. Interestingly, improvement in function among long-stay nursing-home residents is quite common, which reflects the heterogeneity of this population.

NURSING-HOME FINANCING

Nursing-home expenditures currently total more than $120 billion dollars per year. In 2007, the average cost of a private room in a nursing home was $213 per day or $77,745 annually. Public health programs primarily finance this cost; Medicaid and Medicare account for 65% and 14% of nursing-home care payments, respectively (Figure 18.1). With the high annual costs, those paying for nursing-home care out-of-pocket often deplete their personal funds and turn to public funding. While purchase of long-term care insurance has been increasing, at present these policies pay for only a small fraction of nursing-home care.

Medicare funding for nursing-home costs is available for certain limited conditions for beneficiaries who require skilled-nursing or rehabilitation services. In general, to be covered, beneficiaries must receive services from a Medicare-certified skilled-nursing home after a qualifying hospital stay. A qualifying hospital stay is a hospital stay of at least 3 days before entering a nursing home. Medicare covers only those skilled-nursing-facility services rendered to help a beneficiary recover from an acute illness or injury. Medicare pays for skilled care in full for the first 20 days in a skilled-nursing facility. For days 21–100, a co-payment from the resident is required for skilled-nursing-facility services; beyond 100 days, Medicare does not cover skilled-nursing-facility care. As part of the Balanced Budget Act of 1997, Medicare payments to nursing homes are based on an individual's functional needs and potential for rehabilitation. This prospective payment system, also called PPS, requires careful documentation of functional gains, particularly by rehabilitation therapists. Although the PPS has not conclusively limited access to skilled-nursing care for Medicare beneficiaries, it has forced nursing homes to be more diligent with regard to their admission policies. Not unexpectedly, physical, occupational, and speech therapies are commonly prescribed in the nursing home, with half of all patients admitted to nursing homes receiving at least 90 min of these rehabilitation services, according to one study. The PPS requires nursing-home staff to carefully document gains in function to ensure reimbursement. See "Rehabilitation," p 130.

Supplemental increases in reimbursement are made to offset costs of caring for those with HIV/AIDS. Despite the high cost of nursing-home care, resources remain constrained. In general, psychiatric conditions are undervalued with respect to reimbursement in long-term care. Residents with active psychiatric illness often require increased care and staff time, but mechanisms do not exist for increased reimbursement for those efforts. Shortages of psychiatric specialists trained in nursing-home care, combined with relatively low reimbursement rates for care in nursing homes, adds to the challenge of providing optimal mental health care in this setting.

STAFFING PATTERNS

Patient care and evaluation in the nursing home largely depend on nurses and nursing assistants. Nursing facilities are required to provide nurse staffing sufficient to provide the care outlined in its care plans. According to federal guidelines, every nursing home must have the following on staff: a licensed nurse that acts as charge nurse on each shift; a registered nurse who is on duty at least 8 consecutive hours, 7 days a week; and a registered nurse who is designated as the director of nursing. Studies have confirmed the correlation between the provision of quality care to total nursing hours and the ratio of professional nurses (ie, registered nurses) to nonprofessional nursing staff. A 2001 Institute of Medicine report recommended increasing nurse staffing levels to enhance the quality of nursing-home care, spurring Congress to debate the merits of mandatory minimal staffing ratios. Although recom-mendations for minimal and optimal staffing at nursing facilities have been made by the CMS based on links to quality of care, current federal regulations do not mandate specific nurse-to-resident staffing ratios. The total direct care staffing averages 3.4 hours per resident day (HPRD) or roughly 204 minutes per resident per day. Nursing assistants contribute most direct staff time, at 2.3 HPRD. Licensed nurses and registered nurses contribute 0.8 and 0.3 HPRD, respectively. Despite the increasing medical acuity and care needs of nursing-home residents, staff ratios have been relatively stable. It has been estimated that 9 of 10 nursing homes are inadequately staffed, and nearly 8 billion dollars would be needed to bring staffing to adequate levels.

Of note, many states set staffing requirements for nursing facilities that are higher than federal recommendations. Federal guidelines set minimal educational training for nurse aides at 75 hours.

Recruiting and retaining staff, particularly nursing assistants who constitute the bulk of the nursing-home workforce, also continues to be difficult. Turnover rates of >70% for nurse assistants and >50% each for directors of nursing, registered nurses, and licensed practical nurses have been reported. Turnover rates have been associated with increased rates of hospitalization for nursing-home residents and have been linked to the organizational culture within the nursing facility.

FACTORS ASSOCIATED WITH NURSING-HOME PLACEMENT

Although there is a significant chance of being admitted to a nursing home with increasing age, other factors, such as low income, poor family supports (especially lack of spouse and children), and low social activity have been associated with institutionalization (SOE=B). Cognitive and functional impairments have also predicted nursing-home placement. Interestingly, for patients with dementia, education and caregiver support have been shown to delay the need for nursing-home placement for up to a year (SOE=B). Not surprisingly, older adults with more positive attitudes toward nursing homes are more likely to use skilled-nursing facilities than are adults with less favorable attitudes. The range of long-term care services that are now available (ie, skilled nursing, home care, assisted living) further increases the complexity of placement decisions. The use of formal (ie, paid-for) community services does not necessarily reduce the likelihood of nursing-home placement for patients with severe disabilities.

THE INTERFACE OF ACUTE AND LONG-TERM CARE

Most admissions to nursing facilities come from acute-care hospitals (62%), followed by private residences (23%), assisted-living facilities (9%), and other nursing homes (5%). Conversely, nursing-home residents have high rates of hospitalization, ranging upward of 549 admissions per 1,000 nursing-home beds per year. In a 2002 survey by the CDC, nursing-home residents constituted 2% of all emergency department visits. Each year, >25% of nursing-home residents are transferred at least once to an emergency department for evaluation. Infection is the most common reason for transfer of nursing-home residents to short-stay hospitals, accounting for one-fourth of all such admissions. Unfortunately, the transition from acute to long-term care is often complicated by suboptimal information transfer. Illegible or nonexistent transfer summaries, omission of prescribed medications, and the lack of documentation of advanced directives, psychosocial information, and behavioral issues are but a few of the information gaps commonly reported. See also transitions from hospital care in "Hospital Care," p 119; and "Perioperative Care," p 92.

QUALITY ISSUES AND LEGISLATION INFLUENCING CARE IN THE NURSING HOME

In 1983, the Institute of Medicine published a report documenting significant deficiencies in the care of nursing-home residents. The findings of that report influenced the passage of the Omnibus Budget Reconciliation Act (OBRA) in 1987. As the first major revision of nursing-home legislation in over 20 yr and the first detailed source of clinical expectations for nursing-home care, OBRA has had significant impacts on medical care in nursing homes. OBRA set new, higher standards for quality of care provided in nursing facilities certified for reimbursement under Medicare and Medicaid (which includes most skilled-nursing facilities) by the CMS. (See "Financing, Coverage, and Costs of Health Care," p 32.) CMS pays Medicare claims and interprets legislation into written regulations for skilled-nursing facilities. CMS interprets federal statutes and also writes regulations for Medicaid that are administered by each state's Medicaid program. Federal regulations, including those pertaining to long-term care, are compiled in the *Code of Federal Regulations*. Each federal regulation is given a tag number, often called "F-tags." To qualify for federal reimbursement under Medicare and Medicaid, facilities must comply with these CMS regulations. OBRA regulations targeted many residents' rights issues, including setting limits on restraint use and regulating use of psychoactive medications. Assisted-living facilities do not operate under such all-inclusive mandates, which some believe contribute to the significant variability of care practices and quality of care in that setting.

OBRA also mandates comprehensive periodic assessments of all nursing-home residents. This is accomplished by the Minimum Data Set (MDS), which surveys a host of clinical issues thought to directly relate to the quality of resident care and thus considered pertinent to effective care planning. A resident's medical regimen must be consistent with the assessment compiled in the MDS. CMS also uses the MDS for individual facilities to compile nursing-facility quality measures data, which are reported publicly on the CMS Web site. Measures include outcomes data such as prevalence of pain, pressure ulcers, weight loss, and depression, as well as rates of vaccination, restraint use, and urinary tract infection. While publication of these measures is intended to offer a route by which to compare facilities, it has been criticized for lack of standardization of data to account for the substantial variability in disability and medical acuity between different facilities. For quality measures for nursing homes that are publicly reported by CMS, see Table 18.2.

Adherence to regulations is assessed by mandatory site visit surveys. These surveys are mandated every 15 mo, but occur on average every 12 mo. During the survey, facility procedures and records are reviewed, and quality of care and quality of life for residents are observed. Failure to meet regulatory standards for care is cited in a "deficiency." Penalties imposed for deficiencies depend on the nature and severity of the deficiency and can range from implementation of a corrective action plan to monetary fines, limits on facility admissions, or even facility closure. Inspections can also occur at any time in between mandated surveys as a result of a complaint received by the state. In the years since OBRA was instituted, restraint use in nursing homes has decreased significantly, registered nurse staffing has increased, and training requirements for certified nursing assistants has been established.

OBRA mandates that each individual in a nursing facility receive and be provided the necessary care and services to achieve and maintain "the highest practicable physical, medical, and psychological well-being" that can be obtained. The facility must ensure that the resident optimally improves or deteriorates only within the limits of that resident's right to refuse treatments, and within the influence of their illnesses and normal aging. When a resident declines (or does not improve), a survey team may investigate whether the decline was avoidable. A decline may be determined unavoidable if the resident has been given a careful and thorough assessment, which directs the resident's care plan. The interventions included in the care plan should be evaluated and revised as necessary.

OBRA requires that a state agency must screen and preapprove the admission of individuals with mental retardation or serious mental illness to a nursing facility (F285). This screening is done to ensure that the facility can provide appropriate programs and services to meet the individual's needs. Residents readmitted to a nursing facility from a

Table 18.2—Quality Measures for Nursing Homes Based on the Minimum Data Set and Publicly Reported by CMS

Quality Measures	Time Frame for Minimum Data Set Observation*
For Long-Stay Residents	
Percent given influenza vaccination during flu season	October 1 thru March 31
Percent assessed and given pneumococcal vaccination	5 years
Percent whose need for help with ADLs has increased	7 days
Percent with moderate to severe pain	7 days
Percent who were physically restrained	7 days
Percent who are more depressed or anxious	30 days
Percent who have/had an indwelling catheter inserted	14 days
Percent who spent most of their time in bed or in a chair	7 days
Percent whose ability to move about in and around their room worsened	7 days
Percent with a urinary tract infection	30 days
Percent who lose too much weight	30 days
For Low-Risk Long-Stay Residents	
Percent who lose control of their bowels or bladder	14 days
Percent who have pressure sores	7 days
For High-Risk Long-Stay Residents	
Percent who have pressure sores	7 days
For Short-Stay Residents	
Percent given influenza vaccination during flu season	October 1 thru March 31
Percent assessed and given pneumococcal vaccination	5 years
Percent with delirium	7 days
Percent with moderate to severe pain	7 days
Percent with pressure sores	7 days

* If multiple minimum data set items with different timeframes of observation are used to calculate the quality measure, the longest observation period is presented.

SOURCE: Adapted from Department of Health and Human Services, Medicare. *Nursing Home Compare.* http://www.medicare.gov/NHcompare (accessed Jan 2011).

hospital, or those admitted from a hospital with an anticipated stay of <30 days who require treatment at the nursing facility for the same problem for which they were hospitalized, are exempt from screening.

CMS requires that every skilled-nursing facility designate a licensed physician to serve as medical director (F501). The medical director has many roles, including coordination of medical care that meets current standards for care in the nursing home. Integral to the medical director's role is providing guidance in development and implementation of resident-care policies.

Additional regulations require medication review at regular intervals and that each resident's medication regimen includes no unnecessary drugs. Clinical documentation must demonstrate the indication for all drugs, especially psychoactive medications. Unnecessary medications are those given without indication, at excessive dosages, for excessive duration, without adequate monitoring or when there has been a significant adverse event. Residents without a history of antipsychotic drug use should not be treated with antipsychotic medication unless the drug is required to treat a specific diagnosed condition that is docu-

mented in the medical record. For those residents receiving psychoactive medications, gradual dosage reductions and behavioral interventions are mandated unless a clinical contraindication exists and is documented in the medical record. To date, the impact on quality of care from these guidelines has not been well described in the clinical research literature.

A thorough evaluation of medication regimens, done monthly by a pharmacist, is also required. This monthly medication review is intended to minimize adverse events and unnecessary medication use and to ensure proper medication monitoring. A facility must ensure that the medication error rate is <5% and that no significant medication errors occur. No errors should occur that cause a resident discomfort or jeopardize their health and safety.

Care in assisted-living facilities often resembles care given in other outpatient venues, including traditional primary care practices. Care in assisted-living facilities does not have the same regulations that guide care in nursing homes. For a brief summary of selected regulations influencing medical and psychiatric care in the skilled-nursing facility, see Table 18.3.

Table 18.3— Brief Summary of Selected Medicare and Medicaid Requirements for Long-Term Care Facilities

Tag Number	Subject	Regulation	Guideline
F285	Preadmission screening for mental illness or retardation	CFR 483.20(m)	A state agency must screen and approve the admission to a nursing facility of anyone with mental retardation or serious mental illness and ensure that a facility can provide the appropriate programs and services to meet the individual's needs.
F309	Quality of care	CFR 483.25	Each resident must receive and the facility must provide the necessary care and services to attain or maintain the highest practicable physical, mental, and psychological well-being, in accordance with the comprehensive assessment and plan of care. "Highest practicable" is defined as the highest level of functioning and well-being possible, limited only by the individual's presenting functional status and potential for improvement or reduced rate of functional decline.
F319–320	Quality of care: mental and psychosocial functioning	CFR 483.25(f)	Based on the comprehensive assessment of a resident, a facility must ensure that a resident who displays mental or psychosocial adjustment difficulty receives appropriate treatment and services to correct the assessed problem and a resident whose assessment did not display a pattern of decreased social interaction and/or withdrawn, angry, or depressive behaviors, unless that residents' clinical condition demonstrates that such a pattern is unavoidable.
F329–331	Medications, appropriate and unnecessary	CFR 483.25(I)(1)	Residents' medications regimens must be free of unnecessary drugs. These are defined as "those given without indication, at excessive doses, for excessive duration, without adequate monitoring, or in the setting of significant adverse reaction."
F385–386	Physician services	CFR 483.40	It is the attending physician's responsibility to participate in the resident's assessment and care planning, monitoring changes in the resident's medical status and providing consultation or treatment when called by the facility. At scheduled visits, the physician must review the total plan of care; write, sign, and date a progress note; and sign and date all orders.
F428–430	Medications, medication regimen review	CFR 483.60(c)	The medication regimen of each resident must be reviewed at least once a month by a pharmacist. The pharmacist must report irregularities to the attending physician and director of nursing, and reports must be acted upon.
F501	Medical director, required duties	CFR 483.75(i)	Each facility must designate a physician to serve as medical director. The medical director is responsible for implementation of resident care policies and the coordination of care in the facility.

SOURCE: Adapted with permission from the American Medical Directors Association, Synopsis of Federal Regulations in the Nursing Facility. Copyright 2010.

MEDICAL CARE ISSUES

The care of nursing-home residents has become more complex over the past several years, commensurate with an increasing level of medical acuity in an environment continually constrained by lack of adequate resources. Comprehensive, ongoing assessment within an interdisciplinary framework works to restore function, when possible, and almost always to enhance quality of life.

Clinical challenges abound in the nursing home, created, in part, by the atypical and subtle presentation of illness so characteristic of patients with profound physical and psychologic frailty. Families of nursing-home residents often remain an integral part of the overall care plan and may require specific educational and psychosocial supports. Ethical and legal concerns are also very common, particularly those regarding end-of-life, feeding, hydration, and resident rights issues. (See "Legal and Ethical Issues," p 23.) Finally, the heterogeneity among nursing-home residents demands an individualized, thoughtful, and reasoned approach to each individual.

Problems in nursing homes that commonly require unique diagnostic and treatment strategies include infections, falls, malnutrition, dehydration, incontinence, behavioral disturbances, the use of multiple medications, and prevention and screening. (See "Prevention," p 61; "Pharmacotherapy," p 72; "Malnutrition," p 195; "Urinary Incontinence," p 207; "Falls," p 224; "Behavioral Problems in Dementia," p 256; and "Infectious Diseases," p 479.) For example, determining the risks and benefits of tube feedings for frail nursing-home patients must be predicated not only on underlying illness but also on the resident's and the family's value system, the resources available in the nursing facility, and staff acceptance of the intervention. Given that the evidence for and against enteral feeding in nursing-home patients is controversial (ie, benefits are not well established), therapy must be individualized. (See "Eating and Feeding Problems," p 203.) Many of the problems commonly encountered in the nursing home result when multiple comorbidities interact with a host of environmental factors, all of which may be only partially remediable. Unfortunately, expectations of family, as well as state regulators, often do not account for these complexities and commonly engender "risk-averse" behavior that is counter to autonomy and optimal quality of life.

CLINICAL PRACTICE IN THE NURSING HOME

The medical care of nursing-home residents is challenging and fulfilling, requiring excellent clinical skills as well as sensitivity to a variety of ethical, legal, and interdisciplinary issues. Medical interventions, whether they are curative, preventive, or palliative, demand an individualized approach that recognizes the complex interplay among resident, family, and staff needs. Further, the evidence on which to base treatment may be nonexistent.

The comorbidity present in most nursing-home residents commonly creates the need for multiple drug therapies, with attendant risk of complications. Even though residents receiving more than nine medications (32% of all nursing-home residents) are "flagged" by state survey teams as reflecting potential quality concerns, the use of multiple medications cannot always be avoided. In fact, on average, nursing-home residents receive between seven and eight medications each month. The most common health conditions found in the nursing home for those ≥65 yr old, after dementia, are heart disease, hypertension, arthritis, and stroke. The approaches to these and other illnesses have evolved dramatically in recent years and complicate treatment decisions when cost-effectiveness is increasingly considered a desirable goal. Clear documentation of the rationale for a given medication or intervention is the best way to protect against potential scrutiny; frequent discussion with the facility's consultant pharmacist is also helpful. See "Pharmacotherapy," p 72.

Nurse practitioners and physician assistants have become increasingly involved in the primary care of nursing-home residents. Studies suggest that nurse practitioners and physician assistants who collaborate with the primary care physician as a coordinated team provide more intensive care to the nursing-home resident and may decrease hospitalization rates while maintaining cost neutrality (SOE=A). Regulations mandate that the initial comprehensive visit for the

purpose of certifying that a newly admitted nursing-home resident requires a skilled level of care be done by a physician. During this visit, physicians perform a thorough assessment, develop a plan of care, and write appropriate orders for the nursing-home resident. Nurse practitioners may perform initial history and physical visits for long-term care residents who do not require skilled level of care. Regulations mandate that nursing-home residents be seen for subsequent face-to-face medical visits every 30 days for the first 90 days after admission and then at least every 60 days thereafter. For these subsequent visits, a visit by a nonphysician provider may be substituted for every other physician visit. Additional medical visits should occur if acute medical needs or changes in condition develop. Medicare allows for clinician reimbursement for evaluation and management activities for both nursing-home regulatory visits and medically necessary visits to provide acute care. Availability of on-site medical providers can improve timeliness of acute medical care and decrease hospitalization rates. Several studies have documented misdiagnoses, inappropriate interventions, and poor preventive care practices in nursing homes. For example, in a study of nursing-home patients with nonmalignant pain, 25% were found to be receiving no analgesics.

Vaccination rates for eligible chronic-care nursing-home residents vary. Nationally, current vaccination rates in nursing homes are 87% for influenza and 81% for pneumococcus. Intensive research is currently being done to understand the processes necessary to integrate validated care guidelines into nursing homes in an effort to improve quality of care.

Certain care strategies have been developed that may enhance care quality. The commonly used special-care units, although conceptually attractive, have not consistently been shown to enhance quality of care apart from the involvement of individual professionals. Specific consultation services in the nursing home, however, may improve care practices and condition-specific patient outcomes such as the reduction of falls (SOE=A). In addition, interactive educational programs for physicians and nursing staff may improve practice, as has been demonstrated in programs to promote appropriate psychoactive drug use (SOE=B). Clinical practice guidelines for the care of nursing-home residents have been developed by the American Medical Directors Association (http://www.amda.com/) and the American Geriatrics Society (http://www.americangeriatrics.org).

Understanding each nursing-home resident's preference for care in the context of his or her underlying value system will undoubtedly improve overall quality. Basic advanced directives such as do-not-resuscitate orders are present for 37% of nursing-home residents at admission and for 55% after 1 yr of residence. Durable power of attorney for healthcare documentation is present for 26% of nursing-home residents at admission and for 39% after 1 yr of residence. Less than 5% of nursing home residents have "do-not-hospitalize" orders, which document that the resident is not to be hospitalized even after developing a condition that is generally treated in the hospital. While ongoing discussion of care preferences appears to be present in the nursing home, there likely remain ongoing opportunities for improved understanding of nursing-home resident preferences for care. When ethical dilemmas do arise, institutional ethics committees can provide important guidance. The multidisciplinary nature of these committees ensures a spectrum of opinion and insight critical for nursing-home residents. See also "Legal and Ethical Issues," p 23.

REFERENCES

- Kappas-Larson P. The evercare story: reshaping the health care model, revolutionizing long-term care. *J Nurs Practitioners.* 2008;4(2):132–136.

- Kasper J, O'Malley M. Changes in Characteristics, Needs, and Payment for Care of Elderly Nursing Home Residents: 1999 to 2004. Washington, DC: Kaiser Family Foundation; 2007. Available at www.kff.org/medicaid/7663.cfm.

- Mor V. Defining and measuring quality outcomes in long-term care. *J Am Med Dir Assoc.* 2007;8:E129–E137.

- Weiner JM, Freiman MP, Brown D. Nursing home care quality: twenty years after the Omnibus Reconciliation Act of 1987. Washington, DC: Kaiser Family Foundation; 2007. Available at www.kff.org/medicare/7717.cfm.

CHAPTER 19—COMMUNITY-BASED CARE

KEY POINTS

- Home care has changed dramatically since the introduction of prospective payment for services; the number of recipients has declined by 20%, and many home-health agencies have closed because of financial constraints, limiting access to home-care services in some areas.

- Health care providers often find home care rewarding; reimbursement charges for home visits have improved, making home visits more financially viable for clinicians.

- Community-based services that do not require a change of residence (eg, adult day care, day hospitals, home hospitals, Program of All-Inclusive Care for the Elderly, telemedicine) may be a useful alternative to inpatient services. However, the availability of these services strongly depends on financial reimbursement.

- Community-based services requiring a change of residence (eg, assisted living, group homes, adult foster care, and continuing-care retirement communities) offer a wide range of services. These are regulated at the state level and vary considerably in availability, cost, and services provided.

HOME CARE

The 2000 U.S. census data revealed that almost 10 million older adults living in the community require help with ADLs. For a large number of these people, home care has the potential to improve their quality of life and avoid unnecessary institutionalization.

Under a cost-based reimbursement system, home care grew rapidly in the 1980s and 1990s. This growth coincided with the initiation of the prospective payment system (diagnostic-related groups [DRGs]) for hospitals, which resulted in patients being discharged sooner from hospitals, and an increased need for home services. New technologies created the possibility of providing therapies in the home that were previously available only in hospitals or nursing homes. Because of an explosive increase in costs, Congress placed limits on Medicare spending as mandated in the 1997 Balanced Budget Act, which led to the development of a prospective payment system (PPS) for home-care services. Since enactment of the PPS, the number of recipients of home-care services and the number of visits for patients receiving home care have declined by >20%. Many home-care agencies have adjusted to these changes and developed more efficient, targeted home care, but hundreds have closed because of financial pressures.

Table 19.1—Codes, Reimbursement, and Requirements in Home-Care Certification

Code	Reimbursement[a]	Requirements[b]
G0179	$37	Physician recertification for Medicare-covered home-health services. This includes reviewing and signing Home Health Care Plan of Care (form 485), contacts with agency personnel, review of reports per 60-day certification period. Documentation (copy of form 485) must be present in patient medical record.
G0180	$49	Physician certification for Medicare-covered services. As above, the physician affirms the implementation of the care plan and affirms that it meets the patient's needs as documented in form 485, and a copy exists in patient record.
G0181	$96	Physician supervision of a patient receiving Medicare-covered services requiring complex and multidisciplinary care involving regular physician involvement or revision of care plans, review of subsequent reports of patient status, review of diagnostic tests, and discussions with family. This must be 30 min or more within a calendar month. Documentation must be present in the patient medical record or log.
G0182	$98	Same as G0180 but with a patient in a Medicare-approved hospice program.

[a] Reimbursement as of 2009 may vary with different health maintenance organizations and will change with continued enactment of the Balanced Budget Act.

[b] The patient is not present for these activities.

Rural agencies have closed at a higher rate than urban ones. The Outcome and Assessment Information Set (OASIS) is a tool meant to set fees for home-health–related groups (HHRGs). The OASIS instrument is completed by the home-care agency and tracks several domains of the patient's functional status and medical needs. Like the DRGs, the HHRGs provide the basis for agency reimbursement and are based on severity of the patient's illness, disabilities, and nursing needs; they include an adjustment for location in the United States. The instrument is also intended to provide a uniform means of measuring quality of care across all home-care agencies. Refinements to the Medicare PPS were introduced January 1, 2008. The number of HHRGs was increased to 10, and comorbid conditions are considered in the ultimate reimbursement. The OASIS assessment and the International Classification of Diseases (ICD-9) codes must be accurate to ensure that reimbursement matches the needs of the patient being served. Like other sectors of our healthcare system, home-care agencies are charged with developing cost-effective, high-quality care despite diminishing reimbursement. Another major challenge facing home-care agencies is recruiting and retaining qualified nurses and aides. Developing community-wide systems of care between hospitals, home care, nursing homes, and practitioners' offices may help meet these challenges and ensure that patients receive timely and appropriate care.

STRENGTH-OF-EVIDENCE (SOE) RATING DEFINITIONS

A = consistent and good quality patient-oriented evidence
B = somewhat inconsistent or limited quality patient-oriented evidence
C = very inconsistent or very limited patient-oriented evidence, disease-oriented evidence, and/or consensus from professional organizations
D = unstudied common practice or opinion

See inside front cover for detailed information regarding the SOE classification.

The Primary Provider's Role in Home Care

Home care often requires an interdisciplinary team that is generally composed of nurses, therapists (speech, physical, occupational, and respiratory), social workers, personal care aides, home medical equipment suppliers, and most importantly, informal caregivers. Currently, physicians certify and recertify the plan of care and need for individual therapy services for Medicare-covered home-health services.

Physicians are reimbursed for certification of the home-care plan and for oversight of complex cases in skilled home care and hospice. For billing codes and requirements for these services, see Table 19.1. The documentation requirements for billing allow activities over multiple days in a month to be combined. Reimbursement can vary in different parts of the country by as much as 20% based on a Medicare adjustment called "Geographical Practices Cost Indices."

Nurse practitioners are authorized by law to provide both primary care and registered nurse services; however, reimbursement depends on the type of care provided. If the nurse practitioner provides a service described by a CPT code made necessary by an ICD-9 diagnosis to a homebound patient, then this is billable to Medicare Part B as a medical service. It does not require a physician's order and could be billed directly using the nurse practitioner's provider number. If the nurse practitioner is providing nursing care that is billable under Medicare Part A, then the nurse is working as an employee of a certified home care agency that would bills for these services using their Medicare provider number.

House calls can add an important dimension to the primary provider's knowledge of the patient's circumstances and environment. Home evaluation can identify additional problems not readily apparent in office-based assessment. Barriers to maximal functioning can be identified and addressed. House calls have the additional benefit of reducing the burden for patients who have difficulty getting transportation outside the home. Changes in Medicare have increased reimbursement for home visits, making home visits more financially feasible for clinicians.

Patient Assessment

Homebound patients have significant functional impairment. Comprehensive geriatric assessment is particularly valuable in this setting to establish a baseline, monitor the course of illness, and evaluate the effects of intervention. However, assessment in the home has some important differences from office-based assessment.

During a home visit, the patient's actual environment can be assessed to determine whether the home is safe and supportive, given the particular patient's abilities and disabilities. Performance-based functional assessment can focus on the practical aspects of performing ADLs by directly observing the environment for bathing, dressing, and transferring. Difficulties can be identified, and the assessor can evaluate the caregiver's abilities to address the patient's needs. The caregiver's needs for counseling, training, support, and education can also be identified and addressed.

Environmental modifications can be recommended to improve function. For example, modifications of the bathtub, a hand-held shower, a shower seat, grab bars, and a bedside commode can improve the patient's quality of life and functioning. Barriers to wheelchairs and walkers (eg, door sills) can be identified and removed. Chair lifts and outdoor ramps can help patients circumvent stairs. Occupational therapy consultation can be particularly useful in identifying other personal care and assistive devices for performing ADLs and housekeeping chores. A number of home safety checklists are available to help a reviewer assess the home. Additional technological additions to improve home safety, including necklace or wrist radio devices to call for help, can be considered. Some types of emergency response systems require that a person push a button by a specified time each day to avoid triggering an emergency response or telephone call to check on the owner of the device.

Healthcare providers are finding that home diagnostics, including radiology and electrocardiography, are available in most areas, and hand-held laboratory devices are becoming more common. These home diagnostics allow for a much more comprehensive medical evaluation to take place in the home.

Developing an Office-Based House-Call Program

Medical care in the home may be provided as part of an ongoing office-based program, as an extension of hospitalization through a postacute care program, or as a freestanding entity. Regardless of the method chosen, the organization of the home-care program must be well conceived to maximize effectiveness and efficiency and to remain financially viable. Current regulations allow house calls to be provided by physicians, nurse practitioners, and physician assistants. Regardless of the primary care medical provider, appropriate links to other providers of home-based services are necessary to develop an interdisciplinary team. Consistency and familiarity among all members of the interdisciplinary team are essential to a smoothly functioning house-call program.

Choosing the Right Patients

To qualify for Medicare home-care benefits, a patient must meet two criteria to establish homebound status. First, the patient must be absent from the home for reasons other than obtaining medical treatment infrequently (≤3 times per month) or for short periods of time. Second, leaving home must require considerable and taxing effort on the part of the patient or the caregiver, or both (eg, if the patient is bedbound or has a severe mobility impairment).

Patients who are likely to be good candidates for house calls are those with mobility impairments that make transportation to the office difficult; disruptive behaviors; terminal illnesses; and multiple medical, psychiatric, and social problems. For some patients, house calls are needed for a limited amount of time, but others require house visits on an ongoing basis. Home visits may be particularly useful for patients who are either not responding to adequate therapy or responding inconsistently. A diagnostic home visit may reveal caregiver burnout, mistreatment of the patient, or the use of medications from other sources that may be interfering with the expected response. See also "Pharmacotherapy," p 72; and "Mistreatment of Older Adults," p 87.

Equipment for House Calls

For suggested equipment and medications for house calls, see Table 19.2. A small bag with key equipment is particularly useful. A supply of forms needed for common diagnostic tests and orders, educational material for common problems, and community referral information is also useful.

Financial Considerations

House calls are now more financially feasible for clinicians; documentation remains the key to receiv-

Table 19.2—Suggested Equipment and Supplies for House Calls

Basic Equipment and Supplies

Cerumen curette	Sharps container
Cotton tip applicators	Snellen chart
Fecal guaiac cards and developer	Sphygmomanometer
Gloves	Stethoscope
Intravenous starting kit and fluid	Tape measure
Lubricating jelly	Toenail clippers
Oto-ophthalmoscope	Tongue depressors
Phlebotomy equipment	Tuning fork
Reflex hammer	Urine dipsticks
Scalpel	

Additional Supplies

Emergency medications (protect from heat and cold)	Specimen cups
Foley and coudé catheter	Wound debridement kit
Genitourinary syringe	Wound dressing materials
Nasogastric tube	

Also Consider

Handheld audioscope	Portable oxygen
Home glucose monitor, lancets, strips	Pulse oximeter
Portable ECG machine	Voice amplifier

ing reimbursement. There are no specific restrictions on the number of visits as long as sufficient justification is included in the progress notes. As with most documentation, it is necessary that the primary care provider identify historical data, physical examination findings, diagnostic test results, and an assessment that reflects all the active diagnoses. Further, an evaluation of the patient's functioning, caregiver issues, and documentation of the medical plan of care are important elements to include in the house-call progress note. Physician assistants and nurse practitioners can also bill for home-care services under Medicare regulations adopted in January 1998. For codes and reimbursement for home visits, see Table 19.3. When visits become prolonged, time codes can be used that justify an enhanced reimbursement. Insurers sometimes demand copies of the documented visit when time codes or extended visits are billed. Reimbursement can vary in different localities, particularly where health maintenance organizations act as intermediaries for Medicare.

Caregiver Support

Family caregivers provide most of the care received by patients in the community. In the United States, three-fourths of caregivers are women, either wives or daughters. Caregiving is often intense, time consuming, and stressful. The caregiver's physical and emo-

tional health may be affected, resulting in depression and a worsening of his or her own health problems. Attention to caregiver support and issues are essential to allow caregivers to continue to provide care. Caregiver support groups can be particularly helpful.

For discussions of specific issues concerning caregiving, see "Psychosocial Issues," p 18; "Mistreatment of Older Adults," p 87; "Dementia," p 251; "Behavioral Problems in Dementia," p 245; and "Depression and Other Mood Disorders," p 295.

Limitations of Home Care

Most older adults would prefer to remain in their own home, but certain situations and conditions arise that make institutional care a more appropriate choice than in-home care. For example, caregivers may not be available to adequately address the needs of the patient. Relatively unstable medical situations that require frequent laboratory testing, respiratory interventions, or intravenous medications can also make institutional care a better choice than home care. Caregiver burnout and stress can prevent continued safe care for the patient in the home.

Further, the home environment itself may be a barrier to continuing in-home care. Unsafe neighborhoods, ongoing household social disruptions from alcohol or drug abuse, and inadequate room for equipment or environmental modifications may make in-home care a poor or risky option.

Finally, home care can be prohibitively expensive for the patient. It is not always the least expensive alternative, and out-of-pocket expenses can make ongoing home care unaffordable. Insurance coverage is more likely to cover care provided in a nursing facility or other institutional setting.

Liability and Legal Issues

As elsewhere, clinicians are potentially liable for adverse outcomes; however, malpractice suits related to home care are relatively uncommon. It is important to maintain appropriate documentation for medical purposes, to support provider compensation, and to support payment requests for other providers of in-home services. In addition, physicians should be aware that inaccurate certificates of medical necessity could lead to charges of Medicare fraud. These forms should be reviewed carefully before they are signed.

It is important to be sensitive to potential conflicts of interest. Federal legislation prohibits providers from receiving financial benefit, compensation, or rebate for referring a patient to a home-care provider. Further, providers may not refer patients to home-care companies in which the physician or the physician's family has a "substantial" financial interest. Legal advice should be sought for any question of a potential conflict of interest.

Table 19.3—Billing Codes and Reimbursement for Home Visits

| New Patients | | Established Patients | | |
Codes	Reimbursement	Codes	Reimbursement	Requirements
99341	$52	99347	$51	Problem-focused history and examination, straightforward medical decision making
99342	$75	99348	$76	Expanded problem-focused history and physical examination with medical decision making of low complexity; about 30 min spent with patient and/or family
99343	$122	99349	$111	Detailed history and examination; medical decision making of moderate complexity; about 45 min
99344	$160	99350	$155	Comprehensive history and examination with medical decision making of moderate complexity; about 60 min
99345	$192			Above plus medical decision making of high complexity; about 75 min

SOURCE: Data from *CPT—Current Procedural Terminology.* American Medical Association; 2009.

Ethics and Decisions about Institutionalization

Two ethical themes arise commonly in home care. The first is the balance between patient autonomy and patient safety. The second involves issues surrounding mistreatment and neglect of older adults.

Respect for patient autonomy often dictates that the patient remain in the home as a result of the patient's (or surrogate decision maker's) choice. Conflict arises when a patient's medical care or safety cannot be adequately maintained in the home, yet the patient insists on staying at home. It is difficult to balance respect for patient autonomy with the desire to prevent patient neglect. In some situations, the outcome is likely to be terminal, regardless of whether the patient is maintained at home or in an institution. In such situations, a hospice referral can help provide additional services in the home and support for both the patient and family. In situations in which there is a clearly neglectful or abusive situation, Adult Protective Services should be contacted (see "Mistreatment of Older Adults," p 87).

COMMUNITY-BASED SERVICES NOT REQUIRING A CHANGE IN RESIDENCE

Adult Day Care

Adult day care is a community-based option that provides a wide range of social and support services in a congregate setting. Adult day care has become increasingly common. Providers of adult day care may offer a variety of services, ranging from simple nonskilled custodial care to more advanced skilled services. The availability of a registered nurse allows for on-site health services, clinical assessment and monitoring, and assistance with medication management. Adult day care is used commonly for patients with dementia who need supervision and assistance

with their ADLs while primary caregivers work. Adult day care can also serve as a form of respite for caregivers. Most adult day-care centers are community based, either in churches or community centers. In general, custodial adult day care is not covered by Medicare, although some costs may be covered by Medicaid or other insurers.

Day Hospitals

Day hospitals provide a broad range of skilled nursing care services, including parenteral antibiotic treatment, chemotherapy, and intensive rehabilitation. Most programs are housed in chronic-care hospitals or rehabilitation centers. This arrangement allows for the provider to take advantage of in-house professional expertise and resources, while allowing the patient to return to his or her own home or alternative living site after day treatment is complete. Services are covered under Medicare, with similar requirements to those surrounding home-health care.

Day hospitals are most often used for two groups of patients: those needing multidisciplinary rehabilitation and those with psychiatric illnesses. A systematic review of day hospital care found no significant differences between day hospitals and alternative sources of care with respect to death, disability, or use of health services, but that among those receiving care in a day hospital, there was a trend toward less functional decline and less hospital and institutional care (SOE=B).

The Program of All-Inclusive Care for the Elderly (PACE)

PACE is a capitated model of care that provides comprehensive care services to frail community-dwelling older adults by a single organization. The program provides all inpatient, outpatient, and long-term care services to frail older adults. (See also "Financing, Coverage, and Costs of Health Care," p 40.) Participants in the PACE program must be

≥55 yr old and meet state-defined requirements regarding their need for a nursing-home level of care. Most will also qualify for Medicaid and Medicare; pooling funds from Medicare and Medicaid allows for comprehensive care to be planned and coordinated by the PACE interdisciplinary team. Without Medicaid and Medicare coverage, out-of-pocket expenses are high. Few private insurance plans provide a PACE benefit as part of their policies. The average PACE enrollee is 80 yr old and has an average of eight medical conditions and three ADL limitations; half of PACE participants have dementia.

The goal of the PACE program is to keep the participant in the community for as long as it is medically, socially, and financially feasible. The system, designed to be seamless, uses an interdisciplinary team of healthcare providers who know the patient and caregivers well and who provide care across the spectrum of hospital, home, alternative living situations, and institutional care. This team includes a physician (often a geriatrician), nurse practitioner, clinic and home-health nurses, social workers, physical therapist, pharmacist, dietitian, and transportation workers. The hub of care is the PACE center, which provides adult day health care. Other care includes respite, transportation, medication coverage, rehabilitation (including maintenance physical and occupational therapy), hearing aids, eyeglasses, and a variety of other benefits. The program, at the discretion of the interdisciplinary team, has the flexibility to pay for nonmedical costs in unusual circumstances (eg, paying a person's electric or gas bill). Care by the interdisciplinary team provides for the complex social needs as well as the medical needs of the participant. PACE has been described as one of the few truly integrated systems of care in the United States.

Although the effectiveness of PACE has not been directly tested by a randomized controlled trial, research has shown that PACE provides high-quality care, albeit with significant site-to-site variation (SOE=B).

In 1997, legislation was passed that changed the status of PACE from a demonstration program to a permanent provider under Medicare. PACE is an optional program under state Medicaid. There are more than 3 million dually eligible and nursing-home–certifiable older adults in the United States that might benefit from PACE, but only a small fraction have enrolled.

Home Hospital

The home hospital focuses on providing more complex care at home to older adults who would have been hospitalized for an acute-care need. Patients receiving home-hospital care have access to nurses and physi-cians on a regular basis and for episodic care through an on-call system that allows problems to be addressed promptly. The concept can be viewed as an evolution of home care, which it resembles, although it is more intense. Studies conducted outside the United States suggest that care is comparable for selected patients and that patient satisfaction is high. See also "Hospital Care," p 119.

COMMUNITY-BASED SERVICES REQUIRING A CHANGE OF RESIDENCE

Assisted Living

Assisted-living facilities continue to grow as the U.S. population ages. They have different names, including personal care homes, residential care homes, domiciliary care, sheltered care, and community residences. Even though these facilities are based on a social (not medical) model, they are caring for more frail people with significant medical needs. The transitional nature of assisted living is suggested by the average length of residency, about 2 yr in 2002. The most common reason for discharge is need for nursing-home care.

Assisted-living residences are characterized by some level of coordination or provision of personal care services, social activities, health-related services, and supervision services in a home-like atmosphere that maximizes autonomy and privacy. The services provided under assisted living vary considerably, both within and between states.

In one national survey of assisted-living facilities, privacy options ranged from private rooms to apartment units; about half of the facilities would not admit residents with moderate to severe cognitive impairment, and about two-thirds did not have a registered nurse on staff but did provide 24-hour staff oversight, housekeeping, two meals, and personal assistance with ADLs. One example of the difference between state licensing requirements is in the area of medication administration. Depending on licensing requirements, medication administration and management can be directed by nonskilled, skilled, or fully licensed nursing staff.

In states where regulations do not require skilled care in assisted-living facilities, home-health skilled care is often provided as an external or independent service to the individual patient who happens to be living in an assisted-living facility. In this context, the boundary between assisted-living and skilled-nursing facilities often becomes blurred. Because care in assisted living is generally less costly than in a nursing home, there has been a trend to use assisted living as a lower-cost alternative to nursing-home care. Part of the reason assisted-living care is usually less expensive is that there are fewer regulations governing assisted-living facilities. However, as these facilities have come to care for more people with increasing disability and more medical needs, the pressure to regulate them has been increasing.

Costs for assisted-living residences vary greatly (from $800 to $4,000 per month) and depend on the size of units, services provided, and location. Assisted living is covered in a growing number of long-term care insurance policies. The Health Insurance Association of America reports that all 11 of the leading insurance companies that sell long-term care insurance offer assisted-living coverage. However, most people in assisted-living residences or their families pay for care themselves because most older Americans do not carry long-term care insurance.

Assisted living is not covered by Medicare, but certain services are paid under Supplementary Security Income and Social Services Block Grant programs. Thirty-eight states reimburse or plan to reimburse for assisted-living services as a Medicaid service. In addition, states have the option to pay for assisted living under Medicaid by including services in the state's Medicaid plan or by petitioning the U.S. Department of Health and Human Services for a waiver.

Group Homes

Group homes (including domiciliary care, single-room occupancy residences, board-and-care homes, and some congregate living situations) are houses or apartments in which two or more unrelated people live together. Group homes vary in types of residents and often serve patients with chronic mental illness or dementia. Residents share a living room, dining room, and kitchen but usually have their own bedrooms. Advantages of this arrangement include a lower cost of living and socialization with peers. Independence and functional status are supported through the interdependence and relationships of the residents. Resident-to-staff ratios may be higher than in other supported-living environments. Opportunities for socialization are increased, reducing social isolation. Most group homes are run as for-profit businesses, and some states require licensing.

Adult Foster Care

Foster care homes generally provide room, board, and some assistance with ADLs by the sponsoring family or by paid caregivers, who customarily live on the premises. Perhaps the longest experience with adult foster care is in the state of Oregon, where it is used as an alternative to long-term care and institutional-ization. Adult foster care has the advantages of maintaining frail older adults in a more home-like environment. Regulations for foster care vary by state, and some states require licensing. Some states provide coverage of adult foster care through their Medicaid programs.

Sheltered Housing

Sheltered housing is funded through the Older Americans Act and is offered as an option for housing subsidized through section 8, Housing and Urban Development programs for seniors and disabled residents. Often these arrangements are sheltered homes offering personal care assistance, housekeeping services, and meals. Programs may be supplemented by social work services and activities coordinators. Charges to clients are based on a sliding scale, which may cost up to 30% of income.

Continuing-Care Retirement Communities (CCRC)

More affluent seniors may choose a CCRC. CCRCs usually have a variety of living options, ranging from apartments or condominiums, to assisted living, and skilled nursing-home care. Often, residents enter the more independent living areas and progress through assisted living and into skilled care as they age.

Three financial models are common: the all-inclusive model, which provides total healthcare coverage, including long-term care; the fee-for-service model in which payments match the level of care; and the modified coverage model, which covers long-term care to a predetermined maximum. Most CCRCs require an entry fee, which may or may not be refundable, plus a variable monthly fee to pay for rent and supportive services. Monthly fees vary, depending on the level of care being provided. Funding is largely private, although some facilities have Medicare- or Medicaid-funded beds for skilled care.

See also "Financing, Coverage, and Costs of Health Care," p 32.

REFERENCES

■ Program of All-Inclusive Care for the Elderly. Center for Medicare and Medicaid Services. Available at: http://www.cms.gov/QualityInitiativesGenInfo/10_PACE.asp

■ North L, Kehm L, Bent K, et al. Can home-based primary care: cut costs? *Nurse Pract.* 2008;33(7):39–44.

■ Wieland D, Boland R, Baskins J, et al. Five-year survival in a Program of All-Inclusive Care for Elderly compared with alternative institutional and home- and community based-care. *J Gerontol A Biol Sci Med.* 2010;65(7):721–726.

CHAPTER 20—OUTPATIENT CARE SYSTEMS

KEY POINTS

- Outpatient interventions that improve the quality and outcomes of care of older adults include personalized care that is provided by a team in accordance with best practice, coordination among all providers and settings of care, coordination of the resources and environment of older adults, and inclusion of them as active partners in their care.

- For optimal cost-effectiveness, outpatient programs need to be targeted to patients identified in advance who are likely to be active participants in an intervention that is known to better meet their specific clinical needs.

- Broad dissemination of effective models of outpatient care for older adults is limited by current payment mechanisms and the shortage of healthcare professionals in geriatrics.

INTRODUCTION

Traditional outpatient care in the United States does not deliver the recommended standard of care to older adults for preventive services, chronic disease management, and geriatric syndromes. Realizing that a more proactive, patient-centered, and population-based approach is needed to improve the overall quality of geriatric care, several innovative outpatient care systems have been developed over the past two decades. This chapter describes new system approaches having evidence from clinical trials of improved processes and/or outcomes of care, including those that involve geriatric specialty care and others that integrate geriatrics in primary care. Current methods for targeting these approaches most likely to benefit older adults will also be reviewed.

GERIATRIC SPECIALTY CARE

Senior Health Clinic

The Senior Health Clinic (SHC) care model is a specialized ambulatory clinical service center for older adults providing primary care using an interdisciplinary team approach to developing and implementing a plan of care. All SHC providers have

---

STRENGTH-OF-EVIDENCE (SOE) RATING DEFINITIONS

A = consistent and good quality patient-oriented evidence
B = somewhat inconsistent or limited quality patient-oriented evidence
C = very inconsistent or very limited patient-oriented evidence, disease-oriented evidence, and/or consensus from professional organizations
D = unstudied common practice or opinion

See inside front cover for detailed information regarding the SOE classification.

---

competency in geriatrics, and care is provided and/or coordinated throughout the continuum of care, including hospital, skilled nursing facility (SNF), assisted living, and home care. Team members work with patients, families, and caregivers, and link patients with needed community-based services and information. The chronic care model has recently offered an organized framework to provide the comprehensive resources and processes needed to deliver evidence-based primary care within an integrated healthcare system that supports the interactions between the informed, activated patient and a prepared, proactive team. Patients new to the SHC are screened for risk status, and a comprehensive geriatric-focused evaluation is completed.

The core interdisciplinary clinical practice team consists of a geriatrician, nurse practitioner, and social worker. An extended team may include other professionals such as a pharmacist, physical therapist, dietician, and home-health nurse. Provider teams share a common medical record and meet at least weekly to review complex care plans and discuss new or anticipated patient issues. When SHC patients are admitted to the hospital or SNF, care is delivered directly and/or coordinated by providers from the SHC.

Studies in community settings and Veterans Affairs medical centers have demonstrated that geriatric patients cared for in the SHC model have improved mental health status and better maintained health-related quality of life over time than patients in traditional care (SOE=A). Financially, SHCs may be a cost center when viewed in isolation, but these clinics are more likely revenue generators when viewed from the perspective of an integrated health system because of the associated "downstream" fee-for-service revenues generated from hospital inpatient, hospital outpatient, and professional fees (SOE=B). Broad uptake of the SHC model is limited by health system administration considering the clinic in isolation and as a cost center, and the limited number of specialty trained geriatrics healthcare professionals available to staff such clinics.

Program of All-Inclusive Care for the Elderly

See "Community-Based Care," p 150.

GERIATRICS IN PRIMARY CARE

Outpatient Consultation

Comprehensive geriatric assessment (CGA) is a process intended to determine a patient's medical, psychosocial, and functional capabilities and limitations, with the goal of developing an overall plan for treatment and long-term follow-up. Because CGA typically requires a highly trained team of geriatricians, geriatric nurse clinicians, physical and occupational therapists, geriatric psychiatrists, and social workers, it is expensive and time consuming. Success generally requires the geriatric team to take over the direct care of the patient. An extended period of intensive team involvement with ongoing care is essential to ensure the efficacy of the intervention. When the geriatric team assumes a purely consultative role (ie, without a role in implementing the recommendations), CGA is unlikely to be successful in improving patient outcomes (SOE=A). However, CGA coupled with an adherence intervention to improve primary care physician (PCP) and patient adherence with recommendations has demonstrated improved outcomes. In a randomized controlled trial, CGA coupled with adherence strategies was associated with less decline in physical functioning, less fatigue, and better social functioning among community-dwelling older adults with at least one of four conditions (functional impairment, falls, urinary incontinence, or depressive symptoms). In this care model, patients undergo an in-depth, standardized CGA from a social worker, a geriatrics nurse practitioner/geriatrician team, and a physical therapist (when indicated by falls or impaired mobility), after which the evaluation team holds a short interdisciplinary case conference and forms its recommendations for care. The adherence intervention includes the geriatrician contacting the patient's PCP to convey the recommendations and also sending a letter describing the recommendations along with a copy of the dictated consultation and copies of full-text references specific to the patient's conditions. In addition, the patient receives a written list of recommendations at the time of the CGA and is subsequently mailed a copy of the dictated consultation and list of recommendations along with a "How to Talk to Your Doctor" booklet. Approximately 2 weeks later, a health educator telephones the patient to review the team's recommendations and help prepare the patient for discussion of the proposed recommendations with his or her PCP.

Forms of CGA may also be attempted in the home setting. Accumulating evidence suggests that preventive home visitation programs, based on CGA with extended follow-up of patients at lower risk of death, can reduce functional decline and nursing-home placement (SOE=A).

A more intensive outpatient consultation model is short-term geriatric evaluation and management (GEM). In GEM, a geriatrics interdisciplinary team diagnoses *and treats* problems, including adjusting medications, providing counseling and health education, and making referrals to other health professionals and community services. In addition, monitoring and coordination of care between visits is provided through regular telephone calls. In one trial, community-dwelling adults ≥70 yr old and found to be at high risk of hospital admission by mailed screening questionnaire underwent CGA followed by interdisciplinary primary care by the GEM team (geriatrician, geriatrics nurse practitioner, nurse, and social worker) for an average of 6 mo before being discharged for care by their original PCP. This GEM model prevented functional decline, improved patients' satisfaction with their health care, and lessened caregiver burden. Other trials of GEM have shown similar positive results (SOE=A). However, fully implementing the above GEM model was more expensive than usual care. Other GEM trials have produced different results on costs, some costing more than usual care, some costing the same, and some costing less.

Enhanced Primary Care

A variety of new models of primary care aimed at improving the quality and outcomes of care for older adults have been studied and have contributed to an emerging vision of optimal healthcare delivery for those with chronic diseases. Key features of this new vision include 1) personalized care to meet each patient's goals, values, and resources; 2) care that is provided in accordance with best practices; 3) team care that is integrated within the practice and has physician oversight; 4) care that is coordinated among those caring for patients including information linkages such as an electronic health record; 5) care that considers the resources and environment of the person; and 6) care that includes older adults as active partners in their care when possible.

The Geriatric Resources for Assessment and Care of Elders (GRACE) model of primary care includes each of these core principles. GRACE provides patients with home-based CGA and long-term care management by a nurse practitioner and social worker (GRACE support team) who collaborate with the PCP and a geriatrics interdisciplinary team involving a geriatrician, pharmacist, physical therapist, mental health social worker, nurse practitioner, and community-based services liaison. Individualized care planning during weekly team meetings is guided by 12 care protocols for common geriatric conditions, including "advanced care planning" and "health maintenance" protocols used in all patients. The nurse practitioner and social worker (employees of the primary care practice) review and prioritize the care plan with the patient's PCP, and then implement the care plan in collaboration with the PCP and consistent with the patient's goals. The GRACE support team provides ongoing home-based care management, including coordination and continuity of care among all healthcare professionals and sites of care facilitated by an electronic medical record and Web-based tracking system.

Low-income seniors enrolled in a trial of the GRACE intervention, compared with usual care, received better quality of care for the geriatric conditions and general health processes targeted, had improvements in health-related quality-of-life measures, and had fewer emergency department visits over 2 yr. In addition, hospital admissions were significantly reduced in the second year among GRACE patients identified at baseline as being at high risk of future hospitalization (SOE=A). Cost analysis of the GRACE intervention revealed that in the high-risk group, increases in chronic and preventive care costs were offset by reductions in acute-care costs such that the intervention was cost neutral in the first 2 yr.

Other successful models of enhanced primary care demonstrating reduced acute-care utilization have also involved a geriatrics interdisciplinary team that provides ongoing care management (usually including home visitation) in support of and integrated with the PCP (SOE=A). Guided Care was designed to improve the quality of life and the efficiency of resource use for older adults with multiple morbidities. Guided Care aims to enhance primary care by infusing the operative principles of seven chronic care innovations: disease management, self-management, case management, lifestyle modification, transitional care, caregiver education and support, and geriatric evaluation and management. Preliminary results demonstrate improved patient and physician satisfaction with care, and a trend toward less use of expensive health services in the first 8 mo. Final results of a randomized controlled trial of the Guided Care model will be available in 2011.

Disease Management

Disease management programs focus healthcare delivery around a single disease with the goal of optimizing patient care for this disease. The most effective disease management programs are those that are integrated with the patient's primary and/or specialty care provider. Heart failure and depression interventions are examples of disease management programs that lead to better outcomes in older adults and that are potentially cost saving. One notable heart failure program that was nurse-directed and multidisciplinary (geriatrician, cardiologist, nurse, dietitian, and social worker) reduced readmission rates and costs in hospitalized older adults with heart failure (SOE=A). Key components included comprehensive education of the patient and family, a prescribed diet, social-

service consultation and planning for an early discharge, a review of medications, and intensive follow-up.

In the disease management program for late-life depression called Improving Mood—Promoting Access to Collaborative Treatment (IMPACT), patients had access to a depression care manager, supervised by a psychiatrist and a primary care expert, who offered education, care management, and support of antidepressant management by the patient's PCP or a brief psychotherapy for depression. In a large multicenter clinical trial, depressed patients who received the IMPACT intervention were more likely than patients who receive usual care to be given guideline-concordant depression care and to recover from depression (SOE=A).

Finally, a collaborative care model developed for older adults with Alzheimer's disease has demonstrated improvements in the quality of care and in behavioral and psychological symptoms of dementia among primary-care patients and their caregivers (SOE=A). In this program, an advanced practice nurse supported by an interdisciplinary team (psychologist, neuropsychologist, geriatrician, and geriatric psychiatrist) served as the care manager working with the patient's family caregiver and PCP. The team used standard protocols to initiate treatment and to identify, monitor, and treat behavioral and psychological symptoms of dementia with an emphasis on nonpharmacologic management.

PATIENT SELECTION FOR OUTPATIENT INTERVENTIONS

Programs described above have been developed to better address the multiple healthcare needs of older adults with chronic conditions and in response to rising costs. For these interventions to be successful, they must target patient populations having clinical needs that are addressed by the intervention and/or at risk of high healthcare expenditures in the future. Ideally, identifying individuals in advance who are also likely to engage in the intervention program is also desirable. Patient selection for intensive outpatient interventions is one of the major challenges facing healthcare organizations that serve older adults.

Three complementary approaches have been used to identify high-risk older adults: referral by clinicians, screening by mail or telephone, and analysis of administrative data (predictive modeling). The ideal system for identifying high-risk individuals would rely on multiple sources of information. Clinicians in primary care settings are perhaps well positioned to identify some high-risk older adults, especially when provided with objective criteria on which to base referral. However, they may lack the time, skills, and incentives to do so. Surveys can be administered systematically by mail or telephone to a defined population of older adults. The Probability of Repeated Admission Questionnaire (Pra) has been used extensively in managed-care settings to identify high-risk older adults upon enrollment. A risk score is calculated based on age, sex, perceived health, availability of an informal caregiver, heart disease, diabetes, physician visits, and hospitalizations. A score above a certain threshold indicates that the member is at high risk of hospital admission and use of other health-related services during the following year. The Pra has been found to be valid in many different populations of community-dwelling older adults, including Medicaid, fee-for-service, and managed-care patients (SOE=B). Due to the associated expenses and <100% response rates, an administrative proxy has been developed as a close substitute to the Pra. The Vulnerable Elders Survey-13 (VES-13), another risk screening instrument, is a 13-item questionnaire that produces a vulnerability score from 0 to 10 based on age, self-reported health, and function. Patients with a VES-13 score of ≥3 are at four times the risk of functional decline or death over the next 2 yr and are therefore defined as vulnerable (SOE=B). Finally, predictive modeling approaches use administrative data for identifying high-risk older adults and are usually proprietary and not described in the peer-reviewed literature. They typically analyze health insurance enrollment records and claims data with predictions based on age, gender, diagnoses, prior use of health services and associated costs, and pharmacy data.

ACOVE–3* QUALITY INDICATORS PERTAINING TO OUTPATIENT CARE SYSTEMS

Comprehensive Geriatric Assessment (CGA)

- All vulnerable older adults new to a primary care practice should receive the elements of a CGA within 3 mo.
- If a vulnerable older adult receives the elements of a CGA that identifies a problem, then the problem should be addressed within 3 mo.

CONTINUITY AND COORDINATION OF CARE

Identify source of care

- All vulnerable older adults should be able to identify a clinician or a clinic to call for medical care or know the telephone number or other mechanism to reach this source of care.

Medication continuity

- If an outpatient vulnerable older adult is prescribed a new medication for a chronic disease and he or she has a follow-up visit with the prescribing clinician, then one of the following should be noted at the follow-up visit:
- Medication is being taken.
- Patient was asked about the medication (eg, adverse events, adherence, availability).
- Medication was not started, because it was not needed or changed.
- If a vulnerable older adult is under the outpatient care of two or more clinicians and one clinician prescribed a new medication for a chronic disease or changed prescribed medication, then the nonprescribing clinician should acknowledge the medication change at the next visit.

Consultation continuity

- If an outpatient vulnerable older adult was referred to a consultant and revisited the referring clinician, then the referring clinician's medical record should acknowledge the consultant's recommendations, include the consultant's report, or indicate why the consultation did not occur.

Test continuity

- If an outpatient vulnerable older adult was given an order for a diagnostic test, then one of the following should be documented at the follow-up visit:
  - Result of the test initialed or acknowledged
  - Note that the test was not needed or reason why it will not be performed
  - Note that the test is pending

Prevention reminders

- If a vulnerable older adult misses a required preventive care event that is recurrent with a specific periodicity, then there should be medical record documentation of a reminder that the preventive care is needed within one full interval since the missed event.

Outside medical records

- If a vulnerable older adult is new to a primary care practice, then the medical record should contain medical records from a prior care source, a request for such medical records, or an indication that such records are unavailable.

Related quality indicators for Outpatient Care Systems

- Discharge planning in the hospital and post-hospitalization care transitions (see "Hospital Care," p 119)

Assessing Care of Vulnerable Elders – 3rd Set. See inside front cover for explanation.

REFERENCES

- Boyd CM, Boult C, Shadmi E, et al. Guided care for multimorbid older adults. *Gerontologist.* 2007;47(5):697−704.

- Counsell SR, Callahan CM, Clark DO, et al. Geriatric care management for low-income seniors: A randomized controlled trial. *JAMA.* 2007;298(22):2623−2633.

- Hendrix CC, Wojciechowski CW. Chronic care management for the elderly: an opportunity for gerontological nurse practitioners. *J Am Acad Nurse Pract.* 2005;17(7):263–267.

CHAPTER 21—FRAILTY

KEY POINTS

- Frailty appears to be a clinical syndrome of dysregulated energetics, with definable clinical manifestations that become apparent when physiologic dysregulation reaches a critical threshold, and with recognizable causes at the level of both altered physiology and potentially altered genetic, cellular, and molecular processes.

- A validated frailty syndrome is manifested when multiple components are present: weakness, low energy or exhaustion, slowed walking speed, low physical activity, and weight loss.

- Frailty identifies patients at high risk of adverse clinical outcomes, including falls, disability and dependency, and mortality.

- Frailty develops along a continuum of severity, likely including a latent phase of vulnerability that is not clinically apparent in the absence of stressors, early stages likely most responsive to intervention, and a late end-stage that indicates high risk of short-term mortality. The most effective preventive approach appears to be maintaining muscle mass and strength through resistance exercise.

EVIDENCE-BASED FINDINGS

Frailty As a Core Clinical Concept

Care of frail older adults is a central focus of geriatric health care. Frail older adults are a subset of the older population who are at high risk from stressors such as extremes of heat and cold, acute infection or injury, or the stress of hospitalization or surgery. In the face of such stressors, frail older adults are more likely to have delayed recovery from illness and/or are more likely to fall; to develop greater functional impairment, including becoming disabled or dependent; or to die. As a group, frail older adults are at high risk of needing to be hospitalized, and risk worse outcomes once hospitalized, including functional decline.

Frailty is clinically observed to be a chronic, progressive condition, with a spectrum of severity. The most severely frail older adults appear to be in an irreversible, predeath phase with high mortality over 6–12 mo. Earlier phases may be responsive to treatment, either to prevent or ameliorate the clinical manifestations of frailty. Frailty may result from intrinsic aging processes, ie, primary frailty. It also appears that a similar phenotype and vulnerability, thought of as secondary frailty, is associated with the end-stages of several chronic diseases, such as cancer associated with inflammation and wasting, heart failure, COPD, and HIV/AIDS. The similarity of presentation between primary and secondary frailty suggests that, clinically, frailty is actually a physiologic entity unto itself that can be triggered by disparate causes and, ultimately, represents a final common pathway resulting from these causes.

Frailty and Associated Vulnerability

Frailty is associated with heightened vulnerability to adverse outcomes, and this vulnerability may most likely manifest in the face of stressors. Frailty theories suggest that, regardless of the causes, those who are frail have decreased reserves with which to compensate for, or recover from, stressors. Aggregate loss of physiologic function is the process thought to underlie the high risk of adverse outcomes. An emerging research agenda is focused on developing approaches that can identify those with this vulnerable physiologic status before frailty becomes clinically apparent.

Frailty As a Clinical Syndrome

Beyond the consensus that frailty is a physiologic state of heighted vulnerability, current definitions of who is frail fall into two major categories. One is that the vulnerability of frailty is the outcome of the accumulation of a number of likely unrelated abnormal health conditions in an individual. This multimorbid state is associated with increased risk of mortality; the number of conditions predicts this vulnerability, ie, high numbers of conditions mark an individual as frail.

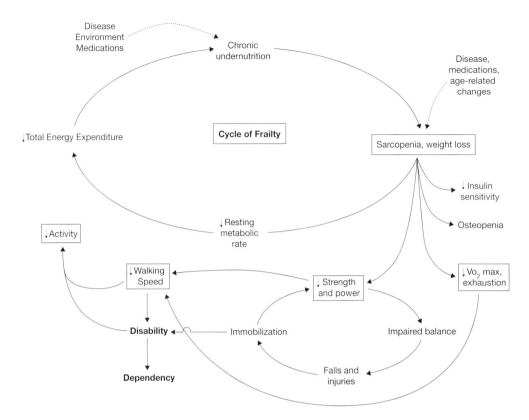

Figure 21.1—The Cycle of Frailty

The second conception of frailty is that it is a distinct physiologic process resulting from dysregulation of multiple physiologic systems; many of these systems interact with each other and together also contribute to clinical manifestations. The aggregate impact of too many dysregulated systems is a decreased ability to maintain homeostasis in the face of stressors, resulting in vulnerability to adverse outcomes. This physiologic (or pathophysiologic) process appears to lead to an observable clinical phenotype. The consensus is that clinical manifestations of frailty are seen in specific domains: strength, balance, motor processing, nutrition, endurance, physical activity, mobility, and possibly cognition. A phenotype has been developed and validated that links all but cognition, based on the hypothesis that the clinical presentation of frailty results from a vicious cycle of dysregulated energetics, leading to 1) decreased muscle mass, or sarcopenia, with resulting loss of strength, 2) worsened exercise tolerance (or low energy or fatigue), 3) slowed motor performance (such as walking speed), 4) decreased physical activity, and

5) inadequate nutritional intake (even when physical activity is low); the latter two result in further sarcopenia and, when nutritional intake is severely inadequate, weight loss as well (Figure 21.1). Identifying the presence of multiple manifestations (formally defined as 3 or more of these 5) provides specificity to defining an individual as frail (Table 21.1). Research has shown this definition to be consistent with that of a clinical syndrome that is primarily chronic and progressive with early stages predicting progression to more severe frailty, but that frailty can also improve. Early stages are likely most amenable to intervention. Earliest presentations tend to be weakness, slowed walking speed, and/or decreased physical activity. Notably, abnormalities in multiple physiologic systems are associated with this clinical presentation (see below). These findings support frailty being a clinical syndrome with definable manifestations that become apparent when physiologic dysregulation reaches a critical threshold, and with recognizable causes at the level of both altered physiology and potentially altered genetic, cellular, and molecular processes.

EVIDENCE AS TO CAUSE

Primary Frailty

Mounting evidence suggests that frailty as a distinct clinical syndrome can be precipitated by a number of

Table 21.1—Criteria that Define Frailty (≥3 indicates frailty)

Characteristic	
Weight loss	**Meets criteria for frailty if:** Lost >10 pounds unintentionally last year
Exhaustion	**Meets criteria for frailty if answer:** Felt that everything I did was an effort in last week or could not get going in last week Self-report of "moderate or most of the time" for either: **1) I felt that everything I did was an effort in the last week:** Rarely or none of the time (<1 day) ☐ Some or little of the time (1 to 2 days) ☐ Moderate amount of the time (3 to 4 days) ☐ Most of the time ☐ **2) I could not get going in the last week:** Rarely or none of the time (<1 day) ☐ Some or little of the time (1 to 2 days) ☐ Moderate amount of time (3 to 4 days) ☐ Most of the time ☐
Slowness	**Meets criteria for frailty if time to walk 15 feet (4.57 meters) is:** *Men* ≥7 seconds for height ≤173 cm ≥6 seconds for height >173 cm *Women* ≥7 seconds for height ≤159 cm ≥6 seconds for height >159 cm *Equipment: 4-meter course in walkway of ≥4.5 meters, a stopwatch.* *Participant will walk 15-foot length twice at his or her usual place. Use average of 2 trials.*
Low activity level	**Meets criteria for frailty if:** ≤270 kcal of physical expenditure on activity scale per week (18 items*)
Weakness	**Meets criteria for frailty if grip strength (average of 3 trials, dominant hand) is:** *Men* ≤29 kg for BMI ≤24 ≤30 kg for BMI 24.1–26 ≤30 kg for BMI 26.1–28 ≤32 kg for BMI >28 *Women* ≤17 kg for BMI ≤23 ≤17.3 kg for BMI 23.1–26 ≤18 kg for BMI 26.1–29 ≤21 kg for BMI >29 *Equipment: Jamar hand dynamometer* *Participant attempts to squeeze the dynamometer maximally 3 times with the dominant hand.*

NOTE: BMI=body mass index

* Walking for exercise, moderately strenuous household chores, mowing or raking the lawn, gardening, hiking, jogging, biking, exercise cycle, dancing, aerobics, bowling, golf, singles or doubles tennis, racquetball, calisthenics, swimming

To compute kcals expended per week, use the formula:

kcal/week = [activity-specific MET (kcal/(kg × hour))] × [(duration per session (min)) / (60 min)] × [body weight (kg)] × [(number of sessions in the last 2 wk) / 2] × [number of months per year activity was done]

SOURCE: Data from Fried LP, Tangen CM, Walston J, et al. Frailty in older adults: evidence for a phenotype. *J Gerontol Med Sci.* 2001;56A:M146–M156.

factors. Sarcopenia, or loss of lean body mass, is a central component of frailty and a key predictor of the other clinical manifestations. Predictors of loss of muscle mass and strength with aging include anabolic factors such as testosterone and IGF-1, as well as the amount of physical activity the individual engages in, his or her nutritional intake (eg, protein, energy, vitamin D and other micronutrients), and age itself.

While the most basic underlying cause of frailty is still unknown, the intermediate process, and precipitant of the clinical manifestations, may be aging-associated dysregulation of multiple physiologic systems. Systems abnormal in frailty include inflammation (indicated by increased IL-6 and C-reactive protein), decreased immune function, anemia, increased insulin resistance, low levels of DHEA-S and IGF-1, and low levels of a number of vitamins and carotenoids (in which the number of micronutrient deficiencies is associated with increased risk of frailty), as well as sarcopenia. The number of abnormal systems is a stronger predictor of frailty than any one abnormal system, and there is evidence for interactions between abnormal systems with synergistically increased frailty risk. It is unknown whether intervention on any one system modifies frailty risk.

Overall, research indicates that the vulnerability and clinical presentation of the frailty syndrome results from an aging-associated dysregulation of the

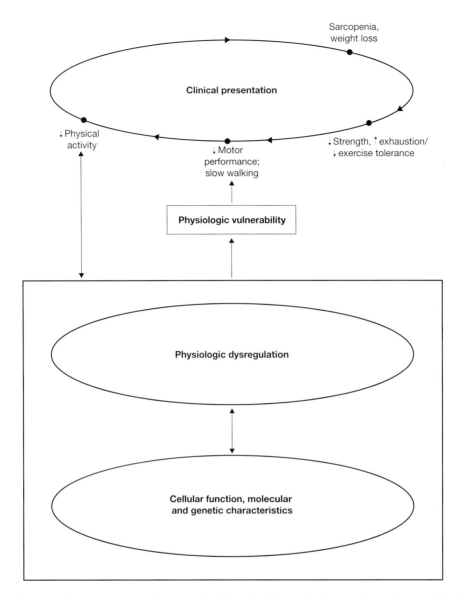

Figure 21.2—Conceptual representation of the multiple levels of contribution to the syndrome of frailty: clinical phenotype, physiologic and biologic etiologies, and resulting vulnerability in the face of stressors

complex biology of interacting systems that maintain a robust organism. When this complex systems biology is compromised, because too many systems are not functioning effectively, there is, theoretically, a loss of both reserves and resilience and diminished ability to maintain homeostasis in the face of stressors. This aggregate dysregulation likely is the combined result of decreased function at multiple levels, including clinical symptoms and signs, physiologic communication systems and other functions, as well as ultimate biologic causes (Figure 21.2).

Secondary Frailty

Inflammatory and wasting diseases independently predict frailty, potentially through inflammation and/or their effect on cardiopulmonary function (eg, heart failure, COPD), immune diseases (eg, HIV/AIDS),

and chronic cytomegalovirus infection. Secondary frailty theoretically develops as a result of the core wasting process of these illnesses, perhaps precipitating an independent, final common process that is frailty. Data on HIV-positive men indicate that HIV infection, even in the absence of clinical AIDS, is associated with rates of a frailty-like presentation that would be found in HIV-negative men who are 10 yr older. Additionally, frailty in association with HIV/AIDS predicts a lower response to therapy and a worse prognosis than AIDS alone.

ASSESSMENT OF FRAILTY

The presence of frailty can be assessed by several established methods. The approach used may differ depending on the setting and goal. However, the consensus is increasing that frailty should be understood as an entity distinct from disability, which is an outcome of frailty. In the clinical setting, if frailty is assessed as a clinical syndrome that has a definable cause and high risk of a range of adverse outcomes due to vulnerability to stressors, then using a screening method might be appropriate to characterize the presence of the syndrome and to consider those who may benefit from risk amelioration as well as treatment (Table 21.1). A clinical global impression of change in frailty has also been validated. This draws on clinical judgment and incorporates assessment of the status of the clinical syndrome plus outcomes and precipitants into one score. Finally, an approach for screening older adults for intervention trials has been published. This suggests quickly excluding those who are too well and those who are too frail, so as to find those most likely to benefit from a certain intervention. Outcome measures such as disability, falls, and mortality can be assessed to characterize the impact of frailty. This predominately involves assessing falling and development or progression of disability; the latter can be measured as difficulty or dependency in ADLs.

PREVAILING MANAGEMENT STRATEGIES

Comprehensive geriatric assessment and management is a clinical care model designed to optimize outcomes for frail older adults, particularly to prevent loss of independence. This team-based, multidisciplinary approach has been shown to have positive effects on polypharmacy, falls, functional status, nursing-home admission, and mortality. The assessment should be coupled with accurate screening for frailty and ongoing, expert geriatric care. The focus of care should be 1) to exclude any modifiable precipitating causes of frailty, including causes that are treatable or environmental; 2) to improve the core manifestations of frailty, especially physical activity, strength, exercise tolerance, and nutrition; and 3) to minimize the consequences of the vulnerability of frail older adults, whether in terms of environmental risks, risks from low social support, or the risks from stressors such as acute illness or injury, hospitalization, or surgery. The impact of each of these stressors is worsened when homeostatic systems and resilience are compromised in frailty. Resistance, or strengthening, exercise, with added nutritional support, appears to be a key management approach for both frailty and its prevention; this can be supplemented by aerobic and balance training. The approach that older adults use to adapt to age-related psychosocial losses and behaviors can also be applied to physical health and to frailty in particular. In the face of diminished resources or reserves, older adults must carefully choose their goals, focus on optimizing the abilities needed to reach their goals, and then compensate for diminished competencies by increased reliance on other functions or by replacement. Clinical management needs to include such approaches for care of frail older adults, as well as more standard medical approaches, as described above. Further, decreasing the stress of environments such as hospitals and maximizing supportive care during acute illness and recovery may be effective clinical approaches. See "Hospital Care," p 119; and "Outpatient Care Systems," p 157.

POTENTIAL APPROACHES TO PREVENTION OF FRAILTY

Points of Vulnerability and Precipitants

Exposure to any of a variety of stressors appears to put frail older adults at risk of adverse outcomes and is thought to potentially precipitate clinically apparent frailty in those already at risk. Frail older adults are more vulnerable to stressors, including hospitalization, surgery, and extremes of heat and cold, likely because of predisposing decrements in function in multiple physiologic systems. A key precipitant is immobility, whether caused by pain, acute illness, and/or in the context of hospitalization. Immobility is likely a trigger causing frailty to develop or worsen, as well as exacerbating onset of adverse outcomes such as dependency. Given the association of depression with decreased activity, energy, and nutritional intake, as well as with inflammation and worsened social isolation, depression may well be a precipitant of frailty. Overall, attention needs to be paid to minimizing these precipitants and/or the stress associated with them. Screening for risk assessment, diagnosis, and early detection can be done using the screening approaches described above.

Potential Pharmacologic Treatments

It has not been demonstrated that replacement of deficiencies of any one hormone can prevent or ameliorate frailty. Theoretically, this is understandable, given that the combined effects of deficits in multiple physiologic systems appear to most strongly predict frailty, much more than any one deficit alone, therefore suggesting that improving only one system may not be clinically effective. Notably, geriatric assessment and management is reported to reduce serious adverse medication events and suboptimal prescribing in frail older adults (SOE=A), who may be at higher risk of these adverse events and of polypharmacy.

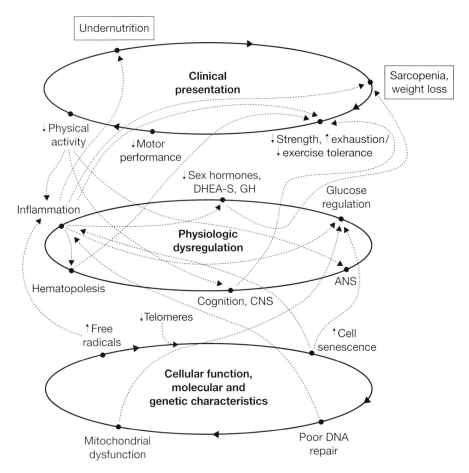

Figure 21.3—Systems Biology of Frailty

Examples of dynamics within and across multiple levels (clinical presentation, physiologic dysregulation, cellular function, and molecular and genetic characteristics), which are theorized to result in the aggregate loss of resilience and ability of the organism to compensate for stressors that is frailty. This multilevel network emphasizes the complexity of an intact system and visually suggests the loss of complexity in response to challenges for the organism as a whole that are likely to result from dysregulation of multiple systems.

NOTE: DHEA-S=dehydroepiandrosterone sulfate; GH=growth hormone; ANS=autonomic nervous system

Behavioral Prevention or Treatment

Preventing or minimizing immobility, and maintaining physical activity and muscle mass, is critical in older adults at risk of frailty. Evidence is substantial that resistance, or strengthening, exercise is effective in increasing muscle mass, strength, and walking speed in frail older adults, such as nursing-home residents (SOE=A). Other forms of exercise, including stretching, Tai Chi, and aerobic exercise, are also helpful. Prehabilitation approaches may be beneficial for frail older adults to prevent decline in physical function. Overall, exercise has notable beneficial physiologic effects on sarcopenia, inflammation, and other systems associated with frailty (Figure 21.3), making maintenance of physical activity as well as strength a cornerstone of prevention and treatment. See "Physical Activity," p 54.

Attention to preventing nutritional inadequacy is likely of import; nutritional supplementation appears to be effective only when added to resistance exercise, at least in nursing-home patients. Preventing and treating depression may also well be important in preventing and ameliorating frailty.

Frailty and Failure to Thrive

A clinical concept that is one antecedent of current conceptualizations of frailty is that of failure to thrive. In geriatrics, this was historically used as a blanket diagnosis at admission to a hospital or long-term care setting, in the setting of an older patient with nonspecific symptoms, including fatigue, poor nutritional intake, weight loss, social withdrawal and/or decline in cognitive and physical function, and without an apparent cause. It was often thought that depression was a key component as well. This diagnosis was found to be associated with poor response to treatment or rehabilitation, increased rates of pressure sores, infection, diminished cell-mediated immunity, and high surgical and short-term mortality rates. Some experts have argued that the term should be abandoned because it does not assist thoughtful evaluation, while others have expressed concern that the application of a term initially used for delayed development in children appeared pejorative when applied to older adults. However, conceptually there may well be overlap between the concept of failure to thrive and very severe, or end-stage frailty.

Frailty and Palliative Care

There is evidence that frailty has its own pattern of functional decline at the end of life, involving substantial disability and dependency in the final year of life. Severe frailty, with a score of 4–5 and metabolic abnormalities of low cholesterol and albumin, is associated with particularly high short-term mortality rates in frail older adults (SOE=B). Additionally, clinical case series suggest a poor response to treatment in those with end-stage frailty. Therefore, it may be appropriate to consider palliative approaches for these patients.

REFERENCES

■ Bortz WM 2nd. A conceptual framework of frailty: a review. *J Gerontol A Biol Sci Med Sci.* 2002;57(5):M283–M288.

■ Chen KM, Fan JT, Wang HH, et al. Silver yoga exercises improved physicial fitness of transitional frail elders. *Nurs Res.* 2010;59(5):364–370.

■ Ferrucci L, Guralnik JM, Studenski S, et al. Designing randomized, controlled trials aimed at preventing or delaying functional decline and disability in frail, older persons: a consensus report. *J Am Geriatr Soc.* 2004;52(4):625–634.

■ Fried LP, Ferrucci L, Darer J, et al. Untangling the concepts of disability, frailty and comorbidity: implications for improved targeting and care. *J Gerontol A Biol Sci Med Sci.* 2004;59(3):255–263.

■ Fried LP, Hadley EC, Walston JD, et al. From bedside to bench: research agenda for frailty. *Sci Aging Knowl Environ.* 2005;(31):pe24.

CHAPTER 22—VISUAL IMPAIRMENT

KEY POINTS

■ Visual impairment affects 20%–30% of older adults ≥75 yr old.

■ Cataracts and refractive error are common; both are correctable, and correction improves quality of life.

■ Age-related macular degeneration (ARMD) is common; the wet form, the major complication of ARMD leading to blindness, may respond to laser surgery or intravitreal antiangiogenesis injection. Antioxidant multivitamins can slow progression to the wet form.

■ Glaucoma is common, and increased intraocular pressure is no longer required to meet diagnostic criteria. Screening for glaucoma should be done every 1–2 yr after age 50 and more often in high-risk individuals.

■ Control of blood glucose, and more importantly, blood pressure, in type 2 diabetes reduces retinopathy. However, approximately 2–3 yr are needed to show benefit for blood pressure control, and approximately 7–8 yr are needed to show benefit for glycemic control.

Visual impairment, defined as visual acuity less than 20/40, increases exponentially with age such that 20%–30% of the population ≥75 yr old is affected. Blindness, defined as visual acuity of 20/200 or worse, affects 2% of the population ≥75 yr old. Those ≥65 yr old make up 12% of the total U.S. population but 50% of the blind population. Refractive error, cataracts, ARMD, diabetic retinopathy, and glaucoma are the most common causes of blindness (Table 22.1). The respective order of importance varies according to the region and race surveyed.

Visual impairment has considerable impact on the medical system and older age groups. Chronic eye conditions are one of the most common reasons for office visits to the clinician among those ≥65 yr old. Of all office visits by older adults, 14% are to ophthalmologists, one of the highest rates of all specialty visits. Falls and car crashes, each associated with impaired vision in older adults, consume considerable medical resources. Moreover, impaired vision has been linked to a significant deterioration in the quality of life and the ADLs of older adults.

The American Academy of Ophthalmology recommends a comprehensive eye examination every 1–2 yr for adults ≥65 yr old. Prophylactic and therapeutic ocular management can effectively alter the course of various conditions causing visual impairment. About one-third of all new cases of blindness can be avoided with effective use of available ophthalmologic services.

Table 22.1— Symptoms and Treatment of Most Common Eye Diseases of Older Adults

Condition	Comments	Signs and Symptoms	Treatment
Cataracts	*Reversible* cause of blindness	Decreased vision; cause refractive shifts, reduced visual acuity, reduced contrast sensitivity, glare	Change eyeglasses to match changing refractive error. Surgical cataract extraction when eyeglasses no longer improve vision: extremely successful in improving vision in those without other ocular pathology; can also be helpful in those with other ocular pathology.
Age-related macular degeneration	Most common cause of *irreversible* blindness		
Dry form		Slow onset, vision loss not severe, usually asymptomatic	To decrease rate of conversion to wet form: vitamin supplements (vitamins C, E, zinc, β-carotene)
Wet form		Sudden onset of vision loss or distortion of vision; central vision loss can be severe, peripheral vision maintained.	Intravitreal injections of vascular endothelial growth factor inhibitors and laser
Glaucoma	Second leading cause of *irreversible* blindness	Peripheral vision lost first, but in advanced stages all vision can be lost; early glaucoma typically asymptomatic	
Open angle		Typically asymptomatic until advanced; may note contrast sensitivity loss or night vision problems	Lowering of intraocular pressure with medications, laser trabeculoplasty, and/or incisional surgery
Narrow angle	Drug warnings apply to this type of glaucoma. Avoid medications that can dilate the pupil.	Acute: painful, red eye, decreased vision, nausea, vomiting, headache. Chronic: usually asymptomatic until vision loss advanced or central vision affected	Acute: pilocarpine 2% ophthalmic solution (2 drops in affected eye) and immediate laser treatment needed; may require continued medical and/or surgical treatment. Chronic: lowering of intraocular pressure with medications, laser, and/or incisional surgery
Diabetic retinopathy	Vision loss is caused by macular edema and ischemia, vitreous hemorrhage, and retinal detachments.	Decreased/blurred vision, sudden loss of vision, floaters	Laser treatment and intravitreal injections; tight control of blood glucose and blood pressure

COMMON EYE CONDITIONS IN OLDER ADULTS

Older adults with eye complaints frequently first seek care from their primary care provider. Common complaints include red eye, ocular swelling or discomfort, blurred or sudden loss of vision, diplopia, and floaters. A key question to differentiate a patient who can be treated by his or her primary care provider versus one that needs an ophthalmologist is "Has your vision changed?" A decrease in vision can indicate a serious condition. For this reason, it is vitally important to check visual acuity in each eye separately with the patient's current corrective aid (eg, eyeglasses) in place for any eye complaint. Significant vision loss can also be indicated by the presence of a relative afferent pupillary defect, which can be checked for using a "swinging flashlight test." While in a dark room, the patient is asked to stare into the distance. A bright flashlight is then placed in front of one eye to check the pupillary light reflex; the other eye should also constrict because of the consensual light reflex. The flashlight is then quickly swung over to the second eye. If this eye dilates, there is an afferent pupillary defect (ie, the second eye is not detecting the light as the first eye detects it).

For serious eye conditions that require immediate attention from an ophthalmologist, see Table 22.2. All of the listed conditions are usually associated with a decrease in vision that can be profound but masked

---

STRENGTH-OF-EVIDENCE (SOE) RATING DEFINITIONS

A = consistent and good quality patient-oriented evidence
B = somewhat inconsistent or limited quality patient-oriented evidence
C = very inconsistent or very limited patient-oriented evidence, disease-oriented evidence, and/or consensus from professional organizations
D = unstudied common practice or opinion

See inside front cover for detailed information regarding the SOE classification.

Table 22.2—Common Signs and Symptoms of Eye Conditions Requiring Immediate Referral to Ophthalmologist

Condition	Symptoms and Signs
Retinal detachment	Flashes, floaters, decreased vision
Acute angle-closure glaucoma	Eye pain or headache, ocular hyperemia, dilated pupil, decreased vision, nausea, vomiting
Ischemic optic neuropathy	Sudden loss of vision (complete or partial) in one eye
Central artery occlusion or giant cell arteritis	Sudden painless loss of vision in one eye; if from giant cell arteritis, then review of symptoms may reveal accompanying jaw claudication, headache, transient diplopia, etc.
Bacterial keratitis	Decreased vision, eye redness, pain, discharge
Scleritis	Eye redness, pain, decreased vision
Posterior uveitis	Floaters, decreased vision
Corneal ulcers	Eye redness, pain, decreased vision, corneal infiltrate
Uveitis	Photophobia, eye redness, decreased vision
Herpes zoster ophthalmicus	Eye redness, pain, burning, rash, decreased vision, light sensitivity

Table 22.3—Treatment of Eye Conditions Commonly Seen by Primary Care Providers

Condition	Treatment and/or Cause
Red eye	
Subconjunctival hemorrhage	Supportive treatment with artificial tears
Dry eye	Artificial tears, cyclosporin 0.2% eye drops
Blepharitis	Lid scrubs, ophthalmic antibiotic ointment qhs, oral doxycycline
Lid malposition/exposure	Ocular lubricant, refer for surgical repair
Allergic conjunctivitis	Cold compresses, allergen avoidance, topical/systemic antihistamines
Viral conjunctivitis	Supportive treatment with artificial tears; refer to ophthalmologist if vision significantly affected
Chalazion	Warm compresses, may refer for excision
Herpes simplex keratitis	Trifluridine eye drops, refer to ophthalmologist
Herpes zoster ophthalmicus	Tear drops, refer to ophthalmologist immediately
Angle-closure glaucoma	Pilocarpine 2% ophthalmic solution, refer to ophthalmologist immediately
Floaters, flashes	Refer to ophthalmologist immediately; may be retinal detachment or vitreous hemorrhage
Sudden decrease in vision	Refer to ophthalmologist immediately; may be secondary to a number of vision-threatening problems
Diplopia	
Monocular	Refractive error, cataract
Binocular	Microvascular infarct to cranial nerve, giant cell arteritis, compressive tumor

by good vision in the other eye. The symptoms of a retinal detachment include new floaters in one eye along with photopsias (the perception of flashes of light), distorted peripheral vision, or decreased vision. Ocular pain and hyperemia do not accompany a retinal detachment; the only signs a primary care provider may detect are a relative afferent pupillary defect, decreased vision, or a monocular visual field deficit. Signs and symptoms of acute angle-closure glaucoma include an injected eye with fixed, dilated pupil and cloudy cornea; the patient is often in severe pain, nauseous, and vomiting. In ischemic optic neuropathy, vision in one eye is lost suddenly, usually in the upper or lower hemifield. Giant cell arteritis must be excluded quickly in patients with ischemic optic neuropathy to prevent bilateral blindness. Diplopia and central retinal artery occlusion can also

be the result of giant cell arteritis. Bacterial keratitis usually presents with pain and a corneal infiltrate. Scleritis is frequently associated with significant autoimmune disease; symptoms include boring pain, decreased vision, and a red eye. Posterior uveitis presents with decreased vision and floaters.

Red eye is an extremely common eye complaint, the cause of which may be benign or malignant (Table 22.3). Hyperemia of the eye can accompany any inflammation or infection. Causes of red eye that require referral include corneal ulcers, which are usually accompanied by a visible white infiltrate on the cornea, anterior and posterior uveitis, herpes simplex and herpes zoster ophthalmicus, scleritis, angle-closure glaucoma, ocular surface tumors, and postoperative infections. The reason for referral is to prevent permanent vision loss, which can be the end point of any of these conditions. While it is sometimes difficult to differentiate one cause from another without a slit lamp ophthalmologic examination, signs and symptoms that should prompt referral are decreased vision, severe pain, photophobia, recent intraocular surgery, or even distant surgery (especially if glaucoma surgery).

Relatively benign causes of red eye include blepharitis or inflammation of the Meibomian glands in the eyelids, dry eye, allergic conjunctivitis, corneal exposure due to lid malposition, viral conjunctivitis, and subconjunctival hemorrhages. Blepharitis and dry eye often present together because blepharitis affects the integrity of the tear film, which then evaporates more readily. Tears serve several important functions, including corneal lubrication, debris clearance, and immune protection. With age, tear production decreases, and older adults are prone to develop keratitis sicca, characterized by redness, foreign body sensation, and reflex tearing. Patients may complain of severe eye discomfort and blurred vision, which usually improves with blinking or eye rubbing because these two maneuvers spread the remaining tear film over the cornea. Dry eye can be especially problematic in older women, in whom hormonal changes are thought to play a role. Keratitis sicca can also be associated with autoimmune disease; conditions such as Sjögren's syndrome should be excluded. Management of dry eye includes tear replacement with artificial tears during the day (preservative-free tears if being used more than four times daily) and a lubricant ointment at bedtime. Topical cyclosporin A (0.2%) eye drops can be used for more severe cases of dry eye to combat the underlying ocular inflammation that affects tear production; however, caution is warranted in patients with a history of ocular herpetic infections. Treatment for accompanying blepharitis includes lid hygiene consisting of gentle scrubbing of the lash bases with nontearing baby shampoo twice daily and applying topical antibiotic ointment to the eyelids nightly. Oral doxycycline can also be a useful adjunct, especially when blepharitis is associated with acne rosacea. If symptoms continue despite these conservative measures, referral is warranted.

Viral conjunctivitis (or pink eye) is associated with severe tearing, mucous discharge, and matting of the eyelids, especially in the morning. Symptoms include eye irritation and blurred vision. Viral conjunctivitis is distinguished from bacterial conjunctivitis by history and, because it is highly contagious, patients frequently report either an upper respiratory tract infection or recent contact with someone suffering from a red eye. It is treated conservatively with warm compresses and artificial tears. Topical antibiotics are not indicated. If viral conjunctivitis is accompanied by severely reduced vision, the patient should be referred for an ophthalmologic examination, because corneal infiltrates can (rarely) develop, requiring steroid eye drops. Viral conjunctivitis is extremely contagious (by contact), and patient education is necessary to limit spread of the infection to the other eye or to contacts (including office staff).

Allergic conjunctivitis is a common benign condition; its hallmark is ocular pruritus. Patients should be advised to avoid known precipitants (eg, pet dander or cosmetics). Management of allergic conjunctivitis includes cool compresses, systemic antihistamines, topical antihistamines or decongestants, and ophthalmic corticosteroids for limited periods of time. Allergic conjunctivitis can also be an adverse event of some topical glaucoma medications. Usually, the conjunctivitis is accompanied by dermatitis of the eyelids. This problem should prompt referral to the ophthalmologist treating the glaucoma.

The use of ophthalmic corticosteroids merits comment. Ophthalmic steroid drops or ointment can have serious potential adverse events, including risks of ocular hypertension and glaucoma development (which can be asymptomatic for a long period of time), secondary infections, cataract formation, and corneal thinning if used in undiagnosed infections. Because of these risks, the prescription of ophthalmic corticosteroids is best limited to practitioners with the tools to monitor for these adverse events. The risk of adverse events increases greatly with prolonged use of steroid (months to years), and therefore prescriptions for any steroid-containing eye medication should never be refilled without ophthalmic evaluation. Ocular hypertension that can lead to glaucoma can develop within 2–3 wk with daily use of topical steroid in susceptible individuals (those with glaucoma, either diagnosed or undiagnosed, or with a family history of glaucoma). Low-potency steroids given for 7–10 days will not be problematic for the vast majority of patients, but patients and caregivers should be warned of the risks of prolonged and unmonitored use of steroids in and around the eyes.

Lid abnormalities are a common problem for older adults. Because of the gradual loss of elasticity and tensile strength that develops with age, secondary degenerative changes can develop. Blepharochalasis (drooping of the brow) and blepharoptosis (drooping of the eyelid) can cause cosmetic deformity and, if severe, can impair vision. Lid ectropion or entropion, eversion and inversion of the lid margins, respectively, can disrupt the ocular surface and cause discomfort. Various surgical procedures can be performed to address these conditions. Ocular lubricant ointments (those without antibiotics) can be recommended to minimize discomfort from exposure of the globe. Older adults can also develop squamous cell and basal cell carcinomas of the eyelids. Ulcerations or chronic irritation, especially if associated with loss of eyelashes, should be evaluated by an ophthalmologist.

Herpes zoster ophthalmicus, or shingles, is a painful reactivation of varicella zoster virus that not uncommonly affects older adults. Dermatomal distribution of weeping vesicles affecting the ophthalmic branch of the trigeminal nerve is the classic presentation. Ocular involvement can be signaled by lesions on the tip of the nose (Hutchinson's sign) and can include dendritic keratopathy or uveitis. Oral acyclovir can shorten the course of disease. Trifluridine eye drops are indicated for herpes simplex dendriform corneal ulcers (not for herpes zoster). Post-herpetic neuralgia can be quite debilitating; systemic medications (narcotics, tricyclic antidepressants[OL], gabapentin, pregabalin) can reduce pain, and less often, topical agents such as capsaicin and lidocaine patches can be tried (these should not be used near the eye—capsaicin can be extremely irritating to the eye and lidocaine can anesthetize the eye, placing the patient at risk of eye injury while the eye is numb). See also "Dermatologic Diseases and Disorders," p 334.

Subconjunctival hemorrhages are very common and, despite being benign, elicit worried responses from patients. Many patients are on a blood thinner, and minor trauma such as eye rubbing, which usually is not recalled by the patient, can cause a small blood vessel to tear and bleed. Artificial tears are recommended for comfort until the hemorrhage clears. If the patient is on warfarin, it may be prudent to check an INR if this has not been done recently.

Other common conditions seen in older adults include cataracts, macular degeneration, glaucoma, and ischemic optic neuropathy, which are discussed more fully in the following sections.

REFRACTIVE ERROR AND CATARACTS

The leading causes of visual impairment worldwide are refractive error and cataracts, for which eyeglasses and surgical cataract extraction, respectively, are mainstays of treatment. Despite the considerable successes of these therapeutic options, many populations do not receive adequate treatment for these problems.

Refractive error can be categorized as emmetropia (neutral refraction), ametropia, or presbyopia. Three forms of ametropia exist: myopia (nearsightedness), hyperopia (farsightedness), and astigmatism (distorted vision). Typically, older adults have increasing hyperopia, unless a cataract is present, which can induce a myopic shift. Although contact lens wear and laser refractive surgery are available for myopic and hyperopic refractive errors, younger people have

traditionally used these forms of refractive treatment. Corneal refractive surgery, such as LASIK, is not the best remedy for refractive problems in older adults who usually have some degree of cataracts. Removal of the cataract and replacement with an artificial intraocular lens, the power of which can be chosen to eliminate refractive error, is a better option in older adults. Toric intraocular lenses can correct astigmatism, and multifocal lenses can decrease the need for eyeglasses after surgery. After the age of approximately 40, emmetropic individuals begin to develop progressive presbyopia, impaired ability to focus on near objects that is caused by gradual hardening of the lens and decreased muscular effectiveness of the ciliary body. Reading glasses can be obtained OTC, or bifocal eyeglasses can be prescribed.

Approximately 20% of adults ≥65 yr old and 50% of adults ≥75 yr old have cataracts, a lens opacity that reduces vision. Cataracts can be associated with increased glare, decreased contrast sensitivity, and decreased visual acuity. The most important risk factor is increased age; other risk factors include decreased vitamin intake, light (ultraviolet B) exposure, smoking, alcohol use, long-term corticosteroid use, and diabetes mellitus.

Cataract extraction is one the most successful surgeries in medicine (90% of patients achieve vision of 20/40 or better). Approximately 1.5 million cataract procedures are performed each year in the United States. The benefits of cataract surgery include not only improved vision but also a decreased rate of falls (SOE=B) and improved vision-related quality of life (SOE=A).

Cataract extraction is safe and can be completed in <30 min under local or topical anesthesia. The surgery involves the breakdown of the lens by ultrasound energy and its aspiration (phacoemulsification). An artificial implant (intraocular lens) is placed in the capsular bag, which is the only remnant of the native lens retained. A secondary laser procedure (capsulotomy) may be necessary to ablate subsequent capsular opacification that can develop in ≥15% of patients.

AGE-RELATED MACULAR DEGENERATION

Age-related macular degeneration (ARMD) is the most common cause of irreversible blindness in older adults throughout the developed world. Increasing age is the most important risk factor, although a genetic predisposition is also contributory. Currently, there is no role for genetic screening as a clinical tool, because it is not yet clear how to use this information. Other risk factors include smoking and hypertension. Fair-skinned individuals are at greater risk of developing this disease than are black individuals, in

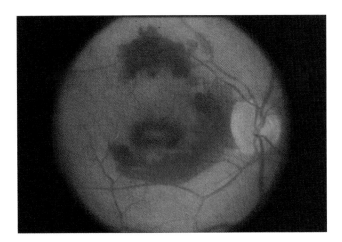

Figure 22.1—Choroidal neovascularization in a patient with the wet form of age-related macular degeneration, demonstrating a gray-green membrane associated with subretinal hemorrhage

whom pigment may serve as a protective element. Exposure to ultraviolet light is a debated risk factor.

ARMD is classified into two forms, dry and wet. The dry form is much more common and is characterized by deposits of macular drusen. Drusen, submacular yellow lipoprotein deposits composed of metabolic by-products, do not typically cause vision loss but are a marker for the wet form of ARMD, which is characterized by angiogenesis or choroidal neovascularization (CNV). The presence of larger, more numerous drusen conveys the greatest risk of development of CNV. The Age-Related Eye Disease Study (AREDS) found that the risk of CNV development could be decreased by 25% when patients with high-risk drusen are treated with high-dose oral multivitamin therapy (SOE=A). Combination multivitamins containing β-carotene 25,000 IU, vitamin E 400 IU, vitamin C 500 mg, and zinc 80 mg are available OTC. Supplements are recommended indefinitely or until the wet form of ARMD develops, which then necessitates other treatment. This vitamin therapy, however, is contraindicated in smokers because of the higher risk of lung cancer with use of β-carotene supplements. High-dose vitamin A and β-carotene are also associated with risk of osteoporosis. The formulation of the combination multivitamins used in AREDS (listed above) is not recommended for patients with less than high-risk drusen (because they have a low baseline risk of progressing to wet ARMD). A follow-up study, AREDS II, is now assessing the prophylactic benefit of other vitamin A derivatives, lutein and zeaxanthine, in preventing progression to the wet type of ARMD. Patients with the dry form of ARMD should be examined periodically by an ophthalmologist for the development of early signs of CNV. CNV in wet ARMD is marked by the presence of subretinal fluid and blood that may appear as a gray-green membrane (Figure 22.1). The development of CNV is signaled by sudden vision loss or distortion of vision and requires urgent evaluation, because untreated CNV can lead to severe central vision loss. The natural history of CNV is progressive subfoveal growth and leakage with eventual fibrotic scarring and central blindness.

Recently, angiogenesis inhibition has proved to be a major breakthrough in the treatment of CNV. Various inhibitors of vascular endothelial growth factor (VEGF) have been approved by the FDA for treatment of wet ARMD. Serial intravitreal injections (9 per year) of pegaptanib sodium, an anti-VEGF aptamer or mRNA oligonucleotide that inhibits mRNA synthesis, are approved for the treatment of all subtypes of wet ARMD. These injections do not typically improve vision, but they do reduce the risk of further vision loss. Another antiangiogenesis inhibitor, ranibizumab, is a fragment antibody that exhibits broad-spectrum inhibition of VEGF. In a multicenter, prospective randomized clinical trial, visual acuity improved by approximately 2 lines in those patients with CNV treated with ranibizumab compared with those given sham treatments (absolute risk reduction [ARR]=33%, number needed to treat [NNT]=3 [SOE=A]). Serial intravitreal injections of ranibizumab are now the gold standard of care for all subtypes of wet ARMD (ANCHOR and MARINA trials). Ranibizumab costs $2,000 per vial, and one vial is needed per eye. The manufacturer has recommended an injection every month for 2 yr ($48,000). However, most clinicians are giving 3 or 4 injections per eye, monitoring, and not reinjecting until neovascularization recurs. Bevacizumab is another VEGF inhibitor related to the ranibizumab molecule that has shown promise as being equally efficacious and is significantly less expensive than ranibizumab, although it is not approved by the FDA for treatment of wet ARMD. The National Institutes of Health has embarked on a comparative study to determine if there is any difference in efficacy or safety between these two related anti-VEGF inhibitors.

DIABETIC RETINOPATHY

Duration of disease, control of blood glucose, and control of blood pressure are the most important variables in the development and progression of diabetic retinopathy. After 10 yr, 70% of those with type 2 diabetes have some form of retinopathy, and nearly 10% show proliferative disease. Diet control, exercise, blood pressure control (target <130/80 mmHg), and maintaining glycosylated hemoglobin concentrations at <7% are general recommendations approved by the American Diabetes Association that can be reasonably applied to older adults without preexisting vascular disease who have a remaining life expectancy of >5−7 yr. The Diabetic Control and Complications Trial demonstrated that tight control of blood glucose in individuals with type 1 diabetes resulted in a long-lasting decrease in the rate of development and progression of diabetic retinopathy. The United Kingdom Prospective Diabetes Study (UKPDS) validated these results in an older population with type 2 diabetes. Tight blood glucose control was shown to decrease the need for the studies' primary outcome measures (ie, the need for laser) and the level of retinopathy; therefore, it was indirectly shown to influence and benefit vision, although some authors have questioned this surrogate measure. For example, a patient with poor control of blood glucose is more likely to progress to preproliferative and proliferative levels of retinopathy and need surgery, which is more likely to result in poor vision. The benefit of tight glucose control reduced the need for phototherapy within 3–4 yr in the groups with no baseline retinopathy and within 2–3 yr in the groups with mild to moderate retinopathy at baseline; however, most other studies and guidelines indicate that 7–8 yr of tight control are needed to show microvascular benefits. However, tight control of blood pressure (≤130/80 mmHg) is an important factor in decreasing microvascular complications, and becomes evident within 2–3 yr.

More recent data from the ACCORD, ADVANCE, and VADT studies have raised the question of whether intensive glycemic control is of enough benefit to outweigh the risks of hypoglycemia. The ACCORD study was stopped early because of excessive mortality in the intensive control group (relative risk increase 20%, absolute risk increase 1.0%, number needed to harm 100) and showed no significant benefit for macro- or microvascular disease in a group of patients of average age 62 yr old and longstanding diabetes. The ADVANCE study showed reductions in microvascular disease (relative risk reduction [RRR]=14%, ARR=1.5%, NNT=67); however, the significant benefits were in reductions of albuminuria rather than retinopathy. In contrast to the ACCORD study, a follow-up of UKPDS found evidence of a "legacy effect," of benefits of intensive control early in the course of the disease. In a group of patients followed for 10 yr after the end of the trial, intensive control during the trial reduced microvascular disease (RRR=25%, ARR=0.37%, NNT=270 in the group treated with sulfonylureas plus insulin; RRR=7%, ARR=0.1%, NNT=1,000 in the group treated with metformin) even though patients had not maintained the low target hemoglobin A_{1c} levels. The results of these studies prompted significant controversy in both the lay press and the medical literature, and led the American Diabetes Association, the American Heart Association, and the American College of Cardiology to issue a revised position statement in 2009 about the value of intensive control in type 2 diabetes mellitus. In this statement, the recommended hemoglobin A_{1c} target remains <7%; however, it notes that targets should be individualized and that patients with limited life expectancy, those with longstanding diabetes mellitus, and those with preexisting vascular disease are less likely to benefit from intensive control. Many, and probably most, geriatric patients fall into the latter categories; thus, the benefits of intensive control need to be very carefully weighed against the potential for harm. The risk of hypoglycemia is significantly greater in those who are frail, demented, or otherwise unable to comply with medical regimens and merit particular attention.

Other systemic risk factors, including kidney function and serum cholesterol, can also influence the course of diabetic retinopathy and should be optimized. ACE inhibitors decrease progressive nephropathy in diabetic patients and may have similar benefits on the retina.

Patients with type 2 diabetes require baseline ophthalmologic screening at diagnosis of systemic disease and annually thereafter. Subsequent follow-up depends on the grade of retinopathy. Nonproliferative diabetic retinopathy, the earliest stage of retinopathy, can first be manifested by retinal microaneurysms. Intraretinal hemorrhages and exudates, with or without associated macular edema, can ensue. Progressive ischemia characterized by increasing hemorrhages, venous caliber changes or intraretinal microvascular abnormalities or both, and capillary nonperfusion on fluorescein angiography characterize the preproliferative stage of diabetic retinopathy. About 40% of patients with preproliferative retinopathy develop proliferative diabetic retinopathy within 1–2 yr, characterized by neovascularization or new blood vessel growth of the retina or disc, or both.

Visual loss in patients with diabetes can occur as a result of macular nonperfusion or macular edema. The Early Treatment Diabetic Retinopathy Study demonstrated the benefit of focal or grid laser photocoagulation in stabilizing and improving vision in diabetic patients with clinically significant macular edema (Figure 22.2). Neovascularization (Figure 22.3) can cause severe vision loss or blindness in proliferative diabetic retinopathy as a result of vitreous hemorrhage or tractional retinal detachment. Proliferative diabetic retinopathy is amenable to treatment by panretinal laser photocoagulation to inhibit the growth stimulus for neovascularization. In the Diabetic Retinopathy Study, incidence of severe visual loss in patients treated with panretinal photocoagulation was 11%, but the incidence in those who did not receive laser during a 2-yr follow-up was 26%

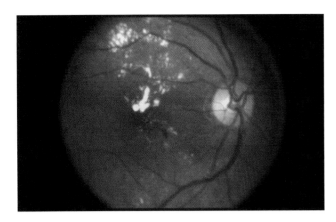

Figure 22.2—Intraretinal edema and exudate in the superior macular region consistent with clinically significant macular edema in a patient with type 2 diabetes mellitus

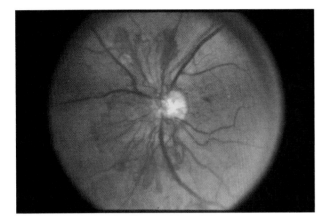

Figure 22.3—Florid neovascularization of the disc in a patient with high-risk proliferative diabetic retinopathy

(ARR=15%, NNT=7). Pars plana vitrectomy, membrane peeling, and endolaser can address nonclearing vitreous hemorrhage or tractional macular detachment surgically.

Although not approved by the FDA for the care of diabetic retinopathy, intravitreal anti-VEGF or steroid therapy is an important adjunct to laser therapy that is not uncommonly used to treat recalcitrant or cystoid diabetic macular edema. Intravitreal bevacizumab therapy has also been used for high-risk proliferative retinopathy.

GLAUCOMA

Glaucoma is the second most common cause of irreversible blindness worldwide and, in the United States, the most common cause of blindness in black Americans. It affects more than 2.25 million Americans ≥40 yr old and results in >3 million office visits each year. The financial burden is considerable because of the prevalence and chronicity of glaucoma and the debilitation that results. Glaucoma-related

Medicare and Medicaid payments and disability are reported to reach as high as $1 billion.

The definition of glaucoma has evolved considerably, and it is now defined as characteristic optic nerve head damage and visual field loss. Increased intraocular pressure (IOP) is no longer considered an absolute criterion, although it is a very important risk factor. There are many different types of glaucoma, of which primary open-angle glaucoma (POAG) is the most common. Adults >50 yr old should be screened for glaucoma every 1–2 yr. Older adults with a family history of glaucoma, black ethnicity, or other risk factors may need more frequent screening.

POAG is a chronic disease most commonly affecting older adults. Aqueous humor can access the eye's drain, but the "clogged" drain results in impaired passage out of the angle. Slow aqueous drainage leads to chronically increased IOPs. This is in contrast to acute angle-closure glaucoma, in which the eye's drain is suddenly blocked off, IOP increases precipitously, and the patient has considerable redness and pain with acute vision loss. Pain may be so severe as to cause headache, nausea, and vomiting. Emergent ophthalmologic referral is required to reverse the angle closure and decrease the IOP through the use of aqueous suppressants, miotics, and laser iridotomy. Conversely, the increase in IOP in POAG is slow and much less severe. Individuals with POAG are asymptomatic and can suffer substantial field loss before consulting an ophthalmologist, which underscores the importance of regular ophthalmologic screening of older adults. Development of POAG is most likely multifactorial and polygenic. Initial pedigrees demonstrated linkage to the *1q* locus. Subsequent investigations have more precisely defined the *GLC1A* gene that encodes for myocilin, the trabecular meshwork-induced glucocorticoid response protein. Several other chromosomal loci, including those mapped to chromosomes 2, 3, 7, and 10, are also associated with the development of glaucoma.

The management of POAG can be approached by the ophthalmologist in a stepwise manner. A variety of IOP-lowering medications, both local and systemic, are available. Mechanisms of action include decreased aqueous production or increased aqueous outflow. Various eye drop formulations are available; α_2-adrenergic agonists that decrease aqueous production and prostaglandin analogs that increase uveal-scleral outflow are two relatively new and effective drugs, but they may have adverse events (Table 22.4). In the face of visual field progression despite maximal medications, intolerance to medications, or inability to comply with eye drop administration (because of problems such as rheumatoid arthritis or dementia), argon laser trabeculoplasty (application of laser energy to the trabecular meshwork) can

Table 22.4—Adverse Events of Selected Eye Drops for Glaucoma

Class	Adverse Events
Aqueous suppressants	
α-Agonists (eg, brimonidine)	Allergic conjunctivitis, dry mouth/nose, mental status changes occasionally
β-Blockers (eg, timolol)	Bradycardia, dyspnea, asthma, heart failure exacerbations, impotence, exercise intolerance, hypoglycemia masking
Carbonic anhydrase inhibitors (eg, dorzolamide)	Blurry vision, stinging, bad taste in mouth
Aqueous outflow facilitators	
Epinephrine (eg, dipivefrin)	Palpitations, angina, cystoid macular edema
Miotics (eg, pilocarpine)	Brow ache, blurriness, detached retina, small pupils
Prostaglandins (eg, latanoprost)	Hyperemia, increased length and thickness and darkness of eyelashes, increased iris and eyelid pigmentation, cystoid macular edema, exacerbation of herpetic eye disease

be effective in lowering IOP in approximately 50% of patients for 3–5 yr after treatment. Intraocular surgery involves the creation of a fistula or filtration site to allow an alternative route of aqueous egress (trabeculectomy). Adjunctive antimetabolite use with 5-fluorouracil[OL] or mitomycin-C[OL] has increased the success of this procedure in those patients at high risk of surgical failure because of fibrosis and scarring of the filtration site. Alternative surgeries for glaucoma include drainage devices or aqueous shunts. Drainage devices, which are made of a foreign material such as plastic, shunt fluid from the anterior chamber to the subconjunctival space. Cryotherapy or laser procedures to destroy the ciliary body (cyclocryoablation or cyclophotocoagulation) can be used when the prognosis for vision in the eye is poor.

The strength of evidence is high in support of treating ocular hypertension to prevent the onset of glaucoma and of treating prevalent glaucoma to slow down progression of disease. Based on a meta-analysis of the literature, 12 ocular hypertensive patients need to be treated to prevent 1 patient from developing visual field defects or optic nerve changes consistent with glaucoma (SOE=A). From a meta-analysis of literature on treatment of established glaucoma patients, the NNT to prevent 1 glaucoma patient from progressive vision damage within 5 yr of treatment is 7. The ARR is 14.2%.

ANTERIOR ISCHEMIC OPTIC NEUROPATHY

Anterior ischemic optic neuropathy (Figure 22.4) can result in acute vision or field loss. Microvascular occlusion of the blood supply to the optic nerve can be attributed to atherosclerotic vascular disease or inflammation in the setting of giant cell (temporal) arteritis. The nonarteritic form typically affects patients with vasculopathic risk factors such as diabetes mellitus and hypertension; the latter, the arteritic form, tends to occur in older adults with a history of myalgias, headaches, and weight loss. An increased

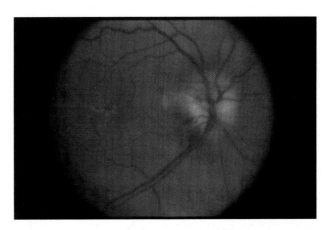

Figure 22.4—Pallid swelling of the optic nerve head in a patient with anterior ischemic optic neuropathy

Westergren erythrocyte sedimentation rate and a positive temporal artery biopsy are diagnostic. Systemic corticosteroid treatment is crucial to avoid visual loss in the other eye.

LOW-VISION REHABILITATION

Despite considerable advancements in the medical treatment of ocular conditions, many patients, especially those with the wet form of ARMD, can ultimately sustain permanent visual loss. Visual training and the provision of visual aids are indispensable services for those with low vision (visual acuity <20/60).

Patients with low vision can develop useful adaptive skills with proper instruction. Eccentric viewing by ARMD patients with central macular pathology uses the principle of off-center fixation. The patient can benefit from formal training to find and use the most effective eccentric viewing points. Instruction in scanning and tracking and other skills can help the patient integrate his or her visual environment.

Various low-vision aids are available to improve the ability to see both near and far. The fine detail required for reading is the most common indication for visual aids. Improved lighting is a simple modification that can enhance visualization of print. Selection of reading material using bold, enlarged fonts and accentuated black-on-white contrast can also be helpful. Magnification also is commonly used. Various devices such as high-plus spectacles, hand-held magnifiers, stand magnifiers, and closed-circuit television can also enhance reading. Distance magnification can be achieved with the use of telescopic devices that can be hand-held for spot viewing or spectacle mounted for continual viewing. Talking devices, which are computers used to create voice synthesis such as those used at stoplights, or Braille can be especially helpful for those who have completely lost vision.

REFERENCES

■ Gandhewar RR, Kamath GG. Acute glaucoma presentations in the elderly. *Emerg Med J.* 2005;22(4):306–307.

■ Jain A, Sarraf D, Fong D. Preventing diabetic retinopathy through the control of systemic risk factors. *Curr Opin Ophthalmol.* 2003;14(6):389–394.

■ Vedula S, Krzystolik M. Antiangiogenic therapy with anti-vascular endothelial growth factor modalities for neovascular age-related macular degeneration. *Cochrane Database Syst Rev.* 2008;(2):CD005139.

CHAPTER 23—HEARING IMPAIRMENT

KEY POINTS

■ Hearing loss is among the most common chronic diseases among older adults: 10% of adults 65–75 yr old and 25% of those >75 yr old have hearing loss.

■ Treatment of hearing loss and attention to communication strategies can improve quality of life for individuals with hearing impairment.

■ Important issues when considering hearing aids for an older adult with hearing loss are the nature and degree of hearing loss, the person's ability to manipulate the aid and adapt to its use, and the person's social support and financial resources.

Hearing loss is the fourth most common chronic disease among older adults. Hearing impairment is often assumed to be benign, but it has profound effects on quality of life. The psychologic effects of hearing loss include family discord, social isolation, loss of self-esteem, anger, and depression. Epidemiologic studies suggest an association between hearing loss and cognitive impairment, and between hearing loss and reduced mobility. Hearing loss can also affect an older adult's interaction with clinicians, making history taking and patient education difficult. Treatment of hearing loss and attention to communication strategies can improve quality of life for individuals with hearing impairment by facilitating interaction with family, friends, and caregivers. Studies indicate that use of a hearing aid can relieve symptoms of depression that are associated with hearing loss.

NORMAL HEARING AND AGE-RELATED CHANGES IN THE AUDITORY SYSTEM

The normal ear is an efficient transducer of sound energy into nerve impulses. Sound energy is transmitted through the external ear to the tympanic membrane and the auditory ossicles. The malleus, incus, and stapes in series transmit vibrations to the oval window of the cochlea. Fluid waves within the cochlea stimulate the outer hair cells of the scala tympani. These cells stimulate the inner hair cells, which generate sensory potential. In turn, an excitatory postsynaptic potential is generated. When threshold is reached, impulses are sent via cochlear neurons to the cochlear nuclei and then to auditory pathways elsewhere in the brain.

Age-related changes in the auditory system can interfere with its function. The walls of the external ear canal become thin. Cerumen becomes drier and more tenacious, increasing the likelihood of cerumen impaction. The tympanic membrane becomes thicker and appears duller in older adults than in younger people. The ossicular joints undergo degenerative changes, but this generally does not interfere with sound transmission to the cochlea. Cochlear changes include loss of sensory hair cells and fibrocytes in the organ of Corti, stiffening of the basilar membrane, calcification of auditory structures, and cochlear neuronal loss. Changes in the stria vascularis include thickening of capillaries, decreased production of endolymph, and decreased Na$^+$/K$^+$-ATPase activity. These degenerative changes occur to varying degrees in different individuals. It is currently not possible to fully correlate the degree of hearing loss with histologic changes in the aging ear.

Changes in central auditory processing also occur with aging. In one study, when competing speech stimuli were presented to each ear, the right ear had a 5%–10% advantage over the left ear in younger people (the effect of right- and left-handedness was not assessed; all the participants were right-handed). In people 80–89 yr old, this difference increased to >40%. This difference may be related to a loss of efficiency of interhemispheric transfer of auditory information through the corpus callosum.

EPIDEMIOLOGY

Hearing loss can result from dysfunction of the auditory system at any point from the external ear to the brain. This loss can be described in terms of the loss of ability to hear pure tones across the range of audio frequencies important for understanding speech, but in practical terms, impairment of the ability to understand spoken language and to perceive environmental sounds significantly affects quality of life. The prevalence of hearing loss increases with age. Ten percent of adults 65–75 yr old and 25% of those >75 yr old have hearing loss. In nursing homes, estimates of prevalence vary from 50% to 100%, depending on the criteria used to define hearing loss.

Hearing loss can be caused by pathology in the external ear canal, the middle ear, the inner ear, the auditory nerve, central auditory pathways, or a combination of these.

Conductive hearing loss is caused by disease in the external ear, such as ceruminosis or a foreign body in the canal, or by middle-ear pathology, such as otosclerosis, cholesteatoma, tympanic membrane perforation, or middle-ear effusion.

Sensorineural hearing loss is most often caused by cochlear disease. Noise is the most common factor in cochlear damage. Hearing loss is less common among people in quiet rural environments than among those in industrialized communities. Other causes of hearing loss include ototoxic medications, genotype, vascular disease, and rarely, occupational and environmental chemical exposures. Smokers have higher rates of hearing loss than nonsmokers. Autoimmune disease and auditory nerve tumors are rare causes of sensorineural hearing loss. Neuronal loss can affect the brain stem and cortical ascending auditory pathways, including the cochlear nuclei, superior olivary complex, lateral lemniscus, inferior colliculi, and medial geniculate complex. The resulting deficits in central auditory processing can affect perception of sound and the ability to understand speech. These deficits would not be apparent on a simple audiogram.

PRESBYCUSIS

Most hearing loss in older adults is categorized as presbycusis (literally, "older hearing"). Presbycusis is a sensorineural, usually symmetrical hearing loss that may have central components. Presbycusis can be classified as sensory, neural, strial, cochlear conductive, combined, or indeterminate, depending on cochlear pathology. Many people with presbycusis can be helped by amplification.

Sensory presbycusis results in a steeply sloping audiogram. It is often slowly progressive, beginning with the higher frequencies of 8,000 Hz, 6,000 Hz, and 4,000 Hz. It can involve the 3,000 and 2,000 Hz range, which is the higher portion of the range of frequencies in human speech. People with this type of hearing loss often have trouble hearing in the presence of background noise but are able to hear adequately in quiet settings. Amplification often helps these patients, because speech discrimination is satisfactory. This loss of auditory acuity can begin when people are in their twenties but may not become clinically evident until later decades. Sensory presbycusis is attributed to a loss of sensory hair cells in the basal end of the cochlea.

Strial presbycusis is considered a metabolic form of hearing loss. The stria vascularis maintains high potassium concentrations in the endolymph. Strial presbycusis, pathologically defined as atrophy of ≥30% of the stria vascularis, is a form of cochlear dysfunction. This disorder typically begins between the ages of 20 and 60 yr old and is characterized by mild to moderate hearing loss in most frequencies. People with strial presbycusis usually have good speech discrimination and do well with amplification.

Neural presbycusis is caused by a cochlear neuronal loss of ≥50% compared with the normal number in neonates. Despite preserved pure-tone thresholds, which are not affected until >90% of cochlear neurons have been lost, individuals with neural presbycusis show very poor speech discrimination. Successful use of amplification is difficult for this form of presbycusis.

Cochlear conductive presbycusis is caused by changes in cochlear mechanics produced by mass or stiffness changes or spiral ligament atrophy. It has a unique audiogram, which gradually descends over at least five octaves with no more than a 25-dB difference between any two adjacent frequencies. Speech discrimination can also be impaired. Patho-

---

STRENGTH-OF-EVIDENCE (SOE) RATING DEFINITIONS

A = consistent and good quality patient-oriented evidence
B = somewhat inconsistent or limited quality patient-oriented evidence
C = very inconsistent or very limited patient-oriented evidence, disease-oriented evidence, and/or consensus from professional organizations
D = unstudied common practice or opinion

See inside front cover for detailed information regarding the SOE classification.

logically, this form is defined by the absence of histologic changes seen in the other forms of presbycusis.

Most presbycusis is probably a mixture of these forms. The shape of the audiogram and speech discrimination scores depends on the extent of injury to various components of the cochlea.

DIAGNOSIS

Partly because of the slowly progressive nature of hearing loss, many older adults are unaware of their hearing deficit. In some cases, the perceived stigma of wearing a hearing aid causes the patient to deny the problem. The hearing loss may be brought to medical attention by family members, who complain that the patient does not hear them or plays the television or radio too loudly. Clinicians may notice that the patient does not respond when spoken to by someone out of the patient's field of view, or seems to misunderstand questions. Hearing loss can also be interpreted as cognitive impairment. Caregivers and physicians may not recognize the presence of hearing loss or may assume it is a benign component of aging.

Tinnitus, or "ringing in the ears," can be an early sign of hearing loss. Individuals with tinnitus or buzzing should be evaluated by an otolaryngologist. Medical treatment for tinnitus is often unsuccessful, but hearing aids for those with hearing loss, or the use of devices that provide background white noise, may be useful to reduce the impact of tinnitus.

Screening programs to identify hearing loss are important. Fitting hearing aids early in the course of hearing loss can help the person adjust to their use (SOE=B), and treatment can reduce psychologic morbidity for helping to adjust to use (SOE=A). A handheld otoscope with a tone generator can be used by primary care providers to screen for the presence of hearing loss at selected frequencies (0.5, 1, 2, and 4 kHz) and two loudness levels (25 and 40 dB hearing loss). This device should be used in a quiet environment. When set at 40 dB hearing loss, testing at 1 and 2 kHz has a sensitivity of 94% and a specificity between 82% and 90% for detecting hearing loss. The Hearing Handicap Inventory for the Elderly—Screening Version is a 10-item questionnaire that asks about difficulty with communication in various settings. It can be useful to determine the impact that hearing loss has on a patient's daily activities. When a screening test is consistent with hearing loss and the patient is willing and able to pay for a hearing aid, referral to an audiologist should be discussed.

The ear canals should be examined with an otoscope to exclude the presence of obstruction before referral for audiologic testing. Cerumen impaction can cause a clinically significant hearing loss, as much as 40 dB. If the patient has a history of tympanic membrane surgery or perforation, referral to an otolaryngologist for removal of the impaction is advisable. Otherwise, cerumen can be removed by manual extraction in cooperative patients. Cerumenolytics alone, used for several days, are effective about 40% of the time in treating cerumen impaction. Alternatively, cerumenolytics or saline can be applied to soften the wax 15–30 min before irrigating the ear with warm water. If irrigation fails, using a cerumenolytic for several days may clear the impaction or soften it enough that repeat irrigation is successful. If the impaction remains, the patient should be referred to an otolaryngologist.

The otolaryngologist will further evaluate the hearing loss and identify treatable causes. An asymmetrical hearing loss demands thorough investigation. Auditory nerve tumors are rare, but tumors of the posterior pharynx can obstruct the eustachian tube, causing a middle-ear effusion with conductive hearing loss.

The audiologist will assess hearing to determine the presence and type of hearing loss. A comprehensive audiologic assessment consists of pure-tone thresholds for both air and bone conduction, speech-recognition thresholds, speech discrimination, and middle-ear function. This information, along with the medical evaluation, is used to determine appropriate treatment. Audiologists recommend and fit hearing aids and provide auditory rehabilitation. Medicare will pay for an audiologic examination if it is ordered by a physician.

TREATMENT

Some causes of hearing loss are amenable to medical or surgical treatment. Paget's disease of the bone can affect the middle ear, causing conductive loss, or the inner ear, leading to sensorineural loss. Bisphosphonate therapy rarely restores hearing, although it may stabilize hearing loss (SOE=C). Otosclerosis or tympanosclerosis may be correctable with surgery (SOE=C). Otosclerosis may respond to bisphosphonate therapy (SOE=C). Sudden hearing loss may be autoimmune in nature and sometimes responds to corticosteroids (SOE=B) or immunosuppressant therapy (SOE=C). Most older adults with hearing loss are treated with communication strategies or amplification, or both. Hearing aids often improve ability to understand speech, particularly soft speech and conversational loud speech (SOE=B).

Strategies to Enhance Communication

Hearing-impaired individuals should be encouraged to let others know about their hearing loss and to suggest strategies that will help them communicate more easily (Table 23.1). In addition to using these strategies, clinicians should provide options for pa-

Table 23.1—Strategies to Improve Communication with Hearing-Impaired People

- ***Ask the listener what is the best way to communicate with him or her.***
- Obtain the listener's attention before speaking.
- Eliminate background noise as much as possible.
- Be sure the listener can see the speaker's lips:
  - Speak face-to-face in the same room.
  - Do not obscure the lips with hands or other objects.
  - Make certain that light shines directly on the speaker's face, not from behind the speaker.
- Speak slowly and clearly, but avoid shouting.
- Speak toward the better ear, if applicable.
- Change phrasing if the listener does not understand at first.
- Spell words out, use gestures, or write them down.
- Have the listener repeat back what he or she heard.

tients with hearing loss, such as sign language interpreters, the use of writing materials (eg, pen and paper, dry-erase board, or computer screen), or assistive devices. Office and hospital staff should be alerted to a patient's hearing loss. Background noise from the environment can interfere with hearing and should be reduced as much as possible.

Lipreading can be a useful adjunct to listening, but it requires thoughtfulness on the part of the speaker. When speaking to a hearing-impaired person who lip-reads, it is important to face him or her and to obtain the person's attention before speaking; a gentle touch on the hand or arm will usually suffice. Each word should be spoken clearly and distinctly. Shouting not only distorts lip movements so they are harder to read but also can make the speaker sound angry even when not. It is best to speak in complete sentences; single words are hard to lip-read because the listener often needs cues from context to identify meaning. It is helpful to make certain the person knows the topic of conversation. The language used should be appropriate for the listener's educational level. Unlike deaf persons who have usually had hearing impairment all or most of their lives, most older adults with hearing loss do not know sign language. Sometimes, amplification and lipreading are not enough. Gestures can aid communication even with cognitively impaired individuals.

For patients with hearing impairment, it can also be helpful to write words down. For those with both hearing and visual impairment, large printing with a marker pen or a laptop computer screen with magnified print may be necessary. These patients may benefit from correction of the visual problem, if possible (eg, cataract removal or use of eyeglasses). In any case, providing written instructions generally improves understanding and retention of important information.

The clinician should be alert to misunderstandings, which are common. If a reply does not make sense, repeating the idea of what was said using different words can help, as can asking the patient to express what he or she heard.

Assistive Listening Devices

For some people with hearing impairment, a personal amplifier may be more useful than hearing aids. These pocket-sized devices are considerably less expensive than hearing aids and are harder to misplace. Headphones stay on the head better than earbuds and provide sound to both ears. The volume and microphone placement of the amplifier should be adjusted to find the best combination for a given user. At least one or two of these devices should be available in every healthcare facility; these devices are not personalized and so can be used by different people.

Adaptive equipment can facilitate telephone use. State agencies may provide amplified telephones, vibrating and flashing ringer alert devices, and text telephones (TTY) at no cost to hearing-impaired people. This equipment is available from electronics and telephone equipment stores.

Many other assistive devices are available. Television listening devices can spare others from overly loud volume levels. FM loop systems can be used for groups of people with FM receivers or telecoil switches in their hearing aids. Wireless FM transmitters and receivers are also available for indoor or outdoor use. Infrared group listening devices are primarily useful indoors. Vibrating and flashing devices such as alarm clocks and timers, smoke alarms, doorbell alerts, and motion sensors can improve quality of life and safety for hearing-impaired people. These items can be purchased through the agencies mentioned above, or from catalog retailers of assistive listening devices.

Hearing Aids

Hearing aids are the most common form of amplification. Many factors need to be considered in deciding whether to fit an individual with a hearing aid. In addition to the nature and degree of hearing loss (Table 23.2), the person's motivation and ability to adapt to use of the aid and to physically manipulate the aid (Table 23.3), the degree of his or her social support, and his or her ability to afford the aid (Table 23.4) must be considered. Although hearing aids can be purchased from numerous sources, including over the Internet, working with an audiologist or other individual who has master's level training in audiology is advisable because of his or her expertise in hearing-aid fitting and adjustment.

Not everyone benefits from a hearing aid. The pattern of sensorineural damage can be such that speech discrimination is poor even with amplification. Some individuals are unable to tolerate the presence of the hearing aid in the ear. It is important to be

Table 23.2—Effects and Rehabilitation of Hearing Loss, by Degree of Loss

Degree of Loss	Hearing Loss (db)	Difficult Sounds to Hear	Effect on Communication	Amplification or Other Assistance Needed
Mild	25–40	Whisper	Difficulty understanding soft speech or normal speech in presence of background noise	Hearing aid needed in specific situations
Moderate	41–55	Conversational speech	Difficulty understanding any but loud speech	Frequent need for hearing aid
Severe	56–80	Shouting, vacuum cleaner	Can understand only amplified speech	Amplification needed for all communication
Profound	≥81	Hair dryer, heavy traffic, telephone ringer	Difficulty understanding amplified speech; may miss telephone calls	May need to supplement hearing aid with lipreading, assistive listening devices, sign language

SOURCE: Data in part from *A Report on Hearing Aids: User Perspectives and Concerns*. Washington, DC: American Association of Retired Persons; 1993:2.

Table 23.3—Advantages and Disadvantages of Styles of Hearing Aids

Style	Degree of Hearing Loss	Advantages	Disadvantages
CIC	Mild to moderate	Almost invisible Less occlusion of ear canal allows more natural sound Easier to use with headphones and telephone	Dexterity may be a problem. Small size may limit available features. May cost more than canal or in-the-ear aids Shorter battery life
Canal	Mild to moderate	More cosmetic than larger aids Telecoil available in some modes May be able to use with headphones	Dexterity may be a problem. Small size may limit available features.
In the ear	Mild to severe	Ease of handling Comfortable fit Available options: telecoil, directional microphone More power than CIC or canal aid	More conspicuous than CIC or canal aid May be difficult to use with headphones
Behind the ear	Mild to profound	Greatest power Available options: telecoil, direct audio input, directional microphone Earmold can be changed separately	More conspicuous May be more difficult to insert than in-the-ear aids Difficult to use with headphones
Body aid	Severe to profound	Greatest separation of microphone from receiver reduces feedback	Most conspicuous Body-level microphone is subject to noise from clothing. Microphone is on chest or at waist, but speech is usually directed at ear level.
Bone conduction aid	Mild to severe	Bypasses middle ear; used if ear canal is unable to tolerate aid or earmold	Receiver causes pressure on the scalp, which can be uncomfortable; does not correct sensorineural loss

NOTE: CIC = completely in the canal

sure that the aid can be returned during an initial trial period, usually 30 days, without having to pay the full cost of the aid. It is equally important not to give up on the aid too soon, because the audiologist often can adjust it to improve comfort and sound quality. The audiologist should provide counseling for optimal use of the aid. In general, two hearing aids are more beneficial than one. The first aid provides the most gain; the second one helps with speech discrimination and with localizing the source of sounds. However, the presence of asymmetrical hearing loss or significant difficulty in understanding competing speech stimuli may mean that the use of a single hearing aid is more appropriate.

Many different styles of hearing aids are available (Table 23.3). Behind-the-ear aids hang behind the ear and are connected directly to an earmold. The earmold is custom made to fit each person's ear. Some behind-the-ear aids can be connected to assistive listening devices via a "boot," which fits over the end of the aid to provide direct audio input. Body aids are worn on the belt or in a pocket or harness, and they are connected to a custom-made earmold by a wire. These are rarely used. All-in-the-ear aids and canal aids have cases that are custom fit to the user. The smaller hearing aids may have remote controls.

Table 23.4—Approximate Costs of Assistive Listening Devices and Hearing Aids

Type of Technology	Cost	Comments
Assistive listening devices (eg, personal amplifiers, telephone amplifiers, television listening devices)	$150–$200	Useful for specific situations (see text for details)
Hearing aids		
Analog	$1,000–$1,100	Smaller aids are more expensive
Analog programmable	$1,150–$1,600	Smaller aids are more expensive
Digital, low end	$1,200–$2,000	Similar to analog aid but with better sound quality
Digital, mid-range	$1,800–$2,500	Some sound processing included, eg, a second program, feedback control, telecoil
Digital, premium	$2,500–$3,000	Multiple features available, eg, background noise suppression, feedback management, multiple programs, telecoil
Bone conduction	$400–$900	Available as all-in-one headpiece or as body aid; used only if in-the-ear aid or earmold is not tolerated

NOTE: Assistive listening devices and hearing aids are not covered by Medicare.

Selection of aid style for each individual depends on the degree of hearing loss, available features, and the person's dexterity and motivation.

The telecoil is an induction coupling coil that can be built into the hearing aid. It detects the magnetic field produced by telephones that are compatible with hearing aids. The telecoil is used to listen to the telephone with less distraction from noise in the same room. It can also be used with many assistive listening devices. The amount of coupling, and therefore the volume of the signal, depends on the angle of the telecoil with respect to the magnetic field. Users may need to experiment to find the right angle. Strongly magnetic devices such as computer monitors often produce interference, which also depends on the angle and the distance of the telecoil from the device. These drawbacks aside, the telecoil is a useful feature and can be added to hearing aids at relatively low cost. Individuals with moderate to severe hearing loss should be encouraged to consider purchasing an aid with a telecoil.

The choice of analog or digital hearing aids depends on the individual. Analog aids are less expensive than digital aids and may provide acceptable sound quality. However, newer digital technology has allowed improved sound quality, reduced size, and increased ability to customize the amplification of the aid to the needs of the user. Programmable aids are adjusted for each individual while he or she is wearing the aid. Often, two or more programs are available within a single aid. Using a computer, the audiologist makes adjustments to gain, response in different frequency ranges, and loudness balance for each program. One program may be most useful in the presence of background noise, whereas another works better in a quiet environment, and a third works with a telecoil. Patients with Meniere disease can have their aids reprogrammed to accommodate fluctuating hearing loss. Some hearing aids automatically adjust the volume to increase amplification of soft sounds while avoiding uncomfortable loudness, reducing the need for the user to manipulate the aid. In a study comparing different methods of limiting loudness, consumers with mild to moderate hearing loss were more likely to prefer compression-limiting or wide dynamic range compression circuitry to peak-clipping circuitry, although the absolute differences in consumer preference and speech comprehension between these methods were small.

Background noise is a significant problem for hearing-aid users. Traditional hearing aids amplify sound indiscriminately, so that background noise, eg, papers rustling or water running, can be very distracting. For new hearing-aid users, this problem can be addressed by having the audiologist gradually increase the gain of the hearing aid as the listener adjusts to being able to hear environmental sounds over the course of weeks. However, background noise in the presence of speech is a problem even for experienced hearing-aid users. The use of multiple microphones in the hearing aid, combined with digital signal processing, can decrease the effects of background noise. This can significantly improve the user's ability to understand speech and increase satisfaction with the aid.

Unfortunately, the cost of hearing aids is often a significant barrier to their use and can affect the purchaser's choice of features (Table 23.4). The cost of a hearing aid ranges from $950 to $3,000 per device. The expected life span of a hearing aid is 3–5 yr, although with care, some aids may last longer. Although hearing aids are covered by Medicaid in most states, the amount of reimbursement often does not cover aids with advanced features. Hearing aids are not covered by Medicare or by private health insurance in many states, except in rare circumstances. Federal programs such as the Department of Veterans Affairs may pay for hearing aids, depending

Table 23.5—Characteristics of Older Candidates for Cochlear Implants

Severe to profound sensorineural hearing loss in both ears

Functional auditory nerve

Short duration of severe hearing loss

Good speech, language, and communication skills

Not benefiting enough from other kinds of hearing aids

No medical contraindication to surgery (eg, active infection, inability to tolerate general anesthesia)

Realistic expectations about results

Appropriate support services available for aural rehabilitation after cochlear implant

Adequate motivation and cognition to participate in aural rehabilitation

on the recipient's eligibility for services. Some charitable organizations assist in providing hearing aids to low-income persons.

Caring for Hearing Aids

Hearing aids are delicate devices and should not be dropped, chewed on by pets, or allowed to go through the laundry. They should be stored with the battery compartment door open; this may be the only way to turn the hearing aid off. They should be wiped with a dry cloth daily (earmolds of behind-the-ear aids should be cleaned according to manufacturer's instructions). Wax may plug the sound outlet of a hearing aid, and the manufacturer's instructions should be consulted before trying to clean it.

Patients may need assistance to insert the hearing aid. First it should be noted whether the hearing aid goes into the right ear (the aid may be marked with red) or the left ear (marked with blue). The battery door faces the outside of the ear. If there is a vent or a removal string, these are usually at the bottom. The following instructions apply to all except behind-the-ear aids:

The aid should first be turned on to be sure it is working. If so, a high-pitched squeal (feedback) should be heard; if no squeal is heard when the volume is set at maximum, the battery should be replaced. The hearing aid should be oriented right side up, with the canal portion of the aid or earmold facing toward the canal. The wide, flat portion of an in-the-ear aid or earmold should be posterior. This part of the aid may need to be rotated so that it fits

into the external ear, and the helix lifted gently to ease this part in. If there is feedback, the aid may be gently pushed back to seat it more firmly into the ear. Turning the volume down may also reduce feedback.

Patients with dementia may remove and dispose of the aid. To reduce this risk, it can be helpful to order a loop attached to the hearing aid case; a piece of fishing line can be attached to the loop and the other end of the line pinned to the patient's clothing to catch the aid when the patient removes it. In long-term care institutions, a system for collecting the aids each night and placing them in the patients' ears each morning may facilitate use of the aids, while reducing the number that are lost.

Cochlear Implants

For patients with severe to profound hearing loss who gain little or no benefit from hearing aids yet who are motivated to participate in the hearing world, cochlear implants can provide useful hearing (Table 23.5). A cochlear implant is an electronic device that bypasses the function of damaged or absent cochlear hair cells by providing electrical stimulation to cochlear nerve fibers. A receiver-stimulator and an intracochlear electrode array are surgically implanted. A headset is worn behind the ear. The headset microphone transmits signals to the speech processor, which filters and digitizes the sound into coded signals. The coded signals are sent to the cochlear implant, which then stimulates auditory nerve fibers in the cochlea. Nerve signals are then sent through the auditory system to the brain. Patients must be able to tolerate general anesthesia and to participate in extensive pre-implant testing and post-implant training. Meningitis is a rare complication of cochlear implants.

The cochlear implant procedure is covered by most Medicare carriers and insurance companies, although prior authorization is generally required. In general, outcomes of cochlear implantation in adults ≥65 yr old have been comparable to those of younger adults, with many patients obtaining excellent results by both audiologic and quality-of-life measures. Cochlear implants do not restore normal hearing, but users can sense environmental sounds and are able to understand speech more easily. Many can use a telephone, and some can even enjoy music.

ACOVE-3* QUALITY INDICATORS PERTAINING TO HEARING IMPAIRMENT

Screening for hearing loss

- All vulnerable older adults should have an annual evaluation of hearing status.
- All vulnerable older adults should have an evaluation of hearing status as part of the initial evaluation.

Formal audiologic evaluation

- If a vulnerable older adult has a self-reported hearing problem or does not pass a hearing screening, then he or she should be referred for formal evaluation by an otolaryngologist or audiologist within 3 mo.

Hearing rehabilitation

- If a vulnerable older adult is a candidate for a hearing aid (according to audiometry), then he or she should be offered rehabilitation with a hearing aid.

Conductive hearing loss

- If a vulnerable older adult has conductive hearing loss (according to audiometry), then he or she should be offered a referral to an otolaryngologist.

Cochlear implantation

- If a cognitively intact vulnerable older adult has profound bilateral sensorineural hearing loss that has not responded to hearing aid rehabilitation, then he or she should be offered referral for cochlear implantation.

Assistive listening device

- If audiometry and formal evaluation reveal that a vulnerable older adult's hearing loss would not benefit from a hearing aid (or he or she cannot afford it) or treatment from an otolaryngologist or that he or she has a persistent hearing handicap, then he or she should be offered hearing rehabilitation or an assistive listening device (eg, telephone amplifiers, TTY/TDD devices, television headphones, infrared systems, lighted telephones, door knock alert systems, vibrating clocks, smoke detectors with strobe lights).

*Assessing Care of Vulnerable Elders – 3rd Set. See inside front cover for explanation.

REFERENCES

- Bagai A, Thavendiranathan P, Detsky AS. Does this patient have hearing loss? *JAMA.* 2006;295(4):416−428.

- Demers K. Hearing Screening in Older Adults: A Brief Hearing Loss Screener. *Try This: Best Practices in Nursing Care to Older Adults.* 2007;(12). Available at: http://consultgerirn.org/uploads/File/trythis/try_this_12.pdf

- McCarter DF, Courtney AU, Pollart SM. Cerumen impaction. *Am Fam Physician.* 2007;75(10):1523−1528, 1530.

- Newman CW, Sandridge SA. Hearing loss is often undiscovered, but screening is easy. *Cleve Clin J Med.* 2004;71(3):225−232.

CHAPTER 24—DIZZINESS

KEY POINTS

- The classification of dizziness into vertigo, presyncope, disequilibrium, mixed, or others may be useful in guiding patient evaluation; however, precise classification is often difficult, and multiple causes of the same symptoms are common.

- Dizziness is associated with increased fear of falling, functional disability, and depressive symptoms.

- Multiple factors can contribute to chronic dizziness.

- Expensive tests like electronystagmography, rotational chair testing, posturography, and neuroimaging, such as CT or MRI, are not often needed in the evaluation of dizziness.

- Multifactorial interventions can help in ameliorating chronic dizziness.

Dizziness ranks among the most common symptoms presented by older adults to primary healthcare providers. The various and often nonspecific terms—lightheadedness, wooziness, vertigo, spinning, floating, and imbalance—that patients typically use to de-scribe dizziness add to the diagnostic and management challenge. Dizziness that continues >1–2 mo is considered chronic. The prevalence of dizziness in adults ≥65 yr old ranges from 4% to 30%. The prevalence of dizziness increases 10% for every 5 yr of age. Dizziness is more common in women than in men.

Acute dizziness, which is independent of age, has causes and interventions similar to those of chronic dizziness. However, chronic dizziness, which is much more common in older adults, has a larger variety of contributing causes and requires additional skill and patience to evaluate and manage successfully. This chapter focuses on chronic dizziness in older adults, which is commonly seen with increasing fear of falling, depressive symptoms, fall risk, and general functional disability.

CLASSIFICATION

Drachman and Hart classified dizziness into four types of sensations: vertigo, presyncope, disequilibrium, and other. A fifth type—mixed—results from a combination of two or more of the above, and is the most common type of dizziness reported by older adults (Table 24.1).

Vertigo

Vertigo is an often episodic spinning or rotational sensation; objective vertigo ("the room is spinning") versus subjective vertigo ("I am spinning") results from disturbances in the vestibular system. The most common causes of vertigo are benign paroxysmal positional vertigo (BPPV) and Meniere disease. BPPV, an inner ear disorder, is characterized by sudden onset, seconds-long bouts of vertigo precipitated by certain changes in the head position (rolling over in bed, gazing up or down). BPPV probably results from changes in endolymphatic pressure during head movements resulting from dislodged otoconia in the semicircular canal. Meniere disease, an idiopathic inner ear disorder, is characterized by episodic vertigo, tinnitus, fluctuating hearing loss, and a sensation of fullness in the inner ear. Other causes of vertigo include idiopathic recurrent vestibulopathy and central vestibular lesions such as cerebrovascular disease and acoustic neuroma. Absence of spinning sensation does not exclude vestibular diseases because patients with vestibular problems can describe dizziness as an imbalance or disequilibrium or other sensation. Patients with cervical dizziness secondary to cervical arthritis can also present with vertigo.

Presyncope

Presyncope, a feeling of faintness or lightheadedness, usually results from a cardiovascular problem causing brain hypoperfusion through postural hypotension. There is no specific definition of postural hypotension in older adults, but it is commonly defined as a drop in systolic arterial blood pressure of at least 20 mmHg and/or a drop in diastolic blood pressure of 10 mmHg after standing up from a supine position. However, older adults commonly describe dizziness on standing from a supine position without any orthostatic changes in blood pressure. Another common condition, postprandial hypotension, is defined as a decrease in systolic blood pressure of ≥ 20 mmHg in a sitting or standing posture within 1–2 hours of eating a meal.

Disequilibrium

Disequilibrium, a feeling of imbalance or unsteadiness on standing or walking, usually results from

visual or proprioceptive system abnormalities, with or without vestibular system involvement. Common contributing conditions include vision problems (eg, refractory errors, cataract, macular degeneration), musculoskeletal disorders (eg, arthritis, muscle weakness, deconditioning after prolonged illness), proprioceptive disorders (eg, neuropathies), and gait disorders (eg, cerebrovascular stroke, Parkinson's disease, cerebellar disorders).

Other Forms of Dizziness

Others include a vague feeling other than vertigo, presyncope, or disequilibrium. The patient may describe "floating," "lightheadedness," "wooziness," "spaciness," "whirling," and other nonspecific sensations. Patients with psychogenic dizziness commonly report anxiety or depressive symptoms. The psychiatric symptoms can primarily cause or contribute to the dizziness complaint in older adults.

Mixed Dizziness

Mixed dizziness, a combination of two or more of the above types, is the most common type of dizziness reported by older adults. It most likely results from combinations of diseases affecting the vestibular, CNS, visual, or proprioceptive systems. Systemic disorders like anemia, heart failure, diabetes mellitus, and hypothyroidism can contribute to instability or dizziness by affecting the sensory, central, or effector components. Although less commonly reported, carotid sinus hypersensitivity or carotid sinus syndrome can also cause dizziness.

Many medications can contribute to chronic dizziness through various mechanisms. Important classes of medications to consider in the dizziness evaluation include anxiolytic, antidepressants, antihistaminics, antihypertensives, aminoglycosides, anticholinergics, and NSAIDs.

Research data indicate that chronic dizziness often has a multifactorial etiology. Chronic dizziness is associated with risk factors such as angina, myocardial infarction, stroke, arthritis, diabetes, syncope, anxiety, depressive symptoms, impaired hearing, and the use of several classes of medications. In a study of a large community sample and in another study in which patients attended a geriatric clinic, an association was found between the complaint of chronic dizziness and factors such as anxiety, depressive symptoms, postural hypotension, use of five or more medications, and impaired gait and balance (SOE=B). Complaints of chronic dizziness were more common in patients who had more than five of these risk factors than in those having less than two of these risk factors. Similar to delirium and falls, chronic dizziness can be thought of as a geriatric syndrome that prompts a multifactorial assessment

---

STRENGTH-OF-EVIDENCE (SOE) RATING DEFINITIONS

A = consistent and good quality patient-oriented evidence
B = somewhat inconsistent or limited quality patient-oriented evidence
C = very inconsistent or very limited patient-oriented evidence, disease-oriented evidence, and/or consensus from professional organizations
D = unstudied common practice or opinion

See inside front cover for detailed information regarding the SOE classification.

Table 24.1—Classification of Dizziness

Type	Common Causes or Coexisting Conditions	Diagnostic Features	Treatment
Vertigo	Benign paroxysmal positional vertigo	History of episodic vertigo; rotational nystagmus; Dix-Hallpike maneuver confirms diagnosis	Epley's maneuver is treatment of choice
	Meniere disease	Episodic vertigo lasting for few hours; tinnitus; fluctuating hearing loss; sensation of fullness in ears; audiogram reveals sensorineural hearing loss (at low more than high frequencies)	Salt restriction, diuretics; vestibular suppressants may be helpful during acute attacks; in severe cases, may need surgical interventions, including endolymphatic decompression, vestibular nerve resection, and labyrinthectomy
	Ototoxic medications, eg, aminoglycosides, diuretics, NSAIDs	Presence of nystagmus, bedside vestibular function tests (eg, head thrust test can be abnormal)	Discontinue, substitute, or reduce the dosage of offending medication
Presyncope	Cerebral ischemia secondary to orthostatic hypotension, cardiac causes, dehydration, medications, vasovagal attack, autonomic dysfunction secondary to diabetes, parkinsonism	Near fainting/lightheaded when getting up from lying down or sitting position; orthostatic changes in blood pressure; investigations relevant to predisposing diseases	Treatment of specific cause, eg, proper hydration; dosage adjustment or removal of the offending medications; slow rising from sitting or lying down position; graduated support stockings; physical therapy and/or occupational therapy; medications (eg, fludrocortisone, midodrine) as needed
	Postprandial hypotension	Near fainting/lightheaded when getting up from lying down or sitting position; orthostatic hypotension usually within 45–60 minutes of eating	Frequent small meals; avoid exertion after meals; slow rising from sitting position; avoid antihypertensive drugs with or near meal time
Disequilibrium	Vertebrobasilar ischemia and/or cerebellar infarcts/hemorrhages	History of dizziness usually associated with slurred speech; visual changes; one-sided weakness and/or gait ataxia; truncal ataxia; CT or MRI or magnetic resonance angiography scan may be helpful	Low-dose aspirin, clopidogrel, or extended-release dipyridamole; rehabilitation
	Cerebellopontine angle tumor, eg, acoustic neuroma	History of vertigo or disequilibrium, unilateral hearing loss, tinnitus; audiometry reveals sensorineural hearing loss more for higher frequencies; MRI is diagnostic	Surgery
	Parkinson's disease	Bradykinesia; muscular rigidity; tremor; orthostatic hypotension	Drug therapy, rehabilitation therapy
	Peripheral neuropathy secondary to diabetes; vitamin B_{12} deficiency; idiopathic, etc	Decreased vibration or position sense; gait abnormality; hyperglycemia; low vitamin B_{12} level	Treatment of the underlying disease
	Cervical spine degenerative arthritis, spondylosis	Limitation of range of motion of neck; decreased vibratory or joint position sense; signs of radiculopathy or myelopathy; cervical spine radiologic abnormalities	Cervical or vestibular rehabilitation; cervical collar; surgery if needed
Other	Anxiety, depression, or psychosomatic disorders	Usually continuous nonspecific dizziness; fatigue; poor appetite; sleep problems; somatic complaints; positive results on anxiety or depression screening scales	Psychotherapy and/or antidepressant therapy
Mixed	Medications: antianxiety drugs, antidepressants, anticonvulsants, antipsychotics, antihypertensives, anticholinergics	History of fatigue; dizziness often vague and can be continuous, postural, or associated with confusion	Discontinue, substitute, or reduce the dosage of offending medication
	Combination of any of the above causes	Combination of any of the above features	Multifactorial intervention

and intervention strategy, which is likely more effective at alleviating symptoms than a standard disease-oriented approach.

EVALUATION

The evaluation of dizziness is challenging and can lead to extensive diagnostic evaluation. Patients present with vague sensations, which generates a broad differential diagnosis. An expansive evaluation can often be avoided by taking a more detailed history and conducting a more directed physical examination.

History

The clinical history begins with helping patients to describe their symptoms as precisely as possible, which is potentially daunting for those with multiple sensations. Patients should be encouraged to use their own words and to try distilling the symptoms into specific sensations such as spinning, imbalance or unsteadiness, or fainting. It is also important to document the frequency and duration of dizziness, and whether changing head position exacerbates the dizziness. It is useful to establish whether symptoms peak at any specific time of day, such as after meals or first thing in the morning. Patients should be asked about associated symptoms such as hearing loss, ear fullness, diplopia, dysarthria, and tinnitus. It is also important to elicit the impact on the patient's quality of life. Patients with Meniere disease complain of recurrent dizziness associated with ear fullness and/or tinnitus along with fluctuating hearing loss. Patients with acoustic neuroma complain of hearing loss and tinnitus but not of ear fullness. Patients with Meniere disease, CNS diseases, and BPPV complain of recurrent dizziness, while patients with psychogenic and central dizziness usually complain of continual dizziness. Inquiring about precipitating factors such as after eating meals (postprandial hypotension), looking down or rolling over in bed (vestibular conditions), or standing from supine position (orthostatic hypotension) can suggest interventions, as well as corroborate timing of symptoms. Any evaluation must include a critical review of medications, including OTC medications.

Physical Examination

The physical examination should begin with measurements of orthostatic changes in blood pressure. Nystagmus should be evaluated; horizontal or rotatory nystagmus usually indicates a peripheral vestibular lesion, while vertical nystagmus is seen in central lesions. Hearing and vision tests should be done, and the cranial nerves examined if vertebrobasilar ischemia or infarction is suspected. The Timed Up and Go test can be performed to look for gait and balance problems (see "Gait Impairment," p 218).

The following provocative tests of the vestibular system can be done at the bedside:

Head-thrust test: Ask the patient to fixate on the examiner's nose. The examiner then rotates the head rapidly about 10 degrees to the left or right. In patients with a vestibular deficit, the eyes move away from the target along with the head, followed by a corrective saccade back to the target, while normal eyes remain fixed on the target without a saccade.

Fukuda stepping test: Draw a circle on the floor, and ask the patient to stand in the center. Blindfold the patient and ask him or her to take a few steps forward as if walking on a straight line with outstretched arms. The examiner notes the patient's body sway as the patient takes the steps. In a unilateral vestibular lesion or acoustic neuroma, the patient's body will sway by >30 degrees toward the affected side.

Dix-Hallpike maneuver: This is a useful test for the diagnosis of BPPV. Ask the patient to sit on the examination table with the head rotated 30–45 degrees to one side. Instruct the patient to fix his or her vision on the examiner's forehead. The examiner holds the patient's head firmly in the same position, and moves the patient from a seated to a supine position with the head hanging below the edge of the table and the chin pointing slightly upward. The examiner notes the direction, latency, and duration of the nystagmus, if present. The diagnostic criteria for BPPV include 1) paroxysmal vertigo along with a rotatory nystagmus, 2) latency for 1–2 seconds between the completion of the maneuver and the onset of vertigo and nystagmus, and 3) fatigability (decrease in the intensity of the vertigo and nystagmus with repeated testing).

Diagnostic Testing

A small battery of laboratory tests, including hematocrit, glucose, electrolytes, BUN, vitamin B_{12}, folic acid, and thyrotropin, should be performed on all patients with chronic dizziness. An ECG should be done if a cardiac cause is suspected, and a Holter and event monitor only if suspicion of arrhythmia is strong. Tilt-table testing should be done only for select patients with postural hypotension or syncope. Audiometry assists in the evaluation of patients with tinnitus or hearing loss, and helps differentiate between acoustic neuroma and Meniere disease.

Suspected vestibular disorders can be evaluated with vestibular function tests such as electronystagmography, rotational testing, and dynamic posturography. These tests are not needed in every patient.

Likewise, neuroimaging is not needed in all patients with dizziness. MRI provides better resolu-

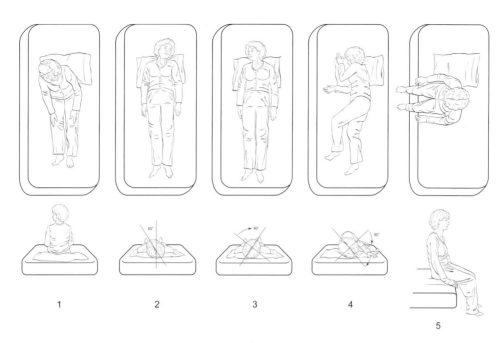

Figure 24.1—Self-treatment of benign positional vertigo using Epley's maneuver

Perform the maneuver three times a day until free of positional vertigo for 24 hours. Use the positions shown here when the right ear is affected. Reverse all positions (left instead of right) when the left ear is affected. The affected ear is the ear that when turned downward during the Dix-Hallpike maneuver triggers vertigo or nystagmus, or both.

Each maneuver consists of the following steps (numbered to match the illustration):

1. Sit on the bed with a pillow far enough behind you to be under your shoulders when you lie back. Turn your head 45 degrees to the left.

2. Holding your head in the turned position, lie back quickly so that your shoulders are supported on the pillow and your head is reclined on the bed. Hold this position for 30 seconds.

3. Remain supine on the bed and turn your head 90 degrees to the right. Hold this position for 30 seconds.

4. Turn your head and body another 90 degrees to the right; you should now be looking down at the bed. Hold this position for 30 seconds.

5. Sit up, facing to the right.

SOURCE: Data from Radtke A, Neuhauser H, von Brevern M, et al. A modified Epley's procedure for self-treatment of benign paroxysmal positional vertigo. *Neurology.* 1999;53(6):1358–1360.

tion than CT for posterior fossa lesions. However, in a community-based study of adults ≥65 yr old, the similar prevalence of MRI abnormalities in the dizzy and nondizzy group led to the conclusion that routine MRI will not identify a specific cause of dizziness in most patients (SOE=B).

MANAGEMENT

Medical therapy of acute dizziness depends on its cause, and patients with chronic dizziness, especially older adults, can have multiple comorbid conditions or impairments. Multifactorial interventions can help treat chronic dizziness and reduce the impact on day-to-day functioning. Treatment of coincident symptoms from depression, anxiety, hearing loss, and vision loss can help reduce the disability arising from dizziness. Dizziness from medication responds to dosage adjustment or to withdrawal of the offending medication.

Vestibular suppressants, including antihistamines (eg, meclizine), provide effective symptomatic relief for acute dizziness but generally do not provide benefit in management of chronic dizziness. Long-term use of meclizine should be avoided be cause it suppresses central and vestibular adaptation and can thus eventually worsen or exacerbate dizziness.

Vestibular rehabilitation therapy can help suppress symptoms in patients with peripheral and central vestibular causes of dizziness. It includes a combination of exercises designed to provoke dizziness; the movements are repeated until they can no longer be tolerated. Initially, the exercises can worsen the dizziness, but over time (weeks to months) movement-related dizziness improves, likely because of central adaptation.

The canalith repositioning procedure, introduced by Semont as well as Epley, can provide quick relief for those patients with BPPV (Figure 24.1).

A small subset of patients need surgical intervention. Surgical excision remains the treatment of choice for cerebellopontine angle tumors. Surgery should be reserved for disabling unilateral peripheral disease that is unresponsive to medical therapy. Surgical procedures are ablative or nonablative. Surgeons select ablative procedures, including transmastoid labyrinthectomy and partial vestibular neurectomy, for uncontrolled Meniere disease. Nonablative procedures, such as posterior canal occlusion, provide benefit to those patients whose BPPV remains refractory to repeated attempts of canalith repositioning procedures.

REFERENCES

- Kwong EC, Pimlott NJ. Assessment of dizziness among older patients at a family practice clinic: a chart audit study. *BMC Family Pract.* 2005;6(1):2.

- Polat S, Uneri A. Vertigo, dizziness and imbalance in the elderly. *J Laryngol Otol.* 2008;122(5):466–469.

- Sloane PD, Coeytaux RR, Beck RS, et al. Dizziness: state of the science. *Ann Intern Med.* 2001;134(9 Pt 2):823–832.

CHAPTER 25—SYNCOPE

KEY POINTS

- The incidence of syncope increases with age.

- In older adults, the cause of syncope is often multifactorial. In nearly one in five cases, the cause of syncope is not determined but the prognosis is generally favorable.

- Although many diagnostic procedures are available to search for the cause of syncope, most of them are expensive and have a low yield unless findings from the history or physical examination suggest a particular cause.

- Bradycardia is the single most common cardiac cause of syncope.

- The treatment of syncope often requires treatment of multiple possible underlying causes in geriatric patients.

Syncope—a sudden, transient loss of postural tone and consciousness not due to trauma and with spontaneous full recovery—is common. Annually it accounts for approximately 3% of emergency department visits and 2%–6% of hospital admissions. The incidence of syncope doubles in those ≥70 yr old, and rates among those ≥80 yr old is three to four times that seen among younger people. Approximately 80% of the patients hospitalized for syncope are ≥65 yr old. Syncope is a clinically important condition that is challenging to evaluate. Its potential causes range from those that are benign and self-limited to those that are life threatening. In older adults, the cause of syncope can often be multifactorial, adding to the diagnostic difficulty. Because syncope encompasses a wide range of potential causes (Table 25.1), its diagnostic evaluation can be complex and expensive. Although a wide variety of diagnostic tools can be used, in many cases the patient's history provides the best clues to the cause and helps direct the evaluation.

NATURAL HISTORY

Syncope is generally caused by reduced cerebral perfusion. Hemodynamic disturbances that can decrease cerebral perfusion include changes in systemic blood pressure or increased cerebral vascular resistance. Common causes of transient decreases in blood pressure include the following:

- Cardiac arrhythmias, such as atrial fibrillation with a rapid ventricular response, ventricular tachycardia, sick sinus syndrome with sinus pauses, and atrioventricular block

- Alterations in the peripheral vasculature due to arterial vasodilation or increased venous pooling

- Cardiopulmonary obstruction, such as that due to pulmonary emboli, aortic stenosis, hypertrophic obstructive cardiomyopathy, and atrial myxoma

Syncope can also occur as a consequence of increased cerebrovascular resistance. In hyperventilation syndrome and panic attacks, cerebrovascular vasoconstriction can occur without a change in systemic vascular resistance. In this situation, syncope can occur as a result of the relative decrease in cerebral blood flow without systemic hypotension. In rare instances, localized atherosclerotic disease can predispose a person to syncope by decreasing cerebral perfusion without a decrease in systemic blood pressure (vertebral basilar insufficiency and subclavian steal).

Syncope occurs most commonly while a person is standing. When a person assumes the standing posi-

Table 25.1—Common Causes of Syncope in Older Adults

Arrhythmia

Aortic stenosis

Carotid sinus hypersensitivity

Dehydration

Hypoglycemia

Medications (eg, β-blockers, diuretics, vasodilators, tricyclics)

Myocardial infarction

Orthostatic hypotension

Postprandial hypotension

Psychogenic causes

Postmicturition

Pulmonary embolism (large)

Unknown

Vasovagal faint

tion, the effects of gravity cause up to one-third of the blood volume to pool in the legs. Unopposed, this reduces cardiac output by reducing venous return and decreases cerebral blood pressure. A number of reflex pathways involving the autonomic and endocrine systems are responsible for rapid compensation of the gravitational effects of standing. The baroreceptor reflex is triggered by carotid and aortic baroreceptors, which act to increase autonomic sympathetic tone, resulting in peripheral vasoconstriction and an increase in heart rate. Increased sympathetic activity of the renal nerve stimulates renin release from the juxtaglomerular apparatus. The activation of the renin-angiotensin system leads to direct vasoconstriction by the action of angiotensin II and the secretion of aldosterone from the adrenal cortex to retain sodium, thereby raising the extracellular fluid volume. A postural change to a standing position also rapidly reduces the level of atrial natriuretic factor, which is a vasodilator and inhibitor of the renin-angiotensin system. The reduction in atrial natriuretic factor facilitates vasoconstriction, and the activity of the volume effects of the renin-angiotensin system contributes to vasoconstriction.

In aging, many of these reflex mechanisms are less responsive. The cardiac response to β-adrenergic stimulation (cardiac acceleration and increased contractility) decreases with advancing age. As a result of this and perhaps other mechanisms, the baroreflex (ie, increasing heart rate and vasoconstriction) is also less effective with advancing age. In addition, comorbid conditions that can affect postural responses, such as

diabetes mellitus, are prevalent among older adults. Medications such as α-blockers, β-blockers, calcium channel blockers, ACE inhibitors, and tricyclic antidepressants can also impair postural reflexes. The effects of age-related decline in adaptive reflexes, comorbid conditions, and medications may combine, becoming factors in syncopal events in older adults. Because older adults have a decreased ability to increase heart rate in response to sympathetic stimulation, maintaining blood volume and vasoconstriction become more important in maintaining postural blood pressure. Thus, older adults can be particularly sensitive to the effects of dehydration, diuretics, and vasodilator medications.

The prognosis of syncope depends on the underlying cause. The major issue is whether a cardiac cause is responsible. The 1-yr mortality for patients with syncope due to cardiac causes is 18%–33% (deaths are chiefly due to underlying disease, not syncope), while that for patients with syncope due to noncardiac causes is approximately 6%. Vasovagal syncope, which has a benign prognosis in the young, was once thought to be an unusual cause of syncope in older adults. However, recent reports from syncope evaluation centers have found vasovagal mechanisms as the cause of syncope in approximately 30%–50% of patients >65 yr old. However, it has not been established that vasovagal syncope in older adults has the same benign prognosis observed in younger individuals. There has been some suggestion that vasovagal syncope in older adults is frequently associated with comorbid illness that can increase overall mortality. In one-third to one-half of syncopal patients, no cause can be found. The prognosis for these patients is intermediate but generally favorable.

EVALUATION

For a general approach to the evaluation of syncope, see Figure 25.1.

History

The clinical history obtained from the patient and, if possible, from witnesses to the event can provide a diagnosis in up to 50% of cases in which a diagnosis can be established. First, it is important to establish whether the patient suffered a true syncopal event, as opposed to dizziness (disequilibrium) or lightheadedness. Falls are common in older adults (estimated annual incidence up to 30% in ambulatory community-dwelling older adults); it is important to consider syncope when assessing falls. Key elements to obtain from the history follow:

- Was there a precipitant? Could the patient's activities around the time of the event have triggered it? Such activities include eating, urinating, coughing, using medication, and

Transient Loss of Consciousness

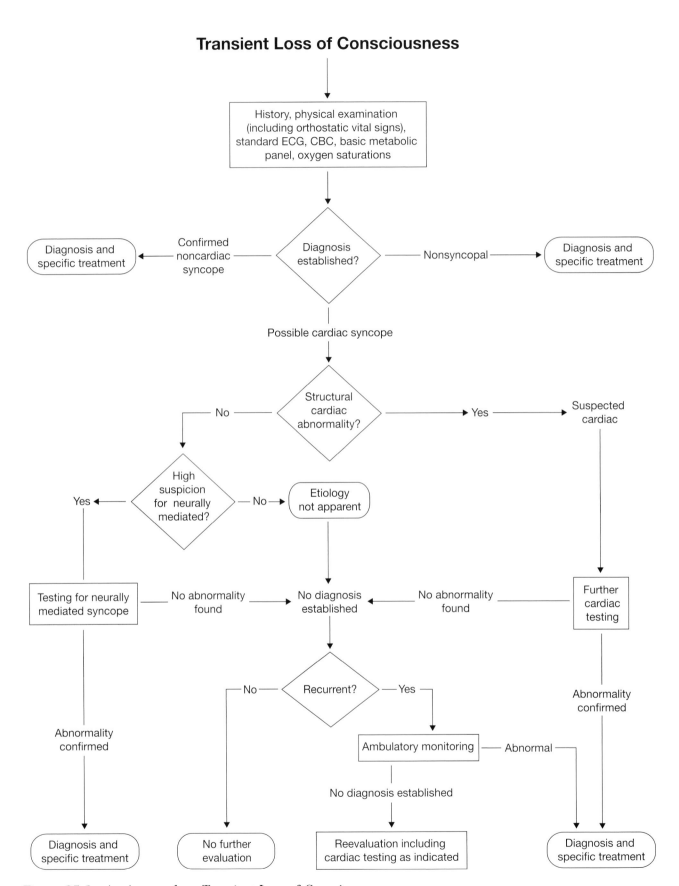

Figure 25.1—An Approach to Transient Loss of Consciousness

experiencing emotional stress. Syncope occurring while sitting or supine suggests a profound hemodynamic disturbance and should raise a concern about a significant cardiac arrhythmia. Syncope occurring during physical exertion should raise the possibility of myocardial ischemia or aortic stenosis. A history of syncope after turning motions of the head should raise the possibility of carotid sinus hypersensitivity.

- Were there prodromal symptoms before the event? Chest pain, palpitations, or shortness of breath suggests a cardiac or pulmonary cause. Diaphoresis, presyncope, and GI symptoms, such as nausea or vomiting, can be associated with vasovagal syncope. Sudden onset of syncope with <5 seconds of warning is characteristic of syncope due to a cardiac arrhythmia and should be evaluated as such. However, in older adults, vasovagal syncope can present with short or no prodrome. Thus, if the initial evaluation for arrhythmia in an older patient with syncope without a prodrome is unrevealing, a vasovagal mechanism should also be considered.

- What medications are being used? It is important to establish how medications were taken with relationship to meals and other activities, and whether the medication regimen was recently changed. Specifics about dosage times should be obtained. Most antiarrhythmic medications and other commonly used medications can increase the propensity for ventricular arrhythmias by prolonging the QT interval (eg, erythromycin, haloperidol, thioridazine; for a full current list, see www.qtdrugs.org).

- What did witnesses observe? They should be queried about the duration of the event and the appearance of the patient during the event. Patients with cardiac causes of syncope are generally flaccid in tone and motionless while unconscious, unless the event lasts for >15 seconds, when myoclonic jerks and truncal extension can be seen. In contrast, increased body motion, tone, and head turning to one side with loss of consciousness are more common with seizure activity.

- Are there significant comorbid conditions? A history of coronary artery disease or its associated symptoms is particularly important. Approximately 5% of myocardial infarctions present as syncope. Sustained ventricular tachycardia resulting in syncope is most common in patients with prior myocardial infarction. Patients with diabetes mellitus are

at increased risk of coronary atherosclerosis as well as autonomic dysfunction predisposing to syncope.

For a summary of the characteristics of three classes of syncope, see Table 25.2. A scoring system has recently been shown to be useful in distinguishing cardiac from noncardiac syncope (Table 25.3). The probability of cardiac syncope increases with higher scores, with scores of ≥3 being associated with 95% sensitivity and 61% specificity for cardiac syncope. Mortality was 17%–21% in those with a score ≥3, and 2%–3% in those with a score <3 after 600 days of follow-up.

Physical Examination

A physical examination should focus on elements raised by the history. It is estimated that of those patients in whom a cause of syncope can be established, 20% are identified by features found during physical examination. Blood pressure should be measured in both arms, as well as with postural changes. The pulse should be taken with the patient in both supine and standing positions. Blood pressure with the patient in the standing position should be obtained after 1 minute and 3 minutes of standing. Although any definition of postural hypotension is arbitrary, a decrease in systolic blood pressure of >20 mmHg is the definition used most frequently (SOE=C).

The character of the carotid pulse should also be assessed for the delayed upstroke and low volume characteristic of significant aortic stenosis. The presence of a carotid bruit, a history of cerebrovascular disease, and recent myocardial infarction are relative contraindications to carotid sinus massage. Even in the absence of contraindications, carotid sinus massage should be performed only under continuous ECG monitoring (to detect induced atrioventricular block or other arrhythmias) in a setting where resuscitation equipment is available.

The physical examination of the patient with syncope should include cardiac examination for evidence of murmurs characteristic of valvular abnormalities or extra heart sounds suggestive of cardiomyopathy. Fecal examination for occult blood and neurologic examination for focal deficits are also important.

An ECG is indicated for all patients presenting with syncope. Although an ECG establishes a diagnosis in only 5% of those with syncope, approximately 50% have an abnormal ECG. Abnormalities on an ECG can provide clues for further cardiovascular evaluation; a normal ECG is associated with a more favorable prognosis. Key features to assess on an ECG include evidence of acute or remote myocardial infarction. Conduction abnormalities, especially block

Table 25.2—Characteristics of Three Common Classes of Sudden Loss of Consciousness

Phase	Sign/Symptom	Cardiac Syncope Due to Arrhythmia	Vasovagal Syncope	Seizure
Before	Position	Any	Aborted if person lies flat	Any
	Warning/prodrome	<5 seconds	Seconds to minutes	None
	Precipitant	Absent	Present	Usually absent
	Palpitations	Sometimes	Absent	Absent
	Nausea/diaphoresis	Absent	Common	Rare
	Visual changes	None	Common	None
During	Tone	Flaccid	Motionless, relaxed	Rigid
	Pulse	Absent or faint	Slow, faint	Rapid
	Color	Blue, ashen	Pale	Pale or normal
	Incontinence	Rare	Very rare	Common
	Eye findings	Variable pupils	Dilated, reactive pupils	Tonic eye deviation common
	Oral frothing	Absent	Absent	Common
After	Type of recovery	Rapid, complete	Fatigue common	Slow, incomplete
	Mental status	No retrograde amnesia	No retrograde amnesia	Disorientation
	Nausea/diaphoresis	Absent	Common	Rare
	Focal neurologic findings	Absent	Absent	Common

Table 25.3—EGSYS Score: Predictors of Cardiac Syncope

Variable	Score[a]
Palpitations preceding syncope	4
Heart disease or abnormal ECG	3
Syncope during effort	3
Syncope while supine	2
Precipitating or predisposing factors or both[b]	-1
Autonomic prodromes (nausea/vomiting)	-1

[a] Scores ≥3 are associated with higher rates of cardiac syncope and higher mortality.

[b] Warm or crowded place, prolonged orthostasis, fear, pain, or emotional distress

in the AV node or below, and preexcitation, such as Wolff-Parkinson-White, can be detected as well; inappropriate sinus bradycardia can also be found. A prolonged QT interval can predispose to ventricular arrhythmias, including torsade de pointes.

Ambulatory Electrocardiographic Monitoring

An ambulatory ECG recording can establish or exclude many causes of syncope if the patient experiences syncopal or presyncopal symptoms during the recording. Unfortunately, the occurrence of symptoms during ambulatory ECG monitoring is relatively rare in most patients with syncope that remains unexplained after a history, physical examination, and ECG. On average, studies examining the diagnostic yield of ambulatory ECG report an arrhythmia correlating with symptoms in approximately 4% of patients. In another 15% of patients studied, an arrhythmia was excluded by the presence of symp-

toms during the recording, but without evidence of an arrhythmia; in approximately 14% of patients, arrhythmias were found to be present but without concomitant symptoms. These patients can represent a diagnostic dilemma. However, certain arrhythmias, even asymptomatic ones, such as nonsustained ventricular tachycardia, second- and third-degree AV block, and sinus pauses >3 seconds, are rare in people without heart disease. Their presence, even if asymptomatic, in a patient with a history of syncope indicates the need for further evaluation.

Ambulatory loop recorders that can be worn for many days or weeks at a time are commonly used to capture ECG recordings of symptoms that occur infrequently. These devices constantly record an ECG tracing on a 5- to 10-minute loop; the patient presses a button to stop the recording after an event has occurred and then transmits this by telephone to a monitoring center. Among patients who are able to operate the recorder, the diagnostic yield is approximately 25%.

Implantable Loop Recorders

Subcutaneous implantable loop recorders have been developed; these devices are placed in the prepectoral region under local anesthesia. The devices have long-term memories and a battery life of approximately 14–18 mo. Generally, no patient intervention is required for the device to store recordings, but the patient can also trigger the device to record and retain an ECG if symptoms occur. In a randomized study of patients with recurrent syncope who did not have evidence of structural heart disease, implantable loop recorders significantly increased the ability to establish a diagnosis (SOE=B).

Echocardiography

Two-dimensional echocardiography has a low yield in the absence of features suggestive of heart disease by history, physical examination, or ECG (SOE=C). It is most useful in confirming a specific diagnosis suspected by other assessment. However, unsuspected findings on echocardiography are reported in approximately 5%–10% of unselected patients. Thus, echocardiography has been advocated for the evaluation of syncope. Occult coronary artery disease is also prevalent among older adults, and stress testing is often used to screen for this. In some patients, particularly those with the suggestion of structural cardiac abnormalities and ischemia by history, physical examination, or ECG, it is efficient to perform stress echocardiography as a single procedure.

Tilt-Table Testing

Head-up tilt-table testing results in pooling of blood in the legs and, in susceptible individuals, can trigger syncope mediated by neurocardiogenic mechanisms. Tilt-table testing is useful for patients suspected of having vasovagal syncope and those with unexplained syncope who are not suspected of having a cardiac cause. In tilt-table testing, the patient reclines on a table that then rotates the patient from supine to head up slowly and passively. The patient is secured on the surface, usually with straps and a foot rest, to minimize muscle contraction and maximize venous pooling in the legs. The patient is continuously monitored for symptoms with an ECG and blood-pressure monitor. The test is considered positive if the patient has a cardioinhibitory or vasodepressor response to tilting, or both. Various protocols are available for this testing, and some include administration of intravenous medications. The sensitivity and specificity of tilt-table testing vary considerably, depending on the protocol used and the patient population. A positive tilt-table result occurs in approximately 11% of healthy older adults (SOE=B). Thus, a positive tilt-table result alone does not ensure that a vasovagal event is the cause. It is generally recommended that men >45 yr old and women >55 yr old have stress testing before tilt-table testing, so that a positive result on a tilt-table test does not delay diagnosis of coronary ischemia when that is the true culprit (SOE=C).

Responses to tilt testing performed for syncope evaluation tend to differ by age among adults without significant structural heart disease. Those ≥65 yr old tend to have far higher rates of symptoms due to pure vasodilatation without significant change in heart rate than individuals ≤35 yr old. In contrast, individuals ≤35 yr old tend to have more profound cardioinhibitory responses, characterized by profound bradycardia or asystole induced by tilt testing, than those ≥65 yr old. The different pattern of responses induced by tilt studies between younger and older adults suggests that different mechanisms for neurocardiogenic syncope predominate at different ages. Exaggerated autonomic response is common in younger people, whereas attenuated autonomic responses become predominant with advancing age.

Electrophysiologic Studies

Guidelines suggest that invasive electrophysiologic (EP) testing should be used in the evaluation of patients with structural heart disease with unexplained syncope. There is also agreement that EP testing should not be used in situations in which the results of the test would not influence subsequent treatment or in which a cause of the syncope has been established. The role of EP testing in patients with recurrent syncope with no structural heart disease and negative tilt-table studies remains undefined. EP testing is most sensitive for detecting ventricular arrhythmias in the setting of ischemic heart disease and is less sensitive for detecting ventricular arrhythmias in dilated nonischemic cardiomyopathies. The sensitivity of EP testing for detecting most bradyarrhythmias is low.

Neurologic Testing

Neurologic testing, including imaging of the head by CT or MRI and electroencephalographic recording, is appropriate in situations when focal neurologic signs or symptoms are present or when the history suggests seizure.

TREATMENT

The treatment of syncope depends on the underlying cause. Therapeutic interventions should concentrate on a single underlying cause if established. This is particularly important for cardiac causes. Myocardial ischemia causing syncope can require revascularization (percutaneous or surgical) or aggressive medical therapy. Valvular heart disease causing syncope, particularly aortic stenosis, is typically managed surgically. Treatment of symptomatic supraventricular tachyarrhythmias, such as atrial flutter or fibrillation, can involve antiarrhythmic medication or electrophysiology ablation procedures. Most bradyarrhythmias causing syncope require pacemakers, unless adverse events of medications or metabolic disturbances are the principal factors.

Significant ventricular tachyarrhythmias are often treated with implanted cardiac defibrillators (ICDs) or antiarrhythmic medications. Candidates for an ICD include individuals with arrhythmias or significant left ventricular dysfunction who did not respond to treatment for underlying ischemia or heart failure. ICD therapy is recommended for the primary prevention of sudden cardiac death in those who have an ejection fraction ≤30% and are at least 40 days after myocardial infarction. In patients with unexplained syncope due to nonischemic dilated cardiomyopathy who despite optimal medical therapy have significant left ventricular dysfunction, ICD implantation has been shown to improve survival (SOE=A). ICD therapy in dilated cardiomyopathy could be considered for those who have good functional status and a reasonable expectation of survival of >1 yr. Antiarrhythmic medications, particularly amiodarone or β-blockers may be considered for those with arrhythmias who are not ICD candidates.

Orthostatic hypotension is common among older adults and often responds to modifications in medication regimens. In particular, avoiding vasodilator drugs may help. An important measure is to ensure that patients have adequate fluid volume by reducing or discontinuing diuretics and, if necessary, by liberalizing salt intake. Other nonpharmacologic measures that can help include the use of waist-high compression stockings, squatting, sleeping in a head-up position, exercise, and consuming small meals and caffeinated beverages in the morning. Avoiding excessively warm environments and activities associated with straining (Valsalva) can also be beneficial. If nonpharmacologic measures are not sufficient, pharmacologic approaches include the use of caffeine or midodrine to increase the heart rate or medications that expand plasma volume such as fludrocortisone. Fludrocortisone can be used if hypertension, heart failure, and hypokalemia are not concerns.

When vasovagal syncope occurs as the result of a specific trigger (eg, sights, smells), avoidance is best if feasible. Counterpressure maneuvers, including leg crossing and handgrip and arm tensing, can reduce syncope burden in patients with recurrent syncope.

Because these maneuvers have been shown to be safe, training in these maneuvers should be initial therapeutic approach for patients found to have vasovagal syncope. A number of pharmacologic therapies have been proposed, including β-blockers, clonidine, paroxetine, midodrine, and others. The pharmacologic approach to the treatment of vasovagal syncope remains somewhat controversial and may require sequential trials of several agents. In a randomized double blind trial, pacing was not effective in reducing the risk of recurrent vasovagal syncope (SOE=B).

Carotid sinus hypersensitivity is best treated by avoiding stimulating factors (tight collars or rapid neck motions). If these measures are ineffective, pacemaker implantation may be useful.

Postprandial hypotension can be improved by avoiding alcohol and large carbohydrate meals. Caffeine consumption and remaining recumbent after meals can also help.

When syncope in an older adult has several causes, addressing a single factor in isolation may be only partially effective, and a broader approach addressing several contributing causes is required. Careful review of medications, as well as discontinuation of medications that increase the risk of syncope, is always a useful early step.

For patients with recurrent syncope without an identifiable cause, care must be taken to help them avoid harming themselves or others if they remain at risk of syncope. The issue of driving may need to be addressed. Guidelines from the American Heart Association recommend that driving be restricted for several months and that, if the patient does not have recurrences, driving be resumed. However, physicians should be aware that many states have reporting or restricting laws regarding driving with a history of syncope.

REFERENCES

■ Kuriachan V, Sheldon RS, Platonov M. Evidence-based treatment for vasovagal syncope. *Heart Rhythm.* 2008;5(11):1609−1614.

■ Strickberger SA, Benson DW, Biaggioni I, et al. AHA/ACCF scientific statement on the evaluation of syncope. *Circulation.* 2006;113(2):316−327.

■ Tan MP, Parry SW. Vasovagal syncope in the older patient. *J Am Coll Cardiol.* 2008;51(6):599−606.

CHAPTER 26—MALNUTRITION

KEY POINTS

- Aging is associated with changes in body composition such that well-standardized nutrient requirements for younger or middle-aged adults cannot be generalized to older adults.

- The Mini-Nutritional Assessment—Short Form is a brief and simple instrument useful for nutritional screening in geriatric patients.

- Identification of the presence of undernutrition or obesity can be facilitated by determining a person's body mass index (BMI).

- Many medications have anorexia as a major adverse event or can reduce nutrient availability in older adults.

- Various appetite stimulants and anabolic agents are being used in older adults and are the focus of intensive investigation.

Malnutrition in older adults spans the spectrum from under- to overnutrition. Nutritional problems accompany many chronic disease processes of older adults. Moreover, age-related changes in physiology, metabolism, and function can alter the older adult's nutritional requirements. Better understanding among clinicians of the aging process and of nutritional screening, assessment, and interventions could potentially improve the health and independence of older adults.

AGE-RELATED CHANGES

Body Composition

Aging is associated with notable changes in body composition: bone mass, lean mass, and water content all decrease, while fat mass generally increases. The volume of distribution of many medications changes as a result of these changes in body composition, and creatinine-based determinations can overestimate renal clearance in older adults. The increase in total body fat is commonly accompanied by greater intra-abdominal fat stores. The consequence of these changes in body composition is that well-standardized

nutrient requirements for younger or middle-aged adults cannot be generalized to older adults. The aging process also affects organ functions, although the degree of change observed is highly variable among individuals. Decline in organ functions can affect nutritional assessment and intervention.

Energy Requirements

Reduced basal metabolic rate in older adults reflects loss of muscle mass. The basal metabolic rate is the principal determinant of total energy expenditure; energy expenditure in relation to physical activity is the most variable component. The Harris-Benedict equations can be used to predict basal energy expenditure. A simple method for estimating the total daily energy needs of older adults is based on body weight alone (Table 26.1). In any determination of energy needs for older adults, care must be taken to avoid overfeeding while still meeting basal requirements.

Macronutrient Needs

A modified food guide pyramid for older adults based on the 2005 U.S. Department of Agriculture food pyramid, now known as MyPyramid, has been released (http://nutrition.tufts.edu/docs/pyramid.pdf [accessed Jan 2010]). The food selections are more relevant to the target audience, and appropriate intakes of water and fiber are emphasized. A flag at the top of the food pyramid highlights the potential need for older adults to discuss possible supplementation of calcium, vitamin D, and vitamin B_{12} with their healthcare providers. MyPyramid is an Internet-based program that offers nutrition information and opportunities for tailored recommendations for older adults (http://www.mypyramid.gov [accessed Jan 2011]).

The Food and Nutrition Board of the Institute of Medicine has released macronutrient guidelines that recommend a prudent diet, with 20%–35% of calories as fat, and reduced intakes of cholesterol, saturated fat, and trans-fatty acids. Carbohydrates should constitute 45%–65% of total calories; complex carbohydrates are the preferred fiber source. More specifically, the recommended fiber intake for those ≥60 yr old is 30 g for men and 21 g for women. Protein intake is recommended at 0.8 g/kg/d at approximately 10%–35% of total calories. With stress or injury, protein requirements are typically estimated at 1.5 g/kg/d, but underlying renal or hepatic insufficiency may warrant protein restriction (Table 26.1).

Table 26.1—Nutritional Requirement Calculations

Estimation of energy needs on basis of body weight

25–30 kcal/kg body wt/day

For obese individuals, use a reduced body weight that approximates 120% of ideal body weight.

Estimation of energy needs using the Harris-Benedict equation for basal energy expenditure (BEE)

Men: BEE = 66 + (13.7 × weight in kg) + (5 × height in cm) – (6.8 × age)

Women: BEE = 655 + (9.6 × weight in kg) + (1.8 × height in cm) – (4.7 × age)

Adjust BEE with empiric stress factors (1 for nonstressed and 1.5 for stressed) to estimate total energy expenditure of ill older adults.

Estimation of protein needs on basis of body weight

Protein = (0.8–1.5) g/kg body wt/day reflects a range of protein values to meet the perceived degree of stress

For obese individuals, use ideal body weight.

NOTE: 1 lb = 0.453 kg; 1 in = 2.54 cm

Micronutrient Requirements

Revisions of the Dietary Reference Intakes include recommended dietary allowances (RDAs) with more specific guidelines for older adults; those for the group ≥71 yr old are shown in Table 26.2.

Fluid Needs

Dehydration is the most common fluid or electrolyte disturbance in older adults. Normal aging is associated with a decreased perception of thirst, impaired response to serum osmolarity, and reduced ability to concentrate urine after fluid deprivation. A decline in fluid intake can also result from disease states that reduce mental or physical ability to recognize or express thirst, or that result in decreased access to water. In general, fluid needs of older adults can be met with 30 mL/kg/d or 1 mL/kcal ingested. Fluid needs may be different during episodes of fever or infection, as well as with diuretic or laxative therapy. Common signs of dehydration are decreased urine output, confusion, constipation, and mucosal dryness.

NUTRITION SCREENING AND ASSESSMENT

Anthropometrics

Anthropometric measurements are often used for nutritional assessment of older adults. An unintended weight loss of 10 pounds in the preceding 6 mo is a useful indicator of morbidity; this degree of weight loss is predictive of functional limitations, healthcare charges, and the need for hospitalization (SOE=B). The Minimum Data Set (MDS) used by Medicare-certified nursing homes defines weight loss as ≥5% in the past month or ≥10% in the past 6 mo as significant. Body mass index (BMI)—weight in kg/

Table 26.2—Recommended Dietary Allowances of Micronutrients for Adults ≥71 Yr Old

Nutrient	Recommended Daily Allowance	
	For Men	*For Women*
Calcium	1,200 mg	1,200 mg
Magnesium	420 mg	320 mg
Vitamin D	800 IU	800 IU
Thiamine	1.2 mg	1.1 mg
Riboflavin	1.3 mg	1.1 mg
Niacin	16 mg	14 mg
Vitamin B_6	1.7 mg	1.5 mg
Folate	400 mcg	400 mcg
Vitamin B_{12}	2.4 mcg	2.4 mcg
Pantothenic acid	5 mg*	5 mg*
Vitamin A	900 mcg	700 mcg
Vitamin K	120 mcg*	90 mcg*
Iron	8 mg	8 mg
Zinc	11 mg	8 mg
Vitamin C	90 mg	75 mg
α-Tocopherol	15 mg	15 mg
Selenium	55 mcg	55 mcg
Potassium	4,700 mg*	4,700 mg*

*Adequate intake, not recommended dietary allowance.

SOURCES: Data from Standing Committee on the Scientific Evaluation of Dietary Reference Intakes, Food and Nutrition Board, Institute of Medicine, *Dietary Reference Intakes for Calcium, Phosphorus, Magnesium, Vitamin D, and Fluoride.* Washington, DC: National Academy Press; 1997; Standing Committee on the Scientific Evaluation of Dietary Reference Intakes, Institute of Medicine, *Dietary Reference Intakes for Thiamin, Riboflavin, Niacin, Vitamin B₆, Folate, Vitamin B₁₂, Pantothenic Acid, Biotin, and Choline.* Washington, DC: National Academy Press; 1999; Standing Committee on the Scientific Evaluation of Dietary Reference Intakes, Food and Nutrition Board, *Dietary Reference Intakes for Vitamin C, Vitamin E, Selenium, and Beta Carotene, and Other Carotenoids.* Washington, DC: National Academy Press; 2000; Standing Committee on the Scientific Evaluation of Dietary Reference Intakes, Food and Nutrition Board, *Dietary Reference Intakes for Vitamin A, Vitamin K, Arsenic, Boron, Chromium, Copper, Iodine, Iron, Manganese, Molybdenum, Nickel, Silicon, Vanadium, and Zinc.* Washington, DC: National Academy Press; 2000; Standing Committee on the Scientific Evaluation of Dietary Reference Intakes, Institute of Medicine, *Dietary Reference Intakes for Water, Potassium, Sodium, Chloride, and Sulfate.* Washington, DC: National Academy Press; 2004. Available at http://www.nal.usda.gov (accessed Jan 2011).

(height in meters)^2—is a useful measure of body size and indirect measure of body fatness that does not require the use of a reference table of ideal weights. National Institutes of Health guidelines regarding body size classification based on BMI have been released (Table 26.3). The risk threshold for low BMI is set at 18.5 but should be interpreted in the context of the individual's lifelong habits. Other anthropometric tools include skin-fold and circumference measurements, but these have had limited practical application because of the difficulty of achieving acceptable reliability among those taking the measurements.

Nutritional Intake

Generally, inadequate nutritional intake has been defined as average or usual intake of servings of food

Table 26.3—Body Size Classification

Body Size	Body Mass Index (kg/m^2)
Underweight	<18.5
Normal weight	18.5–24.9
Overweight	25–29.9
Obesity	≥30
Extreme obesity	≥40

NOTE: 1 lb = 0.453 kg; 1 in = 2.54 cm

SOURCE: Data from NHLBI Obesity Education Initiative Expert Panel. *Clinical Guidelines on the Identification, Evaluation, and Treatment of Overweight and Obesity in Adults: The Evidence Report.* Bethesda, MD: National Institutes of Health, National Heart, Lung and Blood Institute; September 1998: xiv. Pub. No. 98-4083.

groups, nutrients, or energy below a threshold level of the RDA. Poor intake is often an indication of illness. The limited reliability of accurately assessing dietary intake measures is well known, so thresholds of 25%–50% below the RDA have generally been selected. In one study, energy intake (<50% of calculated maintenance energy requirements) was reduced in 21% of a sample of hospitalized older adults. This subset of patients had higher rates of in-hospital mortality and 90-day mortality than did those with energy intakes above the threshold. Surveys of nutritional status conducted among chronically institutionalized older adults suggest that 5%–18% of nursing-home residents have energy intakes below their recommended average energy expenditure. However, evidence is generally lacking to support any benefits of nutritional supplementation in this population.

Energy intakes of men and women 65–98 yr old have been estimated in a nationwide food consumption survey; 37%–40% of the men and women studied had energy intakes lower than two-thirds of the RDA, and many reported skipping at least one meal each day. Estimated intakes by consumption surveys, however, may be unreliable because some studies suggest that older adults under-report energy intakes by 20%–30%.

Food security issues are prevalent contributors to inadequate nutritional intakes among older adults. It is important to ascertain whether limitations in resources, transportation, or functionality may limit access to food or the ability to prepare food.

Laboratory Tests: Albumin, Prealbumin, Cholesterol

Serum albumin has been recognized as a risk indicator for morbidity and mortality. Hypoalbuminemia lacks specificity and sensitivity as an indicator of malnutrition; however, it can be associated with injury, disease, or inflammatory conditions. As a negative acute-phase reactant, albumin is subject to cytokine-mediated decline in synthesis and to in-

creased degradation and transcapillary leakage. Longitudinal studies of serum albumin suggest a modest decline in levels with aging that may be independent of disease. The prognostic value of hypoalbuminemia may be largely because of its use as a proxy measure for injury, disease, or inflammation. In the community setting, hypoalbuminemia has been associated with functional limitation, sarcopenia, increased healthcare use, and mortality (SOE=B). In the hospital setting, it has also been associated with increased length of stay, complications, readmissions, and mortality (SOE=B).

Other protein markers of nutritional status have clinical significance. Prealbumin has a considerably shorter half-life (48 hours) than albumin (18−20 days) and may therefore more adequately reflect short-term changes in protein status. Although prealbumin appears to have the same limitations as albumin as a diagnostic tool for nutritional status, in the absence of an inflammatory state, it can be used to measure the effectiveness of nutritional interventions or as an indicator of recovery (SOE=B). In addition to a shorter half-life, prealbumin has a small serum pool that allows for easier detection of small changes in nutritional status over a shorter time period if inflammation is not present. Serum cholesterol has also been linked to nutritional status. Low cholesterol levels (<160 mg/dL) are often detected in adults with serious underlying disease, such as malignancy. Poor clinical outcomes have been observed among hospitalized and institutionalized older adults with hypocholesterolemia. In a study of community-dwelling older adults, nutrient intakes were not different in those in the lowest quartile of serum cholesterol levels and in others. It appears likely, again, that acquired hypocholesterolemia is a nonspecific feature of poor health status that is independent of nutrient or energy intakes, and that it may better reflect a pro-inflammatory condition. Of interest is the observation that community-dwelling older adults with both hypoalbuminemia and hypocholesterolemia have higher rates of adverse functional and mortality outcomes than those with hypoalbuminemia or hypocholesterolemia alone (SOE=B).

Drug-Nutrient Interactions

Medications can modify the nutrient needs and metabolism of older adults. Certain medications, such as digoxin and phenytoin, even at therapeutic levels, can cause anorexia in older adults. Additional agents that have anorexia as a major potential adverse event include SSRIs, calcium channel blockers (eg, dihydropyridines), H$_2$-receptor antagonists, proton-pump inhibitors, narcotic and nonsteroidal analgesics, furosemide, potassium supplements,

Table 26.4—Drug-Nutrient Interactions

Drug	Reduced Nutrient Availability
Alcohol	Zinc, vitamins A, B_1, B_2, B_6, B_{12}, folate
Antacids	Vitamin B_{12}, folate, iron, total kcal
Antibiotics, broad-spectrum	Vitamin K
Colchicine	Vitamin B_{12}
Digoxin	Zinc, total kcal (via anorexia)
Diuretics	Zinc, magnesium, vitamin B_6, potassium, copper
Isoniazid	Vitamin B_6, niacin
Levodopa	Vitamin B_6
Laxatives	Calcium, vitamins A, B_2, B_{12}, D, E, K
Lipid-binding resins	Vitamins A, D, E, K
Metformin	Vitamin B_{12}, total kcal
Mineral oil	Vitamins A, D, E, K
Phenytoin	Vitamin D, folate
Salicylates	Vitamin C, folate
SSRIs	Total kcal (via anorexia)
Theophylline	Total kcal (via anorexia)
Trimethoprim	Folate

Table 26.5—Risk Factors for Poor Nutritional Status

Alcohol or substance abuse

Cognitive dysfunction

Decreased exercise

Depression, poor mental health

Functional limitations

Inadequate funds

Limited education

Limited mobility, transportation

Medical problems, chronic diseases

Medications

Poor dentition

Restricted diet, poor eating habits

Social isolation

ipratropium bromide, theophylline, and many others. Many medications are known to interfere with taste and smell (see "Oral Diseases and Disorders," Table 44.2, p 352), and others can reduce the availability of specific nutrients (Table 26.4). Some can reduce intake by causing inattention, dysphagia, dysgeusia, or xerostomia. Medications that precipitate significant constipation can also reduce appetite.

Multi-Item Tools for Nutrition Screening

The nutritional status of older adults can be influenced by a variety of factors (Table 26.5). The absence of single assessment measures that are valid indicators of comprehensive nutritional status has prompted the development of multi-item tools. Older adults in acute- or chronic-care facilities have been extensively studied to identify indicators and predictors of nutritional status; those in the community setting have been subject to less investigation. Nutritional screening tools for older adults have been widely disseminated. Their effectiveness remains to be demonstrated—specifically, whether these tools can identify undernourished individuals whose problems are amenable to intervention.

The Nutrition Screening Initiative is a collaborative effort of the American Dietetic Association, the American Academy of Family Practitioners, and the National Council on Aging, Inc. Three interdisciplinary tools to screen for nutrition risk were developed by the Nutrition Screening Initiative to aid in the evaluation of the nutritional status of older adults. The DETERMINE checklist was created to raise public awareness about the importance of nutrition to the health of older adults (see http://www.aafp.org/afp/980301ap/edits.html). This self-report questionnaire is composed of 10 items and is intended to identify potential risks but not to diagnose malnutrition. The Level I screen, intended for use by healthcare professionals, incorporates additional assessment items regarding dietary habits, functional status, living environment, and weight change, as well as measures of height and weight. The Level II screen, for use by more highly trained medical and nutrition professionals and suggested for use in the diagnosis of malnutrition, contains all the items from Level I with additional biochemical and anthropometric measures, as well as a more detailed evaluation of depression and mental status.

The Mini-Nutritional Assessment tool was developed to evaluate the risk of malnutrition among frail older adults and to identify those who may benefit from early intervention (SOE=B). This assessment tool requires administration by a trained professional and consists of 18 items, including questions about BMI, mid-arm and calf circumferences, weight loss, living environment, medication use, dietary habits, clinical global assessment, and self-perception of health and nutrition status. A shortened screening version that contains only 6 items, the short form Mini-Nutritional Assessment (MNA-SF) is now available (see http://www.mna-elderly.com [accessed Jan 2011]).

NUTRITION SYNDROMES

Undernutrition

Attempts to subdivide the group of nutritional syndromes characterized by loss of weight and/or compromised protein status have been challenging. The nomenclature used implies that these syndromes are

Table 26.6—Examples of Lactose-Free Oral Products

Product	Kcal/mL	mOsm	Protein (g/L)	Water (mL/L)	Sodium (mEq/L)	Potassium (mEq/L)	Fiber (g/L)
Routine use formulations							
Boost Drink[a]	1.00	625	42.2	850	24.1	43.5	0
Boost Plus	1.50	630–670	59.1	780	31.3	41.0	0
Ensure[b]	1.06	620	38.0	784	36.7	40.1	12.7
Ensure Plus	1.50	680	54.9	720	40.5	54.0	12.7
Carnation Instant Breakfast lactose-free	1.00	480–490	35.0	848	38.0	32.0	0
Carnation Instant Breakfast lactose-free Plus	1.50	620	52.0	776	50.8	48.0	0
Low volume (packaged as 45-mL supplement; nutrients are provided per serving)							
Resource Benecalorie	330	NA	7.0	0	0	0	0
Clear liquid							
Resource Breeze	1.06	750	38.0	827	15.0	2.2	0
Enlive	1.04	796	37.6	768	8.2	5.0	0
Diabetes formulations							
Boost Glucose Control	1.06	400	58.2	847	47.8	28.2	14.8
Glucerna shake[c]	0.93	530	41.8	800	38.4	40.1	11.8

NA = not available

[a] Also has "pudding" product that has 240 kcal/5 oz and 0 fiber

[b] Also has "pudding" product that has 170 kcal/4 oz and 3 g fiber/serving

[c] Institutional formulation (also available in retail bottle)

Source: Adapted with permission. Reuben DB, Herr KA, Pacala JT, et al. *Geriatrics At Your Fingertips*. New York: American Geriatrics Society; 2010.

distinct, while in practice it is often quite difficult to distinguish one from another, and the syndromes commonly overlap. Inflammation permeates the syndromes of cachexia, protein energy undernutrition, sarcopenia, failure to thrive, and obesity, such that an inflammatory continuum may be a more appropriate model. The presence (cachexia) or absence (wasting) of cytokine-mediated response to injury or disease is at times used, but in examples such as the weight loss from AIDS, there appears that some, but not all, of the loss is the result of inflammation. Some authors note that with cachexia, resting energy expenditure is increased whereas with wasting it is decreased, but this measure is not generally available to most practicing clinicians. Also confusing is the term *protein-energy undernutrition*, which is meant to encompass the spectrum of protein and energy undernutrition but is often erroneously applied to individuals with reduced albumin or prealbumin levels from an inflammatory response.

Obesity

The growing prevalence of obesity in America extends to older adults in their 60s and 70s. According to National Health and Nutrition Examination Surveys (NHANES), the prevalence of obesity (BMI ≥30 kg/m^2) has climbed from 14% to 32% between 1976

and 2004. Trends were similar for all ages, both genders, and all racial or ethnic groups.

Excess body weight and modest weight gain (≥5 kg) in middle age can be associated with medical comorbidities in later life that include hypertension, diabetes mellitus, cardiovascular disease, and osteoarthritis. Adverse outcomes associated with obesity include impaired functional status, increased use of healthcare resources, and increased mortality (SOE=B). A BMI ≥35 kg/m^2 is associated with increased risk of functional decline among older adults. Of interest, poor diet quality and micronutrient deficiencies are relatively common among obese older adults, especially obese older women living alone. Many homebound older adults are also obese. The National Institutes of Health has suggested: "Age alone should not preclude weight loss treatment for older adults. A careful evaluation of potential risks and benefits in the individual patient should guide management." The focus must be on achieving a more healthful weight to promote improved health, function, and quality of life. A combination of prudent diet, behavior modification, and activity or exercise may be appropriate for selected candidates. For frail, obese older adults, the emphasis may better be placed on preservation of strength and flexibility, rather than on weight reduction.

NUTRITIONAL INTERVENTIONS

Oral Nutrition and Supplements

Preventing undernutrition is much easier than treating it. Food intake can be enhanced by catering to food preferences as much as possible and by avoiding therapeutic diets unless their clinical value is certain. Patients should be prepared for meals with appropriate hand and mouth care, and they should be comfortably situated for eating. Assistance should be provided for those who need help. Placing two or more patients together for meals can increase sociability and food intake. Foods should be of appropriate consistency, prepared with attention to color, texture, temperature, and arrangement. The use of herbs, spices, and hot foods helps to compensate for loss of the sense of taste and smell often accompanying old age and to avoid the excessive use of salt and sugar. (See "Oral Diseases and Disorders," p 352.) Hard-to-open individual packages should be avoided. Adequate time should be taken for leisurely meals. Title III C of the Older Americans Act has provided for congregate and home-delivered meals for older adults, regardless of economic status. This service is available in most parts of the country, albeit with a waiting list in some locations. Adequate access to nutritious and appetizing food should be assured for patients of various cultural backgrounds and in all settings.

Dietary supplements have been widely used in an effort to enhance nutrient intake, often when patients eat only small amounts. The use of such supplements often decreases food intake, but overall nutritional intake usually increases owing to the nutrient quality and density of the supplements. Standard supplements contain macro- and micronutrients. Many different oral formulations are available in both liquid and bar forms. They can be chosen based on patient preferences, chewing ability, or product cost. Oral formulas can also be selected based on their caloric density, osmolality, protein, fiber, or lactose content (Table 26.6). Most formulas provide 1–1.5 calories/mL and many are lactose- and gluten-free. However, it has yet to be demonstrated that any supplement is superior to regular food intake.

Interest is also growing in the use of micronutrient supplements in health promotion. Many vitamin and mineral supplements are commonly available in supermarkets and drugstores. New recommendations for older adults include higher intakes of calcium and vitamin D to prevent osteoporosis (SOE=B) (Table 26.2). Vitamin D deficiency is more prevalent than previously realized, and repletion is associated with reduced falls, improved bone healing, and response to bisphosphonates (see "Endocrine and Metabolic Disorders," p 491). Folic acid, B_6, and B_{12} can lower homocysteine levels, theoretically reducing the risk of coronary artery disease and helping to prevent decline in cognitive function. However, results to date from randomized controlled trials with folic acid, B_6, or B_{12} supplementation have been inconsistent. Insufficient evidence exists to determine whether immune function can be improved by supplementation of protein, vitamin E, zinc, or other micronutrients. Whether the effects of antioxidants are beneficial is the subject of controversy. While it has previously been suggested that antioxidants can help in preventing age-related cataracts and macular degeneration, more recent evidence indicates that they may have little or no effect. Although naturally occurring dietary antioxidants can reduce cardiovascular disease and mortality, supplementation with specific antioxidants, namely β-carotene, vitamin A, and vitamin E, can increase mortality in some settings (SOE=C). In addition, vitamin E supplementation has not been shown to slow the progression of Alzheimer's disease or prevent cardiovascular disease, and it may be associated with higher risk of hemorrhagic stroke. Further, among individuals with diabetes or vascular disease, supplementation with vitamin E can increase risk of heart failure (SOE=C).

Nonetheless, oxidative stress associated with micronutrient deficiencies can result in DNA damage that contributes to cancer promotion. Because approximately 60% of older adults take self-prescribed dietary supplements, it is imperative that the clinician obtain information about the patient's use of all supplements. The appropriateness and safety of each supplement should be evaluated, because consumers are often unaware of potential risks and adverse events of many OTC supplements, and solid evidence in favor of these purported benefits is currently lacking.

Drug Treatment for Undernutrition Syndromes

A number of agents have been suggested to promote increased appetite or to serve as anabolic aids. Appetite stimulants include the antidepressant mirtazapine, the serotonin and histamine antagonist cyproheptadine, the progestin megestrol, and the cannabinoid dronabinol. Anabolic aids include human growth hormone, testosterone, and oxandrolone. However, the use of all these drugs for the treatment of undernutrition syndromes is not FDA approved and adverse effects in older adults are an issue. Although appetite and weight gain have improved with megestrol acetate, this weight gain is primarily fat and clinical benefits to the patient have not been demonstrated (SOE=A). In addition, the small amount of research that has been done on the anabolic aids has not demonstrated clinically meaningful benefits to date.

LEGAL AND ETHICAL ISSUES

In the nursing home, unacceptable weight loss, as defined by the Omnibus Budget Reconciliation Act of 1987, is any loss ≥5% in the past month or ≥10% in the past 6 mo. Sections of the MDS (see "Nursing Home Care," p 142) that are related to nutritional status include those assessing cognitive function, mood and behavior, physical function, health condition, oral and nutritional status, dental status, skin condition, and special treatments and procedures, including restorative care for eating and swallowing. Resident Assessment Protocols ensure prompt identification of problems focused on by the MDS. The MDS uses intake of <75% of food provided as the threshold to trigger nutrition assessment. Standards of care dictate the following:

- Acceptable parameters of nutritional status such as body weight and protein levels should be maintained, unless the resident's clinical condition demonstrates that this is not possible.
- A resident should receive a therapeutic diet when there is a problem.

Food and fluid should always be offered to all patients; however, the decision to start or to discontinue artificial nutrition or hydration must be considered very carefully. Competent adults may choose to forgo artificial feeding, just as they have the right to decline any invasive procedure. Some adults have advance directives that were executed at a time when the individual was competent prohibiting the use of feeding tubes. These should be honored unless there is compelling evidence that the individual would have changed his or her mind in the current situation. Incompetent adults without advance directives pose a greater challenge. The decision to start or to discontinue artificial feeding should be considered carefully with the surrogate, taking into account the risks and burdens of such an action, the risks and burdens of alternative actions, and the evidence to support likely benefits of the various actions. To date, evidence supporting the use of feeding tubes in patients with end-stage cancer, dementia, and COPD are lacking. See "Eating and Feeding Problems," p 203.

After total cessation of nutrition, depending on underlying conditions, several weeks may ensue before death, and some patients who consume very little may survive much longer. In this setting, palliative care, including emotional support, is extremely important and complex. See "Palliative Care," p 102; and "Legal and Ethical Issues," p 23.

ACOVE-3* QUALITY INDICATORS PERTAINING TO MALNUTRITION

Weight measurement
- All vulnerable older adults should be weighed at each primary care visit and weights documented in the medical record.

Vitamin D
- All vulnerable older adults in stable health states should take 800 IU (or equivalent) of vitamin D supplementation daily.

Oral intake evaluation in hospital
- If a vulnerable older adult is hospitalized, then evaluation of oral intake should be documented during the hospitalization.

Document weight loss
- If a vulnerable older adult has involuntary weight loss of ≥10% body weight in 1 yr or less, then weight loss (or a related disorder) should be documented in the medical record as recognition of undernutrition as a potential problem.

Evaluate weight loss
- If a vulnerable older adult has involuntary weight loss of ≥10% in 1 yr or less or hypoalbuminemia (<3.5 g/dL), then he or she should be evaluated for potentially reversible causes of poor nutritional intake, including assessment of:
  - Dental status (eg, dentition, gum health, dental referral)
  - Food security (eg, financial status, social work referral)
  - Food-related functional status (eg, ability to feed, prepare meals)
  - Appetite and intake (eg, 72-hour calorie count, dietitian referral)
  - Swallowing ability (eg, bedside swallowing study, swallowing study referral)
  - Dietary restrictions (eg, low-salt or low-protein diet)

Evaluate comorbid conditions
- If a vulnerable older adult has involuntary weight loss of ≥10% in 1 yr or less or hypoalbuminemia (<3.5 g/dL), then he or she should be evaluated for potentially relevant comorbid conditions, including assessment of:

Chapter 26: Malnutrition **201**

- Medications associated with decreased appetite
- Depression
- Cognitive impairment
- Thyroid function
- Screen for cancer
- Diabetes mellitus
- Malabsorption

Alternative alimentation

- If a hospitalized vulnerable older adult is unable to take food orally for >48 hours, then alternative alimentation (eg, enteral or parenteral) should be implemented or documented why not.

Supplementation

- If a hospitalized vulnerable older adult is malnourished or at risk, then he or she should receive oral protein and energy supplementation of ≥400 kcal/d for 35 days or longer.

Related quality indicators for Malnutrition

- Evaluate weight loss for depression (see "Depression," p 295)
- Gastrostomy tube placement (see "Eating and Feeding Problems," p 203)
- Nutritional assessment for patient with pressure ulcer (see "Pressure Ulcers and Wound Care," p 283)
- Dysphagia documentation after stroke (see "Neurologic Diseases and Disorders," p 464)

*Assessing Care of Vulnerable Elders – 3rd Set. See inside front cover for explanation.

REFERENCES

- Amella EJ. Assessing Nutrition in Older Adults. *Try This: Best Practices in Nursing Care to Older Adults.* 2007;(9). Available at http://consultgerirn.org/uploads/File/trythis/try_this_9.pdf

- Guigoz Y. The Mini Nutritional Assessment (MNA) review of the literature—What does it tell us? *J Nutr Health Aging.* 2006;10(6):466−487.

- Jensen GL. Obesity and functional decline: epidemiology and geriatric consequences. *Clin Geriatr Med.* 2005;21:677−687.

- Lichtenstein AH, Rasmussen H, Yu WW, et al. Modified MyPyramid for Older Adults. *J Nutr.* 2008;138(1):5−11.

- Rocchiccioli JT, Sanford JT. Revisiting geriatric failure to thrive: a complex and compelling clinical condition *J Gerontol Nurs.* 2009;35(1):18–24.

CHAPTER 27—EATING AND FEEDING PROBLEMS

KEY POINTS

- Several age-related changes in older adults contribute to a slowed ability to swallow.

- Dementia is the most common cause of oral dysphagia.

- Most healthy people aspirate without any important clinical consequences.

- Aspiration pneumonia is believed to occur when contaminated oral secretions arrive in the lungs in a high enough inoculum to overcome host defenses.

- No studies demonstrate that feeding tubes reduce the occurrence of aspiration, but rather, many studies identify feeding tubes as major risk factors for aspiration.

- The assessment of swallowing function is controversial. Data correlating specific findings from any type of swallowing examination with clinically meaningful outcomes are lacking.

Swallowing is an important and complex task that can be affected by both normal aging and by diseases that are common in older adults. Treatment of eating and feeding problems depends on the identified cause or causes and contributing factors.

SWALLOWING IN HEALTH AND DISEASE

Swallowing and Aging

Swallowing can be divided into three phases on the basis of anatomy. First is the preparatory or oral phase, which includes the complex activities of mastication and propelling the food bolus to the back of the mouth toward the pharynx. This stage is under voluntary control. The second or pharyngeal phase is involuntary and involves the initiation of the swallow reflex with propulsion of the food bolus past the laryngeal vestibule and into the esophagus. Execution of the oral and pharyngeal phases of swallowing requires the complex coordination of five cranial nerves and a large number of small muscles in the head and neck, with regulation from cortical input to the medullary swallow center, all in the appropriate sequence, usually within 1 second. The third stage of swallowing is the esophageal phase, during which food is propelled down the esophagus by the action of skeletal muscle proximally and smooth muscle distally; this phase is regulated by its own intrinsic innervation.

Normal aging is associated with several changes in eating. With advanced age, taste sensation decreases, but not taste discrimination (older adults may be able to distinguish sweet from salty but may need to add more salt to food to taste it sufficiently). Further, olfactory function declines with advancing age, further impairing taste sensation. Salivary function is not clearly reduced with aging, but xerostomia is a common complaint of older adults, usually because of adverse events of medication. Loss of teeth greatly reduces chewing efficiency (ie, chewing is needed for a longer period of time and with more chewing strokes to achieve the same level of food maceration), which is only partly ameliorated with dental prostheses. Sarcopenia, or age-related loss of lean muscle mass, can contribute to loss in chewing efficiency and to pharyngeal muscle weakness demonstrated on videofluoroscopic deglutition examination (VDE) of asymptomatic older adults. Whether aging alone contributes to esophageal dysmotility (so-called *presbyesophagus*) remains a subject of debate. Esophageal function is probably well preserved, except perhaps in very advanced age. In total, these changes with age result in a prolonged duration of each swallow. Further, many diseases that produce dysphagia are more common in older adults.

Dysphagia

Dysphagia, or difficulty swallowing, can occur when a disease affects any level of swallowing function. Dysphagia is usually classified as oral, pharyngeal, or esophageal. In oral dysphagia, there is difficulty with the voluntary transfer of food from the mouth to the pharynx. This might be diagnosed, for example, when scrambled eggs are discovered in the cheeks of a demented patient shortly before lunch. The most common cause of oral dysphagia is dementia.

In pharyngeal dysphagia, there is a problem with reflexive transfer of the food bolus from the pharynx to initiate the involuntary esophageal phase of swallowing while simultaneously protecting the airway from misdirection of food. The affected person may notice coughing, choking, or nasal regurgitation while eating and localize the symptoms to the throat. The most common cause of pharyngeal dysphagia is stroke, but any disease that impairs the swallowing

---

STRENGTH-OF-EVIDENCE (SOE) RATING DEFINITIONS

A = consistent and good quality patient-oriented evidence
B = somewhat inconsistent or limited quality patient-oriented evidence
C = very inconsistent or very limited patient-oriented evidence, disease-oriented evidence, and/or consensus from professional organizations
D = unstudied common practice or opinion

See inside front cover for detailed information regarding the SOE classification.

center in the brain stem or the cranial nerves involved (eg, Parkinson's disease, CNS tumor), the oropharyngeal striated muscle (eg, myasthenia gravis, amyotrophic lateral sclerosis), or the local structures involved (eg, retropharyngeal abscess, tumor) can lead to pharyngeal dysphagia. Management of both oral and pharyngeal dysphagia involves treating the underlying disorder and devising an individualized, often labor-intensive, feeding program.

In esophageal dysphagia, the patient has the sensation that food has gotten "stuck" after a swallow. Dysphagia for both solids and liquids suggests an esophageal motility disorder (eg, achalasia, scleroderma), whereas progressive dysphagia for solids suggests a mechanical obstruction (eg, cancer, esophageal ring, stricture from mucosal irritation). None of these diseases is unique to the geriatric population, though older adults tend to take more medications and are therefore more likely to experience medication-induced esophagitis (which manifests initially as odynophagia, followed by dysphagia). Common causes of medication-induced esophagitis in older adults are potassium, NSAIDs, oral bisphosphonates, and tetracycline-related antibiotics. See also the section on dysphagia in "Gastrointestinal Diseases and Disorders," p 392.

Aspiration

The misdirection of pharyngeal contents into the airway is termed *aspiration*. Generally, there are two major sources of aspiration: oropharyngeal flora or gastric contents. However, despite this relatively straightforward definition, controversy persists over the definition of *aspiration pneumonia*. Aspiration pneumonia is believed to occur when bacteria arrive in the lungs from the pharynx in a large enough inoculum to overcome host defenses. For more viru-lent organisms, smaller inocula are required to overwhelm defenses. Pneumococcal pneumonia arisesfrom aspiration of *Pneumococcus* from a colonized oropharynx, however, and is usually not considered an aspiration pneumonia. Aspiration of gastric contents, or Mendelson's syndrome, usually results in a chemical pneumonitis; the usefulness of antibiotics in this situation is questionable. Most often, local host defense mechanisms clear the lung of the offending aspirate, without serious clinical effect. Many healthy individuals episodically aspirate without any important clinical consequences.

Aspiration of neither contaminated oral contents nor gastric contents is prevented by placement of a feeding tube. Tube feeding is universally cited as a risk factor for major aspiration, and some patients who have never previously aspirated begin to do so after a feeding tube has been placed. A 1996 review found no evidence that tube feeding of any sort would reduce the risk of aspiration pneumonia (SOE=B). A common misconception is that jejunostomy tube feeding has lower rates of associated aspiration of gastric contents than gastrostomy does. Most studies do not demonstrate reduced aspiration with jejunostomy compared with gastrostomy (SOE=C). Whether hand feeding (personal assistance with oral intake) is safer than tube feeding is also unclear. In a single nonrandomized prospective comparison of hand with tube feeding in patients with oropharyngeal aspiration, hand feeding resulted in lower rates of pneumonia. No prospective randomized trials comparing hand with tube feeding to reduce aspiration have been published. An active area of clinical research is focused on the role of substance P in swallowing and aspiration and the potential benefit of ACE inhibitors (which prevent the breakdown of substance P) in patients who aspirate.

Assessment of Oropharyngeal Dysphagia

Several tools can be used to assess swallowing function when oropharyngeal dysphagia is suspected clinically. The most common are the full bedside evaluation, of which there are many variations, the VDE, a variant of the modified barium swallow, and nasopharyngeal laryngoscopy performed by an otolaryngologist. There is considerable controversy regarding the relative efficacy of these tools.

VDE is usually performed by a speech-language pathologist who videotapes the patient swallowing several consistencies of barium-impregnated foods while the patient maintains various head positions. This can permit identification of the food consistency or compensatory mechanisms that minimize fluoroscopic evidence of aspiration. Depending on the results of the VDE, the therapist may recommend swallow therapy or diet modifications, or both. Swallow therapy may be compensatory (eg, turn head toward weaker side while swallowing), indirect (eg, exercises to improve the strength of the involved muscles), or direct (ie, exercises to perform while swallowing, such as swallowing multiple times per bolus). Dietary recommendations generally consist of altering bolus size or consistency of food or of restricting foods of certain consistencies.

Data conflict regarding the usefulness of VDE and nasopharyngeal laryngoscopy have been derived from small, historically controlled studies rather than from larger prospective randomized trials. A systematic review of studies of dysphagia secondary to stroke published by the Agency for Healthcare Research and Quality concluded that evidence was insufficient to recommend one type of swallowing study over another and that data correlating specific findings from any type of examination with clinically meaningful outcomes are lacking (SOE=C).

FEEDING

When an older adult experiences difficulty eating, the two main therapeutic approaches are careful feeding by hand or tube. The first requires extraordinary patience and is labor intensive; the latter is an invasive intervention associated with its own risks. Data about either approach are limited, and randomized comparisons have not been done. The role of dietary supplements, if any, in augmenting the caloric intake of hand-fed persons has not been clearly defined. One systematic review suggested that mortality was less with the use of oral protein and energy supplements in acutely hospitalized or community-dwelling adults >65 yr old, although the quality of the studies reviewed were not optimal. Functional status does not appear to be improved with oral nutritional supplements in any of the studies evaluating this outcome.

The number of percutaneous endoscopic gastrostomy feeding tubes placed in patients ≥65 yr old has grown at an astonishing rate over the past two decades. Low procedure-related complication rates are often cited; however, long-term studies reveal substantial mortality among tube-fed patients. Despite the popularity of feeding tubes, studies have not demonstrated improved survival, reduced incidence of pneumonia or other infections, improved symptoms or function, or reduced pressure ulcers with the use of feeding tubes of any type in demented persons who have eating difficulties. A 2009 Cochrane review of tube feeding in patients with advanced dementia found no evidence of a decrease in mortality (SOE=B). Median survival after placement of a feeding tube is well under a year, but it is unknown whether this results from tube feeding or if the need for tube feeding is a marker that death is near.

Complications described with feeding tubes are numerous and include an increased risk of aspiration pneumonia, metabolic disturbances, diarrhea, and local cellulitis. Monitoring for these complications should be meticulous. In a study that used a large administrative data set, 1-yr mortality was higher in 5,266 nursing-home residents with chewing or swallowing difficulties who were fed with a tube than in those who were not, even when statistically accounting for potential confounding variables (SOE=B). No prospective randomized studies comparing tube and hand feeding have been published, and information

on quality-of-life outcomes is sorely needed. Tube feedings may interfere with the absorption of some medications, eg, levodopa/carbidopa and phenytoin. Time-released medications cannot be crushed to administer them through the tube.

Placement of a percutaneous endoscopic gastrostomy or jejunostomy bypasses the oropharynx and the esophagus, allowing nutrients and medications to be instilled directly into the stomach or the jejunum to be absorbed by a functioning gut. It is clear that neither gastrostomy nor jejunostomy feeding tubes reduce aspiration in comparison with a program of hand feeding, but no randomized trials comparing these interventions have been published. The only disease for which feeding tubes have been shown to be of clinical benefit to the patient is esophageal obstruction, such as from malignancy. For most other disease states, their use remains unproved (SOE=D).

Contraindications to gastrostomy include the inability to pass an endoscope into the stomach, uncorrectable coagulopathy, massive ascites, peritonitis, and bowel obstruction. After successful placement of a gastrostomy, tube feedings of commercially available canned nutritional supplements can be started either as slow gravity boluses for gastrostomy tubes over 30–60 min or as a continuous infusion for gastrostomy or jejunostomy tubes. The feeding tube should be flushed with water before and after each feeding or at least four times a day in cases of continuous feedings.

Consideration of feeding tube placement requires careful examination of the data, with a focus on whether there is evidence of clinical benefit to support this invasive and potentially burdensome approach.

Not all feeding problems, of course, are related to dysphagia, and many contributing factors are quite amenable to therapy. Other approaches to consider in older adults who demonstrate eating or feeding problems are evaluation for depression, elimination of unduly restrictive diets, consideration of individual food preferences, consideration of the environment in which the person eats to improve socialization and reduce disruptive stimuli, examination of the condition of the oral cavity, determination of the needs for personal assistance with feeding, and reduction or elimination of medications that can cause inattention, xerostomia, movement disorders, or anorexia. Small studies have documented improved clinical outcomes in nursing-home residents with the use of flavor enhancers, increased food variety, and attention to the meal ambiance.

REFERENCES

- Amella EJ, Evans LK. Eating and Feeding Issues in Older Adults with Dementia: Part I: Assessment. *Try This: Best Practices in Nursing Care to Older Adults.* 2007;(D11.1). Available at http://consultgerirn.org/uploads/File/trythis/try_this_d11_1.pdf

- Amella EJ. Eating and Feeding Issues in Older Adults with Dementia: Part II: Interventions. *Try This: Best Practices in Nursing Care to Older Adults.* 2007;(D11.2). Available at http://consultgerirn.org/uploads/File/trythis/try_this_d11_2.pdf

- Hill M, Hughes T, Milford C. Treatment for swallowing difficulties (dysphagia) in chronic muscle disease. *Cochrane Database Syst Rev.* 2004(2):CD004303.

- Metheny N. Preventing Aspiration in Older Adults with Dysphagia. *Try This: Best Practices in Nursing Care to Older Adults.* 2007;(20). Available at http://consultgerirn.org/uploads/File/trythis/try_this_20.pdf

- Sampson EL, Candy B, Jones L. Enteral feeding for older people with advanced dementia. *Cochrane Database Syst Rev.* 2009(2):CD007209.

- Watson R, Green SM. Feeding and dementia: a systematic literature review. *J Adv Nurs.* 2006;54(1):86–93.

- White GN, O'Rourke F, Ong BS, et al. Dysphagia: causes, assessment, treatment, and management. *Geriatrics.* 2008;63(5):15–20.

CHAPTER 28—URINARY INCONTINENCE

KEY POINTS

- The prevalence of urinary incontinence (UI) increases with age and ADL dependence, affecting 15%–30% of all adults ≥65 yr old and 60%–70% of long-term care residents.

- UI in older adults can be caused or worsened by medical conditions, functional and cognitive impairment, or medications, with or without concomitant lower urinary tract dysfunction. Therefore, assessment of comorbidity and function are essential components of evaluation.

- Even in frailer older adults, UI is treatable through a stepped approach starting with lifestyle interventions and behavioral therapy, followed by medications and surgical interventions as appropriate.

INTRODUCTION

UI is the involuntary leakage of any amount of urine. Even when UI is distinguished by type of leakage (eg, urge or stress), it does not represent a specific diagnosis, pathophysiologic entity, or syndrome. In younger people, the etiology of UI often can be attributed after evaluation to specific pathophysiology in the lower urinary tract (LUT) and/or pelvic floor. In older adults, however, UI can be caused or worsened by comorbid conditions, medications, or functional and cognitive impairments, either alone or in combination with LUT dysfunction.

The most common types of UI symptoms are as follows:

- Urge UI — occurs with urgency, a compelling and often sudden need to void
- Stress UI — leakage coincident with increases in abdominal pressure, eg, cough, sneeze, laugh, physical activity
- Mixed UI — leakage occurs with both urgency and increases in abdominal pressure
- UI from incomplete emptying – associated with increased postvoid residual (PVR). Associated symptoms include those of urge and stress UI, and/or intermittent small dribbling leakage

STRENGTH-OF-EVIDENCE (SOE) RATING DEFINITIONS

A = consistent and good quality patient-oriented evidence
B = somewhat inconsistent or limited quality patient-oriented evidence
C = very inconsistent or very limited patient-oriented evidence, disease-oriented evidence, and/or consensus from professional organizations
D = unstudied common practice or opinion

See inside front cover for detailed information regarding the SOE classification.

and/or other lower urinary tract symptoms (LUTS) such as frequency, but they are non-specific. Frail patients with urge UI and an increased PVR (in the absence of bladder outlet obstruction) have detrusor hyperactivity with impaired contractility (DHIC).

UI may be accompanied by other LUTS (eg, frequency, nocturia, slow stream, hesitancy, sense of incomplete emptying, intermittent stream), all of which are nonspecific for a specific etiology. "Overactive bladder" is a term applied to a symptom complex of urgency, with or without urge UI, often accompanied with frequency and nocturia. However, in any individual patient these symptoms may not be due to a single cause or even relate directly to bladder dysfunction.

The terms transient UI and functional UI have been used to describe UI in older adults that is caused or exacerbated by factors outside of the LUT, such as comorbid conditions, medications, and impaired mobility. However, such UI will not be transient unless the underlying cause is addressed. People with functional UI may have factors other than impaired mobility, as well as LUT dysfunction, that contribute to UI, and comorbidity outside of the LUT can also cause LUT dysfunction. There is no widely accepted alternative term, although some authors suggest "UI due to potentially reversible factors."

PREVALENCE AND IMPACT

UI increases with age and affects women more than men (ratio 2:1) until age 80, after which men and women are equally affected. The prevalence is 15%–30% in community-dwelling adults ≥65 yr old, and 60%–70% in those in long-term care. In most studies, rates of UI are higher in white women than in black, Hispanic, and Asian women, with stress UI more common in white and Hispanic women than in black women. Racial and ethnic differences among older men are less clear. The few longitudinal studies in older women suggest annual UI incidence rates of 5%–11% in the community and 22% in long-term care, with remission rates that nearly match incidence.

Morbidity associated with UI includes cellulitis, pressure ulcers, urinary tract infections, falls with fractures, sleep deprivation, social withdrawal, depression, and sexual dysfunction. UI is not associated with increased mortality. UI significantly impairs quality of life, including emotional well-being, social function, and general health. Older adults with UI may maintain social activities, but do so with an increased burden of coping, embarrassment, and poor

Table 28.1—Medications That Can Cause or Worsen Urinary Incontinence

Medication	Effect on Continence
Alcohol, any amount	Frequency, urgency, sedation, delirium, immobility
α-Adrenergic agonists	Outlet obstruction (men)
α-Adrenergic blockers	Stress leakage (women)
ACE inhibitors	Associated cough worsens stress and possibly urge leakage in older adults with impaired sphincter function
Anticholinergics	Impaired emptying, retention, delirium, sedation, constipation, fecal impaction
Antipsychotics	Anticholinergic effects plus rigidity and immobility
Calcium channel blockers	Impaired detrusor contractility and retention; dihydropyridine agents can cause pedal edema, leading to nocturnal polyuria
Cholinesterase inhibitors	Urinary incontinence, potential interactions with antimuscarinics
Estrogen	Worsens stress and mixed leakage in women
GABAergic agents (gabapentin, pregabalin)	Pedal edema causing nocturia and nighttime incontinence
Loop diuretics	Polyuria, frequency, urgency
Narcotic analgesics	Urinary retention, fecal impaction, sedation, delirium
NSAIDs	Pedal edema causing nocturnal polyuria
Sedative hypnotics	Sedation, delirium, immobility
Thiazolidinediones	Pedal edema causing nocturnal polyuria
Tricyclic antidepressants	Anticholinergic effects, sedation

self-perception. UI increases caregiving time and burden, which can contribute to decisions for long-term care placement. Estimated annual costs related to UI in older adults total more than $26 billion.

RISK FACTORS

The evidence-based risk factors for UI include lifestyle factors (smoking; consumption of carbonated beverages, alcohol, caffeine), comorbidity (diabetes, constipation, neurologic disease), obesity, recurrent urinary tract infections, functional status (ADL and cognitive impairment), and medications (estrogen, diuretics, antidepressants). The association of vaginal delivery and parity with UI attenuates with age. The data pertain primarily to white women; much less is known about UI risk factors in men (other than prostate disease) and in other racial and ethnic populations.

COMORBIDITY AND UI

Especially in older adults, continence depends not only on LUT function but also on the ability to toilet, which requires sufficient physical function (mobility and manual dexterity), cognition, motivation, and available toilets. Medications (Table 28.1) and medical conditions (Table 28.2) can cause or worsen UI by their effects on toileting, LUT function, and/or urine output.

Not all older adults with a comorbid condition or taking a medication that is associated with UI will develop UI, and the presence of such factors in an individual person with UI does not imply that they are causative. The best example of this is the relationship between UI and dementia. Although older adults with dementia may have impairment in central inhibitory pathways that could result in urge UI, impaired functional status and mobility are at least as strong or stronger predictors of UI than cognitive status. Older adults with advanced dementia may remain continent if they can transfer and ambulate with minimal to moderate assistance. Furthermore, older adults with dementia may have other LUT dysfunction: one-third of incontinent nursing-home residents have stress UI or bladder outlet obstructions on urodynamic testing.

PATHOPHYSIOLOGY

Age-Related LUT Changes

A number of age-related physiologic changes in LUT function predispose older adults to UI. These include atrophic vaginitis, benign prostatic hypertrophy (BPH), decreased ability to postpone voiding, decreased detrusor contractility, decreased total bladder capacity, detrusor overactivity, increased PVR, and more urine output later in the day. Why some older adults develop UI and others do not remains unclear; differences in LUT function and other compensatory mechanisms may play a role.

LUT Pathophysiology in UI

Specific UI symptoms and LUT pathophysiology overlap substantially. However, some general associations (with caveats) are possible:

Table 28.2—Comorbid Conditions That Can Cause or Worsen Urinary Incontinence

Comorbidity	Effect on Continence
Cardiovascular disease	
Arteriovascular disease	Detrusor underactivity or areflexia from ischemic myopathy or neuropathy
Heart failure	Nocturnal polyuria
Gastrointestinal disease	Retention and overflow UI from constipation; fecal and urinary incontinence commonly coexist
Metabolic diseases	
Diabetes mellitus	DO with urge UI; detrusor underactivity due to neuropathy osmotic diuresis; altered mental status from hyper- or hypoglycemia; retention and overflow from constipation
Hypercalcemia	Diuresis; altered mental status
Vitamin B_{12} deficiency	Impaired bladder sensation and detrusor underactivity from peripheral neuropathy
Musculoskeletal disease	Mobility impairment; DO from cervical myelopathy in rheumatoid arthritis and osteoarthritis
Neurologic conditions	
Cerebrovascular disease, stroke	DO with urge UI from damage to upper motor neurons; impaired sensation to void from interruption of subcortical pathways; impaired function and cognition
Delirium	Impaired function and cognition
Dementia	DO with urge UI from damage to upper motor neurons; impaired function and cognition
Multiple sclerosis	DO, areflexia, or sphincter dyssynergia (depending on level of spinal cord involvement)
Normal-pressure hydrocephalus	DO from compression of frontal inhibitory centers; impaired function and cognition
Parkinson's disease	DO from loss of inhibitory inputs to pontine micturition center; impaired function and cognition; retention and overflow from constipation
Spinal cord injury	DO, areflexia, or sphincter dyssynergia (depending on level of injury)
Spinal stenosis	DO from damage to detrusor upper motor neurons (cervical stenosis); DO or areflexia (lumbar stenosis)
Obstructive sleep apnea	Nocturnal polyuria
Peripheral venous insufficiency	Nocturnal polyuria
Pulmonary disease	Conditions with chronic cough can worsen stress UI.
Psychiatric disease	
Affective and anxiety disorders	Decreased motivation
Alcoholism	Functional and cognitive impairment; rapid diuresis and retention in acute intoxication
Psychosis	Functional and cognitive impairment; decreased motivation

NOTE: UI = urinary incontinence; DO = detrusor overactivity

- **Urge UI and uninhibited bladder contractions, called detrusor overactivity (DO):** Up to 40% of continent healthy older adults demonstrate DO on urodynamic testing, suggesting that urge UI requires not just DO but impaired compensatory mechanisms (eg, CNS control) as well. DO may be idiopathic, age-related, secondary to lesions in cerebral and spinal inhibitory pathways, due to bladder outlet obstruction, or (less commonly) result from local bladder irritation (eg, infection, stones, tumor). Recent evidence suggests that increased afferent signaling from the detrusor can also contribute to urge UI.

- **Stress UI and impaired urethral sphincter support, from damage to pelvic muscles and/or connective tissues:** Another cause of stress UI is sphincter damage impairing urethral closure, which can occur from surgical scarring, radical prostatectomy, and some spinal cord injuries. DO can cause apparent "stress" UI, when a cough triggers an uninhibited detrusor contraction. In such cases, leakage usually occurs after and not coincident with the cough, is large in volume, and difficult to stop.

- **Mixed UI and both DO and impaired sphincter support/function, with the same caveats as above**

- **UI with impaired bladder emptying (increased PVR) and bladder obstruction and/or detrusor underactivity:** The most common cause of obstruction in men is prostate disease, and in women urethral scarring or a large cystocele that kinks the urethra. Detrusor underactivity can be caused by intrinsic bladder smooth muscle damage (eg, from ischemia, scarring, fibrosis),

Table 28.3—Causes of Nocturia

Nocturnal polyuria (nocturnal output >35% of total 24-hour output)	Late day/evening fluids, especially with caffeine or alcohol
	Pedal edema (eg, due to medications, venous stasis, heart failure)
	Heart failure
	Obstructive sleep apnea
Sleep disturbance	Medications
	Cardiac or pulmonary disease
	Pain
	Restless legs syndrome
	Depression
	Obstructive sleep apnea
	Sleep partner
Lower urinary tract	Detrusor overactivity
	Benign prostatic hyperplasia
	Impaired bladder emptying

peripheral neuropathy (diabetes mellitus, vitamin B_{12} deficiency, alcoholism), or damage to the sacral cord and spinal bladder efferent nerves by disc herniation, spinal stenosis, tumor, or degenerative neurologic disease. Neurologic diseases affecting the sacral spinal cord can cause detrusor underactivity and/or neurally mediated obstruction, depending on the exact level and extent of damage.

■ **Nocturia is a nonspecific symptom, even in older men, and causes other than urge UI and prostate disease should be considered (Table 28.3).**

EVALUATION

Similar to other geriatric syndromes, UI requires multifactorial evaluation with a focus on comorbidity, function, and medications as potential causes or contributing factors. Evaluation and management of UI in nursing-home residents is discussed in a separate section below.

Screening

All older patients should be asked at least every 2 yr about UI, because 50% of those affected do not voluntarily report their symptoms to a provider.

History

The history should include the type(s) of UI symptoms; UI onset, frequency, volume, and timing; and precipitants (eg, medications, amount and timing of fluid intake, caffeine, alcohol, physical activity, cough). UI may be the herald symptom of neurologic disease and cancer. "Red flag" symptoms that require prompt evaluation and referral are abrupt onset of UI, pelvic pain (constant, worsened, or improved with

voiding), and hematuria. Other LUTS that can be present are frequency, nocturia, slow urine stream, hesitancy, interrupted voiding, straining, and terminal dribbling. Medical conditions, their status, and medications should be reviewed for association with onset or worsening of UI. Review of systems should include a question about fecal incontinence, which is common in older adults with UI. Ask patients (and/or caregivers) specifically about UI-associated bother and impact on quality of life, starting with simple questions (eg, "What bothers you most about your leakage?" or "How does leakage affect your life?"), followed by more specific probes, as appropriate, regarding ADLs, social role, emotional and interpersonal relations, sexual function and relations, self-concept, general health perception, and financial burden.

Physical Examination

The general examination should include cognition and functional status, if not recently assessed, and focus on comorbidity associated with UI (eg, pedal edema). Abdominal palpation is insensitive and nonspecific for bladder distension. Assessments should be made of anal sphincter tone (rest and volitional, tightening around examiner's finger), the rectum for masses, and the prostate (in men) for nodules or firmness. Prostate sizing by digital examination is inaccurate (see "Prostate Disease," p 420). Neurologic evaluation is especially important in patients with new onset or worsening of UI, or who have motor and sensory symptoms. This should include evaluation of sacral cord integrity with perineal sensation, anal "wink" (lightly scratch the perianal area and look for anal sphincter contraction), and bulbocavernosus reflex (lightly touch the clitoris or glans and look for rectal contraction). The vaginal mucosa and pelvic support should be assessed in women (see "Gynecologic Diseases and Disorders," p 415). Uncircumcised men should be checked for phimosis, paraphimosis, and balanitis.

A clinical stress test should be done in patients with stress UI symptoms. The patient should have a full bladder and a relaxed perineum and buttocks, and the examiner positioned to observe or catch any leakage when the patient imparts a single vigorous cough. The test is specific for stress UI if leakage is instantaneous and most sensitive when the patient is upright. It is insensitive if the patient cannot cooperate, is inhibited, or the bladder volume is low.

Additional Testing

The only recommended test for all patients is urinalysis to look for hematuria (and glycosuria in diabetics). Pyuria or bacteriuria likely represents asymptomatic bacteriuria—not cystitis—in women without dysuria, fever, or other signs of urinary tract infection, especially if UI is not acute (see "Infectious Diseases," p 479). Other tests to consider are serum calcium concentration in patients with marked frequency and nocturia, and vitamin B_{12} concentration in patients with increased PVR or peripheral neuropathy.

Bladder diaries can be helpful to determine whether urine volume and timing contribute to frequency and nocturia symptoms, and can assist in evaluation of UI frequency, timing, and circumstances. The diary entails recording the time and volume of all continent voids and UI episodes typically longer than 3 days. For a sample diary, see http://www.healthinaging.org/public_education/bladder_control.php (accessed Jan 2011).

Although some guidelines suggest testing of PVR in all older patients with UI, supporting evidence is scant. Even older men with LUTS and/or known prostate disease do not require routine PVR testing (see "Prostate Disease," p 420). PVR should be done in patients with severe constipation; complex neurologic disease (eg, Parkinson's disease); women with marked pelvic organ prolapse or who have had prior surgery for incontinence; patients using medications known to decrease detrusor contractility; and frail patients, especially those in long-term care, who may have DHIC and in whom PVR testing would affect management (SOE=C). PVR can be measured in the office with ultrasound or catheterization. For patients with a PVR volume of >300 mL, see Table 28.4 for management. Women with a markedly increased PVR have a very low risk of hydronephrosis and do not require further imaging; the PVR volume cut-off at which men should be screened for hydronephrosis is uncertain, but ≥200 mL is reasonable.

Routine urodynamic testing is not necessary. Urodynamics should be considered when the etiology of UI is unclear and knowing it would change management (eg, a man with severe urge UI who may have bladder outlet obstruction), or when empiric treatment has failed. It should be done in patients considered for invasive treatment. Cystometry can determine only bladder proprioception, capacity, and detrusor stability; carbon dioxide cystometry is unreliable. Simultaneous measurement of abdominal pressure is necessary to exclude abdominal straining and detect DHIC. Fluoroscopic monitoring, abdominal leak-point pressure, and/or profilometry are necessary to diagnose physiologic stress UI. Pressure-flow studies are required to diagnose outlet obstruction.

TREATMENT AND MANAGEMENT

Correction of medical illnesses, medications, and other precipitating factors often improves UI, and should be addressed in all patients. Treatment should proceed stepwise, from correcting contributory factors and lifestyle modification, to behavioral therapy, medications, and then minimally invasive procedures and surgery as appropriate. Not all steps will be needed or appropriate for all patients, and some patients may want to proceed directly to surgery (eg, women with severe stress UI). Some treatments are effective for several UI symptoms (see below and Table 28.4 for SOE). Management should focus on relieving the aspect of UI that is most bothersome for the patient; eg, treatment that only decreases daytime UI episodes may not be sufficient for those most bothered by the timing of UI, nocturia, or leakage with exercise.

Lifestyle Modification

Weight loss significantly reduces stress incontinence in obese, younger-old women (SOE=A). Other lifestyle interventions lack confirmatory evidence but may be helpful: avoiding extremes of fluid intake, caffeinated beverages, and alcohol; minimizing evening intake for nocturia; and quitting smoking for patients with stress UI.

Behavioral Therapies

Bladder training and pelvic muscle exercises (PME) are effective for urge, mixed, and stress UI, and are often used in combination (SOE=A). Prompted voiding may be effective in cognitively impaired patients with urge UI; its efficacy in other types of UI is unknown.

Bladder training uses two principles: frequent voluntary voiding to keep bladder volume low, and urgency suppression using CNS and pelvic mechanisms. The initial toileting frequency can be every 2 hours or based on a bladder diary. When urgency occurs, patients should stand still or sit down, do several pelvic muscle contractions, and concentrate on making the urgency decrease (eg, by taking a deep breath and letting it out slowly, or visualizing the urgency as a wave that peaks and then falls). Once patients feel more in control, they should walk to a bathroom and void. After 2 days without leakage, the time between scheduled voids can be increased by 30–60 min, until the person is dry when voiding every 4 hours. Successful bladder training usually takes several weeks, and patients need reassurance to proceed despite any initial failure.

PME strengthen the muscular components of urethral support and are effective for urge, mixed, and stress UI. PME also are effective for prevention and treatment of UI after prostatectomy (see "Prostate Disease," p 420). PME requires patient instruction and motivation, although simple instruction booklets alone have had moderate benefit.

To do PME, the patient 1) performs an isolated pelvic muscle contraction, without contracting buttocks, abdomen, or thighs (this can be checked during a bimanual examination in women), and holds it for 6–8 seconds (initially, only shorter durations may be possible); 2) repeats the contraction 8 to 12 times (one set), relaxing the pelvis between each contraction; 3) completes three sets of contractions starting 3 to 4 times a week, and continuing for at least 15 to 20 weeks. As patients progress, they should try to increase the intensity and duration of the contraction, perform PME in various positions (sitting, standing, walking), and alternate fast and slower contractions. Many experts believe biofeedback can improve bladder retraining and PME teaching and outcomes, but the marginal benefit is unproved. Medicare covers biofeedback for patients who do not improve after 4 weeks with conventional instruction.

The only behavioral treatment with proven efficacy in cognitively impaired patients is prompted voiding. A caregiver monitors the patient and encourages him or her to report any need to void, prompts the patient to toilet on a regular schedule during the day (usually every 2–3 hours) and leads the patient to the bathroom, and gives the patient positive feedback when he or she toilets. Patients most likely to improve void ≤4 times during the day (12 hours) and are able to accept and follow the prompt to toilet at least 75% of the time in an initial 3-day trial. Toileting routines without prompting, such as habit training (based on a patient's usual voiding schedule) and scheduled voiding (using a set schedule) are not effective.

Medications

Antimuscarinic agents are effective for urge UI, urgency, and mixed incontinence. There is good evidence that antimuscarinics should always be combined with behavioral therapy for maximal efficacy. Antimuscarinics are safe and effective in men with BPH-associated urgency and urge UI (see BPH in "Prostate Disease," p 420); it should be noted,

Table 28.4—Efficacy of Incontinence Treatments

Treatment	Target Population	Efficacy	SOE
Behavioral[a]			
Bladder training	Cognitively intact; urge incontinence or urge-predominant mixed incontinence	For urge incontinence, ≥5% decrease in episodes; patient perception of cure at 6 mo, RR 1.69% [95% CI 1.21, 2.34]; for stress incontinence, ≥50% decrease in 75% of patients; all UI, ARR 0.51 [0.36, 0.66]	A
Prompted voiding	Urge incontinence or urge-predominant mixed incontinence; cognitively impaired	Average reduction 0.8–1.8 episodes/day, cure rare	A
Pelvic muscle exercises with bladder training	Urge, stress, or mixed incontinence	For urge incontinence, up to 80% decrease; for stress incontinence, 56%–95% decrease; all UI, mean weighted effect size, −0.54 episodes/day [−0.71, −0.37], ARR 13% [7%, 20%]	A
Pelvic muscle exercises with bladder training and biofeedback	Urge, stress, or mixed incontinence	All UI, 50%–87% improvement, ARR 24% [8%, 39%], RR for continued UI 0.74 [0.6, 0.93]	A
	Men: stress incontinence after prostatectomy	Continence achieved in 57% at 1–2 mo (relative benefit 1.54 [1.01, 2.34])	A
Electrical stimulation	Stress incontinence, mixed incontinence	No marginal benefit over pelvic muscle exercises with bladder training and biofeedback	A

Table 28.4—Efficacy of Incontinence Treatments (continued)

Treatment	Target Population	Efficacy	SOE
Pharmacologic			
All antimuscarinics[b]	Urge incontinence	WMD in daily UI, 0.6 [0.4, 0.8]	A
Oxybutynin	Urge incontinence	IR: WMD in daily UI, −0.72 [−1.09, −0.34]; ER: 71% mean reduction weekly UI episodes, cure rate 23%; topical mean WMD in daily UI, −0.55 [−1.05, −0.04]	A
Tolterodine	Urge incontinence	ER: WMD in daily UI, −0.73 [−0.93, −0.53]; cure rate 17%	A
Darifenacin	Urge incontinence	OR for 70% decrease in UI versus placebo, 1.8 for both 7.5-mg and 15-mg doses	A
Solifenacin	Urge incontinence	10 mg, WMD in daily UI −0.69 [−1.19, −0.19]	A
Trospium	Urge incontinence	20 mg q12h: "marked improvement or cure" in 48% versus in 20% with placebo; ER 60 mg, mean change in daily UI −2.4 versus −1.6 with placebo	A
Fesoterodine	Urge incontinence	Mean change in daily UI −1.65 (4 mg) and −2.28 (8 mg) versus −0.96 with placebo	A
Estrogen	Women's Health Initiative trial secondary analysis	Conjugated equine estrogen 0.625 mg plus medroxyprogesterone 2.5 mg: incident stress incontinence, RR 2.1 [1.7, 2.5]; ARR 9% [7%, 11%]; incident urge incontinence, RR 1.84 [1.58, 2.15], ARR 7% [6%, 9%]	A
Duloxetine[OL]	Stress incontinence	Pooled ARR for improvement in stress incontinence, 11% [7%, 14%]	A
Surgery			
Retropubic suspension	Stress incontinence	Short-term cure 69%–88%, 5-yr 70%; cure or improvement 84%	B
Vaginal sling	Stress incontinence	Short-term cure rate with tension-free vaginal tape similar to that of open abdominal retropubic suspension	B/C
Periurethral bulking injections	Stress incontinence, women	Cure 50% (range 8%–100%), cure or improvement 67%	B
	Stress incontinence, men after prostatectomy	Cure 20% (range 0%–66%), cure or improvement 42%	B
Treatment	Target Population	Efficacy	SOE
Artificial sphincter	Stress incontinence unresponsive to other treatment, women	Cure 77%, cure or improvement 80%; revision rate 40%–50%; less data than with men	B
	Stress incontinence unresponsive to other treatment, men	Cure 66% (range 33%–88%), cure or improvement 85% (range 75%–95%); revision rate 40%–50%	B

[a] Except when indicated, evidence applies to women (very few men included in behavioral trials)

[b] Duration of most drug trials 12 weeks

NOTE: UI=urinary incontinence, CI=confidence interval, RR=relative risk, ARR=absolute risk reduction, IR=immediate release, ER=extended release, WMD=weighted mean difference, OR=odds ratio

SOURCES: Data from Abrams P, Cardozo L, Khoury S, et al., eds. *Incontinence: The International Consultation on Incontinence*. Plymouth, UK: Health Publication Ltd; 2009; Cochrane Library; Chapple C, Khullar V, Gabriel Z, et al. The effects of antimuscarinic treatments in overactive bladder: a systematic review and meta-analysis. *Eur Urol*. 2005;48:5–26; Shamliyan TA, Kane RL, Wyman J, et al. Systematic review: randomized, controlled trials of nonsurgical treatments for urinary incontinence in women. *Ann Intern Med*. 2008;148:459–473; Chapple C, Steers W, Norton P, et al. A pooled analysis of three phase III studies to investigate the efficacy, tolerability and safety of darifenacin, a muscarinic M3 selective receptor antagonist, in the treatment of overactive bladder. *BJU Int*. 2005;95:993–1001; Fröhlich G, Bulitta M, Strösser W. Trospium chloride in patients with detrusor overactivity: meta-analysis of placebo-controlled, randomized, double-blind, multi-center clinical trials on the efficacy and safety of 20 mg trospium chloride twice daily. *Int J Clin Pharmacol Ther*. 2002;40:295–303; Dmochowski RR, Sand PK, Zinner NR, et al. Trospium 60 mg once daily (QD) for overactive bladder syndrome: results from a placebo-controlled interventional study. *Urology*. 2008;71:449–454; Nitti VW, Dmochowski R, Sand PK, et al. Efficacy, safety and tolerability of fesoterodine for overactive bladder syndrome. *J Urol*. 2007;178:2488–2494; Meta-analysis of pelvic floor muscle training randomized controlled trials in incontinent women. *Nurs Res*. 2007;56(4):226–234; MacDonald R, Fink HA, Huckabay C, et al. Pelvic floor muscle training to improve urinary incontinence after radical prostatectomy: a systematic review of effectiveness. *BJU Int*. 2007;100(1):76–81.

however, that the Beers criteria lists oxybutynin as contraindicated in men with BPH (SOE=A). These medications are also safe and effective in DHIC if started at the lowest initial dosage and titrated as necessary based on symptom response. Antimuscarinics are contraindicated for patients with narrow-angle glaucoma (not open-angle), impaired gastric emptying, and urinary retention. It is not necessary to routinely monitor PVR with antimuscarinic treatment. Patients who may need to have a PVR checked are those complaining of worsening UI while taking antimuscarinics, because an increased PVR decreases functional bladder capacity and thus increases frequency and UI; those who have other bladder suppressant medications added (eg, calcium channel blocker, other anticholinergic); and those who develop severe constipation.

Antimuscarinics with proven efficacy are oxybutynin (immediate release, 2.5–5 mg q6–12h; extended release 5–20 mg/d; topical patch 3.9 mg applied to abdomen, thighs, or buttocks twice weekly), tolterodine (immediate release 1–2 mg q12h, extended release 2–4 mg/d), trospium 20 mg q12h or q24h, darifenacin 7.5–15 mg/d, and solifenacin 10–20 mg/d. Fesoterodine (4–8 mg/d), the active metabolite of tolterodine, may be approved in the near future.

All of the muscarinics have similar efficacy in reducing UI but differ in adverse events, metabolism, drug interactions, and dosing requirements. Anticholinergic adverse events impact both tolerability and safety. Chronic antimuscarinic use increases the risk of caries and tooth loss, and patients should have regular dental care. Although anticholinergics can cause cognitive impairment, the risk, prevalence, type, and magnitude of cognitive changes from specific antimuscarinic UI medications in an individual patient are unknown. Evidence is insufficient that one drug is "safer" for all patients or those with dementia, or that the cognitive risk outweighs the potential treatment benefit. The impact of concomitant use of antimuscarinics and cholinesterase inhibitors is also uncertain, especially because the latter drugs can cause or worsen UI. All antimuscarinics except trospium are metabolized by cytochrome P-450 pathways, and can interact with drugs that induce CYP2D6 (eg, fluoxetine) or are metabolized by CYP3A4 (eg, erythromycin, ketoconazole). Trospium is cleared by the kidneys and should be given once daily in patients with renal insufficiency; it should be taken on an empty stomach. Therefore, choice of agent for a particular patient should depend on potential adverse events to be avoided, possible drug-drug and drug-disease interactions, dosing frequency, titration range, and cost. A lack of response to one agent does not preclude response to another.

For other agents (propantheline, dicyclomine, imipramine, hyoscyamine, calcium channel blockers, and NSAIDs), efficacy data are scant. Flavoxate is ineffective. Use of vasopressin (DDAVP) for nocturia should be avoided in older adults because of the risk of hyponatremia.

No medications for stress UI that are effective and/or safe in older women are currently available in the United States. The antidepressant duloxetine is not approved by the FDA for use in stress UI. Oral estrogen, alone or in combination with progestins, increases incontinence and should not be used. There is no consensus on whether topical estrogen applied vaginally (cream, vaginal tablet, or slow-release ring) improves UI, but it is helpful for uncomfortable vaginal atrophy and decreases recurrent urinary tract infections (see Urinary Tract Infection in "Infectious Diseases," p 484). Imipramine has been used for mixed UI, but efficacy data are scant and anticholinergic effects are marked.

Minimally Invasive Procedures

Sacral nerve neuromodulation can be effective for both urge UI refractory to drug treatment and urinary retention (idiopathic and neurogenic). The mechanism of action is unknown. The procedure involves the percutaneous implant of a trial electrode at the S3 sacral root, which is connected to an external stimulator. Permanent lead implantation is done in patients who respond to an initial trial, at which time a pacemaker-like energy source is implanted under the skin.

Evidence is increasing that intravesical injections of botulinum toxin are effective for refractory urge UI. However, botulinum toxin is not approved by the FDA for UI, and patients must be willing to do self-catheterization because of the risk of urinary retention.

Pessaries may benefit women with stress and urge UI exacerbated by bladder or uterine prolapse. See "Gynecologic Diseases and Disorders," p 418.

Surgery

Surgery provides the highest cure rates for stress UI in women. The most commonly used procedures are colposuspension (Burch operation) and slings (synthetic mesh, or autologous or cadaveric fascia placed transvaginally). There are few data to assist in procedure and patient selection for older women, especially if they have mixed UI, detrusor underactiv-ity, or significant comorbidity, or if prior surgery for incontinence has not been successful. Periurethral injection of collagen is a short-term (≤1 yr) alternative and usually requires a series of injections. Early short-term reports suggest that suburethral sling placement may be effective in men with persistent UI after prostatectomy.

Artificial sphincters are used for refractory stress UI from sphincter damage (eg, severe persistent stress UI after radical prostatectomy from surgical scarring). These devices are used most often in men, in which a cuff is placed internally around the urethra, and its inflation controlled by the patient squeezing a reservoir device placed in the scrotum. They are effective but require manual dexterity and intact cognition; an alert bracelet should be considered, because catheter insertion through a closed artificial sphincter can cause significant damage. Revision rates can be high (up to 40%). Urodynamics should assist patient selection, because outcomes are worse with severe DO and poor detrusor compliance.

Supportive Care

Pads and protective garments should be chosen based on patient gender and the type and volume of UI. For example, an absorbent sheath may be sufficient for a man with mild UI after prostatectomy. In some states, Medicaid may cover pads; Medicare and private insurance do not. Medical supply companies and patient advocacy groups publish illustrated catalogs to guide product selection. Because these products are often expensive, some patients may not change pads frequently enough.

EVALUATION AND MANAGEMENT OF UI IN NURSING-HOME RESIDENTS

The CMS *Guidance for Surveyors for Long Term Facilities* sets the nursing-home compliance standards, known as the F-tag 315, for the evaluation and management of UI and urinary catheters. The 2006 revision of F-tag 315 changed the focus from documentation of toileting plans to an increased emphasis on screening, the process and documentation of UI assessment, and reevaluation. The Minimum Data Set requires that residents are screened for UI at admission; quarterly; and with any change in cognition, function, or urinary tract function. F-tag 315 guidance suggests an evaluation essentially equivalent to that described above. Instead of bladder diaries, toileting patterns and UI episodes are monitored over several days. Although evaluation is largely a nursing responsibility, physician input is especially important given the emphasis on physical examination, evaluation of medications and comorbidity as a cause of UI, and differential diagnosis.

Nearly all studies of UI treatment in long-term care involve behavioral therapy. Evidence is strong that prompted voiding is effective in reducing daytime UI. Interventions that combine prompted voiding with bedside exercise improve both incontinence and physical function. Prompted voiding should be tried in all eligible patients (ie, able to state their name, can transfer with at most an assist by one), but continued only in those who are able to accept and follow the prompt to toilet at least 75% of the time in an initial 3-day trial. Long-term care residents who do not respond should be managed with "check and change." The revised F-tag 315 supports this targeted approach and the role of patient and family preference in evaluation and treatment. Unfortunately, in most nursing homes, common practice is scheduled toileting without prompting, which is ineffective. Quality improvement efforts focused on staff organization and systems may ultimately be necessary to reduce UI in long-term care.

The only randomized studies of antimuscarinics in nursing-home residents used oxybutynin. Those studies are old, the study populations were small, and only immediate-release oxybutinin was used. Consequently, antimuscarinics are infrequently prescribed, despite evidence that patients may prefer medications over behavioral therapy and "check and change." It is reasonable to consider an antimuscarinic trial for residents with urge UI who respond to prompted voiding but are still incontinent. Given the high prevalence of DHIC in this population, PVR should be checked before and during antimuscarinic treatment.

It is important to remember that up to a third of nursing-home residents with UI have an underlying bladder outlet problem (eg, stress incontinence or bladder outlet obstruction) and may be candidates for alternative medical or surgical treatment.

CATHETERS AND CATHETER CARE

Indwelling catheters cause significant morbidity, including polymicrobial bacteriuria (universal by 30 days), febrile episodes (1 per 100 patient days), nephrolithiasis, bladder stones, epididymitis, chronic renal inflammation and pyelonephritis, and meatal damage. Condom catheters also cause bacteriuria, infection, penile cellulitis and necrosis, and urinary retention and hydronephrosis if the condom twists or its external band is too tight. Indwelling catheters should be used only for short-term decompression of acute urinary retention, chronic retention that cannot be managed medically or surgically, protection of wounds that may be contaminated by urine, and terminally ill or severely impaired patients who cannot tolerate garment changes and who have an informed preference for catheter management despite risks. Inappropriate and/or poorly documented indications for catheter use are a major focus in the revised F-tag 315 guidance for nursing homes. The guidance states that catheters should primarily be used for short-term decompression of acute retention. However,

F-tag 315 allows for catheter use over 14 days for patients with chronic retention (PVR volumes >200 mL who are not candidates for medical or surgical treatment or management with intermittent catheterization; have persistent UI, urinary tract infections, and/or renal dysfunction; have stage III–IV pressure ulcers for which UI impedes healing; or have terminal illness or severe impairment that makes positioning or clothing changes uncomfortable or that is associated with intractable pain).

All patients with acute retention should have decompression with an indwelling catheter for several days while being evaluated and treated for potentially remediable causes, such as medications that impair detrusor contractility or increase urethral tone, outlet obstruction, and constipation. A voiding trial without catheter should follow decompression. To do so, the catheter should be removed (never clamped), the patient adequately hydrated, and a PVR checked after the first void or bladder volume checked if there is no void after about 6 hours. Studies have not confirmed any benefit of bethanechol chloride for patients with retention.

Intermittent clean catheterization is an effective alternative to an indwelling catheter for willing and able patients. Strict sterility is not necessary, although good handwashing and regular decontamination of the catheters is needed. Special stiffer and smoother short catheters are available for use. Bacteriuria can be minimized by a frequency of catheterization that keeps bladder volume <400 mL. Sterile intermittent catheterization is preferred for frailer patients and those in institutionalized settings.

Bacteriuria is universal in catheterized patients and should not be treated unless there are clear symptoms of cystitis or pyelonephritis. Routine cultures should not be done because of the changing flora and failure to accurately indicate infection. In symptomatic patients, urine for culture should not be obtained from the existing catheter; the old catheter should be removed and urine obtained from a newly placed catheter. Institutionalized patients with catheters should be kept in separate rooms to decrease cross-infection. Topical meatal antimicrobials, catheters with antimicrobial coating, collection bag disinfectants, and antimicrobial irrigation are not effective. Although antibiotics decrease bacteriuria and infection, routine use induces resistant organisms and secondary infections (such as with *Clostridium difficile*) and should not be used. Prophylactic antibiotics are recommended only in high-risk patients (eg, those with prosthetic heart valves) during short-term catheterization. For men with chronic obstruction, suprapubic catheters may be preferable to avoid meatal and penile trauma.

Catheters need not be changed routinely as long as monitoring is adequate and catheter blockage does not develop. Risk factors for blockage include alkaline urine, female gender, poor mobility, calciuria, proteinuria, copious mucin, *Proteus* colonization, and preexistent bladder stones. Changing the catheter every 7 to 10 days may decrease blockage in such patients. If patients cannot be monitored, changing catheters every 30 days is reasonable (SOE=D). Possible causes of persistent leakage around the catheter are large Foley balloon, detrusor overactivity, catheter diameter that is too large, bacteriuria, constipation or impaction, or improper catheter positioning. These can be addressed by trials of partial deflation of the balloon, smaller catheter, treatment of constipation, use of an antimuscarinic, or treatment with pyridium.

Catheters coated with silver alloys reduce asymptomatic bacteriuria in hospitalized patients requiring short-term urethral catheterization, but their use in reducing symptomatic bacteriuria is less certain. Data are scant whether silver alloy catheters reduce asymptomatic or symptomatic bacteriuria in other settings (such as long-term care or home care) or with longer-term catheterization. See "Hospital Care," p 119.

ACOVE-3* QUALITY INDICATORS PERTAINING TO URINARY INCONTINENCE

Screening
- All vulnerable older adults should have documentation of the presence or absence of UI during the initial evaluation.
- All vulnerable older adults should have documentation of the presence or absence of UI every 2 yr.

Annual assessment of UI
- If a vulnerable older adult has UI, then there should be documentation annually of whether the UI is bothersome to the patient or caregiver.

Incontinence history
- If a vulnerable older adult has new UI or established UI with bothersome symptoms, then a targeted history should be documented.

Incontinence examination
- If a vulnerable older adult has new UI, then a targeted physical examination should be documented.

Urine evaluation
- If a vulnerable older adult has new UI or established UI with bothersome symptoms, then a urinalysis (or dipstick urinalysis) and a urine culture, if the urinalysis demonstrates pyuria or hematuria, should be obtained.

Postvoid residual (PVR)

- If a vulnerable older adult has a PVR >300 mL, then he or she should have a serum creatinine within 72 hours and (if no reversible causes found) be referred to a clinician with urologic expertise within 2 mo.
- If a vulnerable older adult with UI has a PVR of 200–300 mL, then renal function should be assessed within 3 mo.

Classification of UI

- If a vulnerable older adult has new UI or established UI with bothersome symptoms, and the UI is treated with medication or surgery, then classification of the type of or suspected reason(s) for UI should be documented.

Discussion of treatment options

- If a vulnerable older adult has new UI or established UI with bothersome symptoms, then treatment options should be discussed within 3 mo.

Assess response to treatment

- If a vulnerable older adult is treated for UI, then response to treatment should be documented within 3 mo.

Behavioral and lifestyle treatments

- If a cognitively intact, ambulatory vulnerable older adult has stress, urge, or mixed UI, then behavioral and lifestyle treatment should be offered.

Preoperative urodynamic testing

- If a female vulnerable older adult undergoes surgery for stress UI, then urodynamic investigations should be performed before surgery.

Surgery for stress incontinence

- If a female vulnerable older adult has stress UI and undergoes a procedure or surgery for UI, then surgical correction with open retropubic suspension or a sling procedure (including tension-free vaginal tape) should be performed or a periurethral bulking agent offered.

Chronic urethral catheter

- If a vulnerable older adult has clinically significant urinary retention, and a long-term (>1 mo) urethral catheter is placed, then there should be documentation of justification for its use.

Related quality indicators for Urinary Incontinence

Indwelling bladder catheter (see "Hospital Care," p 119)

Evaluation and management of prostate problems (see "Prostate Disease," p 420)

*Assessing Care of Vulnerable Elders – 3rd Set. See inside front cover for explanation.

REFERENCES

- Dowling-Castronovo A. Urinary Incontinence Assessment in Older Adults Part I—Transient Urinary Incontinence. *Try This: Best Practices in Nursing Care to Older Adults.* 2007;(10). Available at http://consultgerirn.org/uploads/File/trythis/try_this_10.pdf

- Dowling-Castronovo A. Urinary Incontinence Assessment in Older Adults: Part I—Transient Urinary Incontinence. *Try This: Best Practices in Nursing Care to Older Adults.* 2007;(11.1). Available at http://consultgerirn.org/uploads/File/trythis/try_this_11_1.pdf

- Dowling-Castronovo A. Urinary Incontinence Assessment in Older Adults: Part II—Established Urinary Incontinence. *Try This: Best Practices in Nursing Care to Older Adults.* 2008;(11.2). Available at http://consultgerirn.org/uploads/File/trythis/try_this_11_2.pdf

- Johnson TM 2nd, Ouslander JG. The newly revised F-Tag 315 and surveyor guidance for urinary incontinence in long-term care. *J Am Med Directors Assoc.* 2006;7(9):594−600.

- Landefeld CS, Bowers BJ, Feld AD, et al. National Institutes of Health state-of-the-science conference statement: prevention of fecal and urinary incontinence in adults. *Ann Intern Med.* 2008;148(6):449−458.

- Shamliyan TA, Kane RL, Wyman J, et al. Systematic review: randomized, controlled trials of nonsurgical treatments for urinary incontinence in women. *Ann Intern Med.* 2008;148(6):459−473.

CHAPTER 29—GAIT IMPAIRMENT

KEY POINTS

- Gait disorders are common in older adults and are a predictor of functional decline.

- The cause of gait impairment in older adults is usually multifactorial; therefore, a full assessment must include consideration of a number of different causes, as determined from a detailed physical examination and a functional performance evaluation.

- Various interventions, ranging from medical to surgical to exercise, can reduce the degree of impairment, although some residual impairment is often present.

Gait disorders are commonly associated with falls and disability in older adults. This chapter reviews the epidemiology of gait impairments, comorbidities that contribute to these disorders, and office-based clinical assessments and interventions to reduce their functional impact.

EPIDEMIOLOGY

Limitations in walking increase with age. At least 20% of noninstitutionalized older adults admit to difficulty with walking or require the assistance of another person or special equipment to walk. In some samples of noninstitutionalized older adults ≥85 yr old, the prevalence of walking limitations can be over 50%. Age-related gait changes such as slowed speed are most apparent after age 75 or 80, but most gait disorders appear in connection with underlying diseases, particularly as disease severity increases. For example, advanced age (>85 yr old); three or more chronic conditions at baseline; and the occurrence of stroke, hip fracture, or cancer predict catastrophic loss of walking ability (SOE=B).

Determining that a gait is disordered is difficult because there are no clearly accepted general standards of normal gait for older adults. Some believe that slowed gait speed suggests a disorder; others believe that deviations in smoothness, symmetry, and synchrony of movement patterns suggest a disorder. Regardless, a slowed and aesthetically abnormal gait can in fact provide the older adult with a safe, independent gait pattern.

Longitudinal observational studies suggest that certain gait-related mobility disorders progress with age and that this progression is associated with morbidity and mortality. Community-dwelling older adults with gait disorders, particularly neurologically abnormal gaits, are at higher risk of institutionalization and death (SOE=B).

CONDITIONS THAT CONTRIBUTE TO GAIT IMPAIRMENT

Impaired gait may not be an inevitable consequence of aging but rather a reflection of the increased prevalence and severity of age-associated diseases. These diseases, both neurologic and non-neurologic, are the major contributors to impaired gait. In addition, attributing a gait disorder to one disease in an older adult is particularly difficult because similar gait abnormalities are common to many diseases. (For a glossary of gait abnormalities, see Table 29.1.)

Patients in primary care report that pain, stiffness, dizziness, numbness, weakness, and sensations of abnormal movement are the most common causes of their walking difficulties. The most common conditions seen in primary care that are thought to contribute to gait disorders are degenerative joint disease, acquired musculoskeletal deformities, intermittent claudication, impairments after orthopedic surgery and stroke, and postural hypotension. Usually, more than one contributing condition is found. In a group of community-dwelling adults >88 yr old, joint pain was by far the most common contributor, followed by multiple causes such as stroke and visual loss. Factors such as dementia and fear of falling also contribute to gait disorders. The disorders found in a neurologic referral population include frontal gait disorders (usually related to normal-pressure hydrocephalus [NPH] and cerebrovascular processes), sensory disorders (also involving vestibular and visual function), myelopathy, previously undiagnosed Parkinson's disease or parkinsonian syndromes, and cerebellar disease. Known conditions causing severe gait impairment, such as hemiplegia and severe hip or knee disease, are commonly not mentioned in these neurologic referral populations. Thus, many gait disorders, particularly those that are classical and discrete (eg, those related to stroke and osteoarthritis) and those that are mild or may relate to irreversible disease (eg, vascular dementia), are presumably diagnosed in primary care and treated without a referral to a neurologist. Other less common contributors to gait disorders include metabolic disorders (related to

Table 29.1—Glossary of Gait Abnormalities

Term	Description
Antalgic gait	Pain-induced limp with shortened phase of gait on painful side
Circumduction	Outward swing of leg in semicircle from the hip
Equinovarus	Excessive plantar flexion and inversion of the ankle
Festination	Acceleration of gait
Foot drop	Loss of ankle dorsiflexion secondary to weakness of ankle dorsiflexors
Foot slap	Early, frequent audible foot-floor contact with steppage gait compensation
Genu recurvatum	Hyperextension of knee
Propulsion	Tendency to fall forward
Retropulsion	Tendency to fall backward
Scissoring	Hip adduction such that the knees cross in front of each other with each step
Steppage gait	Exaggerated hip flexion, knee extension, and foot lifting, usually accompanied by foot drop
Trendelenburg gait	Shift of the trunk over the affected hip, which drops because of hip abductor weakness
Turn en bloc	Moving the whole body while turning

renal or hepatic disease), CNS tumors or subdural hematoma, depression, and psychotropic medications. Case reports also document reversible gait disorders due to clinically overt hypo- or hyperthyroidism and B_{12} and folate deficiency.

Factors associated with slowed gait speed are also considered contributors to gait disorders. These factors are commonly disease associated (eg, cardiopulmonary or musculoskeletal disease) and include decreased leg strength, vision, aerobic function, standing balance, and physical activity, as well as joint impairment, previous falls, and fear of falling. Combining these factors can result in an effect greater than the sum of the single impairments (as when combining balance and strength impairments). Furthermore, the effect of improved strength and aerobic capacity on gait speed may be nonlinear; that is, for very impaired individuals, small improvements in strength or aerobic capacity yield relatively larger gains in gait speed, whereas these small improvements yield little gait speed change in healthy older adults.

Although older adults can maintain a relatively normal gait pattern well into their 80s, some slowing occurs, and decreased stride length thus becomes a common feature in descriptions of gait disorders of older adults. Some authors have proposed the emer-gence of an age-related gait disorder without accompanying clinical abnormalities, ie, essential

"senile" gait disorder. This gait pattern is described as broad-based with small steps, diminished arm swing, stooped posture, decreased flexion of the hips and knees, uncertainty and stiffness in turning, occasional difficulty initiating steps, and a tendency toward falling. These and other nonspecific findings (eg, theinability to perform tandem gait) are similar to gait patterns found in a number of other diseases, and yet the clinical abnormalities are insufficient to make a specific diagnosis. This "disorder" may be a precursor to an as-yet-undiagnosed disease (eg, related to subtle extrapyramidal signs) and is likely to be a manifestation of concurrent, progressive cognitive impairment (eg, Alzheimer's disease or vascular dementia). Thus, "senile" gait disorder may reflect a number of potential diseases and is generally not useful in labeling gait disorders in older adults.

Subclinical as well as clinically evident cerebrovascular disease is increasingly recognized as a major contributor to causes of gait disorders (SOE=B). Nondemented persons with clinically abnormal gait (particularly unsteady, frontal, or hemiparetic gait) followed for approximately 7 yr were found to be at higher risk of developing non-Alzheimer's, particularly vascular, dementia. Of note, those with abnormal gait at baseline may not have met criteria for dementia but already had abnormalities in neuropsychologic function, such as in visual-perceptual processing and language skills. Gait disorders with no apparent cause (also termed "idiopathic" or "senile" gait disorder) are associated with a higher mortality rate, primarily from cardiovascular causes (SOE=B). These cardiovascular causes are likely linked to concomitant, possibly undetected, cerebrovascular disease.

ASSESSMENT

Gait disorders can be clinically assessed and described (Table 29.1).

Disorders that are the result of pathology of the low sensorimotor level can be divided into peripheral sensory and peripheral motor dysfunction, including myopathic or neuropathic disorders that cause weakness and musculoskeletal diseases. These disorders are generally distal to the CNS. With peripheral sensory impairment, unsteady and tentative gait is commonly caused by vestibular disorders, peripheral neuropathy, posterior column (proprioceptive) deficits, or visual impairment. With peripheral motor impairment, a number of classical gait patterns emerge. Examples of these patterns include Trendelenburg gait (ie, weight shifts over the weak hip, which drops because of hip abductor weakness), antalgic gait (weight bearing is avoided and stance shortens on one side because of pain), and foot drop (due to ankle dorsiflexor weakness and characterized by a frequently audible foot-floor contact with steppage gait compensation, ie, excessive hip flexion). These gait impairments are the result of body segment and joint deformities, pain, and focal myopathic and neuropathic weakness. In general, if the gait disorder is limited to this low sensorimotor level (ie, the CNS is intact), the person can adapt well to the gait disorder, compensating with an assistive device or learning to negotiate the environment safely.

At the middle sensorimotor level, the execution of centrally selected postural and locomotor responses is faulty, and the sensory and motor modulation of gait is disrupted. Gait may be initiated normally, but stepping patterns are abnormal. Diseases causing spasticity (eg, those related to myelopathy, B$_{12}$ deficiency, and stroke), parkinsonism (idiopathic as well as medication induced), and cerebellar disease (eg, alcohol induced) are examples of those that cause this type of impairment. Gait abnormalities appear when the spasticity is sufficient to cause leg circumduction and fixed deformities (eg, equinovarus), when the Parkinson's produces shuffling steps and reduced arm swing, and when the cerebellar ataxia increases trunk sway sufficiently to require a broad base of gait support.

At the high or central level, the gait impairments become more nonspecific. Lesions in the frontal lobe account for most of the gait abnormalities at this level. The severity of the frontal-related disorders runs a spectrum from difficulty with initiation of gait to frontal disequilibrium, in which unsupported stance is not possible. Cerebrovascular insults to the cortex, as well as to the basal ganglia and their interconnections, may contribute to difficulty with initiation of gait and to apraxia.

Dementia and depression are also thought to contribute to an abnormal gait at the high or central level. With increasing severity of the dementia, particularly in patients with Alzheimer's disease, frontal-related symptoms also increase. Gait impairments in this category have been given a number of overlapping descriptions, including *gait apraxia*, *marche a petits pas*, and *arteriosclerotic parkinsonism*.

More than one disease or impairment is likely to contribute to a gait disorder; one example is the longstanding diabetic patient with peripheral neuropathy and a recent stroke who is now very fearful of falling. Certain disorders can actually involve multiple parts of the nervous system, such as Parkinson's disease affecting cortical and subcortical structures. Drug and metabolic causes (eg, from sedatives, tranquilizers, and anticonvulsants) can involve both central and peripheral nervous systems (eg, phenothiazines can cause central sedation and extrapyramidal effects).

History and Physical Examination

A careful medical history can help elucidate the multiple factors contributing to gait impairments in older patients. A brief systemic evaluation for evidence of subacute metabolic disease (eg, thyroid disorders), acute cardiopulmonary disorders (eg, myocardial infarction), or other acute illness (eg, sepsis) is warranted because an acute gait disorder may be the presenting feature of acute systemic decompensation in older adults. The physical examination should include an attempt to identify motion-related factors, eg, by provoking both vestibular and orthostatic responses. The Dix-Hallpike test (see "Dizziness," p 183) can be performed to test for vestibular dysfunction. Blood pressure should be measured with the patient both supine and standing to exclude orthostatic hypotension. Vision screening, at least for acuity, is essential. The neck, spine, extremities, and feet should be evaluated for pain, deformities, and limitations in range of motion, particularly regarding subtle hip or knee contractures. Leg-length discrepancies such as can occur with a hip prosthesis and either as an antecedent or subsequent to lower back pain can be measured simply as the distance from the anterior superior iliac spine to the medial malleolus. A formal neurologic assessment is critical and should include assessment of strength and tone, sensation (including proprioception), coordination (including cerebellar function), station, and gait. The Romberg test screens for simple postural control and whether the proprioceptive and vestibular systems are functional. Some investigators have proposed that one-legged stance time <5 seconds is a risk factor for injurious falls, although even relatively healthy adults ≥70 yr old can have difficulty with one-legged stance. Given the importance of cognition as a risk factor, assessing cognitive function is also indicated.

Laboratory and Imaging Assessments

Depending on the history and physical examination, further laboratory and diagnostic imaging evaluation may be warranted. A CBC, serum chemistries, and other metabolic studies may be useful when systemic disease is suspected. Head or spine imaging, including radiography, CT, or MRI, is not indicated unless history and physical examination identifies neurologic abnormalities, either preceding or of recent onset, that are related to the gait disorder. However, cerebral white matter changes, often considered to be vascular (termed *leukoaraiosis*), have been increasingly associated with nonspecific gait disorders (SOE=B). Periventricular high signal measurements on MRI as well as increased ventricular volume, even in apparently healthy older adults, are associated with gait slowing. White-matter hyperintensities on MRI correlate with longitudinal changes in balance, and the periventricular frontal and occipitoparietal regions appear to be most affected. Age-specific guidelines for these evaluations and their sensitivity, specificity, and cost-effectiveness of these evaluations remain to be determined.

Performance-Based Functional Assessment

Technologically oriented assessments involving formal kinematic and kinetic analyses have not been applied widely in clinical assessments of balance and gait disorders in older adults. Comfortable gait speed and a related measure, distance walked (as measured by the 6-minute walk test), are powerful predictors of a number of important outcomes, such as disability, institutionalization, and mortality (SOE=B). Several studies have found age- and disease-associated deficits in the ability to walk and perform a simultaneous cognitive task (eg, talking while walking) and have linked these deficits with increased fall risk (SOE=B). Gait speed is faster in individuals who are taller, who have a lower disease burden, and who are more active and less functionally disabled. It has been suggested that slow (impaired) walkers can be defined as those who walk at a speed <0.6 meter/second and that fast (unimpaired) walkers walk at >1 meter/second. While slower gait speed can predict decreased cognition in healthy older adults, the opposite is true as well, namely that decreased cognitive function, particularly executive function, are associated with slower speed.

A number of timed and semiquantitative balance and gait scales have been proposed as a means to detect and quantify abnormalities and to direct interventions. Fall risk, for example, can be increased with more abnormal gait and balance scale scores. Perhaps the simplest battery in the clinical setting is the Timed Up and Go (TUG), a timed sequence of rising from a chair, walking 3 meters, turning, and returning to sit in the chair. One study suggests a TUG score of ≥14 sec as an indicator of fall risk. Other investigators have found limitations in TUG in the presence of cognitive impairment and difficulty in completing the test because of immobility, safety concerns, or refusal. Another functional approach that can be useful clinically is the Functional Ambulation Classification scale, which rates the use of assistive devices, the degree of human assistance (either manual or verbal), the distance the person can walk, and the types of surfaces the person can negotiate (see http://www.cebp.nl/vault_public/filesystem/?ID=1330 [accessed Jan 2011]).

INTERVENTIONS TO REDUCE GAIT DISORDERS

Even if a condition can be diagnosed on evaluation, many conditions causing a gait disorder are, at best, only partially treatable. Functional improvement becomes the treatment goal. Achievement of premorbid gait patterns may be unrealistic, but improvement in measures such as gait speed is reasonable as long as gait remains safe. Comorbidity, disease severity, and overall health status tend to strongly influence treatment outcome.

Many of the older reports dealing with treatment and rehabilitation of gait disorders in older adults are retrospective chart reviews and case studies. Gait disorders presumably secondary to B_{12} deficiency, folate deficiency, hypothyroidism, hyperthyroidism, knee osteoarthritis, Parkinson's disease, and inflammatory polyneuropathy improve with medical therapy.

A variety of modes of physical therapy for knee osteoarthritis can result in modest improvements but continued residual disability. For example, a combined aerobic, strength, and functionally based group exercise program increased gait speed approximately 5% in adults with knee osteoarthritis. The focus is on strengthening the extensor groups (especially knee and hip) and stretching commonly shortened muscles (such as the hip flexors). Randomized controlled trials of exercise for osteoarthritis focus primarily on the knee and can involve strengthening, walking, and aerobic training with positive outcomes on physical function that can include improved walking (SOE=A).

Regarding neurologic disorders, one review suggests unclear effects of conventional physical therapy in treating Parkinson's gait disorders, but that cueing, specifically audio and visual, can improve gait speed (SOE=C). For stroke patients, randomized controlled trials of fair to good quality support the use of strength training, electromyographic biofeedback, and Functional Electrical Stimulation as adjuncts to gait training, while there is conflicting evidence to support the use of ankle-foot orthotics, treadmill training, and partial body-weight support (SOE=B). Meta-analyses of several trials support a beneficial effect on gait of repetitive task-specific training and electromechanical assistance to augment physical therapy after stroke (improvements in 6-minute walk distances of 55 meters [95% CI 18–92] and 34 meters [8–60], respectively [SOE=A]).

A few studies of group exercise have shown improvements in gait parameters such as gait speed. Generally, the most consistent effects are with varied types of exercise provided in the same program (SOE=B). In a 12-week combined program of leg resistance, standing balance, and flexibility exercises, usual gait speed increased 8% in minimally impaired life-care community residents. In a similar varied 16-week format with more intensive individual support and prompting, gait speed increased 23% in selected demented older adults (Mini–Mental State Examination mean score of 15). A number of these studies note improvement in functional, gait-oriented measures (although not strictly gait "disorder" measures), such as the distance walked in 6 minutes by knee osteoarthritis patients undergoing either an aerobic or resistance training program.

Modest improvement and residual disability are also the result of surgical treatment for compressive cervical myelopathy, lumbar stenosis, and NPH. Few controlled prospective studies and no well-controlled randomized studies address the outcome of surgical versus nonsurgical treatment for these three conditions. A number of problems plague the available series: outcomes such as pain and walking disability are not reported separately, the source of the outcome rating is not clearly identified or blinded, the criteria for classifying outcomes differ, the outcomes may be subjective and subject to interpretation, the follow-up intervals are variable, the subjects who are reported in follow-up may be a highly select group, the selection factors for conservative versus surgical treatment between studies differ or are unspecified, and there is publication bias (only positive results are published). Many of the surgical series include all ages, although the mean age is usually >60 yr old. A few studies document equivalent surgical outcomes with conservative, nonsurgical treatment.

With regard to lumbar stenosis procedures, many older adults have reduced pain and improved maximal walking distance after laminectomies and lumbar fusion surgery, although they have continued residual disability (SOE=B). In a somewhat younger cohort (mean age 69 yr) and after an average of 8 yr of follow-up after lumbar stenosis surgery, approximately half reported that they were unable to walk two blocks and many attributed their decreased walking ability to their back problem. Some improvement can be found in selected patients >75 yr old (mean age 78); in an uncontrolled study, 45% of patients with preoperative "severe" limitation of ambulatory ability had either "minimal" or "moderate" limitation postoperatively after an average of 1.5-yr follow-up. Part of the problem in determining long-term gait outcomes of surgery for lumbar stenosis is other comorbidity, such as cardiovascular or musculoskeletal disease, that influences mobility. Nonoperative treatment (with a variety of interventions, including oral anti-inflammatory medications, heating modalities, exercise, mobilizations, and epidural injections) can also result in modest improvements such as in walking tolerance (SOE=B). Regarding cervical stenosis, studies involving postoperative gait outcomes in older adults are limited, but in one nonrandomized study, walking speed improved significantly in most of the postcervical myelopathy decompression patients whose mean age was 60 yr old (SOE=B).

The most substantial improvements after shunt surgery for NPH are seen in gait as opposed to dementia or incontinence (SOE=B). In an uncontrolled study after shunt surgery for NPH (follow-up interval not specified), walking speed increased by >10% in 75% of the patients and by >25% in more than 57% of the patients. While there may be initial improvement after shunt placement, long-term results are often disappointing (eg, in one study, gait disorder initially improved in 65% of patients after shunt surgery, but this improvement was maintained in only 26% by 3-yr follow-up). The poor long-term outcomes may be related to concurrent cerebrovascular and cardiovascular disease, a frequent cause of mortality in these cohorts. Gait outcomes after shunt surgery may be better in those in whom the gait disturbance precedes cognitive impairment and in those who respond with improved gait speed after a trial of cerebrospinal fluid removal (SOE=B).

Outcomes for hip and knee replacement surgery for osteoarthritis are better, although some of the same study methodologic problems exist. Multidisciplinary rehabilitation (versus more limited rehabilitation) after hip or knee replacement results in improved global functioning beyond walking measures (SOE=A). Other than pain relief, sizable gains in gait speed and joint motion occur, although residual walking disability continues for a number of reasons, including residual pathology on the operated side and symptoms on the nonoperated side. In one longitudinal cohort study, self-reported walking-related function was improved in osteoarthritis patients undergoing total hip replacement compared to those who received medical therapy (SOE=B). For joint replacements, despite rehabilitation after surgery, some residual weakness, stiffness, and slowed/altered gait and balance may remain. Simple function may be maintained after knee replacement, such as maintaining the ability to safely clear an obstacle, but usually at the expense of additional compensation by the ipsilateral hip and foot.

Finally, the use of orthoses and other mobility aids can help reduce gait disorders (SOE=C). Although there are few data supporting their use, lifts (either internal or external) to correct for limb length inequality can be used in a conservative, gradually progressive manner. Other ankle braces, shoe inserts, shoe body and sole modifications, and their subsequent adjustments are part of standard care for foot and ankle weakness, deformities, and pain but are beyond the scope of this chapter. In general, well-fitting walking shoes with low heels, relatively thin firm soles, and if feasible, high, fixed heel collar support are recommended to maximize balance and improve gait. Mobility aids such as canes and walkers reduce load on a painful joint and increase stability. Note that light touch of any firm surface like walls or "furniture surfing" provide feedback and enhance balance. See also "Rehabilitation," p 130; and "Diseases and Disorders of the Foot," p 456.

ACOVE-3* QUALITY INDICATORS PERTAINING TO GAIT IMPAIRMENT

Gait and balance evaluation

- If a vulnerable older adult has new or worsening difficulty with ambulation, balance, or mobility, then there should be documentation of a basic gait, balance, and strength evaluation within 3 mo of the report.

Assistive device for balance disorder

- If a vulnerable older adult demonstrates decreased balance or proprioception or excessive postural sway and does not have an assistive device, then an evaluation or prescription for an assistive device should be offered within 3 mo.

Exercise program

- If a vulnerable older adult has a problem with gait, balance, strength, or endurance, then there should be documentation of a structured or supervised exercise program offered in the previous 6 mo or within 3 mo of the report.

Related quality indicators for Gait Impairment

Evaluation and management of falls (see "Falls," p 224)

*Assessing Care of Vulnerable Elders – 3rd Set. See inside front cover for explanation.

REFERENCES

- Mehrholz J, Werner C, Kugler J, et al. Electro-mechanical-assisted training for walking after stroke. *Cochrane Database Syst Rev.* 2007;(4):CD006185.

- Persad CC, Jones JL, Asthon-Miller JA, et al. Executive function and gait in older adults with cognitive impairment. *J Gerontol A Biol Sci Med Sci.* 2008;63(12):1350−1355.

CHAPTER 30—FALLS

KEY POINTS

■ A fall is one of the most common events threatening the independence of older adults. Complications resulting from falls are the leading cause of death from injury in men and women ≥65 yr old.

■ The causes of a fall often involve a complex interaction among factors intrinsic to the individual (age-related declines, chronic disease, acute illness, medications), challenges to postural control (environment, changing position, normal activities), and mediating factors (risk-taking behaviors, underlying mobility level).

■ For patients presenting with a fall, important components of the history include the activity of the patient at the time of the fall, the occurrence of prodromal symptoms (lightheadedness, imbalance, and dizziness), and the location of the fall. Older adults with a single fall should be evaluated for gait and balance.

■ For older adults with two or more falls in the past 12 mo or with gait or balance abnormalities, a multifactorial falls risk assessment should be pursued.

■ Interventions shown to be effective in reducing falls include medication review, exercise programs including muscle strengthening and balance training, vitamin D supplementation, use of appropriate footwear, and multifactorial interventions including home hazards assessment for those at high risk of falls.

PREVALENCE AND MORBIDITY

A fall is one of the most common events threatening the independence of older adults. A fall is considered to have occurred when a person comes to rest inadvertently on the ground or lower level. Most of the literature on falls in older adults does not include falls associated with loss of consciousness (eg, syncope, seizure) or with overwhelming trauma, because most falls are not associated with syncope or trauma.

According to a report by the CDC, 5.8 million U.S. adults (16%) >65 yr old report falling in the previous month, and 33% report falling in the previous year. The incidence of falls is more frequent with advancing age and among nursing-home residents, such that one-half of individuals >80 yr old or nursing-home residents will fall each year. Among those with a history of a fall in the previous year, the annual incidence of falls is close to 60%. Almost one-third of those who fall need medical attention related to the fall or need to restrict their activities for at least 1 day as a result of the fall. Women are more likely to experience a fall-related injury than men. Most falls result in minor soft-tissue injury, while 10%–15% of falls result in fracture, and 5% of falls result in more serious soft-tissue injury or head trauma. Among nursing-home residents, the incidence of major soft-tissue injury or fracture related to a fall is twice that in community dwellers. In general, falls are associated with subsequent declines in functional status, greater likelihood of nursing-home placement, increased use of medical services, and the development of a fear of falling. Of those older adults who fall, only half are able to get up without help, thus experiencing the "long lie." Long lies are associated with lasting declines in functional status.

Fall-related injuries are not a common cause of death in older adults; however, complications resulting from falls are the leading cause of death from injury in men and women ≥65 yr old. The death rate attributable to falls increases with age, with white men ≥85 yr old having the highest death rate (>180 deaths per 100,000 population).

The true cost of falls in healthcare dollars is difficult to ascertain. Because many falls result in injury, use of emergency department facilities among those who fall is significant. Studies from the early 1990s indicate that each year almost 8% of adults ≥70 yr old are evaluated in emergency departments because of a fall-related injury, and close to one-third of these adults are admitted to the hospital for a median length of stay of 8 days. In 2000, the direct cost of medical visits for falls and services/therapies for fall-related injuries totaled $19 billion in the United States. Indirect costs from fall-related injuries, such as hip fractures, can be substantial.

CAUSES

Falls, incontinence, delirium, and other geriatric syndromes result from the accumulated effects of multiple impairments. In older adults, falls rarely have a single cause. Rather, there is often a complex interaction among factors intrinsic to the individual (age-related declines, chronic disease, acute illness, medications), challenges to postural control (environment, changing positions, normal activities), and mediating factors (risk-taking behaviors, underlying mobility level).

In multiple prospective cohort studies, several risk factors have been consistently associated with falls, including older age, cognitive impairment, female gender, past history of a fall, leg or gait problems, foot disorders, balance problems, hypovitaminosis D, psychotropic medication use, Parkinson's disease, stroke, and arthritis (SOE=B). These studies differed significantly in the types of risk factors evaluated, the types of population studied (eg, past fall history was sometimes an entry criterion), and the outcome (one fall, two or more falls, rate of falls, injurious falls). The multiple risk factors found across the studies highlight the multifactorial nature of falls and suggest that there may also be unique circumstances surrounding falls that were not accounted for. In general, the risk of falling increases with the number of risk factors, although as many as 10% of falls occur in individuals with no identifiable risk factor for falls.

Successful prevention of falls begins with knowledge of the age-related changes that increase the risk of falls. With aging, there are declines in the visual, proprioceptive, and vestibular systems. For example, the visual system has reduced visual acuity, depth perception, contrast sensitivity, and dark adaptation. The proprioceptive system loses sensitivity in the legs. The vestibular system has a loss of labyrinthine hair cells, vestibular ganglion cells, and nerve fibers.

Despite these age-related changes in sensory systems, quantifying the age-related changes in postural control that are independent of disease is difficult. In general, when postural stability is tested in young and old people with no apparent musculoskeletal or neurologic impairment, age-related differences in measured sway are most pronounced with moderately severe perturbations of stance, such as changing the support surface, changing body position, altering the visual input, or moving the support surface horizontally or rotationally. This occurs because these perturbations stress the redundancy of the sensory systems in their ability to maintain postural stability. This is borne out by the observation that gait speed deteriorates when individuals are presented with a dual task ("walking while talking"). In addition, there may be other age-related changes in the CNS that affect postural control, including the loss of neurons and dendrites, and the depletion of neurotransmitters, such as dopamine, within the basal ganglia.

Because it is difficult to find older adults without at least subtle neurologic findings, studies have been unable to determine whether some of the differences between young and old people may be due to these factors. Some of the most striking postural control differences between young and old people relate to the order or grouping of muscle activation patterns. Thus, in response to perturbations of the support surface, older adults tend to activate the proximal muscles, such as the quadriceps, before the more distal muscles, such as the tibialis anterior. This strategy may not be an efficient way to maintain postural stability. Similarly, in older adults, there may be greater co-contraction of antagonistic muscles, and the onset of the muscle activation and associated joint torque may be delayed. Finally, the ability to recover balance upon a postural disturbance may be compromised by an age-related decline in the ability to rapidly develop joint torque by using muscles of the leg. All these strategies potentially impair maintenance of upright posture.

Another important physiologic contributor to the successful maintenance of upright posture is the regulation of systemic blood pressure. Lack of brain perfusion, which accompanies hypotension, increases the risk of a fall, usually in association with syncope. In addition to the age-related declines in baroreflex sensitivity to hypotensive stimuli manifested as a lack of increased heart rate, everyday stresses (such as changing posture, eating a meal, or suffering an acute illness) can result in hypotension. Because many older adults have a resting cerebral perfusion that is compromised by vascular disease, even slight reductions in blood pressure can result in cerebral ischemic symptoms, such as falls. Finally, with aging, the amount of total body water is reduced, which places older adults at increased risk of dehydration with acute illness, diuretic use, or hot weather. Because with aging, basal and stimulated renin levels progressively decrease and aldosterone production decreases, dehydrating stresses can lead to orthostatic hypotension and falls.

A number of age-related chronic conditions deserve special mention because of their association with fall risk. Parkinson's disease, in particular, increases the risk of falls through several mechanisms, including the rigidity of leg musculature, the inability to correct sway trajectory because of the slowness in beginning movement, hypotensive effects of medication, and in some cases, cognitive impairment. Strokes can also result in an increased risk of falls secondary to visuospatial defects, impaired peripheral sensation, cerebellar dysfunction, and residual dizziness. Another common disease contributing to falls is osteoarthritis. When present in the knee, osteoarthritis can affect mobility, the ability to step over objects and maneuver, and the tendency to avoid complete weight bearing on a painful joint.

One of the most modifiable risk factors for falls that has been repeatedly demonstrated in observa-

Table 30.1—The Role of Setting in the Assessment and Management of Falls Risk

Characteristic	Home	Hospital	Nursing Home
How falls come to clinical attention	Patient or family reports or clinician queries patient	Staff witnesses fall or finds patient on floor	Staff witnesses fall or finds resident on floor
Assessment of falls risk	Age Past history of fall Cognitive impairment Female gender Leg weakness Gait problems, foot disorders Balance problems Hypovitaminosis D Psychotropic medication use Arthritis Parkinson's disease	Age Past history of a fall Impaired mental status Special toileting needs Impaired mobility Visual impairment	Using MDS data: Age ≥87 yr old Past history of fall Cognitive impairment Unsteady gait Wandering Walking aid ADL deterioration Transfer independence Wheelchair independence
Management	Muscle strengthening or balance training prescribed by clinician[a] (SOE=A) Tai Chi (SOE=B) Home-hazard assessment prescribed for those with history of falls[a] (SOE=A) Multidisciplinary, multifactorial health, and environmental risk-factor screening or intervention for:[a] (SOE=A) ▪ unselected community-dwelling older adults ▪ older adults with a history of falling ▪ older adults selected because of known risk factors Withdrawal of psychotropic medications (SOE=B) Vitamin D supplementation at ≥800 IU/d[b] (SOE=A)	No proven interventions have been reported. Many risk assessments have reasonable sensitivity and specificity to be of potential value in targeting high-risk patients if a proven intervention is developed.	No proven interventions have been reported. Reasonable to target resident's most important individual risk factors[c] (SOE=B) Because nursing-home residents are a high-risk population, it is also prudent to apply universal precautions (SOE=C). Vitamin D supplementation at ≥800 IU/d for ambulatory residents[b] (SOE=A)

NOTE: MDS = Minimum data set

[a] Based on Gillespie L, Gillespie W, Robertson M, et al. Interventions for preventing falls in elderly people. *Cochrane Database Syst Rev.* 2003;(4):CD00340.

[b] Based on Bischoff-Ferrari HA, Dawson-Hughes B, Willett WC, et al. Effect of vitamin D on falls: a meta-analysis. *JAMA.* 2004;291(16):1999–2006.

[c] Based on Coussement J, De Paepe L, Schwendimann R, et al. Interventions for preventing falls in acute- and chronic-care hospitals: a systematic review and meta-analysis. *J Am Geriatr Soc.* 2008;56(1):29–36. decreases, dehydrating stresses can lead to orthostatic hypotension and a fall.

tional studies is medication use. Individual classes of psychotropic medications, such as the benzodiazepines, other sedatives, antidepressants, and antipsychotic medications, have been associated with an increased risk of falls or hip fracture. There appears to be no difference in the risk of falling with the use of older antidepressants versus that of SSRIs. An increased risk of falling has also been associated with recent changes of a benzodiazepine or antipsychotic medication. As might be expected, the risk of falls increases in older adults taking more than one psychotropic medication, and among older adults taking more than 3 or 4 medications of any type.

Other medications that have been associated with falls include certain cardiac medications and hypoglycemic agents. A meta-analysis found that digoxin, diuretics, and type 1A antiarrhythmic agents were associated with a small increased risk of falls. It is less clear whether there is an association between falls and other cardiac medications, including nitrates and centrally acting antihypertensive agents. Hypoglycemic agents can also be associated with fall risk during periods of hypoglycemia. Prospective studies are needed to determine whether an independent association between these medications and falls exists, or whether these medications are simply a surrogate marker for older adults with diabetic neuropathy, a chronic risk factor for falls.

The relative importance of environmental factors on the risk of falling appears to be much less than intrinsic factors of the individual; however, the interaction between environmental factors and intrinsic factors has not been well quantified. Most intervention studies have focused on improving the risk-factor profile of the individual or have combined individual interventions with environmental manipulation, making it difficult to isolate the contributions of the environmental factors. Nevertheless, attention to safety hazards in the home environment appears to be worthwhile.

DIAGNOSTIC APPROACH

The evaluation and management of falls in older adults may differ according to the clinical setting (eg, home, hospital, nursing home). For some differences that might be considered according to setting, see Table 30.1.

History and Physical Examination

Many falls never come to clinical attention for a variety of reasons: the patient may never mention the event, there is no injury at the time of the fall, the clinician may neglect to ask the patient about a history of falls, or the patient or the clinician may make the invalid assumption that falls are an inevitable part of the aging process. In institutional settings, despite attention to falls and incident reporting, not all falls come to the attention of the nursing staff. The treatment of injuries resulting from falls commonly fails to include an investigation of the cause of the fall.

In the clinical evaluation of noninstitutionalized older adults who are not being seen specifically for a problem with falling, it is still important that an assessment of fall risk be integrated into the history and physical examination. (For an overview of falls assessment and management in all older adults, see Figure 30.1.) The most important point in the history is asking whether there is a previous history of a fall, because this is a strong risk factor for future falls. Older adults presenting with a single fall should be evaluated for gait and balance. Older adults with two or more falls in the past 12 mo or with gait or balance abnormalities should undergo a multifactorial falls risk assessment.

For patients presenting with a fall, important components of the history include the activity at the time of the incident, the occurrence of prodromal symptoms (lightheadedness, imbalance, dizziness), and the location and time of the fall. Loss of consciousness is associated with injurious falls and should raise important considerations, such as orthostatic hypotension or cardiac or neurologic disease. (See "Syncope," p 188.) Information on previous falls should be collected to identify patterns that may help target strategies to reduce risk factors. A complete medication history should focus particularly on the use of diuretics and psychotropic medications because of their association with falls and their common use in older adults. In addition to inquiring about the circumstances surrounding the fall, the clinician should attempt to identify any potential contributing environmental factors. Information on lighting, floor coverings, door thresholds, railings, and furniture can add important clues. Footwear can also be an important factor. In one small study that evaluated the effect of various shoe types on balance in older men, shoes with thin, hard soles produced the best results, even though they were perceived as less comfortable than thick, soft, mid-soled shoes, such as running shoes. In another nested-case control study of men and women, athletic shoes were associated with the lowest risk of falls, and shoes with increased heel height and decreased surface area between the sole and the floor were associated with a higher risk of falls.

The physical examination of the person who has fallen should focus on risk factors. Much of the examination duplicates that done in a gait assessment (see "Gait Impairment," p 219). Probably the most important part of the physical examination is an assessment of integrated musculoskeletal function, which can be accomplished by performing one or more of the following tests of postural stability. A simple maneuver called the *functional reach test* is a practical way to test the integrated neuromuscular base of support and has predictive validity for falls in older men. This test is performed with a leveled yardstick secured to a wall at the height of the acromion. The person being tested assumes a comfortable stance without shoes or socks and stands so that his or her shoulders are perpendicular to the yardstick. He or she makes a fist and extends the arm forward as far as possible along the wall without taking a step or losing balance. The total reach is measured along the yardstick and recorded. Inability to reach ≥ 6 inches is cause for concern and merits further evaluation. In its initial description, the functional reach correlated with other physical performance measures, such as walking speed ($r=0.71$), tandem walk using an ordinal scale ($r=0.67$), and standing on one foot measured as number of seconds that a one-footed stance could be maintained ($r=0.64$). Another useful test of integrated strength and balance is the Timed Up and Go test, which can be performed with or without timing. It consists of observation of an individual standing up from a chair without using the arms to push against the chair, walking across a room, turning around, walking back, and sitting down without using the arms. This test can demonstrate muscle weakness, balance problems, and gait abnormalities. A third test of integrated musculoskeletal function is the Berg Balance Test. The Berg test includes 14 items of balance, including timed tandem stance, semitandem stance, and the ability of a person to retrieve an object from the floor. Berg scores <40 have been associated with an increased risk of falls. Lastly, the Performance-Oriented Mobil-

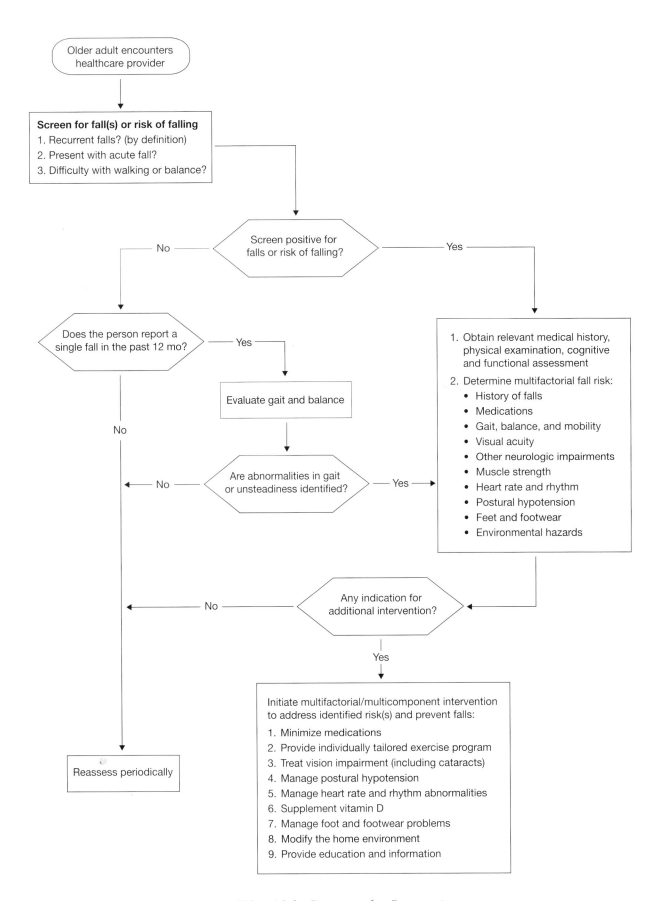

Figure 30.1—Prevention of Falls in Older Adults Living in the Community

SOURCE: Reuben DB, Herr KA, Pacala JT, et al. *Geriatrics At Your Fingertips*, 12th ed. New York: American Geriatrics Society; 2010. Reprinted with permission.

ity Assessment (POMA) tests balance and gait through a number of items, including ability to sit and stand from an armless chair, ability to maintain standing balance when pulled by an examiner, and the ability to walk normally and maneuver obstacles. A reliable cut-point score for predicting falls with the POMA has yet to be established.

Laboratory and Diagnostic Tests

There is no standard diagnostic evaluation of a person with a history of falls or a high risk of falling. Obviously, laboratory tests for hemoglobin, BUN, creatinine, or glucose concentrations can help to exclude anemia, dehydration, or hyperglycemia with hyperosmolar dehydration as the cause of falling. There is no proven value of routinely performing Holter monitoring of individuals who have fallen. Because data demonstrate that carotid sinus hypersensitivity contributes to falls and even hip fracture, some have advocated performing carotid sinus massage with continuous heart rate and phasic blood pressure measurement in older adults with unexplained falls. Similarly, the decision to perform echocardiography, brain imaging, or radiographic studies of the spine should be driven by the findings of the history and physical examination. Echocardiography should be reserved for those with cardiac conditions believed to contribute to the maintenance of blood flow to the brain. Spine radiographs or MRI can be useful in patients with gait disorders, abnormalities on neurologic examination, leg spasticity, or hyperreflexia to exclude cervical spondylosis or lumbar stenosis as a cause of falls.

TREATMENT AND PREVENTION

Multiple studies of preventive interventions have been conducted over the past decade, including programs to improve strength or balance, educational programs, optimization of medications, and environmental modifications in homes or institutions. Some interventions have targeted single risk factors; others have attempted to address multiple factors by either targeting patient-specific risk factors (multifactorial intervention) or by offering the interventions to an entire population (multicomponent intervention).

A Cochrane collaboration systematic review of interventions to reduce the incidence of falling in older adults was performed. Because of the large numbers of fall intervention trials and because interventions may be more effective in certain settings, systematic reviews of fall interventions were divided into two groups: fall prevention interventions among community dwellers and fall prevention interventions among institutionalized persons. The April 2009 update of the Cochrane systematic review of fall interventions among community dwellers included

111 individual trials. As of January 2008, a systematic review of falls interventions in acute and chronic hospital settings included 8 trials.

In 2009, the American Geriatrics Society and the British Geriatrics Society published clinical practice guidelines for the prevention of falls in older adults. These guidelines advocate for initiating multifactorial/multicomponent interventions to address identified risks and to prevent falls; these interventions should include an education component addressing issues specific to the intervention being provided and tailored to the individual's cognitive ability and language. Additionally, offering an exercise program to incorporate balance, gait, and strength training was suggested for older adults at risk of falls. The guidelines place these intervention measures into the following nine groups:

- **Minimize medications:** In one study of 93 community dwellers, a gradual taper of psychotropic medications was associated with a decreased rate of falls (relative hazard 0.34; confidence interval [CI] 95%, 0.16–0.74) (SOE=B). Multifactorial interventions that include education and a review of medications with cessation or dose reduction when possible have also successfully reduced the number of fallers among community dwellers (SOE=B).

- **Initiate an individually tailored exercise program:** As of the 2009 Cochrane review, 43 trials tested the efficacy of exercise as an intervention to prevent falls in the community setting. Exercise classes utilizing more than one type of exercise (eg, gait training, balance, strengthening) were effective in reducing the rate of falls (14 trials; 2,364 participants; relative risk [RR] 0.83; CI 95%, 0.72–0.97) (SOE=A). Tai Chi, which combines both strengthening and balance measures, is effective in reducing the risk of falls among community dwellers (RR 0.65; CI 95%, 0.51–0.82) (SOE=A).

- **Treat vision impairment:** First cataract surgery results in a decreased rate of falls (1 trial; 306 participants; RR 0.66; CI 95%, 0.45–0.95) (SOE=B). Second cataract surgery showed no benefit in reducing the rate of falls or number of fallers. Routine eye screening with correction of visual defects is considered good medical practice. It has not been demonstrated to be effective in reducing falls as a single intervention. Multifactorial interventions that include visual screening and/or treatment have been shown to have a modest effect in reducing the risk of falls.

- **Manage postural hypotension:** A postural fall in blood pressure has not consistently been associated with an increased risk of falls. Nevertheless, the sensation of dizziness is strongly associated with an increased risk of falls, and thus, treating orthostatic hypotension may be prudent among certain groups of older adults at risk of falls. Achieving better control of systolic blood pressure has been associated with a decrease in postural changes in blood pressure. It is unclear whether this might also translate into a decreased risk of falls. While no trial to date has addressed whether a single intervention to reduce orthostasis results in decreased falls, multifactorial interventions that include fluid optimization, medication review and reduction, and behavioral changes have shown a modest effect in reducing the risk of falls among community dwellers (SOE=B).

■ **Manage heart rate and rhythm abnormalities:** One trial demonstrated a reduction in the rate of falls among older adults with carotid sinus hypersensitivity treated with a pacemaker (175 participants; weighted mean difference −5.20; CI 95%, −9.40 to −1.00) (SOE=B).

■ **Supplement vitamin D:** In 2004, a meta-analysis found that higher doses of vitamin D (at least 700–800 IU) have been associated with a 6.7% absolute reduction in the risk of falls among community-dwelling and institutionalized older adults (CI 95%, 0.02–0.13). While the exact mechanism is unknown, it is believed that vitamin D may reduce falls by increasing muscle strength and decreasing body sway. Vitamin D supplementation also improves bone mineral density and reduces the risk of vertebral and nonvertebral fractures (number needed to treat [NNT]=15) (SOE=A).

■ **Manage foot and footwear problems:** One small trial (109 participants) demonstrated a reduction in falls among community-dwelling older adults wearing a nonslip shoe covering during icy conditions (RR 0.42; CI 95%, 0.22–0.78) (SOE=B). Footwear associated with higher heels and decreased surface area has been associated with an increased risk of falls. Although there are limited data to demonstrate that avoiding more risky types of footwear prevents falls, clinicians should advise their patients to use walking shoes with high contact surface area.

■ **Modify the home environment:** When included as part of a multifactorial intervention, home environment assessments with environmental modification performed by a healthcare professional reduces the risk of falling among older adults who have fallen or are at high risk of falling because of visual impairment (2 trials; 491 participants; RR 0.56; CI 95%, 0.42–0.76) (SOE=A).

■ **Provide education and information:** There is little direct evidence to demonstrate that education on falls and fall-related injuries results in a reduction in fall risk. Nonetheless, it may be prudent for clinicians to educate older adults at risk of falls on home hazards, proper choices for footwear, and the importance of regular exercise.

Additionally, several multifactorial interventions in which participants received more than one intervention were effective in reducing the rate of falls (15 trials; 8,141 participants; pooled RR 0.75; CI 95%, 0.65–0.86) (SOE=A). Because these trials were conducted in different populations and used different interventions, it is unclear which combinations of interventions are the most effective.

A number of interventions have not been effective for fall prevention, including group-delivered exercise interventions (SOE=B), nutritional supplementation (SOE=C), isolated modification of home hazards (SOE=B), cognitive-behavioral approach (SOE=B), hormone therapy (SOE=C), and individual strength training (SOE=B).

Fall prevention programs in nursing-home and acute-care settings have been largely unsuccessful to date. Only cluster-randomized trials using a multifactorial intervention including personalized exercises have been successful in reducing falls or in reducing falls within certain subgroups in the long-term care setting (SOE=B). A meta-analysis and systematic review of fall prevention trials in the long-term care setting and acute inpatient setting found a tendency toward a reduction in falls in individual studies that targeted residents' most important risk factors for falls in the long-term care setting. However, the authors found no conclusive evidence that hospital fall prevention programs can reduce the number of falls or fallers.

A practical approach for clinicians who are treating older adults with a high risk of or a history of falls includes targeting risk factors for falls in three major domains: medications, mobility, and medical conditions (Table 30.2). More studies are needed to confirm whether successful fall prevention strategies are also effective in reducing more serious sequelae of falls, such as fractures or other injuries.

HIP PROTECTORS

Systematic reviews have concluded that there is no evidence that hip protectors are effective in reducing hip fractures in studies that randomized individual

Table 30.2—Preventing Falls: Selected Risk Factors and Suggested Interventions

Factors	Suggested Interventions
Medication-Related Factors	
Use of benzodiazepines, sedative-hypnotics, antidepressants, or antipsychotics	Consider agents with less risk of falls Taper dosage and discontinue medications, as possible Address sleep mood problems with nonpharmacologic interventions (see "Sleep Problems," p 272) Educate regarding appropriate use of medications and monitoring for adverse events
Recent change in dosage or number of prescription medications *or* use of ≥4 prescription medications *or* use of other medications associated with fall risk	Review medication profile and reduce number and dosage of all medications, as possible Monitor response to medications and to dosage changes
Mobility-Related Factors	
Presence of environmental hazards (eg, improper bed height, cluttered walking surfaces, lack of railings, poor lighting)	Improve lighting, especially at night Remove floor barriers (eg, loose carpeting) Replace existing furniture with safer furniture (eg, correct height, more stable) Install support structures, especially in bahtroom (eg, railings, grab bars, elevated toilet seat) Use nonslip bath mats
Impaired gait, balance, or transfer skills	Refer to physical therapy for comprehensive evaluation and rehabilitation and for training in use of assistive devices Gait training Balance or strengthening exercises If able to perform tandem stance, refer for Tai Chi, dance, yoga, or postural awareness Provide training in transfer skills Prescribe appropriate assistive devices Recommend appropriate footwear (eg, good fit, nonslip, low heel height, large surface contact area)
Impaired leg or arm strength or range of motion, or proprioception	Strengthening exercises (eg, use of resistive rubber bands, putty) Resistance training 2–3 times/week to 10 repetitions with full range of motion, then increase resistance Tai Chi Physical therapy
Medical Factors	
Parkinson's disease, osteoarthritis, depressive symptoms, impaired cognition, carotid sinus hypersensitivity, other conditions associated with increased falls	Optimize medical therapy Monitor for disease progression and impact on mobility and impairments Determine need for assistive devices Use bedside commode if frequent nighttime urination Cardiac pacing in patiends with carotid sinus hypersensitivity who experience falls due to syncope

Postural hypotension: drop in systolic blood pressure ≥20 mmHg (or ≥20%) with or without symptoms, within 3 minutes of rising from lying to standing	Review medications potentially contributing and adjust dosing or switch to less hypotensive agents; avoid vasodilators and diuretics if possible
	Educate on activities to decrease effect (eg, slow rising, ankle pumps, hand clenching, elevation of head of bed) and to slow rising from recumbent or seated position, grab bars by toilet and bath
	Prescribe pressure stockings
	Liberalize salt intake if appropriate
	Caffeinated coffee (1 cup) or caffeine 100 mg with meals for postprandial hypotension
	Consider medication to increase blood pressure (if hypertension, heart failure, and hypokalemia not serious):
	  ▪ midodrine 2.5–5 mg q8h
	  ▪ fludrocortisone 0.1 mg q8–24h

Table 30.2—Preventing Falls: Selected Risk Factors and Suggested Interventions (continued)

Factors	Suggested Interventions
Vision or hearing impairment	Refraction Cataract extraction Good lighting Home safety evaluation Mobility training for visually impaired Cerumen removal Audiologic evaluation with hearing aid, if appropriate

SOURCE: Adapted with permission from Reuben DB, Herr KA, Pacala JT, et al. *Geriatrics At Your Fingertips*, 12th ed. New York: American Geriatrics Society; 2010.

patients within an institution or among older adults living at home. However, adherence to the use of hip protectors was low in these studies, which many argue could explain the lack of efficacy. Prior studies that found a benefit with hip protectors randomly assigned groups of patients to an intervention based on setting (eg, by ward in a nursing home); thus, these studies were potentially susceptible to bias because unintended "co-interventions" can occur when whole units or facilities participate in trials and are allocated to use hip protectors. A more recent multi-institutional study in which individual nursing-home residents were randomized for use of a right- or left-sided hip protector found no reduction in fractures on the protected hip (SOE=B).

At least a dozen types of hip protectors are commercially available. Many of these hip protectors have not been tested in either the laboratory or in clinical trials. Despite the lack of evidence to date to support the use of hip protectors, it is not unreasonable to consider their use in patients at high risk of hip fractures who are willing to use them.

CLINICAL GUIDELINES

For older adults who have sustained a fall, a multifactorial approach is appropriate, and it should consider known risk factors for falls, include a multidimensional assessment of the patient, and target interventions on the basis of these findings. For older adults who have no history of falling, it is reasonable to use traditional multidimensional geriatric assessment with targeted interventions as risk factors are identified. For a summary of the recommendations of the expert panel on falls prevention assembled by the American Geriatrics Society and the British Geriatrics Society, see www.americangeriatrics.org.

ACOVE-3* QUALITY INDICATORS PERTAINING TO FALLS

Screening for falls

- All vulnerable older adults should have documentation that they were asked annually about the occurrence of recent falls.

Fall history

- If a vulnerable older adult reports a history of two or more falls (or one fall with injury) in the previous year, then there should be documentation of a basic fall history (circumstances, medications, chronic conditions, mobility, alcohol intake) within 3 mo of the report (or within 4 weeks of the report if the most recent fall occurred in the previous 4 weeks).

Fall examination

- If a vulnerable older adult reports a history of two or more falls (or one fall with injury) in the previous year, then there should be documentation of orthostatic vital signs (blood pressure and pulse) within 3 mo of the report (or within 4 weeks of the report if the most recent fall occurred in the previous 4 weeks).

- If a vulnerable older adult reports a history of two or more falls (or one fall with injury) in the previous year, then there should be documentation of receipt of an eye examination in the previous year or evidence of visual acuity testing within 3 mo of the report.

- If a vulnerable older adult reports a history of two or more falls (or one fall with injury) in the previous year, then there should be documentation of a basic gait, balance, and strength evaluation within 3 mo of the report (or within 4 weeks of the report if the most recent fall occurred in the previous 4 weeks).

Cognitive evaluation for fall

- If a vulnerable older adult reports a history of two or more falls (or one fall with injury) in the previous year, then there should be documentation of an assessment of cognitive status in the previous 6 mo or within 3 mo of the report (or within 4 weeks of the report if the most recent fall occurred in the previous 4 weeks).

Home hazard evaluation

- If a vulnerable older adult reports a history of two or more falls (or one fall with injury) in the previous year, then there should be documentation of an assessment and modification of home hazards recommended in the previous year or within 3 mo of the report.

Inpatient fall evaluation

- If a vulnerable older adult falls during hospitalization, then the following should be documented within 24 hours:
  - Presence or absence of prodromal symptoms
  - Review of medications or drugs potentially contributing to the fall

Benzodiazepine discontinuation

- If a vulnerable older adult reports a history of two or more falls (or one fall with injury) in the previous year and is taking a benzodiazepine, then there should be documentation of a discussion of related risks and assistance offered to reduce or discontinue benzodiazepine use.

Assistive device review

- If a vulnerable older adult reports a history of two or more falls (or one fall with injury) in the previous year and has an assistive device, then there should be documentation of an assistive device review in the previous 6 mo or within 3 mo of the report (or within 4 weeks of the report if the most recent fall occurred in the previous 4 weeks).

Related quality indicators for Falls

- Gait and balance evaluation, balance disorders, exercise (see "Gait Impairment," p 218)

*Assessing Care of Vulnerable Elders – 3ʳᵈ Set. See inside front cover for explanation.

REFERENCES

- AMDA – Dedicated to Long Term Care Medicine. *Clinical Practice Guideline: Falls and Fall Risk.* http://www.amda.com/tools/guidelines.cfm#falls

- American Geriatrics Society and British Geriatrics Society. *Clinical Practice Guideline for the Prevention of Falls in Older Persons.* New York: American Geriatrics Society; 2009 (http://www.americangeriatrics.org/).

- Cotter V. Avoiding Restraints in Older Adults with Dementia. *Try This: Best Practices in Nursing Care to Older Adults.* 2007;(D1). Available at http://consultgerirn.org/uploads/File/trythis/try_this_d1.pdf

- Coussement J, De Paepe L, Schwendimann R, et al. Interventions for preventing falls in acute- and chronic-care hospitals: a systematic review and meta-analysis. *J Am Geriatr Soc.* 2008;56(1):29–36.

- Gillespie L, Gillespie W, Robertson M, et al. Interventions for preventing falls in older people living in the community. *Cochrane Database Syst Rev.* 2009;(3):CD00340; 2003 update.

- Gray-Miceli D. Fall Risk Assessment for Older Adults: The Hendrich II Fall Risk Model. *Try This: Best Practices in Nursing Care to Older Adults.* 2007;(8). Available at http://consultgerirn.org/uploads/File/trythis/try_this_8.pdf

- Hartikainen S, Lönnroos E, Louhivuori K. Medication as a risk factor for falls: critical systematic review. *J Gerontol A Biol Sci Med Sci.* 2007;62A(10):1172–1181.

CHAPTER 31—OSTEOPOROSIS

KEY POINTS

- Osteoporosis is a common metabolic bone disorder affecting older women and men (4:1) that is preventable and treatable. The resultant fractures can lead to chronic pain, decreased mobility, loss of independence and function, and mortality.

- Vitamin D deficiency, which can cause bone loss and osteomalacia, is common in older adults and is treatable and preventable; it should be considered in older adults with osteoporosis, myalgias, fatigue, proximal muscle weakness, and fractures.

- Measurement of bone mineral density (BMD) is recommended routinely in women ≥65 yr old, and in younger patients and men with risk factors for osteoporosis.

- Secondary osteoporosis should be excluded in men and women with osteoporosis. Common causes of secondary osteoporosis include medications, hypogonadism, hyperthyroidism, hyperparathyroidism, and osteomalacia.

- Prevention of osteoporosis includes adequate calcium and vitamin D intake, weightbearing exercise, and use of bisphosphonates as first-line pharmacologic treatment. Consideration of teriparatide in severe osteoporosis is also warranted.

- Because osteoporosis is a result of unbalanced bone formation and resorption, and associated fractures usually involve a fall, optimal prevention and treatment include strategies to minimize bone resorption and to reduce falls, as well as measures to reduce risk factors, especially smoking, low physical activity, and poor diet.

DEFINITION

Osteoporosis, the most common metabolic bone disease, is a major cause of morbidity, loss of independence, and mortality in the older population. It was defined in 1993 by a Consensus Development Conference panel as a "disease characterized by low bone mass and micro-architectural deterioration of bone tissue leading to enhanced bone fragility and consequent increase in fracture risk." Prevention of fractures is the main goal of any program of prevention and treatment.

The World Health Organization (WHO) defines osteoporosis in two ways. The first is by BMD measurement performed by dual energy x-ray absorptiometry (DEXA), which allows diagnosis and treatment of osteoporosis before incident fracture. The basis for the WHO-defined DEXA criteria is from analysis of fracture data in postmenopausal white women. The second is by the occurrence of fragility fracture, which is defined as any fracture that occurs from standing height or below, and in a situation in which a pathologic fracture has been excluded.

If a woman has a BMD measurement at any site <2.5 standard deviations below the young adult standard (a T score of less than −2.5), the diagnosis of osteoporosis can be made. Further, DEXA can be used to identify women with osteopenia, or low bone mass (T score of greater than −2.5 but less than −1), and women with normal bone mass (T score of greater than or equal to −1). Thus, the clinician can make the diagnosis of osteoporosis and begin appropriate therapy before a fracture occurs in older adults. In addition, women with osteopenia can be placed on a preventive regimen and then followed carefully for further bone loss. Specific standards for definitions of osteoporosis have not been established for men or for racial and ethnic groups other than whites, although conventional practice applies similar standards universally.

EPIDEMIOLOGY AND IMPACT

Osteoporosis is a major cause of injury, loss of independence, and death in the older population. According to the National Osteoporosis Foundation, the number of U.S. women of menopausal age who have or are at risk of osteoporosis will increase from almost 30 million in 2002 to nearly 41 million in 2020. The estimated numbers of hip and vertebral fractures in women annually are more than 250,000 and 500,000, respectively.

Increased mortality is related primarily to hip fractures; 20% greater mortality occurs in older adults in the year after hip fracture, and approximately 50% of women do not recover prior function (SOE=B). To this number must be added fragility fractures in men, which occur at about one-third the rate seen in women. One in three men dies within the first year after a hip fracture, which may be a surrogate marker of excess comorbidities and frailty. In 1995, 1 million

Americans suffered fragility fractures at a cost of more than $14 billion. With more recent data of 1.5 million osteoporotic fractures occurring in the United States every year, the direct medical costs are estimated to swell to $50 billion by 2040.

The consequences of osteoporosis include decreased quality of life and independence, and increased morbidity and mortality. Pain, kyphosis, height loss, and other changes in body habitus that develop as a result of vertebral compression fractures erode quality of life for both women and men. In addition, the functional status of patients who have had vertebral crush fractures can also decrease. These patients may be unable to bathe, dress, or walk independently. Thus, because the social and economic costs associated with osteoporotic fractures in older adults are great, it is important to prevent as many fractures as possible. Reducing this burden is widely seen as a healthcare policy imperative.

BONE REMODELING AND BONE LOSS IN AGING

Bone is a dynamic tissue that undergoes active remodeling, a coupled process (also called *bone turnover*) of bone resorption followed by bone formation; bone remodeling continues throughout life. Local signals, not yet fully understood, bring osteoclasts to specific areas of bone where resorption is initiated and resorption cavities are formed. Once osteoclasts have completed the resorption process, osteoblasts move into the area and begin to lay down osteoid and, later, to calcify the matrix. Under optimal conditions, once bone remodeling is completed in a specific area, the resorption spaces are completely filled with new bone. However, after menopause in women, and with aging in both sexes, the remodeling cycle becomes unbalanced, and bone resorption increases more than formation does, resulting in net bone loss. Most treatments for osteoporosis act to inhibit bone resorption rather than to increase bone formation.

Bone mass changes over the life span of an individual. In women, bone mass increases rapidly from the time of puberty until approximately the mid-20s to mid-30s, when bone mass peaks. Once women reach peak bone mass, a few years of stability are followed by a slow rate of bone loss, beginning well before the onset of menopause. After menopause, the rate of bone loss is quite rapid—as much as 7% per year—for 5–10 yr, as a consequence of estrogen deficiency. In later life, bone loss continues, albeit at a slower rate, generally 1%–2% per year; however, some older women can lose bone density at a higher rate. Data suggest that decreasing bone loss at any time will decrease fracture risk. It has been estimated that a 4%–5% increase in bone density in 80-yr-old

women would halve the risk of hip fracture. Furthermore, a meta-analysis has shown that oral antiresorptive therapy with alendronate or risedronate in women >75 yr old, based on high risk status rather than bone density measurements, significantly reduces hip fracture incidents. Thus, in addition to maximizing bone density, improving the quality or integrity of bone may be important in reducing fractures.

Although studies thus far have focused mostly on women, it is well documented that men also lose bone with age. It is estimated that men 30–90 yr old lose approximately 1% per year in the radius and spine; some men with risk factors lose as much as 6% per year (SOE=B). Data suggest that older men can lose bone at rates similar to those of older women; however, rates of vertebral fracture are lower in men than in women.

Both men and women lose predominantly cancellous bone, which is concentrated in the vertebral spine. Cortical bone accounts for 45%–75% of the mechanical resistance to compression of the vertebral spine, and men actually gain cortical bone through periosteal bone deposition. The cross-sectional area of the vertebrae of men increases by 15%–20% through adulthood, increasing maximal load levels until the age of 75. The increased bone strength seems to be reversed by thinning of the cortical ring by age 75, the age at which men begin to present with vertebral fractures. Although bone loss at the hip has not been extensively studied in men, in cross-sectional analyses, healthy men lost 40% of femoral neck BMD between the ages of 20 and 90.

PATHOGENESIS

The pathogenesis of osteoporosis in men and women is complex, encompassing factors that affect the level of peak bone mass, the rate of bone resorption, and the rate of bone formation. Peak bone mass appears to be 75%–80% genetically determined, although exactly which genes are involved is not clear. A number of candidate genes that may be important to osteoporosis are currently being studied, including the vitamin D receptor, estrogen receptor, transforming growth factor, interleukin-6, interleukin-1 receptor 2, type I collagen genes, and collagenases.

Estrogen Deficiency in Women

After menopause, the natural decline of estrogen levels is associated with risk of osteoporosis. Increased resorption appears to be the major force for bone loss in estrogen deficiency. Although both markers of bone resorption and formation are increased after menopause, more recent evidence also suggests a role of estrogen in reducing bone formation as well. Fracture risk is inversely related to estrogen levels in postmenopausal women (SOE=A).

Estrogen has both direct and indirect effects on osteoclasts, the cells that are responsible for bone resorption and thus bone loss. It can act on cells of the osteoblastic lineage to decrease the expression of RANK-L, a cytokine that stimulates the differentiation of osteoclasts to mature forms. It can also have direct effects on cells of hematopoietic lineage, including osteoclast precursors, mature osteoclasts, and lymphocytes. Local cytokines and growth factors can mediate these effects and, in rodent models, bone loss after ovariectomy can be prevented by inhibiting interleukin-1 or TNF-α and does not occur in mice deficient in the interleukin-1 receptor or TNF-α.

Calcium and Vitamin D Deficiency and Secondary Hyperparathyroidism

A major mechanism by which older men and women continue to lose bone is likely related to calcium deficiency, which results in secondary hyperparathyroidism. Decreased dietary calcium intake, impaired intestinal absorption of calcium due to disease or aging itself, and vitamin D deficiency can all lead to calcium deficiency and secondary hyperparathyroidism. Aging skin and decreased exposure to sunlight reduce the conversion of 7-dehydrocholesterol to cholecalciferol (vitamin D_3) by ultraviolet light, causing vitamin D deficiency and reduced calcium absorption. The hormonally active form of vitamin D is $1,25(OH)_2D_3$, or calcitriol. It is necessary for optimal intestinal absorption of calcium and phosphorus, and also exerts a tonic inhibitory effect on parathyroid hormone (PTH) synthesis. When vitamin D deficiency occurs with secondary hyperparathyroidism, it not only contributes to accelerated bone loss and increasing fragility, but also to muscle weakness that can increase the risk of falls.

PTH is a potent stimulator of bone resorption when chronically increased. As a result of decreased serum levels of calcium, PTH—acting to maintain serum levels of calcium—increases, which leads to increased bone resorption. In one study, older women (mean age 79 yr) hospitalized with a hip fracture had lower 25(OH)D levels and higher PTH, higher bone resorption, and lower bone formation than women in the control group (mean age 77 yr). Further, data from the Study of Osteoporotic Fractures indicate that women with low fractional absorption of calcium are at increased risk of hip fracture. Trials involving older adults at high risk of calcium and vitamin D deficiency show that supplementation of both can reverse secondary hyperparathyroidism (SOE=A); increase bone mass (SOE=B); and decrease bone resorption (SOE=A), fracture rates (SOE=B), and possibly the frequency of falling (SOE=C). See also

"Endocrine and Metabolic Disorders," p 491, for more on disorders of calcium metabolism.

Hormonal Influences in Men

Hypogonadism is an important risk factor for osteoporosis in men. Androgens are important determinants of peak bone mass in young men. Androgen levels fall gradually as men age. While total testosterone levels remain relatively stable due to an increase in sex-hormone binding globulin levels, a decline in free or bioavailable testosterone levels at a rate of approximately 1% per year has been demonstrated in observational studies. Bioavailable testosterone levels are below the normal reference range of young adult men in approximately half of men >70 yr old.

Several studies have demonstrated that late-onset hypogonadism can also play a role in male osteoporosis. Although it is evident that severe hypogonadism in men (eg, due to pituitary tumors or androgen deprivation treatment) can cause osteoporosis, the effect of moderate decreases in testosterone levels in aging men on rates of bone loss is uncertain. In one study, >60% of men presenting with hip fracture had low testosterone levels compared with about 20% of those in the control group. In several studies in which men with low normal testosterone levels received supplemental testosterone, femoral bone density increased in the testosterone group and leg muscle strength increased in some but not all. For more information on hypogonadism and testosterone supplementation, see Testosterone in "Endocrine and Metabolic Disorders," p 500.

Evidence for the role of estradiol in bone metabolism in men has been demonstrated in observational studies, and also in reports of low bone density and tall stature in men with mutations in the estrogen receptor or in aromatase, the enzyme that converts androgens to estrogens. These genetic defects have also revealed that closure of epiphyses requires estrogen in both men and women. Several studies in men have evaluated the relationship between circulating levels of estrogen and androgen and have found that low levels of both estrogen and androgen are associated with lower bone mass.

Changes in Bone Formation

Osteoblast activity appears to decrease with aging in both men and women, compounding the bone loss that results from increased resorption seen with aging and, for women, with menopause. Growth factors, such as transforming growth factor β and insulin-like growth factor 1, can be impaired with estrogen deficiency or with aging, resulting in decreased osteoblast function.

Table 31.1—Risk Factors for Osteoporosis

- Age (postmenopausal in women, >70 yr in men)
- Female sex
- Low body weight (BMI <20)
- 10% decline in weight (from usual adult body weight)
- Physical inactivity
- Glucocorticoids
- Previous fragility fracture as adult
- Androgen-deprivation therapy
- Current smoking
- Low dietary calcium
- Spinal cord injury
- Alcoholism

Table 31.2—Modifications to Reduce the Risk of Osteoporosis

Exercise: Encourage regular, weightbearing exercise at least 5 times per week for 30 minutes

Nutrition: Encourage adequate intake of calcium (1,200 mg/d in divided doses) and vitamin D_3 (800 IU/d)

Smoking cessation

Medications that can increase risk of osteoporosis—use with caution:
- glucocorticoids
- anticonvulsants
- cyclosporine
- long-term heparin
- excess thyroid hormone replacement
- methotrexate
- GnRH agonists used for prostate cancer
- aromatase inhibitors (eg, anastrozole, letrozole, aromasin) used for breast cancer

DIAGNOSIS AND PREDICTION OF FRACTURE

Data from several studies indicate that patients with hip fractures are often not evaluated and treated for osteoporosis. The diagnosis of osteoporosis should be considered in any older adult with a fracture, and evaluation is indicated if treatment would be considered for the individual patient.

Risk Factors

Risk factors for osteoporosis and osteoporotic fracture have been identified (Table 31.1) and used to determine who should be placed on preventive or therapeutic regimens. However, risk factors are mediocre predictors of low bone density and fractures, and it is more useful to identify modifiable risk factors and to implement change as part of a treatment or preventive program. For modifications of risk factors for osteoporosis, see Table 31.2; all of these risk factors should be addressed as part of the routine care of older adults. Risk factors can also be used to identify women <65 yr old who should have BMD screening.

Secondary Causes

The diagnosis of idiopathic or primary osteoporosis is made by BMD measurement before fracture or by incident fracture. Exclusion of other diseases that can present as fracture or with low bone mass is important in evaluating women and men with osteoporosis, because different treatment would be required. For the major secondary causes of osteoporosis and laboratory tests used to exclude them, see Table 31.3. These laboratory tests should be considered for older adults who present with acute compression fracture or with a diagnosis of osteoporosis by BMD measurement. The most common causes of secondary osteoporosis in women are primary hyperparathyroidism and glucocorticoid use. The most commonly reported secondary causes of osteoporosis in men are hypogonadism and malabsorption syndromes, including gastrectomy. Men are more likely to have a secondary cause of osteoporosis than women; as many as 50% of men with osteoporosis may have a secondary cause. Medications that might have a detrimental effect on bone should be given with adjusted dosages or discontinued. Medications that adversely affect BMD include glucocorticoids, excess thyroid supplementation, anticonvulsants, methotrexate, cyclosporine, and heparin.

Glucocorticoids result in bone loss primarily through direct suppression of bone formation, although they further reduce levels of sex hormone and cause secondary hyperparathyroidism by decreasing intestinal calcium absorption. The prevalence of vertebral fractures in individuals taking glucocorticoids for 1 yr is estimated to be 11%. The rate of trabecular bone loss is dose-dependent and generally occurs in the first 6 mo of therapy. Although inhaled corticosteroids have not been as well studied, high doses of high-potency inhaled steroids can also result in bone loss. The best strategy for older adults who require long-term glucocorticoid therapy is to maximize bone health by a variety of interventions, including using the lowest possible dosage of glucocorticoids and ensuring adequate intake of calcium and vitamin D (see treatment, below). In addition, alendronate and risedronate have successfully prevented bone loss that is caused by glucocorticoid therapy when begun at the same time as the steroids (see treatment, below).

Vitamin D Measurement

Osteomalacia, an impairment of bone mineralization, is less common than osteoporosis and can be definitively diagnosed by bone biopsy. However, bone biopsies are invasive and not performed routinely. The most common cause of osteomalacia in older adults is vitamin D deficiency as a result of inadequate intake, and adequate vitamin D levels are

Table 31.3—Screening for Secondary Osteoporosis[a]

Disease	Recommended Laboratory Tests
Hyperparathyroidism	**Calcium, PTH level**
Hyperthyroidism	**TSH**, thyroxine levels
Hypogonadism (men only)	**Bioavailable testosterone or total testosterone, free testosterone with sex hormone-binding globulin**
Multiple myeloma	**CBC, serum protein electrophoresis**, urine electrophoresis
Osteomalacia	**Bone-specific alkaline phosphatase, 25(OH)D level**
Paget's disease	**Bone-specific alkaline phosphatase**, urine NTx[b]
Cushing's disease	**Electrolytes**, 24-hour urinary free cortisol

[a] Bolded items are recommended routinely.

[b] Type-I collagen N-telopeptide

Table 31.4—Indications for Bone Mineral Density Testing

Women
- All women >65 yr old regardless of other risk factors
- Postmenopausal women <65 yr old who have ≥1 additional risk factor
- Premenopausal women who present with fractures (confirm diagnosis and determine severity)

Men with:
- History of low trauma fractures
- Radiographic evidence of low bone mass
- Low body weight or weight loss >10%
- Men with clinical conditions associated with osteoporosis
  - Low testosterone level
  - Taking chronic steroids or GnRH agonist
  - Malabsorption syndromes

essential for the prevention of osteoporosis fractures. Thus, measurement of vitamin D level is essential in all patients at risk of or with manifest osteoporosis. For a complete discussion of vitamin D deficiency and its management, see vitamin D deficiency in "Endocrine and Metabolic Disorders," p 496.

Bone Density Measurement

BMD is the best predictor of fracture. The relative risk of fracture is 10 times greater in women whose BMD is in the lowest quartile than in women whose BMD is in the highest quartile (SOE=A).

Bone density of the hip, spine, wrist, or calcaneus can be measured by a variety of techniques. The preferred method of BMD measurement is DEXA, which can measure BMD of the hip, anterior-posterior spine, lateral spine, and wrist. Other methods of measuring BMD include quantitative CT, ultrasonography of the calcaneus, single radiographic absorptiometry of the calcaneus, and radiographic absorptiometry. Quantitative DEXA is the best predictor of hip and other osteoporotic fractures.

The National Osteoporosis Foundation, in conjunction with numerous specialty organizations including the U.S. Preventive Services Task Force, recommends BMD testing for all women ≥65 yr old, regardless of risk-factor status; there are no data to determine the frequency of screening or the age to stop screening for osteoporosis in women. For women between 60 and 64 yr old, the presence of additional risk factors, particularly low body weight and no estrogen replacement therapy, makes their risk of osteoporosis and fracture comparable to that of women >65 yr old. For indications for BMD testing, see Table 31.4. Interpretation of BMD involves evaluating the quality of the DEXA as well as the T scores. As previously stated, osteoporosis is defined as 2.5 or more standard deviations below the young adult mean (ie, T score of less than or equal to −2.5). For every standard deviation below the young adult mean (or a 1-unit decrease in T score), fracture risk at the spine and hip approximately doubles. For example, if a woman has a T score of −2, her risk of fracture is four times that of a woman with normal bone density (controlled for height and weight). Several considerations are important when evaluating the BMD of the spine over time. Vertebral or arterial or lymph node calcification or any scoliosis can falsely increase BMD of the anterior-posterior spine DEXA. Thus, a woman with osteoporosis of the spine can have a DEXA T score that is higher than −2.5. Usually, these changes can be seen on the DEXA report if the picture of the scan is included in the report. It is important to evaluate BMD of lumbar vertebrae L1–L4 when making a decision about therapy. Because these changes in and around the spine are common in older adults, hip BMD tends to be the more reliable site for estimating fracture risk. Another important issue when using DEXA over time is measurement variability. Although the DEXA equipment is stable over time, regular testing can allow detection of any drift. More importantly, patient positioning needs to be consistent over multiple measurements. The International Society of Clinical Densitometry offers standardized training courses for technicians and for clinicians interpreting the results. The cost of DEXA testing is $200–$300, and Medicare and Medicaid will cover the cost if indications for its use (eg, estrogen deficiency) are met.

BMD testing can also be used to establish the diagnosis and severity of osteoporosis in men, and it should be considered for men with low-trauma fractures, radiographic criteria consistent with low bone mass, or diseases known to place a person at risk of osteoporosis. Although data relating BMD to fracture risk are derived from studies of women, data also suggest that similar associations may be valid for men.

Vertebral fracture assessment (VFA) is a technology currently available for the diagnosis of vertebral fractures that can be performed as part of a routine DEXA measurement. Vertebral fractures are highly associated with future fracture risk and morbidity (SOE=A), but they are often not clinically apparent and can be present in patients with T scores greater than −2.5. Treatment of patients with vertebral fractures, including those with T scores greater than −2.5, reduces further fracture risk (SOE=A). For diagnosing vertebral fractures, VFA has lower resolution than CT and spine radiographs but has the advantage of less radiation, lower cost, convenience (at time of BMD), and comparable sensitivity and specificity to spine radiographs. VFA can therefore be a useful adjunct to BMD testing, particularly when results can influence clinical decision making. Risk stratification of patients at risk of fracture, who otherwise might not be considered for pharmacologic therapy, is an important benefit of this technology.

The following are suggested indications for VFA:

- When results will influence clinical decision making (eg, regarding beginning medical therapy for bone loss)
- Documented height loss >2 cm or historical height loss >4 cm (1.5 in)
- History of fracture after age 50
- Long-term glucocorticoid use
- History or findings suggestive of vertebral fracture not previously documented

Biochemical Markers of Bone Turnover

Serum and urine biochemical markers can estimate the rate of bone turnover (remodeling) and provide additional information to assist the clinician. A number of markers have been developed that reflect collagen breakdown (or bone resorption) and bone formation. Several markers have been associated with increased risk of hip fracture, decreased bone density, and bone loss in older adults. In addition, markers of bone resorption and formation decrease in response to antiresorptive treatment. However, the use of markers in clinical practice is controversial because of the substantial overlap of marker values in women with different bone densities or rates of bone loss. Further, few studies have investigated the magnitude of decrease of a biochemical marker necessary to prevent bone loss or, more importantly, fracture. Two markers of bone resorption, deoxypyridinoline cross-links and cross-linked N-telopeptides of type I collagen, and one formation marker, bone alkaline phosphatase, can

be used in clinical practice to provide an early assessment of treatment efficacy. A decrease in the level of these markers from baseline after 3–6 mo of therapy indicates successful treatment.

Signs and Symptoms

There are no early signs and symptoms of osteoporosis. Late findings of advanced osteoporosis include back pain, stooped posture with thoracic kyphosis, shortened stature, and protuberant abdomen.

Osteomalacia can present with subtle findings of diffuse bone pain and tenderness, proximal muscle weakness, a waddling gait, and generalized fatigue. Laboratory studies in patients with osteomalacia typically show increased alkaline phosphatase, low phosphate, low or normal calcium, and low 25(OH)D concentrations.

PREVENTION AND TREATMENT

Whom To Treat

General recommendations are to treat older men and women with osteoporosis diagnosed by DEXA or with a history of a fragility fracture. However, some individuals may be at high risk despite not meeting the BMD criteria for osteoporosis or having a history of fracture. Most fractures occur in those with osteopenia (low bone mass) simply because of the greater numbers in that category. Kanis et al analyzed data from 17 cohorts and devised an algorithm based on answers to a 12-item questionnaire to help clinicians assess fracture risk and consider who should be treated for osteoporosis. The algorithm, FRAX™, uses both clinical and BMD information to model the 10-yr fracture probability in men and women (see http://www.shef.ac.uk/FRAX [accessed Jan 2011]). Because FRAX is relatively new, it has not been prospectively validated (nor have other existing algorithms), but it has been retrospectively tested in 11 independent cohorts, with similar geographic distribution of over 1 million patient-years. It should be recognized that FRAX has not been validated in randomized controlled trials focused on fracture prevention and is indicated only for untreated patients; additional risks for fractures (eg, vitamin D deficiency) are not considered.

The Role of Exercise

Exercise is an important component of osteoporosis treatment and prevention, although exercise alone is not adequate to prevent the rapid bone loss associated with estrogen deficiency in early menopause. Regular exercise is positively associated with BMD, and initiating an exercise program even late in life can help to preserve BMD (SOE=A). Further, the effectiveness of high-intensity strength training in maintaining femoral neck BMD as well as in improving

Table 31.5—Calcium-Containing Foods

Food	Serving Size	Calcium (mg) per Serving
Dairy Products		
Milk	1 cup	290–300
Yogurt	1 cup	240–400
Swiss cheese	1 ounce (1 slice)	250–270
American cheese	1 ounce (1 slice)	165–200
Ice cream	½ cup	90–100
Cottage cheese	½ cup	80–100
Parmesan cheese	1 tablespoon	70
Powdered nonfat milk	1 teaspoon	50
Other		
Sardines in oil with bones	3 ounces	370
Calcium-fortified orange juice	1 cup	300
Canned salmon with bones	3 ounces	170–210
Broccoli	1 cup	160–180
Tofu (soybean curd)	4 ounces	145–155
Turnip greens	½ cup, cooked	100–125
Kale	½ cup, cooked	90–100
Cornbread	2 ½-inch square	80–90
Egg	1 medium	55
Other fortified foods (eg, bread, cereal, fruit juices)	1 serving	Varies; read label

muscle mass, strength, and balance in post-menopausal women has been demonstrated, supporting the use of resistance training in helping to maintain BMD and to reduce the risk of falls (SOE=B).

Marked decrease in physical activity or immobilization results in a decline in bone mass; accordingly, it is important to encourage older adults to be as active as possible. Weightbearing exercise, such as walking, can be recommended for all adults. Older adults should be encouraged to start slowly and to gradually increase both the number of days as well as the time spent walking each day. See "Physical Activity," p 54.

Calcium and Vitamin D

Current recommendations for calcium intake to maintain a positive calcium balance for postmenopausal women 51–70 yr old is elemental calcium at a dosage of 1,200 mg/d and for men 51–70 yr old 1,000 mg/d. For women or men >70 yr old, calcium at 1,200 mg/d is recommended. The upper intake level for all groups is 2,000 mg/d. The dietary intake of calcium for postmenopausal women in the United States averages 500–700 mg/d; thus, most American women require calcium supplementation to ensure adequate intake. For information on the amount of calcium in selected foods, see Table 31.5.

The recommended requirement of vitamin D is 600 IU/d for women and men 51–70 yr old, and 800 IU/d for women and men >70 yr old. The upper

intake level for all groups is 4,000 IU/d. See vitamin D deficiency in "Endocrine and Metabolic Disorders," p 496, for information regarding vitamin D supplementation and repletion.

Pharmacologic Options

For dosing and special considerations for the medications used to prevent and treat osteoporosis, see Table 31.6.

Bisphosphonates

The oral bisphosphonates, alendronate and risedronate, are approved for osteoporosis prevention in postmenopausal women and as treatment in both men and women. Both medications increase bone density and decrease fractures at the spine and hip in postmenopausal women with osteoporosis (SOE=A). These medications can be given weekly or monthly (risedronate). Ibandronate, which can be taken orally on a monthly basis or intravenously every 3 mo, is approved for osteoporosis prevention and treatment in postmenopausal women. Ibandronate has shown efficacy in preventing vertebral fractures only (SOE=A). Alendronate and risedronate are also approved to treat osteoporosis in men and glucocorticoid-induced osteoporosis.

The optimal duration of treatment with bisphosphonates is unclear; however, in one study, the greatest increase in vertebral bone mass occurred during the first 5 yr of treatment, and benefit was maintained for 10 yr without undue risk. In another

Table 31.6—Prescription Medications Used to Prevent and Treat Osteoporosis

Medication	Dosage	Special Considerations	Observed Beneficial Treatment Outcomes[a]
Bisphosphonates		Should not be used if CrCl <30 mL/min	
Alendronate	70 mg/wk; 35 mg/wk for prevention	Adherence to dosing instructions required; used in men and women to prevent glucocorticoid-induced osteoporosis	Vertebral fracture: ARR=7.1%, NNT=14 over 3 yr Hip fracture: ARR=1.1%, NNT=91 over 3 yr
Risedronate	35 mg/wk or 150 mg/mo	Adherence to dosing instructions required	Vertebral fracture: ARR=5%, NNT=20 over 3 yr Nonvertebral fracture: ARR=4%, NNT=25 over 3 yr
Ibandronate	150 mg/mo or 3 mg IV every 3 mo	Adherence to dosing instructions required	Vertebral fracture: ARR=4.9%, NNT=20 over 3 yr
Zoledronic acid	5 mg/year IV	Adherence to dosing instructions required	Morphometric vertebral fracture: ARR=7.6%, NNT=13 over 3 yr Clinical vertebral fracture: ARR=2.1%, NNT=48 over 3 yr All nonvertebral fractures: ARR=2.7%, NNT=37 over 3 yr Hip fracture: ARR=1.1%, NNT=91 over 3 yr
Selective estrogen–receptor modulator			
Raloxifene	60 mg/d	Also approved for breast cancer prevention	Vertebral fracture: ARR=3.5%, NNT=29 over 3 yr
Calcitonin			
Nasal spray	200 IU/d	Metered spray; 1 spray gives daily dose; alternate nostrils each day to reduce adverse events	Vertebral fracture: ARR=8.1%, NNT=12 over 5 yr
Injectable (SC or IM)	50–100 IU 3 to 5 times/wk	Injectable can be useful for acute pain syndrome related to vertebral fracture	
Estrogen	See text	Not recommended as first-line choice	See text
Parathyroid hormone (teriparatide injection)	20 mcg SC qd	For use in patients who cannot tolerate other approved treatments for osteoporosis	Vertebral fracture: ARR=9%, NNT=11 over 21 mo Nonvertebral fracture: ARR=3%, NNT=33 over 21 mo
RANK ligand inhibitor			
Denosumab	60 mg SC every 6 mo	For treatment of postmenopausal women at high risk of fractures	New vertebral fractures: ARR=4.9% Nonvertebral fractures: ARR=1.5%

[a] Patient populations were not comparable across studies, so direct comparisons of ARR (absolute risk reduction) and NNT (number needed to treat) may not be valid.

study, the cumulative risk of nonvertebral fractures was not significantly different between women who discontinued alendronate after 5 yr (18.9%) and those who continued (19%), but a higher incidence of vertebral fractures was observed in the discontinued therapy group. These data suggest that while many women may be suitable candidates for shorter term (≤5 yr) bisphosphonate therapy, those at highest risk of vertebral fractures should be considered for longer duration treatment.

The major adverse events of oral bisphosphonates are GI symptoms, which can include abdominal pain, dyspepsia, esophagitis, nausea, vomiting, and diarrhea. Musculoskeletal pain can also occur. Esophagitis, particularly erosive esophagitis, is seen most commonly in patients who do not take the medication properly. The absorption of oral bisphosphonates is very poor; thus, it is extremely important for patients to follow the specific and detailed instructions for taking them.

Bisphosphonate use has been observed to be rarely associated with osteonecrosis of the jaw, a necrotic area of bone, more commonly found in the mandible than the maxilla. The preponderance of cases has been reported in patients receiving parenteral bisphosphonates for malignant bone disorders such as myeloma who have undergone dental procedures such as tooth extraction. There are rare reports of patients contracting osteonecrosis of the jaw on long-term conventional oral bisphosphonates for osteoporosis.

There is concern that long-term use of bisphosphonates could be associated with atypical femur fractures, such as subtrochanteric and diaphyseal femur fractures. These fractures are uncommon, comprising <1% of all femur fractures. It is unclear if bisphosphonates are the cause, but these atypical fractures have been predominantly reported in patients taking bisphosphonates for osteoporosis. Patients taking bisphosphonates are encouraged to report new hip or thigh pain to their health providers.

Zoledronic acid is the most recent addition to the medical regimen of bisphosphonates for osteoporosis. It was approved for osteoporosis treatment in postmenopausal women in 2007, and its indication has been broadened to include fracture prevention after fragility fractures of the hip. It is given as an annual intravenous infusion of 5 mg over 20 minutes. In two randomized trials, one involving 8,000 postmenopausal women and the other over 2,100 patients who were 3 mo after hip-fracture repair, zoledronic acid increased BMD and decreased vertebral fractures (SOE=A). Hip fracture incidence was significantly decreased in one of the trials. The most frequent observed adverse events were transient fever, myalgias, arthralgias, and bone pain. In one of the trials, there was a small number of cases of atrial fibrillation in the treated group (that did not occur within the first few days after infusion); however, the FDA ultimately did not attribute this to zoledronic acid. Ongoing postmarketing surveillance continues regarding this issue with all bisphosphonates.

Selective Estrogen-Receptor Modulators

The selective estrogen-receptor modulators are agents that act as estrogen agonists in bone and heart but act as estrogen antagonists in breast and uterine tissue. These medications have the potential to prevent osteoporosis or cardiovascular disease without increased risk of breast or uterine cancer. Several studies have reported that tamoxifen, an agent used to treat breast cancer, has beneficial effects on bone, but due to stimulatory effects on the uterus, it is not indicated for osteoporosis treatment or prevention.

Raloxifene has been approved for the treatment and prevention of osteoporosis in postmenopausal women. Comparison of raloxifene with placebo in postmenopausal women with osteoporosis found that raloxifene decreases bone turnover, maintains BMD, and reduces incident vertebral fractures (SOE=A). Raloxifene has not, however, been shown to decrease nonvertebral fractures—and it significantly increases the risk of stroke and venous thromboembolism (SOE=A). Additional adverse events with raloxifene include flu-like symptoms, hot flushes, leg cramps, and peripheral edema.

Another important finding with raloxifene was reduced risk of breast cancer in women who participated in the Multiple Outcomes of Raloxifene Trial. When women receiving raloxifene were compared with women receiving placebo, the relative risk of developing breast cancer in women receiving raloxifene was 0.24 (95% CI, 0.13–0.44). Raloxifene is approved by the FDA for the prevention of breast cancer.

Calcitonin

Calcitonin, which inhibits bone resorption, is available as a subcutaneous injection and as a nasal spray for the treatment of osteoporosis in women. The nasal spray is the most widely used. It has fewer reported adverse events and greater patient acceptance but may be less effective.

Although there are no direct comparisons, calcitonin appears to be less effective than other antiresorptive drugs. Compared with placebo, calcitonin modestly improves spine BMD and reduces vertebral fractures but has not been demonstrated to reduce hip or other nonvertebral fractures (SOE=B). There is some evidence that calcitonin produces an analgesic effect in some women with painful vertebral compression fractures, particularly in its subcutaneous injectable form (SOE=C).

Estrogen

Estrogen replacement therapy is an option for osteoporosis prevention (approved by the FDA; indication withdrawn as a treatment); however, it is not recommended as a first-line choice. Multiple studies have demonstrated that postmenopausal estrogen use prevents bone loss at the hip and spine when begun within 10 yr of menopause (SOE=A). Decreased incident vertebral fractures were seen in a small study of postmenopausal women using a transdermal estradiol preparation. The Women's Health Initiative (WHI) trial randomized over 16,000 postmenopausal women to receive estrogen plus progesterone versus placebo. After a mean of 5.2 yr of follow-up, hormone therapy reduced hip fracture number needed to treat, vertebral fracture, and colon cancer. However, hormone therapy also increased the risk of breast cancer, absolute risk, number needed to harm, heart disease, stroke, and venous thromboembolism. Given the WHI findings, recent U.S. Preventive Services Task Force guidelines advise against the routine use of estrogen plus progesterone for the prevention of chronic conditions in postmenopausal women. The estrogen-only arm of the WHI was also stopped a year ahead of schedule and demonstrated an increased risk of stroke but not of coronary heart disease or breast cancer; estrogen alone also decreased hip fracture risk. Previously, hormone therapy was recommended for prevention of osteoporosis; however, given the results of the WHI and the availability of other effective medications for osteoporosis prevention and treatment, the FDA changed its indication for estrogen and estrogen-progestin products: "When these products are being prescribed solely for the prevention of postmenopausal osteoporosis, approved non-estrogen treatments should be carefully considered. Estrogens and combined estrogen-progestin products should only be considered for women with significant risk of osteoporosis that outweighs the risks of the drug."

Other data suggest that lower-than-usual doses of estrogen, when given with adequate calcium and vitamin D, are effective in reducing bone turnover and bone loss in older women. The effect of lower-dose estrogen on fracture incidence and other health outcomes is unknown.

See also estrogen therapy in "Endocrine and Metabolic Disorders," p 501.

Parathyroid Hormone

PTH (teriparatide) is the only anabolic agent approved for the treatment of osteoporosis in men and women. PTH increases both bone formation and resorption. Because formation is increased before resorption, the resultant "anabolic window" leads to increased bone mass, trabecular connectivity, and mechanical strength when PTH is administered in a daily pulsatile manner. This is in contrast to the chronic increases of PTH seen in primary hyperparathyroidism, which lead to increased resorption, bone loss, and osteoporosis.

Teriparatide increases spinal and hip BMD in osteoporotic men and women. It has been shown to reduce vertebral and nonvertebral fractures in postmenopausal women (SOE=A). In men with primary or hypogonadal osteoporosis, PTH also has been shown to increase BMD at all sites. Studies have shown that the most beneficial way to use PTH is on its own for 2 yr followed by bisphosphonate therapy.

PTH, which is given subcutaneously, is approved for men and women who are at risk of osteoporotic fracture and unable to tolerate other approved agents. It is more typically reserved for those with severe osteoporosis (including fracture history). Subcutaneous injections and expense have limited its use. PTH increased the incidence of osteosarcomas in male and female rats; the relevance of these findings to people is unknown. Thus, PTH is approved for use for 18–24 mo duration.

RANK Ligand Inhibitor

Denosumab is a human monoclonal antibody that binds and neutralizes human receptor activator of nuclear factor (NF)-kappaB ligand (RANKL), a critical mediator of bone resorption by cells of osteoclast lineage. In a trial of postmenopausal women with low bone mass or osteoporosis randomized to treatment with denosumab every 3 mo or every 6 mo, to placebo, or to open-label oral alendronate weekly, continual, long-term denosumab treatment increased BMD at the lumbar spine and total hip. Bone turnover was consistently suppressed over 48 mo. This seems to be a promising new therapy for postmenopausal women with low BMD, and the results of long-term trials are pending.

Investigational Agents

Strontium ranelate is an anabolic agent that increases bone formation and decreases bone resorption in animals. In a randomized, placebo-controlled study in postmenopausal women with osteoporosis (at least one vertebral fracture plus lumbar spine T score less than −2.5) at baseline, strontium ranelate increased BMD and decreased the incidence of vertebral fractures at the highest dosage tested (2 g/d). At this dosage, bone alkaline phosphatase increased, and urinary excretion of N-telopeptides of type I collagen decreased. Strontium ranelate is approved in a number of European countries but not in the United States.

Other osteoporosis treatments under study include additional bisphosphonates, cathespin K inhibitors, selective estrogen–receptor modulators, selective androgen–receptor modulators, src inhibitors, vitamin D analogs, calcium receptor antagonist (calcilytic), and integrin inhibitors.

VERTEBRAL FRACTURE MANAGEMENT

Most vertebral compression fractures are asymptomatic and diagnosed by spinal radiographs. Over time, in affected individuals, height may decrease, kyphosis may increase, or clothes may no longer fit properly. Many older adults have chronic back pain caused by changes in the spine that develop with degenerative osteoarthritis or vertebral compression; distinguishing the source of the pain can be difficult. On a practical level, pain should be treated if it interferes with ADLs and quality of life, regardless of cause. However, identifying vertebral fractures is important so that future fractures can be prevented.

In the case of symptomatic vertebral compression fractures, adequate pain control is essential. The pain usually lasts 2–4 weeks and can be quite debilitating.

NSAIDs and subcutaneous calcitonin can be tried; narcotics are commonly required to control the pain. Physical therapy is an important part of osteoporosis treatment programs to manage acute and chronic pain, as well as for patient education. A physical therapist can provide postural exercises, alternative interventions for pain reduction, and information on changes in body mechanics that can help prevent future fractures. See also "Persistent Pain," p 109. Support groups for patients with osteoporosis can also be very helpful.

Vertebroplasty and Kyphoplasty

Vertebroplasty and kyphoplasty have recently been developed as surgical options for treatment of painful vertebral compression fractures. Vertebroplasty was first performed in 1984 for treatment of a cervical vertebral hemangioma by placing surgical cement through a needle into the painful compressed vertebrae. Kyphoplasty was first performed in 1998 using an inflatable balloon tamp to restore vertebral anatomy with subsequent injection of surgical cementinto the newly created space. The number of vertebroplasty procedures has increased dramatically over the past decade in the absence of high-quality data regarding its risks and benefits. In 2009, two randomized trials of vertebroplasty were published, involving 280 patients with painful vertebral fractures. No significant differences in pain reduction were observed between the vertebroplasty and placebo (sham procedure) groups at 1−6 mo of follow-up (SOE=A). Complications were rare.

ACOVE-3* QUALITY INDICATORS PERTAINING TO OSTEOPOROSIS

Preventive advice

- All vulnerable older adults at an initial primary care visit should be counseled about intake of calcium and vitamin D and weightbearing exercises.

Vitamin D

- All vulnerable older adults in stable health states should take 800 IU (or equivalent) of vitamin D supplementation daily.

Screening dual x-ray absorptiometry (DEXA) scan for women

- All female vulnerable older adults without a diagnosis of osteoporosis should have documentation that they were offered a DEXA scan.

Screening DEXA scan for men

- If a male vulnerable older adult without a diagnosis of osteoporosis has any of the following risk factors listed below for osteoporosis, then a DEXA scan should be performed:
  - >3 mo of systemic glucocorticoid treatment
  - Primary hyperparathyroidism
  - Osteoporosis in a first-degree relative
  - Hypogonadism
  - Gonadotropin-releasing hormone antagonist use
  - Osteopenia on radiography

Osteoporosis consideration after fracture

- If a female vulnerable older adult has a new nonpathologic fracture, then she should be treated for osteoporosis, or a DEXA scan should be performed.
- If a vulnerable older adult has a new hip fracture or undergoes kyphoplasty or vertebroplasty, then a DEXA scan should be performed or pharmacologic therapy for osteoporosis should be prescribed within 6 mo.

Osteoporosis prophylaxis for corticosteroids

- If a vulnerable older adult without osteoporosis is taking 7.5 mg/d or more of prednisone (or equivalent) for 1 mo or longer, then he or she should be prescribed calcium and vitamin D supplements.
- If a vulnerable older adult without osteoporosis is taking 7.5 mg/day or more of prednisone (or equivalent) for 3 mo or longer, then he or she should be prescribed bisphosphonate therapy.

Identifying secondary osteoporosis

- If a female vulnerable older adult is newly diagnosed with osteoporosis, then she should receive an evaluation, including the following:
  - Medication use
  - Alcohol use
  - CBC
  - Liver function tests
  - Renal function
  - Calcium
  - Phosphorus
  - 25(OH)D
  - Thyrotropin

Exercise for osteoporosis

■ If an ambulatory vulnerable older adult has a new diagnosis of osteoporosis, then there should be documentation of advice to exercise within 3 mo.

Calcium and vitamin D for osteoporosis

■ If a vulnerable older adult has osteoporosis, then he or she should be prescribed calcium and vitamin D supplements.

Pharmacologic treatment for osteoporosis in women

■ If a female vulnerable older adult has osteoporosis, then she should be treated with bisphosphonates, raloxifene, calcitonin, estrogen therapy, or teriparatide (if this is a new diagnosis, within 3 mo).

Testosterone for osteoporosis in men

■ If a male vulnerable older adult has osteoporosis and is hypogonadal, and has no history of prostate cancer, then he should be prescribed testosterone therapy.

Pharmacologic treatment for osteoporosis in men

■ If a male vulnerable older adult has osteoporosis, then he should be treated with bisphosphonates, calcitonin, parathyroid hormone, or if hypogonadal, testosterone (if this is a new diagnosis, within 3 mo).

Related quality indicators for Osteoporosis

■ Gait and balance evaluation, balance disorders, exercise (see "Gait Impairment," p 218)

■ Evaluation and management of falls (see "Falls," p 224)

*Assessing Care of Vulnerable Elders – 3rd Set. See inside front cover for explanation.

REFERENCES

■ Dawson-Hughes B, Tosteson AN, Melton LJ 3rd, et al; National Osteoporosis Foundation Guide Committee. Implications of absolute fracture risk assessment for osteoporosis practice guidelines in the USA. *Osteoporosis Int.* 2008;19(4):449–458.

■ Giangregorio L, Dolovich L, Cranney A, et al. Osteoporosis risk perceptions among patients who have sustained a fragility fracture. *Patient Educ Couns.* 2009;74(2):213–220.

■ MacLean C, Newberry S, Maglione M, et al. Systematic review: comparative effectiveness of treatments to prevent fractures in men and women with low bone density or osteoporosis. *Ann Intern Med.* 2008;148(3):197–213.

CHAPTER 32—DEMENTIA

KEY POINTS

■ Alzheimer's disease, vascular dementia, and dementia with Lewy bodies are the most common forms of degenerative dementias seen in late life.

■ Cholinesterase inhibitors and N-methyl-d-aspartate antagonists can be modestly helpful in reducing the cognitive symptoms of Alzheimer's dementia.

■ Behavioral symptoms can occur with any type of dementia and tend to respond best to a combination of environmental modifications and medication management of symptoms.

Dementia is a general term used to describe several disorders that cause significant decline in two or more areas of cognitive functioning that are severe enough to result in functional decline. Of those who suffer from dementia, most have Alzheimer's disease (AD), which affects an estimated 5 million people in the United States. Dementia also affects millions more caregivers and relatives, who must cope with the patient's progressive and irreversible decline in cognition, functioning, and behavior. Both caregivers and patients can misinterpret the initial symptoms of dementia as normal age-related cognitive losses; clinicians as well may not recognize early signs or can misdiagnose them. However, dementia and aging are not synonymous. As people age, they usually experience such memory changes as slowing in information processing, but these kinds of changes are benign without affecting function. By contrast, dementia is progressive and disabling and is not an inherent aspect of aging.

Diagnostic and treatment advances have benefited many patients. Early and accurate diagnosis of dementia and its cause can minimize use of costly medical resources and give patients and their relatives time to anticipate future medical, financial, and legal needs. Sustained reversal of the progressive cognitive decline of dementia is not currently possible, but psychosocial and pharmacologic treatments can improve such associated conditions as depression, psychosis, and agitation, and enhance quality of life. See also "Psychosocial Issues," p 17; and "Legal and Ethical Issues," p 23.

EPIDEMIOLOGY AND SOCIETAL IMPACT

Dementia is typically a disease of later life, generally beginning after 65 yr of age. AD is the most common type of dementia, accounting for approximately two-thirds of all cases and affecting 6%–8% of those ≥65 yr old. The disease prevalence doubles every 5 yr after age 60; an estimated 30% or more of those who are ≥85 yr old have AD. Vascular dementia is thought to cause an estimated 15%–20% of cases and often coexists with AD pathology, ie, so-called "mixed dementia." In recent years, dementia associated with Lewy bodies has received increased attention and is now thought to be the second most common cause of dementia. Frontotemporal dementia is also a more recent diagnostic category of dementia and represents a smaller percentage of cases, with a younger age of onset than seen in other dementias. Neurodegenerative diseases such as Huntington's disease, Parkinson's disease, or other causes such as head injury and alcoholism account for other dementia syndromes.

Dementia has a major impact on society. The total costs approach $100 billion annually if the costs of medical and long-term care, home care, and lost productivity for caregivers are included. Medicare, Medicaid, and private insurance pay much of the direct cost, but families caring for patients with dementia bear the greatest burden of expense.

The financial costs of dementia are only one aspect of the total burden. Nearly half of primary caregivers of patients with dementia experience psychologic distress, particularly depression. An accurate economic assessment of the problem underestimates the true cost of the disease to society unless the quality of life of both patients and caregivers is included in the analysis.

RISK FACTORS AND PREVENTION

The two greatest risk factors for AD are age and family history. Studies that account for death from other causes suggest that by 90 yr of age, nearly half of those with first-degree relatives (ie, parents, siblings) with AD develop the disease themselves. Rare forms of familial AD beginning before age 60 have been associated with mutations in one of three genes—amyloid precursor protein (APP), presenilin 1 (PS1), or presenilin 2 (PS2)—and account for approximately 1% of individuals with AD. Most commonly, AD begins late in life, and for such late-onset cases, the apolipoprotein E gene (APOE) on chromosome 19 influences risk. The APOE gene has three alleles: 2, 3, and 4. The risk increases for those carrying two APOE4 alleles, but those with one APOE4 allele are still at greater risk than those with APOE2 and APOE3. The APOE4 allele increases risk and decreases age of onset in a dose-related fashion, whereas the APOE2 allele may have a protective effect. The APOE4 allele may be less common in black Americans than in white Americans. Using APOE genotyping as a prognostic test for asymptomatic older adults is not currently recommended pending results from further studies, and it may be useful only in increasing the diagnostic confidence for AD if a patient already has dementia.

Other possible risk factors include a history of trauma, risk factors for cardiovascular disease, depression, and fewer years of formal education. Head trauma is thought to disrupt neuronal synapses and predispose to β-amyloid formation. Cardiovascular risk factors are thought to increase risk by predisposing individuals to impairment in cognition through ischemic mechanisms, although there is newer evidence linking some vascular risk factors to Alzheimer's pathology. Research suggests that more years of formal education can delay the onset of dementia, which may represent a confounding variable of socioeconomic status or a factor that truly provides protection by supplying a cognitive "reserve."

Prevention of dementia, especially AD, is an active area of research. Drugs associated with reduced risk in epidemiologic studies include NSAIDs[OL], statins[OL], Ginkgo biloba, and possibly antioxidants. Several of these have been studied in randomized clinical trials but to date, none has been shown to be effective. Research in healthy older adults shows a possible protective effect of physical and intellectual activity on the risk of cognitive decline (SOE=B). The onset of dementia can also be delayed by adequate treatment of hypertension (SOE=B).

ASSESSMENT METHODS

Most cases of dementia can be diagnosed on the basis of a general medical and psychiatric evaluation. It is important for primary care clinicians to be alert to the early symptoms, because dementia is often undetected until severe symptoms or an adverse event, such as behavioral disturbances, flags its presence. Subjective complaints are significant and if a patient or family member expresses concerns about cognitive decline, a mental status assessment and probably a dementia evaluation are indicated. Subtle signs of cognitive change can include displaying behavioral changes, missing deadlines or having other problems at work, increasing difficulty managing complex tasks such as finances, or giving up a hobby or interest that may have become too challenging.

The informant interview and clinical assessment are the most important diagnostic tools for dementia. Both the patient and a reliable informant should be interviewed to determine the patient's current condition, medical and medication history, patterns of substance use, and living arrangements. Determination of onset and nature of symptoms can help differentiate clinical syndromes. Useful informant-based instruments, such as the Functional Activities Questionnaire, can help determine whether lapses in memory or language use have occurred and assess the patient's ability to learn and retain new information, handle complex tasks, and demonstrate sound judgment. Any changes are best determined by comparing present with previous performance, because functional decline and multiple cognitive deficits confirm the diagnosis.

A comprehensive physical examination should include a neurologic and mental status evaluation. Brief quantified screening tests of cognitive function, such as the Folstein Mini–Mental State Examination or the Mini-Cog Assessment Instrument for Dementia, can be useful, particularly if they demonstrate change over a 6-mo or 1-yr follow-up period. However, these are screening tests, and full neuropsychologic testing may be necessary to accurately define the character and severity of the deficits, especially in atypical cases or when presentation may be confounded by high education or subtle changes. A laboratory evaluation, generally including a CBC, urinalysis, serum chemistries, liver function tests, rapid plasma reagent test, thyrotropin, vitamin B_{12} level, folate acid level or homocysteine, and methylmalonic acid is also recommended. In addition, the history or physical examination may indicate the need for other tests, such as an ECG or a chest radiograph, or a neurology

consultation. Cognitive and functional assessments should be conducted in the patient's native language, if at all possible. (In the face of cognitive decline, it is common for dementia patients to retain the greatest fluency in their native language.)

Although brain imaging studies are optional, most specialists recommend them. They may be especially useful in the following situations:

- Onset occurs at an age <65 yr old.
- Symptoms begin suddenly or progress rapidly.
- There is evidence of focal or asymmetrical neurologic deficits.
- The clinical picture suggests normal-pressure hydrocephalus (eg, onset has occurred within 1 yr, gait disorder or unexplained incontinence is present).
- There is a history of a recent fall or other head trauma.

In general, a noncontrast CT head scan is adequate to exclude intracranial bleeding, space-occupying lesions, and hydrocephalus. If vascular dementia is suspected, MRI is often performed, but white-matter changes revealed by T2-weighted MRI images should not be overinterpreted.

Cognitive performance is influenced by number of years of formal education. Affected patients with more years of education may have normal scores, while patients with less education may have low scores and no decline in function. This must be considered, especially in patients with more subtle deficits or subjective complaints. In addition, in tests that are most sensitive to language performance, cultural differences can lead to an overinterpretation of dementia in minority patients. One way to improve the accuracy of assessment is to perform serial evaluations (using a medical interpreter if needed), which allow determination of decline in an individual that is consistent with a neurodegenerative process. In addition, measuring changes in everyday memory function by evaluating a person's performance of ADLs, either by direct observation or obtaining information from a reliable informant may be helpful.

The practical use of cognitive measures is that they provide a quantitative baseline against which to compare future assessments. Neuropsychologic testing is helpful in distinguishing normal aging from dementia, as well as in identifying deficits that point to a specific diagnosis, and it is recommended when the diagnosis is unclear or atypical. In general, the diagnosis of dementia is a clinical one, and laboratory assessment and imaging are used to identify uncommon treatable causes and common treatable comorbid conditions.

Table 32.1—Diagnostic Features and Treatment of Dementia Syndromes

Syndrome	Onset	Cognitive Domains, Symptoms	Motor Symptoms	Progression	Imaging	Pharmacologic Treatment of Cognition
Mild cognitive impairment	Gradual	Primarily memory	Rare	Unknown, 12% per year proceed to Alzheimer's disease	Possible global atrophy, small hippocampal volumes	Cholinesterase inhibitor possibly protective for 18 mo
Alzheimer's disease	Gradual	Memory, language, visuospatial	Rare early, apraxia later	Gradual (over 8–10 yr)	Possible global atrophy, small hippocampal volumes	Cholinesterase inhibitors for mild to severe; memantine for moderate to severe stages
Vascular dementia	May be sudden or stepwise	Depends on location of ischemia	Correlates with ischemia	Gradual or stepwise with further ischemia	Cortical or subcortical changes on MRI	Cholinesterase inhibitors; risk factor modifiers
Lewy body dementia	Gradual	Memory, visuospatial, hallucinations, fluctuating symptoms	Parkinsonism	Gradual, but faster than Alzheimer's disease	Possible global atrophy	Cholinesterase inhibitors; +/- carbidopa/levodopa for movement
Frontotemporal dementia	Gradual; age <60 yr	Executive, disinhibition, apathy, language, +/- memory	None	Gradual, but faster than Alzheimer's disease	Atrophy in frontal and temporal lobes	Not recommended by current evidence

DIFFERENTIAL DIAGNOSIS

Dementia is defined as an acquired syndrome of decline in memory and other cognitive functions sufficient to affect daily life in an alert patient. Diagnosis then requires further investigation to identify the cause of the dementia by determining chronology of symptoms along with the pattern and extent of deficits. A general discussion of the most common dementias is provided below; for an overview of diagnostic features, see Table 32.1.

Cognition in aging is now understood to be a continuum ranging from the mild changes of normal aging to the significant impairments that define dementia. Although studies are not conclusive, it appears that normal aging involves some mild decline in memory, usually requiring more effort and time to recall new information. However, this decline does not impair functioning; new learning is slower but still occurs and is usually well compensated with lists, calendars, and other memory supports.

With early identification of cognitive deficits, a disorder referred to as *mild cognitive impairment* has been identified. These patients do not have dementia but do have mild impairment in memory or one cognitive domain without overt impairment in function. These patients often present with subjective complaints of memory loss. Some research suggests that these individuals convert to AD at a rate of about 12% per year. Experts disagree if this is a unique disorder or merely an early prodrome to AD that has been identified with earlier diagnosis of memory impairment. Studies are underway to determine what if any interventions may be beneficial.

AD is characterized by gradual onset and progressive decline in cognitive functioning; motor and sensory functions are spared until middle and late stages. Memory impairment is a core symptom of any dementia, and in AD it is present in the earliest stages. Typically, AD patients demonstrate difficulty learning new information and retaining it for more than a few minutes. In later disease stages, their ability to learn is compromised even more, and patients are unable to access older, more distant memories. Aphasia, apraxia, disorientation, visuospatial dysfunction, impaired judgment, and executive dysfunction are also present. The initial stages of AD are characterized by normal motor, sensory, and cerebellar functioning. If focal motor or sensory signs, except fluent aphasia and apraxia, are present, a diagnosis of vascular dementia or mixed vascular dementia with AD is likely.

Vascular dementia refers to cognitive deficits most often associated with vascular damage in the brain. Vascular dementia is associated with focal neurologic deficits that accompany cognitive loss. Cognitive and neurologic impairments should correlate anatomically with the areas of ischemia, although the often diffuse nature of vascular disease may make this correlation difficult to identify. A history of "small strokes," unless accompanied by a clear demonstration of focal signs of motor or sensory impairment, does not necessarily constitute vascular dementia. Cerebrovascular disease, however, does appear to contribute to the severity of cognitive symptoms in AD.

For a diagnosis of dementia with Lewy bodies, both dementia and at least one of the following must be present: detailed visual hallucinations, parkinsonian signs, and changes in alertness or attention. The diagnosis may overlap with AD and the dementia associated with Parkinson's disease. Poor visuospatial abilities are also often out of proportion to other cognitive deficits. The chronology of symptoms and pattern of cognitive deficits allow differentiation between dementia with Lewy bodies and AD and the dementia associated with Parkinson's disease. Parkinsonian signs, particularly a "pill rolling" tremor that develops before cognitive impairment, generally indicate Parkinson's disease rather than AD. When parkinsonian rigidity and bradykinesia are present during the onset of dementia, a diagnosis of dementia with Lewy bodies should be considered.

Frontotemporal dementia is a disease often seen in patients with onset of cognitive symptoms at a younger age; these patients present most often with executive and language dysfunction and significant behavioral changes. These behaviors include social disinhibition and hyperorality, and they often have had a profound effect on the patient's social functioning. Memory deficits are often not as pronounced in these patients in the early stages as they are in patients with other dementias. The language impairments in frontotemporal dementia may be detected in neuropsychologic tests such as the Boston Naming Test and may progress even early in the course of illness much faster than other cognitive impairments. It is important to recognize the difference between frontotemporal dementia and AD with "frontal" symptoms. The latter refers to social disinhibition and behavioral impulsivity that can be seen with AD. In these patients, the behavioral problems occur much later in the course of illness, after a memory problem is already clearly evident. In contrast, patients with frontotemporal dementia display social disinhibition before prominent memory decline. Pick's disease is a type of frontotemporal dementia characterized by rapid decline and the presence of Pick bodies, balloon-like intracellular inclusions at autopsy.

Common to all types of dementia, cognitive impairment eventually has a profound effect on the patient's daily life. Difficulties in planning meals, managing finances or medications, using a telephone, and driving without getting lost are not uncommon. Such functional impairments may first alert others that a problem is emerging. Numerous functions are maintained in patients with dementia of mild to moderate severity, including such ADLs as eating, bathing, and grooming. The behaviors of many patients remain socially appropriate during the early disease stages.

Behavior and mood changes are common, including personality changes, apathy, irritability, anxiety, or depression. During the middle and late stages of the disease, delusions, hallucinations, aggression, and wandering may develop. These behaviors are extremely troubling to caregivers and often result in family distress and long-term care placement. Although the course of dementia is variable, the progression of dementia often follows a sequential clinical and functional pattern of decline (Table 32.2). See also "Behavioral Problems in Dementia," p 256.

Dementia recognition can be complicated by the presence of either delirium or depression. Delirium has been defined as an acquired impairment of attention, alertness, or perception. Delirium and dementia are in some ways similar: both are characterized by global cognitive impairment. Delirium can be distinguished by acute onset, cognitive fluctuations throughout the course of a day, impaired consciousness and attention, and altered sleep cycles. In hospitalized patients, delirium and dementia often occur together. The presence of dementia increases the risk of delirium and accounts in part for the high rate of delirium in older patients. A delirium episode in an older adult, therefore, should alert the clinician to search for dementia once the delirium clears. See also "Delirium," p 264.

Symptoms of depression and dementia often overlap, presenting additional diagnostic challenges. Patients with primary dementia commonly experience symptoms of depression, and such patients may minimize cognitive losses. By contrast, patients with primary depression can demonstrate decreased motivation during the cognitive examination and express cognitive complaints that exceed objectively measured deficits. Moreover, patients with primary depression usually have intact language and motor skills, whereas patients with primary dementia may show impairment in these domains. As many as half of older adults who present with reversible dementia and depression become progressively demented within 5 yr. See also "Depression and Other Mood Disorders," p 295.

TREATMENT AND MANAGEMENT

The primary treatment goals for patients with dementia are to enhance quality of life and maximize functional performance by improving cognition, mood,

Table 32.2 —The General Progression of Dementia

Stage 1: No cognitive impairment

Unimpaired individuals experience no memory problems, and none is evident to a healthcare professional during a medical interview.

Stage 2: Very mild cognitive decline

Individuals at this stage feel as if they have memory lapses, especially in forgetting familiar words or names or the location of keys, eyeglasses, or other everyday objects. However, these problems are not evident during a medical examination or apparent to friends, family, or coworkers.

Stage 3: Mild cognitive decline

Early-stage Alzheimer's can be diagnosed in some, but not all, individuals with these symptoms.

Friends, family, or coworkers begin to notice deficiencies. Problems with memory or concentration may be measurable in clinical testing or discernible during a detailed medical interview. Common difficulties include the following:

- Word- or name-finding problems noticeable to family or close associates
- Decreased ability to remember names when introduced to new people
- Performance issues in social or work settings noticeable to family, friends, or coworkers
- Reading a passage and retaining little material
- Losing or misplacing a valuable object
- Decline in ability to plan or organize

Stage 4: Moderate cognitive decline (mild or early-stage Alzheimer's disease)

At this stage, a careful medical interview detects clear-cut deficiencies in the following areas:

- Decreased knowledge of recent occasions or current events
- Impaired ability to perform challenging mental arithmetic, eg, to count backward from 100 by 7s
- Decreased ability to perform complex tasks, such as marketing, planning dinner for guests, or paying bills and managing finances
- Reduced memory of personal history

The affected individual may seem subdued and withdrawn, especially in socially or mentally challenging situations.

Stage 5: Moderately severe cognitive decline (moderate or mid-stage Alzheimer's disease)

Major gaps in memory and deficits in cognitive function emerge. Some assistance with day-to-day activities becomes essential. At this stage, individuals may:

- Be unable during a medical interview to recall such important information as their current address, their telephone number, or the name of the college or high school from which they graduated
- Become confused about where they are or about the date, day of the week, or season
- Have trouble with less challenging mental arithmetic, eg, counting backward from 40 by 4s or from 20 by 2s
- Need help choosing proper clothing for the season or occasion
- Usually retain substantial knowledge about themselves and know their own name and the names of their spouse or children
- Usually require no assistance with eating or using the toilet

Stage 6: Severe cognitive decline (moderately severe or mid-stage Alzheimer's disease)

Memory difficulties continue to worsen, significant personality changes may emerge, and affected individuals need extensive help with customary daily activities. At this stage, individuals may:

- Lose most awareness of recent experiences, events, and surroundings
- Recollect their personal history imperfectly, although they generally recall their name
- Occasionally forget the name of their spouse or primary caregiver but generally can distinguish familiar from unfamiliar faces
- Need help getting dressed properly; without supervision, may make errors such as putting pajamas over daytime clothes or shoes on wrong feet
- Experience disruption of their normal sleep-wake cycle
- Need help with handling details of toileting (flushing toilet, wiping, and disposing of tissue properly)
- Have increasing episodes of urinary or fecal incontinence
- Experience significant personality changes and behavioral symptoms, including suspiciousness and delusions (eg, believing that their caregiver is an impostor); hallucinations (seeing or hearing things that are not really there); or compulsive, repetitive behaviors such as hand wringing or tissue shredding
- Tend to wander and become lost

Stage 7: Very severe cognitive decline (severe or late-stage Alzheimer's disease)

This is the final stage of the disease when individuals lose the ability to respond to their environment, to speak, and ultimately to control movement.

- Frequently lose the ability for recognizable speech, although words or phrases may occasionally be uttered
- Need help with eating and toileting, and there is general urinary incontinence
- Lose the ability to walk without assistance, then the ability to sit without support, smile, and to hold up head; reflexes become abnormal, muscles grow rigid, and swallowing is impaired

and behavior. Both pharmacologic and nonpharma-cologic treatments are available, and the latter should be emphasized. However, research has shown only modest effects on cognition, and providers should educate patients and caregivers to have realistic expectations. Patients with dementia often develop significant behavioral symptoms that are a challenge to both family members and professional caregivers. Any acute change requires an evaluation for undiagnosed medical problems, pain, depression, anxiety, sleep loss, or delirium. Other factors that can contribute to behavioral symptoms include interpersonal or emotional issues. Addressing such issues, treating underlying medical conditions, providing reassurance, and attending to the possible need for changes in the patient's environment can reduce agitation. See "Behavioral Problems in Dementia," p 256. The use of pharmacologic treatments for behavioral problems is recommended only after nonpharmacologic ones prove ineffective, or when there is an emergent need such as risk of physical violence or extreme patient distress.

Nonpharmacologic Treatment

Cognitive Rehabilitation

Reality orientation, memory retraining, and cognitive training have all been proposed as possible techniques to perhaps improve cognitive function. A 2006 Cochrane review of cognitive training found no evidence of positive effects in patients with dementia (SOE=B). Given that new learning is a skill lost very early in the course of AD, an overemphasis on quizzing or retraining may lead to anxiety and self-depreciation. In general, a preferred approach is to provide support to accommodate for lost skills.

Supportive Therapy

Emotion-oriented psychotherapy, such as "pleasant events" and "reminiscence" therapy, and stimulation-oriented treatment, including art and other expressive recreational or social therapies, such as exercise or dance, are examples of psychosocial treatments that can minimize depressive symptoms and reduce behavioral symptoms. These interventions can be provided by professionals or informal caregivers who have been specifically trained. Support groups can provide meaningful support and education for both patients and caregivers. Early-onset dementia groups are especially helpful for patients with mild deficits and insight. Well-controlled trials have not demonstrated efficacy for these approaches, but preliminary studies and clinical experience suggest their usefulness for some behavioral and mood symptoms in patients and family members (SOE=C).

Other Therapies

There are some data supporting physical exercise as having effects on functional performance, cognitive function, and behavioral symptoms. Physical activity should be encouraged as part of the treatment plan. Early research also suggests a role for occupational therapy in providing caregiver education strategies and environmental modification.

Regular Appointments

One approach to ensuring optimal health care for patients with dementia is to schedule regular patient surveillance and health maintenance visits every 3–6 mo. During such visits, the clinician should address and treat comorbid conditions, evaluate ongoing medications, and consider initiating medication-free periods. In addition, it is useful to check for sleep and behavioral disturbances and to provide guidance on proper sleep hygiene. Caregiver well-being should also be regularly assessed.

Family and Caregiver Education and Support

Working closely with family members and caregivers will help establish a therapeutic alliance. Education of family and caregivers about diagnosis, clinical course, treatment options, and management strategies is critical. Information about community resources as well as strategies for managing challenging behavioral symptoms can allow families to cope more effectively, reduce institutionalization, and improve quality of life. Relatives are often helpful sources of information about cognitive and behavioral changes, and generally they take the primary responsibility for implementing and monitoring treatment. Often they are also respon-sible for medical and legal assistance. However, early identification of dementia can allow the affected individual to participate in treatment decisions and future planning. Subjects to pursue with family include medical and legal advance directives (also called advance care plans in some contexts). It is often best for a trusted relative to cosign important financial transactions and attend to paying bills. See "Legal and Ethical Issues," p 23.

Discussion about long-term care placement options should be started early rather than late, to provide the individual or family members time to complete arrangements and begin to adjust emotionally. Eventually, almost 75% of patients with dementia need admission to a long-term care facility and to then remain for lifetime care. Caregivers often express concern about their own memory lapses, which should be addressed with counseling or neuropsychologic assessment. Caregiver distress is often reduced with support-group participation, which may relieve common feelings of anger, frustration, and guilt. Respite care is another community resource that offers caregivers relief. Caregiver support interventions involving individual and family counseling combined with regular participation in support groups have demonstrated improvement in caregiver well-being and delay in time to nursing home placement. Use of support groups and counseling services by family caregivers has also been associated with a delay in nursing-home placement of ≥1 yr (SOE=B).

Environmental Modification

Patients with dementia can be extremely sensitive to their environment; in general, a moderate level of stimulation is best. When they experience overstimulation, confusion or agitation can increase, whereas too little stimulation can cause boredom and withdrawal. As deficits change over time, this balance must be reevaluated and activities adjusted regularly. Familiar surroundings maximize existing cognitive functions, and predictability through daily routines is often reassuring. Other helpful orientation and memory measures in early stages include conspicuous displays of clocks, calendars, and to-do lists. Links to the outside world through newspapers, radio, and television can benefit some mildly impaired patients. Adaptive strategies for more impaired individuals can involve providing visual clues to assist patients (eg, picture of a toilet for the bathroom or food for the dining room) or to distract patients from exposure to unsafe situations (eg, STOP sign on door, covering elevator buttons). Simple sentence structure and repeated reminders about conversation content can also enhance communication.

Attention to Safety

In early stages, safety concerns may be minimal because the person with dementia is still able to make appropriate judgments about safety. However, the need for supervision usually increases as the disease progresses and the person becomes more forgetful and is no longer able to anticipate or avoid dangerous situations. Interventions should balance allowing as much independence as possible while ensuring safety, focusing initially on environmental strategies. Door locks or electronic guards prevent wandering, and many families benefit from registering with Safe Return through the Alzheimer's Association (http://www.alz.org). Patient name tags and medical-alert bracelets can assist in locating lost patients.

Cognitive impairment affects driving skills, and the visuospatial and planning disabilities of even mildly demented patients can make them unsafe drivers. Discussions about driving are best started early in treatment. Patients with advanced dementia definitely should not drive, but clinicians disagree about whether mildly demented patients should drive.

Referral for an independent driving assessment is recommended if there is any concern regarding safety. Certainly, when a patient has a history of traffic accidents or significant spatial and executive dysfunction, driving abilities should be carefully scrutinized. See also the older driver in "Assessment," p 47.

Pharmacologic Treatment

General Issues

Several factors should be considered when prescribing medications for older adults with dementia. Patients in the upper age groups vary in their response, so treatments need to be individualized. In addition, age is associated with decreased renal clearance and hepatic metabolism. Older patients often take several medications simultaneously, so drug interactions and adverse events are likely. Medications with anticholinergic effects are a particular problem for patients with dementia because they can worsen cognitive impairment and lead to delirium. Another group of problem medications that can worsen cognition include those causing CNS sedation. Any nonessential medications with CNS adverse events should be considered carefully. The best strategy, in light of such factors, is to start with low dosages and increase dosing gradually ("start low and go slow"). The goal is to identify the lowest effective dosage, thus minimizing adverse events while avoiding subtherapeutic dosing. Before starting any treatment, a thorough medical examination should be conducted to identify and treat any underlying medical conditions that might impair cognition.

Cholinesterase Inhibitors

The primary medications available for stabilizing cognitive function in AD are cholinesterase inhibitors. Currently, four cholinesterase inhibitors approved by the FDA are available: tacrine (rarely prescribed because of adverse events), donepezil, rivastigmine, and galantamine. By slowing the breakdown of the neurotransmitter acetylcholine, these medications are thought to facilitate memory function because of the association of acetylcholine and memory. In clinical trials, these medications demonstrate a modest delay in cognitive decline compared with placebo in patients with AD. Onset of behavioral problems and decline in ADLs is modestly delayed compared with treatment with placebo (SOE=A). In a Cochrane review of 10 randomized, double-blind, placebo-controlled trials, treatment for 6 mo improved cognitive function, on average –2.7 points (95% confidence interval, –3.0 to –2.3, P <.00001), on the 70-point Alzheimer's Disease Assessment Scale-Cognitive Subscale, as well as small improvement on measures of ADLs and behavior. A meta-analysis also suggested modest clinical benefits of cholinesterase inhibitors in AD, with long-term efficacy difficult to assess because of the short duration of the trials. Results of studies of patients with dementing disorders other than AD are also becoming available. Widespread treatment in vascular dementia was not recommended in a meta-analysis because of the limited cognitive benefit and lack of sufficient data (SOE=B). Some studies suggest that cholinesterase inhibitors may be helpful in managing the hallucinations and fluctuations associated with dementia with Lewy bodies (SOE=B). There appears to be no role for cholinesterase inhibitors in treating frontotemporal dementia. Because effects are modest in all disorders, patients and families should be counseled to have realistic expectations, and discontinuation should be considered after a reasonable time period if decline continues at the rate expected without treatment. Clinical evaluation after 6 mo of therapy is suggested.

Donepezil is the most widely prescribed cholinesterase inhibitor. The recommended starting dosage is 5 mg/d; after 4–6 weeks of treatment, an increase to 10 mg/d is recommended. After 3 mo of treatment at 10 mg/d, increasing the dosage to 23 mg/d can be considered. A slower titration may reduce GI adverse events such as nausea and diarrhea if they occur. Rivastigmine is started at 1.5 mg q12h po for 2 weeks and then doubled no faster than every 2 weeks, to a maximum of 6 mg q12h. Rivastigmine is also available as a skin patch, changed daily, which may be associated with fewer GI adverse events. Galantamine is prescribed in initial dosages of 4 mg q12h po for at least 4 weeks, then 8 mg q12h for at least 4 weeks, and then increased to a maximum of 12 mg q12h. An extended-release formulation is also available that permits the option of once-daily dosing. Although the higher dosages are more efficacious for all agents, they are more likely to cause such cholinergic effects as nausea, diarrhea, and insomnia, especially if the dosage is increased too rapidly. Such adverse events also can worsen the patient's behavior. Other cholinesterase inhibitors and cholinergic receptor antagonists are currently under development. There is currently no evidence of any difference in efficacy among the cholinesterase inhibitors because of limited direct comparisons, although one trial showed fewer adverse events with donepezil than with rivastigmine.

Memantine

Memantine, an N-methyl-d-aspartate antagonist, has been used in Europe for many years. It is thought to have neuroprotective effects by reducing glutamate-mediated excitotoxicity. Clinical trials in the United States support the efficacy of memantine in moderate to severe stages of AD (SOE=A). A Cochrane review of two 6-mo studies showed modest beneficial effects on cognition, ADLs, and behavior. Memantine is approved by the FDA for treatment of moderate to severe AD. Research has not supported use in earlier stages of AD, and trials are ongoing to determine efficacy in other dementing diseases. A Cochrane review and a meta-analysis of memantine in vascular dementia found limited effect on cognition and no evidence to recommend widespread use (SOE=A). The recommended dosage of memantine in the management of Alzheimer's type dementia starts at 5 mg/d po, which may then be increased on a weekly basis in 5-mg increments to 10 mg/d, dosed as 5 mg q12h po, then up to 15 mg/d dosed as 5 mg po in the morning then 10 mg po in the evening, and finally arriving at a target dosage of 20 mg/d dosed as 10 mg q12h after a 4-week titration period. For the extended-release formulation, the starting dosage of 7 mg/d can be increased to 14 mg/d, 21 mg/d, and then 28 mg/d all at weekly intervals. The most common adverse events are constipation, dizziness, and headache. Memantine has been used safely as a single agent and in conjunction with cholinesterase inhibitors for moderate to severe AD (SOE=B).

Other Cognitive Enhancers

Ongoing studies are assessing a variety of other agents in AD, including antioxidants and *Ginkgo biloba* extract. In a trial including more than 300 patients with moderately severe AD, treatment with vitamin E (α-tocopherol) or the selective monoamine oxidase B inhibitor selegiline (approved for treatment of Parkinson's disease) lowered rates of functional decline but was not associated with evidence of cognitive improvement. However, this study involved patients with moderate to severe dementia, so effects on cognition earlier in the illness remain unknown. Results from a randomized placebo-controlled trial of vitamin E and donepezil in mild cognitive impairment showed some short-term benefit from donepezil in delaying conversion to AD but no effect of vitamin E. High-dose vitamin E supplementation was associated with increased mortality in a meta-analysis and is no longer recommended for the treatment of AD.

Extract from the leaf of the *Ginkgo* tree has been promoted primarily in Europe for peripheral vascular disease as well as for "cerebral insufficiency." Other studies in Europe and the United States have explored its use in AD. One 52-week double-blind, placebo-controlled study of *Ginkgo* leaf extract in treating AD seemed to show small but statistically significant improvement in some cognitive measures. However, global measures did not improve in the small, limited study. *Ginkgo biloba* has been uncommonly linked to an increase of bleeding. More research is needed before *Ginkgo* can be recommended.

Many patients also use OTC preparations for cognitive enhancement. A complete review of medications should always include questions about use of OTC medications.

Antidepressants

Antidepressant drug treatment is generally considered for AD patients with depressive symptoms, including depressed mood, appetite loss, insomnia, fatigue, irritability, and agitation. (See "Depression and Other Mood Disorders," p 295.) Anecdotal evidence exists that SSRIs can be helpful in managing the disinhibitions and compulsive behaviors associated with frontotemporal dementia.

Psychoactive Medications

Behavioral and psychologic symptoms of dementia such as paranoia, agitation, and irritability are best managed by nonpharmacologic strategies, such as reducing overstimulation, distraction, and redirection. However, when medications are required, target symptoms should be identified and therapy selected accordingly. Although limited evidence exists for effectiveness, antipsychotics can be used to manage delusions, hallucinations, and paranoia as well as some of the significant irritability associated with dementia. Medications such as carbamazapine[OL] and valproic acid are therapeutic options for managing irritability and agitation. The use of benzodiazepines and medications with anticholinergic effects should be avoided. Finally, antidepressants with sedating effects such as mirtazapine and trazodone can be considered in the management of insomnia. For a complete discussion of nonpharmacologic and pharmacologic treatment of behavioral and psychologic symptoms, see "Behavioral Problems in Dementia," p 256.

Other Resources

Most primary care clinicians successfully treat and manage most patients with dementia, but referral to a specialist is sometimes necessary, especially for diagnosis. When the presentation or history is atypical or complex, particularly when the onset begins before age 60, consultation with a specialist in treating dementia patients (eg, geriatric psychiatrist, neurologist) can be useful.

Community support can be informal, in which neighbors or friends help out, or formal, through home-care or family service agencies, the aging or mental health networks, or adult day-care centers. Available specialized services include adult day care and respite care, home-health agencies that can provide skilled nursing, help lines of the Alzheimer's Association, and outreach services offered by Area Agencies on Aging and Councils on Aging, which are mandated and funded under the federal Older Americans Act. Food services for the homebound are available from meals-on-wheels, and many senior citizens' centers, church and community groups, and hospitals offer transportation options.

For organizations providing information and referral for dementia patients and families, see the resources section on the American Geriatrics Society web site at http://www.americangeriatrics.org.

ACOVE-3* QUALITY INDICATORS PERTAINING TO DEMENTIA

Cognitive and functional screening

- If a vulnerable older adult is new to a primary care practice or inpatient service, then there should be a documented assessment of cognitive ability and functional status.
- All vulnerable older adults should be evaluated annually for changes in memory and function.

Cognitive evaluation

- If a vulnerable older adult screens positive for dementia, then a clinician should document an objective cognitive evaluation that tests two or more cognitive domains.

Medication review

- If a vulnerable older adult screens positive for dementia, then the clinician should review the patient's medications (including OTC) for any that may be associated with mental status changes.
- If a vulnerable older adult screens positive for dementia and is taking medications that are commonly associated with mental status changes in older people, then the clinician should discontinue or justify continuing these medications.

Neurologic examination

- If a vulnerable older adult is newly diagnosed with dementia, then a clinician should perform a neurologic examination that includes evaluation of gait, motor function, and reflexes.

Laboratory testing

- If a vulnerable older adult is newly diagnosed with dementia, then a CBC, thyroid testing, electrolytes, liver function tests, glucose, BUN, serum B_{12}, and a syphilis test should be performed.
- If a vulnerable older adult is newly diagnosed with dementia and has risk factors for HIV, then HIV testing should be offered.

Depression screening

- If a vulnerable older adult has newly diagnosed dementia, then he or she should be screened for depression during the initial evaluation period.

Medication discussion

- If a vulnerable older adult has been diagnosed with mild to moderate Alzheimer's disease, mild to moderate vascular dementia, or Lewy body dementia, then there should be a documented discussion with the patient or caregiver about cholinesterase inhibitor treatment.

Stroke prophylaxis

- If a vulnerable older adult has mild to moderate vascular or mixed dementia, then he or she should receive stroke prophylaxis.

Caregiver support and patient safety

- If a vulnerable older adult with dementia has a caregiver, then the patient or caregiver should be given information on the following:
  - Dementia diagnosis, prognosis, and associated behavioral symptoms
  - Home occupational safety
  - Community resources

Behavioral and psychologic symptoms

- If a vulnerable older adult has dementia, then he or she should be screened annually for behavioral symptoms of dementia.
- If a vulnerable older adult with dementia has behavioral symptoms, then specific target symptoms should be documented and behavioral interventions instituted first or concurrently with pharmacotherapy, or if treating first with a pharmacologic intervention, then severe symptoms or safety concerns should be present and documented.
- If a vulnerable older adult with dementia and behavioral symptoms is newly treated with an antipsychotic, then there should be a documented risk-benefit discussion.

Driving

- If a vulnerable older adult has newly diagnosed dementia, then one of the following should occur (consistent with state law):
  - Advised not to drive a motor vehicle
  - Referral to the Department of Motor Vehicles to test driving ability
  - Referred to a driver's safety course that includes assessment of driving ability

Restraints

- If a vulnerable older adult with dementia is physically restrained in the hospital, then the target behavioral disturbance and safety concern justifying the use of restraints must be documented in the medical record and communicated to the patient, caregiver, or guardian.

Related quality indicators for Dementia

- Evaluate memory loss for depression (see "Depression," p 295)
- Goals of care surrogate discussion (see "Legal and Ethical Issues," p 232)
- Delirium evaluation (see "Delirium," p 264)

*Assessing Care of Vulnerable Elders – 3rd Set. See inside front cover for explanation.

REFERENCES

- Carolan Doerflinger D. Mental Status Assessment of Older Adults: The Mini-Cog. *Try This: Best Practices in Nursing Care to Older Adults.* 2007;(3). Available at http://consultgerirn.org/uploads/File/trythis/try_this_3.pdf

- Holsinger R, Deveau J, Boustani M, et al. Does this patient have dementia? *JAMA.* 2007;297(21):2391−2404.

- Mittelman MS, Haley WE, Clay OJ, et al. Improving caregiver well-being delays nursing home placement of patients with Alzheimer's disease. *Neurology.* 2006;67(9):1592−1599.

- Mitty EL. Decision Making and Dementia. *Try This: Best Practices in Nursing Care to Older Adults.* 2007;(D9). Available at http://consultgerirn.org/uploads/File/trythis/try_this_d9.pdf

- Morrris J. Dementia update 2005. *Alzheimer Disease and Associated Disorders.* 2005;19:100−117.

- Raina P, Santaguida P, Ismaila A, et al. Effectiveness of cholinesterase inhibitors and memantine for treating dementia: evidence review for a clinical practice guideline. *Ann Intern Med.* 2008;148:379−397.

- Richards Hall G, Maslow K. Working with Families of Hospitalized Older Adults with Dementia. *Try This: Best Practices in Nursing Care to Older Adults.* 2007;(D10). Available at http://consultgerirn.org/uploads/File/trythis/try_this_d10.pdf

- Vasse E, Vernooij-Dassen M, Spijker A, et al. A systematic review of communication strategies for people with dementia in residential and nursing homes. *Int Psychogeriatrics.* 2010;22(2):189–200.

CHAPTER 33—BEHAVIORAL PROBLEMS IN DEMENTIA

KEY POINTS

- Behavioral disturbances in dementia require evaluation of the specific symptoms, the comfort of the patient, medical comorbidities, the environment of care, the needs of the caregiver, and the degree of distress of all those involved in the life of the demented adult.

- Delirium secondary to an underlying condition such as dehydration, urinary tract infection, or medication toxicity is a common cause of abrupt behavioral disturbances in patients with dementia.

- Medication treatment of behavioral disturbances in dementia is of limited efficacy and should be used only after environmental and nonpharmacologic techniques have been implemented.

- Increased mortality has been identified with the use of both first-generation antipsychotic agents such as haloperidol and perphenazine as well as second-generation antipsychotic agents such as risperidone and olanzapine. All antipsychotic agents now carry an FDA warning regarding increased all-cause mortality in patients with dementia.

- Despite these FDA warnings, antipsychotic medications may be needed for treatment of distressing delusions and hallucinations, and antidepressants may be helpful if symptoms of depression are evident. There is some evidence for considering mood stabilizers for symptoms such as impulsivity and aggression in patients who have a significant behavioral disturbance.

Most dementias are associated with a range of behavioral and psychologic disturbances, with as many as 80%–90% of patients developing at least one distressing symptom over the course of their illness. The development of behavioral disturbances or psychotic symptoms in dementia often precipitates early nursing-home placement and causes significant caregiver burden and distress. These disturbances are potentially treatable, and it is vital that they are anticipated and recognized early. If these symptoms become apparent, it is essential to perform a thorough evaluation of contributing factors, identify the target symptoms of treatment, and implement appropriate interventions for the patient and caregiver.

CLINICAL FEATURES

Behavioral and psychologic symptoms are a common feature of all dementias. These include anxiety, apathy, depression, sleep disturbance, elation, irritability, disinhibition, wandering, hoarding, verbal disruptions, physical aggression, delusions, and hallucinations. Discrete psychiatric symptoms may develop that take on a variety of characteristics resembling mental disorders such as depression or mania; however, the course and features are more difficult to predict, and treatments are less reliably effective than when these disorders occur in younger adults without dementia. Depressive symptoms are common and often manifest as apathy or a lack of interest in previously enjoyable activities. This depressive syndrome can also include a loss of interest in self-care, eating, or interacting with peers. A propensity for irritability and impulsivity can also occur. If these features become progressive, overt hostility or violence may ensue, and patients may be characterized as "agitated," reflecting a loss of the ability to modulate their behavior in a socially acceptable way. This behavior may involve verbal outbursts, physical aggression, resistance to bathing or other care needs, and restless motor activity such as pacing or rocking. Among the behavioral complications of dementia, the most severe disruptions in caregiving occur when patients develop physical behaviors such as hitting, scratching, or pushing, or when they develop paranoid delusions that lead to hostility and altercations with caregivers. This type of overlap across symptoms, in which some are associated with a well-described psychiatric disorder but others such as wandering and hoarding are considered atypical, often creates a significant challenge in diagnostic labeling. In this situation, the fairly non-specific term *agitation* is commonly used to describe the patient, but it may best be accompanied by additional description as to whether the problem is accompanied by irritability, vocal or physical aggression, or motor disturbances. The term *agitation* is too broad and nonspecific to be clinically useful. Assessment of disruptive behavior must include a careful description of the nature of the symptom, when it occurs, and if any precipitants or antecedents are identified. Treatment cannot be provided without adequate assessment of the behavioral disturbance.

In many cases, agitation can occur concomitantly with evidence of paranoia or delusional thinking, such as a fixed false belief that caregivers have stolen possessions or money, or are plotting against the patient. When delusions occur, the patient is then characterized as suffering from "psychotic" symptoms. False perceptions such as hallucinations are another type of psychotic symptom that can accompany episodes of agitated behavior. Depending on the degree of communication deficits in a given patient, the ability to discern the presence of psychosis is variable, and in many cases disruptive behaviors can occur without clear evidence as to whether delusions or other psychoses may be precipitating the disturbance. Antipsychotic medications are commonly used in the management of disruptive behaviors, with the presumption that disturbed perceptions may be the underlying problem.

Occasionally, a behavioral syndrome occurs that includes features of hyperactivity, mood lability, disinhibition, and grandiose beliefs that resemble a manic episode associated with bipolar affective disorder. The features of this "manic-like" syndrome are described below (p 290), and much like other mood symptoms in dementia, the features are similar but less predictable than those seen in younger adults, and treatment strategies are more challenging. One key feature of the manic-like syndromes seen in dementia patients is the tendency to develop additional symptoms outside the typical course of a bipolar manic episode, such as resistance to care, stubbornness, wandering, and hoarding behaviors, as well as a significant degree of fluctuation in symptoms over the course of a single day.

The complaints from family caregivers and professional caregivers in a nursing home or assisted-living facility often arise from behavioral complications occurring during care that involves a resistance to bathing, dressing, feeding, or other routines. Environmental precipitants such as excessive stimuli or a change in the environment (eg, a new roommate) can induce behavioral problems. The presenting complaint may relate to internal cues such as pain, hunger, thirst, or other needs that the patient is not able to express. Family members may feel more overwhelmed than professional caregivers and may consequently attribute more overall distress to these episodes. Overt resistance to care is most often seen in later stages of dementia, but behavioral problems can also be a first sign of an incipient cognitive decline in earlier stages. Neuropsychiatric symptoms such as apathy, poor self-care, or paranoia may be the first indication of dementia before cognitive decline is recognized, such that an evaluation for dementia in any older adult who presents with new behavioral or emotional symptoms may reveal a previously undetected dementia syndrome.

ASSESSMENT AND DIFFERENTIAL DIAGNOSIS

Comprehensive assessment includes a history both from the patient and from an informant or other source. The information should include a clear description of the behavior: temporal onset, course, associated circumstances, and its relationship to key environmental factors such as caregiver status and recent stressors. The problem behaviors and symptoms should then be considered in the context of the patient's family and personal, social, and medical history.

A differential diagnosis of the disturbance should proceed based on findings of a comprehensive geriatric evaluation. The first step is to decide whether the disturbance is a symptom of a new condition, of a preexisting medical problem, or of an adverse drug event. Disturbances that are new, acute in onset, or evolving rapidly are most often due to a medical condition or medication toxicity. An isolated behavioral disturbance in a demented patient can be the *sole* presenting symptom for many acute conditions such as pneumonia, urinary tract infection, acute pain, angina, constipation, or poorly controlled diabetes mellitus. Additionally, the need to satisfy basic physical needs, such as hunger, sleepiness, thirst, boredom, or fatigue, which the patient cannot adequately communicate, can precipitate a behavioral disturbance. Medication toxicity due to new or existing medications might also present as solely behavioral symptoms. Treatment or stabilization of the medical or physical cause is often sufficient to resolve the disturbance. Older adults with dementia may require several weeks longer to recover from routine medical problems than those who are cognitively intact.

The second step is to consider whether the behavioral disturbance is related to an environmental precipitant. These include disruptions in routine, time change (eg, with daylight savings time or travel across time zones), changes in the caregiving environment, new caregivers, a new roommate, or a life stressor (eg, death of a spouse or family member). Other common environmental precipitants include overstimulation (eg, too much noise, crowded rooms, close contact with too many people, too much time spent out of the familiar environment), understimulation (eg, relative absence of people, spending much time alone, use of television as a companion), and the disruptive behavior of other patients. For many disturbances, correcting an environmental precipitant or removing the stressor commonly improves the symptoms.

Another consideration is whether the disturbance results from stress in the patient-caregiver relationship. Caring for dementia patients is difficult and requires a degree of perseverance of which most caregivers are capable if proper guidance and support is provided. Inexperienced caregivers, domineering caregivers, or caregivers who themselves are impaired by medical or psychiatric disturbances can exacerbate or cause a behavioral disturbance. Caregiver burden can be a problem both in community settings and in nursing homes. Assessing the level of stress and burden on the caregiver is an important part of the evaluation of behavioral disturbances. Interventions to improve the patient-caregiver relationship and to provide caregiver education and support are a vital part of treatment of behavioral disturbances in dementia. Providing resources to caregivers such as referral to support groups and respite services is often very helpful. See also "Psychosocial Issues," p 17; and "Dementia," p 245 on family caregiver education and support.

After medical, environmental, and caregiving causes are excluded, it might be concluded that the behavioral problem is a manifestation of the dementia and may not be amenable to a pharmacologic intervention. Such disturbances that are closely linked to the dementia syndrome take on the form of a catastrophic reaction. A catastrophic reaction is an acute behavioral, physical, or verbal reaction to environmental stressors that results from an inability to make routine adjustments in daily life. The reaction might include anger, emotional lability, or aggression when patients are confronted with a deficit, such as the inability to find a word, or confusion about where they are or what they are supposed to do. Catastrophic reactions are best treated by identifying and avoiding their precipitants, by providing structured routines and activities, and by recognizing early signs of the impending catastrophic reaction so that the patient can be distracted and supported before reacting.

If the disturbance is not related to an identifiable cause or environmental precipitant, it may be a consequence of the brain deterioration that occurs during the course of dementia. Disturbances with a more insidious onset or that are persistent are more likely to be symptoms of the underlying disease. Epidemiologic and clinical studies suggest that such disturbances fall into three groups: mood symptoms, psychosis, and specific behavior problems that occur without significant specific psychiatric symptoms. The overlap in the symptoms of these groups can make treatment choices difficult. One approach is to decide whether the predominant symptom of a poly-symptomatic disturbance is psychosis (delusions or hallucinations), mood symptoms (dysphoria, sadness, irritability, lability), aggression, or agitation, and then direct treatment toward the most distressing feature.

Behavioral disturbances can occur in all types of dementias, including Alzheimer's type, vascular, and mixed. Frontotemporal dementia (ie, Pick's disease) is a less common type of dementia often associated with prominent disinhibition, compulsive behaviors, and social impairment due to more advanced frontal lobe degeneration. In severe cases, a syndrome of hyperphagia, hyperactivity, and hypersexuality can occur that is related to bilateral temporal lobe atrophy. Another dementia associated with prominent psychiatric symptoms and behavioral disturbances is dementia with Lewy bodies. This form of dementia may be more common than previously thought. It is characterized by cognitive deterioration and parkinsonian features with prominent psychosis characterized by visual hallucinations. Affected older adults often suffer from distressing hallucinations and a fluctuating clinical course. These patients are extremely sensitive to the extrapyramidal adverse events of antipsychotic medications (eg, muscle rigidity and tremor) and often cannot tolerate even low dosages of second-generation antipsychotic medications.

TREATMENT—BASIC APPROACH

The treatment of the psychiatric and behavioral disturbances in dementia is complex and may require several interventions as part of a comprehensive plan of care. Specialists should be consulted in refractory cases. In general, treatment begins with appropriate environmental and caregiver interventions. Non-pharmacologic interventions should always be used as a first-line treatment in the management of disruptive, aggressive, or agitated behavior. For a list of key behavioral interventions that might ameliorate behavioral symptoms in patients with dementia, see Table 33.1. Having a daily routine and introducing meaningful activities is vital. Behavioral disturbances in patients with dementia may decrease with the use of music, particularly during meals and bathing, and with light physical exercise or walking. Massage, pet therapy, white noise, videotapes of family, and cognitive stimulation programs may also be helpful. If the disturbances persist despite best efforts, pharmacologic interventions for specific target symptoms are often necessary (see next section). Pharmacologic interventions for specific target symptoms are often necessary (see next section).

TREATMENTS FOR SPECIFIC DISTURBANCES

The core of treatment is identifying any possible underlying cause of the behavior change, recognizing

Table 33.1—Behavioral Interventions for Dementia Care

- Evaluate and treat underlying medical conditions
- Correct sensory deficits; replace poorly fitting hearing aids, eyeglasses, and dentures
- Remove offending medications, particularly anticholinergic agents
- Keep the environment comfortable, calm, and homelike with use of familiar possessions
- Provide regular daily activities and structure; refer patient to adult day care programs, if needed
- Monitor for new medical problems
- Attend to patient's sleep and eating patterns; offer regular snacks and finger foods
- Install safety measures to prevent accidents
- Ensure that the caregiver has adequate respite
- Educate caregivers about practical aspects of dementia care and about behavioral disturbances
- Teach caregivers the skills of caregiving: communication skills, avoiding confrontational behavior management, techniques of ADL support, activities for dementia care
- Simplify bathing and dressing with the use of adaptive clothing and assistive devices if needed; offer toileting frequently and anticipate incontinence as dementia progresses
- Provide access to experienced professionals and community resources
- Refer family and patient to local Alzheimer's Association
- Consult with caregiving professionals, such as geriatric case managers

that multiple causes may exist. Managing pain, dehydration, hunger, and thirst is paramount. The possibilities of positional discomforts or nausea secondary to medication effects should be considered because these are common possible culprits. Good lighting, one-on-one attention, supportive care, and attention to personal needs and wants are also important aspects of treatment. If there is sleep-wake cycle disturbance, efforts should be made to stabilize the sleep cycle by maintaining a stable routine, using bright lights, or prescribing short-term use of medications (see the sleep disturbances section, below).

Mood Disturbances

In dementia patients experiencing mood symptoms, measures similar to those used in other behavior disturbances should be implemented, ie, the environment should be optimized by reducing adversive stimuli and physical health should be assessed comprehensively. Recreational programs and activity therapies have shown positive results in improving mood in depressive symptoms in dementia. Criteria for the diagnosis of depression in Alzheimer's dementia have been proposed that note common features of irritability and social isolation or withdrawal. The waxing and waning course of mood symptoms in

dementia is attributed to the cognitive loss and reduced communication skills related to the dementia. Patients with depression that lasts ≥2 weeks and that results in significant distress should be strongly considered for a trial of an antidepressant medication. Similarly, if depressive symptoms last >2 mo after the initiation of behavioral interventions, treatment with antidepressant medications is warranted.

First-line agents are the SSRIs, preferred for their favorable adverse-event profiles. Studies of depression in patients with dementia have demonstrated the efficacy of sertraline and citalopram versus placebo (SOE=B), but other studies using the same medications as well as paroxetine and fluoxetine have been inconclusive. For the antidepressants most commonly used to treat depressive symptoms in dementia, see Table 33.2.

The treatment of depression in dementia requires persistence. If a first agent has failed after administration of an adequate therapeutic dose for 8–12 weeks, an alternative agent should be tried. Venlafaxine, bupropion, mirtazapine, and the tricyclic agents desipramine and nortriptyline might be considered. Tricyclics should be avoided if a bundle-branch block or other significant cardiac conduction disturbance is present. For patients who are partial responders to an antidepressant, augmentation strategies might be considered. The addition of a stimulant such as methylphenidate[OL] (2.5–10 mg/d) may be helpful in some cases (SOE=C), but there is some risk of increasing psychotic symptoms if the patient has a tendency to be suspicious or delusional. Also, the addition of stimulants such as methylphenidate to augment bupropion should be avoided, because bupropion already possesses stimulant effects. If the patient does not improve, the agents should be discontinued. If a patient continues to be significantly depressed after several antidepressant trials and is in danger because of serious weight loss or suicidal ideas, electroconvulsive therapy might be considered. This is the most efficacious and rapidly effective treatment for severe major depression and has a favorable safety profile even in mild dementia (SOE=B).

Manic-Like Behavioral Syndromes

Occasionally mood syndromes may develop in dementia patients that are characterized by pressured speech, disinhibition, elevated or irritable mood, intrusiveness, hyperactivity, impulsivity, and reduced sleep. These syndromes frequently bear a resemblance to the manic episodes observed in the context of bipolar affective disorder in younger adults, although they are generally considered to be secondary

Table 33.2—Medications to Treat Depressive Features of Behavioral Disturbances in Dementia

Medication	Daily Dosage	Uses	Precautions
Selective serotonin-reuptake inhibitors (SSRIs)			
Citalopram	10–40 mg	Depression, anxiety[OL]	GI upset, nausea, insomnia (common among all SSRIs)
Escitalopram	5–20 mg	Depression, anxiety	
Fluoxetine	10–40 mg	Depression, anxiety	Long half-life, greater inhibition of the cytochrome P-450 system
Paroxetine	10–40 mg	Depression, anxiety	Greater inhibition of cytochrome P-450 system, some anticholinergic effects
Sertraline	25–100 mg	Depression, anxiety	
Serotonin norepinephrine-reuptake inhibitors (SNRIs)			
Desvenlafaxine	25–50 mg	Depression, fibromyalgia	Nausea, hypertension, dry mouth, headaches, dizziness
Duloxetine	20–60 mg	Depression, diabetic neuropathy	Nausea, dry mouth, dizziness, hypertension
Mirtazapine	7.5–30 mg	Useful for depression with insomnia	Sedation, hypotension
Venlafaxine	25–150 mg	Useful in severe depression, anxiety	Hypertension may be a problem, insomnia
Tricyclic antidepressants (TCAs)			
Desipramine	10–100 mg	Useful in severe depression, anxiety; high degree of efficacy	Anticholinergic effects, hypotension, sedation, cardiac arrhythmias (conduction delays)
Nortriptyline	10–75 mg	High efficacy for depression if adverse events are tolerable; therapeutic range 50–150 ng/mL	Anticholinergic effects, hypotension, sedation, cardiac arrhythmias (conduction delays)
Other			
Bupropion	75–225 mg	More activating, lack of cardiac effects	Irritability, insomnia
Trazodone	25–150 mg	When sedation is desirable	Sedation, falls, hypotension

Table 33.3—Mood Stabilizers for Behavioral Disturbances in Dementia with Manic-like Features

Medication	Geriatric Dosage	Adverse Events	Comments
Carbamazepine[OL]*	200–1,000 mg/d (therapeutic level 4–12 mcg/mL)	Nausea, fatigue, ataxia, blurred vision, hyponatremia	Poor tolerability in older adults; must monitor CBC, liver function tests, electrolytes every 2 weeks for first 2 mo, then every 3 mo
Lamotrigine[OL]	25–200 mg/d	Skin rash, rare cases of Stevens-Johnson syndrome, dizziness, sedation, neutropenia, anemia	Increased adverse events and interactions when used with divalproex, slow-dose titration required
Lithium[OL]*	150–1,000 mg/d (therapeutic level 0.5–0.8 mEq/L)	Nausea, vomiting, tremor, confusion, leukocytosis	Poor tolerability in older adults; toxicity at low serum concentrations; monitor thyroid and renal function
Divalproex sodium[OL]*	250–2,000 mg/d (therapeutic level 40–100 mcg/mL)	Nausea, GI upset, ataxia, sedation, hyponatremia	Requires monitoring of CBC, platelets, liver function tests at baseline and every 6 mo; better tolerated than other mood stabilizers in older adults

*Approved by FDA for treatment of bipolar disorder

to the dementing disorder. The important distinction in the dementia patient is the frequent co-occurrence with confusional states and a tendency to have more of a fluctuating mood, ie, the patient's mood may be irritable or hostile as opposed to euphoric. The appearance of hypersexual behaviors may be observed in this clinical scenario, although sexual disinhibition frequently occurs with dementia as a consequence of reduced frontal-executive functioning and may not necessarily be part of a manic syndrome. Treatment of manic-like states, emotional lability, disinhibition, or irritability typically begins with the use of mood-

Table 33.4—Antipsychotic Medications for the Treatment of Psychosis (Hallucinations and Delusions) in Dementia

Medication	Daily Dosage	Adverse Events*	Formulations	Comments
Aripiprazole[OL]	5–15 mg	Mild sedation, mild hypotension	Tablet, rapidly dissolving tablet, IM injection, liquid concentrate	
Clozapine[OL]	12.5–200 mg	Sedation, hypotension, anticholinergic effects, agranulocytosis	Tablet, rapidly dissolving tablet	Weekly CBCs required; poorly tolerated by older adults; reserved for treatment of refractory cases
Olanzapine[OL]	2.5–10 mg	Sedation, falls, gait disturbance	Tablet, rapidly dissolving tablet, IM injection	Weight gain
Paliperidone[OL]	3–12 mg	Sedation, fatigue, GI upset, extrapyramidal symptoms	Sustained-release tablet *only*	
Quetiapine[OL]	25–200 mg	Sedation, hypotension	Tablet, sustained-released tablet	Ophthalmologic examination recommended every 6 mo
Risperidone[OL]	0.5–2 mg	Sedation, hypotension, extrapyramidal symptoms with dosages >1 mg/d	Tablet, rapidly dissolving tablet, depot IM injection, liquid concentrate	
Ziprasidone[OL]	40–160 mg	Higher risk of QT_c prolongation	Capsule, IM injection	Warning about increased QTc prolongation; little published information on use in older adults

*NOTE: All listed medications have warning about hyperglycemia, cerebrovascular events, and increase in all-cause mortality in patients with dementia.

stabilizing agents such as divalproex sodium[OL] (Table 33.3). The sustained-release preparation divalproex sodium is commonly recommended (SOE=C). In dementia patients, a typical starting dosage of divalproex is 125 mg q12h. The dosage should be titrated upward slowly while the patient is monitored for sedation, ataxia, and falls. Blood levels in the range of 50–100 μg/dL have been shown to be effective, but individual variability in dose and response is great. Because of the potential adverse effects on the liver and thrombocytopenia, transaminase levels and a CBC with platelets should be taken before therapy is started, rechecked with each dosage increase, and repeated at least every 6 mo while the patient remains on the medication. Alternatives to divalproex sodium are carbamazepine[OL], lamotrigine[OL], or lithium[OL]. Carbamazepine starting at 100 mg q12h (with monitoring of liver enzymes and CBC) is an acceptable alternative for manic-like states, mood lability, or irritability in dementia. Leukopenia is of concern with carbamazepine, and monitoring the CBC with every dose increase and at least every 3 mo while the patient remains on the medication is needed. Lamotrigine is approved by the FDA for the treatment of mania, but no geriatric trials have been conducted. Lithium is valuable as a mood stabilizer, but its use may be a problem in older adults because of enhanced sensitivity to adverse events. Increased lithium concentrations may occur in the context of reduced renal function and dehydration, resulting in ataxia, tremor, GI distress, and confusion.

Delusions and Hallucinations

Delusions (fixed false beliefs) or hallucinations (false perceptions), whether occurring independently or in association with mood syndromes, typically require specific pharmacologic treatment if the patient is disturbed by these experiences, or if the experiences lead to disruptions in the patient's environment that cannot otherwise be controlled. Clinical criteria for the diagnosis of Alzheimer's dementia with psychosis specifies that the presence of delusions or hallucinations occur for at least 1 mo, at least intermittently, and must cause distress for the patient. A sample of antipsychotic drugs are listed in Table 33.4, along with dosing information. The second-generation agents risperidone[OL], olanzapine[OL], quetiapine[OL], and aripiprazole[OL] are being used more commonly than older agents such as haloperidol[OL]. The older agents are more likely to cause extrapyramidal adverse events, such as parkinsonism and tardive dyskinesia. Sedation, hypotension, and falls are common adverse events among all antipsychotic agents. As these medications are more widely used, differences in adverse-event profiles are emerging. The FDA has required that warnings regarding diabetes mellitus, hyperglycemia, ketoacidosis, and hyperosmolar states be included as a risk of therapy with all second-generation antipsychotic agents. Quetiapine is the most sedating of the second-generation agents. Clozapine[OL], the first of the second-generation agents to be introduced, is difficult to use because of the need for weekly CBC

Table 33.5—Behavioral Management of Insomnia

- Establish a stable routine for going to bed and awakening
- Advise and educate caregivers regarding the natural fragmented sleep patterns associated with dementia
- Optimize sleep environment (attention to noise, light, temperature)
- Increase daytime activity, use of regular light exercise and exposure to natural sunlight
- Reduce or eliminate caffeine, nicotine, alcohol
- Reduce evening fluid consumption to minimize nocturia
- Give activating medications (eg, steroids) early in the day
- Control nighttime pain
- Limit daytime napping to periods of 20–30 minutes
- Use relaxation, stress management, breathing techniques to promote natural sleep
- Provide a safe environment for the patient to stay awake if unable to sleep

monitoring, adverse events of sedation and orthostatic hypotension, and the risk of agranulocytosis. Clozapine is still helpful in a small group of patients with psychosis associated with Parkinson's dementia or dementia with Lewy bodies who are unable to tolerate the extrapyramidal adverse events of other agents; quetiapine can also be used in this situation.

An increased risk of cerebrovascular events in patients with dementia was identified with use of second-generation agents in 2002. All such agents, including risperidone, olanzapine, aripiprazole, quetiapine, clozapine, ziprasidone, and paliperidone must carry this warning. It should be noted that most cerebrovascular events were not fatal.

The FDA required in 2005 that the manufacturers of aripiprazole[OL], olanzapine[OL], quetiapine[OL], risperidone[OL], clozapine[OL], and ziprasidone[OL] add a "black box" warning to their labeling describing an increased risk of mortality that has been observed in 17 placebo-controlled studies (SOE=A). In these studies, the rate of death for patients with dementia was approximately 1.6–1.7 times that of placebo. In most cases, the cause of death appeared to be heart related or from infections (eg, pneumonia). All new second-generation agents, including rapid release clozapine and paliperidone, must carry this warning. Based on 2 observational studies, the FDA has required in 2008 that all first-generation (or conventional) antipsychotic agents also add a "black box" warning regarding an increase in all-cause mortality among patients with dementia who are treated with these agents (SOE=B). The mechanism of action of the increase in mortality is not understood, and the FDA has indicated that it is not indicating that clinicians should never use these agents to treat patients with dementia and psychosis. It is strongly suggested that clinicians discuss the risks and benefits of treatment with these agents with families and caregivers before starting therapy. More information on these warnings is available at http://www.fda.gov/.

Although antipsychotic agents have demonstrated efficacy in large controlled trials in the treatment of dementia with psychosis and aggression, overall positive effects have been relatively modest (SOE=B). Controlled studies of geriatric patients have had notorious difficulty with very high placebo responses. Although 45%–55% of patients improved on antipsychotic medications, the response to placebo ranged from 30% to 50% across studies. Phase I outcomes from the CATIE-AD effectiveness trial found that antipsychotic agents may be more effective than placebo for symptoms such as anger, aggression, and paranoid ideation (SOE=B). However, use of antipsychotic agents did not appear to improve functional status, care needs, or quality of life. Antipsychotic agents clearly play an important role in the treatment of delusions, hallucinations, and aggression in dementia, but they must be part of a comprehensive treatment plan.

There is some evidence that cholinesterase inhibitors such as donepezil or galantamine may reduce the onset of psychosis and behavioral disturbances of Alzheimer's disease. Studies comparing these agents with placebo in patients with mild to moderate Alzheimer's disease have suggested that they may reduce the rate of emergence of behavioral disturbances and psychosis (SOE=C). One area in which cholinesterase inhibitors may be likely to improve psychosis is in the case of dementia with Lewy bodies. Reduced visual hallucinations have been reported with cholinesterase inhibitor treatment (SOE=C).

Disturbances of Sleep

Treatment of insomnia and sleep-wake cycle disturbance should begin with improvement of sleep hygiene (Table 33.5). This consists of efforts to get the patient to go to sleep later every day, around 10:00 or 11:00 pm, while keeping the environment calm, comfortable, and conducive to sleep, into the next morning. If the sleep disturbance is associated with depression, suspiciousness, or delusions, those conditions should be treated.

For primary sleep disturbances when good sleep hygiene and increasing daytime activity level are not successful, trazodone[OL] (25–150 mg at bedtime) or mirtazapine[OL] (7.5–15 mg at bedtime) might be used (SOE=D). Benzodiazepines or antihistamines, such as diphenhydramine, should be avoided, because they carry a high risk of falls, hip fractures, disinhibition, and cognitive disturbance when prescribed for patients with dementia. See also "Sleep Problems," p 272.

Zolpidem[OL] and zaleplon[OL] are short-acting nonbenzodiazepine sedative hypnotics that may be helpful for sleep disturbances in older adults, although there have been no controlled trials for their use in sleep disturbances secondary to dementia. Zolpidem has been studied in older patients without dementia and appears to be effective in improving sleep onset, although it does not improve sleep duration because of its short half-life. The recommended dose of zolpidem in older adults is 5 mg, because an increased risk of adverse events appears to be dose related. Zaleplon has been less extensively studied in older patients but appears to have similar properties.

Hypersexuality

If hypersexuality occurs in association with another recognizable syndrome such as a mania-like state, treatment of the specific syndrome, such as with mood stabilizers, should be utilized. In men with dementia who are dangerously hypersexual or aggressive, clinical case reports have suggested a trial of an antiandrogen might be attempted to reduce the sexual drive (SOE=D). Patients have been tried on oral progesterone[OL] 5 mg/d at first. The dosage should be adjusted to suppress serum testosterone well below normal. If the patient responds well behaviorally, 10 mg of depot intramuscular progesterone may be given weekly to maintain a reduction of sexual drive. An alternative treatment to reduce sexual drive is leuprolide acetate[OL] (5–10 mg IM every month), also an antiandrogen. The use of antipsychotic medications is often adopted clinically, given the seriousness of hypersexual behaviors in institutionalized settings such as nursing homes; however, there are no controlled studies supporting this use. Presumably, these medications may enhance the cognitive focus of the individual's perceptions by reducing any psychotic thinking that may in some way be contributing to hypersexual behavior. Studies are needed for this problem.

Intermittent Aggression or Agitation

When disruptive behavior occurs intermittently or episodically, such as once per week or less, behavioral interventions focusing on identifying the antecedents of the behavior and avoiding the triggers are often most useful. Behavior modification using positive reinforcement of desirable behavior has been shown to be helpful, and it also helps encourage the caregiver to focus on times when behavior is not a problem. Caregiver education and support, music therapy, and physical activity appear to show promise in reducing behavioral disturbances (SOE=B). Reminiscence; validation therapy; and environmental modifications of light, sound, and space may all help promote positive behavior. Distraction techniques, activity therapies, and aromatherapy also show promise in reducing troublesome behaviors (SOE=C).

Physical restraint in any form should be avoided if at all possible. If restraining measures are necessary, careful supportive care should be provided to the patient. Over time, it is usually possible to reduce or eliminate the amount of restraint. See also the section on quality issues in "Nursing-Home Care," p 142.

ACOVE-3* QUALITY INDICATORS PERTAINING TO BEHAVIORAL PROBLEMS IN DEMENTIA

Behavioral and psychologic symptoms

■ If a vulnerable older adult has dementia, then he or she should be screened annually for behavioral symptoms of dementia.

■ If a vulnerable older adult with dementia has behavioral symptoms, then specific target symptoms should be documented and behavioral interventions instituted first or concurrently with pharmacotherapy, or if treating first with a pharmacologic intervention, then severe symptoms or safety concerns should be present and documented.

■ If a vulnerable older adult with dementia and behavioral symptoms is newly treated with an antipsychotic, then there should be a documented risk-benefit discussion.

Restraints

■ If a vulnerable older adult with dementia is physically restrained in the hospital, then the target behavioral disturbance and safety concern justifying the use of restraints must be documented in the medical record and communicated to the patient, caregiver, or guardian.

*Assessing Care of Vulnerable Elders – 3ʳᵈ Set. See inside front cover for explanation.

REFERENCES

■ American Psychiatric Association. Practice guideline for the treatment of Alzheimer's disease and other dementias 2nd edition. *Am J Psychiatry*. 2007;164(12 Suppl):1–56.

■ Ayalon L, Gum AM, Feliciano L, et al. Effectiveness of nonpharmacological interventions for the management of neuropsychiatric symptoms in patients with dementia: a systematic review. *Arch Intern Med*. 2006:166(20):2182−2188.

■ Cohen-Mansfield J, Marx M, Dakheel-Ali M, et al. Can agitated behavior of nursing home residents with dementia be prevented with the use of standardized stimuli? *J Am Geriatr Soc*. 2010;58(8):1459–1464.

■ Sink KM, Holden KF, Yaffee K. Pharmacological treatment of neuropsychiatric symptoms of dementia: a review of the evidence. *JAMA*. 2005;293(5):596−608.

CHAPTER 34—DELIRIUM

KEY POINTS

■ The first key step in delirium management is accurate diagnosis, which involves administration of a brief mental status exam that includes testing of attention, and application of the Confusion Assessment Method diagnostic algorithm.

■ All delirious patients require a thorough evaluation for reversible causes; all correctable contributing factors should be addressed.

■ Delirious patients are vulnerable and require an intensive interdisciplinary effort to maximize likelihood of a favorable outcome.

■ Pharmacologic intervention should be reserved for key target symptoms; low-dosage, high-potency antipsychotics are usually the treatment of choice.

■ Proactive, multifactorial interventions have reduced the incidence, severity, and duration of delirium. Interventions begun after the onset of delirium have been less successful.

Delirium remains under-recognized and often inappropriately evaluated and managed. Clinicians call delirium by many different names. *Acute confusional state* is the most common synonym. Other commonly used synonyms include *acute mental status change*, *altered mental status*, *organic brain syndrome*, *reversible dementia*, and *toxic* or *metabolic encephalopathy*.

INCIDENCE AND PROGNOSIS

Delirium is common and associated with substantial morbidity. Approximately one-third of patients ≥70 yr old admitted to a general medical service experience delirium: one-half of these are delirious on admission to the hospital; the other half develop delirium in the hospital. Up to one-third of older adults presenting to the emergency department are delirious. In postacute skilled-nursing facilities, 16% of new admissions meet the full criteria for delirium, and an additional 49% have subsyndromal delirium.

Although delirium is traditionally viewed as a transient phenomenon, there is growing evidence that it may persist for weeks to months in a substantial portion of affected individuals. Recent studies demonstrate that delirium persists through hospital discharge in 25%–50% of those affected. Among those discharged with delirium, persistence rates of up to 50% at 1 mo have been reported. Risk factors for delirium persistence predominantly relate to individual vulnerability, including advanced age, preexisting dementia, multiple comorbidities, and functional impairment, but also include severity of delirium and use of restraints.

Evidence is mounting that delirium is strongly and independently associated with poor patient outcomes (SOE=B). Delirium has been associated with a 10-fold increased risk of death in the hospital and a 3- to 5-fold increased risk of nosocomial complications, prolonged hospital length of stay, and greater need for postacute nursing-home placement. In studies that incorporated follow-up after discharge, delirium was associated with poor functional recovery and increased risk of death up to 2 yr after hospital discharge. These associations persist after adjustment for factors such as patient age, preexisting dementia, and severity of illness. Patients with delirium at discharge and prolonged delirium seem to have the worst outcomes, suggesting that persistence of delirium can play an important role in poor long-term outcomes.

DIAGNOSIS AND DIFFERENTIAL DIAGNOSIS

Under-recognition of delirium is a major problem. The criteria of the *Diagnostic and Statistical Manual of Mental Disorders*, 4th edition, Text Revision (*DSM IV-TR*) although precise, can be difficult to apply in clinical practice. More clinically useful is the Confusion Assessment Method (CAM). By judging the presence or absence of the four key CAM features shown in Table 34.1, the clinician can establish the diagnosis of delirium. Although the CAM can be completed by using observations from routine care, use of a formal mental status evaluation improves detection and reliability of the assessment. A brief formal cognitive assessment such as the Mini–Mental State Examination, with supplemental attentional testing, is recommended before using the CAM. Table 34.2 shows some commonly used tests of attention. In the absence of a formal evaluation or when there is doubt, any older adult with acute change in mental status should be considered delirious, and evaluated and managed as described below.

The Confusion Assessment Method for the Intensive Care Unit (CAM–ICU) is a variant of the CAM that does not require verbal responses from the patient. Although it was designed for ventilated patients in the ICU, it can be used more generally for patients who are unable to speak. It includes the same four features as the CAM diagnostic algorithm but uses mental status testing that requires only yes-no answers, which can be indicated by a nod or raised finger. Attention is tested using the Attention Screening Examination, in which patients are required to immediately recall simple pictures. Disorganized thinking is tested by answers to a series of simple yes-no questions (eg, "Does 1 pound weigh more than 2 pounds?").

The differential diagnosis of delirium includes dementia, depression, and acute psychiatric syndromes. In many cases, it is not truly a "differential" diagnosis, because these syndromes can coexist and indeed are risk factors for one another. Instead, it is better thought of as a series of independent questions: Does this patient have delirium, dementia, depression? Does the patient have more than one disorder? The most common diagnostic issue is whether a newly presenting confused patient has dementia, delirium, or both. To make this determination, the clinician must know the patient's baseline status. In the absence of baseline data, information from family members, caregivers, or others who know the patient is essential. An acute change in mental status from baseline is not consistent with dementia and suggests delirium. In addition, a rapidly fluctuating course (over minutes to hours) and an abnormal level of consciousness are also highly suggestive of delirium. Depression can also be confused with hypoactive

delirium. In one study, one-third of patients who had psychiatric consultations for depression in the acute-care setting actually had hypoactive delirium. Finally, certain acute psychiatric syndromes, such as mania, can present similarly to hyperactive delirium. Hyperactive patients are best initially evaluated and managed as if they have delirium rather than attributing the presentation to psychiatric disease and missing a serious underlying medical disorder.

THE SPECTRUM OF DELIRIUM

The classic presentation of delirium is thought to be the extremely agitated patient. However, agitated or hyperactive delirium represents only 25% of cases. More common is hypoactive or "quiet" delirium, and delirium with mixed features. A recent study of new admissions to postacute facilities demonstrated a 1.6-fold increased risk of death (confidence interval 95%: 1.1, 2.4) among patients with hypoactive delirium relative to delirious patients with normal psychomotor activity. Potentially, one of the reasons for this poorer prognosis is that hypoactive delirium is less frequently recognized. Special case-finding efforts are necessary to detect quiet delirium among high-risk older patients. If agitation is present, behavioral control measures may be necessary (see below), but such measures alone are not adequate treatment for delirium, and in some cases they can exacerbate or prolong the delirium.

RISK FACTORS

In the absence of a clear neuropathophysiologic basis for delirium, the cornerstone of its management focuses on the assessment and treatment of modifiable risk factors. Fortunately, several consistent risk factors for delirium have been identified. These risk factors classify into two groups: baseline factors that predispose patients to delirium, and acute factors that precipitate delirium. Predisposing factors include advanced age, preexisting dementia, preexisting functional impairment in ADLs, and high medical comorbidity. Male gender, sensory impairment (poor vision and hearing), and history of alcohol abuse have also been reported in some studies. Acute precipitating factors include medications, especially those that are sedating or highly anticholinergic, surgery, uncontrolled pain, low hematocrit level, bed rest, and use of certain indwelling devices and restraints. A useful model suggests that delirium is precipitated when the sum of predisposing and precipitating factors crosses a certain threshold. In such a model, the greater the predisposing factors, the fewer precipitating factors are required to initiate delirium. This would explain why older, frail adults develop delirium in the face of stressors that are much less severe than those that

---

STRENGTH-OF-EVIDENCE (SOE) RATING DEFINITIONS

A = consistent and good quality patient-oriented evidence

B = somewhat inconsistent or limited quality patient-oriented evidence

C = very inconsistent or very limited patient-oriented evidence, disease-oriented evidence, and/or consensus from professional organizations

D = unstudied common practice or opinion

See inside front cover for detailed information regarding the SOE classification.

Table 34.1—Comparison of the *DSM IV-TR* Diagnostic Criteria for Delirium and the Confusion Assessment Method

DSM IV-TR Criteria	Confusion Assessment Method	Confusion Assessment Method–Intensive Care Unit Version
1. Acute change in mental status and fluctuating course		
Disturbance of consciousness (ie, reduced clarity of awareness of the environment) with reduced ability to focus, sustain, or shift attention	Is there evidence of an acute change in cognition from the patient's baseline? Does the abnormal behavior fluctuate during the day, ie, tend to come and go, or increase and decrease in severity?	Is there an acute change from baseline? Did the abnormal behavior fluctuate over the past 24 hours? Suggest using the Glasgow Coma Scale evaluations or sedation score ratings over the past 24 hours as well as collateral information from nurse and family.
2. Inattention		
A change in cognition (such as memory deficit, disorientation, language disturbance) or the development of a perceptual disturbance that is not better accounted for by a preexisting, established, or evolving dementia	Does the patient have difficulty focusing attention, eg, being easily distracted, or having difficulty keeping track of what is being said?	Does the patient have difficulty focusing attention? Is there a reduced ability to maintain and shift attention? Suggest using nonverbal examinations such as the picture recognition or Vigilance A letter test because these can be used with mechanically ventilated patients.
3. Disorganized thinking		
Disturbance develops over a short period of time (usually hours to days) and tends to fluctuate during course of the day	Is the patient's thinking disorganized or incoherent, eg, rambling or irrelevant conversation, unclear or illogical flow of ideas, or unpredictable switching from subject to subject?	Was the patient's thinking disorganized or incoherent, such as rambling or irrelevant conversation, unclear or illogical flow of ideas, or unpredictable switching from subject to subject? Was the patient able to follow questions and commands throughout the assesment? Suggest asking the following questions: ▪ Are you having any unclear thinking? ▪ Hold up this many fingers. (Examiner holds up 2 fingers in front of the patient.) ▪ Now do the same thing with the other hand. (Examiner does not repeat the number of fingers.)
4. Altered level of consciousness		
History, physical examination, or laboratory findings provide evidence that the disturbance is caused by the direct physiologic consequences of a general medical condition or a drug, or both	Is the patient's mental status anything other than alert, eg, vigilant, lethargic, stuporous, or comatose	Any level of consciousness other than alert: ▪ Vigilant (hyperalert) ▪ Lethargic (drowsy but easily aroused, unaware of some elements in the environment) ▪ Stuporous (difficult to arouse, unaware of some or all elements in the environment) ▪ Comatose (unarousable, unaware of all elements in the environment)

The diagnosis of delirium requires the presence of features 1 and 2 and either 3 or 4.

SOURCES: Data from *Diagnostic and Statistical Manual of Mental Disorders*. 4th ed. Washington, DC: American Psychiatric Association; 1994; Inouye SK, van Dyck CH, Alessi CA, et al. Clarifying confusion: the Confusion Assessment Method: a new method for detection of delirium. *Ann Intern Med.* 1990;113(12):941–948; and Ely EW, Margolin R, Francis J, et al. Evaluation of delirium in critically ill patients: validation of the Confusion Assessment Method for the Intensive Care Unit (CAM-ICU). *Crit Care Med.* 2001;29(7):1370–1379.

Table 34.2—Commonly Used Tests of Attention

Test	Patient Is Asked To:	Comments
Digit span	Repeat random sequence of numbers, repeat sequence of numbers in reverse order	Should be able to do at least 5 forward, 4 backward
Days, months	Recite the days of the week backward, recite the months of the year backward	Advantage: not much affected by poor memory, hearing, education, knowledge of English
Continuous performance task	Raise hand whenever he or she hears a certain letter or number in a list	Does not require verbal response
Attention screening examination	Show 5 pictures; ask patient to remember them and to recall them in a series of 10 pictures shown subsequently	Used in the CAM–ICU Does not require verbal response
MMSE items	Subtract 7 from 100, then subtract 7 from each remainder ("serial sevens")	Requires ability to calculate
World backward	Spell *world* backward	Requires knowledge of English

NOTE: CAM–ICU = Confusion Assessment Method for the Intensive Care Unit; MMSE = Folstein's Mini–Mental State Examination

Table 34.3—Mnemonic for Reversible Causes of Delirium

Drugs	Any new additions, increased dosages, or interactions
	   Consider OTC drugs and alcohol
	   Consider especially high-risk drugs (Table 34.5)

Electrolyte disturbances	Especially dehydration, sodium imbalance Thyroid abnormalities
Lack of drugs	Withdrawals from chronically used sedatives, including alcohol and sleeping pills Poorly controlled pain (lack of analgesia)
Infection	Especially urinary and respiratory tract infections
Reduced sensory input	Poor vision, poor hearing
Intracranial	Infection, hemorrhage, stroke, tumor Rare; consider only if new focal neurologic findings, suggestive history, or diagnostic evaluation otherwise negative
Urinary, fecal	Urinary retention: "cystocerebral syndrome" Fecal impaction
Myocardial, pulmonary	Myocardial infarction, arrhythmia, exacerbation of heart failure, exacerbation of COPD, hypoxia

can cause delirium in younger, healthy adults. For a mnemonic for reversible risk factors for delirium, see Table 34.3.

DELIRIUM AND DEMENTIA

While dementia is an established risk factor for delirium, evidence is increasing that the relationship may be bidirectional. A series of studies demonstrated that nondemented patients who develop delirium are at increased risk of incident dementia over the next 1–5 yr. Most of these studies did not involve detailed testing of neuropsychologic performance before the onset of delirium, so it remains unclear whether delirium was the herald of previously unrecognized cognitive impairment (or other brain vulnerability), or whether the delirium itself set forth a CNS process that initiated or accelerated onset of dementia. In either case, these findings suggest that previously intact patients who develop delirium need to be monitored closely, even if the acute symptoms of delirium resolve entirely. A related finding suggests that patients with established dementia who develop delirium are at risk of accelerated cognitive and

functional decline. Further studies exploring the interrelationship of delirium with dementia should use serial cognitive testing performed both before and after the episode of delirium, to better define how delirium impacts cognitive trajectory. A more recent study demonstrated that Alzheimer's patients experienced accelerated cognitive decline after an episode of delirium.

POSTOPERATIVE DELIRIUM

Delirium may be the most common complication after surgery in older adults. The incidence is 15% after elective noncardiac surgery, and up to 50% after high-risk procedures such as hip fracture repair, aortic aneurysm repair, and coronary artery bypass grafting. In a prospectively validated clinical prediction rule for delirium after elective noncardiac surgery, seven risk factors could be identified preoperatively: advanced age, cognitive impairment, physical functional impairment, history of alcohol abuse, markedly abnormal serum chemistries, intrathoracic surgery, and aortic aneurysm surgery. Patients with none of these risk factors had a 2% risk of delirium, those with one or two risk factors had a 10% risk, and those with three or more risk factors had a 50% risk.

In addition to baseline risk factors, postoperative management plays an important role in the development of delirium. This is confirmed by the observation that the peak incidence of delirium is not immediately after recovery from anesthesia, but on the second postoperative day. The stresses of surgery and anesthesia are not likely to be the sole precipitants of most cases of postoperative delirium.

Several studies have demonstrated that the route of intraoperative anesthesia, whether general, spinal, epidural, or other, has little impact on the risk of delirium (SOE=B). Postoperative medication management plays a much more important role. Postoperative use of benzodiazepines and certain opioids, especially meperidine, is strongly associated with the development of delirium. Although pain medications can cause delirium, adequate pain management is also important, because high levels of postoperative pain have also been associated with delirium. Strategies to provide adequate analgesia with minimally effective doses of opioids should be used. These include the use of scheduled rather than as-needed dosing, patient-controlled or regional analgesia, and opioid-sparing analgesics and nonpharmacologic approaches, such as ice packs. Low postoperative hematocrit level (<30%) has also been associated with postoperative delirium, although transfusions have not been shown to reduce delirium.

EVALUATION

All patients with newly diagnosed delirium require a careful history, physical examination, and targeted laboratory testing. Most of the treatable causes for delirium lie outside the CNS, and these should be investigated first. Moreover, multiple contributing factors are often present, so the diagnostic evaluation should not be terminated because a single "cause" is identified. For key steps in the evaluation and management of delirium, see Table 34.4.

The history should focus on the time course of the changes in mental status and their association with other symptoms or events (eg, fever, shortness of breath, medication change). Because medications are the most common and treatable cause of delirium, a careful medication history, using the nursing administration sheets in the hospital or a "brown-bag" review in the outpatient setting, is imperative. In the outpatient setting, it is also important to review the patient's use of OTC drugs, herbal or other supplements, and alcohol. The physical examination should include vital signs and oxygen saturation, a careful general medical examination, and a neurologic and mental status examination. The emphasis should be on identifying acute medical problems or exacerbations of chronic medical problems that might be contributing to delirium. Laboratory tests should be selected on the basis of history and examination findings. Most patients require at least a CBC, electrolytes, and kidney function tests. Urinalysis, tests for liver function, serum medication levels, and arterial blood gases, as well as chest radiographs, an ECG, and appropriate cultures are helpful in selected situations. Cerebral imaging is often performed but is rarely helpful, except in cases of head trauma or new focal neurologic findings. In the absence of seizure activity or signs of meningitis, electroencephalograms and cerebrospinal fluid analysis rarely yield helpful results.

MANAGEMENT

Delirious hospitalized patients are particularly vulnerable to complications and poor outcomes. Special care is needed and requires an interdisciplinary effort by health care providers, family members, and others. A multifactorial approach is the most successful because many factors contribute to delirium; thus, multiple interventions, even if individually small, can yield marked clinical improvement (Table 34.4). If delirium is not diagnosed and managed properly, costly and life-threatening complications and long-term loss of function can result.

Modifying the risk factors that contribute to delirium is critically important. Some factors, such as age and prior cognitive impairment, cannot be modified. However, some predisposing factors, such as sensory impairment, can be modified through proper use of eyeglasses and hearing aids. Medications are the most common reversible causes of delirium. Anticholinergics, H_2-blockers, benzodiazepines, opioids, and antipsychotic medications should be replaced with medications that have no central effects. For example, H_2-blockers can be replaced by antacids or proton-pump inhibitors, and regular dosing of 650 mg of acetaminophen three to four times daily can reduce or eliminate the need for opioids in many patients (Table 34.5).

The delirious patient is susceptible to a wide range of iatrogenic complications, and careful surveillance is critical. Bowel and bladder function should be monitored closely, but urinary catheters should be avoided unless absolutely required for monitoring fluids or treating urinary retention. Bowel stimulants and stool softeners can be used to prevent obstipation, particularly in those who are concomitantly using opioids. Complete bed rest should be avoided, because it can lead to increasing disability through disuse of muscles and the development of pressure ulcers and atelectasis in the lungs. Exercise and ambulation prevent the deconditioning often associ-

Table 34.4—Management of Delirium

Step	Key Issues	Proposed Treatment
1. Identify and treat reversible contributors	Medications	Reduce or eliminate offending medications, or substitute less psychoactive medications
	Infections	Treat common infections: urinary, respiratory, soft tissue
	Fluid balance disorders	Assess and treat dehydration, heart failure, electrolyte disorders
	Impaired CNS oxygenation	Treat severe anemia (transfusion), hypoxia, hypotension
	Severe pain	Assess and treat; use local measures and scheduled pain regimens that minimize opioids; avoid meperidine
	Sensory deprivation	Use eyeglasses, hearing aid, portable amplifier
	Elimination problems	Assess and treat urinary retention and fecal impaction
2. Maintain behavioral control	Behavioral interventions	Teach hospital staff appropriate interaction with delirious patients; encourage family visitation
	Pharmacologic interventions	If necessary, use low-dose high-potency antipsychotics (Table 34.6)
3. Anticipate and prevent or manage complications	Urinary incontinence	Implement scheduled toileting program
	Immobility and falls	Avoid physical restraints; mobilize with assistance; use physical therapy
	Pressure ulcers	Mobilize; reposition immobilized patient frequently and monitor pressure points
	Sleep disturbance	Implement a nonpharmacologic sleep hygiene program, including a nighttime sleep protocol; avoid sedatives
	Feeding disorders	Assist with feeding; use aspiration precautions; provide nutritional supplementation as necessary
4. Restore function in delirious patients	Hospital environment	Reduce clutter and noise (especially at night); provide adequate lighting; have familiar objects brought from home
	Cognitive reconditioning	Have staff reorient patient to time, place, person at least three times daily
	Ability to perform ADLs	As delirium clears, match performance to ability
	Family education, support, and participation	Provide education about delirium, its causes and reversibility, how to interact, and family's role in restoring function
	Discharge	Because delirium can persist, provide for increased ADL support; follow mental status changes as "barometer" of recovery

ated with hospitalization. Malnutrition can be avoided through the use of nutritional supplements and careful attention to intake of food and fluids. Some delirious patients may need assistance in feeding.

Managing behavioral problems while ensuring both the comfort and safety of the patient can be challenging. The patient should be placed in a room near the nursing station for close observation. Nonpharmacologic behavioral measures provide orientation and a feeling of safety. Orienting items such as clocks, calendars, and even a window view should be made available. Patients should be encouraged to wear their eyeglasses and hearing aids. Although use of physical restraints in the hospital has not been well studied, evidence from the long-term care setting suggests that such restraints probably do not decrease the rate of falls by confused ambulatory patients, and they may actually increase the risk of fall-related injury. Restraints, although objectionable, may be required because of violent behavior or to prevent the removal of important devices, such as endotracheal tubes, intra-arterial devices, and catheters. Even for patients with these devices, the calm reassurance provided by a family member or sitter may be much more effective than the use of physical restraints or medications. Whenever restraints are used, the indicators for use should be frequently reassessed, and the restraints should be removed as soon as possible.

Medications used as restraints extract a costly toll in accidents, adverse events, and loss of mobility, and they should be avoided if possible. Pharmacologic intervention may be necessary for symptoms such as delusions or hallucinations that are frightening to the patient when verbal comfort and reassurance are not successful. Some delirious patients display behavior that is dangerous to themselves or others and cannot be calmed by a family member or sitter. Indications

Table 34.5—Drugs to Reduce or Eliminate in the Management of Delirium

Agent	Adverse Events	Possible Substitutes	Comments
Alcohol	CNS sedation and withdrawal	If history of heavy intake, careful monitoring and benzodiazepines if withdrawal symptoms	Alcohol history is imperative
Anticholinergics (oxybutynin, benztropine)	Anticholinergic toxicity	Lower dosage; behavioral measures	Rare at low dosages
Anticonvulsants (especially primidone, phenobarbital, phenytoin)	CNS sedation and withdrawal	Alternative agent or none	Toxic reactions can occur despite "therapeutic" drug concentrations
Antidepressants, especially tertiary amine tricyclic agents (amitriptyline, imipramine, doxepin)	Anticholinergic toxicity	Secondary amine tricyclics (nortriptyline, desipramine), SSRIs, or other agents	Secondary amines as good as tertiary for adjuvant treatment of chronic pain
Antihistamines (eg, diphenhydramine)	Anticholinergic toxicity	Nonpharmacologic protocol for sleep; pseudoephedrine for colds	Must take OTC medication history
Antiparkinsonian agents (levodopa-carbidopa, dopamine agonists, amantadine)	Dopaminergic toxicity	Lower dosage; adjusted dosing schedule	Usually with end-stage disease and high dosages
Antipsychotics, especially low-potency anticholinergic agents and second-generation agents (clozapine)	Anticholinergic toxicity; CNS sedation	No agents or, if necessary, low-dosage high-potency agents	See note for Table 34.6 for warnings about second-generation antipsychotics
Barbiturates	CNS sedation; severe withdrawal syndrome	Gradual discontinuation or benzodiazepine	In most cases, should no longer be prescribed; avoid inadvertent or abrupt discontinuation
Benzodiazepines, especially long-acting (eg, diazepam, flurazepam, chlordiazepoxide)	CNS sedation	Nonpharmacologic sleep management; intermediate agents (lorazepam, temazepam)	Associated with delirium in medical and surgical patients
Benzodiazepines: ultra short-acting (eg, triazolam, alprazolam)	CNS sedation and withdrawal	Nonpharmacologic sleep management; intermediate agents (lorazepam, temazepam)	Associated with delirium in case reports and series
Chloral hydrate	CNS sedation	Nonpharmacologic sleep protocol	No better for delirium than benzodiazepines
H$_2$-blocking agents	Possible anticholinergic toxicity	Lower dosage; antacids or proton-pump inhibitors	Most common with high-dosage intravenous infusions
Nonbenzodiazepine hypnotics (eg, zolpidem)	CNS sedation and withdrawal	Nonpharmacologic sleep protocol	Like other sedatives, can cause delirium
Opioid analgesics (especially meperidine)	Anticholinergic toxicity, CNS sedation, fecal impaction	Local measures and nonpsychoactive pain medications around the clock; opioids only for breakthrough and severe pain	Higher risk in patients with renal insufficiency; must consider risks versus benefit
Almost any medication if time course is appropriate			**Consider risks and benefits of all medications in older adults**

for pharmacologic intervention should be clearly identified, documented, and constantly reassessed.

A meta-analysis examined pharmacologic treatment of agitation in delirium. Four studies were included, with the largest having a sample size of 73 participants. One of these studies established the superiority of haloperidol to benzodiazepines. The other studies all demonstrated the equivalence of the

second-generation antipsychotics with haloperidol. Interestingly, none of the studies used a placebo control group. Based on this limited evidence (SOE=B), high-potency antipsychotics are the treatment of choice for agitation in delirium because of their low anticholinergic potency and minimal hypotensive effects. However, they must be used cautiously, because they can actually prolong delirium and increase the

Table 34.6—Pharmacologic Therapy of Agitated Delirium

Agent	Mechanism of Action	Dosage	Benefits	Adverse Events	Comments
Haloperidol[OL]	Antipsychotic	0.25–1 mg po or IM q4h prn agitation	Relatively nonsedating; few hemodynamic effects	EPS, especially if >3 mg/d	Usually agent of choice[a]
Olanzapine[OL]	Antipsychotic	2.5–5 mg po or IM q24h, max dosage 20 mg q24h (cannot be given by IV infusion)	Fewer EPS than haloperidol	More sedating than haloperidol	Small case series only[b];oral formulations less effective for acute management
Quetiapine[OL]	Antipsychotic	25–50 mg po q12h	Fewer EPS than haloperidol	More sedating than haloperidol; hypotension	Small case series[b]
Risperidone[OL]	Antipsychotic	0.25–1 mg po or IV q4h prn agitation	Similar to haloperidol	Might have slightly fewer EPS	Case series only[b]
Lorazepam[OL]	Sedative	0.25–1 mg po or IV q8h prn agitation	Use in sedative and alcohol withdrawal, and history of neuroleptic malignant syndrome	More paradoxic excitation, respiratory depression than haloperidol	Second-line agent, except in specific cases noted

NOTE: EPS = extrapyramidal symptoms

[a] In a randomized trial comparing haloperidol, chlorpromazine, and lorazepam in the treatment of agitated delirium in young patients with AIDS, all were found to be equally effective, but haloperidol had the fewest adverse events.

[b] The FDA has attached warnings to the second-generation antipsychotics because of the increased risk of stroke and mortality associated with their long-term use, primarily for agitation in dementia.

risk of complications by converting a hyperactive, confused patient into a stuporous one whose risk of a fall or aspiration is increased. In older patients with mild delirium, low doses of haloperidol[OL] (0.5–1 mg po or 0.25–0.5 mg parenterally) should be used initially, with careful reassessment before additional dosing. In more severe delirium, somewhat higher doses can be used initially (0.5–2 mg parenterally), with additional dosing every 60 min as required for symptom management. One must be careful to assess for akathisia (motor restlessness), which may be an adverse event of high-potency antipsychotic medications and can be confused with worsening delirium. The treatment for akathisia is less, not more antipsychotic medication. Haloperidol should be avoided in older adults with parkinsonism and Lewy body disease, and a second-generation antipsychotic with less extrapyramidal effects such as quetiapine[OL] can be substituted. For a summary of the pharmacologic management of agitated delirium, see Table 34.6.

It is important to stress to family members that delirium is usually not a permanent condition, but rather that it improves over time. Unfortunately, the persistence of delirium is common. Thus, when counseling families, it is important to point out that many cognitive deficits associated with the delirium syndrome can continue, abating weeks and even months after the illness. Advanced age (≥85 yr old), preexisting cognitive impairment, and severe illness are risk factors for slow recovery of cognitive function. Careful monitoring of mental status and providing adequate functional supports during this period are necessary to give the patient the maximal chance of returning to his or her baseline level. Family members can play an important role in the hospital and postacute setting by providing appropriate orientation, support, and functional assistance. Hospitals are increasingly making provisions for family members to sleep overnight with relatives who are already delirious or at high risk of developing delirium. While symptoms of delirium may persist, acute exacerbation of cognitive dysfunction is not expected during the convalescent period and therefore likely heralds a new medical problem. Families should be counseled to seek prompt medical attention if a patient's mental status acutely worsens.

REFERENCES

- Fick D, Mion L. Assessing and Managing Delirium in Older Adults with Dementia. *Try This: Best Practices in Nursing Care to Older Adults.* 2007;(D8). Available at http://consultgerirn.org/uploads/File/trythis/try_this_d8.pdf

- Fong TG, Jones RN, Shi P, et al. Delirium accelerates cognitive decline in Alzheimer's disease. *Neurology.* 2009;72(18):1570–1575.

- Inouye SK. Delirium in older persons. *N Engl J Med.* 2006;354(11):1157–1165.

- Lundstrom M, Edlund A, Karlsson S, et al. A multifactorial intervention program reduces the duration of delirium, length of hospitalization, and mortality in delirious patients. *J Am Geriatr Soc.* 2005;53(4):622–628.

- Tate J, Happ MB. The Confusion Assessment Method for the ICU (CAM-ICU). *Try This: Best Practices in Nursing Care to Older Adults.* 2008;(25). Available at http://consultgerirn.org/uploads/File/trythis/try_this_25.pdf

- Voyer P, Richard S, Doucet L, et al. Detection of delirium by nurses among long-term care residents with dementia. *BMC Nursing.* 2008;7(4).

- Waszynski C. The Confusion Assessment Method (CAM). *Try This: Best Practices in Nursing Care to Older Adults.* 2007;(13). Available at http://consultgerirn.org/uploads/File/trythis/try_this_13.pdf

CHAPTER 35—SLEEP PROBLEMS

KEY POINTS

- In older adults, insomnia is often accompanied by psychiatric and/or medical conditions, and evidence suggests that comorbid illness, rather than a primary aging effect, is largely responsible for the increased prevalence of insomnia in older adults.

- Compared with younger adults, older adults generally take longer to fall asleep and have more nighttime wakefulness and more daytime napping. An earlier bedtime and earlier wake time are also common.

- Older adults also have less N3 (previously termed stages 3 and 4) sleep (ie, slow-wave sleep, which is the deeper stage of sleep).

- The appropriate treatment of sleep problems must be guided by knowledge of likely causes and potential contributing factors.

- Trials have shown that behavioral interventions can be quite effective for insomnia in older adults.

EPIDEMIOLOGY

Sleep problems are common among older adults, particularly those with other psychiatric and medical conditions. More than two-thirds of older adults with multiple comorbidities have sleep problems. The most common sleep complaints among community-dwelling older adults are difficulty falling asleep (around 40%), nighttime awakening (30%), early morning awakening (20%), and daytime sleepiness (20%). At least one-half of community-dwelling older adults use OTC and/or prescription sleeping medications.

Epidemiologic studies in older adults have demonstrated an association between sleep complaints and risk factors for sleep disturbance (eg, chronic illness, multiple medical problems, mood disturbance, less physical activity, physical disability) but little association with older age, suggesting that these risk factors, rather than aging per se, account for much of the increase in insomnia with age. However, certain sleep disorders do increase in prevalence with age, such as sleep-related breathing disorders (ie, sleep apnea), periodic limb movement disorder, restless legs syndrome, and circadian rhythm sleep disorders.

Table 35.1—Age-Related Changes in Sleep

Sleep Characteristic	Age-Related Change*
Total sleep time	Decrease
Sleep latency (time to fall asleep)	Increase or no change
Sleep efficiency (time asleep over time in bed)	Decrease
Daytime napping	Increase
Stages N1 and N2	Increase
Slow wave sleep (Stage N3)	Decrease
Percent rapid eye movement (REM)	Decrease
Wake after sleep onset	Increase

*Many of these changes seen by middle age

Insomnia is more common in women than in men across the life span (SOE=A). A meta-analysis of several epidemiologic studies from around the world found a risk ratio for insomnia in women compared with men that increased from young adulthood (risk ratio [RR]=1.28) to older age (RR=1.73). Self-reported sleeping difficulties are more common in older black Americans, particularly women and those with depression and chronic illness.

Late-life insomnia is often a chronic problem. In one British study, more than one-third of older adults with insomnia reported persistent severe symptoms at 4 yr follow-up, and one-third of participants who reported use of prescription hypnotics were still using these agents 4 yr later. Even among very old women (≥85 yr old), there is evidence that most report sleeping difficulties, and many regularly use alcohol and/or OTC sleeping agents for sleep. Studies in the United States suggest that around 5% of older adults use sedative hypnotics. Insomnia has been reported as a predictor of death and nursing-home placement (particularly in older men). In addition, in several epidemiologic studies, subjective sleep disturbance was associated with worse health-related quality of life in older adults (SOE=B).

CHANGES IN SLEEP WITH AGING

In general, older adults have decreased sleep efficiency (time asleep divided by time in bed), stable or decreased total sleep time, and increased sleep latency (time to fall asleep) (Table 35.1). Older adults also report an earlier bedtime and earlier morning awakening, more awakenings during the night, more wakefulness during the night, and more daytime

napping. Notable age-related changes in sleep structure as measured by polysomnography include changes in both nonrapid eye movement (NREM) and rapid eye movement (REM) sleep. Older adults have less N3 (previously termed stage 3 and 4) sleep (ie, slow-wave sleep, which is the deeper stage of sleep), while the percentage of stage N1 and N2 sleep (ie, the lighter stages of sleep) increases with age. The decline in slow-wave sleep begins in early adulthood and progresses throughout life, with a notable decline in middle age. Men have more decline in slow-wave sleep than women. Changes in REM sleep with age are less clear, but a decrease in REM sleep and an earlier onset of REM sleep in the night (ie, shorter REM latency) have been reported. Older adults also have a decrease in sleep spindles and K complexes on electroencephalography during sleep. In addition, older adults can have an advance in circadian rhythms of sleep and wake (ie, go to bed earlier, wake up earlier) and a reduced amplitude in circadian rhythms. Of note, new sleep stage scoring criteria and terminology were recommended in 2007 by the American Academy of Sleep Medicine, and these terms will likely be increasingly used in the literature (eg, N1 [NREM1], N2 [NREM2], N3 [NREM3, which includes both stages 3 and 4 sleep], and R [REM] sleep).

Most experts believe that the decreased sleep in older adults is due to a decreased *ability* to sleep, rather than a decreased *need* for sleep. However, after a period of sleep deprivation, older adults show less daytime sleepiness, less evidence of decline in performance measures, and a quicker recovery of normal sleep structure than younger people. Older adults have more sleep disturbance with jet lag and shift work, which may reflect physiologic changes in circadian rhythm with age. In studies comparing good sleepers with poor sleepers, poor sleepers were found to take more medications, make more physician visits, and have poorer self-ratings of health. In addition, as noted above, chronologic age per se does not seem to correlate with higher prevalence of poor sleep.

EVALUATION OF SLEEP

Symptoms of sleep disturbance in older adults can be identified with simple screening questions, such as asking whether the person is satisfied with their sleep, whether sleep or fatigue interferes with daytime activities, and whether a bed partner or others complain of unusual behavior during sleep, such as snoring, interrupted breathing, or leg movements. Having the patient keep a sleep log for 1–2 weeks can be helpful in obtaining a careful description of the sleep complaint. Each morning, the patient should record the time spent in bed the prior night, the estimated amount of sleep, the number of awakenings, the time of morning awakening, and any symptoms that occurred during the night. The time that the patient goes to bed and awakens should be recorded, as well as time spent napping during the day. The patient's sleep log should be supplemented by information from a bed partner (if available) or from others who may have observed unusual symptoms during the night. Several validated sleep questionnaires are available in the literature. The focused physical examination depends on evidence from the history. For example, reports of painful joints should be followed by a careful examination of the affected areas. Reports of nocturia that disrupts sleep should be followed by evaluation for cardiac, renal, or prostatic disease, or diabetes mellitus. Mental status testing should also be considered, with a focus on mood and memory problems. The findings of the history and physical examination should guide laboratory testing.

Polysomnography is indicated when a sleep-related breathing disorder (sleep apnea) or narcolepsy is suspected, or when there are symptoms of violent or injurious behaviors during sleep (SOE=A). Polysomnography may be indicated when other unusual behaviors occur during sleep or if periodic limb movement disorder is suspected (SOE=B). Portable sleep monitoring systems for use in the home have been developed and are used primarily when sleep apnea is suspected. Wrist activity monitors (ie, wrist actigraphy) estimate sleep versus wakefulness based on wrist movement. Wrist actigraphy can be used in identifying circadian rhythm disorders (SOE=A) and in nursing-home residents, in whom traditional sleep monitoring can be difficult because of the setting (SOE=B).

COMMON SLEEP PROBLEMS

Insomnia

Insomnia is defined as difficulty in falling or staying asleep, waking up too early, or experiencing sleep that is nonrestorative or poor in quality, and is associated with daytime impairment (such as fatigue, poor concentration, daytime sleepiness, or concerns about sleep). The prevalence of insomnia increases from about 10% in young adulthood to about 30% in those ≥65 yr old. However, the prevalence of insomnia symptoms is even greater than the prevalence of insomnia using strict diagnostic criteria. Much of the increase in insomnia seen with older age seems to occur by middle age. In older adults in particular, insomnia is generally seen with other conditions, and (compared with good sleepers) older adults with insomnia are more likely to have medical and/or psychiatric illness. In fact, some evidence suggests that much of the increase in insomnia prevalence with older age is due to comorbid insomnia. Other

risk factors for insomnia include female gender, social isolation, low socioeconomic status, and more medications.

Some studies report that an associated psychiatric disorder is present in 30%–60% of patients presenting with insomnia. Depression is the most common and the most strongly associated comorbid psychiatric illness with insomnia, and most patients with depression also have sleep complaints. Common sleep complaints with depression include early morning awakening, increased sleep latency, and more nighttime wakefulness. Chronic insomnia is a risk factor for development of major depressive disorder in older (and younger) adults, and studies suggest that insomnia symptoms commonly precede the onset of depressive symptoms. In depressed older adults with sleep disturbance, treatment of depression can improve sleep complaints. Conversely, lack of attention to sleep complaints in older depressed adults can make depression less likely to respond to treatment. (See also "Depression and Other Mood Disorders," p 295.) After depression, anxiety disorder is the psychiatric condition most commonly associated with insomnia symptoms, particularly difficulty falling asleep and early awakening. See also "Anxiety Disorders," p 307. Caregiving is also associated with insomnia, and older caregivers report more sleep complaints than do noncaregivers of similar age. In one study, nearly 40% of older women who were family caregivers of adults with dementia reported taking a sleeping medication in the past month. See also caregiving in "Psychosocial Issues," p 18; "Mistreatment of Older Adults," p 87; and "Community-Based Care," p 150.

Many medical problems are associated with sleep complaints in older adults. Epidemiologic studies in older adults suggest a greater prevalence of insomnia in those with conditions such as hypertension, heart disease, arthritis, lung disease, gastroesophageal reflux, stroke, neurodegenerative disorders (eg, dementia, Parkinson's disease), and other comorbid conditions. Common symptoms of medical illness that can contribute to sleep disturbance (particularly nighttime awakening) include pain, paresthesias, cough, nocturnal dyspnea, gastroesophageal reflux, and nighttime urination. Older adults with sleeping difficulties who describe pain at night should have their painful condition assessed and managed (see "Persistent Pain," p 109). Nighttime urination is common in both older men and women, and may be associated with sleep disturbance and increased fatigue in the daytime.

Many medications can contribute to insomnia in older adults. Sleep can be impaired by diuretics or stimulating agents (eg, caffeine, sympathomimetics, bronchodilators, activating psychiatric medications) taken near bedtime. Some antidepressants, antiparkinson agents, and antihypertensives (eg, propranolol) can induce nightmares and impair sleep. Required medications that are sedating (eg, sedating antidepressants) should be given at bedtime if possible. Chronic use of sedatives can cause light, fragmented sleep. For some sleeping medications, chronic use can lead to tolerance and the potential for increasing dosages. When chronic use of hypnotics is suddenly stopped, rebound insomnia can occur. Alcohol abuse is associated with lighter sleep of shorter duration. In addition, some older adults try to treat their sleeping difficulties with alcohol. Although nighttime alcohol causes an initial drowsiness, it can impair sleep later in the night. Finally, sedatives and alcohol can worsen sleep apnea; the use of these respiratory depressants should be avoided in older adults with documented or suspected untreated sleep apnea. See also "Addictions," p 322.

Sleep-Related Breathing Disorders

Sleep-related breathing disorders are characterized by disordered respiration during sleep. Central sleep apnea (CSA) syndromes are those in which respiratory effort is absent due to CNS or cardiac dysfunction. Obstructive sleep apnea (OSA) is characterized by an obstruction in the airway resulting in continued breathing effort but inadequate ventilation. In-laboratory polysomnography is the gold standard for diagnosis of these conditions (SOE=A). Portable devices that use cardiac monitoring and oximetry have shown some promise in diagnosing obstructive sleep apnea in the home. These devices are less expensive, and monitoring can be performed more readily than in a sleep laboratory. The sensitivity of home testing is far lower than laboratory polysomnography (SOE=B).

In older adults, CSA can be a primary disorder, secondary to neurodegenerative disease or stroke, or the Cheynes-Stokes breathing pattern of heart failure. CSA is more common in older adults than in younger adults. Treatment of Cheynes-Stokes respiration focuses on management of the heart failure. Current evidence does not support use of continuous positive airway pressure (CPAP) to improve survival in patients with CSA and heart failure (SOE=A). Nighttime oxygen supplementation can reduce the apnea and oxygen desaturation, but effects on important health outcomes are unclear (SOE=C).

Sleep apnea is common among older adults, but reported prevalence varies considerably. Patients with OSA usually present with excessive daytime sleepiness and are typically unaware of their frequent arousals at night. Patients can have morning headache, personality changes, poor memory, confusion, and irritability. A bed partner may report loud snoring, cessation of breathing, and choking sounds during sleep. Patients are generally obese, but there is less association between obesity and OSA in older age. Other reported predictors identified in community-dwelling older adults include falling asleep at inappropriate times, male gender, and napping. The classic sleep apnea patient is the obese, sleepy snorer with hypertension. Large neck circumference has also been reported as a marker for sleep apnea, but this may not be an important predictor of sleep apnea in older adults.

Alcohol abuse and dependence is an important risk factor for sleep apnea, and sleep-disordered breathing is a significant contributor to sleep disturbance in men >40 yr old with a history of alcoholism. Finally, there appears to be an association between sleep apnea and dementia. Of note, evidence suggests that OSA patients with mild-moderate dementia tolerate CPAP well, with acceptable adherence to treatment, improvement in OSA parameters, and some evidence of beneficial effects on cognition (SOE=B).

The importance of mild degrees of sleep-disordered breathing in older adults is unclear. In one study, no association was found between mild or moderate sleep-disordered breathing and subjective sleep-wake disturbance. The long-term consequences of asymptomatic sleep-disordered breathing are also unclear.

Patients suspected of having OSA should be referred to a sleep laboratory for evaluation and, if the diagnosis is documented, treatment. Portable in-home monitoring devices are also available. CPAP reduces sleepiness and improves quality of life in people with moderate and severe OSA (SOE=A). Older adults likely tolerate CPAP as well as younger adults. Careful efforts to use devices (eg, variations in mask, humidification) that improve comfort can improve adherence with CPAP. Early successful adherence with CPAP can predict long-term adherence with CPAP treatment. Unfortunately, clinicians may be prejudiced against the use of CPAP in older adults, perhaps because they assume that the treatment will not be tolerated or successful in this population.

Other mechanical options are available as alternatives to CPAP, eg, bi-level PAP (biPAP), which reduces expiratory pressure in an effort to increase comfort. Evidence suggests that biPAP does not improve efficacy or adherence in the treatment of sleep apnea compared with CPAP (SOE=B), but these alternative devices can be appropriate in certain patients. Oral appliances are also available, but CPAP is more effective in improving OSA. Oral appliances are generally recommended only in patients with mild symptomatic OSA or in those unwilling or unable to tolerate CPAP (SOE=B). Several upper airway surgical approaches have also been used, but evidence of effectiveness from large trials is limited.

Periodic Limb Movements During Sleep and Restless Legs Syndrome

Periodic limb movements during sleep (PLMS) is a condition of repetitive, stereotypic leg movements that generally occur in non-REM sleep. PLMS increases in prevalence with age, but the significance of this is unclear because many studies have found little relationship between PLMS and sleep disruption. In one study, evidence of PLMS was found in more than one-third of community-dwelling older adults. Some authors have suggested that the high prevalence of PLMS with age is associated with delayed motor and sensory latencies noted on nerve conduction testing. When PLMS is associated with clinical sleep disturbance or a complaint of daytime fatigue that is not better explained by another sleep disorder, this is termed periodic limb movement disorder (PLMD). Polysomnography is required to establish a diagnosis of PLMD.

Restless legs syndrome (RLS) is a condition of an uncontrollable urge to move one's legs at night, usually accompanied by an uncomfortable and unpleasant sensation of the legs that worsens with inactivity and improves with movement. The symptoms occur while the person is awake, and symptoms can also involve the arms. The diagnosis is based on the patient's description of the symptoms; polysomnography is not required to make the diagnosis. There may be a family history of the condition (particularly in patients with an earlier age onset of RLS) and, in some cases, an underlying medical disorder (eg, anemia, or renal or neurologic disease). RLS is 1.5 times more common in women than men, and evidence suggests that RLS prevalence increases with age. PLMS occurs in most (80%–90%) patients with RLS, but the presence of PLMS is not specific for RLS. RLS can also be seen in patients with dementia, in which the patient may not be able to adequately describe the symptoms. RLS should be considered in dementia patients who have symptoms such as rubbing or massaging of legs, increased motor activity (eg, pacing, wandering), and evidence of leg discomfort with inactivity and improvement with activity. Many medications can aggravate or induce RLS symptoms, such as antiemetics, antipsychotics, SSRIs, tricyclic antidepressants, and diphenhydramine. These and other medications should be addressed in patients with new or worsening RLS.

If pharmacologic treatment for PLMD or RLS is indicated (because of severity of symptoms or significant effects on quality of life), dopaminergic agents are the initial agent of choice. An evening dose of a dopamine agonist (eg, pramipexole or ropinirole, about 1–2 hours before bedtime) are effective in the treatment of RLS and PLMD (SOE=A). A nighttime dose of carbidopa-levodopa[OL] is also effective (SOE=A) and can be used for patients who need medication infrequently (ie, for as-needed use). Some patients describe a shift of their symptoms to daytime hours with successful treatment of symptoms at night; this appears more commonly with chronic use of carbidopa-levodopa for RLS. RLS can be associated with iron deficiency, in which case RLS symptoms can improve with iron replacement therapy (SOE=B). Patients with RLS should be screened for iron deficiency. Of course, the cause of the iron deficiency should be addressed. Gabapentin[OL] can also be effective (SOE=B), particularly in patients who cannot tolerate dopamine agonists. Benzodiazepines[OL] and opioids[OL] have also been used for RLS but likely have more adverse events in older adults than the dopaminergic agents.

Circadian Rhythm Sleep Disorders

Disturbances in circadian rhythms of the sleep-wake cycle may be more common with advanced age. In particular, older adults are more likely to have an advanced sleep phase (fall asleep early and awaken early) rather than a delayed sleep phase (fall asleep late and awaken late), but a delayed sleep phase can be seen in older adults. Some individuals have extremely irregular sleep-wake cycles, including some patients with dementia and nursing-home residents. Some common changes in sleep pattern seen in older adults (such as increased daytime napping and disrupted nighttime sleep) can be due to alterations in circadian rhythm. Dementia is associated with sleep-wake disturbance and frequent nighttime awakenings, nighttime wandering, and nighttime agitation.

A sleep log can help establish the presence of a circadian rhythm sleep disorder (SOE=B). Wrist actigraphy can also be useful for making a diagnosis (particularly in patients who are unable to complete a sleep log) and in monitoring treatment response in patients with a circadian rhythm sleep disorder (SOE=B), including older patients with dementia and nursing-home residents. Polysomnography is not routinely indicated in patients in whom a circadian rhythm sleep disorder is suspected, but referral to a sleep specialist may be indicated when symptoms do not respond to initial management, when the diagnosis is unclear, or when another sleep disorder is suspected (SOE=C). Treatment depends on the particular circadian rhythm sleep disorder. An advanced sleep phase may respond to appropriately timed (ie, evening) exposure to bright light (SOE=B) (see nonpharmacologic interventions, p 313). A delayed sleep phase may respond to appropriately timed morning bright light and/or evening melatonin (SOE=B).

REM Sleep Behavior Disorder

REM sleep behavior disorder is characterized by excessive motor activities during sleep and a pathologic absence of normal muscle atonia during REM sleep. The presenting symptoms are usually vigorous sleep behaviors associated with vivid dreams, and patients may first present because of injuries (to themselves or their bed partner). The condition can be acute or chronic, and it is much more common in older men (in some series, >85% of cases are older men). There may be a family predisposition. Transient REM sleep behavior disorder has been associated with toxic metabolic abnormalities, primarily drug or alcohol withdrawal or intoxication. The chronic form of the disorder can be idiopathic but is increasingly recognized as associated with neurodegenerative disorders such as Parkinson's disease, Lewy body dementia, multisystem atrophy, and other conditions. Several psychiatric medications have been associated with REM sleep behavior disorder, including tricyclic antidepressants, monoamine oxidase inhibitors, fluoxetine, venlafaxine, cholinesterase inhibitors, and other agents. Polysomnography is indicated to establish the diagnosis. Removal of the offending agent is indicated for drug-induced REM sleep behavior disorder. Clonazepam[OL] is reported to be effective for treatment of REM sleep behavior disorder, with little evidence of tolerance or abuse over long periods of treatment, but some patients (especially older adults) can experience adverse events. There is some evidence for the use of melatonin in the treatment of REM sleep behavior disorder in individuals with coexisting neurodegenerative disorders (eg, Parkinson's disease, dementia with Lewy bodies) (SOE=C). Environmental safety interventions are also indicated, such as removing dangerous objects from the bedroom, putting cushions on the floor around the bed, protecting windows, and in some cases, putting the mattress on the floor.

CHANGES IN SLEEP WITH DEMENTIA

Older adults with dementia have more sleep disruption and arousals, lower sleep efficiency, a higher percentage of stage 1 sleep, and more sleep fragmentation than nondemented older people. Circadian rhythm sleep disorders are more common with dementia, resulting in excessive daytime sleeping and nighttime wakefulness. Cholinesterase inhibitors (often used in treatment of the symptoms of dementia) can exacerbate insomnia and cause vivid dreams; changing dose timing to morning hours can help alleviate this problem. Sedative hypnotic agents have not been adequately tested in patients with dementia. As mentioned above, evidence suggests that those with coexisting OSA and mild to moderate dementia can tolerate CPAP well, with improvement in OSA parameters and beneficial effects on cognition. Results of studies using melatonin for sleep disturbance in dementia have been mixed, but one large randomized controlled trial in patients with Alzheimer's disease suggested melatonin was not effective for sleep disturbance in these individuals (SOE=B). Bright light therapy has also been used in dementia patients, with some beneficial effects on sleep and circadian rhythms (SOE=B), but the most appropriate timing of the light exposure is unclear.

SLEEP DISTURBANCES IN THE HOSPITAL

Acute hospitalization can precipitate transient or short-term insomnia. This insomnia is likely multifactorial in origin and related to illness, medications, change from usual nighttime routines at home, and a sleep-disruptive hospital environment (eg, high noise levels at night). In one small uncontrolled study, nighttime melatonin levels increased in hospitalized older patients treated with daytime bright-light exposure. Another small study implemented "flexible medication times" that allowed inpatients to sleep longer in the morning, and their resulting in-hospital sleeping patterns were more similar to their at-home sleeping patterns. However, adherence with nonpharmacologic interventions can be difficult to achieve in the acute hospital. For example, one large clinical trial of nonpharmacologic interventions to prevent delirium in hospitalized older adults reported only a 10% adherence rate for the sleep protocol portion of the intervention.

Sleeping medications are commonly prescribed in hospitalized older adults. A large Belgian study of consecutively admitted patients at a university hospital found that 45% of patients took a sleeping medication in hospital, with greater use among patients ≥60 yr old. In this sample, >15% of patients who were newly prescribed a sleeping pill while in the hospital reported that they planned to use the medication after discharge to home. In another study of hospitalized older adults in India, among those prescribed a benzodiazepine for sleep during their acute hospitalization, over half were not taking a sleeping pill before their admission. Benzodiazepine receptor agonists are commonly used for insomnia in hospitalized older adults, but prescribers should remember to use smaller dosages (than for younger adults), which are likely effective and safer in older adults. Sedating antihistamines (eg, diphenhydramine) should not be used as a sleep aid in hospitalized older adults because of possible complications related to anticholinergic adverse events (eg, delirium, urinary retention, constipation).

Sleep-related breathing disorders can be common in hospitalized adults, particularly among those with cardiac illness and stroke. In one study of older men on medicine wards in a Veterans Affairs hospital, survival among patients with heart failure and CSA was shorter than among heart failure patients without evidence of this disorder. Sleep apnea among stroke patients is associated with worse survival and less functional recovery.

SLEEP IN THE NURSING HOME

Nursing-home residents often have marked sleep disruption, frequent nighttime awakening, and excessive daytime sleeping. In one study, up to 70% of caregivers reported that nighttime difficulties played a significant role in their decision to institutionalize the older adult, often because the sleep of the caregiver was being disrupted. Once in the nursing home, many residents nap on and off throughout the day and wake up frequently during the night. One study found that 65% of residents reported problems with their sleep and that the use of hypnotic medications was common, but no association was found between the use of sedative hypnotics and the presence, absence, or change in sleep complaints after 6 mo of follow-up. In another study, the average duration of sleep episodes during the night in nursing-home residents was only 20 minutes. Nursing-home residents generally have little or no exposure to outdoor bright light, which likely exacerbates sleep-wake abnormalities. Other common conditions in nursing-home residents that can contribute to sleep disturbance include multiple physical illnesses, the use of psychoactive medications, pain, debility and inactivity, increased prevalence of sleep disorders, and environmental factors (eg, nighttime noise, light, disruptive nursing care).

MANAGEMENT OF SLEEP PROBLEMS

Treatment of sleep problems in older adults must be guided by knowledge of likely causes and potential contributing factors. Sedative hypnotics have a documented association with falls, hip fracture, and daytime carryover symptoms in older adults. However, there is also some evidence that untreated insomnia symptoms are associated with increased risk of falls in older adults. If the initial history and physical examination do not suggest a serious underlying cause for the sleep problem, a trial of improved sleep habits (eg, sleep hygiene techniques) is usually the best first approach (Table 35.2). If the person takes daytime naps, it is important to determine whether these are needed rest periods or due to inactivity, boredom, or sedating medications. It is important to explain that daytime naps will decrease nighttime sleep.

Table 35.2—Measures to Improve Sleep Hygiene

- Maintain regular rising time.
- Maintain regular bed time, but do not go to bed unless sleepy.
- Decrease or eliminate naps, unless necessary part of sleeping schedule.
- Exercise daily but not immediately before bedtime.
- Do not use bed for reading or watching television.
- Relax mentally before going to sleep; do not use bedtime as worry time.
- If hungry, have a light snack (except with symptoms of gastroesophageal reflux or medical contraindications), but avoid heavy meals at bedtime.
- Limit or eliminate alcohol, caffeine, and nicotine, especially before bedtime.
- Wind down before bedtime and maintain a routine period of preparation for bed (eg, washing up, going to the bathroom).
- Control the nighttime environment with comfortable temperature, quiet, and darkness.
- Try a familiar background noise (eg, a fan or other "white noise" machine).
- Wear comfortable bed clothing.
- If unable to fall asleep within 30 min, get out of bed and perform soothing activity such as listening to soft music or light reading (but avoid exposure to bright light).
- Get adequate exposure to bright light during the day.

Short-term hypnotic therapy may be appropriate in conjunction with improved sleep habits in cases of transient, situational insomnia, particularly during bereavement, acute hospitalization, and other periods of temporary acute stress. Sedative hypnotic medication treatment should not be withheld in situations when it is clearly indicated. People generally do not feel well if they do not sleep well. If a decision is reached to use a sedative hypnotic in an older adult, the smallest dosage of the agent with the least risk of adverse events should be chosen. However, in older adults with chronic insomnia, sedative hypnotic agents should be used cautiously because of the complications associated with their long-term use (see chronic hypnotic use, p 281). The chronic use of benzodiazepines can lead to dependence or cognitive impairment. The newer, nonbenzodiazepine hypnotics have been tested in healthy older adults and seem to have less risk of daytime carryover and tolerance to sedative effects. However, there has been little study of these (or other hypnotic) agents in older adults with significant medical comorbidity.

Behavioral and Nonpharmacologic Interventions

Behavioral treatment of insomnia is effective in older adults, including those with insomnia comorbid with other conditions (SOE=A). For a summary of such interventions, see Table 35.3. Several systematic

Table 35.3—Examples of Nonpharmacologic Interventions to Improve Sleep

Intervention	Goal	Brief Description
Stimulus control	To recondition maladaptive sleep-related behaviors	Patient is instructed to go to bed only when sleepy, not use the bed for eating or watching television, get out of bed if unable to fall asleep, return to bed only when sleepy, get up at the same time each morning, not take naps during the day.
Sleep restriction	To improve sleep efficiency (time asleep over time in bed) by limiting time in bed	Patient first keeps a sleep diary for 1–2 weeks to determine average total daily sleep time, then stays in bed only that amount of time plus 15 minutes, gets up at same time each morning, takes no naps in the daytime, gradually increases time allowed in bed as sleep efficiency improves.
Cognitive interventions	To change misunderstandings and false beliefs regarding sleep	Patient's dysfunctional beliefs and attitudes about sleep are identified; patient is educated to change these false beliefs and attitudes, including normal changes in sleep with increased age and changes that are pathologic.
Relaxation techniques	To recognize and relieve tension and anxiety	In progressive muscle relaxation, patient is taught to tense and relax each muscle group; in electromyographic biofeedback, the patient is given feedback regarding muscle tension and learns techniques to relieve it; meditation or imagery techniques are taught to relieve racing thoughts or anxiety.
Cognitive-behavioral therapy	Combines features of several behavioral interventions	Typically combines stimulus control, sleep restriction, and cognitive interventions, with or without relaxation techniques.
Bright light	To correct circadian rhythm causes of sleeping difficulty (ie, sleep-phase problems)	Patient is exposed to sunlight or a light box. Best evidence is from treatment of seasonal affective disorder (from 2,500 lux for 2 hours/day to 10,000 lux for 30 minutes/day). For delayed sleep phase, 2 hours early morning light at 2,500 lux; for advanced sleep phase, 2 hours evening light at 2,500 lux. Appropriate timing of the light exposure is important. Shorter durations may be as effective. Routine eye examination is recommended before treatment; do not use light boxes with ultraviolet exposure.

reviews and meta-analyses of behavioral interventions for insomnia have been published; the strongest evidence currently supports cognitive-behavioral therapy for insomnia (which generally combines stimulus control, sleep restriction, and cognitive therapy). These behavioral interventions produce reliable therapeutic benefits, including improved sleep efficiency, decreased nighttime wakefulness, and greater satisfaction with sleep; treatment is also helpful in reducing chronic hypnotic use. In at least two randomized trials of older adults with insomnia that compared cognitive-behavioral therapy with a prescription sedative-hypnotic agent, participants generally reported better improvement in their sleep patterns and more satisfaction with the cognitive-behavioral therapy (than with the sedative hypnotic), and sleep improvements were better sustained over time with behavioral treatment.

Several small studies have also tested the effectiveness of exposure to bright light (either natural sunlight or with commercially available light boxes) on the sleep of older adults with insomnia (SOE=B). Variable results have been reported for insomnia, with better results seen for circadian rhythm disorders. As mentioned above, appropriately timed morning bright light may be useful in delayed sleep phase, and evening exposure may be useful in older adults with an advanced sleep phase. Even short durations of bright light may be useful. One study reported beneficial effects in older adults using a visor that provided 2,000 lux to each eye worn for only 30 minutes in the evening.

Bathing before sleep enhances the quality of sleep in older adults, perhaps related to changes in body temperature with bathing. Moderate-intensity exercise also improves sleep in healthy, sedentary adults ≥50 yr old who reported moderate sleep complaints at baseline. However, strenuous exercise should not be performed immediately before bedtime, because this can interfere with sleep. Studies have also suggested beneficial effects on sleep with Tai Chi (SOE=B).

Nonpharmacologic interventions have been studied in institutional settings. In a study of institutionalized demented residents with sleep and behavior problems, morning exposure to bright light was associated with better nighttime sleep and less daytime agitation. In a study of ambient bright light therapy (2,500 lux delivered in the morning, evening, or all-day compared with standard lighting) among older adults with dementia in a psychiatric hospital and a dementia-specific residential care facility, nighttime sleep increased significantly in participants exposed to morning and all-day light, with the increase most prominent in those with severe or very severe dementia. In another study of residents with dementia and behavioral problems, social interaction with nurses reduced behavioral problems and sleep-wake rhythm disorders in some residents. In another small trial in the nursing home, nighttime sleep increased and agitation decreased among residents randomized to receive a daytime physical activity program plus nighttime intervention to decrease noise and light disruption. In another trial that combined an enforced schedule of structured social and physical activity for 2 weeks in a small sample of assisted-living residents, treated residents had enhanced slow-wave sleep and improved performance in memory-oriented tasks. Two large multicomponent nonpharmacologic interventions on sleep in nursing-home residents had mixed results, with greatest effects on decreasing daytime sleeping but little effect on nighttime sleep (SOE=B).

Nonpharmacologic interventions can also be important in patients hospitalized for acute care. In a large study that tested the feasibility of a nonpharmacologic sleep protocol for hospitalized older adults (consisting of a back rub, warm drink, and relaxation tapes) administered by nurses, the use of sedative hypnotic medications was successfully reduced; the sleep protocol had a stronger association with improved quality of sleep than the sedative-hypnotic medications.

Environmental modifications, including noise reduction and appropriate use of lighting, may enhance these interventions.

Pharmacotherapy

Pharmacotherapy is generally considered in individuals with transient sleep problems, such as problems associated with an acute stressor, or in individuals with chronic insomnia that has not responded to behavioral therapy. As mentioned above, if a decision is made to use a sedative hypnotic in an older adult, the smallest dosage of an agent with the least risk of adverse events should be chosen and used for the shortest duration necessary. Short-acting sedative hypnotic agents are recommended for patients with problems falling asleep, and intermediate-acting agents are recommended for patients with problems staying asleep (Table 35.4).

Benzodiazepines (eg, the intermediate-acting agents estazolam and temazepam) bind nonselectively to the gamma-aminobutyric acid-benzodiazepine (GABA-BZ) receptor subunits. As a class, these agents have potential adverse events, including confusion, rebound insomnia, tolerance (to treatment effects), and withdrawal symptoms on discontinuation. Older adults can be more sensitive to the sedating effects of benzodiazepines, with greater risk of confusion and falls (SOE=B). Long-acting benzodiazepines (eg, flurazepam, quazepam), in particular, should not be used in older adults. Short-acting agents appear to have less association with falls and hip fractures, presumably due to less daytime carryover, but at least one study demonstrated an association of short-acting agents with falls at night (SOE=B). However, agents with rapid elimination in general also result in the most pronounced rebound and withdrawal syndromes after discontinuation. Rebound insomnia after discontinuation of short-acting agents is dose dependent and can be reduced by tapering the dosage before discontinuing the drug.

The nonbenzodiazepine-benzodiazepine receptor agonists (NBRAs [ie, nonbenzodiazepines such as eszopiclone, zaleplon, zolpidem]) are structurally unrelated to benzodiazepines but bind to the GABA-BZ receptor with relative selectivity for sedative and amnestic properties. These agents also have a relatively shorter duration of action than benzodiazepines with less risk of daytime carryover of sedating effects (SOE=B). Evidence suggests that NBRAs are relatively well tolerated in healthy older adults (SOE=B), but evidence is limited in older adults with significant comorbidity. Zolpidem is a nonbenzodiazepine imidazopyridine. In older adults, studies suggest that zolpidem does not result in rebound insomnia, agitation, or anxiety when discontinued; does not seem to result in impaired daytime performance on cognitive and psychomotor performance tests; and can have a therapeutic effect that outlasts the period of drug treatment. Zaleplon is a nonbenzodiazepine hypnotic from the pyrazolopyrimidine class, which has also been studied for short-term use in older adults with insomnia. Because of their rapid onset of action, zolpidem and zaleplon should be taken only immediately before bedtime or after the individual has gone to bed and has been unable to fall asleep. Eszopiclone is an s-isomer of the cyclopyrrolone zopiclone, and it has a longer duration of action than the other nonbenzodiazepines. In the United States, eszopiclone and extended-release zolpidem are approved for long-term use. Guidelines recommend that

Table 35.4—Prescription Medications Commonly Used for Insomnia in Older Adults

Class, Medication	Starting Dose (mg)	Usual Dose (mg)	Half-Life (hours)	Comments
Intermediate-acting benzodiazepine				
Temazepam	7.5	7.5–30	8.8	Psychomotor impairment, increased risk of falls
Short-acting nonbenzodiazepines				
Eszopiclone	1	1–2	6	Reportedly effective for long-term use in selected individuals; may be associated with unpleasant taste, headache; avoid administration with high-fat meal
Zaleplon (a pyrazolopyrimidine)	5	5–10	1 (reportedly unchanged in older adults)	Reportedly little daytime carryover, tolerance, or rebound insomnia
Zolpidem (an imidazopyridine)	5	5–10	1.5–4.5 (3 in older adults, 10 in hepatic cirrhosis)	Reportedly little daytime carryover, tolerance, or rebound insomnia
Melatonin receptor agonist				
Ramelteon	8	8	1.5 (2.6 in older adults)	Dizziness, myalgia, headache, other adverse events reported; no significant rebound insomnia or withdrawal with discontinuation
Sedating antidepressants				
Mirtazapine[OL]	7.5	7.5–45	31–39 in older adults; 13–34 in younger adults; mean=21	Increased appetite, weight gain, headache, dizziness, daytime carryover; used for insomnia with depression
Trazodone[OL]	25–50	25–150	Reportedly 6 ± 2; prolonged in older adults and obese individuals	Moderate orthostatic effects; administration after food minimizes sedation and postural hypotension; used for insomnia with depression

zolpidem (regular release) or zaleplon, like benzodiazepines, be used only short term (2–3 weeks) and that, if used longer, these agents be used no more than 2 or 3 nights per week. Concerns remain regarding the risks of confusion, falls, and fracture with chronic use of NBRAs in older adults (particularly those who are frail), and caution is warranted even with these newer agents.

The melatonin receptor agonist ramelteon does not act at GABA receptors; rather it is a selective MT1/MT2 receptor agonist. Ramelteon reduces sleep latency (time to fall asleep) and increases total sleep time in older adults (SOE=B), without evidence of significant rebound or withdrawal effects with discontinuation.

Low dosages of sedating antidepressants such as trazodone[OL] or mirtazapine[OL] at bedtime have been used as sleeping aids, particularly for patients with depression, but there is limited evidence to support this practice (SOE=D). Sedating antidepressants have been suggested for use at low dosages as a nighttime aid for sleep in depressed patients receiving another antidepressant at therapeutic dosages during the daytime. Other indications include patients with a history of psychoactive substance use problems, lack of response to other sleeping medications, suspected untreated sleep apnea (in which further respiratory depression is a concern), and fibromyalgia (when

there is some evidence of antidepressant medication treatment effect). However, the adverse effects of sedating antidepressants may limit their usefulness.

Sedating antipsychotics should not be used in the routine management of insomnia in older adults without serious psychiatric illness. Sedating antipsychotics[OL] are sometimes used for sleep complaints in patients with other serious psychiatric conditions that warrant treatment with an antipsychotic medication.

Chronic Hypnotic Use

In European studies, a relatively high prevalence of chronic sedative hypnotic use in older adults (5%–8% in older men, up to 25% in older women) has been reported. There is strong epidemiologic evidence for increased morbidity and mortality with chronic use of prescription sleeping pills; however, much of this literature is older and predates the availability of newer, nonbenzodiazepine hypnotics, so the relationship between the newer hypnotics and morbidity/mortality is not clear. In addition, after tolerance to hypnotics develops, long-term use of these agents can actually make sleep worse. Data reported from a longitudinal study of older adults in Germany indicated a higher rate of sleep-related complaints in those who took sleeping medications than those who did not.

Several studies have shown that the bulk of prescription sleeping medication use is occurring among chronic users, and not those with transient sleeping difficulties.

Methods to help older chronic hypnotic users reduce or eliminate their use of these agents have been reported (SOE=B). Tapering of the hypnotic can be important. One reported strategy involved decreasing the hypnotic dose by one-half for 2 weeks, followed by full withdrawal (perhaps with the use of a substitute pill at night), which was effective in eliminating hypnotic use without adverse events on nighttime sleep, depressive symptoms, or daytime sleepiness. In another small controlled trial in which benzodiazepine use was tapered to complete withdrawal over as many as 6 weeks, more success was seen in those persons randomized to receive a nightly dose of 2 mg of controlled-release melatonin rather than placebo. At follow-up 6 mo later, nearly 80% of those who successfully discontinued benzodiazepines continued to report good sleep quality. Cognitive-behavioral therapy, when combined with gradual tapering of the hypnotic dose, has also been demonstrated to be helpful in reducing or eliminating chronic benzodiazepine use (SOE=B).

Nonprescription Sleeping Agents

Nearly half of older adults report using nonprescription sleeping agents; however, there is little evidence to support this practice. Commonly used nonprescription agents include sedating antihistamines, acetaminophen, alcohol, melatonin, and herbal products. Sedating antihistamines (eg, diphenhydramine) are common ingredients in OTC sleeping agents as well as in combination analgesic-sleeping agents that are marketed for nighttime use. Diphenhydramine has potent anticholinergic effects, and tolerance to its sedating effects develops after several weeks, so it is not recommended for older adults. Individuals with mild nighttime discomfort and sleeping difficulties can have adequate relief with a simple pain reliever (eg, acetaminophen) at bedtime. Although alcohol causes some initial drowsiness, it can interfere with sleep later in the night and can actually worsen sleeping difficulties. Melatonin is available OTC. There is some evidence in older adults with insomnia that melatonin administration decreases sleep latency (time to fall asleep) and wake time after sleep onset, and increases sleep efficiency (time asleep over time in bed), but results are mixed. However, there is evidence for effectiveness of melatonin in certain circadian rhythm sleep disorders. For example, blind people with abnormal circadian sleep-wake rhythms (eg, free-running rhythms not entrained to the external environment due to lack of light perception) may correct with melatonin (SOE=B). Valerian is an herbal product with mild sedative action that has been marketed for insomnia. Its mechanism of action is uncertain, and it contains several potentially active compounds, with risk of adverse events. A systematic review found the existing evidence of valerian's efficacy to be inconclusive (SOE=C). Kava, another herbal product marketed for insomnia, has significant risk of adverse events, including hepatotoxicity, and it should not be recommended.

ACOVE-3* QUALITY INDICATORS PERTAINING TO SLEEP PROBLEMS

Screening
- All vulnerable older adults should be screened annually for sleep problems.

Sleep history
- If a vulnerable older adult reports a sleep problem, then a targeted sleep history should be documented within 6 mo.

Sleep hygiene education
- If a vulnerable older adult has a sleep problem, then a discussion of sleep hygiene should be documented within 6 mo.

Sleep study
- If a vulnerable older adult has daytime sleepiness and observed apneas or loud snoring, then he or she should be referred for sleep evaluation within 6 mo.

Discussion of treatment options
- If a vulnerable older adult has sleep-disordered breathing according to polysomnography, then a discussion of treatment options should be documented within 6 mo.

Nocturnal limb movements
- If a vulnerable older adult has nocturnal limb movements during sleep and frequent awakenings or excessive daytime sleepiness, then treatment or referral to a sleep specialist should occur within 6 mo.

Avoid antihistamines
- If a vulnerable older adult has sleep problems, then he or she should not be treated with sleep aids containing antihistamines.
- If a vulnerable older adult is new to a primary care practice and is chronically (>3 mo) taking an OTC sleep aid containing an antihistamine for sleep problems, then advice to discontinue the medication should be documented within 6 mo.

REFERENCES

■ Bloom HG, Ahmed I, Alessi CA, et al. Evidence-based recommendations for the assessment and management of sleep disorders in older persons. *J Am Geriatr Soc.* 2009;57(5):761–789.

■ Cole CS, Richards KC, Roberson PK, et al. Relationships among disorder sleep and cognitive and functional status in nursing home residents. *Res Gerontol Nurs.* 2009;2(3), 183–191.

■ Irwin MR, Cole JC, Nicassio PM. Comparative meta-analysis of behavioral interventions for insomnia and their efficacy in middle-aged adults and in older adults 55+ years of age. *Health Psychol.* 2006;25(1):3–14.

■ Smyth C. The Pittsburgh Sleep Quality Index (PSQI). *Try This: Best Practices in Nursing Care to Older Adults.* 2007;(6.1). Available at http://consultgerirn.org/uploads/File/trythis/try_this_6_1.pdf

■ Smyth C. The Epworth Sleepiness Scale (ESS). *Try This: Best Practices in Nursing Care to Older Adults.* 2007;(6.2). Available at http://consultgerirn.org/uploads/File/trythis/try_this_6_2.pdf

■ Vaz Fragoso CA, Gill TM. Sleep complaints in community-living older persons: a multifactorial geriatric syndrome. *J Am Geriatr Soc.* 2007;55(11):1853–1866.

CHAPTER 36—PRESSURE ULCERS AND WOUND CARE

KEY POINTS

■ The normal wound-healing cascade comprises four phases: homeostasis, inflammatory, proliferative, and maturation.

■ A pressure ulcer is defined as damage caused to skin and underlying soft tissue by unrelieved pressure when the tissue is compressed between a bony prominence and external surface over a prolonged period of time.

■ Three main factors are believed to play a role in pressure-ulcer formation: pressure, friction, and shear forces. Intrinsic and extrinsic factors determine the tolerance of soft tissue to the adverse effects of pressure.

■ Risk assessment and preventive strategies are required to decrease the incidence of pressure ulcers.

■ The stage of an ulcer determines the appropriate treatment plan.

Wound healing is a complicated process, and it is important to understand the normal function of the wound-healing cascade regardless of the chronic wound type (eg, pressure ulcers, venous stasis ulcers, diabetic foot ulcers, etc). Aging can affect the wound healing phases and thus delay or impede the healing process.

THE WOUND HEALING CASCADE

Homeostasis

Homeostasis is achieved when vasoconstriction of the blood vessels occurs and platelets arrive at the wound. Platelet degranulation provides the first signals that begin the wound-healing cascade. Alpha granules of the platelets contain the following growth factors: 1) platelet-derived growth factors (PDGF), 2) insulin-like growth factor-1, 3) epidermal growth factors, 4) fibroblast growth factor (FGF), and 5) transforming growth factor-β (TGF-β). These growth factors are released from platelets and leave the wound, migrating into the surrounding tissue and blood vessels. Growth factors release signals to inflammatory cells. Growth factors stimulate production, movement, and delineation of wound cells that include epithelial cells, fibroblasts, and endothelial cells. This begins the inflammatory phase of wound healing, which is a catabolic process.

Inflammatory Phase

In the inflammatory phase, polymorphonuclear neutrophils are the first cells initiated to begin the process of phagocytosis. Neutrophils release tumor necrosis factor-α (TNF-α) and the proinflammatory cytokines interleukins IL-2 and IL-4 at the site of injury. Neutrophils also release matrix metalloproteinase eight (MMP-8). MMP-8 removes the damaged extracellular matrix, which is replaced with new extracellular matrix.

Macrophages are the most important wound-healing cells because they are involved in all phases of wound healing. Macrophages replace neutrophils in the wound and are responsible for several actions during the inflammatory phase. They initiate phagocytosis, are bactericidal, and promote angiogenesis. They also secrete more growth factors and signal for additional macrophages and monocytes to respond to the wound. They convert macromolecules into amino acids and sugars, nutrients that are necessary for wound healing. During this phase, mast cells, derived from the dermis, arrive at the site and stimulate local inflammation that increases the sensation of pain.

Proliferative Phase

Macrophages are the mediators for the initiation of the proliferative phase, which is initiated by the stimulation of the movement of fibroblasts, epithelial cells, and vascular endothelial cells to begin the healing of the wound by the formation of granulation tissue. This phase is anabolic and can last for several weeks. Cell movement and production persist as a temporary matrix of fibrin and fibronectin is created. Granulation tissue provides a moist surface for cell migration and replaces the temporary matrix as it fills in the wound cavity. It contains fibroblasts, keratinocytes, macrophages, immature collagen, endothelial cells, and new blood vessels. It is very vascular and easily damaged.

The final step in the proliferative phase is the movement of keratinocytes from the epidermal layer of the wound edge into the wound to begin epithelialization. Keratinocytes form scar tissue as they travel and reproduce across the wound bed only in the presence of healthy granulation tissue. These cells synthesize TGF-β, TNF-α, and IL-1 B, all of which stimulate cell production, extracellular protein formation, and angiogenesis.

Endothelial cells promote development of new blood vessels quickly, which are necessary for nutrition for the new tissue. These cells stimulate fibrinolysis, breaking down the temporary matrix so fibroblast movement and collagen synthesis can occur. The growth factors synthesized by endothelial cells are vascular endothelial growth factors, fibroblast growth factors, and PDGF.

Maturation Phase

The final phase of wound healing is the maturation phase or the remodeling phase. This phase can take months to years and is catabolic. Collagen fibers are the main substance in the wound, and fiber collection increases, creating a thick collagenous arrangement. Fibroblasts, matrix metalloproteinases (MMPs), tissue inhibitors of metalloproteinases (TIMPs), and TGF are vital to organizing, remodeling, and maturing of the collagen fibers. Fibroblasts stimulate production of collagen, elastin, proteoglycans, MMPs, and TIMPs. This action continues until the tensile strength of scar tissue is approximately 80% that of normal tissue. Apoptosis or programmed cell death decrease fibroblast and capillary density. The quality of scar tissue decreases, and the scar becomes less red and flat over time; this is known as remodeling of the scar.

As a person ages, wounds heal more slowly and can become chronic because of a delayed inflammatory phase when one or more chronic diseases are present. This can be attributed to changes within the wound-healing cascade, as well as to the influence of chronic disease and medications that affect tissue perfusion. Malnutrition and infection contribute to slower rates of wound healing in older adults.

The lack of tissue perfusion can significantly affect the rate of wound healing. Diagnoses such as anemia, diabetes, cardiovascular disease, hypotension, COPD; low blood protein levels; high temperature; and smoking can increase demand for oxygen and the metabolic rate. Microvascular changes in the circulatory system in diabetic patients also reduce tissue perfusion.

The use of corticosteroids can impede regeneration of the epidermis and collagen synthesis. Antibiotics, corticosteroids, and hormones can change the skin's protective barrier function. The inflammatory response is affected by other medications such as analgesics, antihistamines, and NSAIDs. Chemotherapeutic agents may interrupt the cell cycle and production of cells.

STRENGTH-OF-EVIDENCE (SOE) RATING DEFINITIONS

A = consistent and good quality patient-oriented evidence

B = somewhat inconsistent or limited quality patient-oriented evidence

C = very inconsistent or very limited patient-oriented evidence, disease-oriented evidence, and/or consensus from professional organizations

D = unstudied common practice or opinion

See inside front cover for detailed information regarding the SOE classification.

Pressure Ulcers

Pressure ulcers are a serious and common problem for older adults, affecting approximately 1 million adults in the United States. The Surgeon General's Healthy People 2010 document has identified pressure ulcers as a national health issue for long-term care, and CMS has designated pressure ulcers as one of the three primary markers of quality of care in the long-term care setting. On October 1, 2008, CMS made the decision to stop paying for hospital-acquired Stage III and IV pressure ulcers. Thus, it is critical for clinicians to be aggressive in both pressure ulcer prevention and treatment programs.

Epidemiology

A pressure ulcer is defined as damage caused to skin and underlying soft tissue by unrelieved pressure when the tissue is compressed between a bony prominence and the external surface over a prolonged period. Because pressure is the major physiologic factor that leads to soft-tissue destruction, the term *pressure ulcer* is most widely used and preferred over the terms *decubitus ulcer* or *bedsore*.

The causes of pressure ulcers are still not fully understood. Most research into the causes of pressure ulcers has been in animal models. Three main factors are believed to play a role in pressure-ulcer formation: pressure, friction, and shear forces. It appears that the amount of pressure, friction, or shear force needed to create a pressure ulcer depends on the quality of tissue, the blood flow, and the amount of pressure applied. Hence, for patients with poor-quality tissue (ie, tissue with inadequate blood perfusion), it may take less sustained pressure over a shorter time to develop a pressure ulcer. Conversely, patients with good-quality tissue may be able to sustain more pressure over a longer time before an ulcer develops. Ulcers caused by shearing forces tend to develop deep in the fascia, whereas ulcers caused by friction tend to be quite superficial, starting in the epidermal and dermal layers. With aging, local blood supply to the skin decreases, epithelial layers flatten and thin, subcutaneous fat decreases, and collagen fibers lose elasticity. These changes in aging skin and the resultant lowered tolerance to hypoxia can predispose older adults to the development of pressure ulcers.

The incidence and prevalence of pressure ulcers vary greatly, depending on the setting. In long-term care, average incidence is 11%, with 50% reported as Stage II; hospitals' average range of incidence was 7%–9% (higher rates are noted in intensive-care units, where patients are less mobile and have severe systemic illnesses) and home health 0%–17%.

The incidence of pressure ulcers differs not only by healthcare setting but also by stage of ulceration.

The Stage I pressure ulcer (persistent erythema) is most common, accounting for 47% of all pressure ulcers. The Stage II pressure ulcers (partial thickness loss involving only the epidermal and dermal layers) are second, at 33%. Stage III (full-thickness skin loss involving subcutaneous tissue) and Stage IV (full thickness involving muscle or bone or supporting structures) pressure ulcers make up the remaining 20%. In several studies, incidence rates of pressure ulcers among black Americans and white Americans differ, with blacks tending to have a greater incidence of Stage III and IV pressure ulcers. Whether this can be attributed to structural skin changes or socioeconomic factors is unknown because of the paucity of pressure-ulcer research among patients in U.S. minority groups.

Risk Factors and Risk-Assessment Scales

The literature abounds with lists of risk factors associated with pressure-ulcer development. However, any disease process that renders an older adult immobile for an extended period of time increases the risk of pressure-ulcer development. Both intrinsic and extrinsic factors determine the tolerance of soft tissue to the adverse effects of pressure. Intrinsic risk factors are physiologic factors or disease states that increase the risk of pressure-ulcer development, eg, age, poor nutritional status, and decreased arteriolar blood pressure. Extrinsic factors are external factors that damage the skin, eg, friction and shear, moisture, and urinary or fecal incontinence or both. Variables that appear to be predictors of pressure-ulcer development include age ≥70 yr old, impaired mobility, use of restraints, current smoking history, low body mass index, altered mental status (eg, confusion), urinary and fecal incontinence, malnutrition, malignancy, diabetes mellitus, stroke, pneumonia, heart failure, fever, sepsis, hypotension, kidney failure, dry and scaly skin, history of pressure ulcers, anemia, lymphopenia, and hypoalbuminemia. Some physiologic risk factors (eg, diabetes mellitus, cerebrovascular accident) have been associated with microcirculatory impairment, thus leading to neural and endothelial compromise and increasing the risk of ulceration (SOE=C).

Because of the myriad risk factors associated with pressure-ulcer development, various scales have been developed to quantify a person's risk by identifying the presence of factors in several categories. The Braden Scale (http://www.bradenscale.com [accessed Jan 2011]) and the Norton Scale are probably the most widely used tools for identifying older adults who are at risk of developing pressure ulcers. Both tools have been validated and are recommended by the Agency for Healthcare Research and Quality (AHRQ). The Braden Scale has a sensitivity of

83%–100% and a specificity of 64%–77%; the Norton Scale has a sensitivity of 73%–92% and a specificity of 61%–94%.

The AHRQ guidelines for preventing pressure ulcers recommend that bed- and chair-bound patients or those with impaired ability to reposition themselves should be assessed on admission to the hospital or the nursing home for additional factors that increase the risk of developing pressure ulcers. Studies have demonstrated that incorporating systematic risk-assessment tools has significantly reduced the incidence of pressure ulcers (SOE=A). To date, the Braden Scale is the only tool to be validated in nonwhite populations. The use of risk-assessment tools does not guarantee that all older adults at risk of pressure ulcers will be identified.

There is no agreement on how frequently risk assessment should be done. However, most clinical guidelines for pressure ulcers indicate that a risk assessment should be done on admission, at discharge, and whenever the patient's clinical condition changes (SOE=D). The appropriate interval for routine reassessment remains unclear. Studies by Bergstrom and Braden found that in a skilled-nursing facility, 80% of pressure ulcers develop within 2 weeks of admission and 96% develop within 3 weeks of admission. Moreover, the Institute for Healthcare Improvement has recently recommended that in hospitalized patients, risk assessment for pressure ulcers be done every 24 hours rather than the previous suggestion of every 48 hours.

Prevention

The AHRQ sponsored the development of recommendations for the prevention of pressure ulcers in adults. These clinical practice guidelines (*Pressure Ulcers in Adults: Prediction and Prevention*, published in May 1992) provide an excellent approach to evidenced-based pressure-ulcer prevention (available at http://www.ncbi.nlm.nih.gov/books/bv.fcgi?rid=hstat2.chapter.4409).

Skin Care

Evidence on the role of skin care in pressure-ulcer prevention is limited. Most recommendations are based on expert opinions and clinical guidelines. Although experts believe that there is a relationship between skin care and pressure ulcer development, there is a dearth of supporting research. How the skin is cleansed may make a difference (SOE=D). One study found that the incidence of Stages I and II pressure ulcers was reduced by educating the staff and by using a body wash and skin protection products. Another study compared hyperoxygenated fatty acid compound in acute-care and long-term care patients and found reduced incidence of ulcers versus

placebo compound (triisotearin). All experts do agree that once an older adult at risk of pressure ulcers has been identified, the goal of skin care is to maintain and improve tissue tolerance to pressure.

All older adults at risk should have a systematic skin inspection at least once a day, with emphasis on the bony prominences. The skin should be cleansed with warm water and a mild cleansing agent to minimize irritation and dryness of the skin. Every effort should be made to minimize environmental factors leading to skin drying, such as low humidity (<40%) and exposure to cold. Decreased skin hydration results in decreased pliability, and severely dry skin damages the stratum corneum. Dry skin should be treated with moisturizers (SOE=D).

Massaging over bony prominences should be avoided. Previously, it was believed that massaging the bony prominences promoted circulation. However, postmortem biopsies showed degenerated tissue in areas that were massaged but no degenerated tissue in areas not massaged. All efforts should be made to avoid exposing the skin to perspiration, wound drainage, or urine and fecal matter resulting from incontinence. When disposable briefs are used to manage incontinence, the patient must be checked and changed frequently, because perineal dermatitis can develop quickly. The use of disposable underpads to control excessive moisture and perspiration can help wick moisture away from skin. The use of moisturizers and moisture barriers should also be considered to protect the skin (SOE=D).

Nutrition

The literature remains unclear about protein-calorie malnutrition and its association with pressure ulcer development. The relationship between nutritional intake and pressure ulcer prevention is not always supported by randomized controlled trials. Some research supports the finding that undernourishment on admission to a healthcare facility increases a person's likelihood of developing a pressure ulcer. In one prospective study, high-risk patients who were undernourished on admission to the hospital were twice as likely to develop pressure ulcers as adequately nourished patients (17% and 9%, respectively). In another study, 59% of residents were undernourished and 7.3% were severely undernourished on admission to a long-term care facility. Pressure ulcers developed in 65% of the severely undernourished residents, but in none of the mild to moderately undernourished or well-nourished residents.

Empirical evidence is lacking that the use of vitamin and mineral supplements (in the absence of deficiency) actually prevents pressure ulcers. Therefore, oversupplementing patients without protein, vitamin, or mineral deficiencies should be avoided. Before enteral or parental nutrition is used, a critical review of overall goals and wishes of the patient, family, and care team should be considered. Despite the lack of evidence regarding nutritional assessment and intervention, maintaining optimal nutrition continues to be part of national pressure ulcer prevention guidelines (SOE=D).

Mechanical Loading

Minimizing friction and shear is important. This can be accomplished through proper repositioning, transferring, and turning techniques. The use of lubricants (eg, cornstarch and creams), protective films (eg, transparent film dressings and skin sealants), protective dressings (eg, hydrocolloids), and protective padding can be used to reduce the possibility of friction and shear. Older adults who are at risk of developing pressure ulcers should be repositioned at least every 2 hours. Research on optimal turning schedules is sparse. The first study—an observational study published in 1975—found that older adults turned every 2–3 hours had fewer ulcers. A more recent study suggests that depending on the support surface used, less frequent turning may be optimal to prevent pressure ulcers in a long-term care facility. Several nurse researchers investigated the effect of four different turning frequencies (every 2 hours on a standard mattress, every 3 hours on a standard mattress, every 4 hours on a viscoelastic foam mattress, and every 6 hours on a viscoelastic foam mattress). They found that the incidence of early pressure ulcers (Stage I) did not differ in the four groups. However, patients being turned every 4 hours on a viscoelastic foam mattress developed significantly less severe pressure ulcers (Stage II and higher) than the three other groups. Although the results of this study may indicate less turning may be appropriate when using a viscoelastic foam mattress, additional studies are needed to examine optimal turning schedules among different populations (SOE=C).

Bed-positioning devices such as pillows or foam wedges should be used to keep bony prominences from direct contact with one another. The head of the bed should be at the lowest degree of elevation consistent with medical conditions. The use of lifting devices, such as trapezes or bed linen, to move the patient in bed also decreases the potential for friction and shear forces. The heel is quite vulnerable to pressure-ulcer development; studies suggest that approximately 20% of all pressure-ulcer development is on the heels. This may be attributed to the limited amount of soft tissue over the heel. Specific clinical interventions to prevent heel pressure ulcers have been developed (SOE=D).

Patients seated in a chair should be assessed for good postural alignment, distribution of weight, and balance. They should be taught or reminded to shift weight every 15 minutes. The use of doughnuts as seating cushions is contraindicated because they increase pressure over the area of contact and can actually cause pressure ulcers (SOE=C).

Mobility

Maintaining or improving mobility is one of the most effective ways to decrease pressure on bony prominences. For bedbound patients, there are benefits of both active and passive range-of-motion exercises. Patients not confined to bed should be encouraged to move from bed to chair to standing to ambulating to minimize the risk of developing pressure ulcers (SOE=C).

Support Surfaces

Any older adult identified as being at risk of developing pressure ulcers should be placed on a pressure redistribution device. The concept of pressure redistribution has been endorsed by the National Pressure Ulcer Advisory Panel (NPUAP). However, if pressure is reduced on one body part, this will result in increased pressure elsewhere on the body. Thus, the goal is to obtain the best pressure redistribution possible. In a systematic review of 49 randomized controlled trials that examined the role of support surfaces in preventing pressure ulcers, no one category of support surface was found to be superior to another; however, use of a support surface was more beneficial than a standard mattress (SOE=A). Two types of devices exist: static (foam, static air, gel or water, or a combination) and dynamic (alternating air, low air loss, or air fluidized). Most static devices are less expensive than dynamic surfaces. For the various types of support surfaces that can guide selection for particular situations, see Table 36.1. Most experts agree that the use of static devices is appropriate for pressure-ulcer prevention (SOE=D). Two conditions warrant consideration of a dynamic surface:

- bottoming-out occurs (the static surface is compressed to <1 inch)
- the patient is at high risk of pressure ulcers, and reactive hyperemia is noted on a bony prominence despite the use of a static support surface

Table 36.1—Support Surfaces for Older Adults at Risk of Pressure Ulcers

Type	Examples	Support Area	Low Moisture Retention	Reduced Heat Accumulation	Shear Reduction	Pressure Reduction	Cost per Day
Static surfaces	Foam	Yes	No	No	No	Yes	Low
	Standard mattress	No	No	No	No	No	Low
	Static flotation—air or water	Yes	No	No	Yes	Yes	Low
Dynamic surfaces	Air fluidized	Yes	Yes	Yes	Yes	Yes	High
	Low-air-loss	Yes	Yes	Yes	?	Yes	High
	Alternating air	Yes	No	No	Yes	Yes	Moderate

SOURCE: Adapted from Bergstrom N, Bennett MA, Carlson CE, et al. *Treatment of Pressure Ulcers. Clinical Practice Guideline No. 15.* Rockville, MD: US Department of Health and Human Services, Public Health Service, Agency for Health Care Policy and Research. December 1994:38. AHCPR Pub. No. 95-0652.

Although effective at reducing pressure, dynamic airflow beds have several potential adverse effects, including dehydration, sensory deprivation, loss of muscle strength, and difficulty with mobilization.

Management

The AHRQ developed evidence-based guidelines on the management of pressure ulcers. This guideline, *Treatment of Pressure Ulcers*, published in December 1994, reviews the foundation for providing evidence-based pressure-ulcer management.

Assessment

A pressure ulcer will not heal unless underlying causes are identified, and effective interventions implemented. When a pressure ulcer has developed, a systematic evaluation is necessary (SOE=D). For an approach to assessment and documentation when a pressure ulcer develops, see Table 36.2.

There is no universal agreement on a single system for classifying pressure ulcers. Most experts do agree that the stage of an ulcer determines the appropriate treatment plan. However, staging alone does not determine the seriousness of the ulcer. Most systems use four stages to classify ulceration. Table 36.3 describes the most commonly used staging system by the NPUAP. This group recently revised the staging system to include deep tissue injury, an ulcer often described as a purple or maroon localized area of discolored intact skin or blood-filled blister due to damage of underlying soft tissue from pressure and/or shear. The NPUAP also reclassified blisters and unstageable pressure ulcers. The new staging system has six stages: suspected deep tissue injury, Stage I, Stage II, Stage III, Stage IV, and unstageable. When eschar (thick brown or black devitalized tissue) is covering the ulcer, the ulcer cannot be accurately staged.

The challenge for most staging systems lies in the definition of the Stage I pressure ulcer. Attempts to classify the first stage of ulcer development are more variable than in any other stage. Most systems define the Stage I pressure ulcer as nonblanchable erythema of intact skin; both the AHRQ prediction and prevention guidelines and the Minimum Data Set (required by CMS for all patients in long-term care facilities) refer to Stage I pressure ulcer in these terms. However, it is difficult (at best) to blanch the skin of people with darkly pigmented skin. Thus, erythema can appear as a defined area of persistent redness in lightly pigmented skin, whereas in darker skin tones, the pressure ulcer can appear with persistent erythema, or blue or purple hues.

Treatment

Debridement

Debridement is necessary when the wound contains necrotic, devitalized tissue (SOE=C). Such tissue supports the growth of pathologic organisms and prevents healing. There are four major types of debridement methods used in the United States: mechanical, enzymatic, autolytic, and sharp. Bio-surgery (ie, maggot or larva therapy), which is used widely in Europe, is another potential debridement option. The debridement method should be selected on the basis of the patient's health condition, the ulcer presentation, the presence or absence of infection, and the patient's ability to tolerate the procedure (Table 36.4).

Dressings

Numerous dressings are used in the healing of pressure ulcers. The use of wet-to-dry gauze has been discouraged by experts; it is actually a debriding technique that can damage the tissue matrix and prolong healing. Many experts advocate the use of hydrocolloid dressings (SOE=B). These dressings,

Table 36.2—Detection, Assessment, and Management of Pressure Ulcers

Evaluate and Document	Consider These Strategies
Location	▪ Examine high-risk sites. ▪ Develop targeted pressure-relieving strategies (eg, positioning and repositioning, padding, seat cushions, heel elevation). ▪ Limit shearing forces by special attention to positioning when the lead of bed is elevated. ▪ Lift rather than slide the patient. ▪ Cleanse and dry regularly if wetted frequently.
Stage	▪ Differentiate between minor Stage I lesions (nonblanchable erythema related to extravasation of RBCs into the interstitium) and deep tissue injuries that can progress to full-thickness lesions. ▪ Discuss with caregivers and families the possibility of significant pressure-ulcer development when deep tissue injury is identified.
Area	▪ Record diameter for circular lesions. ▪ Record lengths of largest perpendiculars for irregular lesions.
Depth	▪ Measure depth from plane of skin. ▪ Probe and measure extent of undermining or depth of sinus tracts.
Drainage	▪ Estimate amount. ▪ Identify degree of odor and purulence. ▪ Monitor hematocrit if more than minor blood loss occurs with dressing changes. ▪ Monitor serum albumin if volume of ulcer drainage is large.
Necrosis	▪ Consider simple blunt debridement of small amounts of necrotic tissue. ▪ Involve general or plastic surgeons for extensive debridement. ▪ Monitor damage to healthy tissue whenever using blunt, enzymatic, or wet-to-dry dressings for debridement. ▪ Monitor use of pressure dressings (which can cause necrosis) after blunt debridement. ▪ Use silver-based dressings to decrease bacterial burden. ▪ Use low-frequency nonthermal ultrasound to remove necrotic tissue.
Granulation	▪ Identify granulation as an indication that wound healing is occurring. ▪ Look for regression if other infections (eg, urinary tract infection or pneumonia) develop. ▪ Develop strategies to protect and enhance growth of granulation tissue (eg, nourishment, vitamins, minerals; use of dressings to ensure moist wound surfaces). ▪ Avoid damage with dressing changes.
Cellulitis	▪ Differentiate from a thin rim of erythema surrounding most healing wounds. ▪ Look for tender, warmth, and redness, particularly if there is progression. ▪ Consider treatment with systemic antibiotics active against gram-positive cocci.
Nonhealing wound	▪ Use negative-pressure wound therapy for excessive exudate. ▪ Consider monochromatic infrared photo energy therapy.

when compared with gauze, have been found to significantly speed the healing process. This is most likely because hydrocolloids require fewer dressing changes (inflicting less trauma), block bacteria from penetrating the wound bed, and maintain a moist wound environment (facilitating increases in the growth factors needed in the healing process). Moreover, studies have demonstrated that the use of hydrocolloids, when compared with the use of gauze, decreases direct and indirect institutional costs. It is essential to select an appropriate dressing, not on the basis of the stage of the pressure ulcer, but rather on the amount of wound exudate. For some of the most common dressings and the indications for their use, see Table 36.5.

Surgical Repair

Surgical repair remains a viable option for Stage III and IV pressure ulcers (SOE=D). However, because many Stage III and IV pressure ulcers eventually heal over a long period of time (if appropriately managed) and the rate of recurrence of surgically closed pressure ulcers is high, the benefits of surgery must be considered carefully. The most common types of surgical repairs are direct closure, skin grafting, skin flaps, musculocutaneous flaps, and free flaps.

Diet and Nutritional Supplements

The importance of diet and dietary supplements in a malnourished patient with a pressure ulcer is controversial. Per AHRQ treatment guidelines, nutritional support that achieves approximately 30–35 calories/kg/d and 1.25–1.5 g of protein/kg/d is recommended (SOE=C). Evidence to support the use of supplemental vitamins and minerals is limited. The use of amino acids such as argine, glutamine, and cysteine have been noted to assist in ulcer healing.

Table 36.3—Staging System for Pressure Ulcers (National Pressure Ulcer Advisory Panel)

Stage	Definition	Comments
Suspected deep tissue injury	Purple or maroon localized area of discolored intact skin or blood-filled blister due to damage of underlying soft tissue from pressure and/or shear. The area may be preceded by tissue that is painful, firm, mushy, boggy, warmer, or cooler than adjacent tissue.	Deep tissue injury can be difficult to detect in individuals with dark skin tones. Evolution can include a thin blister over a dark wound bed. The wound can further evolve and become covered by thin eschar. Evolution can be rapid and expose additional layers of tissue even with optimal treatment.
Stage I	Intact skin with nonblanchable redness of a localized area usually over a bony prominence. Darkly pigmented skin may not have visible blanching; its color may differ from the surrounding area.	The area may be painful, firm, soft, and warmer or cooler than adjacent tissue. Stage I can be difficult to detect in individuals with dark skin tones.
Stage II	Partial-thickness loss of dermis presenting as a shallow open ulcer with a red-pink wound bed, without slough. Can also present as an intact or open/ruptured serum-filled blister.	Presents as a shiny or dry shallow ulcer without slough or bruising (the latter indicates suspected deep tissue injury). This stage should not be used to describe skin tears, tape burns, perineal dermatitis, maceration, or excoriation.
Stage III	Full-thickness tissue loss. Subcutaneous fat can be visible but bone, tendon, or muscle are not exposed. Slough may be present but does not obscure the depth of tissue loss. Can include undermining and tunneling.	The depth of a Stage III pressure ulcer varies by anatomic location. The bridge of the nose, ear, occiput, and malleolus do not have subcutaneous tissue, and Stage III ulcers can be shallow. In contrast, areas of significant adiposity can develop extremely deep Stage III pressure ulcers. Bone/tendon is not visible or directly palpable.
Stage IV	Full-thickness tissue loss with exposed bone, tendon, or muscle. Slough or eschar can be present on some parts of wound bed. Often include undermining and tunneling.	The depth of a Stage IV pressure ulcer varies by anatomic location. The bridge of the nose, ear, occiput, and malleolus do not have subcutaneous tissue, and these ulcers can be shallow. Stage IV ulcers can extend into muscle and/or supporting structures (eg, fascia, tendon, or joint capsule), making osteomyelitis possible. Exposed bone/tendon is visible or directly palpable.
Unstageable	Full-thickness tissue loss in which the base of the ulcer is covered by slough (yellow, tan, gray, green, or brown) and/or eschar (tan, brown, or black) in the wound bed.	Until enough slough and/or eschar is removed to expose the base of the wound, the true depth (and therefore stage) cannot be determined. Stable (dry, adherent, intact without erythema or fluctance) eschar on the heels serves as "the body's natural (biological) cover" and should not be removed.

SOURCE: Adapted with permission by the National Pressure Ulcer Advisory Panel (http://www.npuap.org [accessed Jan 2011]).

New or Unproven Therapies

Throughout the years, a number of treatments have been advocated for the healing of pressure ulcers without sufficient data to support their various claims. Data on the therapeutic efficacy of hyperbaric oxygen, low-energy laser irradiation, and therapeutic ultrasound have not been established. However, areas of promise include the use of recombinant PDGF to stimulate healing and skin equivalents that may prove to heal Stage III and IV pressure ulcers.

Electrical stimulation is the use of electrical current to stimulate a number of cellular processes important to pressure ulcer healing. It influences the migration of neutrophils, fibroblasts, and macrophages into the wound and increases the tensile strength of collagen. Electrical stimulation appears to be most effective on healing recalcitrant Stages III and IV pressure ulcers. In a meta-analysis of 15 studies evaluating the effects of electrical stimulation on the healing of chronic ulcers, the rate of healing per week was 22% for participants receiving electrical stimulation compared with 9% for controls. Thus, electrical stimulation should be considered for nonhealing pressure ulcers (SOE=B).

Negative-pressure wound therapy is widely used, although few randomized controlled trials have been published. This therapy promotes wound healing by applying controlled, localized, negative pressure to the wound bed. In one prospective study of 281 patients investigating the effects of using negative-pressure wound therapy to heal pressure ulcers, those patients using the adjunctive therapy had better healing outcomes than the cohort not using the therapy. Evidence is emerging that this therapy may be helpful in healing pressure ulcers (SOE=C).

Table 36.4—Methods of Debridement

Type	Description	Advantages and Disadvantages
Mechanical	Use of physical forces to remove devitalized tissues; methods include wet-to-dry irrigation (using 19-gauge needle with 35-mL syringe), hydrotherapy, and dextranomer	Can remove both devitalized and vitalized tissues; can cause pain.
Surgical, sharp	Use of scalpel, scissors, and forceps to remove devitalized tissue; laser debridement	Quick and effective if performed by skilled professional; should be used when infection is suspected; pain management is needed.
Enzymatic	Use of topical debriding agent to dissolve the devitalized tissue (chemical force)	Appropriate when there are no signs or symptoms of local infection; some agents can damage surrounding skin.
Autolytic	Use of synthetic dressings to allow the devitalized tissue to self-digest from the enzymes found in the ulcer fluids (natural force)	Recommended for those who cannot tolerate other forms of debridement and when infection is not suspected; may take a long time to be effective.
Biosurgery	Use of larvae to digest devitalized tissue	Quick and effective; good option for those who cannot tolerate surgical debridement.

SOURCE: Data from Bergstrom N, Bennett MA, Carlson CE, et al. *Treatment of Pressure Ulcers. Clinical Practice Guideline No. 15.* Rockville, MD: US Department of Health and Human Services, Public Health Service, Agency for Health Care Policy and Research. December 1994:47–49. AHCPR Pub. No. 95-0652.

The use of growth factors and skin equivalents in healing pressure ulcers remains under investigation, although the use of cytokine growth factors (eg, recombinant PDGF-BB), FGFs, and skin equivalents have been effective in diabetic and venous ulcers. In three small randomized controlled trials, growth factors had beneficial results with pressure ulcers, but the findings warrant further exploration. A greater understanding of the healing cascade may clarify the appropriate use of growth factors in pressure ulcer treatment.

Monitoring Healing

Monitoring the healing of pressure ulcers can pose a challenge. The accurate measurements of a pressure ulcer can provide useful information about the effectiveness of ulcer treatment. However, results obtained using traditional measurements (ie, rulers and tracing paper) are highly variable among raters. In the past 8 yr, two instruments to measure healing of pressure ulcers with some level of validity and reliability have been developed. The Pressure Sore Status Tool and the Pressure Ulcer Scale for Healing (http://www.npuap.org/PDF/push3.pdf [accessed Jan 2011]) are excellent tools for monitoring pressure-ulcer healing. The use of high-frequency portable ultrasound to measure wound healing has been introduced. This technology, which can capture three-dimensional measurements, has been quite beneficial in objectively monitoring healing (SOE=C). Moreover, because ultrasound is "color blind," it can detect Stage I pressure ulcers in darkly pigmented skin.

Expert debate has been considerable regarding the use of reverse staging of pressure ulcers to monitor healing. Staging of pressure ulcers is appropriate only for defining the maximal anatomic depth of tissue damage. Because pressure ulcers heal to a progressively more shallow depth, they do not replace lost muscle, subcutaneous fat, or dermis before they reepithelialize. Instead, pressure ulcers fill with granulation (scar) tissue composed primarily of endothelial cells, fibroblasts, collagen, and extracellular matrix. A Stage IV pressure ulcer cannot become a Stage III, Stage II, and then Stage I; reverse staging does not accurately characterize the physiologic process during healing of the pressure ulcer. When a Stage IV pressure ulcer has healed, it should be classified as a healed Stage IV pressure ulcer, not as a Stage 0. The progress of healing can be documented only by describing ulcer characteristics or by measuring wound characteristics with a validated tool.

Ulcer care should be evaluated for healing progress on a weekly basis. There are no standard healing rates for pressure ulcers. Review of the literature suggests that most Stage I pressure ulcers heal within 1–7 days; Stage II, within 5 days to 3 mo; Stage III, within 1–6 mo; and Stage IV, within 6–12 mo. Some full-thickness pressure ulcers may never heal, depending on comorbidity; however, no clear guidelines exist to determine when a pressure ulcer can be truly defined as recalcitrant or what characteristics must be present to predict that an ulcer will never heal.

Control of Infections

All pressure ulcers become colonized with both aerobic and anaerobic bacteria, and superficial swab

Table 36.5—Common Dressings for Treating Pressure Ulcers

Dressing	Indications	Contraindications	Examples	Comments
Transparent film	Stage I, II Protection from friction Superficial scrape	Draining ulcers Suspected skin infection or fungus	Bioclusive Tegaderm Op-site	Apply skin prep to intact skin to protect from adhesive
Foam island	Stage II, III Low to moderate exudate Can apply as window to secure transparent film	Excessive exudate Dry, crusted wound	Allevyn Lyofoam	
Hydrocolloids	Stage II, III Low to moderate drainage Good periwound skin integrity Autolytic debridement of necrotic tissue	Poor skin integrity Infected ulcers Wound needs packing	DuoDERM Extra thin film DuoDERM Tegasorb RepliCare Comfeel Nu-derm	Left in place 3–5 days Can apply as window to secure transparent film Can apply over alginate to control drainage Must control maceration Apply skin prep to intact skin to protect from adhesive
Alginate	Stage III, IV Excessive drainage	Dry or minimally draining wound Superficial wounds with maceration	Sorbsan Kaltostat Algosteril AlgiDERM	Apply dressing within wound borders Requires secondary dressing Must use skin prep Must control for maceration
Hydrogel				
(amorphous gels)	Stage II, III, IV	Macerated areas Wounds with excess exudate	IntraSite gel SoloSite gel Restore gel	Needs to be combined with gauze dressing Stays moist longer than saline gauze Changed 1–2 times/day Used as alternative to saline gauze for packing deep wounds with tunnels, undermining Reduces adherence of gauze to wound Must control for maceration
(gel sheet)	Stage II	Macerated areas Wounds with moderate to heavy exudate	Vigilon Restore Impregnated Gauze	Needs to be held in place with topper dressing
Gauze packing (moistened with saline)	Stage III, IV	Wounds with depth, especially those with tunnels, undermining	square 2 × 2s, 4 × 4s Fluffed Kerlix Plain NuGauze	Must be remoistened often to maintain moist wound environment
Silver dressings (silver with alginates, gels, charcoal)	Malodorous wounds High level of exudates Wound highly suspicious for critical bacterial load Periwound with signs of inflammation Slow-healing wound	Systemic infection Cellulitis Signs of systemic adverse events, especially erythema multiforme Fungal proliferation Sensitivity of skin to sun Interstitial nephritis Leukopenia Skin necrosis Concurrent use with proteolytic enzymes	Silvercel Silvadene Aquacel Ag Acticoat	

SOURCE: Copyright © 2010 by Rita Frantz. Adapted from Reuben DB, Herr K, Pacala JT, et al. *Geriatrics At Your Fingertips*, 12th ed. New York: American Geriatrics Society; 2010:236–237. Reprinted with permission.

cultures of the wounds have not been helpful in determining the organisms that may be causing the infection. Therefore, routine swab cultures are not recommended (SOE=B). However, some evidence suggests that quantitative tissue swab cultures can be used to determine the wound bioburden. Wound cleansing and dressing changes are two of the most important methods for minimizing the amount of bacterial colonization. Increasing the frequency of wound cleansing and dressing changes is an important first step when purulent or foul-smelling drainage is observed on the ulcer (SOE=C). When ulcers are not healing or have persistent exudate after 2 wk of optimal cleansing and dressing changes, it is reasonable to consider the use of antimicrobials.

Topical antimicrobials have been shown to decrease the bioburden in pressure ulcers (SOE=B). The use of antimicrobials such as silver sulfadiazine and mupirocin ointment can be applied up to three times a day for 1–2 weeks, with careful monitoring for allergic reactions. Because prolonged use of these antimicrobials can result in resistant organisms, they should not be used indefinitely. In the past several years, the use of silver-impregnated dressings to decrease the bioburden has become quite popular. Although the exact mechanism of how silver kills the infecting organisms remains unknown, it is hypothesized that it stops the enzyme that feeds the proliferation of bacteria, viruses, and fungi. These dressings (eg, Aquacel Ag, Acticoat, Actisorb, Arglaes) control bacterial load and ideally control odor caused by the bacteria. The dressing selected determines how the silver is delivered, the length of treatment, the amount of exudate absorption, the incidence of maceration, the ease of dressing removal, and the pain intensity at dressing changes. It is important to select a dressing that meets the needs of the patient and the staff.

Because most topical antibiotics do not penetrate the wound bed, they are not effective for infection control. When ulcers fail to heal despite the treatments described above, it is reasonable to consider the possibility of cellulitis or osteomyelitis. These diagnoses can be established by biopsy of the ulcer for quantitative bacterial cultures or of the underlying bone. Cellulitis, osteomyelitis, bacteremia, and sepsis are all indications for use of systemic antibiotics.

Topical antiseptics (eg, povidone iodine, iodophor, sodium hypochlorite, hydrogen peroxide, acetic acid) reduce bacterial loads; however, most are cytotoxic to healthy granulation tissue needed for the wound to heal.

Bacteria from surrounding skin contaminate the wound within 24 hours. High levels of bacteria in wounds can delay or impede wound healing. An emerging area of interest in wound healing is the role of bacterial biofilms. Bacterial biofilms are bacteria that attach to wound surfaces and aggregate to form communities in a hydrated polymeric matrix of their own syntheses. Although wounds have been shown to have the characteristics that suggest the existence of bacterial biofilms, there remains a paucity of studies investigating the role of bacterial biofilms and wound healing.

Complications From Pressure Ulcers

The development of pressure ulcers can lead to several complications. Probably the most serious complication is sepsis. When a pressure ulcer is present and there is aerobic or anaerobic bacteremia, or both, the pressure ulcer is most often the primary source of the infection. Additional complications of pressure ulcers include localized infection, cellulitis, and osteomyelitis. Quite often, a nonhealing pressure ulcer indicates underlying osteomyelitis. Mortality can also be associated with pressure-ulcer development. Several studies have noted the association of pressure-ulcer development and mortality in both the hospital and nursing-home settings. In fact, the mortality rate has been as high as 60% for those older adults who develop a pressure ulcer within 1 yr of hospital discharge. Finally, other complications of pressure ulcers include pain and depression, both of which have been associated with decreased wound healing.

ACOVE-3* QUALITY INDICATORS PERTAINING TO PRESSURE ULCERS AND WOUND CARE

Risk assessment

- If a vulnerable older adult who is admitted to a hospital is unable to reposition himself or herself or has limited ability to do so, then risk assessment for pressure ulcers using a standardized scale should be performed on admission; if the patient is found to be at risk, the assessment should be repeated at least every 48 hours thereafter.
- If a vulnerable older adult is admitted to a skilled-nursing facility, then risk assessment for pressure ulcers using a standardized scale should be performed on admission, every week during the first 4 weeks, and every 3 mo thereafter.
- If a vulnerable older adult is admitted to a home healthcare organization, then risk assessment for pressure ulcers using a standardized scale should be performed on admission, and if the patient is found to be at risk, then weekly for 4 weeks and every other week thereafter.

Preventive intervention

- If a vulnerable older adult is identified as at risk of pressure ulcer development or presents with a pressure ulcer, then preventive interventions should be instituted that address pressure reduction (or management of tissue loads) and repositioning needs.
- If a vulnerable older adult who is at risk of pressure ulcer development or has a pressure ulcer also demonstrates malnutrition, then a nutritional assessment to identify nutritional deficiencies and nutrition support should be provided.

Pressure ulcer assessment

- If a vulnerable older adult presents with a pressure ulcer, then the pressure ulcer should be assessed for the following wound characteristics:
  - Location
  - Depth and stage
  - Size
  - Wound bed (eg, necrotic tissue, exudates, wound edges for undermining and tunneling, presence or absence of granulation and epithelialization)
- If a vulnerable older adult has a pressure ulcer, then he or she should be assessed for pain caused by the pressure ulcer daily while in the hospital and at each outpatient visit; if present, the pain should be treated.

Pressure ulcer management

- If a vulnerable older adult presents with a full-thickness pressure ulcer covered with necrotic debris or eschar (unless dry eschar is on the heel), then debridement interventions using sharp, mechanical, enzymatic, biosurgery, or autolytic procedures should be instituted within 24 hours.
- If a vulnerable older adult presents with a pressure ulcer that is clean or free of necrotic tissue, then wound cleansing with normal saline or a noncytotoxic cleanser should be instituted at each dressing change.
- If a vulnerable older adult presents with a clean full-thickness or partial-thickness pressure ulcer, then a moisture-retentive topical dressing such as thin-film dressings, hydrocolloids, hydrogels, foams, or alginates should be provided for treatment and not dry gauze in any form.
- If a vulnerable older adult with a full-thickness Stage III or IV pressure ulcer presents with systemic signs and symptoms of infection, such as fever, increased WBC, and confusion and agitation, and it is likely the sepsis is due to the wound, then the pressure ulcer should be debrided to eliminate necrotic debris within 24 hours, and a tissue biopsy, needle aspiration, or quantitative swab after debridement should be obtained for bacterial culture and appropriate systemic antibiotics started.
- If a vulnerable older adult presents with a clean full-thickness Stage III or IV pressure ulcer at 2–4 weeks after treatment with no improvement in pressure ulcer status (eg, decrease in surface area or depth or according to score on standardized wound healing tool), then appropriateness of the treatment plan and presence of complications should be reassessed.
- If a vulnerable older adult presents with a partial-thickness Stage II pressure ulcer at 1–2 weeks after treatment with no improvement in pressure ulcer status, then appropriateness of the treatment plan and presence of complications should be reassessed.

Related quality indicators for Pressure Ulcers and Wound Care

- Mobilization of postoperative patient (see Perioperative Care, p 92)
- Mobilization of hospital patient (see Hospital Care, p 119)

*Assessing Care of Vulnerable Elders – 3rd Set. See inside front cover for explanation.

REFERENCES

- Abel RL, Warren K, Bean G, et al. Quality improvement in nursing homes in Texas: results from a pressure ulcer prevention project. *J Am Med Dir Assoc.* 2005;6(3):181–188.

- American Medical Directors Association. *Clinical Practice Guideline: Pressure Ulcers.* 2004. http://www.amda.com/tools/cpg/pressureulcer.cfm.

- Ayello EA. Predicting Pressure Ulcer Risk. *Try This: Best Practices in Nursing Care to Older Adults.* 2007;(5). Available at http://consultgerirn.org/uploads/File/trythis/try_this_5.pdf

- Baumgarten M, Margolis DJ, Localio AR, et al. Extrinsic risk factors for pressure ulcers early in the hospital stay: a nested case-control study. *J Gerontol A Biol Sci Med Sci.* 2008;63(4):408–413.

- Lyder CH, Ayello EA. Pressure Ulcers: A Patient Safety Issue. In: Hughes RG, ed. *Patient Safety and Quality: An Evidence-Based Handbook for Nurses.* AHRQ Publication No. 08-0043. Rockville, MD: Agency for Health Care Research and Quality. http://www.ahrq.gov/QUAL/nurseshdbk/docs/LyderC_PUPSI.pdf.

CHAPTER 37—DEPRESSION AND OTHER MOOD DISORDERS

KEY POINTS

- Symptoms of depression below the threshold for a diagnosis of major depressive disorder are common in late life and may incur disability, therefore warranting monitoring or intervention.

- SSRIs such as sertraline and citalopram are most commonly used as first-line agents for older adults with depression.

- Bipolar depression in older adults may be more common than previously thought and should be treated with a mood stabilizer rather than an antidepressant.

- Treatment of depression may require up to 12 weeks before remission is complete, but an initial response to medication may be seen within the first 4 weeks.

- In a substantial minority of cases, trials of more than one antidepressant or combination therapy (augmentation) may be required before remission is achieved.

EPIDEMIOLOGY

Depression is a leading cause of disability-adjusted life years lost across the life span and projected to be more so within a generation. Mood disorders were implicated in 10% of all hospitalizations. However, prevalence studies of community residents demonstrate surprisingly low rates of depressive disorders among those ≥65 yr old. Only 1%–2% of women and <1% of men interviewed with standardized instruments met diagnostic criteria for major depressive disorder (SOE=A). Both current and lifetime prevalence rates for older adults are lower than those for middle-aged adults; furthermore, these relatively low rates persist after accounting for possible premature death and institutionalization, both of which can be associated with depression. Similarly, the incidence of first-episode major depressive disorder decreases after age 65. Data demonstrating that older adults are less likely to recognize depression and to endorse depressed mood offer one explanation for the lower prevalence and incidence of depressive syndromes among older community residents.

However, the prevalence of depressive symptoms that do not meet the threshold for a *Diagnostic and Statistical Manual of Mental Disorders, 4th Edition, Text Revision (DSM IV-TR)* clinical diagnosis is substantial in older adults, with most studies reporting rates in the range of 15%. These subsyndromal states are not inconsequential. "Minor" or "subsyndromal" depression has been associated with increased use of health services, excess disability, and poor health outcomes, including higher mortality.

The prevalence rates of both major and subsyndromal depression vary greatly by the setting in which older adults are seen and by methods used to identify cases. Increased rates of depression are found among older adults seen in healthcare facilities and inpatient settings. Major depressive disorder has been identified in 6%–10% of older adults in primary care clinics and in 12%–20% of nursing-home residents. More varied rates of 11%–45% have been reported among older adults requiring inpatient medical care. The reported prevalence rates of minor depression in outpatient medical settings have varied as well, with reported rates of 8% to >40%. In mental health settings, major depressive disorder is the most common disorder seen among older patients and accounts for >40% of outpatient caseloads and inpatient psychiatry admissions.

CLINICAL PRESENTATION AND DIAGNOSIS

The Geriatric Syndrome of Late-Life Depression

Although aging does not markedly affect the phenomenology of depression, older adults are more often preoccupied with somatic symptoms and less frequently report depressed mood and guilty preoccupations. Among those who do not acknowledge sustained sadness, a persistent loss of pleasure and interest in previously enjoyable activities (*anhedonia*) for at least 2 weeks is necessary for a diagnosis of major depressive disorder.

The diagnosis of depression in physically ill older adults is confounded by the overlap among symptoms of major depressive disorder and somatic illness. Patients with advanced physical illness may be preoccupied with thoughts about death or worthlessness because of marked disability, yet not meet criteria for a major depressive episode. The *DSM*

STRENGTH-OF-EVIDENCE (SOE) RATING DEFINITIONS

A = consistent and good quality patient-oriented evidence
B = somewhat inconsistent or limited quality patient-oriented evidence
C = very inconsistent or very limited patient-oriented evidence, disease-oriented evidence, and/or consensus from professional organizations
D = unstudied common practice or opinion

See inside front cover for detailed information regarding the SOE classification.

Table 37.1—The 9-Item Patient Health Questionnaire (PHQ-9): Screening Questions and Complete Assessment

Two-question screening with the "PHQ-2"

Over the last 2 weeks, how often have you been bothered by the following problems?	Not at all	Several days	More than half the days	Nearly every day
A. Little interest or pleasure in doing things?	0	1	2	3
B. Feeling down, depressed, or hopeless?	0	1	2	3

If A + B = 3 or greater, ask the following:

Over the last 2 weeks, how often have you been bothered by the following problems?	Not at all	Several days	More than half the days	Nearly every day
Feeling tired or having little energy?	0	1	2	3
Poor appetite or overeating?	0	1	2	3
Trouble falling or staying asleep, or sleeping too much?	0	1	2	3
Feeling bad about yourself—or that you are a failure or have let yourself or your family down?	0	1	2	3
Trouble concentrating on things, such as reading the newspaper or watching television?	0	1	2	3
Moving or speaking so slowly that other people could have noticed? Or the opposite—being so fidgety or restless that you have been moving around a lot more than usual?	0	1	2	3
Thoughts that you would be better off dead or of hurting yourself?	0	1	2	3

SOURCE: Developed by Spitzer RL, Williams JBW, Kroenke K, et al., with an educational grant from Pfizer Inc. Copyright © Pfizer, Inc. All rights reserved.

Table 37.2—Indications to Start Antidepressant Therapy Based on Patient Health Questionnaire-9

PHQ-9 Score	Depression Severity	Clinician Response
1–4	None	None
5–9	Mild to moderate	If not currently treated, rescreen in 2 weeks. If currently treated, optimize antidepressant and rescreen in 2 weeks.
10–14	Major depressive disorder	Start antidepressant therapy.
≥15	Major depressive disorder	Start antidepressant therapy; obtain psychiatric consultation if suicidality or psychosis suspected.

IV-TR criteria require that the depressive symptoms are not a direct result of a general medical condition or medication used to treat it. The alternative diagnosis of mood disorder due to a general medical condition should be used for patients with depression that appears to result directly from a specific medical condition (eg, hypothyroidism, pancreatic cancer, use of clonidine). In either case, when symptoms are disabling, treatment should be offered.

Screening

Simply screening for the presence of depressed mood and anhedonia identifies most medically ill patients who also meet diagnostic criteria for major depressive disorder. These symptoms are less likely to be confounded by those of a medical illness. When the clinician fears an older adult is minimizing distress or associated disability, it is helpful to obtain further information from involved family members or caregivers.

The 9-item Patient Health Questionnaire (PHQ-9) has been widely used for the more intensive, thorough assessment of depression. The nine items cover the diagnostic criteria for major depressive disorder, and the initial two questions (the "PHQ-2") can be used for screening. In addition, serial administrations of the PHQ-9 can be used to reliably assess response to treatment.

For use of the PHQ-2 and PHQ-9, see Table 37.1. Patients scoring ≥3 on the depressed mood plus anhedonia questions on the PHQ-2 should be assessed with the remaining seven questions of the PHQ-9. For management based on PHQ-9 score, see Table 37.2.

Table 37.3—The Geriatric Depression Scale (GDS, short form)

Choose the best answer for how you felt over the past week.

1. Are you basically satisfied with your life?   yes/**no**
2. Have you dropped many of your activities and interests?   **yes**/no
3. Do you feel that your life is empty?   **yes**/no
4. Do you often get bored?   **yes**/no
5. Are you in good spirits most of the time?   yes/**no**
6. Are you afraid that something bad is going to happen to you?   **yes**/no
7. Do you feel happy most of the time?   yes/**no**
8. Do you often feel helpless?   **yes**/no
9. Do you prefer to stay at home, rather than going out and doing new things?   **yes**/no
10. Do you feel you have more problems with memory than most?   **yes**/no
11. Do you think it is wonderful to be alive now?   yes/**no**
12. Do you feel pretty worthless the way you are now?   **yes**/no
13. Do you feel full of energy?   yes/**no**
14. Do you feel that your situation is hopeless?   **yes**/no
15. Do you think that most people are better off than you are?   **yes**/no

NOTE: Score one point for each bolded answer; 0–5 = normal, >5 suggests depression. For additional information on administration and scoring, refer to the following:

1. Sheikh JI, Yesavage JA. Geriatric Depression Scale: recent evidence and development of a shorter version. *Clin Gerontol.*1986;5:165–172.
2. Yesavage JA, Brink TL, Rose TL, et al. Development and validation of a geriatric depression rating scale: a preliminary report. *J Psych Res.*1983;17:27.

SOURCE: Courtesy of Jerome A. Yesavage, MD. http://www.stanford.edu/~yesavage/GDS.html (accessed Jan 2011).

At a score of ≥10, the nine depression items achieve good sensitivity and specificity for major depressive disorder among primary care patients versus a structured diagnostic interview conducted by a mental health professional. People scoring ≥15 and those with suicidal ideation may require psychiatric consultation. A change of 5 points is considered a minimal clinically important difference and evidence of response to treatment. Remission is best defined as total score of ≤5. When the score has changed by <5 points despite 4 weeks of treatment at recommended dosages, the medication should either be switched or augmented with combination therapy.

Another standardized instrument for evaluating depressive symptoms is the 15-item Geriatric Depression Scale (GDS) (Table 37.3). It offers the advantage of a "yes/no" response format, which older adults may find easier to manage, and it is virtually free of somatic and sleep queries that can be affected by physical illness. However, it lacks a query regarding suicidal ideation. Neither the PHQ-9 nor the GDS are reliable when administered to people with moderate or severe dementia.

Bipolar Disorder

With the increase in the older adult population, clinicians will encounter more patients with bipolar disorder, particularly bipolar depression. Bipolar disorders do not "burn out" in old age. Indeed, few patients with bipolar disorder recover full function despite symptom remission. Among those with bipolar disorder, mania is a more frequent cause of hospitalization than depression, but depression accounts for more disability. Late-onset mania is seen equally among men and women. Age has little impact on the symptom profile except for less sexual preoccupation among older adults. Impaired cognitive processing, executive dysfunction, and changes in subcortical brain structures are common, further reducing the chances of return to full function.

The *DSM IV-TR* criteria for bipolar disorder type 1 (mania with or without depression) and type 2 (major depressive disorder without mania but with hypomania) are unchanged with age. The manic episode often presents with confusion, disorientation, distractibility, and irritability rather than with elevated, positive mood. The clinical interview can be characterized by irrelevant content delivered with an argumentative, emotionally intense yet fluent quality. Grossly unrealistic ideas concerning finances, travel, or plans for the future are common. Inflated self-esteem, grandiosity, and contentious claims of certainty in the face of evidence to the contrary are also seen.

The presence of psychosis, sleep disturbance, and aggressiveness may lead to the mistaken diagnosis of dementia or depressive disorder rather than mania. Because mania in late life is genuinely less frequent than depression or dementia, these patients are often treated with antipsychotics, antidepressants, or benzodiazepines, which provide partial relief.

Late-onset mania is more often secondary to or closely associated with other medical disorders, most commonly stroke, dementia, or hyperthyroidism, and also with medications, including antidepressants, steroids, stimulants, and other agents with known CNS properties. A search for treatable components that contribute acutely to the person's disability should be pursued. Risk factors for cerebrovascular disease, including excessive use of alcohol or tobacco, suboptimal control of hypertension, hyperlipidemia, and other cardiovascular risk factors, should be explored. Careful inquiry of the family may uncover repeated hypomanic episodes that did not seriously impair the individual but in retrospect are clear indications of earlier disease. The difficulty of recognizing the diagnosis, care for contributing conditions, age-related vulnerability to medication adverse events, and the frequency with which structural brain changes are associated all make treatment more difficult.

Occurring in approximately 0.5% of the U.S. population, bipolar disorder type II is characterized by recurrent major depressive episodes interspersed with periods of hypomania. Because interpersonal difficulties can be minimal, and some symptoms can temporarily increase performance with tasks, past episodes of hypomania may be unrecognized by the patient and family. Major depressive episodes also occur in bipolar disorder I, in which the occurrence of one or more manic episodes is the distinguishing diagnostic feature. There are also mixed states in which criteria for both mania and major depressive disorder are present. As a result, the term "bipolar depression" spans the spectrum of bipolar disorders.

TREATMENT

Overview

Although mood disorders are eminently treatable, effective treatment remains a goal not so easily attained. Only 50% of patients with major depressive disorder fully respond to an initial antidepressant treatment (SOE=A). An additional one-third recover when the antidepressant is switched to another agent or augmented with a second antidepressant or psychotherapy. For those who do recover, 40%–60% experience recurrence depending on the severity of the initial episode and persistence of symptoms. Although a substantial number of patients with "subclinical," "subsyndromal," and "minor" depression experience a remission of symptoms without intervention, each category is associated with as much as a 5-fold risk of the subsequent development of a major depressive episode. Poor self-assessed health and perceived lack of social support may be the simplest and most reliable measures to predict a less benign course. The onset of macular degeneration, stroke, and myocardial infarction are reliable indicators of depression risk, especially in the context of a prior history of mood disorder. Although the need to prevent mood disorders is substantial, success to date has been limited

to reducing the progression of minor to major depressive disorder and to preventing recurrent episodes of major depressive disorder.

The current approach to mood disorders in late life includes a more aggressive acute phase of treatment to bring about remission of the current episode, continuation treatment to prevent relapse, and maintenance treatment to prevent recurrence. Continuation treatment to stabilize the recovery involves ongoing treatment for an additional 6 mo after symptom remission. Maintenance treatment (≥3 yr) is provided to patients with bipolar disorders or a history of depression complicated by psychosis, suicidality, or recurrent episodes. The duration of maintenance therapy should be based on the frequency and severity of previous episodes and may need to be lifelong. Combined pharmacotherapy with psychotherapy is recommended for all patients with bipolar disorders and recurrent, severe psychotic or suicidal depression (SOE=B).

The First Weeks of Treatment

Substantial data indicate that 4 weeks is adequate to identify persons who at 12 weeks will be nonresponders or partial responders (SOE=B). The sooner the response occurs, the sooner the remission is likely to be achieved. More severe depression at baseline is associated with slower response; higher self-esteem is associated with rapid response. At 4 weeks, one-third of medicated patients will be nonresponders, one-third will have responded fully, and one-third partially. As the duration of treatment extends, the response rate for both partial and nonresponders decelerates. The longer the patient remains symptomatic, the greater the indication that either the dosage or the medication should be changed. In addition, partial response predicts recurrence of a major episode of depression.

Pharmacotherapy of Single or Recurrent Episodes of Major Depression

For a summary of information about antidepressant treatment for older adults, see Table 37.4. A series of reports from the Sequenced Treatment Alternatives to Relieve Depression (STAR*D) study team offer a genuine advance for older adults in primary care settings with a structured treatment protocol for use by clinicians. When the first SSRI in the STAR*D

Table 37.4—Selected Antidepressants for Older Adults

Generic Name	Initial Dosage (mg)	Final Dosage (mg)	Amnesia, Arrhythmia Potential	Hypotensive Potential	Sedative Potential	Precautions	Comments
Tricyclic Antidepressants (TCA)							
Nortriptyline	10–25	25–100	Moderate	Moderate	Moderate	Lower final dosage, may be fatal in overdose; glaucoma, prostatic disease, diabetes	Therapeutic window 50–150 ng/mL
Desipramine	10–25	25–150	Moderate	Moderate	Low	Can be fatal in overdose; glaucoma, prostatic disease	Therapeutic level 125–300 ng/mL
SSRIs							
Fluoxetine	10 qam; 90 once/wk	20–40	Low	Low	Low	Prolonged half-life, nausea, tremor, insomnia, drug interactions, serotonin syndrome	Adverse events not life threatening; inhibits CYP1A2, -2B6, -2D6, -3A4; liquid preparation available
Sertraline	25 qam	100–200	Low	Low	Low	Nausea, tremor, insomnia, serotonin syndrome	Fewer drug interactions
Paroxetine	10 qhs	20–40	Low	Low	Low	Nausea, tremor, drug interactions; reduce dosage in renal insufficiency; serotonin syndrome	Mild sedative effect; inhibits CYP1A2, -2B6, -2D6, -3A4
Citalopram	10 qam	20–40	Low	Low	Low	Nausea, tremor; reduce dosage in renal insufficiency; serotonin syndrome	Fewer drug interactions, oral solution available
Escitalopram	10 qam	10–20	Low	Low	Low	Nausea, tremor; reduce dosage in renal insufficiency; serotonin syndrome	Single enantiomere, FDA approved for generalized anxiety disorder, oral solution available
Selective Serotonergic and Noradrenergic Reuptake Inhibitors (SSRI/SNRI)							
Venlafaxine	37.5–75 qam	75–300	Low	Low	Low	Mild hypertensive; headache, nausea, vomiting; do not stop abruptly; reduce dosage in renal insufficiency	SSRI and SNRI, fewer drug interactions
Desvenlafaxine	25 qam	25–50	Low	Low	Low	Headache, nausea, hypertension, dizziness; reduce dosage in renal insufficiency	Active metabolite of venlafaxine
Duloxetine	20	30–60	Low	Low	Low	Drug interactions (CYP1A2, -2D6 substrate); chronic liver disease, alcoholism, increased serum transaminase; reduce dosage in renal insufficiency or choose other agent; rare cases of liver toxicity	Equally SSRI and SNRI, narrow dosage range; FDA approved for neuropathic pain, generalized anxiety disorder, maintenance treatment for major depressive disorder

Table 37.4—Selected Antidepressants for Older Adults (continued)

Generic Name	Initial Dosage (mg)	Final Dosage (mg)	Amnesia, Arrhythmia Potential	Hypotensive Potential	Sedative Potential	Precautions	Comments
Monoamine Oxidase Inhibitors (MAOI)							
Tranylcypromine	10–20	30–60	Low	Moderate	Low	Life-threatening diet and drug interactions	When depression resistant to TCA/SSRI; stimulant, short half-life
Selegiline	5 q24h 6 q24h for transdermal patch	5 q12h 12 q24h for transdermal patch	Low	Moderate	Low	MAOI type B with life-threatening diet and drug interactions unlikely at prescribed dosage	Transdermal patch with less risk of adverse events or suicide
Others							
Bupropion	75 q12h 150 qam	150–300 300 extended release qam	Low	Low	Low	Dopaminergic, noradrenergic; agitation, insomnia, seizures; no anxiolytic properties	For apathetic depression, when TCA/SSRI are ineffective; available in immediate-release, sustained-release, and extended-release tablets
Trazodone	25–50	100–400	Low	High	High	Very sedating; rare cases of priaprism with high dosages	Potentially useful for sleep disturbance
Mirtazapine	7.5	15–45	Low	Low	Moderate	Prolonged half-life, dry mouth, weight gain; reduce dosage for renal insufficiency; potential for neutropenia	When depression resistant to TCA/SSRI; sedative, useful for insomnia
Hypericum perforatum (St. John's wort)	300 q12h	900 q8h	Low	Low	Low	Use standardized, freeze-dried extract 0.3% hypericin; drug interactions; little evidence of efficacy	Low adverse-event profile, OTC
Buspirone	5 q12h	30	Low	Low	Low	Only for augmentation, not a benzodiazepine substitute	Antianxiety agent with no dependence
L-triiodothyronine (various T_3)	25 mcg qam	50 mcg qam	Moderate	Low	Low	Anorexia, arrhythmia, hypertension; only for augmentation	Rapid onset of action
Lamotrigine	25–50 q24h	400 q24h	Moderate	Low	Low	Prolonged half-life; can cause fine skin rash, also potential for Stevens-Johnson syndrome	Causes increase in valproate levels when used concurrently; FDA approved for bipolar depression
Stimulants							
Methylphenidate	5 qam	20 q12h	Low	Low	Low	Anorexia, insomnia, daytime use only	Quick results; for the frail and apathetic
Modafinil	100−200 qam	400 qam	Low	Low	Low	Few studies in older adults; potential for drug interactions	Once daily dosing

protocol (citalopram) did not achieve remission, augmentation with a non-SSRI (bupropion or buspirone) reliably achieved remission in one-third of patients. Stopping citalopram because of intolerability or lack of response and switching to bupropion, venlafaxine, or sertraline achieved remission in an additional one-fourth. Of those not well after the first and second trial of monotherapy or augmentation, subsequent augmentation with L-triiodothyronine (T_3) was superior to monotherapy with nortriptyline, mirtazapine, or tranylcypromine and to augmentation with lithium or the combination of venlafaxine plus mirtazapine. In summary, for patients who could tolerate citalopram but did not achieve remission, augmentation with bupropion or buspirone was superior to switching to another agent. However, patients who did not tolerate citalopram did as well with sertraline as with bupropion or venlafaxine.

When psychosis complicates major depressive disorder, the evidence directing choice of pharmacotherapy for older adults is evolving. Electroconvulsive therapy (ECT) is effective for depression complicated by psychosis and is often considered the treatment of choice caused by poor response or adverse events associated with monotherapy or combination therapy with an antidepressant and antipsychotic (SOE=B). Yet, few patients or their family members will consider ECT without having exhausted other alternatives. In the multisite Study of Pharmacotherapy of Psychotic Depression (STOP-PD), remission was achieved in >60% of the geriatric patients who received a combination of sertraline and olanzapine over 12 weeks. Remission rates with combination therapy were substantially better than with sertraline alone. Therefore, while ECT remains an effective treatment option for late-life psychotic depression, intensive combination of antipsychotic and antidepressant pharmacotherapy can be an effective initial strategy.

Pharmacotherapy of Mania

For a summary of treatment of bipolar disorders in older adults, see Table 37.5. Expert opinion, guidelines, and the Systematic Treatment Enhancement Program for Bipolar Disorder (STEP-BD) reports are in agreement that anticonvulsants, called mood stabilizers in this context, are preferable both for acute treatment and for prevention of recurrence in both late-life mania and bipolar depression. The anticonvulsant divalproex is increasingly considered first choice for treatment and prevention of mania. A therapeutic level is available, and while hepatic toxicity is a risk, it is infrequent. Divalproex inhibits hepatic enzymes that metabolize medications frequently used by older adults. Patients taking β-blockers, type 1C antiarrhythmics (eg, flecainide, propafenone), benzodiazepines, or anticoagulants should be monitored more closely until the divalproex dosage has been stabilized. Laboratory tests (including CBC with platelets, AST, ALT, and amylase) to ensure safety are performed when treatment is started, when the dosage is increased, and at least every 6 mo. Dosage reduction is indicated for tremor interfering with self-care, ataxia or unsteady gait, excess sedation, or heart rate <50 beats per minute. Divalproex should be held or discontinued if the following do not remit after dosage reduction or dosage withholding: platelet count <80,000, or AST, ALT, or amylase 2-fold or more above upper limit of normal.

Response to divalproex requires at least a 3-week period, including titration to a therapeutic range. In the interim, individuals whose mania is exhausting or associated with overly aggressive behavior require an antipsychotic or benzodiazepine. A number of second-generation antipsychotics are approved by the FDA for the treatment of mania (Table 37.5). Meta-analyses indicate that these second-generation antipsychotics appear to be equally effective (SOE=A) such that the choice of an individual agent is based on adverse-event profile. However, the available data on the treatment of mania in these studies include few older adults.

Older adults who have had good results with lithium should not be switched to an alternative unless adverse events become disabling. Nonetheless, the use of lithium as initial treatment should be considered cautiously. Structural brain changes that may not be clinically apparent are associated with a higher risk of toxicity. Diabetes insipidus, hyperglycemia, thyroid abnormalities, severe tremor, confusion, heart failure, arrhythmia, and psoriasis are among the more frequent reasons for discontinuing lithium. Manifestations of lithium toxicity include GI complaints, ataxia, slurred speech, delirium, or coma. Toxicity in older adults can occur at plasma concentrations below the therapeutic threshold of 1 mEq/L. Mild tremor and nystagmus without functional consequences frequently accompany lithium treatment and should not be considered signs of toxicity. Dosage reduction is indicated for tremor interfering with self-care or resulting in ataxia or unsteady gait. The onset of diabetes insipidus can also be cause for discontinuing lithium.

Pharmacotherapy of Bipolar Depression

As with the treatment of mania, there is a broad consensus that mood stabilizers are preferable to antidepressants for acute treatment and prevention of

Table 37.5—Medications Used to Stabilize Mood in Mania and Bipolar Depression

Generic Name	Initial Dosage (mg)	Final Dosage (mg)	Sedative Potential	Precautions	Indications
Lithium compounds					
Lithium carbonate Controlled release	300 q24h 450 q24h	300 q8h 450 q12h	Low	Renal clearance is sole route of elimination; toxicity may appear below therapeutic range; mild tremor is a benign universal adverse event but not when excessive or combined with ataxia; polyuria, polydipsia may be signs of diabetes insipidus; nausea, vomiting are signs of toxicity; risk of hypothyroidism, renal impairment	FDA approved for acute and maintenance therapy of mania in bipolar disorder, lowers risk of suicide; therapeutic level 0.6–1 mEq/L
Antipsychotics					
Olanzapine	2.5	15	Moderate	Slightly anticholinergic as dosage increases, weight gain, metabolic syndrome, diabetes	FDA approved for acute manic and mixed bipolar I episodes
Olanzapine/fluoxetine	6/25	12/25		Little data on use in older adults	FDA approved for bipolar depression
Quetiapine	25	750	Moderate	Sedation, weight gain, metabolic syndrome, diabetes	FDA approved for acute manic and bipolar I and II depression; sedative; less extrapyramidal signs, tardive dyskinesia
Risperidone	0.25	6	Low	Extrapyramidal symptoms likely at dosages >2 mg, weight gain, metabolic syndrome, diabetes	FDA approved for acute manic and mixed bipolar I episodes
Aripiprazole	5	15	Low	Prolonged half-life, may produce agitation at high dosages because of D2 dopamine receptor agonist activity	FDA approved for acute manic and mixed bipolar I episodes and for adjunctive treatment of major depressive disorder
Anticonvulsants					
Divalproex sodium Extended-release Delayed-release	250 q12h 250 hs 250 hs	1000 q12h 1000 hs 500 hs	Moderate	Delayed onset of action, drug interactions, GI upset, tremor, weight gain, edema, thrombocytopenia, sedation; CBC and serum chemistries at baseline, then q6mo; inhibits hepatic enzymes and increases other drug concentrations; hepatotoxicity, pancreatitis; reduce dosage in renal insufficiency	FDA approved for acute manic and mixed bipolar I episodes; better tolerated than carbamazepine, therapeutic concentration 50–100 mcg/mL
Carbamazepine	100 q12h 100 qhs	500 q12h 800 hs	Moderate	Delayed onset of action, drug interactions, dizziness, unsteady gait, anemia; CBC and serum chemistries at baseline, then q6mo; enhances cytochrome P450 activity and decreases other drug concentrations	FDA approved for acute manic and mixed bipolar I episodes; therapeutic concentration 4–12 mcg/mL
Lamotrigine	25 hs	100 q12h	Low	Headaches; prolonged half-life; appearance of rash calls for immediate cessation; valproate reduces clearance of lamotrigine	FDA approved for bipolar I depression to prevent recurrence; does not alter cytochrome P450 activity

recurrence of late-life bipolar depression (SOE=B). Indeed, antidepressants should be avoided in bipolar depression because of the risk of a manic reaction as well as other adverse events and lack of efficacy.

Electroconvulsive Therapy

ECT is highly effective for the treatment of major depressive disorder and mania in older adults. ECT is the first-line treatment for patients at serious risk of suicide or life-threatening poor intake due to a major depressive disorder (SOE=B). Patients with delusional depression can demonstrate paranoia about their food or caregivers, precluding pharmacologic treatment because of unreliable oral intake. Also, delusional depression is less responsive to standard medication regimens. Therefore, ECT is generally the first-line treatment for these patients and is associated with response rates that approximate 80%.

The cognitive adverse events of ECT are the principal factor limiting its acceptance. Anterograde amnesia or the inability to learn new information can be pronounced initially, particularly during bilateral ECT, but improves rapidly after treatment is completed. Retrograde amnesia is more persistent, and the recall of events that immediately preceded ECT can be lost permanently. Although patients may complain that ECT has had a long-term effect on their memory, longitudinal studies have not demonstrated lasting cognitive effects; furthermore, improved memory, perhaps owing to recovery from depression, has been reported. There are few absolute medical contraindications other than the presence of increased intracranial pressure or unstable angina. Patients with coronary artery disease or cerebrovascular disease can be administered ECT safely by appropriate pharmacologic management of the autonomic responses that can occur during treatment. Nevertheless, a recent myocardial infarction or cerebrovascular event and unstable coronary artery disease increase the risk of complications. Right unilateral treatment produces fewer cognitive adverse events than bilateral treatment but is less effective unless doses markedly exceeding a patient's seizure threshold are used.

The selection of ECT over aggressive pharmacotherapy is generally made by weighing the risk of waiting for medication to work against the burden of hospital treatment, any medical conditions that can complicate general anesthesia, and fears of the patient and family. After a course of ECT, patients should be treated with continuation of pharmacotherapy after recovery. Patients not responding to intensive antidepressant treatment before receiving ECT have lower acute response rates and are more likely to relapse subsequently, even when antidepressant treatment is continued with a new medication.

Although maintenance ECT is sometimes used to prevent relapse, the burden that maintenance ECT places on patients and their families may limit its usefulness for long-term management of late-life major depressive disorder. However, some patients who respond uniquely well to ECT can tolerate maintenance ECT performed on an outpatient basis.

Psychosocial Interventions

Although evidence-based psychosocial interventions are not accessible to all depressed older adults, many components of the interventions have common sense appeal and can be incorporated into the practices of primary care providers. For psychosocial interventions for older adults with mood disorders, see Table 37.6. Studies demonstrating the efficacy of psychotherapy for major depressive disorder in older adults have included problem-solving therapy (SOE=B), cognitive-behavioral therapy, and interpersonal psychotherapy. Problem-solving therapy involves working with the patient to identify practical life difficulties that are causing distress and providing guidance to help the patient identify solutions. The treatment is delivered generally in six to eight meetings spaced 1–2 weeks apart. Cognitive and interpersonal psychotherapy are also time-limited but less highly structured. Psychotherapy for minor depression has been promising, with efficacy demonstrated particularly in individuals who have suffered a loss; the goal is prevention of progression to major depressive disorder. Also, caregivers of older adults can develop minor or major depressive syndromes that benefit from psychotherapy. Psychosocial interventions can be effective without psychotropic medication. However, psychotherapy combined with an antidepressant has been associated with a longer period of remission after recovery from the acute episode (SOE=A).

Aerobic exercise is also prescribed as a treatment for mild to moderate depression in older adults. Exercise in combination with antidepressants can yield faster, more lasting results than either alone (SOE=B).

For patients with available family, family-focused treatment emphasizes shared planning to prevent relapses, improved listening and communication, and problem-solving skills. In interpersonal and social rhythms therapy, interpersonal problems and difficulties maintaining a physiologically stabilizing schedule of sleep, waking, and activity are examined to minimize destabilizing social and interpersonal situations. In individual cognitive-behavioral therapy, patients and therapists discuss problem solving, cognitive restructuring, and behavioral activation exercises to reverse negative self-attributions and increase rewarding habits.

Table 37.6—Types of Psychotherapy and Other Psychosocial Interventions for Depressed Older Adults

Therapy/Intervention	Distinguishing Attributes
Cognitive-behavioral therapy to prevent recurrent suicide attempts	Thoughts, feelings, images, beliefs leading up to the attempt are addressed, then reprised at end of treatment to assess benefit; flash cards and memory box used to remind oneself why life is worth living
Cognitive bibliotherapy	Self-help format using Burns' *Feeling Good* (1980) as a workbook to identify and challenge maladaptive cognitions; little contact with therapist
Interpersonal	Exploratory, present- rather than past-oriented; focused on interpersonal conflict, role changes, and role deficits
Brief psychodynamic	Problem-focused, transference not examined, identifies conflicts over dependency and independence, intrapsychic locus, insight-oriented
Life review, reminiscence	Recall of personal success and failure to master one's present and future; developed for older adults
Problem-solving	Focused on change, narrow and pragmatic; solutions elicited from the patient not offered by the therapist; can reduce executive dysfunction
Emotionally supportive	Meant to maintain present level of function or symptom control through expression of burdensome feelings without examination of the unconscious or search for insight
Dementia caregiver counseling	Focused on the caregiver role, combines elements of cognitive-behavioral and interpersonal therapy
Bereavement therapy	Restructuring the experience of the lost loved one and restoration of life goals
Complicated grief therapy	Uses retelling and imaging of the death scene; imaginary conversations with the deceased to decrease disbelief, longing, bitterness, and intrusive preoccupations
Behavioral	Educational with focus directed at reducing negative and increasing positive experiences
Social support intervention	Encourages social outreach, network development; counters thoughts that preclude formation of supportive relationships; enhances social communication and assertiveness skills
Control-relevant intervention	Adaptation of behavioral, problem-solving, and social support interventions to provide greater sense of autonomy to depressed nursing-home residents
Behavioral health management	Facilitates treatment of depression in primary care in a disease management model that encourages adherence without directly providing psychotherapy; often includes telephone contact with clinician and patient by a trained mental health counselor
Dialectical behavior therapy	Focus on acceptance of that which cannot be changed, nonjudgmental awareness, distress tolerance, impulse control, acting counter to depressive urges
Social rhythm therapy	Adjunct to interpersonal therapy with focus on maintaining regularity of daily routines and managing precipitants of rhythm disruption to sustain the emotional quality of roles and relationships
Treatment initiation program	Early intervention to address the older adult's attitudes about depression and treatment, including perceived need for care and stigma of illness and treatment
Family-focused therapy	Incorporates psychoeducation with enhancement of communication skills and behaviors along with relapse prevention planning
Depression care management	Promotes treatment of depression in primary care practices through the services of a depression care manager; use of treatment protocols, access to psychotherapy and follow-up regarding compliance with treatment and satisfaction with care

ACOVE-3* QUALITY INDICATORS PERTAINING TO DEPRESSION AND OTHER MOOD DISORDERS

Screening for depression
- All vulnerable older adults should have documentation of a screen for depression during the initial primary care evaluation and annually.
- If a vulnerable older adult is admitted to a nursing home, then the patient should have documentation of a screen for depression within 2 weeks of admission and annually.

Recognizing depression
- If a vulnerable older adult presents with one of the symptoms listed below (and the symptom has not previously been documented as a chronic condition), then the patient should be asked about depression, treated for depression, or referred to a mental health professional within 2 weeks of presentation.
  - Sad mood, feeling down
  - Insomnia or difficulties with sleep
  - Apathy or loss of interest in pleasurable activities
  - Complaints of memory loss
  - Unexplained weight loss of ≥5% in the previous month or ≥10% in the previous year
  - Unexplained fatigue or low energy

Documenting depression symptoms
- If a vulnerable older adult receives a diagnosis of a new depression episode, then the medical record should document at least three of the nine *DSM IV-TR* target symptoms for major depression within 2 weeks of diagnosis.

Suicidality
- If a vulnerable older adult receives a diagnosis of a new depression episode, then the medical record should document on the day of diagnosis the presence or absence of suicidal ideation and psychosis.
- If a vulnerable older adult has thoughts of suicide, then the medical record should document, on the same date, that the patient has no immediate plan for suicide or was referred for evaluation for psychiatric hospitalization.
- If a vulnerable older adult has thoughts of suicide, then the medical record should document, on the same date, that the patient was asked about access to firearms.

Evaluate for comorbid condition
- If a vulnerable older adult receives a diagnosis of a new depression episode, then the medical record should document evaluation of the following within 1 mo or in the prior 3 mo:
  - Hypothyroidism for women
  - Substance dependence or abuse

Initiating depression treatment
- If a vulnerable older adult is diagnosed with depression, then antidepressant treatment, psychotherapy, or electroconvulsive therapy (ECT) should be offered within 2 weeks after diagnosis unless there is documentation within that period that the patient has improved or the patient has substance abuse or dependence, in which case treatment may wait until 8 weeks after the patient is in a drug- or alcohol-free state.

Antidepressant choice
- If a vulnerable older adult is started on antidepressant medication, then the following medications should not be used as first- or second-line therapy: tertiary amine tricyclics (amitriptyline, imipramine, doxepin, clomipramine, trimipramine), monoamine oxidase inhibitors (MAOIs; unless atypical depression is present), benzodiazepines, or stimulants (except methylphenidate).

Psychotic depression
- If a vulnerable older adult has depression with psychotic features, then he or she should be referred to a psychiatrist or should receive treatment with a combination of an antidepressant and an antipsychotic or with ECT.

ECG for tricyclic use
- If a vulnerable older adult with a history of cardiac disease is started on a tricyclic medication, then a baseline ECG should be performed before initiation if one was not performed in the prior 3 mo.

Interactions with MAOI
- If a vulnerable older adult is taking an SSRI, then an MAOI should not be used for at least 2 weeks after termination of the SSRI (and for at least 5 weeks after termination of fluoxetine).
- If a vulnerable older adult is taking an MAOI, then he or she should not receive medications that have the potential for serious interactions with MAOIs or for at least 2 weeks after termination of the MAOI.

Depression follow-up
- If a vulnerable older adult is newly treated for depression, then the following should be documented at the first follow-up visit with the same clinician or with a mental health provider within 4 weeks of treatment initiation:
  - Degree of response to at least two of the nine *DSM IV-TR* target symptoms for major depression
  - Medication adverse events, if he or she is taking antidepressant medications

- If a vulnerable older adult is newly treated for depression and has suicidal ideation at an outpatient visit, then at the next follow-up visit, which must occur within 1 week, documentation should reflect asking about suicide risk.
- If a vulnerable older adult has no meaningful symptom response after 6 weeks of depression treatment, then one of the following treatment options should be initiated by the eighth week of treatment.
  ○ If initial treatment was medication, the dosage should be optimized or changed, or the patient should be referred to a psychiatrist.
  ○ If initial treatment was psychotherapy alone, medication should be initiated, or referral to a psychiatrist should be offered.
- If a vulnerable older adult with depression responds only partially after 12 weeks of treatment, then one of the following treatment options should be instituted by the 16th week of treatment.
  ○ If initial treatment includes medication, switch to a different medication class or add a second medication to the first.
  ○ If the initial treatment was medication, add psychotherapy.
  ○ If initial treatment was psychotherapy without medication, try medication.
  ○ Consider ECT.
  ○ Refer to a psychiatrist.

Continuing depression therapy
- If a vulnerable older adult with depression has responded to antidepressant medication, then he or she should be continued on the medication at the same dosage for at least 6 mo and make at least one clinician contact (office visit or phone) during that period.

Maintenance depression therapy
- If a vulnerable older adult has experienced three or more episodes of depression, then he or she should receive maintenance antidepressant medication with the same type and dosage of medication for at least 24 mo with at least four office or telephone visits for depression during that period.

Related quality indicators for Depression and Other Mood Disorders
- Assessment of caregiver stress, bereavement (see "Palliative Care," p 102)
- Depression evaluation for weight loss (see "Malnutrition," p 195)
- Depression screening in new dementia (see "Dementia," p 245)
- Depression screening for new stroke (see "Neurologic Diseases and Disorders," p 464)

*Assessing Care of Vulnerable Elders – 3ʳᵈ Set. See inside front cover for explanation.

REFERENCES

- Arean P, Hegel M, Vannoy S, et al. Effectiveness of problem-solving therapy for older, primary care patients with depression: results from the IMPACT project. *The Gerontologist.* 2008;43(3):311–323.

- Greenberg S, Kurlowicz L. The Geriatric Depression Scale (GDS). *Try This: Best Practices in Nursing Care to Older Adults.* 2007;(4). Available at http://consultgerirn.org/uploads/File/trythis/try_this_4.pdf

- Lyness JM, Kim J, Tang W, et al. The clinical significance of subsyndromal depression in older primary care patients. *Am J Geriatr Psychiatry.* 2007;15(3):214–223.

- Rojas-Fernandez C, Miller L, Sadowski C. Considerations in the treatment of geriatric depression. *Res Gerontol Nurs.* 2010;3(3):176–186.

- Trivedi M, Rush AJ, Wisniewski SR, et al. Evaluation of outcomes with citalopram for depression using measurement-based care in STAR*D: implications for clinical practice. *Am J Psychiatry.* 2006;16(1)3:28–40.

CHAPTER 38—ANXIETY DISORDERS

KEY POINTS

- Late-life anxiety is often seen with other medical illnesses or depression.

- Comorbid medical problems that commonly lead to anxiety include cardiovascular and pulmonary disorders.

- SSRIs, including citalopram and sertraline, are often used as first-line treatment for anxiety in late life.

- Nonpharmacologic therapies, particularly cognitive-behavioral therapy and other types of psychotherapies, are beneficial in older adults.

The term anxiety disorder encompasses a spectrum of psychiatric illnesses that includes panic disorder, phobias, obsessive-compulsive disorder, posttraumatic stress disorder, and generalized anxiety disorder. Older adults can suffer from the full spectrum of anxiety disorders. A thorough review of the *Diagnostic and Statistical Manual of Mental Disorders, 4th Edition, Text Revision (DSM IV-TR)* should guide the clinician. Older adults can experience a subjective feeling of anxiety that can meet a level of clinical concern that warrants treatment but does not necessarily fulfill the full diagnostic criteria for an anxiety disorder. While such symptoms merit clinical attention, true anxiety disorders are the focus of this chapter.

Because the published literature on anxiety disorders in older adults is limited, some of the characterizations and treatment strategies described here are based on research conducted in younger populations. Such strategies have been modified to take into account the physiologic and psychologic differences between older and younger adults.

Numerous complexities are involved in a proper assessment of anxiety in older adults. Understanding the common issues faced in such an assessment will lead to a more accurate diagnosis and treatment plan. Examples of these complexities include differentiating anxiety disorders from symptoms related to medical conditions or medications; differentiating anxiety disorders from the appropriate ("normal") experience of anxiety associated with the stressors of late life, appropriately attributing the cause of anxiety to an adverse event of medication, and differentiating anxiety from depression. These common challenges are further complicated by the tendency of older adults to resist psychiatric evaluation because of stigma surrounding mental illness or frank denial of illness.

Assessment of anxiety in older adults generally begins with a clinical psychiatric interview to determine the course and nature of symptoms. The interview should include an evaluation of the patient's mental status, including appearance, stated mood, observed affect, and thought process. Consideration of the patient's social context and support systems is particularly relevant in the geriatric population. Assessment of any impairment in functioning related to the anxiety is an important part of the evaluation. A review of all medications, both prescription and OTC, should be done to exclude an alternative medical or pharmacologic explanation for what appears to be an anxiety disorder, or to identify an aggravating condition. Laboratory tests to check for common medical conditions such as renal, thyroid, or hematologic diseases are important. Urine toxicology should be considered in cases in which substance abuse or misuse is suspected.

Anxiety as a symptom and full-scale anxiety disorders are common problems. The ability to recognize and effectively treat anxiety in older adults is important, given the debilitating effects that an unhealthy level of anxiety can have in this population.

CLASSES OF ANXIETY DISORDERS

The types of anxiety disorders as currently defined in the *DSM IV–TR* are discussed in the following section.

Panic Disorder

Panic disorder is characterized by chronic, repeated, and unexpected panic attacks—bouts of overwhelming and irrational fear, terror, or dread when there is no specific cause for it. During a panic attack, the person experiences a constellation of physical and cognitive symptoms that can include palpitations, sweating, trembling, shortness of breath, the feeling of choking, chest pain or discomfort, nausea or abdominal distress, dizziness or lightheadedness, feelings of derealization (ie, that one or others are unreal) or depersonalization (ie, feeling detached from oneself), paresthesias, chills or hot flashes, fear of losing control, "going crazy," or dying. A diagnosis of a true panic attack requires that at least four of the somatic symptoms listed above are experienced. Attacks are brief, lasting typically 10–30 minutes. In between

---

panic attacks, individuals with panic disorder worry excessively about when and where the next attack may occur. A clinically significant degree of panic symptoms exists if the history reveals that recurrent and unpredictable panic attacks have occurred for at least 1 mo and that time is being spent in worried anticipation of possible recurrence. Whether agoraphobia related to the panic attacks is present also needs to be considered. In such cases, agoraphobia involves the persistent fear of situations that can trigger a panic attack, such as when a patient reports remaining at home to avoid an attack. Patients who experience one or more panic attacks may not necessarily warrant a diagnosis of panic disorder. Panic attacks in late life often present with *limited symptoms* often related to one or two organ systems, such as shortness of breath, nausea and diarrhea, overwhelming feelings of pounding in the chest, or dizziness. These limited-symptom panic attacks are accompanied by feelings of doom, dread, or fears of dying. Panic attacks in older adults are commonly associated with other psychiatric diagnoses, including major depressive disorder, as well as with medical illnesses, including pheochromocytoma.

Specific Phobia

A specific phobia is defined as a marked, persistent, excessive, unreasonable fear in the presence of or in anticipation of a particular distinct trigger, such as a specific person, animal, place, object, event, or situation. Commonly, the person's anxiety level increases instantly when the feared trigger is encountered. Interestingly, he or she is able to identify this fear as unrealistic and unsupported, even though the cognitive and physiologic responses persist. Specific phobias often involve a great amount of anticipatory anxiety (ie, thoughts of just the possibility of encountering the feared stimulus), and avoidance behaviors are likely to be reported. The consequence is that the person experiences a variety of personal difficulties as a result of the anxiety. These behaviors interfere with work and daily routines, and they decrease the person's opportunities to experience pleasurable situations (for fear that a trigger might be present). They can also contribute to secondary symptoms, such as frustration, hopelessness, and a sense of lack of control in one's life. The level of anxiety or fear usually varies as a function of both the degree of proximity to the phobic stimuli and the degree to which escape is limited. Examples of simple phobias include fear of mice, dogs, elevators, flying, or heights. Frequently, specific phobias are seen with panic disorder, with or without agoraphobia. Among older adults, especially in urban settings, fear of crime seems to be particularly prevalent. Phobic disorders tend to be chronic and persist into old age.

However, fear of falling is a specific phobia that is increasingly recognized to have an onset in later life.

Obsessive-Compulsive Disorder

Obsessive-compulsive disorder involves persistent thoughts (obsessions) and behaviors (compulsions) that are performed in an effort to decrease the anxiety experienced as a result of the obsessions. Obsessions are thoughts or ideas that come to a person's mind, often while completing a specific task or during a particular type of situation, that are generally experienced as intrusive. Compulsions are either clearly excessive or are not connected in any realistic way with the thought/obsession that they are designed to "neutralize." For example, a person may wash his or her hands repeatedly, for hours at a time, after shaking a stranger's hand; the unwanted thought is that of possibly having been exposed to a serious disease. In this example, the act of washing is the compulsion, and the obsessive-compulsive person may realize that this behavior is excessive. Obsessive-compulsive disorder is chronic and often disabling. Sufferers may spend many hours every day carrying out their compulsions. Depression and other symptoms of anxiety can also be comorbid illnesses in the older population.

Obsessive-compulsive disorder first appearing in late life is unlikely. More commonly, symptoms of obsessions occur along with a depressive syndrome or early dementia. For example, obsessions about paying bills on time can occur in the context of difficulty in estimating time and planning.

Diogenes syndrome, although not coded in the *DSM IV-TR*, is a late-life disorder that is seemingly related to obsessive-compulsive disorder. Also known as senile squalor syndrome, it is characterized by extreme self-neglect. It usually manifests itself with compulsive hoarding and the pathologic collection and storage of objects, often including items collected from garbage cans and dumpsters that the individual believes have value and meaning.

Posttraumatic Stress Disorder

The distinctive feature of posttraumatic stress disorder is that the person has experienced, either as a witness or a victim, a traumatic event to which they have reacted with fear and helplessness. Examples of such events include those that involve actual or threatened death or serious injury, other threats to personal integrity, witnessing an event that involves death or serious injury of another, or even hearing about death or serious injury of a family member or close associate. Commonly observed symptoms include the reexperiencing of the traumatic event, avoidance (both cognitively and behaviorally) of stimuli associated with the event, psychologic numbing, and increased physiologic arousal. Reexperiencing can take the form of recurrent, intrusive recollections or images, thoughts, or even perceptions of the traumatic event. Such experiences are commonly termed flashbacks. Symptoms of hyperarousal include difficulty falling or staying asleep, hypervigilance, and exaggerated startle response. Nightmares, or recurrent distressing dreams of the traumatic event, are evidence of both hyperarousal and reexperiencing. Disorders often seen with posttraumatic stress disorder include depression, panic disorder, and substance-use disorders. Symptoms must be present for at least 1 mo and cause clinically significant distress or impairment in social, occupational, or other important areas of functioning.

For individuals who are experiencing significant symptoms after a recent trauma (from 2 days to 1 mo) and diagnosed with acute stress disorder, posttraumatic stress disorder must be considered if distress persists. While <50% of people exposed to a traumatic event go on to develop posttraumatic stress disorder, those who experience symptoms of acute stress disorder are at higher risk than those who do not develop acute symptoms (SOE=B). In older adults, posttraumatic stress disorder can have a delayed onset, eg, a new presentation of the disorder in a Holocaust survivor. It is postulated that lack of social supports in the context of new stressors in an older adult's life can contribute to such a presentation.

Generalized Anxiety Disorder

The distinctive symptoms of generalized anxiety disorder include feeling easily tired and experiencing other physical symptoms, such as muscle tension, difficulty sleeping through the night, difficulty concentrating on a task, and feeling irritable or on edge. These symptoms need to have occurred for at least 6 mo and must be accompanied by the sense that one cannot control the feelings of anxiety. In addition, these feelings of intense worry must be a result of more than one stressor. For example, intense worry over financial matters or a medical illness alone, even with all the associated symptoms, in and of itself does not indicate a diagnosis of generalized anxiety disorder. Many older adults with generalized anxiety disorder also have symptoms of depression. The clinician must try to distinguish between the two diagnoses. When these symptoms occur in the context of a major depressive disorder, it is the latter diagnosis that must be assigned.

COMORBIDITY

Depression with Marked Anxiety

Anxiety can be a prominent symptom of depression in many older adults. In fact, anxiety can be the presenting symptom that belies an underlying diagnosis of major depressive disorder. It is commonly believed that the expression of anxiety is more culturally acceptable in this cohort of older adults than the expression of depression. Patients presenting with a chief complaint of anxiety should routinely be evaluated for a major depressive disorder. Patients suffering from a combination of depressive and anxious symptoms can have clinically significant levels of distress despite the fact that they do not meet the full criteria for a diagnosis of either disorder.

Anxiety and Medical Disorders

It is common to encounter patients with comorbid anxiety and medical disorders. In many cases, medical illness can mimic an anxiety disorder in its presentation. Medical illness can also exacerbate a concurrent anxiety disorder, or vice versa. Finally, adverse events of medications can produce or contribute to anxiety symptoms.

COPD is a common medical illness that can mimic an anxiety disorder. The common cold or influenza can aggravate a concurrent anxiety disorder. Other common medical illnesses that can cause or contribute to an anxiety disorder include cardiovascular or pulmonary conditions and hyperthyroidism. Medical illnesses that can be exacerbated by high levels of anxiety include angina pectoris or myocardial infarction.

Adverse events of medications, including those commonly encountered with thyroid hormone replacement, antipsychotics, and caffeine can also be the primary cause of anxiety symptoms. Given the complicated clinical picture that results when anxiety and medical disorders coexist, a thorough assessment, including a clinical history, review of both prescribed and OTC medications (with an eye toward possible interactions), appropriate laboratory tests, and measurement of therapeutic medication concentrations when appropriate, is imperative before treatment begins. When medical illness and anxiety symptoms coexist, maximizing potential anxiolytic properties of a medical treatment should be considered. For instance, in the treatment of a patient with diabetic neuropathy and anxiety, it would be appropriate to consider maximizing the dosage of duloxetine to take full advantage of its anxiolytic effects.

PHARMACOLOGIC MANAGEMENT

Numerous drugs have been used over the years as anxiolytics: alcohol, barbiturates, antihistamines, benzodiazepines, antipsychotic medications, and β-blockers. Evidence to support the use of many of these agents is significantly lacking. Although empirical studies of the use of medications in treating older

Table 38.1—Treatment Strategies for Anxiety Disorders in Late Life

Disorder	First-Line Treatments	Second-Line Treatments
Panic disorder with or without agoraphobia	SSRIs[a], SNRIs[a], CBT[a]	Benzodiazepines[b]
Social phobia	SSRIs[a] plus CBT[b]	Benzodiazepines[b]
Social phobia, specific type (eg, public speaking)	β-blockers plus CBT[b]	Buspirone[b]
Specific phobia (eg, rats, blood)	CBT[b] or benzodiazepines[b]	β-Blockers[b]
Obsessive-compulsive disorder	SSRIs[a], SNRIs[b], CBT[b]	Clomipramine[b]
Posttraumatic stress disorder	SSRIs[b], SNRIs[b]	CBT[b]
Generalized anxiety disorder	SNRIs[a], SSRIs[a], CBT[a]	Benzodiazepines[b]
Anxiety and medical disorders	Identify and treat underlying cause, use SSRIs[a] or SNRIs[a] in primary anxiety disorder	Benzodiazepines[b]
Depression with severe anxiety	SSRIs[a], SNRIs[a]	Buspirone[b], benzodiazepines[b], CBT[a]

NOTE: SNRIs = serotonin-norepinephrine reuptake inhibitors; CBT = cognitive-behavioral therapy
[a]SOE=A in studies of the geriatric population
[b]SOE=A in studies of the general adult population; insufficient studies in the geriatric population

adults were initially limited, the body of literature to support this practice is increasing, including several randomized controlled trials of the treatment of late-life anxiety disorders (most often generalized anxiety disorder). For some disorders, the body of literature supporting the efficacy of these medications is gleaned from use in younger patients, modified by age considerations. A brief description of the various classes of compounds currently favored as anxiolytics follows. For a summary of the treatment strategies for anxiety disorders in late life, see Table 38.1.

Antidepressants

Antidepressants have proved efficacious in the treatment of panic disorder, obsessive-compulsive disorder, generalized anxiety disorder, and posttraumatic stress disorder in younger patients. Studies have demonstrated that SSRIs, particularly citalopram, are safe and efficacious in the specific treatment of late-life anxiety disorders. Given their relatively favorable adverse-event profile, the SSRIs or serotonin-norepinephrine reuptake inhibitors (eg, venlafaxine, duloxetine) should now be considered the medications of choice for these disorders (SOE=A). Further, SSRIs should also be considered treatments of choice for treating depression with severe anxiety symptoms. Compounds such as venlafaxine and duloxetine should be considered as alternatives for those patients who do not respond to SSRIs or who develop adverse events.

Benzodiazepines

Over the past several decades, benzodiazepines have been the most commonly prescribed anxiolytics for both younger and older patients, but their use is now discouraged. When needed because symptoms are severe, benzodiazepines with shorter half-lives and without active metabolites, such as lorazepam and oxazepam, are preferable in treating older adults because they are metabolized by direct conjugation, a process relatively unaffected by aging. However, the use of even short-acting benzodiazepines should be limited to <6 mo because long-term use is fraught with multiple complications, such as motor incoordination and falls, cognitive impairment, depression, and the potential for abuse and dependence.

Other Medications

Several studies have suggested that buspirone, an anxiolytic medication with some serotonin-agonist properties, is efficacious for treatment of generalized anxiety disorder (SOE=A), although clinical experience is less positive. Buspirone appears to be a safer choice than benzodiazepines for patients taking several other medications or needing treatment for longer periods of time. One drawback of buspirone is the amount of time required to see a clinical response (approximately 4 weeks). This suggests that concomitant use of a short-acting benzodiazepine in the initial stage of treatment would be useful for some patients. Although antihistamines such as hydroxyzine and diphenhydramine[OL] are sometimes used to manage mild anxiety in younger patients, the anticholinergic properties of these agents can cause serious problems in older adults, in whom their use is not recommended. Second-generation antipsychotics, such as risperidone[OL], olanzapine[OL], and quetiapine[OL], are not appropriate choices for treatment of a nonpsychotic older adult with an anxiety disorder.

PSYCHOLOGIC MANAGEMENT

Although pharmacotherapy is commonly the first-line

The schizophrenia-like psychoses of late life differ from schizophrenia beginning in early life in two ways (SOE=C). First, thought disorder, a sign described as speech in which a series of thoughts are not connected to one another in a logical fashion, is much less common in older adults, comprising only 5% of cases. In early-onset schizophrenia, thought treatment for late-life anxiety disorders, psychologic treatments are often efficacious, either alone or as adjuncts to medication (SOE=A). The psychotherapeutic remedies that have been most rigorously tested all fall under the rubric of cognitive-behavioral therapy. Techniques generally fall into three categories: 1) relaxation training used with music, visual imagery, aromatherapy, and instruction in relaxation techniques; 2) cognitive restructuring to help the patient identify triggers and stimuli that maintain anxiety, gain more control over the effect of such stimuli, and develop a range of coping strategies and tools; and 3) exposure with response prevention (ie, the individual is exposed to the feared stimuli and prevented from performing a compulsive action), which is particularly effective with obsessive-compulsive disorder. Graded desensitization, which is used in panic and phobias, relies on exposure to gradually more anxiety-producing stimuli, with techniques to manage and tolerate the resultant anxiety. Treatment of older adults typically includes a combination of these therapeutic approaches. Success depends on the appropriateness of the patient for psychotherapy; the patient's support system, intellectual functioning, and level of motivation; the degree of coordination of care with medical professionals; and the nature of the disorder. Consultation with a mental health professional can assist in determining the appropriateness of a referral.

REFERENCES

- Ayers C, Sorrell J, Thorp SR, et al. Evidence-based psychological treatments for late life anxiety. *Psychol Aging.* 2007;22(1):8–17.

- Pinquart M, Duberstein P. Treatment of anxiety disorders in older adults: a meta-analytic comparison of behavioral and pharmacological interventions. *Am J Geriatr Psychiatry.* 2007;15(8):639–651.

- Smith M, Ingram T, Brighton V. Evidence-based guideline. Detection and assessment of late-life anxiety. *J Gerontol Nurs.* 2009;35(7):9–15.

CHAPTER 39—PSYCHOTIC DISORDERS

KEY POINTS

- Hallucinations are perceptions without stimuli that can occur in any sensory modality (ie, visual, auditory, tactile, olfactory, gustatory). In late life, multimodal hallucinations are common.

- Delusions are abnormal beliefs that in late life are often paranoid or persecutory, such as a belief that one's safety is in jeopardy or that one's belongings are being stolen.

- Psychosis occurring for the first time in late life is often due to dementia or neurologic conditions such as Parkinson's disease or stroke, as opposed to a primary psychotic disorder, such as schizophrenia.

- Dementia with Lewy bodies is associated with characteristically vivid visual hallucinations, often including people or animals.

- When psychotic symptoms arise in the context of depression, the symptoms are often "mood congruent," such as delusions that one is penniless or that one is already dead.

Psychotic symptoms are defined as either *hallucinations*, ie, perceptions without stimuli, or *delusions*, ie, fixed, false, idiosyncratic ideas. Hallucinations are abnormal perceptions that can be in any of the five sensory modalities (auditory, visual, tactile, olfactory, gustatory). Delusions are unfounded beliefs that can be suspicious (paranoid), grandiose, somatic, self-blaming, or hopeless. This chapter focuses on conditions in which psychotic symptoms are prominent and central to making the diagnosis. It only briefly discusses other disorders, such as dementia, delirium, and the mood disorders, in which psychotic symptoms can occur but whose defining features are in the cognitive or mood realms and which are discussed elsewhere. See "Dementia," p 245; "Delirium," p 245; and "Depression and Other Mood Disorders," p 295.

Hallucinations and delusions occur in a variety of disorders. The evaluation of an older adult with hallucinations and delusions (Figure 39.1) should begin with evaluation for underlying sources such as delirium, dementia, stroke, or Parkinson's disease. An acute onset of altered level of consciousness or

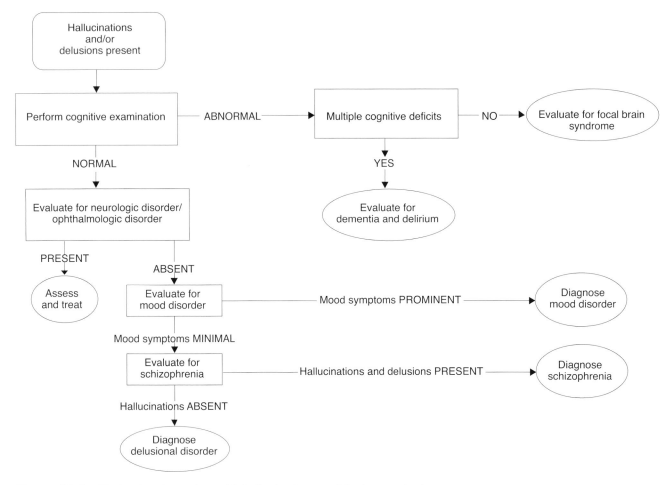

Figure 39.1—Evaluating the patient with hallucinations or delusions, or both

inability to sustain attention suggests delirium. Next, a primary mood disorder should be considered. Only after other causes are excluded should the diagnosis of a schizophrenia-like state be made. Delirium, most often superimposed on an underlying dementia, is the most common cause of new-onset psychosis in late life.

SCHIZOPHRENIA AND SCHIZOPHRENIA-LIKE SYNDROMES

Schizophrenia is defined as a chronic psychiatric disorder characterized by positive symptoms (eg, hallucinations, delusions, and thought disorder) and negative symptoms (eg, social dilapidation and apathy). Mood disorder and cognitive disorder should be excluded before the diagnosis is made. In men,

schizophrenia has a modal onset at age 18; onset after age 45 yr is uncommon. In women, modal age of onset is 28, and 20%–30% of cases begin after age 45. Approximately 85% of older adults with schizophrenia experienced onset of illness in early adult life. However, 10%–15% of cases of schizophrenia first come to clinical attention after patients are 45 yr old. Schizophrenia with onset between the ages of 40 and 60 is called "late-onset schizophrenia," while patients with onset after age 60 are considered to have "very-late-onset schizophrenia-like psychosis."

In older adults, late-onset schizophrenia-like conditions are characterized by onset after age 44, prominent persecutory (paranoid) delusions, and multimodal hallucinations (SOE=C). For example, patients commonly complain that items are being stolen or report that they are being persecuted unjustly. Hallucinations often manifest in complaints, for example, that a neighbor is persistently banging on walls or the roof, that someone is pumping gas under the door, or that electrical sensations are being sent through the walls of the person's home and into his or her body. A schizophrenia-like psychosis can be diagnosed only when cognitive disorder, mood disorder, or other explanatory medical conditions such as delirium or focal brain pathology have been excluded (Figure 39.1).

The schizophrenia-like psychoses of late life differ from schizophrenia beginning in early life in two ways (SOE=C). First, thought disorder, a sign described as speech in which a series of thoughts are not connected to one another in a logical fashion, is much less common in older adults, comprising only 5% of cases. In early-onset schizophrenia, thought disorder is present in approximately 50% of cases. Thought disorder in schizophrenia occurs in the absence of an impaired sensorium (ie, delirium). When illogical speech occurs in late life, a delirium or dementia should be excluded. A second significant difference is the rarity of social deterioration and dilapidation among older adults. Thus, personality is often intact in late-onset cases. However, there is a dearth of long-term follow-up studies, so it is unknown whether social deterioration and personality changes occur after many years of symptoms.

Epidemiology and Clinical Characteristics

Late-onset schizophrenia is more common among women. The population-based incidence of late-onset schizophrenia is unknown, but the lifetime prevalence of schizophrenia is 1% among both men and women.

Late-onset schizophrenia-like psychoses affect predominantly women, with the female:male ratio ranging from 5:1 to 10:1. Many older adults with late-onset schizophrenia-like psychosis have been able to hold responsible jobs and work efficiently, but premorbid isolation and "schizoid" (socially isolated personality) traits are common.

While many individuals with schizophrenia experience fewer hallucinations and delusions as they age, others remain significantly functionally impaired by psychotic symptoms. Moreover, older adults with schizophrenia have an increased risk of suicidal behavior compared with that of their peers without mental illness (SOE=C).

One condition that may be confused with late-onset schizophrenia is frontotemporal dementia, because it can involve features of socially inappropriate and odd behaviors as well as premorbidly odd or "schizoid" personality features. See Dementia, p 245.

Treatment and Management

Nonpharmacologic

Because suspiciousness and paranoid delusions are commonly the most prominent symptoms, the clinician's first task in treating late-onset psychosis is often to establish a trusting therapeutic relationship with the patient. On occasion, the suspicious ideas are plausible (eg, the claim that the patient is being financially abused by a relative), but usually the delusions are bizarre and implausible. It is rarely effective to confront the patient with the unreality or implausibility of his or her ideas. The patient is more likely to respond positively if the clinician empathizes with the distress that the symptoms cause ("I can see how upset you are by all of this"). If patients ask whether the clinician "believes" them, a response such as, "I don't hear anything like that, but I appreciate the fact that you do" is both honest and empathic. The symptoms are usually frightening and distressing to the patients and can lead to unusual behaviors. For example, patients who develop concerns that their food is being poisoned may exhibit unusual eating habits or food avoidance. Furthermore, suspiciousness can isolate the patient from friends and family. Therefore, encouraging patients to maintain important relationships and seeking their permission to discuss the source of symptoms with close family members or friends can help these patients maintain important, supportive relationships.

Pharmacologic

Clinical experience and descriptive case series suggest that antipsychotic medications are as effective in late-onset schizophrenia as in early-onset cases (SOE=C). Second-generation antipsychotic medications are recommended because such agents are less likely to cause tardive dyskinesia (TD), an adverse event for which older age is a predisposing factor. Dosages should be increased at semiweekly or weekly intervals, as needed. While dosages are being titrated, patients should be monitored for the emergence of extrapyramidal adverse events (eg, parkinsonian tremor, rigidity, dystonia) and other movement disorders. (See drug-induced movement disorders in "Neurologic Diseases and Disorders," p 472.) These should be treated by lowering the dosage and switching to an alternative antipsychotic if necessary. Polypharmacy should be avoided by reducing the dosage or switching the antipsychotic medication rather than by adding a medication for extrapyramidal symptoms. The more common adverse events with quetiapine are sedation and orthostatic hypotension; with risperidone, extrapyramidal symptoms; and with olanzapine, weight gain and sedation (Table 39.1).

No studies are available to guide the duration of treatment. Clinical experience suggests that patients who respond to antipsychotic medications should be continued on the minimal effective dosage for at least 6 mo. Patients with early-onset schizophrenia and chronic stable symptoms may be able to tolerate a gradual reduction in dosage of antipsychotic medication. For all patients who relapse on treatment or when the dosage is lowered, maintenance over a longer term (at least 1–2 yr) is recommended (SOE=D). Patients should be monitored for the emergence of TD, a syndrome characterized by repetitive

Table 39.1—Dosing and Adverse Events of Commonly Used Antipsychotic Medications

Medication	Starting Daily Dosage (mg)	Maximal Daily Dosage (mg)	Adverse Events		
			EPS*	Drowsiness	Weight Gain
Aripiprazole	5	15	++ (akathisia)	+	+
Clozapine	12.5	100	+	+++	+++
Haloperidol	0.5–1	5–10	+++	++	+
Olanzapine	2.5	10–15	+	++	+++
Perphenazine	4	32	++	++	++
Quetiapine	25	200–300	+	+++	++
Risperidone	0.5–1	2–4	++	+	++
Ziprasidone	20	120	+	++	+

NOTE: + = uncommon, ++ = somewhat common, +++ = common

*EPS = extrapyramidal adverse signs: rigidity, parkinsonian tremor, dystonia, akathisia

involuntary movements of the oral and limb musculature. Rating scales for TD, such as the AIMS or DISCUS, are clinically useful and easy to administer in the office or institutional setting. If TD develops, the dosage of the antipsychotic medication should be lowered, if possible. Depending on the duration of exposure, TD may worsen or appear when the antipsychotic is discontinued or the dosage is lowered, or when switching from one antipsychotic to another. At the time antipsychotic medications are initiated or as soon as symptoms improve enough so that the patient can understand the risk, he or she should be informed of the risk of TD and the possibility that it can be irreversible.

PSYCHOTIC SYMPTOMS IN DELIRIUM

Hallucinations, particularly visual hallucinations, can be a symptom of delirium, even when it is mild. The onset of delirium is typically acute, and there is usually an identifiable metabolic, pharmacologic, or infectious cause. The mental status examination reveals multiple cognitive impairments and a diminished or waxing and waning level of consciousness. See "Delirium," p 264.

PSYCHOTIC SYMPTOMS IN MOOD DISORDER

Delusions can be seen in major depressive disorder and in the manic phase of bipolar disorder. These delusions are described as "mood congruent." That is, in patients with depression, the delusional content usually reflects self-deprecation, self-blame, hopelessness, or the conviction of ill health. A patient may complain that he or she has no blood or that his or her intestines are not working, for example; another patient may believe that he or she has caused a terrible wrong and deserves to be punished (a

self-blaming delusion). Some patients become convinced that they are dying and that nothing can be done to help them when there is no physiologic evidence to support their concerns. Other common depressive delusions are the conviction that one has no insurance, no clothing, or no money when this is not true (delusion of poverty). Delusions congruent with mania are grandiose. Examples include the person's belief that he or she is infallible, can do impossible physical or intellectual activities, has skills and abilities that no other human being has, or is a special personage such as Jesus Christ. See "Depression and Other Mood Disorders," p 295.

PSYCHOTIC SYMPTOMS IN DEMENTIA

Patients with dementia experience both hallucinations and delusions. These are usually less complex than the delusions seen in schizophrenia or mood disorder. Common delusions in dementia are the belief that one's belongings have been stolen or moved, or the conviction that one is being persecuted. Delusions that one's spouse is unfaithful (delusions of infidelity) are also common. See "Dementia," p 245.

Management of psychosis in dementia is particularly challenging, because the use of antipsychotic medication warrants careful consideration of risks and adverse events. Nonpharmacologic interventions, such as redirection and reassurance, should be tried first. However, if the patient is physically aggressive or severely distressed by the psychotic symptoms, then a trial with low-dose antipsychotic medication is warranted (SOE=C). Both first- and second-generation antipsychotic medications are associated with numerous adverse events, including death, in patients with dementia; for a detailed discussion of this topic, see "Behavioral Problems in Dementia," p 256.

There is also a class warning for second-generation antipsychotics concerning the risk of hyperglycemia in both younger and older patients with schizophrenia. The FDA has asked all manufacturers of second-generation antipsychotic medications to include a warning on the increased risk of developing hyperglycemia and diabetes. The mechanism for these adverse events is unclear, although the fact that weight gain occurs with most of these medications may account for the increased rate of hyperglycemia.

SYNDROMES OF ISOLATED HALLUCINATIONS

Charles Bonnet Syndrome

Between 10% and 13% of patients with significant visual impairment (bilateral acuity worse than 20/60) experience visual hallucinations. These can take the form of shapes such as diamonds or rectangles but more commonly consist of complex hallucinations such as small children, multiple animals, or a vivid scene such as one would see in a movie. This condition, first described more than 200 yr ago, goes by the eponym Charles Bonnet syndrome. The criteria for this syndrome are as follows:

- visual hallucinations
- partially or fully intact insight (the patient is aware that the perceptions cannot be real but still reports that they appear absolutely real and vivid)
- visual impairment
- lack of evidence of brain disease or other psychiatric disorder

It has been suggested that this syndrome is a concomitant of the phantom limb syndrome caused by retinal lesions. However, visual hallucinations have also been reported in individuals with field defects caused by cortical lesions of the visual pathways.

The best treatment for the Charles Bonnet syndrome is information and support. Patients should be informed that the hallucinations are a sign of eye disease, not mental illness. An occasional patient has partial insight or loses insight and becomes very distressed by this symptom. When this distress is significant or leads to dangerous behavior, a cautious trial of low dosages of a second-generation antipsychotic medication is occasionally beneficial.

Psychotic Disorder Caused by a General Medical Condition

Patients with Parkinson's disease, stroke, and other brain disorders occasionally experience delusions and hallucinations without prominent cognitive impairment or other evidence of psychiatric disorder (SOE=C). Delirium caused by a superimposed condition should be excluded. In patients with Parkinson's disease, the symptoms may be secondary to a prescribed dopaminergic agent, but some patients experience visual hallucinations before any medications are started. Education and support should be offered to all patients with these symptoms. If the patients experience significant emotional distress or if the symptoms lead to dangerous or upsetting behavior, cautious use of an antipsychotic medication is appropriate (SOE=B). For patients with Parkinson's disease and hallucinations, quetiapine[OL] 12.5–75 mg/d or olanzapine[OL] 2.5–5 mg/d may be beneficial. Some patients require clozapine[OL] 12.5–75 mg/d. However, patients taking clozapine should have a CBC done once a week for 6 mo and then biweekly thereafter because of the risk of granulocytopenia.

Dementia associated with Lewy bodies is increasingly recognized as an important cause of hallucinations in late life. The clinical scenario typically involves cognitive decline accompanied by motor features of parkinsonism. However, prominent visual hallucinations are a key part of the diagnosis. These hallucinations are often vivid and troubling. See "Dementia," p 245.

Dementia associated with Lewy bodies presents a challenge similar to that of psychosis in Parkinson's disease, because the medications in the class approved to treat psychosis, the antipsychotics, worsen the parkinsonian symptoms. No trial data are available to guide medication choice, but there are case reports of significant improvement through the use of cholinesterase inhibitors[OL] (SOE=B). If an antipsychotic medication must be used, then the treatment strategies outlined above are appropriate if there is careful attention to the risk of extrapyramidal adverse events. Nonpharmacologic treatments include redirection, reassurance, and explanation.

REFERENCES

- Cohen CI, Vahia I, Reyes P, et al. Schizophrenia in later life: clinical symptoms and social well-being. *Psychiatr Serv.* 2008;59(3):232–234.

- Cohen CI, ed. *Schizophrenia into Later Life: Treatment, Research, and Policy.* Arlington, Virginia: American Psychiatric Publishing, Inc.; 2003.

- Folsom DP, Lebowitz BD, Lindamer LA, et al. Schizophrenia in late life: emerging issues. *Dialogues Clin Neurosci.* 2006;8(1):45–52.

- Reeves R, Brister J. Psychosis in late life: emerging issues. *J Psychosoc Nurs Ment Health Serv.* 2008;46(11):45–52.

- Schneider LS, Dagerman KS, Insel P. Risk of death with atypical antipsychotic drug treatment for dementia: meta-analysis of randomized placebo-controlled trials. *JAMA.* 2005;294(15):1934–1943.

- Weintraub D, Hurtig H. Presentation and management of psychosis in Parkinson's disease and dementia with Lewy bodies. *Am J Psychiatry.* 2007;164(10):1491–1498.

CHAPTER 40—PERSONALITY AND SOMATOFORM DISORDERS

KEY POINTS

- Personality disorders persist into late life and pose complex challenges in patients across various medical and psychiatric settings.

- Personality disorders can be more difficult to detect in late life because of age-associated changes in symptoms, comorbid psychopathology, and lack of age-adjusted diagnostic instruments.

- The goal of treatment of personality disorders in late life is not to cure the disorder but to decrease the frequency and intensity of symptoms. To this end, both psychotherapeutic and psychopharmacologic strategies are needed.

- Somatoform disorders represent the presence of physical symptoms without established underlying pathology and with strongly associated psychologic factors. Undifferentiated somatoform disorder and hypochondriasis are the most common forms seen in late life.

- Treatment of somatoform disorders must attend to the affected individual's distress and belief in the veracity of his or her symptoms. Repeated reassuring clinical visits help to build a therapeutic relationship. Both psychotherapy and pharmacotherapy can be helpful for some individuals.

PERSONALITY DISORDERS

Personality disorders are defined in the *Diagnostic and Statistical Manual of Mental Disorders, 4th Edition, Text Revision* (*DSM IV-TR*) by the presence of chronic and pervasive patterns of inflexible and maladaptive inner experiences and behaviors. These patterns lead to significant disruptions in several spheres of function, including cognitive perception and interpretation, affective expression, interpersonal relations, and impulse control. Individuals with personality disorders are often distinguished by repeated episodes of disruptive or noxious behaviors and, as a result, they often receive pejorative labels, depending

on their form. Descriptive terms often applied to those with personality disorders include "difficult," "dramatic," and "strange," to name just a few. The developmental roots of personality disorders are believed to lie in childhood and adolescence, but their features can present clinically at any age in adulthood. Personality disorders are influenced by both genetic and environmental factors.

The *DSM IV-TR* describes ten personality disorders, grouped into three broad clusters that are based on common phenomenology. Depressive and passive-aggressive personality disorders are two additional categories, but they are considered provisional because they appear to lack the empirical support of the other ten diagnoses. For late-life features of all twelve personality disorders, see Table 40.1. Mixed diagnoses and those that do not fit into any existing category are labeled "personality disorder, not otherwise specified."

Many older adults with personality disorders can easily become overwhelmed by age-associated losses and stresses, largely because they lack appropriate coping skills and the personal, social, or financial resources to buffer their losses. In particular, admission to a hospital or long-term care setting poses a unique stress on all individuals with personality disorders in late life. The loss of a familiar environment, personal items, privacy, and the control over one's schedule can lead to a sense of disorganization and displacement. Conflict in an institutional setting begins when patients with personality disorders try to cope with the stresses from their new environment by exaggerating their maladaptive behaviors. An obsessive-compulsive person may attempt to maintain a sense of control by demanding rigid adherence to schedules and rules of hygiene. Dependent individuals may feel helpless and panicked without enough attention to their needs, responding with clinging behaviors and excessive questions or requests for assistance. Paranoid, antisocial, and borderline patients may refuse to cooperate with treatment plans or institutional rules.

Epidemiology

Prevalence rates of late-life personality disorders in the community range from 5% to 13%, which is a slightly lower range than the 10% to 20% prevalence estimates for individuals of all ages in the community. The most common personality disorders in late life are dependent, obsessive-compulsive, paranoid, and not otherwise specified. Although most research has demonstrated fewer diagnoses in older age groups, it

Table 40.1—Features of Personality Disorders

Cluster, Disorder	General Features*	Features Specific to Older Adults
Cluster A: Odd or Eccentric Behaviors		
Paranoid	Pervasive suspiciousness of the motives of others, which often leads to irritability and hostility	Episodes of paranoid psychosis, agitation, and assaultiveness
Schizoid	Disinterest in social relationships, coupled with isolative and sometimes odd behaviors	Poor, strained, or absent relationships with caregivers
Schizotypal	Characteristic appearance, behaviors, and beliefs that are strange, unusual, or inappropriate	Beliefs that can become delusional and lead to conflicts with others; relationships with caregivers can be strained or absent
Cluster B: Dramatic, Emotional, or Erratic Behaviors		
Antisocial	Poor regard for social norms and laws; lack of conscience and empathy for others; frequent reckless and criminal behaviors	Frequent remission of antisocial behaviors with less aggression and impulsivity
Borderline	Impaired control of emotional expression and impulses associated with unstable interpersonal relations, poor self-identity, and self-injurious behaviors	Persistent emotional lability and unstable relationships but less self-injurious and impulsive behaviors
Histrionic	Excessive emotionality and attention-seeking behaviors, sometimes appearing overly seductive or provocative	Behaviors that can become excessively disinhibited and disorganized, appearing manic
Narcissistic	Pervasive sense of entitlement, grandiosity, and arrogance, coupled with lack of empathy	Can present as hostile, enraged, paranoid, or depressed
Cluster C: Anxious or Fearful Behaviors		
Avoidant	Excessive sensitivity to rejection and social scrutiny; social demeanor that can be timid and inhibited	Social contacts that can be extremely limited, providing for inadequate support
Dependent	Excessive dependence on others to help make decisions and provide support	Commonly, comorbid depression; clinical appearance often with demanding or clinging behaviors if dependency needs not met
Obsessive-compulsive	Pervasive preoccupation with orderliness and cleanliness; a perfectionistic, rigid, and controlling approach that can become more inflexible and indecisive under stress	Obsessive-compulsive traits that can become exaggerated in efforts to maintain control over somatic and environmental changes
Provisional Personality Disorders		
Passive-aggressive	Pervasive pattern of passive resistance to demands and authority, such as through procrastination; attitudes toward others and responsibilities that are often critical and resentful	No clear changes in late life
Depressive	Outlook on life that is pervasively gloomy and pessimistic; excessively guilt prone with poor self-esteem	Commonly seen with comorbid depression in late life

* Descriptions of the clusters and of the disorders in each cluster are based on the *Diagnostic and Statistical Manual of Mental Disorders. 4th ed. Text Revision*, Washington, DC: American Psychiatric Association; 2000. The provisional disorders are described in the *DSM IV-TR* appendix.

is unclear whether this represents an actual difference in prevalence or merely reflects the fact that it is more difficult to make a diagnosis in late life.

Diagnostic Challenges

Establishing a diagnosis of personality disorder in older adults can be especially challenging because it requires a detailed, longitudinal psychiatric and psychosocial history. Older patients and their informants are not always able to provide sufficient history, especially when it may span ≥50 yr. The history can be distorted by recall bias (the tendency to present more socially desirable traits) or memory impairment. Furthermore, schizotypal and paranoid individuals may be reluctant to engage in clinical interviews and share personal history, and antisocial and narcissistic individuals who lack insight into their problems may refuse to divulge relevant experiences. Records often do not provide sufficient information to determine prior personality dynamics. Remote diagnoses from previous decades cannot be easily correlated with current ones, because the diagnostic criteria for personality disorders have changed significantly in the past 50 yr. As a result of all of these limitations, clinicians often are unable to make a diagnosis or to make judgments that are based on insufficient information.

Differential Diagnosis

In clinical settings, it is important to remember that not every older patient with prominent or troubling personality features has a personality disorder. Those who demonstrate rigid and maladaptive personality traits but without the pervasiveness or severity as represented by *DSM IV-TR* criteria are better described as suffering from certain personality traits or an adjustment disorder. An adjustment disorder might best characterize previously healthy and well-adjusted individuals who demonstrate acute changes in personality as a result of severe stresses. For example, physical pain and disability can lead to dependent or avoidant behaviors that resemble those seen in personality disorders, but without the pervasive pattern and degree of maladaptiveness. Often, the symptoms of major psychiatric disorders and those of personality disorders overlap considerably, and without longitudinal history it can be difficult to distinguish between them. Diagnosis of a personality disorder becomes more certain when seemingly acute behaviors emerge as enduring and pervasive personality traits. This process depends on the opportunity to observe a person over time and in multiple settings or situations.

Personality disorders as described in *DSM IV-TR* must also be differentiated from the diagnosis of personality change due to a specific medical condition. When personality change is a direct result of brain damage, it has classically been described within the context of an "organic" personality disorder, although this term is no longer used in *DSM* nomenclature. Most often, personality changes with an "organic" source involve impairments in executive functioning, consisting of poor impulse control, poor planning, and greater vulnerability to irritability or agitation. Along these lines, Alzheimer's disease and other dementias are often associated with personality changes, including apathy, egocentricity, and impulsivity. Frontal lobe injury can result in a disinhibited impulsive syndrome, or conversely, an apathetic, avolitional syndrome. Frontotemporal dementia has been associated with distinct personality changes characterized by odd social interactions and compulsive behaviors such as hoarding. (See "Dementia," p 245.) Temporal lobe epilepsy has been associated with personality change, including emotional deepening, verbosity, hypergraphia, hypersexuality, and preoccupation with religious, moral, and cosmic issues. Other disorders found in older adults that are associated with personality disorders include brain tumors, multiple sclerosis, and encephalopathies.

Long-Term Course

Personality disorders can follow one of four possible courses: persist unchanged, evolve into a different form or major psychiatric disorder (eg, depression), improve, or remit. Few disorders have actually been studied over time, and rarely into late life. Several studies have suggested that personality disorders can enter a period of relative quiescence in middle age, with fewer and less intense symptoms and increased adaptation (SOE=C). However, this period may precede their reemergence in late life. Other researchers have proposed that personality disorders characterized by emotional and behavioral lability, including antisocial, borderline, histrionic, narcissistic, and dependent disorders, tend to improve over time, although patients remain vulnerable to depression. Personality disorders characterized by an overcontrol of affect and impulses, including paranoid, schizoid, schizotypal, and obsessive-compulsive personality disorders, are thought either to remain stable or to worsen in late life. Only antisocial and borderline personality disorders have been looked at longitudinally, and both have shown symptom improvement and even remittance into middle and later life for a significant percentage of patients (SOE=B).

Treatment

The treatment of personality disorders in late life is complicated and often has limited success. Given the chronic and pervasive nature of personality disorders, the overall goal of treatment in late life is not to cure the disorder but to decrease the frequency and intensity of disruptive behaviors. The first step should always be to clarify the diagnosis and then to identify recent stressors that may account for the current presentation. The resultant formulation can guide the selection of realistic target symptoms and therapeutic approaches, and allow a treatment team to anticipate future stressors. Treatment of personality disorders in late life uses the same basic approaches as with younger patients, but clinicians must incorporate a much broader understanding of the impact of age-related stressors and comorbid disorders. All forms of psychotherapy have been used to treat personality disorders in older adults. In late life, time and intensity of therapy may be more limited and, as a result, treatment must focus more on short-term approaches. Studies in adults generally find that comorbid personality disorders complicate the treatment of psychiatric illness, but that with consistent treatment, the prognosis is often favorable (SOE=B).

In outpatient settings, control over a patient's environment is limited, and clinicians must therefore rely on one-to-one interventions (if the patient is willing to cooperate with treatment). With some patients, it may be necessary to convey a basic formulation of their behaviors, along with suggested approaches, to caregivers and affiliated healthcare professionals. This communication is important when patients are vulnerable to self-harm or likely to cause significant disruptions in other settings when they are not understood and approached in a therapeutic manner. For some therapeutic approaches that can be used with various personality disorders, see Table 40.2.

Long-term care settings allow more opportunities for intervention. A staff meeting or case conference often provides the best forum to discuss disruptive patients and to coordinate a consistent treatment plan. Disruptive behaviors can sometimes be traced to particular activities or staff interactions, which can be adapted as part of an overall treatment strategy. Sometimes, disengagement from patients reduces the intensity of disruptive interactions. In other situations, the continuity of staffing and of daily schedules is critical. In all situations, a treatment plan should be well documented and conveyed to the patient, as well as to all involved staff and caregivers. All plans must provide appropriate limits to ensure the safety of patients and staff. A written contract, signed by all parties, may be needed with nonadherent patients to eliminate ambiguity. Although it is important to involve family members in the treatment plan, clinicians must recognize that patients with personality disorders often have conflictual relationships with them. Attention should also be given to individual staff members who must work with difficult patients. These staff members need opportunities to discuss feelings of anxiety and frustration, and to feel acknowledged and supported by administrative and other clinical staff.

There have been no studies looking specifically at pharmacologic strategies for personality disorders in late life, so extrapolation from guidelines used for younger people is needed. Psychotropic medications can be targeted at a particular personality disorder; specific symptoms or symptom clusters; or comorbid depression, anxiety, or psychosis. The goal is not to cure the disorder but to reduce the frequency and intensity of targeted symptoms. Antidepressant medication can be helpful for the target symptoms of depression and anxiety found in most personality disorders (SOE=B). Mood stabilizers (eg, lithium carbonate[OL] and divalproex sodium[OL]) and antipsychotic medications can reduce mood lability and impulsivity in borderline patients, and they can be useful with similar symptoms in antisocial personality disorder (SOE=B). Antianxiety agents are commonly used for transient agitation seen in borderline, antisocial, narcissistic, and paranoid disorders, and they may reduce social anxiety and panic in avoidant and dependent patients (SOE=C). Antidepressants are

Table 40.2—Therapeutic Strategies for Personality Disorders in Late Life*

Cluster A: Paranoid, Schizoid, Schizotypal Personality Disorders

- Always assess for and treat comorbid psychosis.
- Do not force social interactions, but offer support and problem-solving assistance in a professional and consistent manner.
- Do not challenge paranoid ideation; instead, solicit and empathize with emotional responses to inner turmoil and fear of paranoid states.

Cluster B: Antisocial, Borderline, Histrionic, and Narcissistic Personality Disorders

- Assess for and treat underlying mood lability, depression, anxiety, and substance abuse.
- Adopt a consistent, structured, and predictable approach with strict boundaries to contain disruptive behaviors.
- Adopt a team approach with all involved clinicians to devise a common plan; avoid staff splits between "supporters" and "detractors" of the patient.
- Use behavioral contracts and authority figures when necessary to address recurrent disruptive behaviors.
- Do not personalize belligerent behaviors directed toward staff members; instead, provide opportunities for staff to discuss frustration and negative thoughts and emotions with professional colleagues.

Cluster C: Avoidant, Dependent, and Obsessive-Compulsive Personality Disorders

- Assess for and treat underlying anxiety, panic, and depression.
- Provide regularly scheduled clinical contacts rather than on an as-needed basis.
- When possible, provide case managers to solicit the needs of avoidant patients and to provide extra reassurance and attention to the needs of dependent and obsessive-compulsive patients.

Depressive and Passive-Aggressive Personality Disorders

- Differentiate between the depressive and negative attitudes and the actual symptoms of a major depressive disorder. Provide appropriate and adequate antidepressant treatment.
- Avoid becoming too pessimistic or exhausted with attempts at providing care; shift focus to a supportive and nonjudgmental therapeutic relationship, with minimal expectations as to outcome.
- Encourage individual psychotherapy to identify underlying emotions and to redirect negative attitudes toward more constructive activities.

*SOE=D

used commonly to treat obsessive-compulsive personality symptoms, although efficacy has not been established for the treatment of these symptoms (as it has been demonstrated for obsessive-compulsive disorder). Antipsychotic agents, both first- and second-generation, can treat the transient psychosis, agitation, and impulsivity seen in dramatic cluster and paranoid disorders, as well as the borderline psychosis and paranoia seen in cluster A disorders (SOE=B).

For personality disorders, psychotropic medications are best used as adjuncts to psychotherapy. In older adults, multiple medications should be avoided in general, and particularly when there is a history of nonadherence, confusion, or impulsivity. Attention must be given to potential interactions with multiple other medications used to treat medical disorders.

Finally, clinicians must recognize that in some cases it is best not to prescribe a psychotropic medication. Such cases include older adults with personality disorders and comorbid substance abuse, chronic nonadherence, or a history of or potential for abusive or self-injurious use of medications. Antisocial and borderline individuals often demonstrate such behaviors. Dependent patients often insist on medications as a means of fostering dependency on the clinician, and obsessive-compulsive patients can perpetuate a maladaptive relationship with the clinician through detailed and controlling discussions of medication management. In each example, medication management is corrupted by dysfunctional interpersonal behaviors that lie at the heart of personality disorders.

SOMATOFORM DISORDERS

Somatoform disorders encompass a heterogeneous group of seven diagnoses that have in common the presence of physical symptoms or complaints without objective organic causes, and that are strongly associated with psychologic factors. *Somatization disorder* is characterized by prolonged, multiple somatic complaints that cannot be explained by medical evaluation; *undifferentiated somatoform disorder* is similar but more limited in duration and range of symptoms. *Conversion disorder* is defined by motor and/or sensory deficits that cannot be explained by medical evaluation. Pain is the central feature of *pain disorder*. Patients with *hypochondriasis* have a pervasive fear of having a serious illness that is resistant to reassurance provided by medical evaluation. In *body dysmorphic disorder*, the patient is overly concerned about an imagined physical defect. Finally, somatoform symptoms that do not fit any of the above diagnoses are classified as *somatoform disorder, not otherwise specified*. Specific diagnostic criteria for these seven conditions can be found in the *DSM IV-TR*.

These disorders are especially relevant to geriatric care because affected older adults are seen in all healthcare settings, and they tend to overuse medical services. Somatoform disorders in late life have not been well studied, and existing research has usually focused on select diagnoses, such as hypochondriasis, in limited or biased samples. Increased somatic preoccupation and symptoms are, however, associated

with depression in late life, and older age of onset for depression may be most predictive. In addition to depression, increased somatic preoccupation is associated with the presence of the personality trait of neuroticism, in which a person displays a tendency to experience more negative emotions. Somatoform disorders are found more commonly in women and in lower socioeconomic groups. Late onset of a somatoform disorder can suggest associated neurologic illness.

Clinical Characteristics and Causes

Somatoform disorders do not represent intentional, conscious attempts by older adults to present factitious physical symptoms. Somatoform symptoms are experienced by the affected individual as real physical pain and discomfort, usually without insight into associated psychologic factors. Somatoform disorders do not represent delusional thinking as seen in psychotic states (although body dysmorphic disorder can be associated with beliefs of delusional quality), and they are different from psychosomatic disorders, which are characterized by actual disease states with presumed psychologic triggers. They also differ from malingering, with its intentional and fully conscious goal of avoiding a specific responsibility such as work, and from factitious disorders (such as Munchausen syndrome), in which the patient's sole, semiconscious intent is to assume the sick role. Rather, somatoform disorders represent a complex interaction between mind and brain in which an affected person is unknowingly expressing psychologic stress or conflict through the body. It is not surprising, then, that depression and anxiety are associated with increased somatic expressions. In late life, somatoform disorders, in particular hypochondriasis, can be a way for a person to express anxiety and attempt to cope with accumulating fears and losses. These may include fears of abandonment by family and caregivers, loss of beauty and strength, financial setbacks, loss of independence, loss of social role (eg, through retirement, loss of spouse, occupational disability), and loneliness. The psychologic distress and anxiety over such losses can be less threatening and more controllable when shifted to somatic complaints or symptoms. In turn, the resultant state of debility might be reinforced by increased social contacts and support.

The causes of somatoform disorders are usually multifactorial and are often rooted in early developmental experiences and personality traits. Psychodynamic approaches suggest that these disorders result from unconscious conflict in which intolerable impulses or affects are expressed through more tolerable somatic symptoms or complaints.

Treatment

People with somatoform disorder do not usually present as such; by definition, they appear to have legitimate somatic complaints with an unknown physical cause. It is only after repeated but fruitless evaluations, multiple and persistent complaints and requests, and sometimes angry and inappropriate reactions to treatment that clinicians begin to suspect a somatoform disorder. In some cases, the manner of presentation and symptom complex is more immediately suggestive of a particular somatoform disorder. In any event, it is important for the clinician to remember that from the perspective of the patient, the symptoms and complaints are quite real and disturbing. It is never wise to challenge the patient or to suggest that the symptoms are "all in your mind," even after diagnostic evaluation has made it obvious that psychologic factors are involved. The typical response to such advice is for the patient to seek additional opinions and medical tests, which in turn can perpetuate a cycle of somatization that never addresses the underlying issues.

Instead, the clinician should attempt to foster an ongoing, supportive, consistent, and professional relationship with the affected patient. Such a relationship serves to provide reassurance as well as to protect the patient from excessive and unnecessary medical visits and procedures. The clinician should focus on responding to individual complaints, perhaps with periodic but regularly scheduled appointments, and to set limits on evaluation and treatment in a firm but empathetic manner. This can be difficult to do when patients become demanding and attempt to consume excessive amounts of time, but the clinician must endeavor to remain professional, without personalizing the situation or feel that he or she is failing the patient. Overall, the role of the clinician is to focus on reducing symptoms and rehabilitating the patient, and not attempting to force the patient to have insight into the potential psychologic nature of his or her symptoms. It would be hazardous to prematurely diagnose a somatoform disorder when there might actually be an underlying medical problem that has eluded diagnosis. For example, disorders such as multiple sclerosis, systemic lupus erythematosus, and acute intermittent porphyria commonly have complex presentations that elude initial diagnostic evaluation. Moreover, many somatoform disorders coexist with actual disease states, eg, many individuals with pseudoseizures also have an actual seizure disorder. At the same time, it is important for the clinician to set limits on what he or she can offer and to make appropriate referrals to specialists and mental health clinicians.

The clinician should have an active role in addressing the somatoform disorder. Unfortunately, no particular treatment for any somatoform disorder has been found to have good efficacy, and most disorders tend to be lifelong. As a result, the goal of treatment is not to cure, but to control symptoms. The clinician first forms a therapeutic alliance based on empathetic listening and acknowledgment of physical discomfort, without trivializing the somatic complaints. Sometimes an offer to review all available medical records can be a tangible way of conveying one's seriousness to the patient. Underlying anxiety and depression must be identified and treated with psychotherapy and, when necessary, antidepressant or antianxiety medications, or both. Cognitive-behavioral therapy focuses on identifying distorted thought patterns and triggers of anxiety, and then replacing them with more realistic and adaptive strategies. A mental health professional can assist in determining whether cognitive-behavioral therapy may be of benefit. In many cases, however, the supportive nature of regular visits to a primary care provider may be sufficient to meet the needs of individuals with somatoform disorders.

REFERENCES

■ Balsis S, Woods CM, Gleason MEJ, et al. The over and underdiagnosis of personality disorders in older adults. *Am J Geriatr Psychiatry.* 2007;15(9):742–753.

■ Escobar JI, Gara MA, Diaz-Martinez AM, et al. Effectiveness of a time-limited cognitive behavior therapy type intervention among primary care patients with medically unexplained symptoms. *Ann Fam Med.* 2007;5(4):328–335.

■ Magoteaux A, Bonnivier J. Distinguishing between personality disorders, stereotypes, and eccentricities in older adults. *J Psychosoc Nurs Ment Health Serv.* 2009;47(7):19–24

■ Zweig RA, Agronin ME. Personality disorders. In: Agronin ME, Maletta GJ, eds. *Principles and Practice of Geriatric Psychiatry.* Philadelphia: Lippincott Williams & Wilkins; 2006:449–470.

CHAPTER 41—ADDICTIONS

KEY POINTS

- Alcohol and other substance-abuse problems can remain undetected when screening questions are omitted during routine medical visits.

- Alcohol use can be an unrecognized cause of falls, cognitive decline, and medical problems (eg, anemia, increased liver function tests, thrombocytopenia).

- It is important to consider a diagnosis of alcohol or benzodiazepine withdrawal in older adults who develop delirium with hospitalization or facility placement.

- Cognitive impairment from chronic alcoholism in older adults can improve with sustained abstinence.

- Abuse of prescription drugs, including benzodiazepines and opioids, is often unrecognized and occurs with alcohol abuse.

- Smoking cessation efforts should persist throughout life.

The abuse and misuse of alcohol, psychoactive medications, illicit drugs, and nicotine have become significant public health concerns for the growing population of older adults. Substance abuse and dependence among older adults is common, and older adults are particularly vulnerable to the cognitive and physical effects of these substances. Typically, substance-use problems are thought to develop only in those who use substances in large quantities and at regular intervals. Among older adults, however, negative health consequences have been demonstrated at consumption amounts previously thought of as light to moderate, and certainly not in the amounts usually associated with a diagnosis of substance dependence. A growing number of effective treatments for these problems lead not only to reduced substance use but also to improved general health. Both the risks and the emergence of new treatments underscore the need to identify problems and provide appropriate treatment for older adults suffering from the effects of substance misuse.

STRENGTH-OF-EVIDENCE (SOE) RATING DEFINITIONS

A = consistent and good quality patient-oriented evidence
B = somewhat inconsistent or limited quality patient-oriented evidence
C = very inconsistent or very limited patient-oriented evidence, disease-oriented evidence, and/or consensus from professional organizations
D = unstudied common practice or opinion

See inside front cover for detailed information regarding the SOE classification.

DEFINITIONS OF SUBSTANCE ABUSE

Establishing valid criteria for determining which older adults would benefit from reducing or eliminating their substance use is the first step in successful intervention. *Substance dependence* has been defined as any use that imparts significant disability and warrants treatment. Many older adults are not recognized as having problems that are related to their substance use, partly because the diagnostic criteria are difficult to interpret and apply consistently to older adults. For instance, many older people drink at home by themselves; thus, they are less likely than younger drinkers to be arrested, get into arguments, or have difficulties in employment. Moreover, because many of the diseases caused or affected by substance misuse (eg, hypertension, stroke, and peptic ulcer disease) are common disorders in late life, the effects of substance use on older adults who have these disorders can be overlooked. The literature indicates that older problem drinkers are identified less often by clinicians and are less often referred for treatment than their younger counterparts.

Because of the difficulties in assessing older adults for substance dependence, many experts advocate screening to identify those who are at risk of problem behaviors or who have at-risk or problem use. *At-risk use* is defined as any use of a substance at a quantity or frequency greater than a recommended level. The level of use is often determined empirically based on association with significant disability. For instance, the recommended upper limit of alcohol consumption for older adults has been established as no more than an average of one standard drink per day and no more than two episodes of binge drinking (four or more drinks in a day) during a 3-mo period. *Problem substance use* is defined as the consumption of any amount of an abusable substance that results in at least one problem related to this use. For example, the use of benzodiazepines by a patient who has a preexisting unsteady gait would be considered problem use.

On the other end of the spectrum, *abstinence* is defined as drinking no alcohol in the previous year. Approximately 60% of older adults are abstinent. If an older adult is abstinent, it can be useful to ascertain why alcohol is not used. Some individuals are abstinent because of a previous history of alcohol problems. For this reason, it is particularly important to obtain a history of both current and past use. Some older adults are abstinent because of recent illness; others have lifelong patterns of abstinence or low-risk use. Individuals who have a previous history of alcohol problems can require preventive monitoring to determine if any new stresses could exacerbate an old pattern. In addition, a previous history of at-risk drinking or alcohol dependence increases the risk of developing other mental health problems in late life, such as depressive disorders or cognitive problems, and can limit treatment response because of brain damage.

Low-risk or *moderate use* of alcohol is that which falls within the recommended guidelines for consumption and is not associated with problems. Older adults in this category not only consume amounts that fall within recommended drinking guidelines but also are able to reasonably limit their alcohol consumption, ie, they do not drink when driving a motor vehicle or boat, or when using contraindicated medications. However, a change in either physical health or prescription medications can increase even low-risk use to a problem level.

The most practical method for identifying individuals who could benefit from intervention is to determine the quantity and frequency of their use of abusable substances. This method has advantages over formal diagnostic interviews because of its brevity, easily interpretable results, and absence of stigmatizing language, such as "addiction," "alcoholism," "alcoholic," or "alcohol dependence." For more on screening, see the section below on identifying substance-use disorders, p 325.

MAGNITUDE OF THE PROBLEM

Drug Use

Little is known about the epidemiology of substance-use disorders among older adults other than alcoholism. The general belief is that older drug addicts are only younger addicts grown old and that few individuals initiate drug use in their later years. In the Epidemiologic Catchment Area study, lifetime prevalence rates of drug abuse and dependence were 0.12% for older men and 0.06% for older women, and lifetime history of illicit drug use was 2.88% for men and 0.66% for women. No active cases were reported in either gender. In contrast, a more recent study of an elder-specific drug program in a veteran population found that one-fourth had either a primary drug problem or concurrent drug and alcohol problems. This study may be a reflection of the growing number of older adults who used drugs during a time of expanded drug experimentation in the United States in the 1960s. Indeed, reports from the National Household survey on drug use suggest a rise in marijuana and cocaine use among individuals ≥50 yr old, whereas use of illicit drugs has decreased in all younger age groups. Recent increases in hepatitis C among those ≥60 yr old can reflect both a history of intravenous drug use, as well as increased risk of nosocomial infection with advanced age. Other studies to determine the prevalence and incidence of substance-use disorders (in later life) involving nicotine, caffeine, benzodiazepines, marijuana, and opioids are needed.

Medication Use

An increasing problem with the older age group is the misuse or inappropriate use of prescription and OTC medications. This problem includes the misuse of substances such as sedatives, hypnotics, narcotic and non-narcotic analgesics, diet aids, decongestants, and a wide variety of OTC medications. Community surveys have found that 60% of older adults are taking an analgesic, 22% are taking a CNS medication, and 11% are taking a benzodiazepine. Many medications used by older adults have the potential for inducing tolerance, withdrawal syndromes, and harmful medical consequences, such as cognitive changes, kidney disease, falls, and liver disease. A growing body of literature demonstrates a concerning increase in morbidity and mortality associated with the misuse of prescription and nonprescription medications, even though this is not considered as a disorder in the *Diagnostic and Statistical Manual of Mental Disorders, 4th Edition, Text Revision*.

Medication use by all older adults needs to be monitored carefully; prescribing potentially hazardous combinations of medications, medications with a high risk of adverse events, and ineffective or unnecessary medications should be avoided. (See "Pharmacotherapy," p 72.) A practical approach to monitoring psychoactive medications is to reevaluate the older patient's use every 3–6 mo. Maintenance treatment should be continued only in those patients who have specific target symptoms and a documented response to the treatment. Patients who have no response or only a partial response should be reevaluated to consider the appropriate diagnosis and further care. In such cases, consultation with a geriatric mental health professional could be advantageous. See also "Depression and Other Mood Disorders," p 295; "Anxiety Disorders," p 307; "Psychotic Disorders," p 311; and "Personality and Somatoform Disorders," p 316.

Alcohol Use

Community-based epidemiologic studies define the extent and nature of alcohol use in the older population by reporting percentages of abstainers, heavy drinkers, and daily drinkers. Abstention from alcohol ranges from 31% to 58%, and daily drinking ranges from 10% to 22% in samples of older adults.

"Heavy" drinking, defined as a minimum of 12 to 21 drinks per week, is present in 3%–9% of the older population; alcohol abuse, as defined clinically, is present in approximately 2%–4%.

Cultural and Demographic Factors

The prevalence of alcohol use and alcohol-related problems among older adults is much higher for men than for women. Among younger adults, however, the ratio of male to female drinkers has changed over the past several decades, with the result that more women present for treatment. These changes are likely to continue to be reflected in the next generation of older women. Similar patterns by gender are seen with illicit drug use, except that benzodiazepines are much more commonly used by older women than by older men.

Conclusions are less clear from the few studies addressing differences among various ethnic groups. Depending on the study, older black Americans and older Hispanic Americans consume amounts of alcohol similar to or lower than the amounts consumed by older white Americans. The Epidemiologic Catchment Area data demonstrated no significant differences in the 1-yr diagnosis of alcohol abuse and dependence among black Americans (2.93% among men and 0.60% among women), white Americans (2.85% among men and 0.47% among women), and Hispanic Americans (6.57% among men and 0.0% among women). Increased leisure time and higher disposable income are more relevant risk factors for alcohol consumption among older adults than race or ethnicity.

RISKS AND BENEFITS OF SUBSTANCE USE

Benefits of Alcohol Consumption

Moderate alcohol consumption among otherwise healthy older adults has been promoted as having significant beneficial effects, especially with regard to cardiovascular disease. Findings from the cardiovascular literature have led to a host of articles in the popular press espousing the benefits of alcohol use.

Alcohol in moderate amounts can promote relaxation and reduce social anxiety. However, even though there are benefits of moderate drinking, the practice of recommending drinking to people who currently do not drink is not advocated. Many older adults do not drink because of past problems with drinking, family problems with drinking, the expense related to drinking, and the adverse effects of intoxication. There is no direct evidence to justify prescribing alcohol for individuals with heart disease or any other health condition.

Excess Physical Disability

Substance abuse has clear and profound effects on the health and well-being of older adults in all spheres of life. Older adults are particularly prone to the toxic effects of substances on many different organ systems because of both the physiologic changes associated with aging and the changes associated with other illnesses common in late life. The social and economic impact is also tremendous. Substance abuse has adverse effects on self-esteem, coping skills, and interpersonal relationships, which may be compounded by losses that are common in the late stages of life.

Levels of alcohol consumption above seven drinks per week, so-called at-risk drinking, have been associated with a number of health problems, including an increased risk of stroke caused by bleeding, impaired driving skills, and an increased rate of injuries such as falls and fractures (SOE=A). Of particular importance to older adults are the potential harmful interactions between alcohol and both prescribed and OTC medications, especially psychoactive medications such as benzodiazepines and antidepressants. Alcohol also interferes with the metabolism of many medications, including warfarin.

Older adults who consume more than an average of four drinks per day or whose drinking has led to a diagnosis of alcohol dependence are at greatest risk of excess physical disability and physical illness related to drinking. The most common problems associated with alcohol dependence are alcoholic liver disease, COPD, peptic ulcer disease, and psoriasis. Moreover, unexplained multisystem disease should alert the clinician to probe more closely for alcohol use. With smoking, the risks are much clearer, including increased rates of pulmonary disease, especially cancer. Medications such as benzodiazepines are also associated with excess physical disability, increased rates of falls, and driving-related impairment. Research is beginning to demonstrate that the disability associated with these problems is also reversible with reduced substance use (SOE=B).

Mental Health Problems

Substance use can be a significant factor in the course and prognosis of nearly all mental health problems of late life. Use of alcohol, benzodiazepines, opioids, and cigarettes has been demonstrated to be related etiologically to mood disturbances, but these substances also complicate the treatment of concurrent mood disorders. Individuals with both alcoholism and depression have a more complicated clinical course of depression with an increased risk of suicide and more social dysfunction than nondepressed individuals with alcoholism. Overall, older adults with alcohol abuse or dependence are nearly three times more likely to have a lifetime diagnosis of another mental disorder. Alcoholism has been implicated in mood disorders, suicide, dementia, anxiety disorders, and sleep disturbances.

As might be expected, patients with alcohol-related dementia who become abstinent do not show a progression in cognitive impairment comparable to that of those with Alzheimer's disease. The complex role of alcoholism in the development of Alzheimer's disease is not fully understood, but alcoholism does lead independently to a syndrome of dementia. Interesting new hypotheses implicate glutamatergic toxicity, but overall, the mechanisms are not well understood. The criteria for alcohol-related dementia are as follows:

- clinically evident dementia at least 60 days after last alcohol use
- a history of significant use for at least 5 yr, ie, at least 35 drinks per week for men and 28 per week for women
- the occurrence of this period of significant use within 3 yr of the onset of cognitive deficits

Clinical features supporting the diagnosis include end-organ damage (eg, liver disease), cognitive stabilization or improvement after abstinence, and evidence of cerebellar atrophy in brain imaging. Further research is needed to understand the potential benefits of long-term abstinence in alcohol-related dementia. Similarly, those with comorbid depression and alcohol use are likely to have better depression outcomes if they become abstinent. Moderate alcohol use has also been demonstrated to have negative effects on the treatment of late-life depression, further underscoring the need for reducing moderate use in the context of chronic health problems in older adults.

IDENTIFYING SUBSTANCE-USE DISORDERS

Although clinical examination remains the most valuable tool for identifying substance-use problems, screening instruments can help increase the sensitivity and efficiency of diagnosis. Several instruments have been developed for identifying alcohol-use disorders, including self-administered questionnaires and laboratory studies. Self-administered questionnaires provide a rapid, sensitive, and inexpensive method of screening for alcohol problems. Two questionnaires have been developed with these principles in mind: the Michigan Alcoholism Screening Test (MAST)—Geriatric Version, and the AUDIT C (Table 41.1). Both of these instruments have high sensitivity and specificity for identifying alcohol misuse in middle-aged and older adults. The CAGE is a brief

clinician-administered screening test that is also useful to identify problem drinking. (Table 41.2).

TREATMENT

Older adults with a substance-use problem often need a variety of treatments. It is therefore important to have an array of services available for older adults that can be tailored to their individual needs and that have the flexibility to adapt to changing needs over time. The most important aspect of treating an older adult who is misusing a substance is to engage the individual in the intervention. Older adults engaged in treatment have been shown to have robust improvement, especially compared with younger cohorts. The spectrum of interventions for alcohol abuse in older adults range from prevention and education for those who are abstinent or low-risk drinkers, to minimal advice or brief structured interventions for at-risk or problem drinkers, to formalized alcoholism treatment for drinkers who meet criteria for abuse or dependence. The array of formal treatment options available includes psychotherapy, education, rehabilitative and residential care, and psychopharmacologic agents. An example of the necessity to tailor care is the contrast between the at-risk drinker or benzodiazepine user and the severely dependent patient. The at-risk user will not likely need the intensity of services required for the severely dependent patient. Indeed, requiring the at-risk drinker to accept a set of rigorous services can be more detrimental than helpful.

Dependency on medications such as benzodiazepines is managed by placing the patient on a 24-hour equivalent of the dosage of the drug on which the patient is dependent; tapering the dosage by 10% every three half-lives; and providing supportive counseling via groups, psychosocial support, and 12-step programs. Symptoms of withdrawal from narcotics can be controlled when necessary with oral clonidine[OL]. Assuring that the patient enters a long-term treatment program increases the likelihood of long-term success. For smoking cessation, it is important to prepare the patient for quitting by discussing management strategies before quitting, setting a quit date, and implementing a monitoring plan for maintaining success.

Detoxification and Stabilization

The assessment of any substance abuser starts with a thorough history, physical examination, and laboratory tests. The patient's potential to suffer acute withdrawal should also be assessed. Severe withdrawal such as that from alcohol use can be life threatening and warrants careful attention. Patients with severe symptoms of dependency or withdrawal potential and patients with significant medical or psychiatric comorbidity can require inpatient hospitalization for

Table 41.1—The AUDIT-C Questionnaire: The Alcohol Use Disorders Identification Test-Consumption Questions

The AUDIT-C is an alcohol screen that can help identify patients who are hazardous drinkers or who have active alcohol-use disorders (including alcohol abuse or dependence).

Read questions as written. Record answers carefully. Begin the AUDIT-C by saying, "Now I am going to ask you some questions about your use of alcoholic beverages during the past year." Explain that "alcoholic beverages" refers to beer, wine, vodka, etc. Code answers in terms of "standard drinks."

Question #1: How often did you have a drink containing alcohol in the past year?

▪ Never	0 points
▪ Less than monthly	1 point
▪ 2–4 times per month	2 points
▪ 2–3 times per week	3 points
▪ 4 or more times per week	4 points

Question #2: In the past year, how many drinks did you typically have when you drank?

▪ I did not drink in the past year	0 points
▪ 1–2 drinks	0 points
▪ 3–4 drinks	1 point
▪ 5–6 drinks	2 points
▪ 7–9 drinks	3 points
▪ More than 10 drinks	4 points

Question #3: How often did you have 6 or more drinks on one occasion in the past year?

▪ Never	0 points
▪ Less than monthly	1 point
▪ Monthly	2 points
▪ Weekly	3 points
▪ Daily	4 points

The AUDIT-C is scored on a scale of 0 to 12 (scores of 0 reflect no alcohol use). In men, a score ≥4 is considered positive; in women, a score ≥3 is considered positive. Generally, the higher the AUDIT-C score, the more likely it is that the patient's drinking is affecting his or her health and safety.

References: Babor TF, Bohn MJ, Kranzler HR. The Alcohol Use Disorders Identification Test (AUDIT): validation of a screening instrument for use in medical settings. *J Stud Alcohol*. 1995;56:423−432; http://www.queri.research.va.gov/tools/alcohol-misuse/alcohol-faqs.cfm#3.

Table 41.2—The CAGE Questionnaire

C	Have you ever tried to **C**ut down on your drinking?
A	Have you ever gotten **A**nnoyed at someone for criticizing your drinking?
G	Do you ever feel **G**uilty about your drinking?
E	Have you ever had an **E**ye-opener to steady your nerves or get rid of a hangover?

NOTE: A positive answer to one or more questions suggests problem drinking.

acute stabilization before implementing an outpatient management strategy. Detoxification is achieved by placing the patient on the minimal amount of drug that suppresses withdrawal symptoms and then decreasing the dosage by 10% every three half-lives. In general, longer-acting formulations of the drug being abused are preferred to shorter-acting formulations, but many clinicians find that prescribing the specific drug that a patient was abusing makes the process more acceptable to the patient and minimizes the time needed to determine the initial dose.

For patients who are hospitalized for an elective surgery or condition unrelated to the substance problem, remaining vigilant for any evidence of withdrawal is extremely important. Unrecognized alcohol withdrawal can result in serious morbidity and mortality in older adults. Early symptoms include tachycardia, diaphoresis, tremulousness, and hypertension. These symptoms can progress to overt delirium, psychosis, and seizures. Intravenous lorazepam[OL] is the most expedient intervention in this scenario, followed by oral lorazepam, in tapering dosages.

Outpatient Management

Traditionally, outpatient substance-abuse treatment has been reserved for specialized clinics focused on substance abuse. However, it is becoming increasingly apparent that this model is inadequate in addressing the broader public health demand, and there is a need to involve a variety of clinicians and clinical settings to deliver substance-abuse treatment. This is particularly important for older adults, who frequently seek medical services but rarely seek specialized addiction services. The traditional addiction clinic is focused on supportive group psychotherapy and encouragement to attend regular self-help group meetings such as Alcoholics Anonymous, Alcoholics Victorious, Rational Recovery, or Narcotics Anonymous. For older adults, peer-specific group activities are considered superior to mixed-age group activities. Clinicians should be wary of focusing on abstinence as the only positive outcome of treatment and should commend patients for making progress in decreasing use as well as stopping. This can be particularly relevant for misuse of medications such as benzodiazepines, because eliminating the use may be more difficult. For benzodiazepines, the risk of adverse events such as falls is greater with higher dosages and medications with a longer half-life such as diazepam or clonazepam. Therefore, using medications with a half-life of 6–12 hours reduces the risks for that patient. If benzodiazepines seem to be indicated for an anxiety condition and treatment is started for the first time, shorter-acting agents that do not have active metabolites (eg, lorazepam) are preferred to long-acting preparations. However, for patients already receiving long-acting benzodiazepines (eg, diazepam at ≥50 mg/d), the risk of withdrawal complications is increased, and the dosage should be reduced very gradually. If the daily dose is greater than the equivalent of 100 mg of diazepam, then the patient should be hospitalized to start withdrawal. Ultimately, a transition to shorter-acting agents is ideal, but this should be done carefully and initially involve an equivalent dosage before any reductions are considered. The use of resources such as day programs and senior centers can be beneficial, especially for cognitively impaired patients. Supervised living arrangements, such as halfway houses, group homes, nursing homes, and residing with relatives, should also be considered.

Pharmacotherapy

The use of medications to support abstinence may be of benefit, but it is not well studied. Small-scale studies have demonstrated that naltrexone for alcohol abuse is well tolerated and efficacious in older adults. Naltrexone is available in both oral and long-acting injectable forms. Studies of antidepressants, including the SSRIs, do not support the widespread use of antidepressants as a treatment for alcohol misuse, although they can be effective in treating concurrent depression. Some of the general principles used in treating younger patients should be applied to older drinkers as well. For example, benzodiazepines are important in the treatment of alcohol detoxification, but they have no clinical place in maintaining long-term abstinence because of their potential for abuse and for fostering further alcohol or benzodiazepine abuse. Disulfiram can benefit some

well-motivated patients, but cardiac and hepatic disease limits its use by older adults who abuse alcohol. Acamprosate has not been studied in older adults. Methadone maintenance has proven efficacy in opioid dependence. Older adults can be started and maintained on methadone, following the same principles of use as in younger patients. Comorbid medical and psychiatric disorders must be identified and properly treated, and they may necessitate the need for referral to, or consultation with, a psychiatrist with expertise in these areas. Buprenorphine and buprenorphine with naloxone have been approved for outpatient treatment of opioid dependence. However, given the complexity of the treatment of opioid dependence, systematic training, practice, monitoring, regulation, and evaluation are necessary in a multidisciplinary treatment setting to optimize outcomes. Guidelines for developing treatment programs using buprenorphine are available on the web site of the Substance Abuse and Mental Health Services Administration (http://buprenorphine.samhsa.gov/index.html [accessed Jan 2011]).

Tobacco Dependence

Tobacco dependence is a chronic disease that typically requires multiple attempts to quit with repeated interventions over the life span. Smoking cessation at any age slows the decline in lung function, and aggressive cessation efforts are appropriate even in the oldest-old patient. There is significant evidence to demonstrate that brief interventions performed at each office visit will promote smoking cessation (SOE=A). The basic elements of the approach are the "Five A's" from the Agency for Health Care Policy and Research:

- **A**sk patients about use of tobacco at every office visit.
- **A**ssess readiness to quit.
- **A**dvise patients to quit.
- **A**ssist patients in the quit attempt with aids such as a local cessation program and pharmacologic agents such as bupropion, nicotine replacement, or varenicline.
- **A**rrange both a quit date and a follow-up visit or contact to discuss the quit attempt.

Establishing abstinence from nicotine follows the same principles as that from other addicting substances. Initially, pharmacologic substitution with either nicotine gum or patch is followed by a gradual decrease in dosage. In several trials, antidepressant medications improved rates of continued abstinence, but only bupropion has been approved for this purpose by the FDA. Varenicline has not received specific attention in older adults but should be considered. As with other abstinence regimens, psychotherapy plus pharmacotherapy is better than pharmacotherapy alone.

Gambling

Gambling in late life is less prevalent than in young adulthood. However, older adults who have engaged in problematic and compulsive gambling behaviors earlier in life often continue this pattern of destructive behavior. Gambling in late life, both recreational and problematic, is associated with a higher prevalence of mental and physical health problems (SOE=B). Many older adults report that gambling is a means of coping with loneliness and boredom. While gambling activities can be a source of socialization, the clinician must be mindful of asking about problematic gambling when taking a history. These include symptoms such as preoccupation with gambling, restlessness or irritability when trying to quit, loss of control, need to bet more money with increasing frequency, "chasing" losses, and continuation of gambling despite negative social or occupational consequences. No medications have been helpful in reducing pathologic gambling behaviors. States that allow legalized gaming activities are required to post toll-free telephone numbers to access assistance with problematic gambling. Many 12-step programs are focused on problematic gambling. Older adults who engage in gambling activities should be screened for alcohol, smoking, and other substance-use disorders. Referrals to community resources and 12-step programs may be useful.

ACOVE-3* QUALITY INDICATORS PERTAINING TO ADDICTION

Smoking cessation

- If a vulnerable older adult with COPD lives with others who smoke, then the patient, smoker, or both should be counseled to eliminate smoking in the home.
- If a vulnerable older adult with COPD is new to a primary care practice, then smoking status should be documented, and if the patient ever smoked, smoking status should be assessed annually.
- If a vulnerable older adult with COPD is a current smoker, then counseling to quit smoking should be documented annually.

*Assessing Care of Vulnerable Elders – 3ʳᵈ Set. See inside front cover for explanation.

REFERENCES

- Fiore MC, Jaen CR, Baker TB, et al. *Treating Tobacco Use and Dependence: 2008 Update.* Clinical Practice Guideline. Rockville, MD: U.S. Department of Health and Human Services. Public Health Service. May 2008.

- Moore AA and the American Geriatrics Society Clinical Practice Committee. Clinical guidelines for alcohol use disorders in older adults. Updated Nov 2003. Available at http:// www.americangeriatrics.org/products/positionpapers/alcohol.shtml.

- Naegle M. Alcohol Use Screening and Assessment for Older Adults. *Try This: Best Practices in Nursing Care to Older Adults.* 2007;(17). Available at http://consultgerirn.org/uploads/File/trythis/try_this_17.pdf

- Oslin DW. Evidence-based treatment of geriatric substance abuse. *Psychiatr Clin North Am.* 2005;28(4):897—911.

- Snow D, Amalu J. Research reviews: older adults and substance abuse. *J Addictions Nursing.* 2009;20(3):153–157.

CHAPTER 42—MENTAL RETARDATION AND DEVELOPMENTAL DISABILITIES

KEY POINTS

- Individuals with mental retardation surviving into adulthood and old age are increasing in numbers.

- Maladaptive and challenging behaviors, as well as difficulties learning and retaining new skills of coping and adaptation, are significant problems for adults with mental retardation and, consequently, for their caregivers.

- Receptive and expressive communication impairments and coexisting cognitive limitations can contribute to diagnostic and treatment difficulties for medical, psychiatric, and behavioral problems.

- Physiologic changes related to age as well as disease states in individuals with mental retardation can exacerbate or attenuate behaviors.

- Therapeutic interventions for maladaptive behaviors or psychiatric illnesses that coexist with mental retardation can include medications and behavioral therapies.

- The term developmental disability can describe a variety of medical conditions that are not defined by mental retardation. However, these conditions can contribute to challenging behaviors and impact an individual's quality of life.

Mental retardation, as used in the *Diagnostic and Statistical Manual, 4th Edition, Text Revision (DSM IV-TR)*, is defined as an IQ of approximately 70 or below based on formal test results and impairment in adaptive functioning with onset before 18 yr of age. Unfortunately, differences over nomenclature for mental retardation continue to exist based on historical, cultural, or geographic issues, or on perceptions of "correctness."

A demographic issue to keep in mind is that not everyone with a developmental disability has mental retardation. This chapter will focus on individuals with mental retardation who may or may not have other comorbid conditions, such as cerebral palsy, epilepsy, and autism spectrum disorders.

PREVALENCE

The number of individuals with mental retardation surviving into old age is increasing because of generally better health care overall, including earlier detection and treatment of some conditions. It is difficult to quantify the prevalence of older individuals with mental retardation because of methodologic considerations. It is even more problematic to consider the issues from the perspectives of other cultures and standards in areas other than Europe and North America. It is certainly safe to say that life expectancy for individuals with mental retardation has increased over time. In the 1930s, the average age at death for males suffering from mental retardation was 15 yr, and for females, 22 yr. In 1932, for children 10 yr old, only 28% were expected to survive to age 60. By the 1990s, that figure increased to >40% for institutionalized as well as community-based individuals.

Various studies on the prevalence of individuals with mental retardation have had some predictable variation in the results. Published estimates of mental retardation have put the number at 1%–1.5% in the United States. Using the 1% estimate of the population, this number would be proposed to double for individuals ≥60 yr old by 2030. In general, longevity decreases with severity of intellectual impairment, certain comorbid conditions (eg, seizure disorders, Down syndrome), and the general health and wealth of the country or culture.

Mental Retardation and Mental Illness

The literature on older adults with mental retardation and mental illness (other than dementia) has been relatively sparse over the last few decades. This makes it even more problematic to determine accurate numbers for a number of reasons: definitions have changed (ie, through various editions of the *DSM* and various versions of the *International Classification of Diseases [ICD]*), health care has improved, studies have been conducted in different countries or regions, standard methodologies are lacking, and the relative numbers of institutionalized versus community-based individuals have changed.

Over the last decades, several studies with diverse methodologies and equally uneven goals have been conducted, but there have been some common general conclusions, notably that the prevalence of psychiatric disorders among adults with mental retardation is much greater than that of age-matched controls (SOE=B). Adults with mental retardation have similar risk factors (biologic, psychologic, and social) for mental illnesses as their "normal" peers but may have additional risks depending on the cause of their mental disability. Older adults who were raised in institutions or who have not benefitted from modern medical care are also at greater risk.

There are many reports of greater than expected rates of certain mental illnesses or behavioral disorders associated with specific physical illnesses or genetic disorders. For example, older adults with autistic spectrum disorders exhibit higher rates of compulsive behaviors requiring psychiatric treatment.

DIAGNOSTIC AND TREATMENT ISSUES

There are many diagnostic and treatment challenges for clinicians when seeing patients with mental retardation with or without comorbid issues of mental illness or challenging behaviors. The best treatment requires an accurate, or at least the most likely, diagnosis, and that requires obtaining the best history. Unfortunately, all too often the patient's history and his or her subjective reporting are limited or unavailable.

Barriers to communication can exist for both the clinician and patient. Under these circumstances, it is up to the clinician to try to be as effective as possible by recognizing the limitations of the patient. For the purposes of this discussion, the problems are grouped within three broad categories: self-awareness, communication abilities, and comorbid overshadowing.

For adult and older adult patients with mental retardation, the clinician needs to estimate the degree to which the patient is aware of his or her problem, condition, or feelings. Barriers to that process of evaluation can come from the organic cause of mental retardation or from the interviewer by asking questions that are too complex or using vocabulary beyond the grasp of the patient. It is almost always desirable to have collateral sources of information, such as family or caregivers who can provide histories, narratives, and other data.

The patient's receptive and expressive abilities need to be considered. These two abilities can be comparable in some individuals with mental retardation or quite different in others with autism or fragile X syndrome. Differences in these abilities can be characteristic features for some conditions. The goal is to adapt the questions to fit the communication abilities of the patient.

An enduring and important concept is that of diagnostic overshadowing. This addresses the idea that the presence of mental retardation itself makes the appropriate diagnosis and treatment of symptoms of mental illness or challenging behaviors more difficult. It exists as a barrier within the critical thinking of the clinician and, therefore, clinicians should remain aware when presented with a difficult situation.

PSYCHIATRIC AND MENTAL DISORDERS IN AGING ADULTS WITH MENTAL RETARDATION

The prevalence of psychiatric disorders among adults with mental retardation is about 5 times that of age-matched control groups. Depending on the exact population studied and the type of diagnoses included, rates range from 10% to 40%. It is, of course, more complicated because human aging and pathologic processes are neither simple nor linear. In older adults with mental retardation, the occurrence and severity of psychiatric disturbances can vary by age and comorbid conditions. For example, in a study of individuals with Down syndrome who subsequently developed Alzheimer's dementia, these individuals were far more likely to suffer from psychologic and behavioral symptoms with more rapid decline in functional status than those who did not develop dementia.

Some symptoms may improve as the patient ages or develops comorbid problems. In adults with Down syndrome, it is not uncommon to have complaints of significant obsessive and compulsive symptoms. This can be the primary focus of concern from young adulthood through the fifth or sixth decade of life or until symptoms of dementia become evident. As the dementia worsens, the anxieties of obsessions and compulsions can wane, and as memory function worsens, those symptoms are often lost or of little concern.

It is also true that some behaviors or conditions can worsen with age through various processes. Individuals with mental retardation have no special immunity from the disorders of aging, and their coping mechanisms may be reduced. For example, they may be more affected by chronic pain conditions or by vision or hearing loss.

In lower-functioning individuals or in those with expressive communication disorders, a new behavioral concern can be a sentinel sign of a physical disorder. As a general rule, before determining that a new problem behavior should be the focus of a psychotropic medication or intervention, physical causes should be excluded. New-onset, self-injurious behavior in particular can be an important clue to occult illness. Self-injurious behavior to the ears can be a sign of otitis externa or media. Self-injurious behavior to the eyes can be a clue to vision loss or changes.

Dementias

Individuals with mental retardation have a higher prevalence of dementias overall than is found in age-matched controls in the general population; this is especially true for dementia associated with Down syndrome (SOE=A). The challenge is to diagnose the condition correctly given the individual's baseline cognitive impairment and diminished reporting skills. All causes of dementia are possible, but some are more likely than others. Similarly, so-called "pugilistic dementia" is higher than might be expected in this population because of repeated self-injuring blows to the head from coup/contracoup effects.

For well over 100 yr, it has been recognized that there is an association and a significantly increased risk of dementia and Down syndrome. Adults with Down syndrome are at increased risk of the early onset of Alzheimer's disease, with nearly 100% already having developed the characteristic histologic neuropathology of plaques and tangles by age 40. However, it is not typical for individuals with Down syndrome to develop overt dementia at that early an age. In a 1989 study, 49 of 96 patients with Down syndrome met criteria for dementia with an average age of onset of about 54 yr ± 6 yr. In general, the prevalence for dementia and Down syndrome is approximately 40% for those ≥50 yr old and approximately 75% for those ≥60 yr old (SOE=B).

The diagnosis of dementia among individuals with mental retardation is made according to the same criteria as in the general population. The evaluation includes establishing presence of cognitive and adaptive deterioration; demonstration of deficits on examination (preferably with longitudinal follow-up showing progression of deficits); and exclusion of other possible causes of deterioration, such as medical or environmental factors, or other mental disorders, such as depression or delirium. See "Dementia," p 245.

Interest has been growing in attempting to demonstrate the efficacy of medications such as cholinesterase inhibitors (donepezil, rivastigmine, galantamine) and the glutamate antagonist memantine in individuals with mental retardation. While case reports have demonstrated the tolerability of these medications in patients with mental retardation, there is no evidence of efficacy in this population.

Behavioral Disorders

Maladaptive behaviors are observable phenomena that are counterproductive or disruptive for the individual. Various other terms are sometimes used to describe these acts, including target behaviors (behaviors targeted for extinction) or challenging behaviors. As many as 50%–60% of adults with mental retardation have a maladaptive behavior (such as withdrawal, self-injury, stereotypy) that is severe or that occurs frequently, and follow-up studies show that these behaviors can persist for years. The proportion decreases with age for various reasons, except in Down syndrome, in which the proportion is higher and the incidence of behavioral problems increases with the degree of mental retardation. Aggression is seen with similar frequency in all age groups and has an extremely variable presentation.

Diagnosis and Treatment

The diagnosis of a mental disorder in an older adult with mental retardation is based on the same principles of history and examination that apply in the general population. However, as discussed above, the patient's presentation or reported symptoms can be different, and the perceptions of the clinician and the criteria used pose additional challenges.

Typically, it is difficult for patients to report their emotional or physical state because of impaired verbal skills or a limited awareness of their internal state. Often, mental disorders present as behavioral changes; therefore, the reports of family or other caregivers are extremely important. Their interpretation of an individual's behaviors or symptoms, as well as any physical or behavioral responses to therapeutic interventions, can be critically important.

It is important to not over-diagnose and therefore over-treat an individual's presentation. Because insight, judgment, and adaptive or coping skills are limited, individuals may be more likely to "act out," which may be incorrectly perceived as a serious symptom of illness when, in fact, it may just be frustration. Medication may not be called for in a situation in which supportive therapy and time could lead to resolution. Medication can be used, however, to create a window of opportunity to make behavioral supports or strategies more effective.

Changes in staff, residential or vocational settings, or family health should be reported and considered as precipitating factors for all behavioral changes. The concepts of applied behavioral analysis are important tools to use in determining cause and effect of problem behaviors.

Maladaptive behaviors, such as aggression, can be common in individuals with mental retardation and can be either a learned response or an impulsive response to a stressor. An appropriate treatment or response, as mentioned earlier, might be instructional or behavioral. Preferred behavior programs reward good behavior.

Table 42.1—Developmental Disabilities and Health Problems

System/Condition	Change with Developmental Disabilities	Management Strategies
Mental retardation	Two-thirds of patients with developmental disabilities suffer from mental retardation, many in the mild-to-moderate range.	Evaluation and referral to specialized services to maximize intellectual potential
Growth retardation	Usually found in patients with moderate to severe disabilities; it may present as short stature, inability to gain weight, lack of sexual development, or failure to thrive.	Medical evaluation for treatable causes
Sensory impairment	Nearly 90% of patients have impairments in hearing, vision, and speech. Strabismus is common, as is dysarthric speech.	Regular evaluation of hearing, vision, and speech; correction of deficits
Dental/oral conditions	Poor dentition and oral health are very common.	Oral hygiene and tooth brushing; regular dental visits
Thyroid	Thyroid problems can be a cause or a result of developmental disability.	Regular testing and treatment as indicated
Spinal deformities	Kyphosis, scoliosis, and lordosis are common among patients with muscle weakness and spasticity.	Monitoring of body habitus; physical therapy
Seizure disorders	Half of patients may suffer from some type of seizure disorder.	Diagnosis; anticonvulsant medications
Degenerative joint disease	Chronic muscle spasticity and mobility limitations often lead to osteoarthritis and joint disease. Strength and functional status may be prematurely impaired.	Physical therapy, occupational therapy, pain management
Osteopenia and osteoporosis	Lack of weight bearing leads to these chronic conditions in patients who are unable to ambulate.	Promotion of mobility (physical therapy); adequate calcium and vitamin D supplementation
Chronic pain syndromes	Muscle abnormalities and associated spinal deformities often result in chronic pain syndromes. Sensory abnormalities can result in the inability to describe the type, location, and source of the pain.	Regular monitoring of function and behavior to detect possible painful conditions; pain management
Functional decline	Aging patients with cerebral palsy and other similar conditions often develop fatigue, pain, weakness, and overuse syndromes that result in premature loss of function. This is referred to as *postimpairment syndrome* and often requires a reduction in work hours, increase in assistance or use of adaptive devices, and sometimes nursing-home placement.	Physical therapy, occupational therapy, pain management
Cardiac and pulmonary conditions	Patients with cerebral palsy and other similar physical disabilities typically require $3-5$ times the energy level of unimpaired adults, predisposing patients to premature conditions of aging, such as hypertension, heart failure, and coronary artery disease.	Monitoring for hypertension, shortness of breath, angina; risk factor management
GI conditions	Gastroesophageal reflux disease and constipation common; constipation can be chronic and severe.	Monitoring; medications, fiber-rich diet, exercise
Incontinence	Many patients are incontinent of bowel and bladder from childhood, but others develop these problems with age.	Screening for treatable causes; identifying functional impairments that can limit toileting
Depression and mood disorders	Patients with cerebral palsy are 4 times more likely to develop depression than age-compared other adults. The stress associated with multiple disabilities is a risk factor, as is the premature decline in functional status associated with the disorder.	Regular screening; counseling and/or medications for those diagnosed with mood disorder

Despite appropriate attempts to control physical aggression through behavioral methods, pharmacologic intervention may be necessary for the safety of the patient or those nearby. Very few medications are approved for the most common and challenging behaviors, and prescribing medications off-label is common. Medication management for symptoms of major mental illnesses in older adults with mental retardation is not much different from that in the general population, keeping in mind the diagnostic caveats already mentioned. See "Dementia," p 245; "Behavioral Problems in Dementia," p 256; "Depression and Other Mood Disorders," p 295; "Anxiety Disorders," p 307; and "Psychotic Disorders," p 311.

MEDICAL DISORDERS

Adults with mental retardation have more medical problems than age-matched individuals (approximately five medical conditions per person; those with more severe mental retardation have more problems). Approximately two-thirds of those in a community setting have chronic conditions or major physical disability. It is estimated that 50% of these medical conditions go undetected. Prompt detection and treatment is associated with better survival. Visual or hearing impairments are more common in individuals with mental retardation; they increase with age and affect approximately 25%.

Life expectancy decreases with increasing severity of mental retardation and with other morbidity, such as inability to ambulate, lack of feeding skills, and incontinence. Life expectancy for adults with mental retardation is about 65 yr, with the most common causes of death being cardiovascular and respiratory disorders, cancer, and dementia (particularly in Down syndrome).

SOCIAL CONDITIONS

At least 80% of adults with mental retardation live at home and are cared for by aging family members; 20% live in residential programs. It is estimated that about 40% of eligible individuals may not be served by the formal service system. This situation often leads to a crisis when the parent is no longer able to provide adequate care or is unable to manage a behavioral problem. It is estimated that about half of developmentally disabled adults with a behavior problem eventually need a different living arrangement. Typically, more than half of families have not made plans for the future care of adult relatives with mental retardation. Clients in day programs or workshops do not typically have pensions or Social Security benefits to allow retirement. Not surprisingly, the degree of mental retardation, physical health, and functional skills of the aging individual correlate with the degree of parental stress and burden, although maternal and family characteristics such as education and income are more correlated with overall life satisfaction and maternal well-being.

REFERENCES

■ Alexander L, Bullock K, Maring J. Challenges in the recognition and management of age-related conditions in older adults with developmental disabilities. *Topics Geriatr Rehab.* 2008;24(1):12–25.

■ Coppus AM, Evenhuis HM, Verbberne GJ, et al. Survival in elderly persons with Down syndrome. *J Am Geriatr Soc.* 2008;56(12):2311–2316.

■ Fletcher R, Loschen E, Stavrakaki C, et al, eds. *Diagnostic Manual—Intellectual Disability (DM-ID): A Textbook of Diagnosis of Mental Disorders in Persons with Intellectual Disability.* Kingston, NY: NADD Press; 2007.

CHAPTER 43—DERMATOLOGIC DISEASES AND DISORDERS

KEY POINTS

- Photoaging increases the fragility of the skin and decreases the elasticity/tensile strength of the skin.

- Older adults are at risk of xerosis and neurodermatitis, or lichen simplex chronicus.

- Venous insufficiency can cause stasis dermatitis and chronic leg ulcers. Treatment should begin by controlling venous hypertension with compression therapy.

- Ultraviolet (UV) light exposure and age are associated with increased incidence of skin cancers, including squamous cell carcinomas, basal cell carcinomas, and melanomas.

AGING AND PHOTOAGING

The incidence and prevalence of skin disease increase with aging and sun exposure. Dermatologic care of older adults requires an awareness of cutaneous changes of aging and the effects of cumulative UV radiation exposure, as well as knowledge of the common tumors, inflammatory diseases, and infections seen in older adults. The skin of older individuals is characterized by a number of changes, including increased fragility, graying of hairs, and increased wrinkles, particularly at rest. Each of the skin layers changes with aging. In normal young skin, the epidermis interdigitates with the dermis. With time, the epidermis becomes flattened with reduced keratinocyte turnover and melanocyte numbers, contributing in part to the decreased rate of wound healing. In the dermis, the fibroblasts are elongated and collapsed. There is a decrease in types I and III collagen and fewer microfibrils of elastin, leading to the appearance of laxity and atrophy. Changes in hair include graying of hairs, which is caused by changes in follicular melanocytes, and a decrease in scalp hair density secondary to a shortened length of anagen (the growth phase of the hair cycle) and an increase in the proportion of hairs in telogen (the resting phase). In aging skin, there is a decrease in the number of immune antigen-presenting cells, such as

Langerhans cells, which may have consequences for cutaneous immune surveillance.

Aging of skin is a result of both intrinsic and extrinsic factors. The largest contributor to aging is the cumulative exposure to UV light. This leads to the clinical appearance of lentigines, guttate hypomelanosis, poikiloderma, laxity, yellow hue, and leathery appearance. Cumulative exposure to sunlight remains the largest contributor to the aging of skin. *Photoaging* refers to the effects of UV exposure on skin. UV light appears to activate signaling pathways that lead to increased matrix metalloproteinase activity and decreased collagen production. In a vicious cycle, the fibroblasts become elongated and collapsed and respond by decreasing collagen production. UV light also causes DNA injury in part via oxidative damage, which likely also contributes to the aging phenotype. Cutaneous malignancies are also more common in photodamaged skin because of photocarcinogenesis and UV light-mediated immunosuppression.

Prevention of photodamage involves using broad-spectrum sunscreens—sunscreens that protect against both UVB and UVA radiation—as well as avoiding direct sunlight and wearing protective clothing along with hats and sunglasses. Although there are claims that various topical agents decrease photodamage, only topical tretinoin has been shown to increase the thickness of the superficial skin layers, reduce pigmentary changes and roughness, and increase collagen synthesis (SOE=A). There are multiple surgical options for treating photodamage, including chemical peeling agents, dermabrasion, and laser resurfacing. All rely on the destruction of surface populations of keratinocytes, followed by repopulation with keratinocytes deep from within the sun-protected follicular structures. Controlled trials to evaluate the effectiveness of these expensive modalities are few and have been inconclusive. Soft-tissue augmentation, via hyaluronic acid fillers, can also reverse the degradation of extracellular matrix in part by reversing the collapse of fibroblasts.

INFLAMMATORY AND AUTOIMMUNE SKIN CONDITIONS

Seborrheic Dermatitis

Seborrheic dermatitis is a chronic inflammatory dermatosis that is characterized by symmetric pink patches with overlying greasy bran-like scaling distributed in the areas where sebaceous glands are

While seborrheic dermatitis can be treated, it cannot be cured or eliminated. Treatment can be in the form of creams (face and body) or shampoos (scalp). Medications that target yeast, including selenium sulfide, ketoconazole, and various tar shampoos, are effective. In an acute flare, patients can be treated with mild topical corticosteroids such as hydrocortisone 1%; if treatment is unsuccessful, a trial of topical calcineurin inhibitors can be tried. Aggressive topical or systemic therapy should be avoided because of risk of rebound.

Rosacea

Rosacea (Figure 43.1) is a common condition in fair-skinned people that has multiple subtypes. In the erythematotelangiectatic subtype, there is persistent erythema of the central convex areas of the face (ie, nose, forehead, cheeks, and chin) with telangiectasias and flushing. In the papulopustular subtype, there are follicular and nonfollicular papules and pustules in addition to the persistent erythema. In the phymatous subtype, there is sebaceous hyperplasia and thickening of the skin, in part due to recurrent flushing and edema. In some cases, this leads to rhinophyma. Rosacea can also involve the eye, causing irritation and burning that can present as conjunctival injection, blepharitis, episcleritis, chalazion, or hordeolum. Other variants include periorificial dermatitis, granulomatous rosacea, and pyoderma faciale.

Incidence of rosacea peaks in the third and fourth decades, but the disease is seen in young and older adults as well. The cause of acne rosacea is likely multifactorial, including contributions from vasodilatation, *Demodex* mites, and propionobacterium. In addition, thermal stimuli, sunlight exposure, and a number of medications can contribute to rosacea, including oral niacin and topical steroids. Often, seborrheic dermatitis and rosacea are seen together.

The treatment of rosacea depends on the subtype and severity. Topical antibiotics such as benzoyl peroxide, erythromycin, and metronidazole can be used to treat papulopustular rosacea. Oral antibiotics such as tetracylines (eg, doxycycline, minocycline) and macrolides are used to treat moderate to severe cases. Alternative therapies include topical azelaic acid, topical tretinoin, and oral isotretinoin for severe cases. For the persistent erythema, nasal decongestants such as oxymetazoline hydrochloride have shown some promise in small case series. For treatment of the telangiectasias, lasers, such as the potassium-titanyl-phosphate laser, intense pulsed light, and the pulsed dye laser, can be used. Rhinophyma can be treated with surgical excision or electrosurgery.

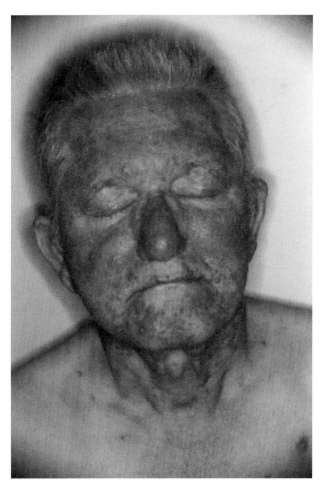

Figure 43.1—Rosacea. Diffuse erythema and erythematous papules and papulopustules are seen on the cheeks, forehead, and chin. The nose shows thickening of the skin and changes consistent with an early rhinophyma.

found, namely on the scalp, the face, and sometimes on the presternal chest and intertriginous areas. On the face, the lesions are found on the forehead, medial portions of the eyebrows, upper eyelids, nasolabial folds and lateral aspects of the nose, retroauricular areas, and occasionally the occiput and neck. At times, the lesions may be arcuate or petaloid, resembling flower petals. Occasionally patients have features of both psoriasis and seborrheic dermatitis, particularly in the hairline and eyebrows, and this condition is therefore known as sebopsoriasis.

The pathogenesis of seborrheic dermatitis is unclear but may be related to the yeast colonies that normally colonize the skin, ie, *Malassezia furfur*. Seborrheic dermatitis tends to be more prevalent in patients with Parkinson's disease. Extensive and severe eruptions of seborrheic dermatitis often warrant an examination of HIV status. Rebound flares of seborrheic dermatitis can follow tapering of corticosteroid medications.

Xerosis

Dryness of the skin, often a concern for older adults, is due to altered barrier function in the aging epidermis and a reduced ability to retain water. It is exacerbated by environmental factors such as decreased humidity; prolonged exposure to water, which can dilute out natural moisturizing factor; and use of harsh soaps, which can further damage the stratum corneum. This condition is often more pronounced on the legs. Depending on the severity of the dryness, xerosis can present as rough, itchy skin or as scales that give the skin a dry, cracked riverbed appearance known as *eczema craquelé* (Figure 43.2).

Treatment usually begins with avoiding the exacerbating factors mentioned above. Patients should be advised to take tepid showers and avoid using washcloths, sponges, or brushes to scrub the skin. Moisturizing agents, especially those containing lactic acid or α-hydroxy acids, can reduce the roughness and scaliness. Moisturizing agents are often most helpful when applied immediately after a bath or shower. When irritation or inflammation is a prominent finding, episodic use of mild topical corticosteroids for a short time provides relief.

Neurodermatitis

Neurodermatitis is a nonspecific term that is used to refer to chronic, pruritic conditions of unclear cause. Another commonly used term is *lichen simplex chronicus*. It is most common in adults >60 yr old. The lesions show signs of chronic scratching, such as hyperpigmentation and lichenification (increased skin markings), along with redness and scaling. Scratching these lesions is often satisfying and leads to a vicious cycle of skin changes and more pruritus. Treatment consists of potent topical corticosteroids (often under occlusion), emollients, and behavior modification. Other causes of pruritus such as irritant or allergic contact dermatitis, drug allergy, or xerosis must be excluded.

Intertrigo

Intertrigo (Figure 43.3) is any infectious or noninfectious inflammatory condition of two closely opposed skin surfaces (intertriginous area). It is more common in older adults because of the increased skin folds secondary to decreased dermal elasticity. Additional contributory factors include decreased mobility, moisture, friction, and poor hygiene. Factors that increase moisture (eg, obesity) and factors that decrease immunity (eg, diabetes or systemic corticosteroids) predispose patients to develop intertrigo. Commonly involved areas, such as the inframammary area, abdominal folds, groin, and axillae, appear erythematous, macerated, moist, and mildly malodor-

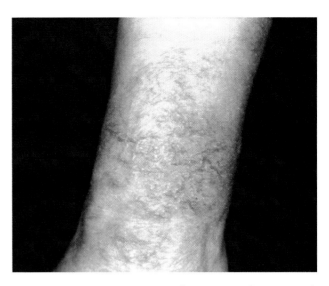

Figure 43.2—Eczema craquelé. Dry, erythematous, fissured, and cracked skin is seen on the lower legs of this patient.

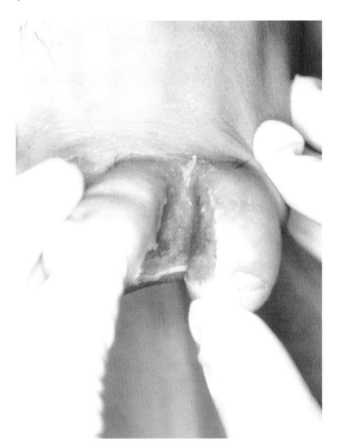

Figure 43.3—Intertrigo and candidiasis. This fungal infection is commonly found in the web space between the fourth and fifth toes. Moist erythema, maceration, and superficial erosion are apparent.

ous. The differential diagnosis includes seborrheic dermatitis and inverse psoriasis. Intertrigo often is associated with superficial infection with bacteria or *Candida*. Successful treatment involves decreasing moisture with topical drying agents, such as corn starch and antifungal powder (eg, miconazole or nystatin powder). Physical means of keeping the area dry include bed sheets/handkerchiefs to separate skin folds and frequent airing, or careful use of a hair dryer. If candidal intertrigo is suspected, treatment involves the topical polyene and azole antifungals, such as topical nystatin or ketoconazole. Occasionally, a very mild topical corticosteroid such as 1%–2% hydrocortisone is needed for a short period to reduce inflammation and irritation (see also candidiasis, p 341).

Bullous Pemphigoid

Bullous pemphigoid (Figure 43.4) is the most common autoimmune subepidermal blistering disease. It is a disease of older adults, with the age of onset commonly >60 yr. Clinically, the disease has diverse manifestations. Typically, bullous pemphigoid presents as an extremely pruritic eruption with widespread blister formation. The blisters are typically tense, often filled with clear fluid. The distribution is symmetrical and widespread, although the flexural areas and lower trunk may be favored. Up to one-third of patients have mucous membrane involvement. The blisters often resolve without scarring. Early or atypical lesions may be nonbullous with primarily urticarial lesions (Figure 43.4).

Bullous pemphigoid is a prototypical organ-specific autoimmune disease with a humoral and cellular immune response targeted against two antigens in the hemidesmosome. BPAg1 and BPAg2 are two proteins that help anchor the basal epidermal cells to the basement membrane zones. With the help of autoreactive T cells, pathogenic B cells produce antibodies that target these two hemidesmosomal antigens. The antibodies trigger an inflammatory cascade of complement activation, the recruitment of neutrophils and eosinophils, and the elaboration of proteases. Bullous pemphigoid has been associated with medications including diuretics, analgesics, antibiotics, and ACE inhibitors.

Diagnosis is made by clinicopathologic correlation. Generally, two biopsies are performed and serum is obtained. Biopsy of the lesion characteristically shows a subepidermal split with associated infiltrating eosinophils and neutrophils. Direct immunofluorescence of perilesional skin demonstrates linear C3 complement and sometimes IgG deposited at the basement membrane zone. Circulating antibodies can be detected by indirect immunofluorescence of salt split skin. In these assays, patient serum binds to and stains the hemidesmosomal side of skin treated with 1M NaCl.

While the disease may last for months to years, it is often self-limited. Treatment should be commensu-

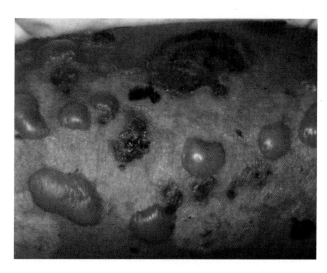

Figure 43.4—Bullous pemphigoid. Tense, fluid-filled, and hemorrhagic bullae on an erythematous base are seen on the trunk and extremities. Some of the bullae have ruptured and left a scab with crusting.

rate to the severity of disease. Limited, localized disease can be treated with potent topical corticosteroids, topical calcineurin inhibitors, and nicotinamide with tetracycline. Systemic corticosteroids are the mainstay of more extensive treatment. Steroid-sparing agents (eg, azathioprine and cyclophosphamide) are often used to avoid the adverse events of corticosteroids.

Pruritus

Pruritus, a very common skin complaint, is associated with many cutaneous and systemic conditions. Severe pruritus can compromise quality of life. Pruritus can be idiopathic, related to a primary skin disease, or secondary to a systemic disease. In older adults, xerosis is the most common cause of chronic pruritus. However, evaluation must exclude other underlying pruritic dermatologic conditions, including infestations such as scabies; genetic/childhood diseases such as atopic dermatitis; and autoimmune blistering diseases, including bullous pemphigoid. Pruritus can be caused by medications (eg, dermal hypersensitivity reactions), related to chemical exposures (eg, irritant dermatitis or allergic contact dermatitis), or a consequence of autosensitization to stasis dermatitis. Pruritus can be secondary to systemic diseases such as renal disease, cholestasis or chronic liver disease, thyroid disease, anemia, and occult malignancies. Finally, generalized pruritus can also be associated with generalized anxiety disorder, depression, and even psychosis, including delusions of parasitosis.

A thorough evaluation of pruritus in an older adult therefore includes a complete history and physical examination to exclude underlying and treatable skin disease. Distribution of the pruritus may help to determine the underlying cause. Involvement of flexural areas suggests atopic dermatitis or bullous pemphigoid, whereas primary involvement of the lower legs suggests an autosensitization to stasis dermatitis. Laboratory evaluation to exclude secondary causes includes a CBC and function tests of the liver, kidneys, and thyroid. It is also important to perform age-appropriate cancer screening, as warranted by the findings of above.

Treatment requires addressing the cause of the pruritus, if known, and relieving symptoms. If there is a primary dermatologic condition or a systemic disease, treatment should be tailored to the underlying disease. For example, prednisone may be warranted for bullous pemphigoid, and topical corticosteroids for atopic dermatitis. In addition, symptomatic relief often requires multiple modalities. Nonpharmacologic measures include open-wet dressings: in brief, a thin, white material such as a bed sheet can be moistened with lukewarm tap water and subsequently placed over the skin for 10–15 minutes. As the water evaporates, it can relieve pruritus. It is important to treat xerosis with frequent uses of emollients. Topical corticosteroids, such as 0.1% triamcinolone ointment, can also relieve xerosis and any underlying inflammation. Topical pramoxine, menthol in calamine preparations, and capsaicin[OL] cream can change the neurologic sensation of pruritus. These topical agents can also be used frequently with minimal adverse events in the short-term. Systemic therapy can include nonsedating oral antihistamines. Most trials investigating their use have used desloratadine in the treatment of chronic idiopathic urticaria. It has significantly improved patient-reported pruritus, sleep disruption, and interference with daily activities with a low incidence of adverse events (SOE=A). Cetirizine, fexofenadine, and levocetirizine are also used for this purpose. In severe, refractory cases, including cases secondary to systemic disease, patients can be referred to a dermatologist for UVB phototherapy or oral thalidomide.

Psoriasis

Psoriasis (Figure 43.5) is a chronic inflammatory skin disease characterized by well-demarcated plaques with overlying silvery scale. Chronic plaque psoriasis is the most common variant, and it characteristically involves the scalp, the gluteal cleft, and extensor surfaces. Hands and feet can be involved, as well as the nails, which may portend psoriatic arthritis. The other psoriatic subtypes are as follows:

- inverse pattern, in which lesions develop in skin folds, such as the neck, axillae, and genital area

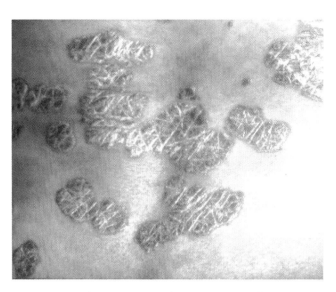

Figure 43.5—Psoriasis. Characteristic well-demarcated beefy red plaques with overlying silvery white scales are evident on the back of this patient.

- guttate, in which small papules (approximately 1 cm) appear over the upper trunk and proximal extremities, usually after an infection
- pustular, which is acute with generalized eruption sterile pustules (2–3 mm) and fever
- palmoplantar pustulosis, in which sterile pustules are confined to the palms and soles
- erythrodermic psoriasis, in which the patient has generalized erythema

Psoriasis is common, affecting 2% of the population. The incidence is bimodal, first in the mid-20s and then at about 50–60 yr of age. The etiology is likely multifactorial. There is a strong genetic predisposition, with multigene mode of inheritance, as well as a role for environmental factors. Triggers that initiate or exacerbate disease include physical trauma (known as Koebner's phenomenon), infections (including streptococcal upper respiratory infections), stress, and medications (eg, oral corticosteroids, lithium, β-blockers, ACE inhibitors, as well as NSAIDs). In psoriasis, the risk factors ultimately lead to the activation and recruitment of autoreactive Th1 and Th17 T cells to the skin. Cytokines such as tumor necrosis factor-alpha (TNF-α) and IL-23 likely lead to the activation of T cells, and IL-22 leads ultimately to increased keratinocyte proliferation.

Five to thirty percent of patients suffer also from psoriatic arthritis, which is characterized by pain, swelling, and stiffness of affected joints. Classically, psoriatic arthritis is an asymmetric oligoarthritis of the small joints of the hands. Alternative patterns of presentation include inflammation restricted to the distal interphalangeal joints, symmetric polyarthritis

Table 43.1—Characteristics of Venous and Arterial Ulcers

Characteristic	Venous Disease	Arterial Disease
Signs and symptoms	Limb heaviness, aching and swelling that is associated with standing and is worse at end of day, brawny skin changes	Claudication (pain in leg with walking), ankle-brachial index <0.9, loss of hair, cool extremities
Risk factors	Advanced age, obesity, history of deep-vein thrombosis or phlebitis	Age >40 yr old, cigarette smoking, diabetes mellitus, hyperlipidemia, hypertension, male gender, sedentary lifestyle
Location of ulcers	Along the course of the long saphenous vein, between the lower medial calf to just below the medial malleolus	Over bony prominences

of the hands, and arthritis mutilans with telescoping of the involved digit. Also, some patients suffer from back pain in the form of spondylitis or sacroiliitis. Because of the wide clinical spectrum of disease, treatment should be tailored to the individual with special attention paid to the risks and benefits for the older patient. Therapies directed at the skin are appropriate for patients with limited disease. These include topical treatments such as topical corticosteroids, vitamin D derivatives (eg, calcipotriene), topical retinoids (eg, tazarotene), salicylic acid, and tar compounds. Long-term use of topical steroids is limited by the risk of cutaneous atrophy. In patients in whom topical therapy is unsuccessful and in those who have extensive disease, phototherapy can be of benefit. UV light therapy, including narrow-band UVB therapy and psoralen with UVA light (PUVA), can be used alone or in conjunction with topical therapies. Patients receiving UV light therapy must be able to stand for the duration of the treatment. Risks include increased incidence of skin cancer.

For those with widespread and recalcitrant disease, systemic agents are available. Oral immunosuppressive agents including cyclosporine and methotrexate are effective but require careful monitoring for adverse events. Toxicities of cyclosporine include hypertension and renal dysfunction. Toxicities of methotrexate include bone marrow suppression, liver fibrosis, and interstitial lung pneumonitis. Oral retinoids such as acitretin can be used in conjunction with other therapies such as UV light. Biologics can be effective in patients in whom traditional systemic therapies are either ineffective or contraindicated. These include agents that block the cytokine TNF, and T-cell surface molecules including adhesion molecules and co-stimulatory molecules. These agents have their own adverse events. In general, anti-TNF agents are contraindicated in those with a history of hepatitis C, multiple sclerosis, heart failure, and lymphoma. Antibodies targeting the common IL-12/IL-23 subunit (uztekinumab) have demonstrated remarkable efficacy and duration of response (up to 16 weeks from each treatment) in phase II and III studies. These antibodies are not FDA approved as of November 2009.

Stasis Dermatitis

Stasis dermatitis can be an early sign of chronic venous insufficiency of the legs. Chronic venous hypertension, caused mostly by incompetency of the venous valves, is the initial trigger for stasis dermatitis. Venous hypertension slows down the flow of blood in the microvasculature, damages the permeability barrier of the small vessels, and allows for the passage of fluid and plasma proteins into the tissue, leading to edema and extravasation of erythrocytes. These processes lead to decreased oxygen diffusion and metabolic exchange and to activation and attraction of inflammatory cells and mediators to the site. Stasis dermatitis typically develops in the medial supramalleolar areas. It is often associated with intense pruritus. Initially, pitting edema to the ankle is noted, which is often worse later in the day. Over time, these events lead to progressive induration and adherence of the skin and subcutaneous tissues. Venous ulcers can develop spontaneously or secondary to trauma, arising most often in the supramalleolar areas.

The goal of therapy is to control the venous hypertension by regularly using compression bandages or stockings and exercising the calf muscles to improve venous return. Topical treatment includes the judicious use of corticosteroids and emollients. Sensitization to ingredients in topical medications and emollients, including topical antibiotics, is common and frequently overlooked. Patch testing to exclude contact sensitization to these agents should be considered before use.

ULCERS

Venous and Arterial Ulcers

An ulcer is a wound with a loss of epidermal and dermal layers. Ulcers of the lower leg are most often caused by vascular disease or neuropathy. Of those caused by vascular disease, 72% of leg ulcers are caused by venous disease, 22% have a mixed arterial and venous cause, and only 6% are caused by pure arterial disease. They have characteristic risk factors, morphologies, and distributions (Table 43.1).

Chronic leg ulcers are defined as open ulcers that fail to heal within a 6-week period. Treatment of the leg ulcers should be selected based on the cause of the ulceration. In addition to clinical criteria, ankle-brachial indices (ABI) can be used to determine the presence of underlying arterial disease; an ABI <0.8 is abnormal, and compression is contraindicated with an ABI <0.5.

For venous ulcers, venous hypertension can be reversed by either elastic compression, ie, compression stockings, or by inelastic compression, ie, by Unna boot. Debridement of necrotic and fibrinous debris is important for reepithelialization and can be achieved by mechanical or chemical methods, eg, collagenase treatment. Occlusive dressings can be used to help the wound heal; the type of dressing used depends on the ulcer type and amount of drainage (Table 36.5). Surgical options include pinch grafts, split-thickness skin grafts, and allografts.

For arterial ulcers, the main goal is reestablishing the blood supply. Revascularization can be achieved with arterioplasty and bypass surgery. To preclude worsening of disease and development of new ulcers, patients should be encouraged to reduce their risk factors for arterial disease, including smoking, hyperlipidemia, hypertension, and diabetes mellitus. See peripheral arterial disease in "Cardiovascular Diseases and Disorders," p 360.

Pressure Ulcers

See "Pressure Ulcers and Wound Care," p 283.

INFECTIONS AND INFESTATIONS

Onychomycosis

See "Diseases and Disorders of the Foot," p 456.

Herpes Zoster

Herpes zoster represents reactivation of the varicella zoster virus (VZV), the virus that is responsible for varicella, ie, chickenpox. Classically, it is a disease of older adults, with more than two-thirds of cases in patients >50 yr old. The lifetime risk of reactivation of VZV is 20% in healthy adults and 50% in immunocompromised individuals. During primary infection, ie, varicella, VZV establishes a latent infection in sensory ganglia. Partly because of the decline in the cellular immune response associated with age or immunosuppressive conditions (Table 58.1), the virus is reactivated and leads to painful ganglionitis.

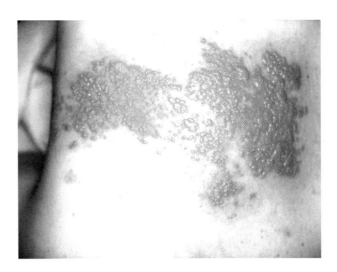

Figure 43.6—Herpes zoster. This patient has clusters of vesicles and pustules on an erythematous base involving a thoracic dermatome.

The infection spreads down the sensory nerve and is released around the sensory nerve endings in the skin, producing the characteristic lesions.

Usually, zoster begins with a prodrome of pain. In some people, the prodrome includes sensations of pruritus, tingling, tenderness, or hyperesthesia. The pain is followed by a painful eruption of grouped vesicles on an erythematous base, usually in a sensory distribution. In the localized form of zoster, the vesicles rarely cross midline (Figure 43.6). Rarely, prodromal pain is not followed by a cutaneous eruption, a condition called zoster sine herpete.

A number of complications have been associated with herpes zoster infection, including post-herpetic neuralgia (PHN), scarring ophthalmic zoster, and Ramsay Hunt syndrome. The incidence and severity of PHN increase with increasing age and an immunocompromised state. In 7% of cases of herpes zoster, the ophthalmic branch of the trigeminal nerve is involved. Involvement of the nasociliary branch, which presents as vesicles on the tip of the nose (known as Hutchinson's sign), requires careful ophthalmic examination to monitor for complications, such as neurotrophic keratitis and ulceration, scleritis, uveitis, and ultimately blindness. In the Ramsay Hunt syndrome, the geniculate ganglion is involved. In addition to producing vesicles on the external ear or tympanic membrane, Ramsay Hunt is associated with facial palsy with or without tinnitus, vertigo, and deafness. Zoster is considered disseminated if it involves two noncontiguous dermatomes. In disseminated zoster, meningoencephalitis, hepatitis, and pneumonitis are also complications.

Although the symptoms of herpes zoster can be confused with a variety of conditions causing localized pain (ie, pleurisy, myocardial infarction, renal colic, cholecystitis, and glaucoma), the combination of the history and the characteristic physical examination, ie, the dermatomal distribution, facilitate the diagnosis. A Tzanck smear from the base of the vesicle can be performed to confirm the diagnosis. Detection of multinucleated giant cells suggests a herpes simplex or herpes zoster infection. Direct fluorescence antibody testing can be performed to confirm the presence of VZV. Polymerase chain reaction and viral cultures are the most sensitive means to confirm the diagnosis.

Early treatment with antiviral therapies, optimally within 72 hours of onset of rash, decreases disease duration and pain (SOE=A). FDA-approved therapies include acyclovir, famcyclovir, and valacyclovir. The addition of oral corticosteroids has not been shown to shorten the duration of complete recovery, although in one randomized controlled trial participants treated with a 3-week tapering dosage of prednisone had a greater chance of being pain-free 1 mo after the onset of the lesions (SOE=B). Intravenous antiviral therapy is reserved for immunocompromised individuals and for those who demonstrate signs of disseminated disease or complications. Most cases of acute herpes zoster are self-limited, but the probability of developing PHN increases with advanced age. PHN occurs in approximately 20% of zoster patients ≥70 yr old and is difficult to treat. Acute herpetic neuralgia refers to pain preceding or accompanying the eruption of rash that persists up to 30 days from its onset. Subacute herpetic neuralgia refers to pain that persists beyond healing of the rash but that resolves within 4 mo of onset. PHN refers to pain persisting beyond 4 mo from the initial onset of the rash. Prevention of PHN can be attempted by vaccinating to decrease the incidence of acute zoster and PHN, by treating the acute zoster infection itself, or by treating acute zoster very early with preventive pain medications such as tricyclic antidepressants or anticonvulsants. Anticholinergic adverse events of tricyclics may limit their use in older adults.

Treatment of PHN can be challenging. Systematic reviews of randomized controlled trials of treatments of PHN with evaluation periods of >24-hour duration found that no single best treatment is known. Tricyclic antidepressants[OL], opioids, topical capsaicin, gabapentin, topical lidocaine, pregabalin, and tramadol can alleviate the pain of PHN, but the long-term benefits of most therapies are not known and adverse events are common. Intrathecal methylprednisolone may relieve pain in patients refractory to the oral and topical measures discussed above.

Because of the high incidence and high morbidity associated with herpes zoster, prophylaxis by zoster vaccination is recommended for patients >60 yr old. Vaccination is associated with a statistically significant decrease in zoster incidence and incidence of PHN (SOE=A). The vaccine is more effective in preventing zoster infection in patients 60–69 yr old than in those ≥70 yr old.

Candidiasis

Candidiasis has a wide spectrum of presentation. Cutaneous candidiasis is often seen in intertriginous areas; it can be superimposed on intertrigo caused by psoriasis or seborrheic dermatitis (see intertrigo, p 336). *Candida* pustules can also develop on the backs of bedridden patients and on other areas prone to moisture and occlusion. In these areas, candidiasis is characterized by red patches, sometimes with erosions. Often, there are peripheral satellite pustules. Candidiasis can also affect the scrotum, the nails, the genital area, and the lips, causing perleche. Oral thrush is an example of mucocutaneous candidiasis, observed most commonly in patients on corticosteroid inhalers, antibiotics, or immunosuppressive medications; or with concomitant systemic illnesses, such as diabetes mellitus. A potassium hydroxide preparation of skin scrapings of the involved site can confirm the diagnosis. The presence of spores and pseudohyphae is consistent with candidiasis.

Topical treatments are generally effective. Most commonly used are topical polyenes such as nystatin, and topical azoles such as miconazole, clotrimazole, ketoconazole, and econazole. Other topical agents that are effective are terbinafine, butenafine, and ciclopirox. Topical therapies can be used twice a day until symptoms resolve and subsequently twice a week for prophylaxis as necessary. In the event of pruritus, pain, and burning, a low-dose topical corticosteroid can sometimes be used in conjunction with topical antifungal therapy, but these symptoms generally resolve with use of topical antifungal medications. In patients with widespread candidiasis, oral therapy with an azole has a response rate of 80%–100%. Effective eradication of candidiasis generally also requires treating the underlying intertrigo by keeping the moist areas dry with drying agents and physical barriers to keep the skin folds separated (eg, bed sheets).

Scabies

Human scabies is a pruritic eruption caused by the mite *Sarcoptes scabei* var *hominis*. The entire 30-day life cycle is confined to the human epidermis. Adult female mites become fertilized and lay their eggs. Eggs mature over 10 days. For first-time infestations, sensitization can take 2–6 weeks; therefore, symptoms may not be seen until a month after infestation, making it difficult to make a diagnosis before disease spread. Scabies is spread primarily by person-to-person contact and is common in institutionalized older adults.

Scabies is characterized by intense pruritus, worse at night, and a symmetrically distributed cutaneous eruption. The eruption is most often characterized by small erythematous papules, sometimes accompanied by linear excoriations. The pathognomic sign is a burrow that is characterized by a wavy, threadlike lesion about 1–10 mm long. The lesions are distributed over the interdigital webs, the flexural wrists, the umbilicus, the wrists, the ankles, and the feet. In men, lesions are also seen on the scrotum and penis. In women, the areolae, nipples, and genital areas are commonly affected. Immunocompromised patients can get crusted scabies, characterized by thousands of mites per gram of epidermis. Other manifestations include vesicles and indurated nodules. The lesions may be nonspecific, and the diagnosis should be considered in anyone with intense pruritus.

Diagnosis can be confirmed by microscopic examination of skin scrapings in mineral oil. This allows direct visualization of the adult mites, nymphs, eggs, or fecal matter (scybala). Occasionally, diagnosis can also be made by skin biopsy. Treatment includes topical creams such as 5% permethrin cream applied head to toe and left on for 8–14 hours, or systemic medications such as ivermectin (200 mcg/kg). Therapies are generally not effective against the eggs; therefore, patients require retreatment in 1–2 weeks after the eggs mature. Clothes, linens, and towels should be either washed in hot water and dried in high heat or left in a closed bag for 10 days to prevent reinfestation by fomites. In the absence of human contact, the mite cannot survive. Caregivers should also be treated because they are usually exposed even though they may not have symptoms.

Louse Infestations

Lice can infest the body (pediculosis corporis), scalp (pediculosis capitis), or pubic hair (pediculosis pubis). With pediculosis corporis or capitis, lice are spread from person to person through physical contact or fomites. Pediculosis pubis is usually spread by sexual contact. In all cases, patients complain of pruritus of the involved areas, and there can be secondary infection. In pediculosis corporis, the lice feed on the body but live on clothing, where they lay eggs, often near the seams. In pediculosis capitis, the lice lay eggs on the proximal part of the hair shaft. The eggs (or nits) are visible as white specks cemented to the hair at an oblique angle. Patients with pediculosis pubis also have nits on the pubic hair and commonly have more organisms.

Treatment involves eradicating the lice and larvae, treating close contacts, and treating the secondary infection. Pyrethrin or its derivatives (permethrin) are ovicidal and can be used as a single 10-minute

topical treatment. People who come into contact with the patient, including caregivers and those who share bedding, should be evaluated for lice and treated. Combs, brushes, hats, clothing, bedding, and towels must be washed with hot water.

BENIGN GROWTHS

Seborrheic Keratoses

Seborrheic keratoses (Figure 43.7) are benign growths that are extremely common in adults >40 yr old. They are tan, gray, or black waxy or warty papules and plaques. They often have a stuck-on appearance with follicular prominence. They can be found anywhere on the body except on mucous membranes, palms, and soles. Occasionally, some lesions are darkly pigmented, and differentiation from a melanoma can be difficult without a biopsy. These growths can be removed for cosmetic purposes with cryosurgery or shave excision if necessary.

Cherry Angiomas

Cherry angiomas are the most common acquired cutaneous vascular proliferations. They usually appear in people in their 20s and increase in number over

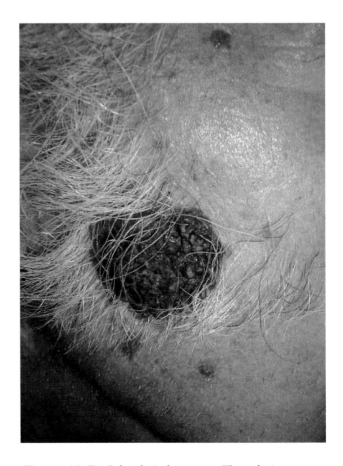

Figure 43.7—Seborrheic keratoses. These lesions present as waxy, warty stuck-on papules in a variety of colors.

time. They are round to oval, bright red, dome-shaped or polypoid papules ranging in size from <1 mm to several millimeters. Cherry angiomas are benign, consisting of dilated, congested capillaries and postcapillary venules. However, they can bleed when traumatized. These lesions can be removed with excision, electrodessication, or laser ablation.

Actinic Keratoses

Actinic keratoses (Figure 43.8) are precancerous lesions caused by chronic UV radiation. They are seen in fair-skinned people and characterized by occasionally tender, rough, poorly circumscribed, erythematous papules with white or yellow scaling. They appear most often in areas with prolonged sun exposure, including the face, neck, ears, arms, and the dorsum of the hands. The scalp of alopecic men is commonly affected. There are a number of clinical variants, including hypertrophic, pigmented, and lichenoid types. Some may have an overlying thick, hard, raised crust known as a *cutaneous horn*. Actinic keratosis or actinic damage of the lips is called *actinic cheilitis*.

Actinic keratoses are considered premalignant growths, precursors of squamous cell carcinoma. It is unclear how many progress to squamous cell carcinoma; reports vary from 0.24% to 20%. Actinic keratoses are treated to prevent progression to squamous cell carcinoma. They may respond to medical and surgical management. They can be easily treated in the office setting with cryotherapy (liquid nitrogen) or photodynamic therapy. Alternatively, they can respond to topical chemotherapeutic agents such as 5-fluorouracil, and immunomodulators such as imiquimod[OL]. When there are numerous lesions, topical treatment with 5-fluorouracil or imiquimod is preferred over cryotherapy. These topical therapies are associated with a transient reaction characterized by bright erythema and discomfort.

SKIN CANCER

Basal Cell Carcinoma

Basal cell carcinoma (Figure 43.9) is the most common cancer in the United States. While the tumors may be locally invasive, the risk of metastasis is low. There are many clinical subtypes, including nodular, superficial, and pigmented (which can be confused for melanoma). The three major clinical subtypes are the following:

- nodular—the most common variant; appears as a waxy, translucent papule with overlying telangiectasias
- morpheaform—has a scar-like appearance and can look atrophic
- superficial—appears as an erythematous macule or papule with fine scale or superficial erosion

Risk factors for basal cell carcinoma include age, UV exposure, immunosuppression, genetic syndromes,

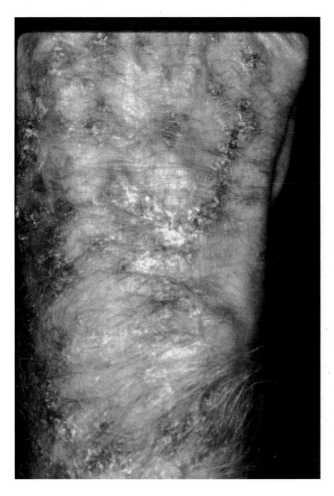

Figure 43.8—Actinic keratoses. These rough, scaly, red-brown macules on sun-exposed skin are premalignant.

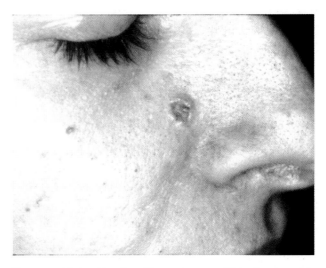

Figure 43.9—Basal cell carcinoma. This is a pearly, fleshy papule but is ulcerated in the center and has a characteristic rolled border.

Chapter 43: Dermatologic Diseases and Disorders   **343**

and chemical exposures. Definitive treatment of basal cell carcinoma is surgical excision. Because of its higher cure rate, Mohs micrographic surgery is warranted for basal cell carcinomas that have indistinct borders, are >2 cm in diameter, are recurrent, or have high-risk histologic features (ie, morpheaform). An additional benefit of Mohs micrographic surgery is that it spares tissues and therefore can provide additional cosmetic benefits. Basal cell carcinomas that develop in poor surgical candidates can also be treated with ablative methods such as cryosurgery and radiation. Superficial basal cell carcinomas can be treated with less invasive techniques such as curettage with electrodessication and topical imiquimod therapy.

Squamous Cell Carcinoma

Squamous cell carcinoma is the second most common form of skin cancer. It generally presents as an occasionally tender, erythematous papule, plaque, or nodule with keratotic scale. The lesions can develop scaling and crusting. Squamous cell carcinomas are locally invasive and can cause subsequent tissue destruction. The risk of metastasis is low but higher than that of basal cell carcinomas. The risk of metastases increases with size of the tumor, high-risk histologic features (eg, poor differentiation, perineural invasion), depth of invasion, and location. Squamous cell carcinomas on the lip and ear can behave more aggressively. Squamous cell carcinomas also have a propensity to develop in longstanding, nonhealing wounds and in burn and radiation scars; these lesions are known as Marjolin's ulcers and are associated with a higher risk of metastasis.

Like other nonmelanoma skin cancers, squamous cell carcinomas are associated with cumulative sun exposure and age. They tend to be found on sites chronically exposed to the sun, such as the face, the dorsum of hands, and arms. Additional risk factors include exposure to arsenic, ionizing radiation, and immunosuppression. Definitive treatment consists of surgical excision. In anatomically sensitive areas or with high-risk tumors, Mohs micrographic surgery is indicated. If surgery is contraindicated, palliative measures with lower cure rates (such as ionizing radiation) can be used.

Melanoma

Melanomas are a malignant tumor of melanocytes. They have a higher risk of metastasis than basal cell carcinomas and squamous cell carcinomas. In addition to spreading locally, they are associated with distant metastases to the skin, brain, lung, and small intestine. The tumors present usually as atypical pigmented lesions. There are four clinical types:

- lentigo maligna—the type seen most commonly on atrophic, sun-damaged skin of an older adult; appears as an irregularly shaped tan or brown macule that has been enlarging slowly

- superficial spreading—this type can occur anywhere and often presents as an irregularly shaped macule, papule, or plaque with great variation in color (Figure 43.10)

- nodular—a papule or nodule, often black or gray, that has been growing rapidly

- acral lentiginous—this type is found on the palms, soles, or nail beds (Figure 43.11); it is found in all skin types and presents as a dark brown or black patch; incidence is highest in adults ≥65 yr old

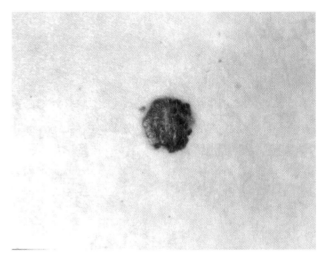

Figure 43.10—Melanoma. This lesion has irregular variegation in pigment (shades of brown and blue-black) as well as irregular borders, suggesting melanoma.

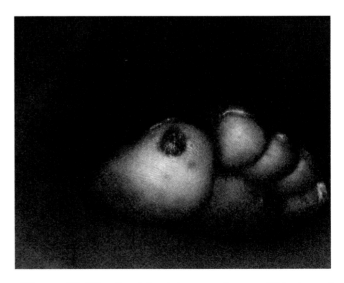

Figure 43.11—Acral lentiginous melanoma. This type of melanoma presents as a dark macular growth with irregular borders on volar surfaces of palms and soles (as in this case), and nails.

The incidence of melanoma continues to increase. Mortality due to melanoma has also increased but at a lower rate, in part because of earlier detection. Risk factors for melanoma include family history, fair skin type, red hair, history of dysplastic or numerous nevi, and sunlight exposure, particularly intermittent blistering sunburns in childhood.

Melanomas are usually asymptomatic. If detected early, they can be associated with a high rate of cure. Therefore, regular skin examinations and early recognition are important. A new pigmented skin lesion or a change in the color, size, surface, or borders of a preexisting mole should be biopsied. A useful mnemonic when examining skin for melanoma or atypical moles is ABCD: **a**symmetry, **b**orders, **c**olor, **d**iameter >6 mm.

Risk factors for metastases and mortality due to melanoma are depth of invasion, ulceration, and number of mitoses. Treatment is tailored to the perceived aggressiveness of the tumor. If caught early with a Breslow depth <1 mm, definitive treatment is surgical excision. If Breslow depth is ≥1 mm, standard treatment is wide excision, and sentinel node biopsy may be indicated. Adjuvant therapy such as interferon is sometimes used in cases with lymph node involvement. If there is evidence of distant metastases, treatment options include immunotherapy such as interleukin-2 and chemotherapy.

REFERENCES

■ Loar, R. Case study #2: Herpes Zoster. In: Auerhahn C, ed. *Geriatrics and the Advanced Practice Curriculum: A Series of Web-Based Interactive Case Studies.* 2007; New York: Hartford Institute for Geriatric Nursing. Available at http://www.hartfordign.org/case_study/

■ Menter A, Griffiths CE. Current and future management of psoriasis. *Lancet.* 2007;370(9583):272−284.

■ Naldi L, Rebora A. Seborrheic dermatitis. *N Engl J Med.* 2009;360(4):387−396.

■ Rabe JH, Mamelak AJ, McElgunn PJ, et al. Photoaging: mechanisms and repair. *J Am Acad Dermatol.* 2006;55(1):1−19.

CHAPTER 44—ORAL DISEASES AND DISORDERS

KEY POINTS

■ Because teeth become less sensitive with age, it is not uncommon to observe profound yet asymptomatic untreated dental disease in older adults, which justifies a need for regular dental evaluation every 6–12 mo.

■ Periodontitis caused by plaque formation within the gingival sulcus that may be controlled with regular oral hygiene can lead to loss of alveolar bone height, decreased support around the tooth, malposition, loosening, and eventual loss of the tooth.

■ Dentures usually aid in speech and restore diminished facial contours, but improved ability to masticate is unpredictable and improved oral intake is a less likely outcome.

■ Oral cancer screening can detect oral cancer early, potentially translating into improved outcomes and better survival rates.

■ Antibiotic prophylactic coverage before invasive dental procedures to avoid infective bacterial endocarditis or infection of implanted prostheses (eg, prosthetic joints) is indicated only for specific high-risk situations. Patients at increased risk of these orally seeded infections should be counseled to maintain excellent oral hygiene to minimize incidence and severity of orally seeded bacteremia.

The oral cavity functions in initiating food intake, producing speech, and protecting the GI tract and upper airway. Dysfunction and disease in the mouth can profoundly affect overall health and social functioning and can be particularly important for older adults who are frail or nutritionally at risk. Findings prevalent in older adults (eg, decay, missing teeth, periodontal disease, salivary hypofunction) do not represent normal aging, and those with such conditions should be urged to seek preventive and therapeutic care.

Table 44.1—Clinical Significance of Selected Age-Related Changes in Oral Tissues

Tissue Affected	Nature of Change	Clinical Significance
Tooth dentin	Increased thickness	Diminished pulp space
	Diminished permeability resulting from sclerosis of dentinal tubules	Diminished sensitivity of dentin; diminished susceptibility to effects of bacterial metabolites; increased tooth brittleness
Dental pulp	Diminished volume	Diminished reparative capacity; diminished sensitivity and change in nature of sensitivity
	Shift in proportion of nervous, vascular, and connective tissues	Diminished reparative capacity; diminished sensitivity and change in nature of sensitivity
Salivary glands	Fatty replacement of acini	Possibly less physiologic reserve

AGING OF THE TEETH

Most age-related changes in teeth are subtle (Table 44.1) but become significant in the presence of environmental factors or disease. For a combination of reasons, the teeth of older adults are typically less sensitive or wholly insensitive to temperature changes and, importantly, to the sensations that commonly herald dental disease in younger adults. It is not uncommon to observe profound yet asymptomatic untreated dental disease in older adults.

DENTAL DECAY

Dental *caries*, or decay, is a bacterially derived demineralization and cavitation that can attack teeth throughout life. *Recurrent caries* refers to decay at the interface between a dental restoration (such as a filling or crown) and the tooth. For the anatomy of the tooth, see Figure 44.1. Older adults have more restored teeth (and usually the restorations are older and more extensive) and thus are more likely to have recurrent caries. The teeth of older adults can have more caries of the root surfaces than are typically seen in younger adults because prior periodontal disease exposes the root surface, thereby predisposing it to demineralization and an increased risk of decay. Both recurrent and root caries are generally asymptomatic and can become advanced before discovery, often resulting in destruction of much or all of the tooth.

Advanced caries commonly results in necrosis of the remaining pulp, which usually leads to an acute or chronic dental abscess. Even if such infections do not cause pain, they should not be ignored, because severe metastatic infections of dental and oral origin have been reported in virtually every organ system. In particular, α-hemolytic (viridans) streptococci of the oral cavity have long been implicated in close to one-third of the cases of bacterial endocarditis reported annually in the United States, and bacteria associated with dental abscesses (eg, *Staphylococcus aureus*) have been cultured from aspirates of infected hip arthroplasties.

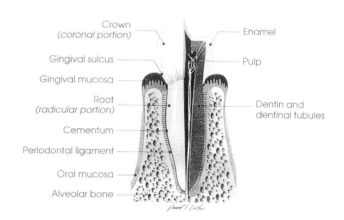

Figure 44.1—Dental and periodontal anatomy

The risk factors for dental caries are the same at any age, but many of the risk factors increase in prevalence with age. A primary risk factor is poor oral hygiene, which often occurs in older adults when visual acuity, manual dexterity, or arm flexibility is impaired, or when salivary flow is diminished. Another risk factor is frequent ingestion of sticky foods with a high content of sucrose, such as cake, candy, and cookies. Other risk factors include infrequent dental visits because of financial, access, or educational barriers; the presence of permanent or removable artificial teeth (more common with increasing age); and limited lifetime exposure to fluoride, widely used in the United States only in the past 40 yr. White older Americans have a higher incidence of root caries than either black or Hispanic older Americans, but they are more likely to have received dental treatment for the lesions. Recurrent caries are also more common in white older Americans because of the greater likelihood that they have received prior dental treatment.

The prevention of caries involves daily oral hygiene with fluoride toothpaste, limitation of sugar intake, and regular dental examinations. The treatment of dental caries includes topical high-potency fluoride for remineralization, removal of demineralized tooth structure ("drilling"), and replacement of removed tooth structure with fillings or crowns. When caries involves the dental pulp, root canal treatment becomes necessary. This in turn usually requires reinforcement of the remaining tooth structure with a crown ("cap").

DISEASES OF THE PERIODONTIUM

The investing tissues of the teeth, termed the *periodontium*, consist of the gingiva, the alveolar bone, and a collagenous sleeve (termed the *periodontal ligament*) located between the tooth root and the surrounding bone. Periodontal disease occurs when microorganic colonies (*plaque*) form on the teeth near the gingiva and between the gingiva and the root surface within the gingival sulcus. The most common form of periodontal disease is gingivitis, in which the inflammatory reaction to plaque is limited to the gingiva. Gingivitis develops more rapidly in older adults than in younger ones, but in both groups the changes—including gingival edema and light bleeding on brushing—are rapidly reversible after removal of plaque. If the inflammatory process extends to the periodontal ligament and alveolar bone, the process is termed *periodontitis*. In periodontitis, there is destruction of the hard and soft tissues of the periodontium. In most adults, the process of periodontitis is marked by long periods of disease quiescence punctuated by bursts of localized destructive inflammation. The prevalence of active periodontitis is 20%–40% of dentate adults. By their 50s, more than 90% of Americans with teeth show ≥2 mm of lost alveolar bone height, the primary marker of prior periodontal disease activity. In advanced cases of periodontitis, the decreased support around a tooth leads to its malposition, loosening, and eventual loss.

Epidemiologic data support the concept that those who reach advanced age without significant periodontal bone loss will not likely experience a worsening of the disease in senescence. In contrast, other adults who have experienced a more rapid rate of bone loss commonly will have lost teeth in their 40s and 50s. In addition to age, risk factors for periodontitis include smoking and poor oral hygiene. Black and Hispanic Americans have a significantly higher prevalence of advanced periodontitis than white Americans. Preventing gingivitis and periodontitis is largely a matter of oral hygiene and regular dental examinations and cleanings. Managing periodontal disease involves debriding the roots below the gingiva, which may require surgical access. Adjunctive therapy with topical antibiotics such as chlorhexidine oral rinse (SOE=B) or systemic antibiotics such as minocycline (SOE=B) or metronidazole (SOE=C) can also be useful in periodontal therapy.

Periodontitis has long been reported to be worse in patients with poorly controlled diabetes mellitus. Investigations also support the contention that periodontitis, as an active infection, impairs diabetic control. Periodontal disease can be rapidly destructive in a patient whose immune system is impaired by disease or immunosuppressive therapy. Epidemiologic data also correlate osteoporosis and tooth loss due to periodontitis. Periodontal disease and the pathogens responsible for it have been linked epidemiologically and immunologically with peripheral vascular disease, cerebrovascular disease, and pneumonia. Similar correlations have been reported for coronary heart disease, although one report disputes this. There is also epidemiologic association between gram-negative pneumonia, gram-negative periodontal pathogens, salivary hypofunction, and impaired swallowing (SOE=C).

The prevention and control of periodontal disease revolve around daily oral care, ie, tooth brushing and flossing to remove bacterial plaque on the teeth, particularly within the gingival sulcus. Properly used, electronic toothbrushes can facilitate oral hygiene for people with impaired manual dexterity, and make plaque removal by caregivers easier and more effective as well. Regular dental evaluation, every 6–12 mo, is important to ensure that the periodontium is healthy or to provide early intervention if it is not.

TOOTHLESSNESS

Advanced age was once considered synonymous with the need for false teeth, but that stereotype is fading. In the early 1960s, more than 70% of adult Americans ≥75 yr old were edentulous. By the 1990s, fewer than 40% of this group were edentulous, most likely because of some level of preventive and restorative dental care in childhood or early adulthood.

Nevertheless, removal of one or more teeth in an older adult may be necessitated by various combinations of physiologic and behavioral factors. The leading cause is inability or unwillingness to access and pay for restorative dental treatment in the face of a symptomatic dental disease, usually stemming from dental caries. A second common cause is loosening of teeth as a consequence of periodontal disease, to the point that mastication becomes painful or ineffective. A third common cause is removal of otherwise healthy teeth that, because of the absence or loss of other teeth for the preceding or other reasons, would hinder the fabrication or function of a dental prosthesis.

Nearly 50% of Americans ≥85 yr old have no natural teeth, and there are unique problems associated with the edentulous state. Functionally, the teeth aid in mastication and enunciation. Aesthetically, the teeth support the lips and cheeks and keep the nose and chin a fixed distance apart. When a person has lost all teeth and there are no prosthetic replacements, the facial appearance is dramatically changed because of the lack of tissue support and diminished vertical height in the lower half of the face. Chewing ability is severely compromised, yet the impact on nutritional intake is difficult to characterize. One longitudinal study using diet diaries demonstrated a correlation between loss of teeth and increased intake of carbohydrates, and decreased intake of protein and selected micronutrients.

Removal dentures can compensate for loss of all of the teeth, aid in speech, and restore diminished facial contours, but they are less predictably successful in restoring the ability to masticate. Edentulous people with dentures can generally eat a wider range of foods than edentulous people without dentures. Yet dentures restore, on average, only about 15% of the chewing ability of the natural dentition. The range of foods regularly eaten by denture wearers is significantly restricted in comparison with the dietary range of people with natural teeth. Denture wearers also have to chew more times before they swallow food, and they swallow their food in larger particles. Older patients and their clinicians who hope that dentures will restore oral intake in cases of malnutrition or unexplained weight loss are usually disappointed, whereas those who hope for a more socially acceptable appearance, clearer speech, and modest improvement in chewing comfort and range of dietary choices are more likely to be satisfied.

Dentures often are a considerable source of discomfort, dysfunction, and embarrassment for older adults. This is because the alveolar processes that originally held the natural teeth continually remodel and diminish in volume once the natural teeth are gone. For most patients, dentures require frequent professional adjustment and periodic replacement. Alveolar ridge resorption is most severe in the oldest patients who have had the longest time without natural teeth; this effect is more pronounced in those with osteoporosis.

For health of the oral mucosa, dentures should be kept clean by removing them and cleaning them after meals and by soaking them in a commercial disinfectant several times each week. Dentures should remain out of the mouth for several hours each day; most people choose to leave their dentures out during sleep. Fractured or broken dentures, as well as denture looseness or soreness, should be brought to a dentist's attention without delay. However, because neither dental services nor dentures are currently covered by Medicare and <10% of older Americans have private dental insurance, many older adults continue to use inadequate or even damaging dentures.

SALIVARY FUNCTION IN AGING

Saliva is critical for protecting the tissues of the oral cavity and maintaining their function in speech, mastication, swallowing, and taste perception. Saliva buffers the intraoral pH, contains a wide spectrum of antimicrobial factors, remineralizes and lubricates the oral surfaces, and keeps the taste pores patent. In the absence of disease, the major salivary glands undergo regressive histologic changes with age. Yet data from the Baltimore Longitudinal Study on Aging and the Veterans Affairs Dental Longitudinal Study have demonstrated that with healthy aging, flow from the parotid glands under both resting and stimulated conditions remains essentially unchanged. In both studies, flow from the submandibular glands did not change with age; in data from other centers, there has been a measurable but clinically minor decrease. It has been suggested that the major salivary glands show "organ reserve," in which the capacity of youthful glands exceeds ordinary demands, but that with age-related changes, functional reserves dwindle. By extreme old age, healthy glands function adequately under normal conditions but are more susceptible to factors that impede function, such as dehydration or drug-induced hypofunction.

Complaints of dry mouth are very common among older adults. The leading causes are medications that have this adverse event. Commonly implicated are medications with anticholinergic effects, including tricyclic antidepressants, opioids, antihistamines, antihypertensives (including diuretics, ACE inhibitors, calcium channel blockers, and both α- and β-blockers), and antiarrhythmic agents. Separate studies have found that 72% of institutionalized older adults received at least one (and some as many as five) potentially xerostomic medications daily and that 55% of >4,000 rural community-dwelling older adults took at least one potentially xerostomic medication daily. Dry mouth can also be due to local disease, such as salivary gland tumors and blocked ducts, or to systemic disease. Sjögren's syndrome affects approximately 3 million Americans, predominantly women, ≥50 yr old. Cevimeline (30 mg q8h) is a medication approved for dry mouth in patients with Sjögren's syndrome. Depression has been reported to diminish saliva flow, as have poorly controlled diabetes mellitus and hypothyroidism.

Dry mouth is also an adverse event of therapeutic irradiation of the head and neck. In the total dosage range administered for oral and oropharyngeal squamous cell carcinoma, salivary flow is commonly obliterated as a consequence of short-term direct effects on the glands and long-term fibrosis of their vascular supply. As a result, patients who have undergone radiation of the head can experience rapidly destructive dental caries and painful oral mucositis, which can affect nutritional status.

Treatment of older adults with dry mouth requires attention to both diagnosis and prevention. Diminished oral secretions increase the risk of serious oral disease. Medications that reduce salivary flow should be decreased, discontinued, or substituted for, if possible. Systemic causes, as well as a history of irradiation of the head and neck, should be excluded. Patients who have had irradiation should be considered for a 3-mo course of oral pilocarpine (5–10 mg q8h), which may restore some salivary function. Saliva substitutes and oral lubricants, available without prescription and used as needed, can provide transient relief but have none of the protective properties of saliva. Patients should be counseled on the greatly increased risk of oral disease and educated on the need to limit dietary sugar and to optimize daily oral hygiene practices.

COMMON ORAL LESIONS

Squamous cell carcinoma accounts for 96% of oral and oropharyngeal malignancies. Of the 28,000 new cases of oral cancer reported in the United States annually, ≥95% occur in people ≥40 yr old; age is the primary risk factor identified in epidemiologic analyses. The 5-yr survival rate for white Americans is approximately 55% and for black Americans, 34%. Carcinoma of the lip, tongue, and floor of the mouth represents >65% of all oropharyngeal cases. Lip cancer affects men eight times more frequently than women; most other sites affect men at a ratio slightly below 2:1. Oral cancer is strongly linked with the use of tobacco, particularly cigarettes (SOE=A). Lip cancer is strongly correlated with pipe and cigar smoking (SOE=A). Alcohol is a potent cofactor that enhances the effects of tobacco. Other potential risk factors—dentures, poor oral care, oral viral disease, oral lichen planus, candidosis—have been suggested, but none has shown the unambiguous associations of age, smoking, and alcohol use.

Oral malignancies appear clinically as painless red, white, or mixed red and white areas of the oral mucosa that may be ulcerated or indurated. Red and mixed lesions (termed *erythroplakia*) (Figure 44.2) display cellular atypia in as many as 93% of cases and should be biopsied immediately. White lesions (*leukoplakia*) (Figure 44.3) are malignant or premalignant <10% of the time and merit close monitoring; biopsy is indicated if a lesion does not resolve in 14 days or is increasing in size. Less invasive diagnostic tools can be used for determining whether a white or red lesion in the mouth merits biopsy, such as scraping (exfoliative cytology) and in situ staining. Early identification markedly improves outcome: 5-yr survival without nodal involvement in

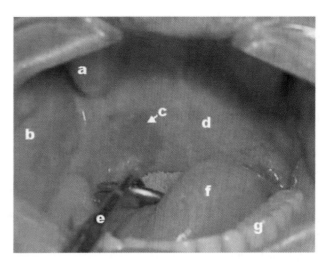

Figure 44.2—Erythroplakia in a 72-yr-old man with a history of cigar smoking and alcohol abuse. Lesion confirmed by biopsy to be invasive squamous cell carcinoma, poorly differentiated.
Key: a = right posterior maxillary alveolar ridge; b = inner aspect of right cheek; c = erythroplakia; d = soft palate; e = tongue retractor; f = tongue dorsum; g = mandibular denture

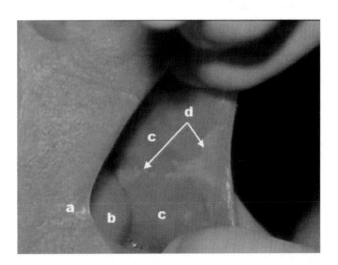

Figure 44.3—Leukoplakia in a 66-yr-old man with a history of smoking. Lesion confirmed by biopsy to be carcinoma in situ.
Key: a = right lip commissure; b = tongue; c = inner aspect of left cheek; d = leukoplakia

white Americans is 80% and in black Americans is 69%, but survival rates decline with nodal involvement (41% and 30%, respectively) and with distant metastases (18% and 12%). A thorough oral cancer screening, which can be completed in <2 minutes, consists of a head and neck nodal assessment followed by inspection of the oral cavity using gauze to retract the tongue and tongue blades to enhance visualization of the cheeks, lips, and vestibules. Although oral cancer screening is easy to learn, straightforward to perform, requires minimal instrumentation, and causes no discomfort to the patient,

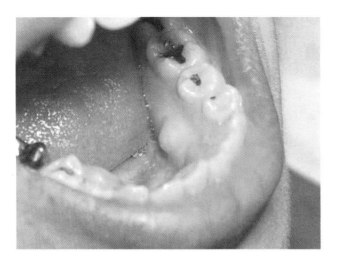

Figure 44.4—Mandibular torus

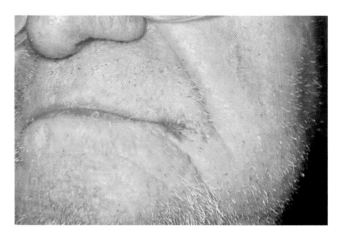

Figure 44.5—Angular cheilitis [7]

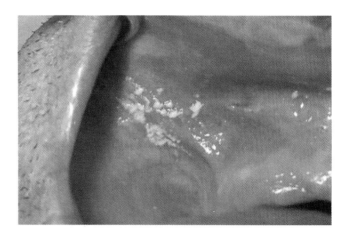

Figure 44.6—Thrush

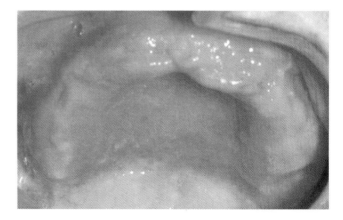

Figure 44.7—Denture stomatitis due to a maxillary complete (ie, replacing all the teeth of the upper jaw) denture

few older smokers receive oral evaluations as part of the routine physical examination.

The treatment of localized oral squamous cell carcinoma is generally surgical, although large but localized tumors can be managed with radioactive implants. More extensive disease necessitates surgery followed by beam irradiation. Concern over the deleterious adverse effects of irradiation (described in the preceding section) has led to the development of techniques that seek to limit destruction of healthy tissues surrounding a tumor. Radiation alone has been used to shrink inoperable tumors. Newer protocols combine surgery and chemotherapy with the goal of a cure.

Certainly not every oral lesion is malignant, but most clinicians have not been trained to distinguish among different oral lesions or even normal oral anatomic structures so a brief overview is provided here. Exostoses can form on either or both sides of the palatal suture at the crest of the roof of the mouth in about 20% of the population. Termed "torus" (plural "tori"), these also are commonly found on the medial aspects of the mandible instead or as well (Figure 44.4). Tori can grow slowly throughout adulthood and sometimes reach dimensions that can predispose to trauma from food and impede swallowing.

The parotid ducts enter the mouth under small flaps of tissue termed Stenson's papillae, which are located lateral to the maxillary second molars. These can be distinguished from pathologic polypoid structures by applying gentle pressure to the preauricular area—saliva will be excreted only if the structure is Stenson's papilla.

The dorsum of the tongue in some individuals displays irregular patterns of hyperkeratotic and denuded reddened areas lacking lingual papillae. This presentation is variously termed geographic tongue (because the pattern looks map-like) and migratory

glossitis (because the patterns change over time) and is no basis for concern.

Candidiasis presents as diffusely erythematous mucositis, cracking at the corners of the mouth (angular cheilitis [Figure 44.5]), curd-like white patches (thrush [Figure 44.6]), or erythema in denture-bearing areas (denture stomatitis [Figure 44.7]); it can be wholly asymptomatic or result in

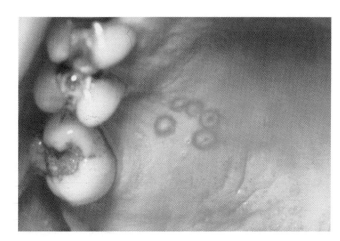

Figure 44.8—Early lesions of herpes simplex, right palate

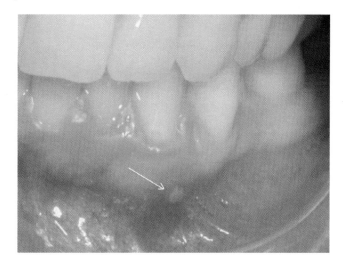

Figure 44.9—Aphthous ulcer

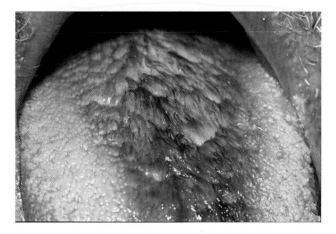

Figure 44.10—Black hairy tongue

taste dysfunction, burning, itching, and pain. Older adults are particularly susceptible to candidiasis because of denture use, salivary hypofunction, the prevalence of diabetes mellitus, and the use of antibiotics for pulmonary and urologic diseases. Use of inhaled corticosteroids places oropharyngeal struc-

tures in the path of the spray, increasing risk of candidal colonization. Management of candidiasis involves first excluding any immunopathic cause for the disease, followed by administering topical or systemic antifungal agents and optimizing oral and denture hygiene.

Herpes simplex is a virus that resides preferentially in the trigeminal ganglion and periodically causes intraoral outbreaks. These outbreaks are limited to the hyperkeratotic areas of the palate (Figure 44.8) and to the gingival and extraoral aspects of the lips. They begin as clusters of small, circular, red-rimmed yellowish blisters that burst and coalesce into irregular denuded lesions. They are highly contagious until healed. Herpes can be readily distinguished from another episodic, painful oral outbreak, aphthous ulcer (Figure 44.9), in that the latter tend to appear as isolated lesions and form only on the parakeratinized tissues of the mouth (ie, inner aspects of the cheeks and lips, floor of the mouth, and lateral border of the tongue).

An idiopathic disruption of the desquamation of tongue filiform papillae (normally about 1 mm long), which seems to become more prevalent with advancing age, results in elongation of the papillae (to ≥3 mm) and the appearance of a "hairy tongue." This condition is prone to staining from a variety of foods (eg, tea, coffee), from tobacco use, and from medications (eg, bismuth). The condition can also serve as a substrate for bacterial and/or fungal growth. Any of these, all of which are exacerbated by salivary hypofunction, can confer on the tongue notable colorations (eg, "black hairy tongue" [Figure 44.10]), but none is associated with symptoms.

Burning mouth syndrome is a chronic orofacial pain disorder usually without other clinical signs. It typically affects women ≥50 yr old, particularly in Asian Americans and Native Americans. The pain most commonly affects the lips, tongue, and palate. Multiple causes have been suggested, including xerostomia, denture use, candidiasis, nutritional deficiencies, and psychiatric disorders. Treatment is symptomatic and empirical.

CHEMOSENSORY PERCEPTION

Olfactory function declines with age. A decreased ability to identify odors and to rank their intensities affects both older men (to the greater extent) and women. Several medications have been implicated in olfactory dysfunction, as has Alzheimer's disease, among other disorders common among older adults. Impaired olfaction in older adults has been anecdotally implicated as a risk factor for eating spoiled food or failing to notice gas leaks or domestic fires.

Taste perception changes with aging. The subjective perception of saltiness and sweetness blunts with

Table 44.2—Medications That Interfere With Gustation (Taste) and Olfaction (Smell)

Gustation[a]

Acyclovir	Enalapril	Pentoxifylline
Allopurinol	Ethacrynic acid	Phenytoin
Amiloride	Ethambutol	Procainamide
Amitriptyline	Fenoprofen	Prochlorperazine
Amphotericin B	Gemfibrozil	Promethazine
Ampicillin	Hydrochlorothiazide	Propafenone
Baclofen	Imipramine	Propranolol
Buspirone	Labetalol	Ritonavir
Captopril	Levamisole	Saquinavir
Chlorpheniramine	Lomefloxacin	Sulfamethoxazole
Desipramine	Mexiletine	Sulindac
Doxepin	Nabumetone	Terfenadine
Dexamethasone	Nelfinavir	Tetracyclines
Diclofenac	Ofloxacin	Trifluoperazine
Dicyclomine	Nifedipine	Zidovudine
Diltiazem	Pentamidine	

Olfaction[b]

Amitriptyline	Enalapril	Pentamidine
Amphetamine	Flunisolide	Pirbuterol
Beclomethasone dipropionate	Flurbiprofen	Propafenone
Cocaine	Hydromorphone	Tocainide
Codeine	Levamisole	Zalcitabine
Dexamethasone	Morphine	

[a] Gustation: source lists >250 agents reported to disturb the sense of taste; agents listed are limited to those for which taste disturbance was determined objectively through threshold or intensity scaling or both, using one or more standardized solutions.

[b] Olfaction: source lists >40 agents reported to disturb the sense of smell; agents listed are limited to those for which olfactory disturbance was determined objectively through experiment or clinical trial.

SOURCE: Data from Schiffman SS, Zervakis J. Taste and smell perception in the elderly: effect of medications and disease. *Adv Food Nutr Res.* 2002;44:247–346.

---

advancing age. This change potentially has clinical significance, possibly playing a role in a person's tendency to oversalt foods or crave sweets.

Complaints of taste and smell dysfunction are common among older adults. Often the complaint derives from medication use, but other causes are possible (Table 44.2 and Table 44.3). Some medications may have no primary effect on taste but reduce saliva flow and lead to impaired taste perception. The sense of "taste" can actually be more accurately termed "flavor," ie, the full range of sensations that accompany eating, including temperature, texture, sound, and smell in addition to the perception of sweet, salt, sour, and bitter. Older adults are prone to impaired flavor perception because of changes in olfaction and oral stereognosis, salivary hypofunction, and the presence of dentures, which present physical

Table 44.3—Nonpharmacologic Causes of Taste and Smell Dysfunction in Older Adults

Gustatory dysfunction

Oral causes:
Burning mouth syndrome
Candidiasis
Laceration
Malignancy
Salivary hypofunction
Therapeutic irradiation of head
Thermal or chemical burn

Other causes:
Alzheimer's disease, other neurodegenerative disorders
CNS tumor
Endocrinopathies (eg, diabetes mellitus, Cushing's syndrome, adrenocortical insufficiency, hypothyroidism)
Head trauma
Nutritional deficiencies (vitamin B_{12}, zinc)
Psychiatric disorder
Stroke

Olfactory dysfunction

Upper aerodigestive and respiratory causes:
Dental infection
Periodontal disease
Poor oral hygiene, including poor denture hygiene
Sinusitis
Tobacco smoking or use of nasal snuff
Tumor of airway or sinus
Upper respiratory infection (bacterial or viral)

Other causes:
Alzheimer's disease, other neurodegenerative disorders
CNS tumor
Exposure to volatile or particulate toxins
Head trauma
Nutritional deficiencies (niacin, zinc)
Psychiatric disorder
Stroke

---

and thermal barriers. Flavor enhancement strategies have had positive effects on both food preference and caloric intake among frail older adults.

COMMON MEDICAL CONSIDERATIONS IN DENTAL TREATMENT OF OLDER ADULTS

The mouth contains about 10^{11}–10^{13} microorganisms, and the rich vascular supply beneath the relatively delicate mucosal covering predisposes to episodes of orally seeded bacteremia. Approximately one-third of the reported cases of infective endocarditis are caused by organisms normally found only in the mouth. Case reports of prosthetic implants infected by organisms originating in infected oral tissues have for years compelled clinicians and dentists to administer antibiotics prophylactically before invasive dental care for patients with such history. However, the recommendations from the American Heart Association in 2007 reflect that tooth brushing and eating in the presence of gingival inflammation are recognized to present, over time, as much as or a greater source of bacteremia than dental care, and that there is growing concern that widespread, short-term antibiotic treatment promotes the emergence of drug-resistant strains of microorganisms. Prophylactic coverage is now recommended only in specific high-risk situations (Table 58.4 and Table 58.5). While those recommendations are directed at preventing infective endocarditis, bacteremia-induced infections of prosthetic implants (such as joint arthroplasties, stents, vascular patches, and shunts) are less common than endocarditis, and the link between their occurrence and dental disease far more tenuous. As such, the case for antibiotic coverage in such situations is also less robust and should be the exception rather than the rule.

Because of the rich vascular supply of the head and neck, invasive dental treatment of a patient on anticoagulants caries particular risk of prolonged bleeding. Generally, if the INR is ≤3.5, the risk of uncontrolled oral hemorrhage is minimized and outweighed by the protective effects of anticoagulation (SOE=B).

The risk of precipitating a hypertensive episode or an ischemic cardiac event in a susceptible patient due to accidental intravascular injection of epinephrine as a part of dental care is quite remote and should not in general be of concern. It is undeniable that the common forms of injectable local anesthetic solutions used by dentists contain some vasoconstricting agent to prolong the anesthetic effect. In general, however, the amount of endogenous epinephrine that might be secreted in response to pain induced by dental treatment (due to inadequate anesthesia) is likely far greater than would be introduced by dental personnel.

REFERENCES

■ Chia-Hui Chen C. The Kayser-Jones Brief Oral Health Status Examination (BOHSE). *Try This: Best Practices in Nursing Care to Older Adults.* 2007;(18). Available at http://consultgerirn.org/uploads/File/trythis/try_this_18.pdf

■ Gil-Montoya JA, de Mello AL, Cardena CB, et al. Oral health protocol for the dependent institutionalized elderly. *Geriatr Nurs.* 2006;27(2):95–101.

■ Scannapieco FA. Pneumonia in nonambulatory patients. The role of oral bacteria and oral hygiene. *J Am Dent Assoc.* 2006;137 Suppl:21S–25S.

■ Schiffman SS, Sattely-Miller EA, Taylor EL, et al. Combination of flavor enhancement and chemosensory education improves nutritional status in older cancer patients. *J Nutr Health Aging.* 2007;11:439–454.

■ Soell M, Hassan M, Miliauskaite A, et al. The oral cavity of elderly patients in diabetes. *Diab Metab.* 2007;33 Suppl 1:S10–S18.

CHAPTER 45—RESPIRATORY DISEASES AND DISORDERS

KEY POINTS

■ With age, forced vital capacity (FVC), forced expiratory volume in 1 second (FEV_1), and PaO_2 all decrease, while the A-a gradient increases.

■ Clinically significant dyspnea is often under-reported and unrecognized in older adults.

■ 5%–10% of people ≥65 yr old meet the criteria for asthma.

■ Smoking cessation will slow the decline in lung function at any age.

■ COPD is the fourth leading cause of death in older adults. Pharmacologic treatment of COPD chiefly consists of inhaled β-agonists and steroids.

AGE-RELATED PULMONARY CHANGES

Studies of age-specific changes in pulmonary function are limited by common, important comorbidities experienced by older adults, which include smoking-related diseases, occupational and industrial exposures, and other significant organ dysfunction such as heart failure, deconditioning, or malignancies. These limitations notwithstanding, decrements in various aspects of pulmonary function occur with aging.

Because of changes in connective tissue, the size of the airways is reduced and the alveolar sacs become shallow. Chest wall compliance is reduced as a consequence of kyphoscoliosis, calcification of the costal cartilage, and arthritic changes in the costovertebral joints. Sarcopenia results in intercostal muscle atrophy, and diaphragmatic strength is reduced by 25%. These processes result in a decline of

FVC and FEV_1 of 25–30 mL/yr in nonsmokers and approximately double that (60–70 mL/yr) in smokers ≥ 65 yr old. The normal A-a gradient increases with age and can be approximated by the following formula: (age / 4) + 4. The PaO_2 decreases with age and can be approximated by the following equation: $PaO_2 = 110 - (0.4 \times age)$.

COMMON RESPIRATORY SYMPTOMS AND COMPLAINTS

There is a common misperception that older adults tend to overestimate or exaggerate respiratory symptoms; however, the opposite is more often true. For example, many older adults and their physicians tend to underestimate the importance of dyspnea, which may go undiagnosed until disease is advanced. This is partly because dyspnea is blamed on deconditioning and age. Older adults often adjust their activity level to compensate for insidiously shrinking lung function and disabling dyspnea. Such changes in lifestyle often go unnoticed by family, the physician, and even the patient. It is not unusual to deny dyspnea because they limit activity such that the symptom does not occur. Pulmonary or cardiac disorders, or both, may underlie such modifications in lifestyle, and testing (eg, pulmonary function tests or chest radiography) can reveal major abnormalities such as asthma, emphysema, or pulmonary fibrosis. Another complicating feature of symptom recognition is that older adults often have more than one explanation for their problems. A patient may have overlapping symptoms of dyspnea, cough, and wheezing because of a combination of diseases such as asthma or emphysema, obstructive sleep apnea, heart failure, and gastroesophageal reflux.

Rhinosinusitis

There are no data to determine if either acute or chronic rhinosinusitis manifests itself any differently in older than in younger adults, so guidelines from the American Academy of Otolaryngology–Head and Neck Surgery do not advise different approaches to diagnosis or treatment based on age. Acute (<4 weeks in duration), subacute (4–12 weeks in duration), and chronic (>12 weeks in duration) rhinosinusitis are further subclassified as uncomplicated when inflammation is restricted to the nasal cavity and sinuses or complicated when inflammation extends beyond these areas (eg, soft-tissue involvement, neurologic involvement). Bacterial rhinosinusitis is associated with purulent nasal discharge and facial pain or pressure. Treatment may focus on pain relief with simple analgesics, as well as relief of nasal obstruction by saline irrigation. Antibiotics may not be prescribed for patients who have mild illness but are generally advised if symptoms persist another 7 days or if the symptoms worsen at any time. Early treatment with antibiotics in patients with mild disease has been shown to be harmful (SOE=B). In patients with clear nasal discharge, the cause of the rhinosinusitis is likely viral, and treatment should be symptomatic only. Although topical α-adrenergic decongestants may be effective, their use should be restricted in older adults, particularly those with hypertension. Chronic rhinosinusitis is treated with a variety of topical agents. A Cochrane review demonstrated that saline irrigation is more effective than placebo and offers a safe approach for many older patients. Topical nasal steroids are more effective than saline irrigation but can cause more epistaxis and local irrigation. Allergic causes of rhinosinusitis are best treated by avoidance of the inciting allergens if possible, although topical nasal steroids are often required.

Dyspnea

Dyspnea can become prominent in malignancies and end-stage lung diseases such as COPD and idiopathic pulmonary fibrosis. Importantly, the level of dyspnea is the best predictor of quality of life, yet it does not correlate with either oxygenation or pulmonary function test results. A thorough history and physical examination can help tailor both testing and empirical treatment choices. For example, in an older adult presenting with dyspnea and associated nocturnal cough, common diseases such as asthma, emphysema, allergic rhinitis with postnasal drip, and gastroesophageal reflux disease should be considered first. Minimal testing (eg, pulmonary function tests only) followed by an empiric trial directed toward the most likely cause would be a reasonable approach. In the same patient, the presence of significant weight loss or constitutional symptoms (eg, fever, night sweats) could suggest other disease, such as malignancy or tuberculosis. At times, the particular language the patient chooses to describe the dyspnea can be revealing, such as "heavy" for cardiac dysfunction or deconditioning or "tight" for angina or asthma. The most common causes of dyspnea to consider in older adults include COPD, cardiac disease, asthma, interstitial lung disease, and deconditioning.

Chronic Cough

Fortunately, most patients can be reassured that chronic cough, although particularly annoying, usually

---

has a benign cause in individuals without a history of chronic lung disease or smoking. By far, the most common causes of chronic cough are postnasal drip, asthma, and gastroesophageal reflux. These three diagnoses account for >90% of the causes identified in most series, and a reasonable approach to the treatment of chronic cough, then, is empiric treatment for these conditions (SOE=C). Not infrequently, a combination of these conditions may contribute, and treatment for multiple causes may be warranted when single therapies are ineffective. In older adults, the possibility of silent aspiration needs to be considered, especially in patients with frequent pneumonias. In these cases, a barium swallow can evaluate oropharyngeal and esophageal aspiration. Less common yet important differential diagnostic considerations of cough in older adults include medication effects (eg, ACE inhibitors), heart failure, laryngeal dysfunction, *Bordetella pertussis* infection, chronic cough after viral upper respiratory tract infection or secondary bacterial infection, recurrent aspiration, or respiratory tract abnormalities such as bronchiectasis or airway tumors. A careful history and physical examination should help direct the diagnostic evaluation or empiric treatment of cough.

Wheezing

Although asthma is a common cause of wheezing in all age groups, it is not the principal etiology in older adults, particularly if the wheezing is not associated with cough or dyspnea. Wheezing in older adults is most commonly caused by COPD or heart failure—called "cardiac asthma." Rates of heart failure rise in the older age groups, and associated pulmonary edema may present as cardiac asthma. Other common causes of wheezing to consider include postnasal drip and chronic bronchitis in older adults with a history of cough, sputum production, and tobacco use.

MAJOR PULMONARY DISEASES

Asthma

After childhood, the prevalence of asthma has a second peak after the age of 65 yr; 5%–10% of older adults meet criteria for obstruction and bronchial hyperreactivity. Asthma deaths in older adults account for >50% of asthma fatalities annually. This is likely due to reduced awareness of bronchial constriction on the part of the patient (with delays in seeking medical attention), as well as under-recognition and undertreatment on the part of clinicians. Methacholine challenge testing is a safe, effective method to identify asthma in older adults. Population studies of asthma in older adults have shown that unlike younger adults, who may need only symptomatic treatment, most older adults require continual treat-

ment programs to control their disease (SOE=B). Overall asthma management does not differ in older and younger people. Inhaled corticosteroids (or other controller drugs such as leukotriene-receptor antagonists) are the mainstay of therapy in both older and younger patients, with use of the lowest effective dosage and counsel regarding rinsing of the oropharynx to avoid thrush. Oral corticosteroids are discussed in COPD, below. The bronchodilator response to inhaled β-agonists declines with age, but β-agonists are still the mainstay as-needed reliever medication for asthma treatment. The potential for adverse events of β-agonists—eg, hypokalemia or possible QT prolongation in cardiac patients on digoxin or other medications—warrants adequate controller use by asthmatic patients to minimize their overreliance on the β-agonist. Use of long-acting β-agonists is helpful for long-term maintenance therapy and nocturnal symptoms. In older adults, theophylline is fraught with adverse events and drug interactions, and it should be considered a third-line medication to be used only once daily in the evening for severe asthma or COPD, targeting a serum level of 5–15 mg/L if tolerated.

Chronic Obstructive Pulmonary Disease

COPD affects approximately 15 million people in the United States and is the fourth most common cause of death after heart disease, cancer, and stroke. The prevalence and mortality rate from COPD is increasing, especially in older adults. Episodes of acute respiratory failure that require mechanical ventilation are associated with mortality rates ranging from 11% to 46%. The National Lung Health Education Program Executive Committee has noted that the morbidity and mortality from COPD accounts for more than $15 billion per year in U.S. medical care expenditures. COPD is a leading cause of hospitalization in the United States and accounts for 19.9% of the total hospitalizations for patients 65–75 yr old and 18.2% of these patients >75 yr old. In one study, patients >65 yr old who were admitted to an intensive care unit with COPD had a hospital mortality of 30% and a 1-yr mortality of 59%.

The diagnosis of airflow limitation is challenging in that no single item or combination of items from the history and clinical examination excludes airflow limitation. For criteria often used to make the diagnosis of COPD, see Table 45.1. FEV_1/FVC decreases with age, so using a fixed FEV_1:FVC ratio to separate normal from obstructive creates a risk of overdiagnosis of COPD in older adults. Up to one-fifth of current smokers and one-seventh of individuals >50 yr old who have never smoked can be misidentified as abnormal when a fixed cut-off is used. Current guidelines recommend against screening asympto-

Table 45.1—GOLD^a Guidelines for COPD

Key Factors for Considering a Diagnosis of COPD

Dyspnea	Progressive or worsens over time Worse with exercise Persistent (present daily) Described as "increased effort to breathe," "heaviness," "air hunger," "gasping"
Chronic cough	May be intermittent and nonproductive
Sputum production	Any pattern of chronic sputum production can indicate COPD
Risk factors	Tobacco smoke Occupational dusts and chemicals Smoke from home cooking and heating fuel

Spirometric Classification of COPD

Mild	FEV_1/FVC <70%^b FEV_1 ≥80% predicted
Moderate	FEV_1/FVC <70% 50% ≤ FEV_1 <80% predicted
Severe	FEV_1/FVC <70% 30% ≤ FEV_1 <50% predicted
Very severe	FEV_1/FVC <70% FEV_1 <30% predicted or FEV_1 <50% predicted and chronic respiratory failure

NOTE: FEV_1 = forced expiratory volume in 1 second; FVC = forced vital capacity

^a GOLD=Global Initiative for Chronic Obstructive Lung Disease

^b Using the criteria FEV_1/FVC <70% may over diagnose COPD in older, nonsmoking adults; some experts recommend using FEV_1/FVC <65% after the age of 70, because the changes seen may be related to structural changes that occur in the airways with increasing age.

matic older adults for COPD. Wheezing noted on physical examination is the most potent predictor of airflow limitation; individuals with obstructive airflow limitation are 36 times more likely to have wheezing than those without this problem. Other findings associated with an increased likelihood of airflow limitation include a barrel-shaped chest, hyperresonance on percussion, and a forced expiratory time of >9 seconds measured during the clinical bedside examination.

Smoking cessation at any age slows the decline in lung function, and aggressive cessation efforts are appropriate even in the oldest-old patient. For a commonly used approach for addressing smoking cessation with patients (The "Five As" method), see "Addictions," p 456.

The chief components of daily medication therapy in emphysema consist of a β-agonist, ipratropium bromide or tiotropium, or both in combination (Table 45.2 and Table 45.3). For more severe disease, the use of long-acting β-agonists such as salmeterol, along with a combined albuterol and ipratropium bromide metered-dose inhaler as needed, can achieve improved adherence and long-term control by reducing the number of inhalers by one (ie, the patient will have only the scheduled long-acting inhaler and the as-needed combination short-acting inhaler rather

than three inhalers). Use of inhaled corticosteroids has been associated with some improvement in lung function, airway reactivity, frequency of exacerbations and respiratory symptoms, but they have not been shown to impact the rate of decline in lung function (SOE=A). Combination therapy with inhaled corticosteroids and a long-acting β-agonist has been associated with better lung function and symptom control but without survival benefit. A landmark investigation documented that use of systemic corticosteroids (intravenous followed by oral) reduces the duration and recurrence of acute exacerbations of COPD for up to 6 mo (SOE=A). Importantly, there is no benefit to a course of systemic steroids for >14 days for acute exacerbation of COPD. For the few patients (5%–10%) who chronically use systemic corticosteroids, the risks of peptic ulcer disease, hypertension, cataracts, diabetes mellitus, osteoporosis, psychosis, seizures, poor wound healing, infections, and aseptic necrosis of the hip must be carefully considered. Appropriate preventive measures should also be taken in circumstances of prolonged use, such as using the lowest possible dosage of corticosteroids and using supplemental vitamin D, calcium, and perhaps a bisphosphonate for those at risk of osteoporosis.

Long-term oxygen therapy benefits patients who have a resting PaO_2 of ≤55 mmHg on room air (SOE=A). Use of oxygen for at least 15 hours per day improves survival, exercise tolerance, sleep, and cognitive function. Other possible beneficial interventions in older adults with emphysema include pulmonary rehabilitation via exercise training and respiratory therapy and education. Both major depressive disorder and anxiety are present in up to 40% of patients with COPD; these diagnoses should be screened for and treated appropriately. In older adults, anxiety is associated with the level of physical functioning and disability and is a major predictor of emergency department visits and hospitalization.

Paramount to the care of older adults with asthma or COPD is adequate instruction in the proper use of peak expiratory flow meters and inhalers. Neurologic, muscular, and arthritic diseases in older adults can lead to suboptimal timing and lack of coordination in the actuation of the inhaler device. Only 60% of older adults have been reported to have adequate technique with a metered-dose inhaler; this number decreases to 36% when objective criteria are used. While the use of spacers improves technique, 85% of older adults do not use the spacer when it is prescribed. Breath-activated dry-powder inhalers require less coordination but do require a certain minimal negative peak inspiratory flow for adequate drug delivery. The clinician should observe the patient actually using the inhaler.

Table 45.2—Inhaled Bronchodilators for COPD

Class	Medication	Duration (hours)	Dosage
Short-acting			
B_2-Agonist	Albuterol sulfate	4–6	2 puffs q6h
B_2-Agonist	Levalbuterol	4–6	2 puffs q6h
B_2-Agonist	Pirbuterol	4–6	2 puffs q6h
Anticholinergic	Ipratropium bromide	4–6	2 puffs q6h
Long-acting			
B_2-Agonist	Formoterol fumarate	8–12	1 puff q12h
B_2-Agonist	Salmeterol xinafoate	8–12	1 puff q12h
B_2-Agonist	Arformoterol	8–12	15 mcg nebulized q12h
Anticholinergic	Tiotropium bromide	>24	1 puff q24h

Table 45.3—COPD Therapy

Class	Treatment
Mild COPD	
FEV_1 ≥80% FEV_1/FVC <70%	Short-acting β_2-agonist when needed
Moderate COPD	
50% ≤FEV_1 <80% FEV_1/FVC <70%	Regular treatment with one or more bronchodilators[a] Long-acting bronchodilator if needed for added benefit or if ≥2 exacerbations per year Rehabilitation
Severe COPD	
30% ≤FEV_1 <50% FEV_1/FVC <70%	Regular treatment with one or more bronchodilators[a] Inhaled steroids[b] or if significant symptoms and lung function response or if ≥2 exacerbations per year Rehabilitation
Very severe COPD	
FEV_1 <30% *or* FEV_1 <50% plus chronic respiratory failure FEV_1/FVC <70%	Regular treatment with one or more bronchodilators[a] Inhaled steroids[b] or if significant symptoms and lung function response or if repeated exacerbations Treatment of complications Long-term oxygen therapy if respiratory failure
COPD exacerbation	
(increased breathlessness, wheezing, cough, and sputum of acute onset and beyond normal day-to-day variation)	Increased dosage and/or frequency of β_2-agonists with or without anticholinergics Add steroid (eg, methylprednisolone 30–40 mg/d po for 7–10 d) Add antibiotics if increased sputum with increased purulence or increased dyspnea (cover *Streptococcus pneumoniae, Heamophilus influenzae, Moraxella catarrhalis*) CBC, chest radiograph, ECG, arterial blood gas; titrate oxygen to 90% saturation and recheck arterial blood gas If two or more of severe dyspnea, respiratory rate ≥25, or PCO_2 45–60, then noninvasive positive-pressure ventilation reduces risk of ventilator use and mortality and length of hospital stay

[a] β_2-agonists, ipratropium, slow-release theophylline (caution in older adults with other conditions and taking other medications)
[b] Consider osteoporosis prophylaxis.
SOURCE: *Global Initiative for Chronic Obstructive Lung Disease (GOLD)*; 2007. www.goldcopd.org (accessed Jan 2011).

Obstructive Sleep Apnea

Sleep-related breathing disorders are very common in older adults, obstructive sleep apnea (OSA) being the most frequent. As with younger patients, OSA in older patients is more common in men. The estimated prevalence of OSA in older men ranges from 13% to 28% and in women from 4% to 20%. Age-related changes of respiratory anatomy and physiology, such as increased upper airway adipose tissue deposition and pharyngeal bony changes, may predispose older adults to sleep apnea. Body habitus as a risk factor for apnea is less important in older patients then in younger patients. OSA has been associated with cerebrovascular accidents, myocardial infarctions, and a 3-fold increase in mortality (SOE=B). Most patients with OSA remain undiagnosed and therefore without treatment of this life-threatening, yet potentially correctable disease. Treatment options include addressing upper-airway obstruction via weight loss, avoiding alcohol and sedatives, sleeping on one's side or upright, correcting metabolic disorders such as hypothyroidism, and using continuous positive airway pressure (CPAP) via a nasal mask. To increase adherence to the use of CPAP, the treatment can be ordered with "nasal pillows" to increase comfort and "ramping technique" to give a delayed rise in the applied pressure after the individual has fallen asleep. Diagnosis and treatment issues are generally the same for both young and old, and the major consideration for the clinician is a high index of suspicion and clinical recognition of this disease. See "Sleep Problems," p 272.

Idiopathic Pulmonary Fibrosis

There are >100 causes of interstitial lung diseases; however, idiopathic pulmonary fibrosis is the most common among older adults. It has a mean onset age of 55 yr and increases in prevalence with age. Pulmonary fibrosis is extremely frustrating for all involved because of its relentless progression. The median survival is 3–5 yr. The presentation is normally one of insidious dyspnea (often unrecognized because of a decrease in the activity level on the part of the patient) and cough with dry inspiratory rales on examination. Clubbing is often a prominent finding on physical examination in pulmonary fibrosis (40%–70%), as opposed to emphysema, which rarely causes clubbing (prompting a search for another disease such as occult lung cancer). Older adults often present with advanced disease because of the insidious onset of symptoms. Idiopathic pulmonary fibrosis should be considered in older adults with a restrictive ventilatory defect and/or a reduced diffusing capacity on pulmonary function testing. Chest radiographs often show reticular opacities in the mid and lower lung zones. High resolution CT scans show characteristic areas of subpleural reticulation and honeycombing.

There is no known curative therapy for idiopathic pulmonary fibrosis. Oral corticosteroids (0.5 mg/kg/d) for 3–6 mo is the most common initial therapy, yet only 10%–20% of patients respond and adverse events are often prominent. Although the current treatment options are limited, early referral to a subspecialist is warranted if the patient wishes to consider further therapeutic attempts or to enroll in a randomized controlled trial of newer pharmacologic agents. The primary care provider may initiate the evaluation by obtaining a history searching for evidence of chemical exposure, asbestosis, connective tissue syndromes, or a family history of lung diseases. Chest CT and pulmonary function tests are helpful in guiding subsequent management decisions.

Pulmonary Thromboembolism

The incidence of pulmonary thromboembolism triples between the ages of 65 and 90 yr and has a reported 10% recurrence rate within 1 yr. Age >70 yr has been independently associated with missed antemortem diagnosis. Importantly, 10%–20% of patients with documented pulmonary embolism have an entirely normal blood-gas profile (ie, normal PaO_2 and normal A-a gradient for age). Age-specific risk factors for pulmonary thromboembolism include hypercoagulability due to increases in fibrinogen, activated protein-C resistance due to factor-V Leiden gene mutation, malignancy, stasis (decreased mobility due to stroke, heart failure, or arthritis), or vessel injury (due to trauma or varicosities). The diagnostic evaluation is not different for young and older patients. Anticoagulants are central to therapy, and their use is generally guided by the same principles in patients of any age. Because of lessened cardiopulmonary reserve in older patients, achieving therapeutic levels of heparin quickly may be even more important to avoid major adverse hemodynamic or oxygenation defects. The trend toward increased use of low-molecular-weight heparin preparations for outpatients, while achieving anticoagulation with warfarin, is supported by large, well-designed randomized controlled trials (SOE=A). There should be an overlap of approximately 1–3 days between heparinization and adequate warfarin therapy with an INR target of 2–3. Long-term anticoagulation (≥6 mo) is preferred to shorter term (eg, 3 mo), unless there are increased risks of bleeding. Indeed, patients with multiple ongoing risk factors for pulmonary thromboembolic disease are to be considered for anticoagulation therapy for up to 2 yr or longer. Recurrent pulmonary thromboembolism is usually treated with lifelong anticoagulation therapy.

INTENSIVE CARE OF THE CRITICALLY ILL

See "Hospital Care," p 119.

ACOVE-3* Quality Indicators Pertaining to Respiratory Diseases and Disorders

Chronic Obstructive Pulmonary Disease (COPD)

Evaluate respiratory symptoms

- If a vulnerable older adult presents with noncardiac exertional dyspnea, chronic cough ($\geq$6 mo), wheeze, or two or more episodes per year of bronchitis, then he or she should have spirometry.

Smoking cessation

- If a vulnerable older adult with COPD lives with others who smoke, then the patient, smoker, or both should be counseled to eliminate smoking in the home.
- If a vulnerable older adult with COPD is new to a primary care practice, then smoking status should be documented, and if the patient ever smoked, smoking status should be assessed annually.
- If a vulnerable older adult with COPD is a current smoker, then counseling to quit smoking should be documented annually.

Screening for hypoxemia

- If a vulnerable older adult with COPD does not use supplemental oxygen and has a postbronchodilator FEV_1 <50% predicted (or unknown), then oxygenation (pulse oximetry or arterial blood gas) should be assessed annually.

Rapid-acting bronchodilator

- If a vulnerable older adult has COPD (GOLD Stage >I), then he or she should be prescribed a rapid-acting bronchodilator.

Inhaler device training

- If a vulnerable older adult with COPD is given a new inhaler device, spacer, or nebulizer, then training to use the device should be documented.

Long-acting bronchodilator

- If a vulnerable older adult with moderate to very severe COPD (GOLD Stage II–IV) has symptoms not controlled by as-needed bronchodilator use or had two or more exacerbations in the previous year, then a long-acting bronchodilator should be prescribed.

Inhaled corticosteroids

- If a vulnerable older adult with severe to very severe COPD (GOLD Stage III–IV) has two or more exacerbations requiring antibiotics or oral corticosteroids in the previous year, then (in addition to a long-acting bronchodilator) inhaled steroids (if not taking oral steroids) should be prescribed.

Long-term oxygen therapy

- If a vulnerable older adult with COPD has an arterial partial pressure of oxygen <55 mmHg or an oxygen saturation <88% (not during an exacerbation), then long-term oxygen therapy should be offered.
- If a vulnerable older adult with COPD is prescribed long-term oxygen therapy, then encouragement to use it for 18 hours per day or longer (including portable oxygen) should be documented.

Related quality indicators for Respiratory Diseases and Disorders

- Goals of care, surrogate discussion, withdrawal of mechanical ventilation (see "Legal and Ethical Issues," p 23)
- Tobacco screening and counseling (see "Addictions," p 322; and "Prevention," p 61)
- Preoperative pulmonary assessment (see "Perioperative Care," p 92)
- Severe dyspnea assessment (see "Palliative Care," p 102)

*Assessing Care of Vulnerable Elders – 3rd Set. See inside front cover for explanation.

References

- Braman SS, Hanania NA. Asthma in older adults. *Clin Chest Med.* 2007;28(4):685–702.
- Nazir SA, Al-Hamed MM, Erbland ML. Chronic obstructive pulmonary disease in the older patient. *Clin Chest Med.* 2007;28(4):703–715.

CHAPTER 46—CARDIOVASCULAR DISEASES AND DISORDERS

KEY POINTS

- Increasing age is associated with extensive changes throughout the cardiovascular system that lead to a progressive decline in cardiovascular reserve capacity and substantive alterations in the clinical presentation, response to therapy, and prognosis of cardiovascular disease in older adults.

- Older adults account for the majority of patients hospitalized with acute coronary syndromes (ACS), and >80% of deaths attributable to ACS occur in patients ≥65 yr old. Although the benefits of current treatments for ACS are generally similar in older and younger patients, older patients are at increased risk of major complications from therapeutic interventions.

- Atrial fibrillation (AF), the most common sustained dysrhythmia in clinical practice, increases in prevalence with age, and >50% of all patients with AF are ≥75 yr old. Most older patients with AF respond to rate-control medications in conjunction with antithrombotic therapy, but some patients require antiarrhythmic drug therapy to maintain sinus rhythm and alleviate symptoms.

- The prevalence of peripheral arterial disease (PAD) increases progressively with age, and PAD is a potent risk marker for concomitant coronary artery disease and cerebrovascular disease. Management of patients with PAD should therefore include appropriate treatment of hypertension, dyslipidemia, diabetes, and tobacco abuse in accordance with existing practice guidelines.

EPIDEMIOLOGY

The prevalence of cardiovascular disease increases progressively with age, exceeding 80% in men and 90% in women >80 yr old (Figure 46.1). Similarly, the annual incidence of cardiovascular disease increases from 1.0% in men 45−54 yr old to 7.4% in men 85−94 yr old, and from 0.4% in women 45−54

yr old to 6.5% in women 85−94 yr old. Due to the high prevalence of cardiovascular disease at older age, adults ≥65 yr old account for 63% of hospitalizations for cardiovascular disease in the United States, including over 50% of percutaneous and surgical coronary revascularization procedures, 55% of defibrillator implantations, 80% of arterial endarterectomies, and 86% of permanent pacemaker insertions. In addition, women comprise an increasing proportion of cardiovascular hospitalizations and procedures with increasing age.

Over the past 50 yr, lifestyle changes and medical advances have led to a progressive decline in age-adjusted mortality rates from cardiovascular disease. However, cardiovascular disease remains the leading cause of death in the United States, accounting for approximately one-third of all deaths in 2004. Notably, cancer is the leading cause of death among adults up to age 75 yr, and it is only after age 75 that cardiovascular disease becomes the dominant cause of death.

EFFECTS OF AGING ON CARDIOVASCULAR FUNCTION

See Table 46.1.

CARDIOVASCULAR RISK FACTORS

Major Risk Factors

In general, the 4 major risk factors for cardiovascular disease—hypertension, diabetes mellitus, dyslipidemia, and smoking—continue to exert significant influence on cardiovascular risk in older adults. In addition, because the incidence and prevalence of cardiovascular diseases are higher in older than in younger individuals, the absolute number of cases attributable to a given risk factor tends to increase with age. Moreover, because the prevalence of hypertension, diabetes mellitus, and dyslipidemia increases with age, older adults are more likely to have multiple risk factors that act in concert with age-related cardiovascular changes to promote the development and progression of heart and vascular disorders.

Other Risk Factors

The importance of obesity as a cardiovascular risk factor among older adults, especially those >80 yr old, is less clear. Indeed, among older adults with

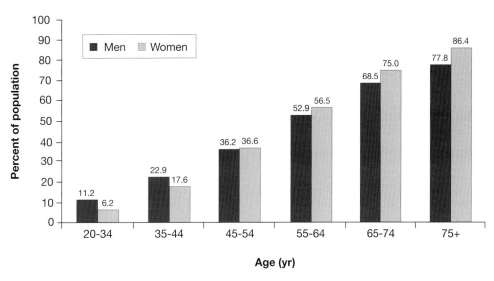

Figure 46.1—Prevalence of cardiovascular disease in Americans by age and sex (NHANES 1999–2002). Data include coronary heart disease, heart failure, stroke, and hypertension.

SOURCE: Centers for Disease Control and Prevention, National Center for Health Statistics, and National Heart, Lung and Blood Institute.

Table 46.1—Principal Effects of Aging on the Cardiovascular System

Age Effect	Clinical Implication
↑ Arterial stiffness	↑ Afterload and systolic blood pressure
↓ Myocardial relaxation and compliance	↑ Risk of diastolic heart failure and atrial fibrillation
Impaired responsiveness to β-adrenergic stimulation	↓ Maximal cardiac output; impaired thermoregulation
↓ Sinus node function and conduction velocity in the atrioventricular node and infranodal conduction system	↑ Risk of sick sinus syndrome, left anterior fascicular block, and bundle branch block
Impaired endothelium-dependent vasodilation	↑ Demand ischemia and risk of coronary artery disease and peripheral arterial disease
↓ Baroreceptor responsiveness	↑ Risk of orthostatic hypotension
↓ Exercise response (↓ maximal heart rate, maximal cardiac output, Vo$_2$ max, coronary blood flow, peripheral vasodilation)	↓ Exercise capacity and ↑ cardiac complications (ischemia, heart failure, shock, arrhythmias, death) with illness

CAD, heart failure, or renal insufficiency, there is evidence that being overweight or mildly obese (ie, body mass index [BMI] 25−35 kg/m^2) exerts a favorable effect on prognosis, while being underweight (BMI <20 kg/m^2) confers the highest mortality risk (SOE=B).

Increased levels of the inflammatory marker C-reactive protein (CRP) are associated with increased risk of incident CAD events and cardiovascular death in older adults, but the clinical utility of CRP in guiding management is undefined and routine measurement of CRP is not currently recommended. Similarly, although increased levels of fibrinogen, D-dimer, and plasmin-antiplasmin complex have been associated with increased risk of myocardial infarction in older adults, use of these markers to identify patients at increased risk is not recommended.

The value of quantitation of coronary artery calcium content by CT scanning is controversial and evolving. Coronary artery calcium scores increase with age, while the correlation of calcium scores with the severity of clinically significant coronary artery stenoses declines with age. Nonetheless, calcium scores ≥100 (Agatston method) are associated with increased risk of incident coronary events in older adults, and higher scores are associated with progressively higher risk. However, the value of routine CT scans to screen for CAD, even in patients with multiple risk factors, remains to be defined.

In the Cardiovascular Health Study, several subclinical markers of cardiovascular disease were found to identify individuals at increased risk of subsequent cardiovascular events. These included increased carotid artery intima-media thickness assessed by carotid ultrasonography, increased left ventricular mass by echocardiography, borderline or decreased left ventricular ejection fraction, and decreased ankle-arm index (the ratio of leg-to-arm systolic blood pressure). As with CT scanning, the clinical use and cost-effectiveness of these measures require further study, but in patients with diabetes or multiple other risk factors, the presence of any of these markers may identify patients likely to benefit from more aggressive management (SOE=C).

CORONARY ARTERY DISEASE

Epidemiology

Autopsy studies indicate that up to 70% of adults ≥70 yr old have significant CAD, defined as ≥50% obstruction of one or more coronary arteries. The prevalence of clinical CAD increases with age in both men and women, while the incidence of angina pectoris peaks between the ages of 65 and 84 and decreases modestly thereafter. Of an estimated 1.2 million fatal and nonfatal myocardial infarctions (MIs) occurring annually in the United States (excluding silent MIs), two-thirds are in adults ≥65 yr old, including 44% in those ≥75 yr old. In addition, the proportion of MIs occurring in women increases from 26% among those 45−64 yr old, to 35% in those 65−74 yr old, and to 55% in those ≥75 yr old. Mortality after acute MI increases exponentially with age, with >80% of MI deaths occurring in adults ≥65 yr old, and approximately 60% occurring among those ≥75 yr old.

ACUTE CORONARY SYNDROMES

The acute coronary syndromes (ACS) comprise unstable angina, non-ST-elevation MI (NSTEMI), and ST-elevation MI (STEMI). Unstable angina and NSTEMI are often considered together because they are pathophysiologically similar and clinically difficult to distinguish at the time of presentation, pending analysis of cardiac biomarker proteins (ie, troponin or creatine phosphokinase).

Presentation

The proportion of patients with ACS who present with chest pain declines with age, especially after age 80, and shortness of breath is the most common initial symptom in patients >80−85 yr old. In addition, older ACS patients are more likely than younger patients to present with altered mental status, confusion, dizziness, or syncope, and the prevalence of these symptoms approaches 20% among patients ≥85 yr old. The time from onset of symptoms to initial presentation at a medical facility also tends to be longer in older patients, in part due to the decreased prevalence of chest pain, although other factors likely contribute to delays in presentation.

The initial ECG is more likely to be nondiagnostic of ACS in older than in younger patients due to the higher prevalence of prior MI, conduction abnormalities (especially left bundle branch block), left ventricular hypertrophy, and paced rhythm. In addition, the proportion of ACS associated with ST elevation declines with age, further reducing the diagnostic accuracy of the ECG. Importantly, the combination of presentation delays, altered symptomatology, and nondiagnostic ECGs often results in substantial delays to initiation of treatment, thereby limiting the potential benefits of current therapies and contributing to higher complication rates and worse outcomes.

Therapy

All patients with suspected ACS should immediately receive aspirin 160−325 mg regardless of age (SOE=A). Oxygen should be administered to maintain an arterial oxygen saturation of at least 92%. Patients with ongoing chest discomfort should receive intravenous nitroglycerin initially, followed by intravenous morphine if nitroglycerin is ineffective. Patients with STEMI should also receive oral metoprolol or atenolol in the absence of contraindications (ie, heart rate <45−50 beats per minute, systolic blood pressure <100 mmHg, advanced heart block, moderate or severe heart failure, active bronchospasm). An ACE inhibitor should be administered to hemodynamically stable patients with adequate renal function (estimated creatinine clearance ≥30 mL/min), especially those with left ventricular (LV) systolic dysfunction and/or clinical heart failure (SOE=A). An angiotensin-receptor blocker (ARB) may be substituted in patients with known intolerance to ACE inhibitors due to cough. Early administration of high-dose statin therapy (eg, atorvastatin 80 mg) has been associated with improved outcomes in some but not all studies, and some experts recommend its routine use; data in patients >75−80 yr old are, however, very limited (SOE=C). In patients with diabetes, glucose control should be optimized.

The role of adjunctive antithrombotic therapy (ie, in addition to aspirin) in patients with ACS continues to evolve. In general, low-molecular-weight heparins (enoxaparin, dalteparin) have been associated with more favorable outcomes than intravenous unfractionated heparin (SOE=B), including in older adults, but appropriate dosage adjustment for renal function is essential to minimize the risk of bleeding. Fondaparinux, a factor Xa inhibitor, and bivalirudin, a direct thrombin inhibitor, have been associated with improved clinical outcomes and fewer major bleeding complications than either unfractionated or low-molecular-weight heparin, with similar benefits in younger and older patients (SOE=A). Fondaparinux[OL] is not currently approved for treatment of ACS in the United States, and it is contraindicated in patients with creatinine clearance <30 mL/min and in individuals weighing <50 kg. Dosage reduction is also required in patients >75 yr old because of reduced clearance. Bivalirudin is currently approved only for treatment of patients with ACS undergoing percutaneous coronary intervention. Dosage reduction is required in patients with impaired renal function. A loading dose of clopidogrel 300−600 mg should be given to patients undergoing early coronary angiography in whom percutaneous coronary intervention (PCI) is anticipated, but it is prudent to withhold clopidogrel in patients who may be candidates for coronary bypass surgery rather than PCI, because perioperative bleeding risks are increased for up to 5 days after even a single dose of clopidogrel. Prasugrel at a loading dose of 60 mg is an alternative to clopidogrel in patients <75 yr old. Glycoprotein IIb/IIIa inhibitors (eptifibatide, tirofiban, abciximab) reduce the risk of ischemic complications in selected patients with ACS, but the value of routine use of these agents in older adults receiving aspirin, clopidogrel (or prasugrel), and heparin is uncertain while the risk of bleeding is increased; therefore, judicious use of these agents is warranted.

Reperfusion therapy with a fibrinolytic agent or PCI is indicated in patients presenting within 6−12 hours of onset of STEMI (or MI associated with new left bundle branch block). Fibrinolytic therapy reduces mortality in a broad range of STEMI patients <75 yr old, as well as in carefully selected patients ≥75 yr old. The risk of intracranial hemorrhage after administration of a fibrinolytic agent increases with age, especially after age 75, and is higher with fibrin-selective agents, such as tissue plasminogen activator or reteplase, than with the nonselective agent streptokinase. PCI has been associated with superior outcomes relative to fibrinolysis in patients up to 85 yr old, provided the procedure can be performed within 90−120 minutes of the patient's arrival at the hospital.

In the setting of non-ST-elevation ACS, early PCI has been associated with improved outcomes in high-risk patients, including older adults, especially those with ongoing ischemia, extensive ECG changes, decreased LV systolic function, or hemodynamic instability (hypotension, tachycardia, heart failure) (SOE=A). In hemodynamically stable patients without active chest pain or major ECG abnormalities, an initial strategy of optimal medical therapy is appropriate.

Routine use of antiarrhythmic agents, including lidocaine and amiodarone, is not recommended in patients with ACS. Similarly, intravenous magnesium and the combination of glucose-insulin-potassium have not been shown to be beneficial. Dihydropyridine calcium channel blockers are contraindicated in patients with acute MI (SOE=A), and the use of diltiazem and verapamil should be limited to the treatment of supraventricular tachyarrhythmias (including atrial fibrillation and atrial flutter) in patients unresponsive or intolerant to β-blockers. Digoxin is not indicated for patients with ACS, including those with heart failure, and it also has limited efficacy in the treatment of atrial fibrillation.

After documented ACS, patients should be maintained on aspirin, a β-blocker, an ACE inhibitor (or ARB), and a statin in the absence of contraindications (SOE=A). Clopidogrel 75 mg (or prasugrel 10 mg for patients <75 yr old) is recommended for at least 9−12 mo for all ACS patients undergoing PCI, as well as for those with non-ST-elevation ACS in whom PCI is not performed. Patients with large anterior MIs associated with apical wall motion abnormalities should receive warfarin for 3−6 mo to maintain an INR of 2−3 to reduce the risk of mural thrombus formation and embolization. In addition, aggressive interventions should be undertaken to control all treatable cardiovascular risk factors, and appropriate recommendations about diet, exercise, and sexual activity should be conveyed before hospital discharge. Whenever feasible, patients should be referred to a structured cardiac rehabilitation program, because such programs have been associated with improved functional, emotional, behavioral, and clinical outcomes, including 25%−30% reduction in mortality, and the beneficial effects are at least as great in older as in younger patients (SOE=A).

CHRONIC CORONARY ARTERY DISEASE

Presentation and Diagnosis

As with ACS, older patients with chronic CAD are more likely than younger patients to present with exertional fatigue or shortness of breath rather than classical angina pectoris. In addition, older patients tend to present later in the course of disease, in part because more sedentary lifestyles result in delays in symptom onset or reduced symptom severity. Coronary angiographic studies and autopsy series indicate that older patients tend to have more severe and diffuse CAD, including more triple-vessel and left main CAD, as well as higher prevalence of prior MI and associated LV dysfunction.

The diagnosis of CAD is similar in older and younger adults, except that older adults have, on average, a higher pretest likelihood of having significant coronary obstructions. As a result, false-positive rates on stress tests tend to be lower in older adults, while false-negative rates tend to be higher. Diminished exercise capacity can also contribute to higher false-negative rates on exercise stress tests (but not pharmacologic stress tests) in older patients.

In most patients with stable symptoms likely to be due to coronary ischemia, a stress test is the initial diagnostic test of choice. When feasible, an exercise test is preferable to a pharmacologic test because it is more physiologic and provides additional information about exercise tolerance and the hemodynamic response to exercise not afforded by pharmacologic testing. In patients unable to exercise due to poor physical conditioning or comorbid illness (especially orthopedic or neurologic disorders), pharmacologic stress tests such as dobutamine echocardiography or adenosine thallium provide equivalent diagnostic sensitivity and specificity relative to exercise tests.

In patients with accelerating symptoms or a markedly abnormal stress test in whom coronary revascularization is a suitable therapeutic option, coronary angiography provides definitive information about the precise location and severity of coronary stenoses. Although the risks of coronary angiography increase slightly with age, in experienced centers the procedure can be performed with very low risk of major complications (<2% combined risk of all major complications, including death), even in patients of very advanced age (ie, nonagenarians and beyond).

Alternative approaches to the diagnosis of CAD include coronary artery calcium scores, CT coronary angiography, MRI scans, contrast echocardiography, and ambulatory ST-segment monitors. Although some of these techniques hold considerable promise and may eventually supplant stress testing and/or coronary angiography in selected situations, none is recommended for routine use at the time of this writing.

Medical Therapy

Control of risk factors is the foundation for reducing CAD progression in patients of all ages. Diabetes, hypertension, and lipid abnormalities should be treated in accordance with published guidelines. If hypertension is present, the blood pressure should be lowered to <140/90 mmHg. The target LDL-cholesterol level in all patients with established CAD is <100 mg/dL, and a goal of <70 mg/dL is a reasonable option in very high-risk patients, especially those with concomitant diabetes (SOE=A). Individuals who smoke should be strongly encouraged to discontinue use of all tobacco products, and behavioral and/or pharmacologic support should be routinely offered to all patients who indicate an interest in smoking cessation (see "Addictions," p 322). A diet low in saturated fat and cholesterol but high in fruits, vegetables, and whole grain products should be prescribed, and patients should be encouraged to engage in at least 30 minutes of aerobic exercise, such as walking, at least 5 days per week. Modest weight reduction is advisable in patients who

are markedly overweight (BMI $\geq$35 kg/m^2), but as noted above, the value of weight loss in older patients with lesser degrees of obesity has not been established.

All patients with chronic CAD should receive aspirin 75–325 mg/d (SOE=A). Lower dosages are associated with decreased incidence of GI intolerance and bleeding complications, but somewhat higher risk of aspirin resistance. Therefore, the optimal dosage of aspirin may vary, but 75–160 mg is appropriate in most patients. In the small percentage of patients with true aspirin allergy or intolerance, clopidogrel 75 mg/d is a reasonable alternative. Although the combination of aspirin with either clopidogrel or warfarin is somewhat more effective than aspirin alone in reducing the risk of ACS in patients with CAD, the additional expense and higher risk of major hemorrhage makes combination therapy less desirable in the absence of specific indications (eg, clopidogrel after PCI or warfarin for atrial fibrillation).

Statin therapy is indicated for all patients with CAD, even in those with untreated LDL-cholesterol levels within the desirable range, because statins have been shown to reduce mortality and major cardiac events regardless of the pretreatment LDL-cholesterol level (SOE=A). Statin doses should be sufficient to induce a 30%−40% reduction in the LDL-cholesterol level and to ensure that the target LDL-cholesterol level is achieved. Statins have been shown to improve clinical outcomes in trials involving patients up to 85 yr old, and observational studies support the use of statins for secondary prevention in older patients as well. Although altered hepatic metabolism and the use of multiple medications may place older patients at increased risk of statin-related adverse events, studies have not consistently shown an increased incidence of major statin toxicity in older individuals.

ACE inhibitors have been shown to reduce mortality and cardiovascular morbidity in patients up to 85 yr old with CAD, peripheral arterial disease, or diabetes, and routine use of ACE inhibitors is recommended for most patients with established CAD in the absence of contraindications (SOE=A). ARBs are an acceptable alternative in patients unable to tolerate ACE inhibitors due to cough. Both classes of agents should be used cautiously, if at all, in patients with estimated creatinine clearance <30 mL/min (unless receiving dialysis). Renal function and serum potassium levels should be monitored closely when starting or titrating ACE inhibitors or ARBs.

All patients with prior MI should be treated with a β-blocker in the absence of contraindications or limiting adverse events (SOE=A). In addition, β-blockers are indicated for all patients with an LV ejection fraction ≤40%, regardless of cause. β-Blockers are also the most effective anti-ischemic agents and should be considered the medications of first choice for treatment of angina pectoris or other ischemic symptoms. The dosage of β-blocker should be titrated to maintain a resting heart rate of 50 to no more than 70 beats per minute. Up to 20%−30% of patients are unable to tolerate β-blockers because of adverse events, but there is no convincing evidence that older patients experience more adverse events than younger patients.

Calcium channel blockers are effective anti-ischemic agents, either as first-line therapy in patients unable to take β-blockers, or in combination with either β-blockers or long-acting nitrates. Calcium channel blockers are relatively contraindicated in patients with heart failure or an LV ejection fraction <40%. Leg edema due to venodilation is a common adverse event of dihydropyridine calcium channel blockers, whereas constipation occurs more commonly with the nondihydropyridines, especially verapamil; both types of adverse events appear to be more common in older patients.

Long-acting nitrate preparations, such as isosorbide mononitrate, are less effective anti-ischemic agents than β-blockers or calcium channel blockers, in part because of the high rate of tolerance that develops during long-term use and the need for a daily nitrate-free interval of at least several hours. These agents are therefore best used as adjunctive therapy in patients with persistent symptoms despite β-blocker and/or calcium channel blocker treatment. Headache is the most common adverse event associated with nitrates, but most cases resolve with continued use. Occasionally patients develop hypotension, dizziness, falls, or syncope, most commonly on initiation of nitrate therapy.

Ranolazine, alone or in combination with conventional antianginal medications, reduces angina and improves exercise tolerance in patients with symptomatic CAD. In addition, the benefits of ranolazine are similar in older and younger patients. Ranolazine is generally well-tolerated, although adverse events, including constipation and dizziness, tend to be more common in patients >70 yr old than in younger patients. Ranolazine increases the QT interval slightly, but a significant proarrhythmic effect has not been reported.

Revascularization

Adults >65 yr old currently account for over half of all PCIs and coronary bypass operations performed in the United States, and both of these procedures are now routinely performed in octogenarians. In patients with chronic CAD, the principal indication for coronary revascularization is relief of symptoms to improve quality of life. In patients <70 yr old, clinical trials conducted more than two decades ago demon-

strated that coronary bypass surgery decreased mortality relative to medical therapy in patients with stenosis of the left main coronary artery, in patients with severe multivessel CAD and LV systolic dysfunction, and in other patient subgroups. The applicability of these findings to the current population of older patients is unclear, especially in light of the availability of more effective medical treatments. In addition, neither coronary bypass surgery nor PCI has been shown to reduce the risk of MI in patients with stable CAD. Conversely, complication rates, including mortality, increase with age after both PCI and coronary bypass surgery, especially among patients >80 yr old. However, despite the failure of revascularization procedures to reduce mortality or major coronary event rates in most patients with stable CAD, more recent trials have demonstrated improved symptoms and quality of life in older patients in whom aggressive medical therapy did not elicit an adequate response (SOE=A). Therefore, it is appropriate to offer revascularization on an individualized basis to older patients with persistent symptoms and impaired quality of life attributable to coronary ischemia.

Several trials have compared PCI and coronary bypass surgery in patients who are suitable candidates for either procedure. In general, long-term outcomes are similar with either approach. Short-term mortality, major complication rates (including cognitive dysfunction), hospital length of stay, and convalescence time are all increased with surgery relative to PCI, but the need for subsequent revascularization procedures and late mortality are higher after PCI; in addition, PCI is somewhat less effective in relieving symptoms (SOE=A). There is also evidence that surgery may be associated with superior outcomes in patients with diabetes. On balance, factors favoring PCI include severe CAD that is amenable to complete revascularization by PCI, increased risk of perioperative complications (eg, multiple comorbid conditions, renal insufficiency, frailty), and personal preference to avoid a major operation if possible. Factors favoring bypass surgery include more severe CAD (especially if complete revascularization by PCI is unlikely), high risk coronary anatomy (eg, left main disease or high-grade stenosis of the proximal left anterior descending artery not suitable for PCI), personal preference to minimize the need for subsequent revascularization procedures, and possibly diabetes. In all cases, the benefits and risks of all major therapeutic options—continued medical therapy, PCI, or bypass surgery—should be discussed in detail with the patient and family before making a determination as to the best course of treatment.

An additional important consideration in assessing the risk of bypass surgery is the potential for postoperative cognitive impairment and functional decline. Up to 50% of older patients undergoing bypass surgery using extracorporeal circulation experience measurable cognitive impairment after surgery (SOE=B). Although complete recovery occurs in most patients within 3−6 mo, a small percentage have persistent cognitive dysfunction. Bypass surgery performed without extracorporeal circulation (so-called "off pump" surgery) has been associated with a lower incidence of postoperative cognitive dysfunction in some but not all studies and should be considered when technically feasible. Functional decline is also common after major cardiac surgery, and return to the preoperative functional status often takes several months, with some patients experiencing persistent irreversible functional decline. To minimize functional deficits, rehabilitation should be started in the hospital as soon as possible after surgery, and patients should be referred to a structured cardiac rehabilitation program after hospital discharge whenever possible.

VALVULAR HEART DISEASE

Valvular heart diseases include aortic stenosis (AS), aortic regurgitation (AR), mitral stenosis (MS), and mitral regurgitation (MR).

Epidemiology

The prevalence of AS increases with age, approaching 15% in octogenarians, as a result of which AS is the most common valvular abnormality requiring surgery in older adults. AS in patients >70 yr old is usually due to fibrosis and calcification of a previously normal trileaflet aortic valve, rather than to a congenitally bicuspid valve or rheumatic disease, which are the most common causes of AS in middle-aged adults.

AR may be acute or chronic, and the incidence of both increases with age. Although up to 30% of older adults have some degree of AR detectable by echocardiography, in most cases it is mild or moderate in severity and only rarely is it severe enough to require surgical intervention. The most common causes of acute AR in older adults include infective endocarditis, dissection of the ascending aorta, malfunction of a previously implanted prosthetic valve (eg, dehiscence or thrombosis), and chest trauma. Chronic AR may be due to pathology of the valvular apparatus (eg, calcific or rheumatic valve disease, prior endocarditis, chronic malfunction of a valve prosthesis) or to dilatation of the aortic root resulting in poor coaptation of the valve leaflets (eg, ascending aortic root aneurysm, sinus of Valsalva aneurysm, chronic ascending aortic dissection).

Rheumatic MS is uncommon in older adults in the United States, but occasionally patients in their 70s or 80s will present with symptoms attributable to previously undiagnosed rheumatic disease. Alterna-tively, the diagnosis may be established incidentally when the patient undergoes echocardiography for another reason (eg, new-onset atrial fibrillation). More commonly, MS in older adults is due to nonrheumatic calcification of the mitral valve annulus and subvalvular apparatus, leading to a narrowed orifice and decreased excursion of the valve leaflets.

MR of at least mild severity is present in up to one-third of older adults, but only a small proportion require surgical intervention. As with AR, MR may be acute or chronic. Causes of acute MR include papillary muscle dysfunction or rupture due to acute myocardial infarction, rupture of a chordae tendinae related to myxomatous degeneration (ie, mitral valve prolapse), and destruction of the valvular apparatus due to infective endocarditis. Chronic MR may be due to myxomatous degeneration, annular dilatation associated with ischemic or nonischemic dilated cardiomyopathy, mitral annular calcification, rheumatic mitral valve disease, or prior endocarditis.

Diagnosis

The echocardiogram is the procedure of choice for diagnosing valvular disorders. For AS, it is essential for assessing disease severity, evaluating left ventricular function, and determining the presence of associated valvular lesions. Moderate AS is indicated by an aortic jet velocity (AJV) of 3−4 meters/second or an aortic valve area (AVA) of 1−1.5 cm^2; severe AS is indicated by an AJV >4 meters/second or AVA <1 cm^2. Occasionally, technical considerations or the presence of severe LV dysfunction preclude accurate echocardiographic assessment of AS severity; in these cases, right and left heart catheterization is definitive.

In patients with acute severe AR, echocardiography demonstrates a short duration AR jet with rapid deceleration and premature closure of the mitral valve. In patients with severe chronic AR, the AR jet is typically more prominent and of longer duration, often persisting throughout diastole. The left ventricle is usually dilated and there are signs of LV diastolic volume overload. In advanced cases, there may be evidence of LV systolic dysfunction, as evidenced by a reduced ejection fraction. Echocardiography is the definitive test for diagnosing MS, quantifying disease severity, and evaluating for the presence of other valvular lesions, especially MR. Severe MS is indicated by a mitral valve area <1 cm^2.

Echocardiography with Doppler assesses the cause and severity of either acute or chronic MR. Echocardiography also provides important information about left ventricular size and function, left atrial size, pulmonary artery pressure, and the presence and severity of other valvular lesions.

Clinical Features and Treatment

See Table 46.3.

Table 46.2—Cardiac Valvular Conditions

Condition	Symptoms	Findings	Treatment
Aortic stenosis (AS)	Angina; DOE; heart failure; presyncope/syncope	*Physical examination*: mid/late systolic ejection murmur radiating to carotids; S4 gallop; left ventricular heave *ECG*: LVH	*Medical*: no known effective therapy *Surgical*: AVR[a] indicated for severe AS with symptoms, bioprosthetic valves preferred in older patients
Aortic regurgitation (AR)	Can be acute or chronic; aymptomatic or minimally symptomatic in mild/moderate AR; DOE, heart failure, angina in severe AR	*Physical examination*: ↑ pulse pressure; bounding/collapsing pulses; early diastolic decrescendo murmur; systolic ejection murmur in acute severe AR *ECG*: LVH (severe chronic AR); tachycardia (acute AR) *Chest radiograph*: cardiomegaly (severe chronic AR); pulmonary congestion (acute AR)	*Medical* (less severe cases): control of hypertension and other cardiac risk factors; vasodilator therapy with nifedipine, hydralazine, or ACE inhibitor as alternative to AVR in severe chronic AR (SOE=D) *Surgical*: AVR[a] indicated for acute severe AR complicated by heart failure or hemodynamic instability and for chronic AR with onset of heart failure, LVEF <50%, or left ventricular end-systolic dimension ≥5.5 cm
Mitral stenosis (MS)	Gradually worsening DOE early; orthopnea and leg edema late; progressive decline in exercise capacity	*Physical examination*: early diastolic opening snap; low-pitched ("rumbling") diastolic murmur at apex; pulmonary hypertension; right heart failure	*Medical*: includes diuretics for volume overload and β-blockers for decreased exercise tolerance *Surgical*: balloon valvuloplasty is safe and effective, but most older adults are not good candidates due to extensive calcification and commissural fusion or concomitant mitral regurgitation; MVR[a] is effective but with 5%−15% operative mortality in older patients
Mitral regurgitation (MR)	Can be acute or chronic; marked shortness of breath, orthopnea in acute, severe MR; progressive DOE in chronic MR	*Physical examination*: pulmonary rales, tachycardia, narrow pulse pressure, S3, and short harsh systolic murmur in acute MR; holosystolic murmur radiating to axilla, S3, pulmonary hypertension, right heart failure in chronic MR	*Medical*: afterload reduction and aggressive control of hypertension *Surgical*: mitral valve repair preferred over MVR[a] (and for MVR, bioprosthetic valves[b] are preferred over mechanical in older patients); all effective but with 5%−15% operative mortality in older patients. Surgical intervention is indicated: ▪ Urgently for acute severe MR with heart failure ▪ At onset of symptoms or with LVEF of <60% or left ventricular end-systolic dimension ≥4 cm for chronic severe MR (SOE=B) ▪ When mitral valve repair is deemed likely to be successful in asymptomatic patients with chronic severe MR and an LVEF ≥60% (SOE=B) ▪ With increased pulmonary artery pressure or new-onset atrial fibrillation in patients with chronic severe MR and an LVEF ≥60% (SOE=C)

NOTE: DOE = dyspnea on exertion; LVH = left ventricular hypertrophy; LVEF = left ventricular ejection fraction; AVR = aortic valve replacement; MVR = mitral valve replacement

[a] Older adults being considered for AVR and MVR should have coronary angiography first because significant CAD is present in >50% of patients.

[b] After MVR with bioprosthetic valve, anticoagulation to maintain INR of 2−3 is recommended for 3 mo, followed by maintenance therapy with aspirin 75−100 mg/d in the absence of risk factors for thromboembolism (SOE=C).

Infective Endocarditis

See Infective Endocarditis in "Infectious Diseases," p 486.

HEART FAILURE

See "Heart Failure," p 376.

CARDIAC ARRHYTHMIAS

Epidemiology

Age-related changes in the cardiac conduction system coupled with the increasing prevalence of cardiovascular diseases at older age lead to a progressive increase in the incidence and prevalence of conduction abnormalities and heart rhythm disturbances in older adults. In a cohort of 1,372 healthy adults ≥65 yr old participating in the Baltimore Longitudinal Study on Aging (BLSA), >90% of men and women demonstrated supraventricular ectopic activity and >75% demonstrated ventricular ectopic activity on 24-hour ambulatory electrocardiographic recordings. In addition, almost 50% of men and women exhibited short runs of supraventricular tachycardia, while 13% of men and 4% of women had three or more consecutive ventricular premature depolarizations. In contrast, <0.5% of men and women in this cohort had runs of five or more beats of ventricular tachycardia. In a related study, approximately 4% of women >60 yr old developed supraventricular tachycardia (SVT) during an exercise test, whereas the proportion of men developing SVT with exercise continued to increase with age, approaching 15% in those ≥80 yr old.

In the absence of structural heart disease, the presence of supraventricular and ventricular arrhythmias had no effect on mortality or the incidence of cardiac events in BLSA participants, except that exercise-induced SVT was associated with an increased risk of developing atrial fibrillation during follow-up. Conversely, in patients with prevalent cardiovascular disease, increased ventricular (but not supraventricular) ectopy was associated with an increased risk of cardiovascular mortality. In addition, although patients with preexisting atrial fibrillation were excluded from the BLSA ambulatory monitoring study, atrial fibrillation, whether paroxysmal or persistent, has been shown to be an independent predictor of increased mortality in both men and women (SOE=A).

Age-related degenerative changes in and around the sinoatrial and atrioventricular (AV) nodes lead to an increase in bradyarrhythmias with advancing age. Although resting heart rate is unaffected by age in healthy individuals, the incidence and prevalence of sinus node dysfunction ("sick sinus syndrome") and AV-nodal block increase progressively with age. As a result, >75% of permanent pacemakers are implanted in patients ≥65 yr old, and approximately half are in patients ≥75 yr old. The prevalence of infranodal conduction disorders, including left anterior fascicular block and left and right bundle branch block, also increase with age.

Atrial Fibrillation

Atrial fibrillation (AF) is the most common sustained arrhythmia encountered in clinical practice. The incidence and prevalence of AF increase exponentially with age, such that the prevalence of AF in octogenarians is approximately 10%. Among older patients with valvular heart disease or HF, the prevalence of AF is even higher, approaching 30%. Currently, >50% of patients with AF are ≥75 yr old, and it is projected that by 2050 half of all adults with AF will be ≥80 yr old. As noted above, AF is an independent predictor of increased mortality in older adults, conferring relative risks of 1.10−1.15 in men and 1.20−1.25 in women. The proportion of strokes attributable to AF also increases exponentially with age, such that AF accounts for about 1.5% of strokes in patients 50−59 yr old but 23.5% of strokes in patients 80−89 yr old. In addition, women with AF are at increased risk of stroke relative to men, especially after age 75, and the relative risk for stroke in women compared with that in men is approximately 1.8 (ie, an 80% greater risk) in this age group.

Clinical Features

Symptoms related to AF are highly variable. Most commonly, patients experience palpitations, shortness of breath, or impaired exercise tolerance. However, some patients are entirely asymptomatic, while others present with acute pulmonary edema. Less commonly, stroke, transient ischemic attack, or an acute coronary syndrome may be the initial manifestation. Physical examination reveals an irregularly irregular rhythm with heart rates ranging from <60 beats per minute (eg, in patients with sinoatrial dysfunction and in those taking a β-blocker) to >150 beats per minute. Increased systolic blood pressure is a common but nonspecific finding. Pulmonary crackles may be present in patients with acute HF, while a heart murmur may be heard in patients with valvular heart disease. Rarely, an enlarged or nodular thyroid may be detected, or signs of deep venous thrombosis may be evident.

Diagnosis

In patients with ongoing AF, the standard 12-lead electrocardiogram is diagnostic. Additional laboratory studies should include evaluation of serum electrolytes (especially potassium and magnesium) and an assessment of thyroid function. A transthoracic echocardiogram is indicated in all patients with new-onset AF to evaluate LV size and function, left atrial size, pulmonary artery pressure, and the cardiac valves. Further evaluation in selected cases might include a chest radiograph, serial cardiac biomarker proteins to exclude acute MI, a brain natriuretic peptide level, a D-dimer level, leg venous Dopplers, and an evaluation for pulmonary embolism.

Management

The objectives of therapy for AF include relieving symptoms and minimizing the risk of thromboembolic events, particularly stroke. The principal strategies for relieving symptoms are control of heart rate and maintenance of normal sinus rhythm. Several clinical trials comparing "rate control" with "rhythm control" have consistently demonstrated that in patients who are asymptomatic or minimally symptomatic, therapy directed at controlling the heart rate with AV-nodal blocking agents such as a β-blocker, diltiazem, verapamil, or digoxin, alone or in combination, is associated with fewer hospitalizations and favorable trends in stroke and mortality rates relative to therapy directed at maintaining sinus rhythm through the use of antiarrhythmic medications (SOE=A). Based on these findings, rate control to maintain a resting heart rate of <80 beats per minute and a peak exercise heart rate of <110−120 beats per minute is the preferred treatment approach for AF patients with minimal or no symptoms.

Patients who experience significant shortness of breath, fatigue, or exercise intolerance attributable to AF may be best managed with antiarrhythmic drug therapy aimed at maintaining sinus rhythm. Selection of an antiarrhythmic agent for maintenance of sinus rhythm is challenging. Amiodarone is the most effective medication available, but it is associated with multiple adverse events, some potentially serious, and numerous drug interactions. Dronedarone, a newer agent, is somewhat less effective than amiodarone but has fewer adverse events. Dronedarone is contraindicated in patients with advanced heart failure. Sotalol is less effective than amiodarone and is contraindicated in patients with significant renal insufficiency. Flecainide and propafenone are contraindicated in patients with CAD or heart failure. Quinidine and procainamide have limited efficacy and are accompanied by relatively frequent adverse events, while disopyramide is generally contraindicated in older adults because of its anticholinergic effects. Alternatives to antiarrhythmic drug therapy for maintenance of sinus rhythm include catheter ablation of the arrhythmogenic foci, usually through pulmonary vein isolation, and the surgical

maze procedure. Pulmonary vein isolation has been associated with "cure" rates of >80% in younger patients with paroxysmal AF, but experience is limited with this procedure in older patients with persistent AF. The surgical maze procedure results in long-term maintenance of sinus rhythm in >90% of cases but requires an open heart procedure; nonetheless, it is a reasonable option in older patients with AF undergoing open heart surgery for other reasons if a surgeon with expertise in performing the procedure is available.

All older patients with paroxysmal or persistent AF require stroke prophylaxis, regardless of whether a rate-control or rhythm-control strategy is adopted. The two main options for stroke prophylaxis are warfarin titrated to maintain an INR of 2−3 and aspirin 75−325 mg/d, alone or in combination with clopidogrel. In patients with nonvalvular AF, warfarin reduces the relative risk of stroke by 65%−70%, whereas aspirin reduces the relative risk of stroke by 20%−25% (SOE=A). Conversely, warfarin is associated with a higher risk of hemorrhagic complications, and older patients may have additional risk factors for major bleeding, such as colonic polyps or GI arteriovenous malformations. In patients who are not considered candidates for warfarin, the addition of clopidogrel to aspirin reduces the risk of stroke but increases the risk of bleeding. For these reasons, the choice of warfarin versus aspirin (with or without clopidogrel) for stroke prophylaxis in older adults is often challenging. To aid in the decision-making process, it is helpful to stratify AF patients according to stroke risk, for which the $CHADS_2$ score is currently the most widely used risk-stratification scheme. $CHADS_2$ assigns 1 point for chronic heart failure, hypertension, age ≥75 yr, and diabetes, and 2 points for prior stroke or transient ischemic attack. Annual stroke risk increases from about 2% in patients with a $CHADS_2$ score of 0 to about 18% in patients with a $CHADS_2$ score of 6. In general, patients with a $CHADS_2$ score of 0 are at low risk of stroke, and the risks of warfarin outweigh the benefits; therefore, aspirin therapy is appropriate in these patients. Patients with a $CHADS_2$ score of ≥2 are at significant risk of stroke, and in most cases the beneficial effects of warfarin in reducing the risk of stroke outweigh the adverse events. In patients with a $CHADS_2$ score of 1, either warfarin or aspirin is acceptable, but warfarin is preferred in older patients in the absence of contraindications. Note that all patients ≥75 yr old have a $CHADS_2$ score of at least 1, and the vast majority will have a score of ≥2 (given the high prevalence of hypertension, diabetes, and heart failure in this age group), so that warfarin is the recommended therapy for stroke prevention in most older AF patients.

Dabigatran

Dabigatran etexilate (Pradaxa), an oral thrombin inhibitor, was approved in late 2010 to reduce the risk of stroke and systemic embolism in patients with nonvalvular atrial fibrillation. Dabigatran may be more convenient in some older patients in that there is no need to monitor the INR and there are less drug interactions than with warfarin. The approved dosage is 150 mg twice daily. In patients with severe renal impairment (creatinine clearance 15–30 mL/min), the dosage is 75 mg twice daily. The major adverse events of dabigatran are increased risk of bleeding and GI disturbances (dyspepsia, gastritis-like symptoms, hemorrhage).

Other Supraventricular Arrhythmias

Atrial flutter most often occurs in older patients with concomitant AF, and for this reason management is similar to that for AF as discussed above. Occasionally patients have incessant atrial flutter without evidence of AF. Patients with symptomatic persistent atrial flutter in whom response to medical therapy is not satisfactory should be considered for catheter ablation of the atrial flutter focus. This procedure is successful in alleviating atrial flutter in >70% of cases, although some patients subsequently develop atrial fibrillation.

Atrial tachycardia, AV-nodal reentrant tachycardia, accessory pathway-mediated SVT, and multifocal atrial tachycardia are less common than AF and atrial flutter in older patients, especially after age 75. Management is similar for older and younger patients with these arrhythmias and generally involves treatment of the underlying condition and pharmacotherapy aimed at rate control. In selected patients with recurrent symptomatic episodes, antiarrhythmic medications or catheter ablation may be considered.

Ventricular Arrhythmias

In general, frequent ventricular premature beats, ventricular couplets, and short runs of nonsustained ventricular tachycardia require no specific therapy unless highly symptomatic, in which case β-blockers are the medications of first choice. Patients with longer episodes of ventricular tachycardia associated with dizziness or syncope should be referred to a cardiologist or electrophysiologist for consideration of antiarrhythmic drug therapy or an implantable cardiac defibrillator. In addition, patients with New York Heart Association class II–III heart failure, an LV ejection fraction of ≤35%, and a life expectancy of at least 1 yr may be considered for an implantable cardiac defibrillator (see "Heart Failure," p 376), regardless of whether ventricular arrhythmias are clinically manifest.

Bradyarrhythmias

Age-related degenerative changes in the sinoatrial node, AV node, and infranodal conduction system result in a marked increase in bradyarrhythmias with increasing age. As a result, >75% of pacemaker recipients in the United States are ≥65 yr old, and half are ≥75 yr old.

Patients with mild bradycardia (resting heart rate 50–60 beats per minute) are often asymptomatic; indeed, bradycardia may protect against the development of angina pectoris in patients with CAD. Patients with more marked bradycardia (resting heart rate 40–50 beats per minute) may experience fatigue, lightheadedness (especially on standing), or reduced exercise tolerance. Presyncope or syncope may occur in patients with profound bradycardia, manifested by a heart rate of <40 beats per minute or asystolic pauses of ≥3 seconds, whether due to sinus node dysfunction or heart block within the AV node or infranodal conduction system.

Diagnostic evaluation of patients with suspected symptomatic bradycardia should start with exclusion of significant electrolyte abnormalities, measurement of the thyrotropin level to exclude hypothyroidism, and a review of the patient's medications (including OTC medications and dietary supplements). The most commonly used medications associated with bradycardia in older adults include β-blockers (including eye drops), diltiazem, verapamil, clonidine, amiodarone and other antiarrhythmic agents, and cholinesterase inhibitors. In patients with orthostatic hypotension, presyncope, or syncope, blood pressure should be measured in the supine, sitting, and standing positions. Detection of significant orthostatic hypotension should prompt a search for potentially treatable causes, including adverse events of medication(s), dehydration, or autonomic dysfunction (eg, due to diabetes, amyloidosis, Parkinsonism, or other neurologic disorders). Patients with presyncope or syncope should undergo carotid sinus massage to evaluate for carotid hypersensitivity. An abnormal response to carotid massage is defined as unequivocal reproduction of the patient's symptoms (eg, syncope), asystole ≥3 seconds, or a decrease in systolic blood pressure ≥50 mmHg in the absence of symptoms or ≥30 mmHg in association with symptoms (eg, dizziness, presyncope).

In patients with intermittent symptoms, it is essential to establish a correlation between symptoms and bradyarrhythmias before considering pacemaker implantation. If symptoms occur daily or almost every day, a 24–48 hour ambulatory monitor may be helpful for confirming or excluding bradycardia (or other heart rhythm disorder) as the proximate cause. In patients whose symptoms occur at least once a month (but not daily), a 30-day event monitor may

Table 46.3—Arrhythmic or Conduction Disturbance Indications for Permanent Pacemaker Implantation

- Symptomatic bradycardia due to sinus node dysfunction (SOE=C), second-degree atrioventricular (AV) block (SOE=B), or third-degree AV block (SOE=C)

- Asystole ≥3 seconds or any escape rate <40 beats per minute in awake patients with advanced second- or third-degree AV block, whether symptomatic or asymptomatic (SOE=B/C)

- Type II second-degree AV block (SOE=B), intermittent third-degree AV block (SOE=B), or alternating bundle branch block (SOE=C) in patients with chronic bifascicular or trifascicular block

- Recurrent syncope caused by carotid sinus stimulation associated with asystole ≥3 seconds in the absence of medications that depress the sinus node or AV conduction (SOE=C)

- Symptomatic chronotropic incompetence (inability to increase heart rate commensurate with increased activity level) (SOE=C)

- Transient or persistent second- or third-degree infranodal block associated with bundle branch block after acute myocardial infarction (SOE=B)

- Third-degree AV block after catheter ablation of the AV junction (SOE=B/C)

- Conditions requiring medications that result in symptomatic bradycardia (SOE=C)

provide a definitive diagnosis. In patients with rare (ie, less than monthly) but recurrent symptoms of a serious nature (eg, syncope with injury), an implantable loop recorder may be considered. These devices, which may be left in place for a year or longer, have been shown to increase diagnostic yield in patients with infrequent syncopal events. Head-up tilt testing may be useful in diagnosing vasovagal (neurocardiogenic) syncope in younger patients, but it is of limited use in older adults because of low specificity and a high prevalence of "false-positive" tests (see "Syncope," p 188).

Invasive electrophysiologic (EP) testing is not usually indicated for the diagnosis of syncope or bradyarrhythmias. However, in patients with recurrent unexplained syncope and a nondiagnostic noninvasive evaluation, EP testing may be helpful, especially in patients with CAD, cardiomyopathy, or with evidence of infranodal conduction system disease (eg, right or left bundle branch block). In such cases, EP testing may distinguish syncope due to bradycardia (eg, high-grade infranodal AV block) from that due to a tachyarrhythmia (eg, sustained monomorphic ventricular tachycardia), thus facilitating appropriate therapy.

Management of bradycardia includes correction of any treatable causes (eg, hypothyroidism) and elimination of potentially offending medications, if possible. In patients with confirmed symptomatic bradycardia not amenable to conservative management, permanent pacemaker implantation is warranted. For class I indications for permanent pacing,

see Table 46.4. In patients with sinus rhythm and preserved atrioventricular conduction (ie, normal PR interval and narrow QRS complex), atrial pacing is the preferred pacing mode. Patients with sinus rhythm but impaired atrioventricular conduction are often best served by dual-chamber (ie, atrial and ventricular) pacing, whereas patients with bradycardia in the context of atrial fibrillation or atrial flutter should receive a single-chamber ventricular pacemaker. Dual-chamber pacemakers (often referred to as DDD or DVI pacemakers in accordance with the universal pacemaker code) have been associated with reduced incidence of atrial fibrillation and heart failure relative to single-chamber ventricular pacemakers (VVI), but beneficial effects on mortality and stroke have not been demonstrated.

Tachy-Brady Syndrome

The tachy-brady syndrome is a common variant of "sick sinus syndrome," in which patients manifest both tachyarrhythmias (most commonly SVT or atrial fibrillation) and bradyarrhythmias, either or both of which can result in symptoms. Treatment of the tachyarrhythmias with AV-nodal blocking agents or antiarrhythmic medications often exacerbates symptoms related to bradycardia, for which pacemaker implantation may be required.

PERIPHERAL ARTERIAL DISEASE

Peripheral arterial disease (PAD) encompasses disorders of the abdominal aorta, renal and mesenteric arteries, and the iliofemoral-popliteal arterial tree. The prevalence of PAD increases with age and is higher in men than in women. In one study, the prevalence of PAD increased from 5.6% in adults 38−59 yr old, to 15.9% in adults 60−69 yr old, and to 33.8% in adults 70−82 yr old. In another study, the prevalence of symptomatic PAD in nursing-home residents with a mean age of 81 yr was 32% in men and 26% in women. In addition to age, risk factors for PAD include hypertension, diabetes, cigarette smoking, and to a lesser extent in older adults, family history.

Abdominal aortic aneurysms (AAA) are usually asymptomatic in the early stages. As the aneurysm enlarges, patients may notice abdominal pulsations or experience back pain or abdominal discomfort; less commonly, neurologic symptoms may be evident. Symptoms of leg PAD include claudication with exertion and skin changes related to chronically impaired circulation. In advanced cases, rest pain, ulcers, or dry gangrene may develop. Physical findings associated with PAD may include a pulsatile abdominal mass, bruits over the renal and/or femoral arteries, diminished or absent peripheral pulses, and skin changes ranging from hair loss and hyperpigmentation to ulcers and gangrene.

Diagnosis

It is estimated that at least 50% of patients with PAD are either asymptomatic or attribute their symptoms to another disorder (eg, arthritis); this proportion is likely even higher in older adults due to a more sedentary lifestyle. Diagnosis of PAD therefore requires a high index of suspicion and a proactive approach. Current guidelines recommend a formal history and physical examination to screen for symptoms and signs of PAD in all adults 50−69 yr old with risk factors for atherosclerosis, as well as all individuals ≥70 yr old with or without risk factors (SOE=C). Men ≥60 yr old with a family history of AAA and men 65−75 yr old who have ever smoked should undergo an abdominal ultrasound to screen for the presence of AAA (SOE=B).

Individuals with symptoms or physical findings suggestive of PAD should undergo assessment of the ankle-brachial index (ABI), the ratio of the systolic blood pressure obtained at the ankle to the blood pressure obtained over the ipsilateral brachial artery. A normal ABI is 0.9−1.3, and an ABI <0.9 has been reported to be 95% sensitive and 99% specific for leg PAD. Older patients with stiff, noncompressible arteries may have artifactually high systolic blood pressure readings using conventional blood pressure cuffs, thereby leading to falsely normal or even increased ABI. An ABI <0.40 is generally associated with critical PAD and severely impaired perfusion of the distal limb.

Patients with moderate or severe symptoms and an abnormal ABI should undergo additional evaluation if percutaneous or surgical revascularization is being contemplated. Imaging procedures that may be useful in selected cases include Doppler flow velocity measurements, ultrasonic duplex scanning, magnetic resonance angiography, and CT angiography. If revascularization is indicated based on symptoms and the results of noninvasive testing, contrast angiography is usually required before performing the revascularization procedure.

Treatment

PAD is considered a CAD risk-equivalent, indicating that patients with PAD have a ≥20% risk of experiencing a new coronary event within 10 yr (SOE=A); in patients with comorbid diabetes or established CAD, the risk is even higher. Indeed, most deaths in patients with PAD are attributable to CAD or its complications (eg, heart failure, arrhythmias) rather than to PAD per se. The importance of PAD as a risk marker for CAD provides the rationale for the proactive approach to diagnosis described above, as well as for the aggressive treatment of prevalent cardiovascular risk factors. Thus, the target LDL-cholesterol level in patients with PAD is <100 mg/dL, and blood pressure should be treated in accordance with current guidelines (see "Hypertension," p 384). Smoking cessation should be strongly encouraged, and patients who indicate an interest in quitting should be offered counseling in combination with drug therapy. See "Addictions," p 322.

In addition to risk factor management, patients with significant leg PAD should engage in a regular exercise program, preferably under supervision (SOE=A). Exercise should include walking for at least 30−45 minutes at least 3 times a week for a minimum of 12 weeks (SOE=A). Data from multiple randomized trials and at least one large meta-analysis indicate that the beneficial effects of exercise on maximal walking capacity exceed those of available pharmacotherapies. In addition, the greatest improvements in walking ability occur in individuals who exercise to near maximal pain threshold for a period of at least 6 mo.

Pharmacotherapy for PAD includes aspirin 75−325 mg to reduce the risk of MI, stroke, or vascular death (SOE=A). Clopidogrel 75 mg is more effective than aspirin in reducing cardiovascular risk in patients with PAD, but it is also considerably more expensive and there is no evidence that the combination of aspirin and clopidogrel is superior to either agent alone. For these reasons, clopidogrel is recommended as a reasonable alternative to aspirin in selected patients (SOE=A). In addition to antiplatelet therapy, routine treatment with an ACE inhibitor or ARB for the prevention of cardiovascular events is reasonable in patients with symptomatic PAD (SOE=B).

Currently, the only pharmacologic agent that has been convincingly shown to improve symptoms and walking distance in patients with claudication is the phosphodiesterase inhibitor (type III) cilostazol. At dosages of 100 mg q12h, cilostazol increases maximal walking distance by 40%−60%, and a therapeutic trial of this agent is recommended for all patients with lifestyle-limiting claudication (SOE=A). Although cilostazol is generally well tolerated, it is not recommended in patients with heart failure because of its phosphodiesterase inhibitor effects. Pentoxifylline is another agent approved for use in patients with symptomatic PAD, but the clinical effectiveness of this drug is marginal and not well established (SOE=C).

Revascularization is indicated for patients with severe symptoms attributable to PAD that have not responded to a reasonable trial of aggressive risk factor modification, exercise, and pharmacotherapy. Revascularization is also indicated for patients with critical-limb ischemia, defined as rest pain, ulceration, or gangrene; in this context, revascularization has been shown not only to improve symptoms but also to reduce the likelihood of subsequent amputation. The choice of revascularization procedure, ie, percutaneous transluminal angioplasty with or without stenting versus surgical revascularization, depends on lesion location and severity, likelihood of success, risk of major complications, and experience and technical expertise of the interventionalist and surgeon. Importantly, these two therapeutic approaches should be viewed as complementary rather than competing strategies, and the choice of revascularization procedure should be tailored to individual patient circumstances and preferences.

Indications for AAA repair include development of symptoms, rapid aneurysmal dilatation detected during serial assessments (≥ 1 cm in 1 yr), and aneurysms ≥ 5.5 cm in diameter. Patients with asymptomatic AAAs $4-5.4$ cm in diameter should undergo repeat evaluations at intervals of $6-12$ mo. The choice of open or endovascular surgical repair of AAAs is based on location of the lesion and patient comorbidities and prognosis. Open repair is favored for suprarenal AAAs and for patients with fewer comorbidities and life expectancy >10 yr, because this procedure has reduced rates of long-term leakage and rupture (SOE=B). Endovascular repair is suitable for patients with infrarenal AAAs, higher surgical risks, and lower life expectancy, because it is associated with lower perioperative complications and mortality (SOE=B).

VENOUS THROMBOEMBOLIC DISEASE

Older adults are at markedly increased risk of developing venous thromboembolic disease (VTED), including deep venous thrombosis (DVT) and pulmonary embolism (PE), due to age-related changes in the hemostatic system that predispose to thrombosis; venous stasis related to illness, injuries (eg, hip fracture), and immobility (especially hospitalization and residence in long-term care); incompetency of the superficial and deep veins, including failure of the venous valves; and the high prevalence of systemic illnesses associated with thrombogenesis (eg, heart failure, cancer, neurologic diseases). As a result, the incidence and prevalence of both DVT and PE increase exponentially with age.

Symptoms and signs of VTED are similar in older and younger patients, but it is important to recognize that most patients with DVT and/or PE are asymptomatic; therefore, a high index of suspicion for these conditions must be maintained, particularly in hospitalized patients and in residents of transitional-care facilities and nursing homes. The utility of most routine tests, including blood tests, arterial blood gases, chest radiograph, and ECG, for diagnosing VTED is quite low, and the presence of "normal" findings on each of these tests does not exclude a diagnosis of DVT or PE. The plasma D-dimer level, when performed using ELISA, has a high sensitivity for VTED but very low specificity in older adults; therefore, a normal D-dimer level in an older patient with low to intermediate clinical suspicion for VTED essentially excludes the diagnosis. Noninvasive tests for DVT include leg venous Dopplers, impedance plethysmography, and CT of the legs; rarely, contrast venography may be required to establish the diagnosis. When positive, noninvasive tests provide presumptive evidence for DVT, but negative tests do not exclude DVT or PE, especially in patients for whom the clinical suspicion is high. Similarly, ventilation/perfusion lung scanning and spiral CT of the chest are useful when the findings are unequivocally normal or abnormal. However, indeterminant ventilation/perfusion scans are common in older patients, and 10%−20% of patients with PE have false negative spiral CT scans. Therefore, in patients with high clinical suspicion for PE but negative noninvasive evaluations, pulmonary angiography should be performed as the definitive diagnostic procedure. Although clinicians are often reluctant to recommend pulmonary angiography, data from the PIOPED study indicate that this procedure is generally well tolerated by older adults, and that the risks of the procedure are lower than either empiric anticoagulation in patients without PE, or of not anticoagulating patients with PE.

Management

VTED prophylaxis with subcutaneous unfractionated or low-molecular-weight heparin or intermittent pneumatic compression of the calves is indicated in all hospitalized older adults who are not fully ambulatory, as well as in transitional care and nursing-home residents at increased risk of VTED because of disability, immobilization, or chronic medical conditions (Table 13.4). Treatment of acute DVT or PE includes intravenous unfractionated heparin to maintain the activated partial thromboplastin time in the range of $50-70$ seconds ($1.5-2$ times the control value), or full-dose low-molecular-weight heparin adjusted for weight and renal function. Warfarin should be started and heparin continued until the INR is $2-3$ with at least 24-hour overlap. Patients who are not candidates for anticoagulation should be considered for an inferior vena caval filter, recognizing that although such devices reduce the risk of PE, the risk of recurrent DVT and postphlebotic syndrome may be increased. The duration of warfarin therapy depends on the risk of recurrent VTED. In patients with a first episode of DVT or PE due to a reversible factor (eg, immobilization in the hospital), warfarin should be continued for 3 mo. In patients who develop DVT or PE in the absence of an identifiable or reversible cause, warfarin therapy should be continued for at least $6-12$ mo (SOE=B), and possibly indefinitely (SOE=C). Ultrasonography can be used to document recanalization of the vein after a limited course of anticoagulation; if no recanalization is observed, a longer course of anticoagulation should be strongly considered. Because the efficacy of warfarin for the prevention of recurrent VTED is reduced in patients with cancer, low-molecular-weight heparin is recommended for the first 3−6 mo of therapy, followed by warfarin indefinitely (or until the cancer is resolved). In patients with recurrent VTED, long-term treatment with warfarin is recommended, and placement of an inferior vena caval filter should be considered in patients with recurrent VTED despite therapeutic anticoagulation. In addition to the above measures, regular exercise, such as walking, is recommended to reduce the risk of recurrent DVT, and elastic compression stockings are recommended for up to 2 yr after an episode of DVT to reduce the risk of the postphlebotic syndrome.

For those in long-term care settings, screening for risk every 5−7 days is recommended. VTED risk factors include age >60 yr old, active cancer, acute infectious disease, catheter in a central vein, COPD, dehydration, history of VTED, having a first-degree relative with VTED, heart failure, hypercoagulable state, immobility, inflammatory bowel disease, obesity, rheumatoid arthritis, and treatment with erythroid-stimulating agents to a hemoglobin concentration of >12 g/dL, aromatase inhibitor, hormone therapy, megestrol acetate, or selective estrogen-receptor modulators. Immobility is defined as the presence of ≥1 of the following: being bedridden or bedridden except for bathroom privileges, unable to walk at least 10 feet, recent reduction in ability to walk at least 10 feet for at least 72 hours, and having a lower limb cast. For some risk factors (eg, fractures), the recommendation is for prophylaxis for 35 days. If the individual has ≥2 risk factors and is immobile, prophylaxis for 10 days or until the immobility resolves is recommended. If there is immobility but only a single risk factor, consideration should be given to pneumatic compression, and ongoing assessment continued.

ACOVE-3* QUALITY INDICATORS PERTAINING TO CARDIOVASCULAR DISEASES AND DISORDERS

Cardiovascular risk factors

■ If a vulnerable older adult has a body mass index of ≥25, then risk factors for cardiovascular disease should be assessed.

Early aspirin therapy

■ If a vulnerable older adult has an acute coronary syndrome, then he or she should be given aspirin within 1 hour of presentation.

Aspirin and clopidogrel (or prasugrel)

■ If a vulnerable older adult has non-ST-elevation acute coronary syndrome (unstable angina pectoris or non-ST-elevation acute myocardial infarction), and coronary artery bypass graft surgery is not planned, then he or she should be treated with aspirin and clopidogrel (or prasugrel if <75 yr old) for at least 3 mo.

Early β-blocker therapy

■ If a vulnerable older adult has an acute coronary syndrome, then he or she should be given a β-blocker within 12 hours.

Early ACE inhibitor therapy for MI and heart failure

■ If a vulnerable older adult has an MI (ST-segment elevation myocardial infarction [STEMI] or non-ST-elevation MI [NSTEMI]) complicated by heart failure or LVEF <40%, then he or she should be given an ACE inhibitor or angiotensin-receptor blocker (ARB) within 36 hours of presentation and advised to continue this treatment for ≥4 weeks.

Assess left ventricular function

■ If a vulnerable older adult is hospitalized with an acute MI (STEMI or NSTEMI), then an assessment of left ventricular function (LVEF) should be performed in the hospital or within 7 days of discharge.

Noninvasive stress testing

■ If a vulnerable older adult is hospitalized with acute coronary syndrome, did not undergo angiography, and does not have contraindications to revascularization, then he or she should be offered noninvasive stress testing before or within 2 weeks of discharge.

Depression screening

■ If a vulnerable older adult has a diagnosis of acute MI, then he or she should be screened for depression within 3 mo.

Reperfusion therapy

■ If a vulnerable older adult has an acute STEMI, then he or she should be offered reperfusion therapy.

Revascularization

■ If a vulnerable older adult has significant left main or three-vessel coronary artery disease and LVEF <50%, then he or she should be offered revascularization.

Cholesterol evaluation

■ All vulnerable older adults with coronary artery disease (CAD) should have a fasting cholesterol evaluation (LDL-C, HDL-C, and triglycerides) at least every 2 yr.

Medication for elevated cholesterol

■ If a vulnerable older adult with CAD has an LDL-C >100 mg/dL, then he or she should be offered cholesterol-lowering medication.

Antiplatelet therapy

- If a vulnerable older adult with CAD is not taking warfarin, then he or she should be offered daily aspirin or other antiplatelet therapy.

β-blocker therapy

- If a vulnerable older adult has had an MI (STEMI or NSTEMI), then he or she should be offered a β-blocker and advised to continue treatment for 2 yr or longer after infarction.

ACE inhibitor therapy

- If a vulnerable older adult has CAD, then he or she should be offered ACE inhibitor or ARB therapy and advised to continue the treatment indefinitely.

Warfarin therapy

- If a vulnerable older adult receives a new prescription for warfarin, then he or she should receive education about diet and drug interactions and the risk of bleeding complications, or should be referred to an anticoagulation clinic.

- If a vulnerable older adult is prescribed warfarin, then an INR should be determined within 4 days after initiation of therapy and at least every 6 weeks thereafter.

Avoid ticlopidine

- If a vulnerable older adult has had a recent stroke or MI or has peripheral arterial disease or acute coronary syndrome that will be treated medically or with a percutaneous angioplasty, and he or she requires antiplatelet therapy, then clopidogrel (or prasugrel) should be prescribed rather than ticlopidine.

Smoking cessation

- If a vulnerable older adult with CAD smokes, then there should be documentation of smoking cessation counseling annually.

Cardiac rehabilitation

- If a vulnerable older adult has had an MI (STEMI or NSTEMI) or coronary artery bypass graft surgery in the past year, then he or she should be offered cardiac rehabilitation (formal program or its components).

Estrogen and progesterone counseling

- If a female vulnerable older adult with CAD is currently taking combination estrogen and progesterone therapy, then she should be counseled about possible increased cardiovascular risk, or this therapy should be discontinued.

Anticoagulate atrial fibrillation

- If a vulnerable older adult has chronic atrial fibrillation and is at medium to high risk of stroke, then anticoagulation should be offered.
- If a vulnerable older adult has chronic atrial fibrillation, medium to high risk of stroke, and has a contraindication to anticoagulation, then antiplatelet therapy should be prescribed.
- If a vulnerable older adult is prescribed anticoagulants for atrial fibrillation, then there should be documentation that the goal for the INR is 2–3 or reason for other goal.

Related quality indicators for Cardiovascular Diseases and Disorders

- ECG for tricyclic use (see "Depression," p 504)
- Aspirin therapy and hypercholesterolemia treatment in patients with diabetes mellitus (see "Diabetes Mellitus," p 504)
- Preoperative cardiovascular risk assessment and management (see "Perioperative Care," p 92)

*Assessing Care of Vulnerable Elders – 3ʳᵈ Set. See inside front cover for explanation.

REFERENCES

- Bonow RO, Carabello BA, Chatterjee K, et al. ACC/AHA 2006 guidelines for the management of patients with valvular heart disease. *Circulation.* 2006;114(5):e84–e131.

- Coke L. Cardiac Risk Assessment of the Older Cardiovascular Patient: The Framingham Global Risk Assessment Tools. *Try This: Best Practices in Nursing Care to Older Adults.* 2010;(SP3). Available at http://consultgerirn.org/uploads/File/trythis/try_this_sp3.pdf

- Coke L. Vascular Risk Assessment of the Older Cardiovascular Patient: The Ankle-Brachial Index (ABI) *Try This: Best Practices in Nursing Care to Older Adults.* 2010;(SP4). Available at http://consultgerirn.org/uploads/File/trythis/try_this_sp4.pdf

- Fuster V, Ryden LE, Cannom DS, et al. ACC/AHA/ESC 2006 Guidelines for the management of patients with atrial fibrillation. *J Am Coll Cardiol.* 2006;48(4):854–906.

- Hirsch AT, Haskal ZJ, Hertzer NR, et al. ACC/AHA 2005 Practice guidelines for the management of patients with peripheral arterial disease (lower extremity, renal, mesenteric, and abdominal aortic). *J Am Coll Cardiol.* 2006;47(6):1239–1312.

- McLennan SN, Mathias JL, Brennan LC. Cognitive impairment predicts functional capacity in dementia-free patients with cardiovascular disease. *J Cardiovasc Nurs.* 2010;25(5):390–397.

- Zarowitz BJ, Tangalos E, Lefkovitz A, et al. Thrombotic risk and immobility in residents of long-term care facilities. *J Am Med Dir Assoc.* 2010;11(3):211–221.

CHAPTER 47—HEART FAILURE

KEY POINTS

- Heart failure (HF) is the leading cause of hospitalization in older adults and a major source of chronic disability.

- Compared with younger patients, older patients with HF are more likely to be women and more likely to have preserved left ventricular systolic function.

- ACE inhibitors, angiotensin-receptor blockers, β-blockers, and aldosterone antagonists reduce morbidity and mortality from HF with reduced ejection fraction (systolic HF). Optimal medical therapy for HF with preserved ejection fraction (diastolic HF) is undefined.

- Optimal management of HF in older patients often requires a multidisciplinary approach.

EPIDEMIOLOGY

Heart failure (HF) affects more than 5 million Americans, and >550,000 new cases are diagnosed each year. The incidence and prevalence of HF increase progressively with age, and HF is the leading cause of hospitalization and rehospitalization in older adults. The median age of patients hospitalized with HF is 75 yr, and approximately two-thirds of deaths attributable to HF occur in this age group. In addition, HF is a major cause of chronic disability and impaired quality of life in older adults, and it is a common factor contributing to loss of independence and admission to a long-term care facility. Although the incidence of HF is somewhat higher in men, women comprise slightly over half of prevalent HF cases.

ETIOLOGY AND PATHOPHYSIOLOGY

HF in older adults is often multifactorial in origin. Hypertension is the most common antecedent cardiovascular condition in both men and women with HF, and it is the principal cause of HF in 60%–70% of women. In men, 30%–40% of HF is attributable to hypertension, and a similar proportion is attributable to coronary artery disease (CAD). Other common causes of HF in older adults include valvular heart disease and nonischemic dilated cardiomyopathy. Less common causes include hypertrophic cardiomyopathy, restrictive cardiomyopathy (eg, amyloid), and pericardial disease.

The rising prevalence of HF with increasing age reflects the combination of age-related changes in cardiovascular structure and function that serve to diminish cardiovascular reserve, in conjunction with the rising prevalence of cardiovascular diseases with increasing age (especially hypertension and CAD) that predispose to HF. While up to 90% of HF patients <65 yr old have low left ventricular (LV) ejection fraction (LVEF; ie, HF with reduced ejection fraction, henceforth referred to as systolic HF), approximately 40% of men and two-thirds of women >65 yr old with HF have an LVEF ≥50% (ie, HF with preserved ejection fraction, henceforth referred to as diastolic HF). The rising prevalence of diastolic HF in older patients is due to age-associated alterations in LV diastolic function coupled with the increasing importance of hypertension as the etiologic mechanism for HF in older adults, particularly women.

CLINICAL FEATURES

As in younger patients, exertional shortness of breath, fatigue, orthopnea, and leg edema are the most common symptoms of HF in older adults. However, exertional symptoms may be less prominent in older adults because of a more sedentary lifestyle. Conversely, the prevalence of atypical symptoms increases with age, and older HF patients may present with decreased mental acuity, confusion, lethargy, irritability, anorexia, abdominal discomfort, or altered bowel function.

Classical physical findings of HF in younger patients include tachycardia, narrowed pulse pressure, increased jugular venous pressure, hepatojugular reflux, an S_3 gallop, moist pulmonary crackles, diminished breath sounds at the lung bases (due to pleural effusions), and pitting edema of the legs. However, many or even all of these findings may be absent in older HF patients, especially those with diastolic HF, in whom an S_3 gallop and signs of right-heart failure are not usually present. In addition, pulmonary crackles in older patients may be due to comorbid chronic lung disease or atelectasis, and peripheral edema may be due to hepatic or renal disease, venous insufficiency, hypoalbuminemia, or medications (especially calcium channel blockers).

In summary, the symptoms and signs of HF in older adults are often atypical and nonspecific, and it is therefore important for the clinician to maintain both a high index of suspicion and a healthy measure of skepticism when evaluating an older patient for possible HF.

DIAGNOSIS

The diagnosis of HF can usually be established on clinical grounds in patients who present with a constellation of classical symptoms and signs. Often, however, the diagnosis is uncertain, and additional supporting evidence is required.

The standard chest radiograph remains the most useful initial test for determining the presence of pulmonary congestion and pleural effusions, as well as for excluding pneumonia as a cause of shortness of breath in older adults. However, the chest radiograph may be difficult to interpret in older adults with chronic lung disease, kyphoscoliosis, or poor inspiratory effort, and the absence of pulmonary congestion on chest radiograph does not preclude a diagnosis of HF.

The ECG may show LV hypertrophy, acute ischemia or prior myocardial infarction (MI), left atrial enlargement, or atrial fibrillation—all of which predispose to the development of HF—but the ECG is not usually helpful in establishing a diagnosis of either acute or chronic HF. Similarly, although it is appropriate to obtain a CBC, routine chemistry panel, thyroid studies, a urinalysis, and in selected cases, cardiac biomarker proteins (ie, troponin, creatine kinase) in patients with suspected HF, in most cases these tests are insufficient for confirming the diagnosis.

In recent years, B-type natriuretic peptide (BNP) and its precursor N-terminal pro-BNP (nt-proBNP) have proved to be of value in establishing the presence of HF and, in particular, in distinguishing shortness of breath due to HF from that attributable to noncardiac causes. However, BNP and nt-proBNP levels increase with age, especially in women, as well as with decreasing renal function. As a result, the specificity of increased levels of these peptides decreases with age, and the clinical significance of an isolated increased BNP or nt-proBNP level in an older adult may be difficult to interpret. Despite these caveats, a BNP level <100 pg/mL in an older adult with suspected acute HF makes the diagnosis very unlikely (likelihood ratio negative approximately 0.1), whereas a BNP level ≥500 pg/mL is consistent with active HF (likelihood ratio positive approximately 6).

Once a diagnosis of HF has been established, it is important to determine the cause and to assess LV function, because these factors often affect management. In most patients with recently diagnosed HF, an echocardiogram with Doppler is indicated for the assessment of LV and right ventricular (RV) size, systolic and diastolic function, atrial size, LV and RV wall thicknesses, valve function, and the pericardium. In patients with suspected CAD who are suitable candidates for revascularization, a stress test should be performed, followed by coronary angiography if the stress test indicates severe CAD, especially in a multivessel distribution.

MANAGEMENT

The goals of HF management are to decrease symptoms and improve quality of life, reduce acute exacerbations requiring hospitalization, and increase survival. Hypertension, hyperlipidemia, and diabetes should be treated in accordance with current guidelines. Smoking cessation should be strongly encouraged and supported if indicated, and alcohol intake should be limited to no more than 2 drinks/day in men and 1 drink/day in women. NSAIDs should be avoided because they promote water and sodium retention and antagonize the effects of diuretics and renin-angiotensin system inhibitors. CAD should be treated with anti-ischemic medications and, if indicated, percutaneous or surgical revascularization. Similarly, valvular lesions should be managed in accordance with established practice guidelines. Patients should be screened for anemia and thyroid dysfunction, and appropriate therapy should be initiated if indicated.

Nonpharmacologic Therapy

Patients should be counseled to restrict dietary sodium intake to no more than 2 g/d (SOE=C). Fluid restriction is not usually necessary except in patients with advanced HF, but patients should be advised to avoid excess fluid intake (ie, the oft-quoted dictum to drink 8–10 glasses of water every day does not apply to individuals with HF, renal insufficiency, or other fluid-retaining states). Most patients with HF should also be advised to engage in regular exercise such as walking, stationary cycling, swimming, or water aerobics. Exercise duration and intensity should be adjusted to the individual patient's level of conditioning, severity of HF, and comorbidities but should be gradually increased over time, if possible, to achieve 30–60 minutes aerobic exercise most days of the week. These activities should be complemented by stretching and strengthening exercises, as well as by gait and balance exercises if indicated.

Patients should be instructed to keep an ongoing record of their daily weight. Weights should be obtained in the morning without clothes after going to the bathroom but before eating. A "dry weight"

Table 47.1— Recommended Dosages of ACE Inhibitors, Angiotensin II Receptor Blockers, and β-Blockers in Patients with Heart Failure

Agent	Starting Dosage	Target Dosage
ACE Inhibitors		
Benazepril[a]	2.5 mg/d	40 mg/d
Captopril	6.25 mg q8h	50–100 mg q8h
Enalapril	2.5 mg/d	20 mg q12h
Fosinopril	5 mg/d	40 mg/d
Lisinopril	2.5 mg/d	20–40 mg/d
Moexipril[a]	3.75 mg/d	15 mg/d
Perindopril[a]	4 mg/d	8 mg/d
Quinapril	5 mg/d	10–20 mg q12h
Ramipril	1.25 mg/d	10 mg/d
Trandolapril	1 mg/d	4 mg/d
Angiotensin II Receptor Blockers		
Candesartan	4 mg/d	32 mg/d
Eprosartan[a]	400 mg/d	400 mg q12h
Irbesartan[a]	75 mg/d	150–300 mg/d
Losartan[a]	12.5–25 mg/d	50 mg q12h
Olmesartan[a]	20 mg/d	40 mg/d
Telmisartan[a]	20 mg/d	80 mg/d
Valsartan	20–40 mg q12h	160 mg q12h
β-Blockers		
Bisoprolol[b]	1.25 mg/d	10 mg/d
Carvedilol	3.125 mg q12h	25–50 mg q12h
Carvedilol ER	10 mg/d	80 mg/d
Metoprolol XL	12.5–25 mg/d	200 mg/d

[a] Not approved for HF by the FDA

[b] Not approved for HF by the FDA but has been shown to be effective in HF

should be established (based on the home scale, not the office scale), and the patient should be instructed to contact the health care provider if the weight varies by more than 2–3 pounds above or below the dry weight. Alternatively, selected patients may be provided with detailed instructions for self-adjustment of diuretic dosages based on daily weights.

Older patients with moderate or advanced HF, multiple comorbidities, or a recent HF exacerbation requiring hospitalization may benefit from participation in a structured HF disease management program. Such programs offer enhanced education and follow-up, usually by an HF nurse specialist or multidisciplinary team, in some cases supplemented by telemonitoring devices, and have been shown to reduce hospitalizations and inpatient costs, as well as to improve quality of life in older HF patients.

Pharmacotherapy of Systolic HF

ACE inhibitors, angiotensin-receptor blockers (ARBs), and β-blockers have been shown to improve outcomes and reduce mortality in multiple large prospective trials involving a broad range of HF patients with decreased LV systolic function (SOE=A), and these agents are now considered the cornerstone of therapy for systolic HF. Although older patients, especially those with multiple comorbid conditions, have been markedly under-represented in these trials, the available evidence indicates that the beneficial effects of these agents likely extend to older patients.

For ACE inhibitors approved for the treatment of HF along with recommended initial and maintenance dosages, see Table 47.1. In general, treatment of older HF patients should be started at the lowest dosage and gradually titrated to the maintenance dosage as tolerated. Contraindications to ACE inhibitors include known intolerance to these agents, hyperkalemia (serum potassium ≥5.5 mEq/L), and severe renal insufficiency (estimated creatinine clearance <30 mL/min) in patients not currently undergoing dialysis. Common adverse events include cough in 5%–10% of patients during long-term treatment, mild worsening of renal function (often transient), hyperkalemia, hypotension, and GI distress. Renal function and potassium concentrations should be monitored closely during initiation and titration of ACE inhibitor therapy.

ARBs are indicated as an alternative to ACE inhibitors in HF patients unable to tolerate the latter class of medications because of cough, allergic reactions, or GI disturbances. Contraindications and adverse events associated with these agents are otherwise similar to those of ACE inhibitors. In particular, the incidence of renal insufficiency, hyperkalemia, and hypotension are comparable with equivalent dosages of ACE inhibitors and ARBs. Combination therapy with an ACE inhibitor and ARB is not currently recommended because of an increased incidence of adverse events in the absence of a clear clinical benefit.

β-Blockers counteract the deleterious effects of chronic activation of the adrenergic nervous system in HF patients, and β-blockers have been shown to improve ventricular function and symptoms while reducing the risk of both sudden and nonsudden cardiac death (SOE=A). As with ACE inhibitors and ARBs, treatment should be started at the lowest available dosage and gradually titrated to the maintenance dosage over several weeks (Table 47.1). Contraindications to starting β-blocker therapy include severe decompensated HF, active bronchospastic lung disease, marked bradycardia (heart rate <45–50 beats per minute), relative hypotension (systolic blood pressure <90–100 mmHg), significant atrioventricular nodal block (PR interval ≥240 msec or higher degrees of block), and known intolerance to β-blockers. Occasionally, HF symptoms will worsen on initiation or titration of a β-blocker (and patients should be warned about this possibility), but in most cases this is a transient phenomenon and the vast majority of HF patients (>80%) are able to tolerate long-term β-blocker therapy when judiciously initiated and titrated.

Diuretics are an essential component of HF therapy in most patients, and they remain the most effective agents for relief of congestion and edema. In general, the diuretic dosage should be adjusted to maintain euvolemia, manifested by the absence of pulmonary rales, an S_3 gallop, increased jugular venous pressure, hepatojugular reflux, and peripheral edema. Some clinicians recommend obtaining serial BNPs as a means of assessing volume status, with a BNP level <100–200 pg/mL indicative of optimal intravascular volume. Some patients with mild HF respond satisfactorily to a thiazide diuretic, but most require maintenance therapy with a loop diuretic, such as furosemide, bumetanide, or torsemide. Patients with advanced HF and/or concomitant renal insufficiency may be resistant to conventional dosages of loop diuretics; in these patients, the addition of metolazone at 2.5–10 mg/d is often effective, but close monitoring of electrolytes is required. The principal adverse events associated with diuretic therapy are electrolyte disturbances, including hypokalemia, hyponatremia, and hypomagnesemia; close monitoring of these electrolytes, as well as renal function, is therefore warranted. Thiamine deficiency may occur during long-term treatment with loop diuretics and can contribute to apparent diuretic resistance. Although routine monitoring of thiamine levels is not currently recommended, supplemental thiamine in the form of a multivitamin is reasonable in older patients requiring long-term therapy with a loop diuretic (SOE=D). Older patients are also at increased risk of dehydration during diuretic treatment due to attenuation of the thirst response and diminished oral fluid intake, especially during periods of illness. Therefore, clinicians should remain vigilant for possible signs of dehydration, including excess weight loss during daily weight monitoring.

The aldosterone antagonist spironolactone has been shown to reduce mortality and hospitalizations in patients with New York Heart Association (NYHA) class III–IV HF and an LVEF <30% (SOE=A), with similar benefits in older and younger patients. Likewise, the selective aldosterone antagonist eplerenone has been associated with improved outcomes in patients with recent MI complicated by HF or an LVEF <40% (SOE=A). Based on these studies, spironolactone at 12.5–25 mg/d is recommended in patients with severe LV dysfunction and persistent advanced HF symptoms despite triple-drug therapy

with an ACE inhibitor (or ARB), β-blocker, and diuretic. Spironolactone and eplerenone are contraindicated in patients with serum creatinine ≥2.5 mg/dL or serum potassium ≥5 mEq/L. Older adults are at increased risk of worsening renal function and hyperkalemia during spironolactone therapy, and frequent monitoring of electrolytes and creatinine is necessary. Up to 10% of patients develop painful gynecomastia during long-term treatment with spironolactone; this adverse event is much less frequent with eplerenone.

Digoxin improves symptoms and reduces HF hospitalizations in patients with chronic systolic HF but has no effect on mortality (SOE=B). Digoxin remains a reasonable therapeutic option in patients with persistent limiting symptoms and/or recurrent hospitalizations who have not had a satisfactory response to the measures discussed above. Retrospective analyses based on a large randomized trial suggest that the optimal digoxin concentration for improving clinical outcomes is 0.5–0.9 ng/mL, which is substantially lower than the "therapeutic range" previously reported by most clinical laboratories. Therefore, digoxin should be dosed to maintain the digoxin concentration <1 ng/mL, and a dosage of 0.125 mg/d is likely to be sufficient in most older patients with relatively preserved renal function, while a lower dosage might be indicated in patients with moderate or severe renal insufficiency. Adverse events of digoxin include nausea, visual disturbances, and cardiac arrhythmias (bradyarrhythmias as well as supraventricular and ventricular tachyarrhythmias). However, with appropriate monitoring of the serum digoxin concentration, serious digoxin toxicity is infrequent, and there is no convincing evidence that older patients are at increased risk of life-threatening digitalis intoxication. Amiodarone, quinidine, and verapamil, as well as several other medications, are associated with up to a 2-fold increase in serum digoxin concentrations, and the dosage of digoxin should be reduced by 50% in patients receiving these medications.

In a small study conducted >20 yr ago (ie, before the advent of ACE inhibitors and β-blockers for the treatment of HF), the combination of hydralazine and isosorbide dinitrate reduced mortality relative to placebo in patients with systolic HF. More recently, this combination was shown to improve outcomes in black Americans with advanced HF symptoms and severe LV systolic dysfunction, most of whom were also receiving ACE inhibitors and β-blockers (SOE=A). Based on these studies, the combination of hydralazine-nitrates is recommended for HF patients with contraindications to ACE inhibitors and ARBs (eg, severe renal insufficiency), and in black American patients with advanced HF as an adjunct to

ACE-inhibitor and β-blocker therapy. The starting dosage of hydralazine is 25–50 mg q8h, titrating to a maximal dosage of 100 mg q8h. The starting dosage of isosorbide dinitrate is 10 mg q8h, titrating to a maximal dosage of 30–40 mg q8h. Common adverse events associated with hydralazine include palpitations, nausea, and dizziness; rarely, a drug-lupus syndrome may occur during prolonged therapy at high dosage (≥300 mg/d). The most common adverse event from isosorbide dinitrate is headache; this usually resolves with continued use.

In summary, optimal treatment of systolic HF usually requires a minimum of three medications and, in some cases, up to seven. In addition, because HF in older patients almost never occurs as an isolated disease process, almost all patients are taking one or more additional medications for other coexisting illnesses. Thus, pharmacotherapy of the older HF patient is problematic from the perspective of adherence, high potential for drug interactions and adverse events, and cost. Therefore, it is essential that therapy be individualized, taking into consideration the multiple and often competing factors that influence quality of life and other desirable clinical outcomes in older adults with multiple chronic illnesses and limited life expectancy.

Pharmacotherapy of Diastolic HF

In contrast to systolic HF, few clinical trials have been directed at treatment of diastolic HF, and to date no trials have demonstrated a beneficial effect on mortality with any intervention in patients with this form of HF. However, several agents have been shown to reduce hospitalizations due to diastolic HF, including the ARB candesartan (SOE=A), the ACE inhibitor perindopril (SOE=B), and the β-blocker nebivolol (SOE=B). Digoxin also reduces hospitalizations due to HF in patients with HF and preserved LV systolic function, but at the expense of increased hospitalizations for unstable angina (SOE=B). The I-PRESERVE trial, completed in 2008, showed no effect of the ARB irbesartan on mortality, hospitalizations, or other cardiac outcomes in older adults with diastolic HF. Results for the NHLBI-sponsored TOPCAT trial, which is comparing spironolactone to placebo in patients with diastolic HF, are anticipated in late 2010 or early 2011. Based on the available evidence, optimal therapy for diastolic HF remains undefined. Current recommendations include aggressive treatment of hypertension and other risk factors, appropriate management of comorbid CAD, and maintenance of sinus rhythm or effective rate control in patients with atrial fibrillation (SOE=D). Diuretics should be used judiciously to maintain euvolemia while avoiding overdiuresis, because patients with diastolic HF are often "volume-sensitive." The addition of an ACE inhibitor or ARB, and possibly a β-blocker (especially in patients with CAD), is appropriate to reduce the risk of hospitalization, recognizing that the impact of these agents on other clinically relevant outcomes is unproved.

Device Therapy

The implantable cardiac defibrillator (ICD) has been shown to reduce mortality from sudden cardiac death in patients with systolic HF and an LVEF of ≤35%, including patients with either ischemic or nonischemic HF (SOE=A). Although few older patients were enrolled in the ICD randomized trials, subsequent observational studies indicate that the benefits of ICDs are similar in older and younger patients (SOE=B). In addition, approximately 40%–45% of ICDs in the United States are implanted in patients ≥70 yr old. Conversely, ICDs have not been shown to improve survival in patients with NYHA class I or IV HF, and there is no survival benefit within the first 12–18 mo after implantation. Also, quality of life is impaired in patients who receive one or more ICD shocks, and up to 20% of shocks are inappropriate, ie, occurring in the absence of a life-threatening tachyarrhythmia.

Based on available evidence, prophylactic ICD placement is recommended in patients with NYHA class II or III HF, an LVEF ≤35%, and a remaining life expectancy of at least 1 yr. ICD implantation should be deferred for at least 40 days after acute MI and for at least 90 days after a new diagnosis of dilated cardiomyopathy, in the latter case because LV function often improves after initiation of β-blocker and ACE inhibitor therapy.

Recognizing that HF patients >75–80 yr old have limited remaining life expectancy, especially if they have multiple comorbid illnesses or frailty, selection of older patients for ICD therapy must be individualized. Patients should be advised about the potential benefits and risks of ICD implantation, including the possibility of an adverse effect on quality of life. Although many older patients elect to forego ICD implantation after an informed discussion, those who choose to undergo the procedure should not be denied solely on the basis of age, assuming that appropriate indications for ICD therapy are present. In these patients, it is, however, appropriate to discuss circumstances under which the patient would want to have the device disabled, especially at end of life because of progressive HF or other terminal illness.

Cardiac resynchronization therapy (CRT) has been shown to improve symptoms, exercise tolerance, quality of life, and survival in selected patients with advanced systolic HF and persistent severe symptoms (NYHA class III or IV) despite conventional medical therapy (SOE=A). CRT involves placement of a biventricular pacemaker with one lead in the right ventricle and a second lead inserted retrograde intothe coronary sinus to stimulate the left ventricle. CRT is indicated in patients with dyssynchronous LV contraction, most commonly related to left bundle branch block, which is present in up to 30% of patients with systolic HF. The basis for CRT, as the name implies, is to "resynchronize" LV contraction, thereby increasing myocardial efficiency, stroke work, ejection fraction, and cardiac output. Although few older patients have been enrolled in the CRT trials, observational studies indicate that appropriately selected older patients derive significant benefit from CRT (SOE=B). Therefore, because the main objective of CRT is to improve symptoms and quality of life, and the only significant risk is modest and related to insertion of the device, it seems reasonable to offer CRT to older patients with severe LV dysfunction, advanced HF symptoms, and evidence of LV dyssynchrony.

RECURRENT HOSPITALIZATION

Multiple studies indicate that up to 50% of patients with HF are readmitted within 3–6 mo after an initial hospitalization for HF. The most common cause of readmission is nonadherence to the medication regimen and/or to dietary sodium and fluid recommendations. Other causes include inadequate follow-up, poor social support, and failure to seek medical attention promptly when symptoms worsen. Intercurrent cardiac events, such as an acute coronary syndrome or recurrent atrial fibrillation, are less common causes of repetitive hospitalizations.

Patients who experience recurrent HF hospitalization within 3–6 mo after an index admission should be questioned carefully about adherence to the medication regimen, use of OTC medications (especially NSAIDs and "dietary supplements"), recent dietary choices, and daily fluid intake. Patients should also be asked if they have been monitoring their weight and if there have been any recent changes. In patients who acknowledge nonadherence to the medication regimen or sodium restriction, reasons for nonadherence should be explored; in the case of medications, these often include concerns about adverse events, cost, efficacy, and excess number of pills. Nonadherence to sodium restriction often involves lack of knowledge about the salt content of foods, inability to acquire low-sodium foods, frequent eating out, and poor sense of taste. If possible, strategies should be developed to overcome these barriers, and the importance of future adherence as a means to prevent subsequent admissions emphasized. A multidisciplinary team approach, including the physician, an HF nurse specialist (if available), dietitian, social worker, pharmacist (preferably with expertise in geriatric drug prescribing), and home-health representative is most likely to result in significant changes in health behavior, thereby fostering improved adherence and self-efficacy, ultimately leading to decreased risk of early readmission (SOE=A). When feasible, the patient's family or spouse/partner should be actively engaged in the evaluation and teaching process.

PROGNOSIS

The prognosis of older patients with HF is poor, with median survival rates of 2–3 yr. However, the prognosis is also heterogeneous, with 25%–30% of patients dying within 1 yr after initial diagnosis, 50% surviving 1–5 yr, and 20%–25% surviving >5 yr. Women and patients with diastolic HF have somewhat better survival rates than men and patients with systolic HF, respectively, but other outcomes, including hospitalization rates, functional status, and quality of life, do not differ significantly among these subgroups. Other factors that adversely affect prognosis include older age, more severe symptoms (eg, higher NYHA functional class), lower systolic blood pressure, the presence of CAD (an important factor contributing to worse outcomes in men), diabetes (especially in women), peripheral arterial or cerebrovascular disease, cognitive impairment or dementia, renal insufficiency, anemia, and hyponatremia. Patients with higher BNP also have a worse prognosis, especially if the BNP remains substantially increased despite aggressive therapy.

END-OF-LIFE CARE

In light of the poor prognosis of older HF patients, which is worse than for most forms of cancer, it is appropriate to initiate discussions about end-of-life care early in the course of treatment, and to readdress these issues as clinical circumstances evolve. Patients should be counseled to develop an advance directive, designate a durable power of attorney, and explicitly indicate what interventions they would or would not wish to undergo in the event that their condition worsened and death appeared imminent. Patients with ICDs should be asked to indicate under what conditions they would want the ICD turned off to avoid repetitive painful shocks at the end of life. In patients with particularly poor prognosis and remaining life expectancy of <6 mo, frank but empathetic discussions should be undertaken with the patient and family, during which information about prognosis and likely disease trajectory should be conveyed, and transition to palliative care and hospice should be offered.

ACOVE-3* Quality Indicators Pertaining to Heart Failure

ACE inhibitor

- If a vulnerable older adult has a left ventricular ejection fraction (LVEF) <40%, then he or she should receive an ACE inhibitor (or an angiotensin-receptor blocker [ARB] if ACE inhibitor intolerant).
- If a vulnerable older adult is prescribed an ACE inhibitor, then he or she should have serum creatinine and potassium monitored within 2 weeks after initiation of therapy and at least yearly thereafter.

Heart failure (HF) history

- If a vulnerable older adult is newly diagnosed with HF, then he or she should have a history taken at diagnosis or hospitalization that documents the following:
  - Symptoms of volume overload
  - Current symptoms of chest pain or angina pectoris
  - Prior myocardial infarction, coronary artery disease, or revascularization
  - Hypertension
  - Diabetes mellitus
  - Hypercholesterolemia
  - Valvular heart disease
  - Thyroid disease
  - Alcohol use
  - Smoking
  - Current medications
  - New York Heart Association functional class or other description of functional status

HF examination

- If a vulnerable older adult is newly diagnosed with HF, then he or she should have a physical examination at diagnosis or hospitalization that documents the following:
  - Weight
  - Blood pressure and heart rate
  - Lung examination
  - Cardiac examination
  - Abdominal examination
  - Lower extremity examination

HF diagnostic testing

- If a vulnerable older adult is newly diagnosed with HF, then he or she should undergo the following studies within 1 mo of diagnosis if not done in the prior 3 mo:
  - Chest radiograph
  - ECG
  - CBC
  - Serum electrolytes
  - BUN
  - Creatinine
  - Glucose
  - Albumin
  - Liver function tests
  - Thyrotropin
  - Urinalysis

Left ventricular function evaluation

- If a vulnerable older adult is newly diagnosed with HF or has known HF with an unexplained clinical deterioration, then he or she should have an evaluation of left ventricular function.

Inpatient laboratory testing

- If a vulnerable older adult is hospitalized with HF, then he or she should have serum electrolytes, creatinine, and BUN determined within 1 day.

Selective β-blocker

- If a vulnerable older adult has HF and an LVEF <40%, then he or she should be treated with a β-blocker known to prolong survival (carvedilol, metoprolol, or bisoprolol).

Calcium channel blocker use

- If a vulnerable older adult has HF, LVEF <40%, and no atrial fibrillation, then he or she should not be treated with a first- or second-generation calcium channel blocker.

Laboratory monitoring for loop diuretic

- If a vulnerable older adult is prescribed a loop diuretic, then he or she should have electrolytes checked within 2 weeks after initiation and at least yearly thereafter.

Antiarrhythmic use

- If a vulnerable older adult has HF and an LVEF <40%, then he or she should not be treated with a type I antiarrhythmic agent unless an implantable cardiac defibrillator is in place.

Digoxin toxicity

- If a vulnerable older adult with HF is taking digoxin and has signs of toxicity, then a digoxin level should be checked or digoxin discontinued within 1 week.

HF education

- If a vulnerable older adult is newly diagnosed or hospitalized with HF, then patient counseling in the following areas should be provided and documented:
  - Medication use, dosage, intervals, adverse events
  - Low-salt diet
  - Exercise and physical activity
  - Smoking cessation
  - Weight monitoring
  - Symptom management
  - Avoiding or minimizing use of NSAIDs
  - Prognosis/end-of-life issues

HF outpatient visit: volume status

- If a vulnerable older adult has HF, then the following physical examination elements should be documented at each primary care or cardiology outpatient visit:
  - Weight
  - Blood pressure
  - Heart rate
  - Assessment of volume overload

Related quality indicators for Heart Failure

- Dyspnea assessment and management (see "Palliative Care," p 102)
- Preoperative cardiovascular risk assessment (see "Perioperative Care," p 92)

*Assessing Care of Vulnerable Elders – 3rd Set. See inside front cover for explanation.

REFERENCES

- Hodges P. Heart failure: epidemiologic update. *Crit Care Nurs Q.* 2009;32(1):24–32.

- Hunt SA, Abraham WT, Chin MH, et al. ACC/AHA 2005 Guideline Update for the Diagnosis and Management of Chronic Heart Failure in the Adult. *Circulation.* 2005;112(12):e154–e235.

- Gohler A, Januzzi JL, Worrell SS, et al. A systematic meta-analysis of the efficacy and heterogeneity of disease management programs in congestive heart failure. *J Card Fail.* 2006;12(7):554–567.

CHAPTER 48—HYPERTENSION

KEY POINTS

- Physiologic age-related changes in systems that regulate blood pressure lead to greater variability in blood pressure. Multiple blood pressure readings are needed to accurately diagnose hypertension.

- Treating hypertension is beneficial in older adults—including the very old—resulting in reductions in stroke, heart failure, and cardiovascular and overall mortality.

- Choice of initial antihypertensive drug therapy should be individualized according to the patient's comorbidities. In uncomplicated patients, thiazide diuretics are the preferred first-line agents.

- Caution is needed in treating frail, older adults with antihypertensives. "Start low and go slow." Monitoring for falls, orthostatic hypertension, and other adverse drug events is essential.

EPIDEMIOLOGY AND PHYSIOLOGY

Blood pressure, particularly systolic pressure, increases with increasing age. The risks associated with hypertension do not decline with age, and the criteria that define hypertension, outlined in the Seventh Report of the *Joint National Committee on Prevention, Detection, Evaluation, and Treatment of High Blood Pressure* (*JNC 7*; see references at end of chapter and Table 48.1), are not age adjusted. Epidemiologic studies, including the National Health and Nutrition Examination surveys, suggest that the prevalence of hypertension in adults ≥65 yr old is between 50% and 70%; the prevalence is highest among older black Americans (SOE=A). In contrast to younger hypertensive populations, among whom men predominate, in the older hypertensive population the prevalence rate is higher for women, particularly for those >75 yr old. Over the past 50 yr, the use of antihypertensive medications has increased, and the prevalence rates of increased blood pressure, left ventricular hypertrophy, and cardiovascular and stroke mortality have all declined. However, these trends have been delayed among the older population, and blood pressure remains poorly controlled in many

Table 48.1—Classification of Blood-Pressure Levels

Category	Systolic (mmHg)		Diastolic (mmHg)
Normal	<120	*and*	<80
Prehypertension	120–139	*or*	80–89
Hypertension			
Stage 1	140–159	*or*	90–99
Stage 2	>160	*or*	> 100

NOTE: Diagnoses should be based on the average of two or more readings taken at each of two or more visits after an initial screening.

SOURCE: Data from *JNC 7 Express: The Seventh Report of the Joint National Committee on Prevention, Detection, Evaluation, and Treatment of High Blood Pressure*. Bethesda, MD: National High Blood Pressure Education Program, National Heart, Lung and Blood Institute, National Institutes of Health, US Department of Health and Human Services; May 2003:3 (Table 1).

older adults despite treatment for hypertension. Many factors contribute to poor rates of blood pressure control. These factors include a lack of both awareness of having hypertension and knowledge of what normal blood pressure goals should be; these issues appear to be particular barriers among older black-American and Hispanic women.

Many of the physiologic changes that occur with aging contribute to the increase in blood pressure, but lifestyle factors such as obesity and physical inactivity and the presence of comorbid diseases are also important contributors. Several physiologic changes combine to increase peripheral vascular resistance, the physiologic hallmark of hypertension in older adults. Several mechanisms contribute to the age-associated increase in arterial vascular stiffness. Arterial stiffness, or reduced vascular compliance, provides the best explanation for the relatively greater increase in systolic pressure and the increase in pulse pressure (the difference between systolic and diastolic pressure) seen with aging. Decreased sensitivity of the baroreflex, perhaps related to decreased arterial distensibility, contributes to an increase in blood-pressure variability and sympathetic nervous system activity. The dynamic regulation of vascular tone is affected by impairments in vasodilator systems (eg, production of nitric oxide by vascular endothelial cells and vasodilation mediated by β-adrenergic receptors) and by heightened vasoconstriction mediated by α-adrenergic receptors. Changes in kidney function as well as in neurohumoral systems that are involved in sodium balance combine to increase the proportion of older hypertensive adults whose blood pressure increases with increased sodium intake. Approximately two-thirds of older hypertensive adults have sodium-sensitive hypertension.

The regulation of blood-pressure homeostasis may be impaired in older hypertensive adults, making older adults with increased systolic blood pressure more likely to develop both orthostatic and postprandial hypotension. Maintaining normal blood pressure and cerebrovascular and coronary perfusion in the face of hypotensive stimuli related to postural challenge, meals, or medications requires the integrated coordination of multiple compensatory mechanisms. The age-associated decline in baroreflex sensitivity and changes in sympathetic nervous system function impair the dynamic regulation of blood pressure. Because of the blunted sensitivity of the baroreflex, a greater decrease in blood pressure occurs before the increase in heart rate and other compensatory mechanisms are activated. Other pathophysiologic changes that impair blood-pressure regulation include arterial and cardiac stiffness and a decrease in early diastolic filling.

CLINICAL EVALUATION

Accurate measurement of blood pressure is the most critical aspect of the diagnosis of hypertension in older adults. Because variability in blood pressure increases with age, the diagnosis of hypertension requires using the average of several blood-pressure readings taken on each of three separate visits. Ambulatory blood-pressure monitoring is recommended for patients with extreme blood-pressure variability or possible "white-coat" hypertension. It is also recommended for the evaluation of resistant hypertension, and when there is concern regarding hypotensive episodes including postural hypotension. Additional clinically useful information derived from ambulatory blood pressure monitoring is the mean blood pressure over an entire 24-hour period and the diurnal blood pressure rhythm. A diminished nocturnal fall in blood pressure (<10% of waking values)— the nondipping pattern—has been associated with higher cardiovascular risk.

Indirect, or cuff, blood pressures correlate very well with direct, intra-arterial measures in most older adults. In rare individuals, extreme rigidity of the peripheral arteries may prevent complete compression of the brachial artery when the cuff is inflated, resulting in a falsely high blood pressure measurement. This is referred to as pseudohypertension and should be considered in cases of what appears to be resistant hypertension or when there are marked adverse events—especially hypotension—when antihypertensive therapy is started. Clinicians should also be aware of an auscultatory gap, which can lead to underestimation of the true systolic blood pressure and can indicate arterial stiffness. Determining the true systolic blood pressure by palpation avoids this problem.

Once hypertension has been diagnosed, the remainder of the clinical evaluation centers on excluding secondary forms of hypertension (using an approach similar to that used in younger patient populations), identifying target organ damage, and determining cardiovascular risk factors and the presence of comorbid conditions. Although most older patients have essential hypertension, secondary forms of hypertension should be suspected in the presence of malignant hypertension, a sudden increase in diastolic blood pressure, worsening level of control, or poorly controlled blood pressure on a regimen of three antihypertensive medications. Renovascular disease is the most common secondary form of hypertension among older adults (see "Kidney Diseases and Disorders," p 404). Treatment decisions should be made considering cardiovascular disease, target-organ damage (eg, left ventricular hypertrophy), diabetes mellitus, and other comorbid diseases. Finally, the patient's smoking history, dietary intake of sodium and fat, alcohol intake, and the level of usual physical activity should be determined to allow the clinician to individualize advice about lifestyle modifications to help control blood pressure as well as to reduce overall cardiovascular disease risk factors.

TREATMENT

The overwhelming consensus derived from the results of numerous randomized placebo-controlled clinical trials is that treatment of hypertension in older adults is safe and effective. Meta-analyses of more than forty randomized clinical trials of antihypertensive therapy have provided compelling evidence that treatment is effective in reducing cardiovascular (eg, chronic heart failure) and cerebrovascular (eg, stroke) morbidity and mortality (SOE=A). A meta-analysis of outcome trials in systolic hypertension among older adults demonstrated that treatment was associated with significant reductions in overall mortality, cardiovascular events, and stroke (SOE=A). The treatment effect was largest in men, in those ≥70 yr old, and in those who had greater pulse pressures.

Until the Hypertension in the Very Elderly Trial (HYVET) study was completed in 2007, few participants in randomized controlled trials of hypertension treatment were >80 yr old and almost none were >85 yr old. This randomized controlled trial of 3,845 participants >80 yr old ended early when its data safety monitoring board identified a significant 21% reduction in total mortality (10.1% versus 12.2%, absolute risk reduction 2.2%, number needed to treat = 45 over a median of 1.8 yr) in the intervention (extended-release indapamide plus perindopril if needed to achieve a goal systolic blood pressure of 150 mmHg) relative to the placebo control group (relative risk [RR] 0.76; confidence interval [CI] 95%, 0.62–0.93; P=.007). The treatment group also demonstrated improvements in fatal and nonfatal stroke (RR 0.59; CI 95%, 0.40–0.88; *P*=.009) and heart failure and reported fewer adverse events. It is important to note that the participants in this trial were generally healthy, community-living older adults—those with dementia, living in nursing homes, or an inability to walk were excluded. The study design also required participants to have a standing blood pressure above 140 mmHg at entry into the trial. For these reasons, the HYVET study results cannot be generalized to apply to frail, very old individuals. A HYVET substudy that assessed cognitive function and the rate of dementia developing in study participants, HYVET-COG, identified similar rates of incident dementia in the treatment and control groups.

As with other chronic conditions in older adults, it is important to balance the recognized beneficial effects of antihypertensive therapy with the potential impact on the individual's functional status and quality of life (eg, with the development of orthostatic hypotension). A treatment approach using modalities least likely to result in adverse events and that target a reduction in systolic blood pressure to 135–140 mmHg and diastolic blood pressure to <90 mmHg should be developed. For individuals with type 2 diabetes, a systolic blood pressure goal of <130 mmHg is recommended (SOE=A). For patients with markedly increased systolic blood pressure, an intermediate target, such as <160 mmHg, may be an appropriate initial goal in the absence of target-organ damage.

Although it is clear that any increase in blood pressure above normal (>115/80 mmHg) is positively and linearly associated with morbidity and mortality, concerns have been expressed that reducing blood pressure below a given threshold level may be linked to adverse outcomes. Some studies have shown increased mortality with blood-pressure reduction—especially diastolic blood pressure—below a certain threshold, creating a J-shaped curve in relation to mortality (SOE=B). The significance of these concerns remains controversial. This relationship has been evaluated in older participants enrolled in the Systolic Hypertension in the Elderly Trial. This post hoc analysis suggested that an on-treatment diastolic blood pressure <70 mmHg was associated with more cardiovascular events only in those with a history of underlying coronary heart disease. While cardiovascular mortality was not increased as a function of lower diastolic pressures to as low as 55 mmHg, hazard ratios for noncardiovascular mortality were higher. It therefore seems reasonable to attempt to avoid excessive reductions in diastolic blood pressure (eg, diastolic levels <70 mmHg), especially in individuals with coronary heart disease.

Treatment should focus on the systolic blood pressure and pulse pressure, because among older

Table 48.2—Nonpharmacologic Therapies for Stage 1 Hypertension

- Weight reduction
- Aerobic and strength-training exercise programs
- Smoking cessation
- Moderation of alcohol intake
- Dietary changes to decrease sodium, saturated fat, and cholesterol while maintaining adequate intake of potassium, magnesium, and calcium

hypertensive adults, these are stronger predictors of adverse outcomes than the diastolic blood pressure. The systolic blood pressure alone correctly classifies the blood-pressure stage of >99% of older hypertensive adults. In addition, analysis of data from the Systolic Hypertension in the Elderly Trial demonstrates a significant relationship between pulse pressure and the risk of stroke and overall mortality that is independent of the level of mean arterial pressure.

Lifestyle Modification

Nonpharmacologic therapy may be effective for older adults with Stage 1 hypertension (140–159 mmHg systolic or 90–99 mmHg diastolic blood pressure) and is an important adjunct to drug treatment in all patients because of synergistic effects with antihypertensive drugs and the benefits realized through the reduction in other cardiovascular risk factors (Table 48.2). Lifestyle modifications that target the typical characteristics of the older hypertensive adult—overweight, sedentary, and salt-sensitive—are likely to be effective. The randomized Trial of Nonpharmacologic Interventions in Elderly study, which evaluated the effects of dietary sodium restriction and weight loss in older adults, demonstrated that relatively modest reductions in dietary sodium intake (40 mmol/d) and in body weight (4 kg) are accompanied by a 30% decrease in the need to reinitiate pharmacologic treatment. A meta-analysis of randomized trials assessing the effects of dietary sodium restriction demonstrated a significant reduction in systolic (a mean decrease of 3.7 mmHg for each decrease of 100 mmol/d in sodium intake) but not in diastolic blood pressure (SOE=A). This differential reduction in systolic pressure is particularly well suited for the older hypertensive patient. Older adults with Stage 1 hypertension who do not have diabetes mellitus should complete a 6-mo trial of nonpharmacologic therapy before adding an antihypertensive medication if the target blood pressure is not achieved. See also "Physical Activity," p 54; and "Malnutrition," p 195.

Pharmacologic Treatment

The general approach to pharmacologic management of older hypertensive adults is presented in the JNC 7

Table 48.3—General Treatment Recommendations for Stage 1, Simple Hypertension

- Begin with a nonpharmacologic approach (Table 46.2).
- Base drug selection or combination therapies on individual patient characteristics.
- Use a low-dose diuretic as the first choice for initial pharmacologic therapy in uncomplicated patients.
- When starting drug therapy, begin at half the usual dosage, increase dosage slowly, and continue nonpharmacologic therapies.
- Treatment goals should be gauged by systolic blood pressure, and based on patient's comorbidity profile.
- Avoid excessive reduction in diastolic blood pressure (<70 mmHg).
- Do not treat aggressively when adverse events (eg, postural hypotension) cannot be avoided.

and modified by more recent findings. General principles regarding drug selection are reviewed here and summarized in Table 48.3. Whether the patient has simple hypertension or hypertension complicated by any of several comorbid conditions (eg, diabetes mellitus, coronary artery disease or history of myocardial infarction, heart failure, prostatism) can influence the choice of drug. Racial and ethnic background likely has an effect on an individual's response to antihypertensive drug therapy; for example, the blood-pressure reduction resulting from monotherapy with ACE inhibitors or angiotensin receptor blockers is somewhat attenuated among blacks.

Given the available evidence to date, for those with simple, uncomplicated hypertension, the initial antihypertensive drug choice is a low-dose thiazide-type diuretic (SOE=A). This recommendation was confirmed in a 2009 Cochrane review. This review also found that ACE inhibitors may be similarly effective as initial treatment, but the amount of evidence is less than that for diuretics (SOE=B). Most patients will not reach their systolic blood pressure goal on a single drug; JNC 7 recommends starting patients on two drugs if their initial blood pressure is >20 mmHg above the target level. Evidence is accumulating that blood pressure reductions are greater with a lower incidence of adverse events by combination therapy consisting of low dosages of multiple antihypertensive medications than with the typical full dosage of any one of the individual agents (SOE=B).

Beyond these general recommendations for initial therapy, there is no universally accepted approach to choosing alternative agents or combination therapies; these decisions should be made on an individual basis that considers the advantages and disadvantages of the medication together with the patient's comorbidities. Finally, centrally acting agents (eg,

clonidine, methyldopa) and those more likely to produce orthostatic hypotension should be avoided in most older adults.

Diuretics

Therapy with low-dose thiazide-type diuretics (eg, hydrochlorothiazide ≤25 mg/d, or the equivalent) has demonstrated significant benefits in mortality, stroke, and coronary events in randomized clinical trials in older hypertensive adults (SOE=A). These beneficial effects, combined with their relative safety, favorable adverse-event profile (their adverse metabolic effects—hypokalemia, hyperuricemia, and glucose intolerance—are attenuated at lower doses), once-daily dosing, and low cost have led to the recommendation that diuretics are preferred for initial therapy in uncomplicated cases. Another advantage is that diuretic therapy leads to a disproportionate reduction in systolic blood pressure relative to diastolic, and diuretics are better than other agents at reducing systolic blood pressure. Thiazide diuretics are also well suited for use in combination therapies because of synergistic effects with other classes of antihypertensive medications. The importance of maintaining a normal potassium concentration during therapy with thiazide-type diuretics deserves emphasis. Adequate potassium replacement during diuretic-based treatment has been shown to prevent the risk of arrhythmias as well as to decrease the impairment in glucose tolerance.

ACE Inhibitors

ACE inhibitors have been demonstrated to be effective in lowering blood pressure in older hypertensive adults. Results from three randomized controlled trials support use of ACE inhibitors as initial monotherapy for simple hypertension in older hypertensive patients, especially in men. Medications in this class are generally well tolerated (except for cough during ACE inhibitor therapy), and they do not adversely affect the CNS or metabolic profile. There are compelling benefits from using ACE inhibitors in those patients with coexisting diabetes mellitus (particularly when there is microalbuminuria), as well as in those with left ventricular systolic dysfunction (SOE=A).

Angiotensin-Receptor Blockers

No randomized controlled trials have compared outcomes from treatment with angiotensin-receptor blockers (ARBs) with diuretics among older hypertensive patients. Results from a network meta-analysis suggest that diuretic therapy is superior to ARBs for most outcomes. In the absence of data from randomized controlled trials to support their benefit with respect to cardiovascular events and mortality, ARBs generally should not be considered as initial monotherapy for simple hypertension (SOE=B). ARB therapy may be considered in patients with underlying diabetes, heart failure, or chronic kidney disease, especially if they are not able to tolerate ACE inhibitor therapy (SOE=B).

Calcium-Channel Antagonists

Therapy with calcium-channel antagonists (CCAs), particularly long-acting agents in the dihydropyridine (nifedipine-like) class, has been shown in the Systolic Hypertension in Europe and China Trials to lead to significant reduction in stroke risk in older hypertensive patients (SOE=A). The pathophysiologic (reduction in peripheral vascular resistance) and adverse-event (absence of central or metabolic effects) profiles of the CCA class are other factors that support their use in this patient population. In a subject population selected to be at high cardiovascular risk because of a history of coronary events, stroke, impaired renal function, LVH or diabetes (two-thirds of whom were >65 yr old), the ACCOMPLISH trial results identified superiority of an ACE–CCA (amlodipine) to an ACE–thiazide combination with respect to reduction in cardiovascular events even though the achieved blood pressure was similar between groups. Because of age-related changes in the pharmacokinetics of CCAs, lower dosages should be used. Short-acting CCAs should not be used to treat hypertension.

β-Receptor Antagonists

β-Receptor antagonists are recommended in the JNC 7 report as another option for second-line drug therapy. β-Receptor antagonists should not be considered as first-line monotherapy for simple hypertension in older adults. Analysis of evidence from randomized controlled trials has questioned the efficacy of β-blockers in older hypertensive adults. Results from these studies suggest that initial antihypertensive therapy with a β-receptor antagonist is less effective than therapy with low-dose thiazide diuretics with respect to reducing blood-pressure and preventing cardiovascular events, stroke, and death (SOE=A). In addition, β-blockers are more likely to be discontinued because of adverse events. Because of their effectiveness in the management of symptomatic coronary artery disease, in secondary prevention after myocardial infarction, and in certain heart failure settings, β-receptor antagonists should be considered for older adults whose hypertension is complicated by these comorbid conditions (SOE=A).

α-Receptor Antagonists

Although the reduction in peripheral vascular resistance that occurs with therapy using an α-receptor antagonist is particularly appropriate for the pathophysiologic profile of geriatric hypertension, and although these agents are effective in blood-pressure reduction, the development of postural hypotension has limited their widespread use for treating hypertension. The treatment arm that included participants randomized to therapy with the α-receptor antagonist doxazosin in the ALLHAT study was stopped early because of a higher rate of cardiovascular end points, including a 2-fold greater likelihood of being hospitalized for heart failure. α-Receptor antagonist therapy, usually in combination with another medication, might be considered for treating older hypertensive men with prostatism because these drugs have been shown to be efficacious in improving obstructive urinary symptoms.

Follow-Up Visits

The frequency of follow-up visits should reflect the patient's degree of blood-pressure increase at presentation, with closer follow-up indicated for those with a systolic blood pressure >180 mmHg. Except for hypertensive emergencies (discussed below), attempts to reduce blood pressure to target levels too rapidly are unnecessary and likely deleterious. For most patients, an interval of 1–2 mo between visits is appropriate to determine the need for dosage adjustment.

Given the age-related changes in systems that regulate blood pressure and impaired blood-pressure homeostasis, overtreatment of hypertension can result in situational (eg, postural or postprandial) hypotension. At all follow-up visits, it is imperative to determine both supine and standing blood pressure measurements (Table 48.4). It is good practice to adjust antihypertensive drug dosages to achieve the target (seated) blood pressure only after determining whether postural hypotension is present.

The patient's adherence to the current antihypertensive medication regimen should be assessed before an increased dosage is recommended or an alternative medication is considered. For some patients, additional information derived from blood-pressure measurements taken at home or another nonclinical setting may be important; home blood-pressure monitoring may also aid in promoting adherence to therapy. Because hypertension is usually

Table 48.4—Hypertension Management: Follow-up Visits

- Assess adherence to therapy.
- Monitor for adverse events, especially postural hypotension.
- Measure supine and upright blood pressure.
- Encourage self-monitoring of blood pressure.
- Reinforce lifestyle modifications (eg, diet, exercise).
- Adjust dosage cautiously.
- Evaluate for refractory hypertension.

asymptomatic, patient education regarding the significant benefits to be gained from adequate blood-pressure control is of particular importance. The interdisciplinary geriatric team is well suited to promote this approach (eg, nurses to provide feedback on the degree of blood-pressure control, dietitians to review dietary information and adherence, pharmacists to promote adherence to the medical regimen, and social workers to review and [when possible] alleviate the financial burden associated with medical therapy). Evaluation should also include a careful review of the patient's other medications to identify those (eg, NSAIDs and corticosteroids) that can worsen blood-pressure control.

When a patient's blood pressure has not been successfully reduced to the target level, cautiously increasing the dosage, adding another medication (particularly a thiazide diuretic, if the patient is not already taking one), or switching to another class of medication should be considered. Patients also should be counseled to continue their lifestyle modifications. Many months may be needed to achieve the target blood-pressure goal. When this goal is not attained despite adherence to a three-drug regimen, an evaluation for refractory or resistant hypertension (especially renovascular disease, hyperaldosteronism, and sleep apnea) should be considered. After more than a year of appropriate stable blood-pressure control, step-down treatment may be considered; dosages may be decreased cautiously, with close blood-pressure monitoring. Patients who have been successful at lifestyle modifications (eg, weight loss) are most likely to be able to reduce their dosage or eliminate antihypertensive medications.

SPECIAL CONSIDERATIONS

Hypertensive Emergencies and Urgencies

Increased blood pressure per se in the absence of signs or symptoms of target-organ damage does not constitute a hypertensive emergency or urgency. Rapidly and too aggressively decreasing blood pressure in a patient with incidentally discovered increased blood pressure is potentially harmful and can cause complications, such as coronary or cerebral hypoperfusion syndromes (SOE=B).

Examples of true hypertensive emergencies in older adults include hypertensive encephalopathy, acute heart failure with pulmonary edema, dissecting aortic aneurysm, and unstable angina. These patients present with symptoms and signs of vascular compromise of affected organs. The management of these emergencies requires an acute hospital setting, with the parenteral administration of an antihypertensive agent and continuous blood-pressure monitoring to

immediately reduce blood pressure, although not initially to a normal target level. Blood pressure should not be lowered emergently more than 25% within the first 2 hours, with a goal of achieving 160/100 mmHg gradually over the first 6 hours of therapy (SOE=D).

Hypertensive urgencies, situations in which blood pressure should be lowered within 24 hours to prevent the risk of target-organ damage, are more common than true emergencies. Most can be managed with oral administration of antihypertensive medications to gradually reduce blood pressure.

Hypertension in the Long-Term Care Setting

Approximately one-third to two-thirds of residents in long-term care facilities have hypertension. Special considerations are warranted in the care of residents with respect to making the correct diagnosis and defining the goals of therapy and its effects on quality of life. Blood-pressure measurements in long-term care settings may not be accurate because of measurement errors and the temporal variability in blood pressure, particularly in relation to meals. Blood pressure appears to be highest in the morning before breakfast. Postprandial hypotension is common among long-term care residents, affecting about one-third of this population. It has been associated with otherwise unexplained syncope and found to be a significant independent risk factor for falls, syncope, stroke, and overall mortality.

Several factors should be considered in the management of hypertension in this setting. First, the advanced average age and comorbidity of residents in long-term care facilities raises controversy surrounding the question whether the benefits of antihypertensive therapy extend to this population. If the beneficial effects of treatment are less evident, the potential adverse events and risks of therapy should be weighed more heavily in defining the goals of therapy. Even an intervention as seemingly innocuous as a sodium-restricted diet needs to be evaluated in the context of the high prevalence of protein-energy malnutrition among nursing-home residents. Second, the average resident in long-term care takes 9 to 10 medications, and most have three or more comorbid conditions. The addition of an antihypertensive medication increases the possibility of an adverse event in this frail, at-risk group. Third, several studies have identified the use of antihypertensive medications, particularly vasodilators, as a risk factor for falls in this high-risk population, who experience an average of two falls each year (SOE=B). It is therefore important to assess both postural and postprandial blood pressure in this population. Randomized controlled trials that could provide clear risk-benefit evidence to support an approach to antihypertensive management in the long-term care population have not yet been conducted. Available data suggest that diuretic therapy is effective in controlling systolic blood-pressure elevations and that blood-pressure reduction with diuretics lowers the prevalence of postural hypotension.

ACOVE-3* QUALITY INDICATORS PERTAINING TO HYPERTENSION

Confirm increased BP measurement

■ If an asymptomatic vulnerable older adult without a diagnosis of hypertension has an increased systolic blood-pressure measurement, then a blood-pressure measurement should be repeated as follows:
  ○ 140–159 mmHg: within 6 mo
  ○ 160–179 mmHg: within 2 mo
  ○ ≥180 mmHg: within 1 mo

Diagnose hypertension

■ If a vulnerable older adult without a diagnosis of hypertension has a systolic blood pressure of ≥140 mmHg on two consecutive visits, then the diagnosis of hypertension should be documented or home or 24-hour ambulatory blood-pressure monitoring should be ordered within 2 mo or documented as done in the previous 2 yr.

Evaluation of new hypertension

■ If a vulnerable older adult is newly diagnosed with hypertension, then the risk of cardiovascular disease should be assessed within 3 mo (if not done in the prior 3 mo), including:
  ○ History: myocardial infarction, angina pectoris, cardiomyopathy, aortic aneurysm, peripheral arterial disease, stroke, transient ischemic disease, hypercholesterolemia, family history of early coronary artery disease, smoking
  ○ Examination: murmurs or gallops, peripheral arterial examination, peripheral edema, weight, body mass index, waist circumference
  ○ Review of systems: chest pain, shortness of breath, transient vision or neurologic symptoms, nocturnal dyspnea, leg pain
  ○ Laboratory: blood glucose and serum lipids
  ○ ECG

Renal function check

■ If a vulnerable older adult is newly diagnosed with hypertension, then renal function should be assessed within 3 mo (if not done in the prior 3 mo).

Alcohol intake check

■ If a vulnerable older adult is newly diagnosed with hypertension, then the quantity and frequency of alcohol intake should be documented within 3 mo (if not done in the prior 3 mo).

NSAID reduction

■ If a vulnerable older adult is newly diagnosed with hypertension and is taking an NSAID or cyclooxygenase-2 inhibitor, then there should be documentation within 6 mo of dose reduction, an attempt to use an alternative medication, or justification for continued use.

Discussion of goal blood pressure

■ If a vulnerable older adult is newly diagnosed with hypertension, then a discussion of goal blood pressure or risks of prolonged hypertension should be documented within 3 mo.

Nonpharmacologic intervention

■ If a vulnerable older adult is newly diagnosed with hypertension, then a nonpharmacologic intervention (eg, diet, exercise, weight loss, reduced alcohol) should be recommended within 3 mo (if not done in the prior 3 mo).

Intervening for persistent hypertension

■ If a vulnerable older adult with hypertension has persistent (on 2 consecutive visits) systolic blood pressure above goal (see below), then an intervention (eg, pharmacologic, lifestyle, compliance) should occur, or there should be documentation of a reversible cause or other justification for the increase.

■ *Goal systolic blood pressure:*
  ○ Diabetes mellitus or chronic renal disease: 130 mmHg
  ○ Home ambulatory monitoring: 135 mmHg
  ○ All other patients: 140 mmHg, or other specified goal

Refractory hypertension

■ If a vulnerable older adult with hypertension has persistent (on 2 consecutive visits) systolic blood pressure above goal (see below) continuously for >6 mo, then there should be documentation of the suspected reason why the target was not reached and efforts to address the limitation.

- *Goal systolic blood pressure:*
  - Diabetes mellitus or chronic renal disease: 130 mmHg
  - Home ambulatory monitoring: 135 mmHg
  - All other patients: 140 mmHg, or other specified goal

Hypertensive urgency

- If a vulnerable older adult without target organ damage has a diastolic blood pressure of ≥ 120 mmHg, then immediate therapy or referral to the emergency department or hospital should occur.

Orthostatic hypotension check

- If a vulnerable older adult's medication regimen for hypertension is changed (new medication or dosage change) and within 1 week he or she reports dizziness, syncope or near syncope, or fall or near fall, then he or she should be evaluated for orthostatic hypotension at the time of the report (or within 1 week if outside the office), or the medication regimen should be changed.

β-blocker for hypertension and ischemic heart disease

- If a vulnerable older adult with hypertension has ischemic heart disease, then treatment with a β-blocker should be recommended, or there should be documentation of why such treatment is not provided.

ACE inhibitor for comorbid vascular disease

- If a vulnerable older adult with hypertension has a history of heart failure, left ventricular hypertrophy, ischemic heart disease, chronic kidney disease, or cerebrovascular accident, then he or she should be treated with an ACE inhibitor or angiotensin-receptor blocker, or there should be documentation of why such treatment is not provided.

Related quality indicators for Hypertension

- Blood pressure control for diabetic patients (see "Diabetes Mellitus," p 504)
- Laboratory follow-up of ACE inhibitor, loop diuretic (see "Cardiovascular Diseases and Disorders," p 360)

*Assessing Care of Vulnerable Elders – 3ʳᵈ Set. See inside front cover for explanation.

REFERENCES

- Beckett NS, Peters R, Fletcher AE, et al. Treatment of hypertension in patients 80 years of age or older. *N Engl J Med.* 2008;358(18):1887−1898.

- Chobanian AV, Bakris GL, Black HR, et al. The Seventh Report of the Joint National Committee on Prevention, Detection, Evaluation, and Treatment of High Blood Pressure; The JNC 7 Report. *JAMA.* 2003;289(19):2560–2572. Available at http://www.nhlbi.nih.gov/guidelines/hypertension.

- Wright JM, Musini VM. First-line drugs for hypertension. *Cochrane Database Syst Rev.* 2009;July 8(3):CD001841.

CHAPTER 49—GASTROINTESTINAL DISEASES AND DISORDERS

KEY POINTS

- Although physiologic changes of aging can affect GI function, most GI symptoms and signs are due to pathologic conditions.

- Medications used to treat many of the illnesses affecting older adults can cause GI symptoms and disorders.

- Colon cancer is a common and often preventable cause of death.

The structure and function of the GI tract are affected both by physiologic changes of aging and by the effects of accumulating disorders involving many body systems. In association with advancing age, changes in connective tissue can limit the elasticity of the gut, and changes in the nerves and muscles can impair motility. Disturbances of epithelial, muscle, or neural function may all result from age-related enteric neurodegeneration and loss of excitatory enteric neurons. Accumulating disorders and diseases are often associated with increased use of medications by older adults, many of which have direct effects on intestinal mucosa and motility. Some disease states, such as atherosclerosis and diabetes mellitus, can adversely influence GI function and lead to symptoms and complications. GI problems can quickly compromise the older adult's ability to maintain adequate nutrition and lead to fatigue and weight loss.

ESOPHAGUS

Dysphagia

Dysphagia implies either the inability to initiate a swallow, or a sensation that solids or liquids do not pass easily from the mouth into the stomach; it is a common problem among older adults and always requires immediate evaluation and therapy. Patients with oropharyngeal dysphagia complain of foods getting stuck shortly after they swallow, inability to initiate a swallow, impaired ability to transfer food from the mouth to the esophagus, nasal regurgitation, and coughing. Cerebrovascular accidents, Parkinson's disease and other neuromuscular disorders, Zenker's

diverticulum, oropharyngeal tumors, and prominent cervical osteophytes are the most common causes of oropharyngeal dysphagia in older adults.

In particular, hesitancy in swallowing and defects in swallowing related to tremor of the tongue occur in patients with Parkinson's disease. In contrast, patients with esophageal dysphagia usually point to the sternum when asked to localize the site. Dysphagia for both solids and liquids from the onset usually implies a motility disorder of the esophagus. In contrast, dysphagia for solids that progresses later to involve liquids suggests mechanical obstruction. Progressive dysphagia results from either cancer or peptic stricture, whereas intermittent dysphagia is most often related to a lower esophageal ring or esophageal dysmotility, such as achalasia or diffuse esophageal spasm. It is particularly important to obtain a detailed review of medications, because anticholinergics, antihistamines, and certain antihypertensive agents can reduce salivary flow. Slurred speech can indicate weakness or incoordination of muscles involved in articulation and swallowing. Dysarthria and nasal regurgitation of food suggest weakness of the soft palate or pharyngeal constrictors. Food regurgitation, halitosis, a sensation of fullness in the neck, or a history of pneumonia accompanying dysphagia may be the result of a pharyngoesophageal (or Zenker's) diverticulum, which may be associated with a poorly relaxing or hypertensive upper esophageal sphincter. Painful swallowing (odynophagia) typically results from infection due to fungi or viruses, drug-induced esophagitis, or malignancy. Esophagitis (gastro-esophageal reflux disease [GERD]) causes heartburn but not odynophagia, which results from viruses, medications, or cancer. While common in AIDS patients, esophageal candidiasis occurs in debilitated older adults on broad-spectrum antibiotics, immunosuppressive medications, and both oral and inhaled corticosteroids, and among those with hematologic malignancies. This disorder may or may not be accompanied by oropharyngeal candidiasis.

Endoscopy is the best first test to evaluate dysphagia; it allows biopsies and therapeutic interventions, such as dilation. However, lower esophageal rings or extrinsic esophageal compression can be overlooked during endoscopy (SOE=C). In such cases, radiologic evaluation with a 13-mm barium tablet or a solid bolus with barium, such as a marshmallow or bread, can identify the level and nature of obstruction. If results of these tests are normal, an esophageal motility study should be performed. For patients with oropharyngeal dysphagia, videofluoroscopy allows detailed analysis of swallowing mechanics, identifies whether aspiration is present, and evaluates the effects of different barium consistencies. Nasopharyngolaryngoscopy is a bedside procedure that evaluates the oropharynx, vallecula, and piriform sinuses, as well as the larynx and perilaryngeal regions, for pooled secretions or retained food; its utility is uncertain.

The treatment of dysphagia depends on its underlying cause. Esophageal cancer requires resection, chemotherapy, or radiation therapy. For patients who are poor surgical candidates, palliative endoscopic techniques, such as endoscopic mucosal resection for early esophageal cancer, radiofrequency or photodynamic therapy for high-grade dysplasia in Barrett's esophagus, and stent placement in obstructing esophageal cancer, may be considered. After stroke or head or neck surgery, or in degenerative neurologic diseases, swallowing rehabilitation and dietary modifications to facilitate oral intake are required. In some cases, feeding with a cup, straw, or spoon may improve swallowing. Endoscopic dilation is performed in patients with esophageal webs or strictures. Cricopharyngeal myotomy may benefit patients who have inadequate pharyngeal contraction, pharyngoesophageal diverticulum, or lack coordination between the pharynx and the upper esophageal sphincter. Endoscopic incision of the septum between the pharyngoesophageal (Zenker's) diverticulum and the esophagus with a flexible endoscope and needle-knife may also be performed. Botulinum toxin injection to the cricopharyngeus muscle is an alternative to surgery for patients with cricopharyngeal achalasia. (See also "Eating and Feeding Problems," p 203.) Similarly, endoscopically administered botulinum injection[OL] of the lower esophageal sphincter is an effective treatment for esophageal achalasia, a condition in which the incompletely relaxing sphincter is matched with loss of esophageal body peristaltic function to cause dysphagia and postural regurgitation. Unfortunately, the effect of botulinum toxin injection is transient, and repeat injections are needed months to years after initial therapy (SOE=A).

Gastroesophageal Reflux Disease

GERD is defined as chronic symptoms or mucosal damage produced by the abnormal reflux of gastric contents into the esophagus. Highly specific symptoms of GERD include heartburn, regurgitation, or both, which occur often after meals and are aggravated by recumbency and relieved by antacids. Among adults ≥65 yr old, symptoms of heartburn or acid regurgitation occur at least weekly in 20% of the population and at least monthly in 59%, rates similar to those observed in younger adults. Because of degradation of the gastroesophageal junction, reduced

visceral sensitivity, and impaired esophageal clearance, age is associated with an increase in esophageal acid exposure and reduced severity of reflux symptoms.

In >80% of patients, GERD is caused by transient inappropriate lower esophageal sphincter relaxations that lead to acid reflux into the esophagus. Some patients may have reduced lower esophageal sphincter tone, which permits reflux when intra-abdominal pressure rises. Sliding hiatal hernia occurs in about 30% of patients ≥50 yr old and may contribute to acid reflux and regurgitation. Poor esophageal peristalsis leads to delayed clearance of the refluxate and increased acid exposure time. In patients receiving anticholinergic medications, reduced salivary secretion decreases the buffering capacity of the esophagus against refluxed acid and can aggravate mucosal injury.

Patients with uncomplicated heartburn or regurgitation should be treated empirically with acid-suppressing medications. If such therapy is unsuccessful, or if there are symptoms suggesting complicated disease, an upper endoscopy should be performed. Individuals, particularly white men, who have longstanding symptoms or who require continuous therapy for reflux, need endoscopic screening for Barrett's esophagus, a premalignant condition to esophageal adenocarcinoma. The frequency and severity of reflux symptoms are poorly predictive of the presence of Barrett's esophagus, particularly in patients ≥65 yr old.

The presence of anemia, dysphagia, GI bleeding, recurrent vomiting, and weight loss suggests complicated GERD. Patients with these signs and symptoms should be considered for endoscopy. This is the procedure of choice to evaluate mucosal integrity and confirm the diagnosis of dysplasia or cancer in cases of Barrett's esophagus (SOE=B). However, many patients with reflux symptoms do not have esophagitis. In such cases, 24-hour ambulatory esophageal pH testing helps to confirm the diagnosis. This noninvasive test is also useful for patients with noncardiac chest pain or reflux-associated pulmonary and upper respiratory symptoms or to monitor the esophageal acid exposure in patients with refractory symptoms. Esophageal manometry is used to document the presence of effective esophageal peristalsis in patients in whom antireflux surgery is being considered and to exclude underlying esophageal motility disorder, such as achalasia, as the cause of the symptoms. In patients with resistant reflux symptoms, a recently introduced technology, ambulatory esophageal pH-impedance monitoring, allows for measurement and quantification of both acid and nonacid reflux.

Proton-pump inhibitors (PPIs) are the treatment of choice for patients with GERD, but they are expensive. One of them, omeprazole, is available OTC. PPIs heal esophagitis in 85% of cases and eradicate heartburn and regurgitation in 80%. In comparison, H_2 antagonists ameliorate symptoms and heal esophagitis in only 60% of cases. For dysphagic older adults, various formulations of PPIs, such as orally disintegrating tablets, are available. Regardless, therapy should be maintained for at least 8 weeks. After acute medical therapy alleviates symptoms, the patient should be given a trial off medication. Endoscopy, esophageal motility, and ambulatory 24-hour pH monitoring should be performed if the most potent medical therapy still results in a poor response. Bravo™, a wireless pH recording device, is a convenient method (SOE=B) for ambulatory pH monitoring; it is easily placed in the distal esophagus and is well tolerated by patients, who can continue their usual activity and diet over the duration of the 48-hour study.

Recurrence of symptoms is common after therapy is stopped, and lifelong therapy is commonly needed. Intermittent therapy with an H_2 antagonist or PPI may be successful in some patients with mild to moderate symptoms without severe esophagitis. Depending on the initial therapy rendered, the medical regimen is adjusted in a step-up or step-down fashion to the most cost-effective regimen. The need for maintenance medical therapy is determined by the rapidity of recurrence. Among patients whose symptoms recur <3 mo after stopping therapy, their disease may best be managed with continual drug therapy. Patients whose symptoms recur ≥3 mo after stopping treatment may be adequately managed with intermittent use of medication. The induction of hypergastrinemia and gastric carcinoid tumors in rats treated with omeprazole has raised safety concerns about the long-term safety of PPIs. However, although patients treated with omeprazole for up to 5 yr have shown gastritis and gastric atrophy, no neoplastic changes have been seen. Because gastric acidity normally protects against ingested pathogens, another concern with gastric-acid inhibition is an increased risk of enteric infections, particularly *Clostridium difficile*. In a similar fashion, acid-suppressive therapy also allows pathogen colonization of the upper GI tract with an increased risk of community-acquired pneumonia.

While a single case-control study suggested that chronic PPI use may slightly increase the risk of hip fractures (possibly via decreased absorption of calcium) in patients >50 yr old, a 2008 update by the American Gastroenterological Society Institute found the current evidence insufficient to support recommendations regarding bone density measurements and calcium replacement in long-term PPI users (SOE=B). PPIs can cause arthralgias, myalgias, and progressive weakness due to myopathy that may be mistakenly attributed to other diseases in older adults. Care of patients with GERD must weigh benefits and risks of PPI use.

Older adults with large hiatal hernia, with persistent regurgitation despite PPI therapy, or who do not wish to take PPIs long term, should be considered for antireflux surgery. This can be performed laparoscopically, with success rates of >90%.

Drug-Induced Esophageal Injury

Decreased esophageal peristaltic clearance, which is common among older adults, may be associated with pill retention. Esophageal injury can then occur as a result of prolonged contact of the caustic contents of the medication with the esophageal mucosa. The site of injury is commonly at the level of the aortic arch, of an enlarged left atrium, or of the esophagogastric junction. Because salivation and swallowing are markedly reduced during sleep, pill intake immediately before lying down and without adequate fluid bolus leads to pill retention and injury. Taking medications with at least 8 ounces of water or other fluid helps dissolve tablets or capsules and can also reduce the risk of injury or GI complaints. Patients with medication-induced esophageal injury present with sudden odynophagia to a degree that even swallowing saliva is difficult. A classic example is the older patient in a nursing home given a number of medications with a small amount of water while recumbent before sleep.

Tetracyclines, particularly doxycycline, are the most common antibiotics that induce esophagitis. Aspirin and all of the NSAIDs can also damage the esophagus. Other offenders include potassium chloride, quinidine, iron, and alendronate, an agent used for osteoporosis treatment. Because of this, alendronate should be used cautiously in patients with esophageal dysfunction and taken with at least 8 ounces of water to minimize the risk of the tablet getting stuck in the esophagus and causing damage. In addition, patients should stand or sit upright for at least 30 minutes and should not eat during this interval. Etidronate is another bisphosphonate used to treat Paget's disease that has not been associated with esophageal injury. Other bisphosphonates, such as risedronate and ibandronate, which are available for both prevention and treatment of osteoporosis, have less esophageal and GI toxicity, although they also need to be taken with at least 8 ounces of water followed by the patient remaining upright for at least 30 minutes. Intravenous formulations of bisphosphonates (eg, zoledronic acid) are now available and provide an alternative in very high-risk patients.

Upper endoscopy, the most sensitive diagnostic tool, may reveal a discrete ulcer of variable size with normal surrounding mucosa. These lesions typically heal spontaneously within a few days, and it is unclear whether therapy is needed. Suspension of sucralfate provides a protective coat on the esophageal mucosa and promotes healing. (Sucralfate is approved only for treating duodenal ulcers; its use for treating stomach or esophageal ulcers is off-label.) Strictures may be noted in those who use NSAIDs. Endoscopic dilation may be needed if a stricture is found. If possible, potentially caustic oral medications should be discontinued or a liquid preparation substituted.

Esophageal Cancer and Endoscopic Palliation

Esophageal cancer is commonly diagnosed at an advanced, incurable stage in older patients who are not candidates for tumor resection. These patients are plagued by symptoms of esophageal obstruction or fistula formation, dysphagia, aspiration, and weight loss. In such instances, endoscopic palliation can be achieved with either laser therapy or a single, permanent, metal stent placement. Laser therapy with neodymium-yttrium-aluminum-garnet (Nd:YAG) laser fulgurates the malignant obstructing tissue and restores luminal patency in >90% of cases, with a 5% risk of perforation. Relief can last for up to several months; treatments may be repeated. Photodynamic therapy uses a photosensitizing agent in combination with endoscopic laser exposure. It is more effective than Nd:YAG laser for palliation and has fewer complications, but it can cause skin photosensitivity.

Stenting with self-expanding metal stents is preferable therapy for patients with a malignant stricture or an esophagobronchial fistula, because it relieves dysphagia and aspiration in up to 95% of patients and has a low complication rate (SOE=B). The disadvantages of stents include their high cost, tumor ingrowth, and stent migration.

STOMACH

Dyspepsia

Dyspepsia implies chronic or recurrent pain or discomfort in the upper abdomen. The major causes of dyspepsia are gastric or duodenal ulcer, gastroesophageal reflux, and gastric cancer. Because symptom pattern is inadequate for accurate diagnosis, endoscopy is the test of choice. Endoscopy is normal in up to 60% of patients, who are then classified as having functional dyspepsia. It is unclear whether Helicobacter pylori gastritis causes symptoms of dyspepsia.

Because the incidence of gastric cancer increases with age, upper endoscopy should be considered in older adults presenting with new onset of dyspepsia.

Helicobacter pylori testing should be performed using a 13C-urea breath test or fecal antigen test. Treatment is then targeted at the underlying diagnosis. For patients with ulcer and documented H pylori infection, a trial of H pylori therapy should heal the ulcer and abolish the ulcer diathesis. For most patients with functional (or nonulcer) dyspepsia, reassurance and a course of antisecretory therapy using either H$_2$-receptor antagonists or PPIs is recommended.

Treatment of H pylori can lead to or possibly exacerbate reflux esophagitis. One possibility is that ammonia production by H pylori buffers acid. Alternatively, reversal of H pylori–induced gastritis (and associated hypochlorhydria) can increase gastric acid secretion and precipitate previously asymptomatic reflux. Despite this association, eradication of H pylori should not be avoided solely to prevent the development or exacerbation of reflux esophagitis.

Those who are H pylori negative should be given a 2-mo empirical trial of a PPI. Such empirical PPI therapy is also the most cost-effective approach in populations with a prevalence of H pylori infection of <10% (SOE=A).

NSAID-Induced Gastric Complications

NSAID-induced injury results from both local effects and systemic prostaglandin inhibition. The risk of ulcers and their complications is three times greater in those who use NSAIDs than in those who do not. Most of these ulcers are asymptomatic and uncomplicated. For those ≥60 yr old, the relative risk increases even more, to 5-fold. Older patients, particularly women, are two to four times more likely than younger patients to be hospitalized with peptic ulcer disease. Older adults with a prior history of bleeding ulcer are at increased risk of recurrent ulcer and complications. NSAIDs also have been implicated as an important factor in nonhealing ulcers. The presence of H pylori infection can have a synergistic effect on NSAID-induced ulcer disease. Older adults with NSAID-induced ulcers tend to present with anemia, bleeding, or perforation without the warning symptoms of dyspepsia or abdominal pain. In addition, older NSAID users commonly require emergency surgery for serious complications and have higher rebleeding rates, greater transfusion requirements, longer hospital stays, and higher mortality rates than do younger patients. When NSAIDs are used in older patients, the concomitant use of misoprostol or a PPI may reduce the risk of gastric bleeding by approximately 50% (SOE=A). In one trial, more patients remained in remission during maintenance treatment with omeprazole (61%) than with misoprostol (48%, P=.001), and with either drug than with placebo (27%, P<.001; absolute risk reduction [ARR] 12.7%). Risk factors for upper GI complications of

NSAID use are indicated in Table 49.1. COX-2 inhibitor therapy with celecoxib may be substituted for selected patients at risk of gastric complications from conventional NSAIDs, but a careful evaluation of underlying cardiovascular risk and risk-to-benefit assessment is mandatory. High-risk patients, particularly those who have experienced a GI complication, such as ulcer bleeding or perforation, should be placed on long-term PPI therapy; this approach reduces the risk of further bleeding (ARR approximately 9% over 13 mo of treatment) (SOE=B).

Peptic Ulcer Disease

In the United States, *H pylori* infection is responsible for about 80% of duodenal ulcers and approximately 60% of gastric ulcers. Most older adults with ulcers complain of dyspepsia, although bleeding, anemia, and acute abdominal pain can also occur. Typically, the diagnosis of peptic ulcer is made by upper GI radiography or endoscopy. Endoscopy is more sensitive and specific than double-contrast barium study (92% versus 54%, and 100% versus 91%, respectively). It is important to differentiate benign gastric ulcers from gastric cancer by obtaining multiple endoscopic biopsies and by repeating the endoscopic examination 2 mo after therapy to verify complete ulcer healing.

The goal in evaluating an older patient with upper GI symptoms is to quickly establish a definitive diagnosis, avoiding costly and risky diagnostic procedures. Medications that can cause dyspepsia, especially NSAIDs, should be eliminated when possible. If early satiety, weight loss, occult GI bleeding, or otherwise unexplained anemia is present, an endoscopy should be performed to exclude malignancy.

Among patients with dyspepsia who test positive for *H pylori*, antibiotic therapy may be beneficial for up to 30% of those with underlying peptic ulcer, but those with nonulcer (functional) dyspepsia will have a variable response. *H pylori* testing should not be performed in asymptomatic people. All PPIs are effective in inducing ulcer healing with rates of 80%−100% at 8 weeks.

Biliary Disease

Gall stones primarily form in the gallbladder and can obstruct the cystic or common bile duct, causing biliary pain, cholecystitis, and cholangitis. When stones obstruct the ampulla, pancreatitis may occur. Biliary pain is acute, severe upper abdominal pain, usually in the epigastrium or right upper quadrant, and it may last for >1 hour. The pain may radiate to the back or scapula and is often associated with restlessness, nausea, or vomiting. Older patients with complicated cholelithiasis may not have fever or

Table 49.1—Risk Factors for Upper GI Adverse Events in Patients Treated with NSAIDs

Age ≥60 yr old

Comorbid medical conditions

Higher NSAID dosage

Past history of peptic ulcer disease or ulcer complication (bleeding, perforation)

Past history of gastroduodenal toxicity from NSAIDs

Concurrent use of anticoagulants, corticosteroids, bisphosphonates, aspirin or other NSAIDs

leukocytosis; their pain may be nonspecific rather than in the right upper quadrant, or they may experience no pain, only vomiting. Episodes are typically separated by several weeks. Postprandial epigastric fullness, fatty food intolerance, and regurgitation are nonspecific symptoms and are not related to gall stones. If biliary disease is suspected in older patients, ultrasonography should be the initial imaging modality. Abdominal CT scanning may be used if common bile duct stones or ductal obstruction are suspected. Magnetic resonance cholangiography and endoscopic ultrasonography are two new, very accurate imaging modalities to detect common bile duct pathology, including gall stones. However, for patients with obstructive jaundice, cholangitis, or suspected biliary pancreatitis in whom the probability of common bile duct stones is high, therapeutic endoscopic retrograde cholangiopancreatography is preferred.

Gall stones can be found in 35% of women and 20% of men by 70 yr of age because of an aging-related increase in the lithogenicity of bile. While many older adults with cholelithiasis are asymptomatic, biliary disease is the predominant indication for urgent abdominal operations in this population; in adults >80 yr old, hepatobiliary disease accounts for 20% of all abdominal surgeries. An isolated increase in alkaline phosphatase without jaundice may be a presenting manifestation of biliary obstruction in older patients and should always be evaluated. If cholelithiasis is detected in patients with biliary pain, laparoscopic cholecystectomy is the procedure of choice. However, this procedure is not indicated in patients with gall stones without biliary pain or complications. In the rare older patient who is unable to undergo surgery, treatment with ursodeoxycholic acid or lithotripsy, or both, may be attempted. In patients with common bile duct obstruction due to gall stones, endoscopic sphincterotomy and bile ductal drainage is adequate in preventing recurrent cholangitis, and the gallbladder may be left *in situ*. In any older patient with gall stones, the possibility of gallbladder cancer should be considered. In older adults presenting with biliary pain who have had a cholecystectomy, a retained common bile duct stone should be suspected and evaluated by endoscopic retrograde cholangiopancreatography, magnetic resonance cholangiography, or endoscopic ultrasonography. In patients with abnormal liver function tests, right upper quadrant pain, and an increased common bile duct diameter, biliary manometry should also be considered. If sphincter of Oddi dysfunction is confirmed, endoscopic sphincterotomy should be performed. For patients with malignant jaundice, treatments are mostly palliative, with either surgery or percutaneous or endoscopic stenting. Such drainage improves quality of life, decreases pruritus, and improves nutritional state, but it does not improve survival.

COLON

Constipation

Chronic constipation affects about 30% of adults ≥65 yr old, more commonly women. Although it commonly occurs as an adverse event of medication, it may be a manifestation of metabolic or neurodegenerative disease resulting from loss of excitatory (eg, cholinergic) enteric neurons and interstitial cells of Cajal. Regardless, colonic obstruction must always be excluded. Constipation has been defined as a fecal frequency of <3 times per week. However, some individuals may complain of straining at defecation or a sense of incomplete defecation despite a daily bowel evacuation. A more objective diagnosis of constipation is based on colonic transit times. Estimation of the colonic transit time is accomplished by having the patient ingest a gelatin capsule containing radiopaque markers, followed by a plain abdominal film 5 days later. Normally, all markers should have passed by that time point. If not, their distribution on the plain film may suggest either colonic inertia or pelvic floor dyssynergia (outlet delay), or both.

Patients with irritable bowel syndrome often complain of constipation that alternates with periods of diarrhea or normal bowel evacuation. Such patients have normal colonic transit times. Lumbosacral spinal disease can lead to colonic hypomotility (inertia) and dilatation, decreased rectal tone and sensation, and impaired defecation. Older adults with Parkinson's disease may have constipation worsened by physical inactivity or medication use. In middle-aged and older women, the pelvic floor muscles that contribute to the external sphincter of the rectum may acquire laxity that contributes to problems with fecal incontinence.

Most patients with prolonged colonic transit have colonic inertia, defined as the delayed passage of radiopaque markers through the proximal colon. Outlet delay is a form of idiopathic constipation in which markers move normally through the colon but stagnate in the rectum. This is typically seen in older women with fecal impaction and megarectum, and in women with pelvic floor dyssynergia who demonstrate abnormal responses of the pelvic floor muscles during defecation. Older patients with megacolon or megarectum have chronic fecal retention, increased rectal compliance and elasticity, and blunted rectal sensation, all leading to fecal impaction and soiling.

Defecography is a technique in which thick barium simulating feces is introduced into the rectum, and evacuation is monitored by fluoroscopy while the patient sits on a commode. Assessment of the anorectal structure and function is then made at rest and during barium expulsion. Anorectal manometry evaluates rectal sensation and compliance, reflex relaxation of the internal anal sphincter, and the competence of the anal sphincters.

For most patients with constipation and normal colonic transit time, fluids, dietary fiber, and bulk laxatives, such as psyllium seed or calcium polycarbophil, are effective in increasing the frequency and softening the consistency of feces with a minimum of adverse events. Patients who respond poorly or who do not tolerate fiber may require laxatives. Chronic use of stimulant laxatives such as bisacodyl and senna can lead to hypokalemia, protein-losing enteropathy, and impaired bowel motility. Fecal softeners, such as docusate sodium, have few adverse events but are less effective than laxatives (SOE=C). Constipation among patients with dementia is common, especially if psychotropic medications are being used. Because the patient cannot be relied on to describe symptoms, a proactive approach is needed (Table 49.2 and Table 49.3).

Management of slow-transit constipation requires daily osmotic laxatives, such as sorbitol, lactulose, or a polyethylene glycol solution. Lubiprostone, a locally acting chloride channel activator that enhances chloride-rich intestinal fluid secretion, is also effective. Severe intractable colonic inertia with megacolon may require subtotal colectomy and ileorectostomy. Pelvic floor dysfunction requires biofeedback, relaxation exercises, and the use of suppositories.

Patients with fecal impaction should first have their colon evacuated with enemas or polyethylene glycol electrolyte solution until cleansing is complete. Recurrence of fecal impaction is then prevented with a fiber-restricted diet together with cleansing enemas twice weekly or daily oral intake of 12−16 fluid ounces of polyethylene glycol solution.

Fecal Incontinence

Fecal incontinence, defined as the recurrent uncontrolled passage of fecal material for at least 1 mo, is a disturbing disability because it affects quality of life and can lead to social isolation. Fecal incontinence may be minor, with inadvertent passage of flatus or soiling of underwear with liquid feces, or it may be major, with involuntary leakage of feces. Fecal incontinence affects 2%−7% of adults, mostly older adults in poor general health.

Fecal continence depends on many factors, such as physical and mental function, fecal consistency, colonic transit, rectal compliance, internal and external anal sphincter function, as well as anorectal sensation and reflexes. Normal defecation is a complex sequential process that starts with the entry of feces into the rectum, leading to reflex relaxation of the internal anal sphincter. If defecation is desired, the anorectal angle is voluntarily straightened, and abdominal pressure is increased by straining. This results in descent of the pelvic floor, contraction of the rectum, and inhibition of the external anal sphincter, which causes evacuation of the rectal contents.

Decreased anal sphincter tone can result from trauma (eg, anal surgery) or neurologic disorders (eg, spinal cord injury or a secondary effect of diabetes mellitus). Vaginal delivery associated with anal sphincter tears or trauma to the pudendal nerve can result in fecal incontinence immediately or after many years. Decreased rectal compliance resulting from ulcerative or radiation proctitis leads to increased fecal frequency and urgency. Impaction is a common cause of fecal incontinence in older adults because it inhibits the internal anal sphincter tone, permitting leakage of liquid feces. Idiopathic fecal incontinence caused by denervation of the pelvic floor musculature occurs most commonly in middle-aged and older women.

The history and physical examination often provide clues to the cause of fecal incontinence. A flexible sigmoidoscopy may be considered to exclude inflammation or tumor. The next step is anorectal manometry, which measures resting anal sphincter tone, the squeeze pressure, the rectoanal inhibitory reflex, rectal sensation, and rectal compliance. Abnormalities of the anal sphincters, the rectal wall, and the puborectalis muscle can be further evaluated by use of endorectal ultrasound. Typically, a defect in the internal anal sphincter is associated with low resting sphincter pressure, whereas defects in the external sphincter are associated with lower anal squeeze pressure.

Medical therapy is aimed at reducing fecal frequency and improving fecal consistency. The former is achieved with antidiarrheal drugs, such as loperamide; the latter, by supplementing the diet with a bulking agent, such as methylcellulose. Older adults with incontinence related to cognitive impairment or physical debility may benefit from a regular defecation program. Biofeedback therapy is a pain-

Table 49.2—Management of Chronic Constipation

Step 1.	Stop all constipating medications, when possible.
Step 2.	Increase dietary fiber to 6–25 g/d, increase fluid intake to ≥1,500 mL/d, and increase physical activity; or add bulk laxative provided fluid intake is to ≥1,500 mL/d. If fiber exacerbates symptoms or is not tolerated, go to Step 3.
Step 3.	Add 70% sorbitol solution (15–30 mL q12–24h, max 150 mL/d.
Step 4.	Add stimulant laxative (eg, senna, bisacodyl), 2–3 times per week. (Alternative: saline laxative, but avoid if creatinine clearance <30 mL/min.)
Step 5.	Use tap water enema or saline enema 2 times per week.
Step 6.	Use oil-retention enema for refractory constipation.

less, noninvasive method of retraining the pelvic floor and the abdominal wall musculature, and is recommended for patients with fecal incontinence associated with a structurally intact sphincter (SOE=A). Surgery may involve sphincter repair or implantation of an artificial sphincter. Colostomy may be needed for patients with intractable symptoms in whom other treatments have failed. A synthetic sphincter device, consisting of an inflatable cuff with a valve that allows the cuff to deflate for defecation, can maintain continence (SOE=C).

Diverticular Disease

The prevalence of diverticular disease is age dependent, increasing to 30% by age 60 and to 65% by age 85. Although most patients remain asymptomatic, 20% develop diverticulitis, and 10% may develop diverticular bleeding. Therefore, the mere presence of diverticulosis does not require specific therapy. A diet high in fiber appears to be associated with a reduced risk of developing diverticular disease and may reduce the risk of subsequent complications.

Uncomplicated diverticulosis is often an incidental finding on screening sigmoidoscopy, colonoscopy, or barium enema. Some patients may complain of nonspecific abdominal cramping, bloating, flatulence, and irregular bowel habits. Diverticular bleeding is usually painless and self-limited, and it rarely coexists with acute diverticulitis. Diverticulitis usually presents with left lower quadrant pain, although nausea, vomiting, constipation, diarrhea, and dysuria or frequency may occur. The physical examination usually reveals left lower quadrant tenderness, a tender mass, and abdominal distention. Generalized tenderness suggests perforation and peritonitis. Low-grade fever and leukocytosis are common, but their absence in older adults does not exclude the diagnosis. Urinalysis may reveal sterile pyuria induced by adjacent colonic inflammation; the presence

Table 49.3—Medications that May Relieve Constipation

Medication	Onset of Action	Starting Dosage	Site and Mechanism of Action
Bulk laxatives—not useful in managing opioid-induced constipation			
Methylcellulose[a] (Citrucel[a])	12–24 h (up to 72 h)	2–4 caplets or 1 heaping tablespoon with 8 oz water q8–24h	Small and large intestine; holds water in feces; mechanical distention
Psyllium[a] (Metamucil[a,b])	12–24 h (up to 72 h)	1–2 capsules, packets, or teaspoons with 8 oz water or juice q8–24h	Small and large intestine; holds water in feces; mechanical distention
Polycarbophil[a] (FiberCon[a], others)	12–24 h (up to 72 h)	1250 mg q6–24h	Small and large intestine; holds water in feces; mechanical distention
Chloride channel activator			
Lubiprostone (Amitiza)		24 mcg q12h with food	Enhances chloride-ion intestinal fluid secretion; does not affect serum sodium or potassium concentrations; for idiopathic chronic constipation.
Osmotic laxatives			
Lactulose[a] (Chronulac)	24–48 h	15–30 mL q12–24h	Colon; osmotic effect
Polyethylene glycol[a] (Miralax[a])	48–96 h	17 g powder q24h (approximately 1 tablespoon) dissolved in 8 oz water	GI tract; osmotic effect
Sorbitol 70%[a]	24–48 h	15–30 mL q12–24h; max 150 mL/d	Colon; delivers osmotically active molecules to colon
Saline laxatives			
			Class effect: potential hyperphosphatemia in patients with renal insufficiency
Magnesium citrate[a] (Citroma[a])	30 min–3 h	120–240 mL × 1; 10 oz q24h or 5 oz q12h followed by 8 oz water × ≤5 d	Small and large intestine; attracts, retains water in intestinal lumen
Magnesium hydroxide[a] (Milk of Magnesia[a])	30 min–3 h	30 mL q12–24h	Osmotic effect and increased peristalsis in colon
Sodium phosphate/biphosphate emollient enema[a] (Fleet[a])	2–15 min	14.5 oz enema × 1, repeat prn	Colon; osmotic effect
Stimulant laxatives			
Bisacodyl tablet[a] (Dulcolax[a])	6–10 h	5–15 mg × 1	Colon; increases peristalsis
Bisacodyl suppository[a] (Dulcolax[a])	15 min–1 h	10 mg × 1	Colon; increases peristalsis
Senna[a] (Senokot[a])	6–10 h	2 tablets or 1 teaspoon qhs	Colon; direct action on intestine; stimulates myenteric plexus; alters water and electrolyte secretion
Surfactant laxative (fecal softener)			
Docusate[a] (Colace[a])	24–72 h	100 mg q12–24h	Small and large intestine; detergent activity; facilitates admixture of fat and water to soften feces (effectiveness questionable); does not increase frequency of bowel movements

[a] Available OTC

[b] Psyllium caplets and packets contain ≥3 g dietary fiber and 2–3 g soluble fiber each. A teaspoonful contains approximately 3.8 g dietary fiber and 3 g soluble fiber.

SOURCE: Reuben DB, Herr KA, Pacala JT, et al. *Geriatrics At Your Fingertips*, 12th ed. New York: American Geriatrics Society; 2010. Reprinted with permission.

of mixed colonic flora on urine culture suggests a colovesical fistula. Other potential complications include perforation, obstruction, and abscess formation.

CT scanning is the optimal imaging method in acute diverticulitis. CT features of acute diverticulitis include increased density of soft tissue within pericolic fat and colonic diverticula, thickening of the bowel wall, soft-tissue masses (phlegmon), and pericolic fluid collections (abscess formation). CT can also identify peritonitis; obstruction; and fistula to the bladder, vagina, and abdominal wall. However, in approximately 10% of patients, diverticulitis cannot be distinguished from colon cancer, because both may show focal thickening of the bowel wall. In such cases, on resolution of the acute inflammation, a colonoscopy is indicated. In older adults, CT-guided percutaneous drainage of localized abscesses may obviate emergent surgery and permit single-stage elective surgical resection.

Most (85%) patients with simple diverticulitis respond to medical therapy. In contrast, all patients with complicated diverticulitis require surgery. Indications for emergency surgery are free perforation with peritonitis, obstruction, clinical deterioration or lack of improvement with conservative management, and an abscess that cannot be drained percutaneously. Indications for elective surgical intervention are recurrent or intractable symptoms, persistent mass, obstruction, and fistula or abscess formation.

Mild diverticulitis with left lower quadrant pain, low-grade fever, and minimal physical findings is often treated on an outpatient basis, with clear liquids and oral antibiotics, such as ciprofloxacin 500 mg q12h or metronidazole 500 mg q8h, or both. Hospitalization is needed only if no improvement is seen. Once the episode resolves, solid food is reintroduced and the colon is evaluated, preferably by colonoscopy. For patients with moderate to severe symptoms, treatment with bowel rest, fluids, and intravenous antibiotics is initiated, with the aim to avoid urgent surgery. Antibiotics should be active against gram-negative rods and anaerobes. Possible regimens include cefoxitin, piperacillin-tazobactam, or gentamicin plus clindamycin. If there is no improvement, either the diagnosis is incorrect or an abscess, peritonitis, fistula, or obstruction is present. Older immunosuppressed patients with multiple underlying medical conditions may present with minimal symptoms or signs even with frank peritonitis, and the diagnosis is commonly delayed. In such cases, early surgical intervention should be considered. Diffuse peritonitis requires fluid resuscitation, broad-spectrum antibiotics, and emergency laparotomy. Colonic resective surgery removes the septic focus, corrects the obstruction or fistula formation, and restores bowel continuity. In most elective cases, resection and primary anastomosis are possible if the disease is well localized or has significantly resolved.

After successful medical therapy of the first episode of diverticulitis, one-third of patients will remain asymptomatic, another third will have episodic abdominal cramps (painful diverticulosis), and the remaining third will proceed to a second attack of diverticulitis. Therefore, elective surgery is not necessary for all patients with diverticulitis who respond to medical therapy. If surgery is performed, progression of diverticulosis in the remaining colon occurs in only 15%, and the need for further surgery is reduced to <10%.

Irritable Bowel Syndrome

Irritable bowel syndrome (IBS) is a functional GI disorder with remissions and exacerbations, characterized by abdominal pain, bloating, and either constipation or diarrhea, or both. IBS results from altered bowel motility, visceral hypersensitivity, and enhanced perception by the brain of many visceral stimuli. A common mediator for all these abnormalities is serotonin, and serotonin-receptor agonists and antagonists are used in the management of IBS. Although psychosocial factors are commonly involved in IBS, they are not known to have a causative role.

Because the clinical symptoms characteristic of IBS are not specific, it is important to be mindful of features that are not consistent with IBS. These include weight loss, first onset of symptoms after age 50, nocturnal diarrhea, family history of cancer or inflammatory bowel disease, rectal bleeding or obstruction, and laboratory abnormalities (eg, anemia, leukocytosis, abnormal chemistries, positive fecal cultures, or the presence of parasites in the feces). In older patients, the diagnosis should be made only after other conditions (ie, ischemia, diverticulosis, colon cancer, or inflammatory bowel disease) have been carefully excluded. An appropriate evaluation of an older adult with symptoms consistent with IBS should include a colonoscopy to exclude structural abnormalities of the colon. A CT scan of the abdomen and a small-bowel series may also be useful. If the history, physical examination, and laboratory or imaging studies are negative, the diagnosis of IBS can then be made and subcategorized as IBS with constipation, IBS with diarrhea, or IBS with alternating constipation and diarrhea.

Depending on the IBS subtype, treatment includes reassurance, antispasmodics, antidiarrheals, fiber supplements, and serotonin-receptor agents, such as alosetron. Although quite effective, the latter medications may precipitate intestinal ischemia and should be used with caution, particularly in older patients. Access to alosetron is strictly limited to physicians enrolled in the Prometheus Prescribing

Program (1-888-423-5277 or www.lotronex.com). It is important to establish a definitive diagnosis of IBS, avoid repetitive investigations, and clarify that although IBS is not life threatening, it can certainly negatively impact quality of life. It is also important that clinicians listen actively to patients' symptoms, validate their feelings, provide empathy, set realistic shared goals, negotiate treatment strategies instead of issuing directives, help patients take responsibility for treatment decisions, establish limits on the duration and frequency of visits and phone calls, and maintain a continuing relationship as part of chronic disease management.

Occult Gastrointestinal Bleeding

Older patients are commonly noted to have a positive fecal occult blood test and/or are diagnosed with unexplained iron-deficiency anemia. Although colorectal cancer is a leading concern in such patients, other causes (of which there are many) include esophagitis, peptic ulcers, esophageal and gastric malignancies, intestinal or colonic angiodysplasia, benign colon polyps, inflammatory bowel disease, or hemorrhoids. A positive fecal occult blood test should not be attributed to esophageal varices or colonic diverticula, because it is rare for such lesions to bleed in an occult fashion. The presence of fecal occult blood should not be attributed to aspirin or warfarin use or to alcohol ingestion.

Detection of fecal occult blood has a low sensitivity and a high rate of false-positive results, leading to more invasive and expensive tests. Despite these limitations, annual fecal occult blood testing is currently recommended as one method of screening for colon cancer and has been associated with up to a 33% reduction in mortality from colon cancer (SOE=A). Because of the high prevalence of colorectal cancer and adenomatous polyps in older adults with a positive fecal occult blood test, colonoscopy is performed and, if negative, is followed by an upper endoscopy. If symptoms of upper GI disease are present, there is a high likelihood for a positive endoscopy. However, in older patients at risk of colon cancer, the presence of a proximal lesion should not preclude evaluation of the colon. Patients with normal upper and lower tract may require evaluation for a small-bowel source using video capsule endoscopy, followed if necessary by balloon enteroscopy. The most common cause of bleeding from the small bowel is angiodysplasia, followed by tumors or ulcers that are commonly caused by NSAIDs. Unrecognized gluten-sensitive enteropathy can result in iron-deficiency anemia, because iron is absorbed in the proximal small bowel, and multiple biopsies should always be taken from the duodenum to confirm this diagnosis histologically.

In one prospective study in which patients with iron-deficiency anemia were evaluated with colonoscopy, endoscopy, and if these tests were negative, radiographic examination of the small intestine, a source of bleeding was identified in 62% of cases. A lesion was seen on colonoscopy in 25%, on upper endoscopy in 36%, and on both in 1% of patients. Peptic ulcer disease was the primary abnormality in the upper GI tract, but cancer was detected on colonoscopy in 11% of patients. In cases in which the source is not found, video capsule endoscopy, simple and noninvasive and with a higher diagnostic yield than radiography, should be considered.

Colonic Angiodysplasia

The terms *angiodysplasia*, *arteriovenous malformation*, and *vascular ectasia* have been used interchangeably. Angiodysplasias occur most often in the cecum and ascending colon, where they may cause bleeding, particularly in patients ≥60 yr old. However, angiodysplasias occur throughout the GI tract and may be multiple or coexist in several different regions of the GI tract. They may be asymptomatic or cause occult or clinically overt GI bleeding.

Angiodysplasias are dilated, thin-walled vessels in the mucosa and submucosa that are lined by endothelium or by smooth muscle. Although they are mostly tortuous veins, arteriovenous communications or enlarged arteries may be present, leading to brisk bleeding. The pathogenesis of angiodysplasias is not well understood. They may result from local ischemia associated with cardiac, vascular, or pulmonary disease. More recently, increased expression of angiogenic factors, ie, basic fibroblast growth factor and vascular endothelial growth factor, has been detected in segments of colon with angiodysplasia.

Angiodysplasias are usually diagnosed during endoscopy or colonoscopy, appearing as 5- to 10-mm cherry-red, ectatic blood vessels radiating from a central vascular core. Angiodysplasias can also be diagnosed by angiography. If they are serendipitously detected during routine endoscopy or colonoscopy, angiodysplasias should not be treated. However, an actively bleeding angiodysplasia should be treated. Whether angiodysplasias were the cause of bleeding in patients who have stopped bleeding and, in particular, in patients who are found to have both angiodysplasias and diverticula is a more difficult problem. In such cases, bleeding from angiodysplasias is almost always from the cecum or ascending colon.

Many endoscopic ablation techniques have been used in the treatment of angiodysplasias. Although acute bleeding can be successfully controlled with these approaches, rebleeding is common. Angiography may localize the site of active bleeding and allows embolization or infusion of vasopressin. Surgical resection is definitive for lesions that have been clearly identified as the source of bleeding. However, recurrent bleeding may occur from other proximal or distal lesions in >30% of cases. Hormonal therapy with estrogen (with or without progesterone) has also been used in women, but its benefit should be weighed against the potential risks of thromboembolic disease, estrogen-dependent tumors, or uterine bleeding.

Colonic Ischemia

Ischemic colitis is typically encountered in patients ≥65 yr old who have atherosclerosis or atrial fibrillation or who have had surgical bypass or vascular grafting procedures. The main symptoms at presentation are abdominal pain and lower GI bleeding. Colonoscopy reveals segmental edema, hemorrhages, gray-black pseudomembrane formation, and focal ulcers, mostly in the region of the splenic flexure and typically sparing the rectum. Treatment is mostly supportive, but even with treatment colonic strictures can ensue. The development of peritoneal signs calls for surgical intervention with colonic resection of the involved segment.

Clostridium difficile Infection and Pseudomembranous Colitis

Clostridium difficile infection is becoming increasingly recognized among hospitalized patients and as the source of epidemics in hospitals and long-term care facilities for older adults. A new, hypervirulent strain, NAP1/BI/027, has been implicated as the responsible pathogen in selected C difficile outbreaks and is capable of enhanced production of toxins A and B. The infection is often precipitated by the use of antibiotics, such as cephalosporins, penicillins, or clindamycin. Clinically the disease presents with watery diarrhea, crampy abdominal pain, fever, abdominal tenderness and distention, and an increased WBC count. Serious complications, such as ileus with dehydration and electrolyte abnormalities, toxic megacolon, perforation, and death, may occur. Clostridium difficile infection should be considered when acute abdominal distention occurs in older hospitalized adults without diarrhea but with associated severe leukocytosis; it carries high mortality. Clostridium difficile infection can be recognized endoscopically by the appearance of diffuse or segmental pseudomembranes coating an edematous mucosa, but the diagnosis is often made by the detection of C difficile cytotoxins in the feces either by cytotoxin tissue culture assay, latex agglutination, or enzyme-linked immunoassays. Metronidazole 250 mg po q6h is effective in 85% of cases, and it may be given intravenously in severe cases of ileus or megacolon. Vancomycin (125 mg q6h) is also highly effective but only if given orally. Antibiotic treatment for C difficile colitis should be for 10 to 14 days to reduce the risk of relapse. Relapses may occur in up to 20% of cases and require repeat treatment with metronidazole, vancomycin, or a combination of vancomycin and rifampin (SOE=D). To prevent the disease in predisposed individuals and to avoid relapses, restitution of the colonic flora with lactobacilli or Saccharomyces boulardii has been used (SOE=D).

Acute Colonic Pseudo-Obstruction

Acute colonic pseudo-obstruction is manifested by acute massive dilation of the colon without evidence of mechanical obstruction. In older adults, it is often related to neurologic disease, such as Parkinson's or cerebrovascular disease, trauma, recent orthopedic surgery, or use of narcotics. Infections, particularly C difficile, and colonic ischemia need to be excluded. Urgent colonoscopy not only can assist with the diagnosis but also allows placement of a decompression colonic tube. Parenteral fluids and supportive measures, discontinuation of narcotics, and the use of neostigmine intravenously often lead to rapid resolution.

Colonic Polyps and Colon Cancer

Polyps are usually asymptomatic, but they may bleed or predispose the patient to cancer. Colonic polyps are usually classified as neoplastic (adenomas) or non-neoplastic (hyperplastic). Approximately 40% of the U.S. population ≥50 yr old has one or more adenomas. Detection and removal of adenomas significantly decrease the morbidity and mortality associated with colorectal cancer. Old age and male gender are major risk factors. First-degree relatives of patients with adenomas are also at increased risk of colorectal cancer and should undergo screening. Adenomas are most often detected by colon cancer screening tests, primarily sigmoidoscopy. Because adenomas do not typically bleed, the fecal occult blood test is an insensitive screening method. Older age, villous histology, and size are independent risk factors for malignancy within an adenoma. The risk of colon cancer also increases with the number of high-risk adenomas that are present.

Colorectal cancer is the third leading cause of cancer in the United States and the second leading cause of cancer death. The risk of colorectal cancer increases dramatically with age, with >90% of cases occurring in people >50 yr old. Women are more likely than men to harbor right-sided colonic adenomas. The risk of colorectal cancer in patients with rectal bleeding is age related and may reach 25% in patients ≥80 yr old. Up to 40% of colorectal

Table 49.4—Follow-Up Recommendations Based on Polyp Characteristics

Polyp Characteristics	Relative Risk of Malignancy in Subsequent 5–6 Years	Repeat Colonoscopy Recommendation (yr)
Non-neoplastic		
Hyperplastic	1 (reference)	10
Neoplastic		
Tubular adenoma (1–2) <1 cm	1–2	5–10
Tubular adenoma (>3) <1 cm	1.5–6	3
Advanced neoplastic		
Tubular adenoma >1 cm	2–6	3
Villous adenoma	1.5–6	3
Adenoma with high grade dysplasia	1.5–6	3

SOURCE: Data from Winawer SJ, Zauber AG, Fletcher RH, et al. Guidelines for colonoscopy surveillance after polypectomy; a consensus update by the US Multi-Society Task Force on Colorectal Cancer and the American Cancer Society. *Gastroenterology.* 2006;130(6):1872–1885.

cancer arises proximal to the splenic flexure, and <10% is within the reach of the digital rectal examination. Because it is impossible to identify the source of bleeding by clinical criteria, a colonoscopy should be performed in all cases of hematochezia, occult GI bleeding, iron-deficiency anemia, or even melena after a negative upper endoscopy (SOE=C). Other symptoms, such as abdominal pain, altered bowel habits, or pencil-thin feces are less predictive of colorectal cancer but do require thorough investigation, starting with a colonoscopy. Typically, right-sided cancers present with iron-deficiency anemia and occult GI bleeding, whereas left-sided cancers lead to obstructive symptoms, changes in bowel habits, and overt hematochezia.

Colonoscopy with endoscopic polypectomy is the ideal examination for the detection and removal of adenomatous polyps. The examination should be meticulous with emphasis to mucosal detail to not miss flat or depressed adenomatous lesions. In addition, a minimum of 6 minutes of colonoscopic withdrawal time is associated with increased polyp yield. Large adenomas that cannot be safely or completely resected endoscopically should generally be removed by segmental colectomy. If a polyp is detected by barium enema, colonoscopy is recommended to establish the histology, remove the polyp, and search for other lesions. If a single polyp is detected by sigmoidoscopy, it should be biopsied. If the polyp is hyperplastic, colonoscopy is not required. If the polyp is adenomatous, full colonoscopy is warranted. In patients with a known history of polyps, discontinuation of surveillance should be considered in those >75 yr old in whom a follow-up examination is normal or shows only small tubular adenomas. For follow-up colonoscopy recommendations based on polyp characteristics, see Table 49.4.

A 3-yr interval for surveillance colonoscopy is safe and cost-effective for most patients with adenomas. If only a small tubular adenoma is found, the interval may be extended to 5 yr; in contrast, after removal of a large villous adenoma, a 1-yr follow-up is recommended. After a negative screening or surveillance colonoscopy, an examination interval of 5 yr appears to be safe. Patients with colorectal cancer should also have regular colonoscopic surveillance for adenomas starting 1 yr after surgery, because these patients have adenoma or cancer recurrence rates of 25%–30% at 3 yr.

ACOVE-3* QUALITY INDICATORS PERTAINING TO GASTROINTESTINAL DISEASES AND DISORDERS

MEDICATION USE

NSAIDs and aspirin

- If a vulnerable older adult is prescribed an NSAID (nonselective or selective), then GI bleeding risks should be discussed and documented.
- If a vulnerable older adult is prescribed daily aspirin (including low-dose, ≤325 mg/d), then GI bleeding risks should be discussed and documented.
- If a vulnerable older adult with a risk factor for GI bleeding (age ≥75 yr old, peptic ulcer disease, history of GI bleeding, warfarin use, chronic glucocorticoid use) is treated with a nonselective NSAID, then he or she should be treated concomitantly with misoprostol or a proton-pump inhibitor.
- If a vulnerable older adult with two or more risk factors for GI bleeding (age ≥75 yr old, peptic ulcer disease, history of GI bleeding, warfarin use, chronic glucocorticoid use) is treated with daily aspirin, then he or she should be treated concomitantly with misoprostol or a proton-pump inhibitor.

REFERENCES

■ Crane SJ, Talley NJ. Chronic gastrointestinal symptoms in the elderly. *Clin Geriatr Med.* 2007;23(4):721−734.

■ Eisenstadt SE. Dysphagia and aspiration pneumonia in older adults. *J Am Acad Nurse Pract.* 2010;22(1):17−22.

■ Tariq SH, Mekhjian G. Gastrointestinal bleeding in older adults. *Clin Geriatr Med.* 2007;23(4):769−784.

■ Whitlock EP, Lin JS, Liles E, et al. Screening for colorectal cancer: a targeted, upated systematic review for the U.S. Preventive Services Task Force. *Ann Intern Med.* 2008;149(9):638−658.

CHAPTER 50—KIDNEY DISEASES AND DISORDERS

KEY POINTS

■ The aging kidney is less able to maintain homeostasis in response to physiologic stress.

■ Serum creatinine is a poor marker of kidney function. Kidney function is best measured by the glomerular filtration rate (GFR).

■ Prerenal azotemia causing acute intrinsic renal damage is more common in older adults than in younger ones.

■ Chronic kidney disease (CKD) is very common in the older population and is classified into five stages based on GFR. Preventing progression of CKD is important at any age.

■ Referral to a nephrologist for patients with advanced CKD is helpful for assisting with management and for discussing the options and likely outcomes of dialysis or a kidney transplant.

THE AGING KIDNEY

Age-related anatomic, hemodynamic, and hormonal changes in the kidneys affect crucial functions that maintain homeostasis of fluids, electrolytes, volume, and acid-base balance. Under normal conditions, the aging kidney is able to maintain homeostasis; however, under stress, the adaptive response of the kidney to maintain homeostasis is impaired. For some of the changes seen in renal tubular functioning with aging, see Table 50.1.

Monitoring Kidney Function

The most important indicator of kidney function to be monitored with aging is the GFR. Cross-sectional studies have shown a progressive decline in GFR after the age of 30–40 yr in both men and women. Traditionally, BUN and serum creatinine have been monitored to assess kidney function. However, these are notoriously insensitive indicators of loss of renal function, typically not increasing until 75% of function has been lost. Muscle mass, the main source of serum creatinine, declines with age, especially in frail older adults. Because the decline in muscle mass tends to parallel the decline in kidney function, most older adults maintain a stable serum creatinine, frequently leading to overestimation of kidney functioning through creatinine measurement. Figure 50.1 illustrates how kidney function can be profoundly impaired even though serum creatinine concentration is normal. As shown in Figure 50.1, an 80-yr-old woman with a serum creatinine of 1 can have an estimated GFR of around 30 mL/min, a level at which almost all medications need significant dosing adjustment.

Because direct measurement of GFR is both expensive and time consuming, formulas for estimat-

Table 50.1—Declines in Kidney Function with Aging

Function	Mechanisms	Clinical Significance
Glomerular filtration rate (GFR)	Numerous	Increased susceptibility to acute and chronic kidney disease
Sodium conservation	Decrease in distal tubular sodium reabsorption, renin levels and activity, and aldosterone levels	Increased susceptibility to hyponatremia from salt loss caused by excessive diaphoresis, GI losses, etc
Sodium excretion	Decrease in GFR and response to atrial natriuretic peptide	Increased percentage of nocturnal sodium load excretion contributing to nocturia and susceptibility to hypernatremia
Renal concentrating capacity	Decrease in tubular water transport in response to arginine vasopressin release	Decreased response to hyperosmolar and volume-deprived conditions
Renal diluting capacity	Unclear; may be due to decrease in GFR	Decreased response to hypoosmolar and volume-overloaded conditions
Acid and ammonium excretion	Decrease in GFR and renal mass	Increased susceptibility to metabolic acidosis

ing GFR have been developed. These formulas predict GFR far more accurately than measures of serum creatinine, but they tend to become less accurate in the oldest and frailest patients. The most commonly used and practical method for estimating GFR is to calculate creatinine clearance by using the Cockcroft-Gault equation:

Creatinine clearance =

$$\frac{(140 - \text{age})(\text{weight in kg})(0.85 \text{ if female})}{(72)(\text{stable serum creatinine in mg/dL})}$$

Many clinical laboratories now provide estimates of GFR based on the Modified Diet in Renal Disease (MDRD) formula, and this information can be requested when submitting samples for a basic or comprehensive metabolic panel. However, the MDRD formula has not been validated in adults >70 yr old, and it is unreliable at extreme weights and extreme age. Determining the actual GFR by performing a 24-hour creatinine clearance can be useful for sensitive medication dosing and for assessing the risk of ischemic, toxic, or metabolic events in the aging kidney.

ELECTROLYTE DISORDERS

Older adults are vulnerable to dehydration and/or volume overload. For age-related changes that predispose older adults to osmolar abnormalities, see Table 50.1. Precipitants of osmolar disturbances include the following:

- Decreased thirst sensation in older adults, especially with concomitant cognitive impairment
- Impaired access to fluids and/or sodium, especially in institutionalized patients
- Fluid and/or sodium loss from diarrhea, vomiting, or diaphoresis
- Volume and pressure changes related to surgery
- Increased fluid intake, especially from injudicious administration of intravenous fluids
- Medications, especially diuretics (particularly thiazides) and NSAIDs
- Conditions and medications that cause syndrome of inappropriate antidiuretic hormone secretion (SIADH), such as pulmonary malignancies, infections, and antidepressant medications
- Comorbidities, especially cardiac and hepatic dysfunction

Disorders of Sodium Balance

Serum sodium concentrations are abnormal in >25% of older adults presenting acutely to the hospital. Increasing age is a strong independent risk factor for both hyponatremia and hypernatremia.

Hyponatremia

Hyponatremia has been reported to occur in 11.3% of hospitalized geriatric patients and in as high as 22.5% of older adults in long-term care facilities. Enhanced osmotic release of antidiuretic hormone (ADH) and impaired diluting ability predispose older adults to a higher incidence of hyponatremia.

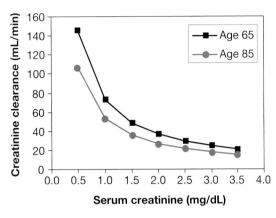

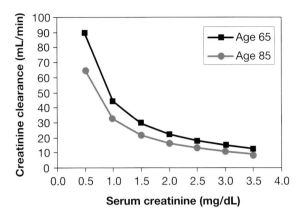

Figure 50.1—Calculated creatinine clearance versus serum creatinine for a 70-kg man and a 50-kg woman. Clearances were calculated using the Cockcroft-Gault equation.

Thiazide diuretics have also been implicated in up to 30% of cases in older adults. When administered with other medications such as sulfonylureas or NSAIDs, thiazides potentiate the peripheral action of ADH and impair free water excretion.

Patients with hyponatremia are generally asymptomatic until the serum sodium concentration falls below 125 mEq/L. The osmotic shift of water from the extracellular to the intracellular space with hyponatremia can cause brain edema, leading to symptoms of apathy, disorientation, lethargy, muscle cramps, anorexia, nausea, agitation, headache, and seizures. If hyponatremia develops rapidly, muscular twitches, irritability, and convulsions can occur. The only manifestations of chronic hyponatremia may be lethargy, confusion, and malaise. Recognizing hyponatremia, discerning its primary cause, and instituting therapy is important to avoid severe neurologic sequelae, including central pontine demyelinolysis. Urgent or emergent treatment of hyponatremia is indicated with the appearance of the above symptoms or with acute severe hyponatremia (serum sodium concentration <120 mEq/L).

Hyponatremia can develop when plasma osmolality is increased (hypertonic hyponatremia usually caused by hyperglycemia), normal (isotonic hyponatremia usually presenting as pseudohyponatremia in hyperlipidemic or hyperproteinemic states), or most commonly, decreased (hypotonic hyponatremia). Hypotonic hyponatremia results from three major causes related to extracellular fluid (ECF) volume status:

■ Contracted ECF volume (primary salt depletion)

■ Expanded ECF volume (dilutional hyponatremia)

■ Normal ECF volume (SIADH)

Hypotonic Hyponatremia with Contracted ECF Volume (Primary Salt Depletion)

Older adults who have lost both salt and water caused by concurrent illness are frequently hypovolemic and hyponatremic because of excess (sodium) losses and oral replacement with water only. A urine sodium concentration of <10 mEq/L indicates extrarenal salt depletion; possible causes include the following:

■ Decreased salt intake

■ Excessive sweating and replacement with hypotonic fluid

■ Excess GI losses

■ Third spacing

A urine sodium concentration of >20 mEq/L indicates renal salt loss; possible causes include the following:

■ Use of diuretics, particularly thiazides and/or ACE inhibitors

■ Adrenal insufficiency

■ Pituitary insufficiency

■ Intrinsic renal disease with salt wasting

In older adults with hyponatremia and ECF volume depletion, the urgency for correction of serum sodium depends on the magnitude and rate of development of hyponatremia (see treatment of hyponatremia, below).

Hypotonic Hyponatremia with Expanded ECF Volume (Dilutional Hyponatremia)

In this condition, both free water and sodium excretion are impaired. Common conditions include heart failure, hepatic cirrhosis, and renal disease, including nephrotic syndrome. In these conditions, a decrease in effective arterial volume stimulates the renin-angiotensin-aldosterone axis, thus promoting salt and water retention. The urine sodium concentration is typically <10 mEq/L.

Hypotonic Hyponatremia with Normal ECF Volume (SIADH)

In this condition, ADH is released inappropriately when neither serum hyperosmolality nor volume depletion is present. Urine sodium concentration is usually >40 mEq/L, and serum uric acid is usually <4 mg/dL. Pulmonary pathology, including infections and malignancy, is prominent among many conditions associated with SIADH. In addition, several agents potentiate the action of ADH, including angiotensin, nicotine, vincristine, morphine, cyclophosphamide, histamine, and sulfonylureas. Centrally acting drugs such as antidepressants and anticonvulsant medications can also cause SIADH.

Treatment of Hyponatremia

Treatment depends on the pathogenesis of the hyponatremia and the severity of symptoms. Asymptomatic patients with hypovolemic hyponatremia and those with hypotension are best treated by the administration of isotonic saline to replenish the intravascular volume. Water restriction is indicated in asymptomatic patients with hypervolemic hyponatremia or SIADH. The addition of loop diuretics can be effective in prompting both salt and water excretion in hypervolemic states or severe SIADH.

Symptomatic hyponatremia warrants treatment with intravenous hypertonic saline. Patients treated with either isotonic or hypertonic saline should be reassessed frequently for adequacy of volume repletion by monitoring skin turgor, jugular venous pressure, and urine sodium concentration. Care must also be taken not to induce fluid overload and pulmonary vascular congestion. The administration of normal saline at 75 mL/h should raise serum sodium concentration by approximately 0.3–0.4 mEq/h. If there are concerns about heart disease, a slower rate of 50 mL/h is advisable. The serum sodium concentration should be determined as necessary and regulated as dictated by the clinical situation.

The amount of sodium required to increase the plasma sodium concentration to a desired value can be more carefully determined using the following formula:

Sodium deficit = lean body weight in kg × (desired Na − measured Na) × 0.6 [in men] or 0.5 [in women]

In patients with serum sodium concentrations <120 mEq/L or in those with neurologic symptoms, the sodium deficit to increase plasma sodium concentration to 120 mEq/L is calculated and administered as 3% hypertonic saline. As an example, a 60-kg woman started on a thiazide diuretic presents 5 days later with lethargy, confusion, and a serum sodium of 110 mEq/L. The amount of sodium required to increase the plasma sodium concentration to a safe level of 120 mEq/L is:

Sodium deficit = 60 × (120–110) × 0.5 = 300 mEq

Because 3% hypertonic saline contains 513 mEq/L of sodium, 600 mL of this solution will provide the required amount of sodium.

The rate of administration should be adjusted to provide enough sodium to raise the plasma sodium concentration by 0.3–0.4 mEq/h (7–10 mEq/24 h), because correction at a rate >0.5 mEq/h has been associated with severe neurologic complications, including osmotic demyelinating syndrome. For the example noted above, 600 mL of hypertonic saline administered at a rate of 25 mL/h over 24 hours should raise plasma sodium from 110 mEq/L to 120 mEq/L. Once a safe serum sodium concentration is reached (120 mEq/L), the sodium and volume deficit can be corrected with isotonic saline.

Conivaptan is a nonselective ADH-receptor antagonist that has been approved by the FDA as an intravenous infusion for inpatient treatment of euvolemic or hypervolemic hyponatremia. In initial studies, conivaptan effectively raised plasma sodium concentration up to 9 mEq/L in the acute setting over 4 days, but plasma sodium concentrations were not maintained at the higher level over several additional days. While nonselective ADH-receptor antagonists look promising, their role remains unclear for treatment of hyponatremia in older adults.

Hypernatremia

Serum sodium concentration can increase from either a net loss of water or a gain of sodium from ingestion. The impaired ability of the aging kidney to concentrate urine and conserve sodium can predispose older adults to hypernatremia. Further risks of hypernatremia in older adults stem from impaired thirst and decreased fluid consumption. Patients with a depressed level of consciousness or immobility with decreased ability to obtain access to free water are at greatest risk of hypernatremia; mortality can be as high as 70%.

Older adults with systemic illnesses, infections, fever, dementia, and neurologic disorders are at significant risk of dehydration and hypernatremia. Medications that inhibit the action of ADH (eg, lithium, demeclocycline) should be avoided in older adults. In addition, medications that can cloud the sensorium, osmotic diuretic agents, tube feedings containing high protein and glucose, and bowel cathartics should be limited in older adults to minimize risk of hypernatremia.

Cellular dehydration can lead to severe neurologic sequelae, including obtundation, stupor, coma, and death. Free water deficits should be corrected by administering intravenous dextrose solution or enteral free water. Free water deficit should be replaced over 72 hours and can be calculated as follows:

Free water deficit (L) = (serum sodium/140 − 1) × weight in kg × 0.6 [in men] or 0.5 [in women]

Ongoing losses should also be included in the replacement.

Disorders of Potassium Balance

Hypokalemia in older adults generally results from renal loss of potassium through the use of diuretics and GI loss from vomiting, diarrhea, fistula drainage, and the use of enemas. Inadequate intake of potassium can also contribute to the development of hypokalemia. Treatment is most commonly accomplished by administration of oral potassium.

Several factors contribute to the increased risk of hyperkalemia in older adults, including the following:

- An age-related decline in aldosterone levels, leading to decreased potassium excretion in the distal tubule

- A defect in distal renal acidification, possibly leading to increased incidence of type 4 renal tubular acidosis or hyporeninemic hypoaldosteronism

- Medications that interfere with the renin-angiotensin-aldosterone axis, including ACE inhibitors, angiotensin-receptor blockers (ARBs), potassium-sparing diuretics, eplerenone, heparin, NSAIDs, and β-blockers. The concomitant use of sodium channel blocking drugs (eg, trimethoprim, pentamidine) has similar effects.

Hyperkalemia is most commonly seen in the setting of CKD. It is also seen in acute conditions causing acidosis. It is advisable to repeat potassium measurement when hyperkalemia is found, because potassium concentrations can be falsely increased from acidosis being produced by repeated fist clenching and unclenching during a blood draw. Restricting potassium-rich foods, discontinuing medications that cause hyperkalemia (see above), and using loop diuretics are effective for minor cases of hyperkalemia. Adding sodium polystyrene sulfonate orally or rectally is useful for more severe (eg, potassium concentration ≥6 mEq/L) or refractory cases, and emergent treatment is indicated for signs of cardiac toxicity or severe increases of serum potassium.

Nephrotic Syndrome

Nephrotic syndrome consists of urinary excretion of >3 g of protein per day, with associated hypo- albuminemia, hyperlipidemia, edema, and a hypercoagulable state. Hypertension and renal failure are also seen in about one-third of cases in older adults. Nephrotic syndrome can result from primary glomerular disease or from secondary glomerular disease caused by infection, malignancy, exposure to allergens or medications, or multisystem disease.

The histologic lesions of nephrotic syndrome in order of approximate frequency in the older population (based on cumulative data from several studies) are as follows:

- Membranous nephropathy, 54%
- Minimal change, 19%
- Amyloidosis, up to 10%
- Mesangial and membranoproliferative glomerulonephritis, 9% each
- Focal segmental glomerulosclerosis, 7%

The histopathology of nephrotic syndrome is unpredictable based on only clinical data; therefore, renal biopsy is essential for early diagnosis and appropriate therapy.

Renovascular Disease

Renovascular disease is primarily an illness of the older population. Most risk factors for renovascular disease increase with age and include smoking, atherosclerosis, thromboembolic disease, hypertension, hyperlipidemia, diabetes mellitus, dissecting aortic aneurysms, vasculitis, and neurofibromatosis. Renovascular disease is closely associated with other vascular disease and is present in 24% of those undergoing coronary angiography (SOE=A). In patients with renovascular disease, mortality is typically related to cardiovascular events rather than to renal impairment. Stenosis of the renal artery needs to be >70%–80% of the luminal area to cause changes in pressure and blood flow. These changes in turn activate the renin-angiotensin system in an attempt to restore renal perfusion.

Renal artery stenosis should be suspected in cases of new onset diastolic hypertension, inability to control hypertension despite therapy with maximal doses of 3 antihypertensive agents, abruptly worsening hypertension that was previously stable, azotemia induced by treatment with an ACE inhibitor or an ARB, or hypertension accompanied by widespread vascular disease. Diagnostic test options include renal artery duplex ultrasonography, CT angiography, or magnetic resonance angiography.

Atherosclerosis is a progressive disorder, and management of renovascular disease needs to address the underlying process as well as the stenotic lesion. Therapy is based on aggressive management of the above risk factors. Antihypertensive regimens should include angiotensin blockade. Although 2%–6% of patients treated with an ACE inhibitor or an ARB may have an increase in serum creatinine concentration as an expected complication of therapy, modest increases in creatinine should not deter prescribing these medications, which reduce morbidity and mortality in patients with hypertension and vascular disease (SOE=A for ACE inhibitors, SOE=B for ARBs).

Renovascular angioplasty, with or without stenting, carries significant risks, particularly in patients with abdominal aortic atherosclerosis. Renal function declines abruptly in about 25% of patients after revascularization. Numerous case series of angioplasty with stenting show complication rates of 0–8% for embolization, 0–3% for dialysis, 0–4% for death, and 11%–26% for restenosis over an average of 10 mo, while hypertension was significantly improved or cured in an average of 57% of cases (SOE=B). Invasive procedures should be limited to those in whom medical management has been unable to satisfactorily control blood pressure, those who develop heart failure, and those with progressive decline in renal function.

ACUTE RENAL FAILURE (ARF)

More than half of patients with ARF are >60 yr old. Changes in renal function with aging (Table 50.1) create a progressive decline in renal reserve and compromise the kidney's ability to respond to sudden excesses or deficits of salt or water. Older adults are thus particularly vulnerable to superimposed renal complications during acute illnesses. Chronic conditions such as hypertension accelerate this age-related loss of renal reserve, and increased vulnerability to ARF in these patients should be anticipated.

Predisposing factors for ARF are more common with aging and include the following:

- Reduced renal blood flow and GFR
- Volume contraction
- Medications, especially NSAIDs, ACE inhibitors, ARBs, and diuretics
- Surgery
- Arrhythmias
- Sepsis
- Toxins, including intravenous contrast dyes
- Thromboembolic disease
- Urinary obstruction

ARF has three primary causes: prerenal azotemia, intrinsic renal damage, and postrenal ARF. The BUN-to-creatinine ratio is useful in determining the cause but may not always be applicable in older adults. In prerenal and postrenal failure, the BUN-to-creatinine ratio is generally greater than 20:1, but in intrinsic renal damage, the ratio remains close to normal at 10:1. Hypovolemic prerenal azotemia, acute tubular necrosis, obstructive uropathy, and renal embolic syndromes are much more common in older patients than in younger ones.

Even though older adults may be at higher risk of developing ARF and renal recovery can take longer, age is not an important determinant of survival in patients with ARF. Therefore, age should not be used as a discriminating factor in making therapeutic decisions. Most patients respond well to treatment of ARF with dialysis. Therefore, prompt therapy with dialysis should be started to treat uremic symptoms and to prevent complications, including infection, heart failure, and bleeding.

Prerenal Azotemia

Prerenal azotemia is due to hypoperfusion of the kidney. The aged kidney's impaired ability to retain sodium and concentrate urine, along with age-related impairment of thirst and declines in renal plasma flow, GFR, and autoregulation of renal plasma flow can render the kidney more susceptible to prerenal failure.

Several clinical conditions can cause renal hypoperfusion. Hypovolemia, frequently from dehydration, excessive diuresis, or GI fluid loss, is a major cause of prerenal failure in older adults. The use of ACE inhibitors, ARBs, NSAIDS, and α-adrenergic blockers can further exacerbate prerenal azotemia by compromising renal blood flow due to increased vascular resistance. Reduced cardiac output, most commonly from exacerbations of heart failure, is another common cause of hypoperfusion.

Prompt identification of prerenal ARF and treatment of its underlying causes are critical, because restoration of perfusion often results in recovery of renal function. If uncorrected, prerenal ARF can result in intrinsic renal disease, namely acute tubular necrosis, which has a prerenal cause in >50% of older patients.

Intrinsic Renal Disease

Intrinsic renal disease results from three pathologic processes: acute tubular necrosis, acute interstitial nephritis, and acute glomerulonephritis.

Acute Tubular Necrosis (ATN)

Ischemia is the most common cause of ATN in older adults. Evolution of prerenal azotemia to frank ATN is more common in older patients with ARF (23%) than in younger ones (15%). Renal hypoperfusion leading to ATN is generally due to systemic hypotension in which the normal autoregulation of renal blood flow and GFR are interfered with by therapeutic interventions or by preexisting renovascular disease in situations such as:

- Complications of surgery, accounting for about 30% of cases
- Vasodilation and hypotension from infection and sepsis, accounting for about 30% of cases
- Antibiotic use for treatment of sepsis, particularly aminoglycosides
- Radiocontrast agents
- Atheroembolic renal disease as a complication of arterial cannulation

The differentiation between prerenal azotemia and established ATN generally depends on the analysis of urinary electrolytes, urine osmolality, and careful inspection of urinary sediment for the presence of granular "muddy brown" casts. Typically in prerenal azotemia, the fractional excretion of sodium (FE_{Na}) is <1%, the urinary sodium concentration (U_{Na}) is <20 mEq/L, the urine osmolality is >500 mOsm/kg, and muddy brown casts are absent. In ATN, usual values are FE_{Na} >3%, U_{Na} >20 mEq/L, urine osmolality <300 mOsm/kg, and muddy brown casts are more likely to be present.

Treatment of patients with ATN is generally supportive. Early management of patients with established ATN should include investigating the cause, assessing volume status and systemic hemodynamics, and instituting appropriate therapeutic measures designed to prevent or reduce worsening kidney function. Interventions should include maintaining adequate hemodynamic status to ensure renal perfusion and avoiding further injury by removing or decreasing the effect of any nephrotoxins. Medication dosing needs to be adjusted to the level of renal function to prevent toxicity and further renal injury. Careful attention should be paid to nutritional status and correction of fluid and electrolyte abnormalities. When required, older patients respond well to treatment with dialysis to alleviate uremic symptoms and complications of ARF such as volume overload, bleeding, disorientation, catabolic state, and electrolyte disturbances.

Acute Interstitial Nephritis

Acute interstitial nephritis induced by medication is becoming increasingly common in older adults. Medications such as NSAIDs and ACE inhibitors can cause interstitial inflammation and acute interstitial nephritis. In addition, more than forty other commonly used medications have been implicated in causing acute interstitial nephritis. Commonly implicated antibiotics include β-lactam antibiotics, particularly methicillin, and fluoroquinolones, particularly ciprofloxacin. Therapy consists of discontinuing the offending agent. Rarely, a short trial of oral corticosteroids may be necessary when the interstitial inflammation is severe.

Acute Glomerulonephritis

The clinical features of hematuria, proteinuria, sodium and fluid retention, decreased renal function, and hypertension seen in acute glomerulonephritis are seen in all age groups. The diagnosis may be delayed in older adults because of incorrectly attributing symptoms to preexisting conditions, to common conditions found in older adults (particularly heart failure), or to "normal" aging.

Rapidly progressive glomerulonephritis is the most common form of acute glomerulonephritis in older adults. Many patients have systemic vasculitis, a group of disorders characterized by inflammation and necrotizing lesions of the blood vessel walls, including Wegener's granulomatosis and polyarteritis nodosa. Rapidly progressive glomerulonephritis should be considered in patients with ARF and fever, weight loss, arthritis, abdominal pain, myopathy, cardiac disease, or CNS dysfunction. Clinically, renal function declines rapidly and is accompanied by hematuria, pyuria, moderate to severe proteinuria, and RBC casts in the urine sediment. Histologic examination reveals severe crescentic involvement, commonly affecting more than half of the glomeruli. A pauci-immune crescentic glomerulonephritis is frequently diagnosed on immunofluorescence, but antiglomerular basement membrane disease has also been reported. Often, these patients have sera that are antineutrophil cytoplasmic antibody (ANCA)-positive but no immune deposits on renal biopsy. Therapy for rapidly progressive glomerulonephritis includes pulse steroids, cyclophosphamide, and plasmapheresis. While successful treatment has been reported in small, uncontrolled case series, the overall prognosis for older adults with rapidly progressive glomerulonephritis is poor.

Diffuse poststreptococcal acute glomerulonephritis is associated with streptococcal infection of the throat and skin in older adults, with an incidence as high as 22.6% in patients >55 yr old. The prognosis is generally favorable.

Postrenal Acute Renal Failure

Postrenal obstruction is a common and often treatable cause of ARF in older adults. Symptomatic obstructive uropathy with rising BUN and creatinine concentrations is often seen in older men with prostatic hypertrophy. Ureteric obstruction in women can arise from pelvic tumors of the ovary, uterus, or cervix. In addition, other retroperitoneal malignancies, such as lymphoma, bladder carcinoma, and rectal tumors can also present with ARF in the geriatric population. The typical symptoms of urinary tract obstruction, such as urinary frequency and voiding difficulties, may not be readily apparent in older adults. Careful review of medications, particularly anticholinergic

Table 50.2—Stages of Chronic Kidney Disease

Stage	Description	GFR (mL/min/1.73 m²)
1	Kidney damage with normal or increased GFR	>90
2	Kidney damage with mild decrease in GFR	60–89
3	Moderate decrease in GFR	30–59
4	Severe decrease in GFR	15–29
5	Kidney failure	<15 (or dialysis)

agents, can be useful. Measurement of postvoid residual urine volumes as well as renal ultrasonography may be necessary to establish the diagnosis. Prompt urologic evaluation is warranted in cases of documented urinary tract obstruction.

CHRONIC KIDNEY DISEASE

Kidney function as measured by GFR declines 10% per decade after age 40 in 70% of the population. Glomerulosclerosis (fibrosis of the kidney) increases with age, leading to CKD. CKD has many causes in older adults, including glomerulopathies (especially diabetic nephropathy), tubulointerstitial nephritis (often medication-induced), obstructive nephropathies, and renovascular disease. Progression of medical illnesses, especially chronic hypertension, often leads to development of CKD late in life. Clinical progression of CKD in older adults frequently manifests as a decompensation of preexisting medical illness such as heart failure, diabetes mellitus, hypertension, or dementia.

NHANES III data suggest that 6.6 million people >60 yr old have CKD. The incidence varies between ethnic and racial groups. Diabetes and hypertension, both important causes of CKD, are more common in black, Hispanic, and some Native American populations. Blacks with diabetes or hypertension are more than twice as likely to develop kidney failure than other ethnic or racial groups, and the odds increase for individuals with a first-degree relative on dialysis for any reason.

Chronic Kidney Disease Classification

In 2002, The National Kidney Foundation issued clinical practice guidelines and established the current classification nomenclature for chronic renal disorders. Chronic renal insufficiency, the term that had been used traditionally, was renamed chronic kidney disease, classified into five stages based on GFR regardless of underlying diagnosis (Table 50.2). CKD is defined as either kidney damage or decreased kidney function for ≥3 mo. CKD progresses from Stage 1, kidney damage with preserved GFR, to Stage

5, kidney failure defined as a GFR of <15 mL/min/ 1.73 m² or the need to start renal replacement therapy.

Management

Emphasis in older adults should be on preserving residual renal function using the same approaches as in younger people. Basic treatment principles include correcting reversible causes; aggressively controlling blood pressure; using ACE inhibitors, ARBs, and aldosterone antagonists; optimally controlling blood glucose; treating hyperlipidemia; minimizing proteinuria; aggressively managing phosphorous concentration; and moderately restricting dietary protein. Detailed clinical guidelines are available on the National Kidney Foundation Web site at http://www.kidney.org (accessed Jan 2011).

Declines in GFR are accompanied by a broad range of complications, including hypertension, anemia, malnutrition, metabolic bone disease, neuropathy, depression, impaired functional status, and increased cardiovascular morbidity and mortality. Early recognition of impaired kidney function allows screening for and managing these complications, thus preventing comorbidities and reduced quality of life. National Kidney Foundation Guidelines recommend referral to a nephrologist when a patient reaches Stage 4 CKD for management of the complications of impaired function such as acidosis, phosphorous retention, and anemia. Preparation for renal replacement therapy should also begin during Stage 4, so referral should be made to a nephrologist when the GFR falls to <30 mL/min/1.73 m².

Medication Use in Chronic Kidney Disease

Prescribing medications in the CKD population is complicated by age-associated changes in pharmacokinetics and pharmacodynamics (see "Pharmacotherapy," p 72), and compounded by diminished renal clearance. Most medications or their metabolites are renally excreted. Adjustments in dosage or dosing frequency may be needed once the estimated GFR falls to <50 mL/min/1.73 m². Almost all dosages need to be adjusted after the GFR falls to <30 mL/min/1.73 m². This is particularly true of medications likely to cause complications in older adults, including the following:

- Analgesics, including NSAIDs
- Barbiturates
- Antihistamines, including diphenhydramine
- Decongestants containing ephedrine-related compounds
- Muscle relaxants
- Cardiac drugs, including antiarrhythmics, amiodarone, short-acting calcium channel blockers, and digoxin

Management of Anemia

Screening for anemia should start when patients reach Stage 3 CKD. The anemia is typically normochromic and normocytic and is primarily caused by reduced production of erythropoietin by the kidneys. It is important to exclude other causes before treatment is started. In older adults, vitamin B_{12}, folate, thyrotropin, and iron studies (including transferrin saturation) should be checked. In case of iron deficiency, a bowel evaluation should be performed.

Approximately 50% of patients who reach end-stage kidney disease are iron deficient for dietary reasons by the time renal replacement therapy is needed. Iron should be replaced before starting other therapy for anemia. The goal is to raise the transferrin saturation to >20%. Giving erythropoietin to replace lost RBC mass requires adequate iron stores to support accelerated erythropoiesis. Most patients can tolerate oral iron, and stores can be replenished over a period of time. If the patient has severe or symptomatic anemia, iron can be given intravenously using iron sucrose, which is better tolerated than older iron preparations and much less likely to cause flu-like symptoms.

Once iron deficiency is corrected, treatment with human recombinant erythropoietin can be started. This medication is expensive, and Medicare requires the health care provider to certify that the anemia is due to kidney failure and that iron stores are adequate. Current Medicare guidelines require a hemoglobin concentration of <12.5 g/dL with a hematocrit of <39% to qualify for erythropoietin therapy. Some controversy exists over the goal of replacement hemoglobin; two large, randomized controlled trials of erythropoietin treatment support a target hemoglobin concentration of 11.3–11.5 mg/dL without exceeding 12 mg/dL (SOE=A).

Calcium, Phosphorus, and Renal Bone Disease

Abnormalities of calcium, phosphorus, and parathyroid hormone (PTH) are common in patients whose GFR is <60 mL/min/1.73 m². All patients with impaired renal function should be screened regularly for these abnormalities. Phosphorous retention begins early in CKD, with serum phosphorous concentrations often remaining normal while PTH will increase. Restriction of dietary phosphorus should start if the PTH is increased, even if serum phosphorus remains normal. Phosphorous concentrations should be maintained between 2.7 and 4.6 mg/dL in patients with Stage 3 or 4 CKD. Phosphorous binders should be used as soon as the PTH concentration starts to increase. Hyperphosphatemia leads to secondary hyperparathyroidism and consequent ectopic calcification and renal osteodystrophy. The PTH values will help to distinguish between high turn-over bone disease and adynamic bone disease. Some patients also need supplementation with vitamin D, but care needs to be taken if serum calcium concentration starts to increase. Calcium and phosphorous concentrations need to be carefully monitored when vitamin D supplementation is prescribed; referral to a nephrologist should be done to manage renal failure and response to treatment.

In the older population, renal osteodystrophy is often complicated by osteoporosis. CKD is one of many risk factors for osteoporosis. The incidence of fractures in patients with kidney failure is 4 times that of age-matched controls. Dual-energy x-ray absorptiometry (DEXA) scanning can be used to diagnose osteoporosis. Although data on their use in the CKD population are sparse, bisphosphonates are the recommended treatment of choice for osteoporosis in the early stages of renal impairment. Small studies have shown measurable increases in bone mineral density and reductions in fractures in the dialysis population (SOE=C). Bisphosphonates are also efficacious in the transplant population. They are contraindicated in adynamic bone disease because they inhibit osteoclastic bone resorption. Calcitonin is probably safe in patients with adynamic bone disease, but no efficacy data are available (SOE=D). No safety or efficacy data are available on the use of estrogens and their derivatives in CKD.

Depression

Depression is very common in any population suffering from chronic disease, but it has been under-recognized in the CKD population, especially those on dialysis. In one study, 13% of dialysis patients had been diagnosed with depression, while 43% tested positive on a randomly administered depression screening test, suggesting that the true rate of depression is three times that of the recognized rate. Therefore, screening for depression in patients with CKD and in those on dialysis is warranted. Depression can be difficult to diagnose in the dialysis population, because the vegetative symptoms can be similar to those of uremia or insufficient dialysis. Functional and cognitive decline are particularly common presenting symptoms in older adults with kidney disease.

Most depression screening instruments have been validated in the kidney failure population. Very low doses of SSRIs can safely be used for treatment. Long-acting medications such as fluoxetine and paroxetine should be avoided, while the shorter-acting sertraline and citalopram are safer in this population. See "Depression," p 295.

Nutrition

Dietary requirements for patients with CKD are complex. Intake of protein, phosphorus, and potas-

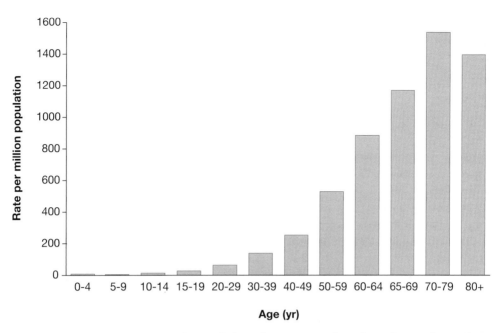

Figure 50.2—Annual incidence rates of treated end-stage kidney disease. Data from the U.S. Renal Data System (USRDS): USRDS 2007 Annual Data Report, Bethesda, MD, National Institutes of Health, National Institute of Diabetes and Digestive and Kidney Diseases, 2007.

sium ideally should be controlled while maintaining adequate energy intake. Once a patient reaches Stage 4 CKD, an experienced renal dietician should be involved in the patient's nutritional management. The recommended protein intake for patients with Stage 4 CKD is 0.6 g/kg/day. This diet is unpalatable to most people, and a goal of 0.75 g/kg/d is frequently prescribed to increase compliance. Adequate dietary energy intake is easier to achieve at this level of protein restriction. Protein restriction also helps with control of phosphorus and reduces metabolic acidosis. Dietary phosphorus should be limited to 800–1,000 mg/d. Such restrictions may not be realistic in the adult living or nursing home setting.

Adequate nutrition and dietary therapy in older adults with advanced kidney disease is complicated by many common age-related factors. Lack of transportation, lower income, and loss of social/family support can compromise access to therapeutic food choices. Loss of teeth, impaired sensory function, and medications that reduce appetite or cause nausea can also impede adequate nutritional intake. Comorbid conditions such as depression, cognitive deficits, mobility impairment, or loss of function from stroke, arthritis, or Parkinson's disease pose obstacles to appropriate food preparation.

END-STAGE KIDNEY DISEASE

Epidemiology

End-stage kidney disease, requiring dialysis or transplant for survival, is primarily a disease of the older population. The mean age at the start of renal replacement therapy is 62.3 yr for men and 63.4 yr for women. The incidence of treated end-stage kidney disease in the age group 70–79 yr old is 1,543 per million person-years and is increasing (Figure 50.2). More than 55% of end-stage kidney disease patients are >60 yr old. Increases in renal replacement therapy for the older population likely indicate a greater willingness to offer treatment to older adults as well as lengthening life expectancy with attendant progression of CKD.

Renal Replacement Therapy

Advanced renal failure with no identifiable reversible cause necessitates renal replacement therapy, ie, dialysis or renal transplant, before uremic symptoms develop. Older patients become symptomatic at lower concentrations of serum creatinine. Increasing numbers of older patients are being accepted for renal replacement therapy. Age should not be the sole exclusion criterion from dialysis.

Most older patients with established end-stage kidney disease are treated with hemodialysis. Hemodialysis does not provide normal life expectancy, but it can provide meaningful extension of life (Table 50.3). The median survival time for octogenarians on hemodialysis is about 24 mo. The overall mortality in older adults on hemodialysis is influenced by several factors, including comorbid vascular disease, infection, malnutrition, or malignancy, and voluntary withdrawal from dialysis. Although older adults are more likely to suffer hypotension and silent ischemia during hemodialysis treatments, many older patients can be rehabilitated and have a quality of life that is comparable to that of their age-matched counterparts without end-stage kidney disease.

Guidelines of the National Kidney Foundation call for referral to a nephrologist when a patient develops Stage 4 CKD. Early referral ensures adequate time for discussing options for renal replacement therapy and for creating adequate access to dialysis. For patients opting for hemodialysis, creation of a native arteriovenous fistula, the optimal dialysis access, can require up to 6 mo before use.

Hemodialysis and continuous ambulatory peritoneal dialysis appear to be about equally effective in older adults. Therefore, the mode of renal replacement therapy should be individualized in older patients, especially with regard to underlying medical conditions and psychosocial factors. Hemodialysis can be appropriate for debilitated older patients because less self-care is involved. In-center hemodialysis can also have a social benefit for those who are living alone or depressed. Patients with severe cardiovascular disease and blood pressure that is difficult to control might benefit from continuous ambulatory peritoneal dialysis.

Offering dialysis to patients with dementia is controversial. Sometimes, distinguishing between cognitive impairment related to uremia and progressing dementia can be difficult. It is certainly reasonable to offer a trial of dialysis for 4–6 weeks to see if cognition improves with correction of the electrolyte abnormalities. It should be made clear that the decision to continue dialysis is contingent on improvement in cognition, and families should be helped to prepare for withdrawal of dialysis if that should be the ultimate course.

Kidney Transplantation: Older Donors, Older Recipients

About 60,000 patients are currently on the kidney transplant wait list, and the list grows every year with an average wait time of 5 yr. Older patients are increasingly considered for transplantation. As in younger patients, mortality rates in older patients with transplants are considerably less than in those maintained on dialysis. Remaining life expectancy doubles for a dialysis patient once moved from the wait list to transplantation. Transplantation is routinely considered for patients in their seventies, who generally do well with suitable donors. Living donor transplants are growing at about 4% per year, eliminating the need to be on the wait list for a deceased donor kidney. Older patients and their families should be encouraged to explore the option of transplantation as soon as the need for renal replacement therapy arises.

Table 50.3—Remaining Life Expectancy (yr) on Dialysis in the United States

Age (yr)	Dialysis Population	General Population
40–44	6.7–9.2	30.1–40.8
50–54	5.1–6.9	22.5–31.5
60–64	3.7–5.1	16.0–22.8
70–74	2.7–3.5	10.8–15.2
80–84	2.0–2.4	6.9–8.8

Older patients undergo the same transplantation evaluation process as younger patients. However, older patients are more likely than younger patients to have vascular contraindications to transplantation, as well as other contraindications such as metastatic cancer and advanced dementia. Older renal transplant recipients demonstrate lower acute rejection rates, lower incidence of chronic rejection, and higher risk of infection and sepsis than younger recipients, and they have greater survival probability than patients remaining on dialysis even when corrected for levels of comorbidity (SOE=A). Both donor and recipient age are independent additive risk factors for chronic allograft failure. Immunosuppressive therapy should be adjusted in older recipients.

Hospice

Most people who choose to withdraw from dialysis are >65 yr old. The decision to withdraw can be precipitated by a catastrophic insult such as a major stroke or myocardial infarction, but in almost half of cases, failure to thrive is the driving reason. About 20% of the dialysis cohort withdraws from dialysis in any given year. Of the patients who do choose to withdraw from dialysis, less than half use hospice. Patients enrolled in hospice are far more likely to die at home; in a 2006 study, only 22.9% of patients enrolled in hospice who withdrew from dialysis died in the hospital versus 69% of nonhospice patients. Once a patient on chronic dialysis withdraws, death within 7–14 days is almost certain. The patient's primary clinician has a unique role in educating nephrologists and patients about the value of hospice and the opportunity to end life outside the hospital.

REFERENCES

■ Hodak SP, Verbalis JG. Abnormalities of water homeostasis in aging. *Endocrinol Metab Clin North Am.* 2005;34(4): 1031–1046.

■ Coresh J, Selvin E, Stevens LA, et al. Prevalence of chronic kidney disease in the United States. *JAMA.* 2007;298(17): 2038–2047.

■ National Kidney Foundation. K/DOQI clinical practice guidelines for chronic kidney disease: evaluation, classification, and stratification. *Am J Kidney Dis.* 2002;39(2 Suppl 1):S1–266.

CHAPTER 51—GYNECOLOGIC DISEASES AND DISORDERS

KEY POINTS

- Many older women do not spontaneously discuss gynecologic problems, yet many of these problems are treatable.

- Symptomatic urogenital atrophy is common in postmenopausal women and is readily reversed with the administration of local estrogen.

- Half of all cases of invasive cancer of the vulva are in women >70 yr old.

- Pessaries can improve comfort and bladder function in some older women with pelvic organ prolapse.

- Any abnormal genital bleeding in a postmenopausal woman should be evaluated.

Most older women do not seek regular gynecologic care, maybe in part because they believe these are normal age changes and they are reticent about discussing personal gynecologic problems. Consequently, important and treatable disorders often go undiagnosed until they become severely disabling. For example, although urinary incontinence affects 16 million adults in the United States, the average time between onset and reporting to a physician is 8.5 yr; gynecologic problems such as genital prolapse and atrophic vaginitis often exacerbate urinary incontinence. Full gynecologic examination should be a routine part of a complete history and physical examination for all older women who are amenable to screening.

HISTORY AND PHYSICAL EXAMINATION

The American College of Obstetrics and Gynecology recommendations for primary care of women ≥65 yr old include inquiring not only about routine gynecologic issues but also about involuntary loss of urine or feces, sexual behavior patterns and potential exposure to sexually transmitted diseases, and use of alternative medical treatments.

Nongynecologic medical problems that can have significant gynecologic effects should be noted in the history. For example, breast cancer therapy typically leads to severe urogenital atrophy. Obesity can result in hyperestrogenic states due to peripheral conversion of androgens to estrogen. Osteoporotic lordosis causes increased intra-abdominal pressure and resultant predisposition to genital prolapse. Previous obstetrical events can cause neuromuscular damage to the pelvic floor and eventual development of urinary incontinence and genital prolapse.

If a woman is on hormone therapy (HT), the regimen should be reviewed annually to ensure adherence, need for continued therapy, and absence of adverse events. If the uterus is present, estrogen must be combined with a progestin to prevent development of endometrial hyperplasia (see estrogen therapy in "Endocrine and Metabolic Disorders," p 501). The history should also include inquiry about abdominal distention (sign of ovarian cancer) and abnormal vaginal discharge or bleeding (signs of endometrial, cervical, or vaginal cancer).

The pelvic examination also presents an opportunity to discuss sexual function with the patient. Although the lack of available, sexually capable men may limit an older woman's sexual activities, many older women are interested in maintaining sexual relationships. Issues related to sexual activity such as atrophy-related dyspareunia, postcoital bleeding, and sexually transmitted diseases should be addressed. Many women require reassurance that enjoyable sexual activity is possible and normal at their age. Also, women who maintain regular sexual activity are less likely to have significant vaginal atrophy. See "Disorders of Sexual Function," p 430.

Most ambulatory older women can assume the lithotomy position for a pelvic examination. The dorsal position, in stirrups for a pelvic examination, requires flexion and external rotation of the hips. Patients with osteoarthritis who find the lithotomy position uncomfortable or impossible to assume will need to use an alternative position. The left lateral decubitus position is one alternative. The patient lies on her left side, with knees flexed. The upper hip (right) is flexed to a greater degree and the right leg is elevated, exposing the perineum. An adequate speculum and bimanual examination can usually be done in this position. A bedbound patient can be examined by positioning an inverted bedpan under the sacrum to elevate the pelvis. Because the vaginal introitus can be small and stenotic, smaller speculums may be needed. Water-based lubricants facilitate the examination and can be used if a Pap smear will be performed.

STRENGTH-OF-EVIDENCE (SOE) RATING DEFINITIONS

A = consistent and good quality patient-oriented evidence
B = somewhat inconsistent or limited quality patient-oriented evidence
C = very inconsistent or very limited patient-oriented evidence, disease-oriented evidence, and/or consensus from professional organizations
D = unstudied common practice or opinion

See inside front cover for detailed information regarding the SOE classification.

The pelvic examination of older women should include the following:

- examination of the vulva for abnormal pigmentation, erythema, or raised lesions
- examination for signs of urogenital atrophy, including urethral caruncle, vaginal dryness, pale vaginal mucosa, loss of rugae, and reduced vaginal caliber and depth
- Valsalva's maneuver performed by the patient to evaluate for pelvic organ prolapse and urinary incontinence
- careful palpation for pelvic masses or ovarian enlargement on bimanual examination
- a Pap smear if indicated (see cervical cancer in "Prevention," p 65)

The presence of significant vaginal mucosal atrophic changes can lead to inadequate or abnormal Pap smear interpretation. In this situation, the Pap smear should be repeated after 2–3 mo of local estrogen therapy. Bimanual examinations and perineal inspection performed annually can detect vulvar, vaginal, or ovarian pathology. A rectal examination can also be performed at the same time to identify masses, detect occult bleeding, and evaluate the anal sphincter.

Ovaries become smaller with aging, and any palpable adnexal tissue should prompt consideration of malignancy. Although uterine fibroids are common, any increase in uterus size should be investigated. An ovarian or uterine mass could be evaluated by abdominal or pelvic ultrasound (using a vaginal probe) to determine location and character. Sonography, however, cannot definitively establish the nature (benign or malignant) of the mass, so further evaluation with laparoscopy ultimately depends on clinical judgment.

TREATMENT OF MENOPAUSAL SYMPTOMS

Estrogen is labeled by the FDA for treatment of menopausal symptoms and urogenital dryness and for prevention of osteoporosis, but HT has historically been used for other reasons as well.

Menopause on average occurs at age 51 in the United States. With a life expectancy of 78 yr, the average American woman is postmenopausal for one-third of her life. In light of the risks and benefits of HT found in the Women's Health Initiative Trial, many women and their physicians choose to treat or prevent the sequelae of estrogen deficiency in menopause. Individualization of therapy is essential.

Vasomotor symptoms or hot flushes are the most common symptom of the climacteric, occurring in up to 80% of perimenopausal women. Symptoms persist for >5 yr in 25% of women and are lifelong in a small minority. Although the cause of the vasomotor response remains unknown, vasomotor symptoms are usually relieved within the first cycle of HT (SOE=A). Low-dose therapy can be started, and estrogen dosages titrated until symptoms improve. When estrogen is contraindicated or not acceptable, SSRIs[OL] or progestins are considered the second most effective therapies (SOE=B). Clonidine[OL], methyldopa[OL], vitamin E, or herbal remedies such as yams and black cohosh have also been tried with little evidence to support their use (SOE=C). Recently, the FDA has warned against the use of "bio-identical" hormonal products because of lack of beneficial evidence.

See also estrogen therapy in HT and osteoporosis prevention in "Osteoporosis," p 234 and "Endocrine and Metabolic Disorders," p 501.

TREATMENT OF UROGENITAL SYMPTOMS

Estrogen deficiency causes atrophy of both the vaginal and urethral mucosa. Both have a high density of estrogen receptors. A Cochrane Database Review concluded that estrogen can improve urinary urgency and urge incontinence more than placebo (SOE=A). See also "Disorders of Sexual Function," p 430; and "Urinary Incontinence," p 207.

UROGENITAL ATROPHY

The lower genital tract is exquisitely sensitive to estrogen. Urogenital atrophy occurs in all postmenopausal women. Proliferation and maturation of the vaginal epithelium depends on adequate estrogen stimulation. With reduced estrogen production, genital blood flow decreases, leading to further decline in delivery of estrogen to those tissues. This reduction in microvascularity leads to vaginal dryness, mucosal pallor, decreased rugation, mucosal thinning, inflammation with discharge, and ultimately decreased vaginal caliber and depth. With progressive atrophy, the vaginal Pap smear–maturation index shows atrophic changes with a decrease in mucosal superficial cells and an increase in intermediate and basal cells. Vaginal pH can be measured using pH paper; a reading >5.0−5.5 usually denotes significant atrophy. Many women experience dyspareunia, burning, and even vaginal bleeding in some cases (Figure 51.1).

These changes are readily reversed by administration of local estrogen (SOE=A). The intravaginal use of estrogen cream, one-quarter to one-half an applicator (1 g) as infrequently as two nights per week, allows topical estrogen therapy with minimal (if any) absorption into the circulation, endometrial proliferation, or other systemic effects. The available prescription estrogen creams appear to be therapeutically equivalent. The estrogen ring can be used for 3 mo per ring, and vaginal tablets are available for

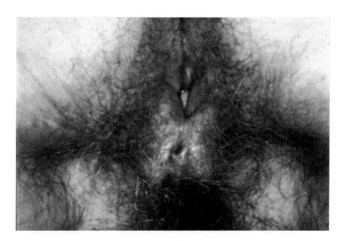

Figure 51.1—Severe vulvovaginal atrophy, including labial fusion secondary to lichen sclerosus.

use twice a week. Estrogen cream is also an excellent lubricant for use during intercourse or for pessary insertion. See also "Disorders of Sexual Function," p 430.

VULVOVAGINAL INFECTION AND INFLAMMATION

Postmenopausal women are susceptible to a broad range of vulvovaginal infections. Candidal infection, common in diabetic and obese patients who are plagued with moisture and irritation, can be treated with oral, intravaginal, and topical antifungal agents. Women should be questioned about their ability to insert a vaginal applicator before beginning therapy. Topical corticosteroids can be used to hasten relief of symptoms of vulvar irritation. Combination therapy with a steroid and antifungal cream may be necessary, because older women commonly have more chronic, untreated candidal infections that spread from the vulva to the inguinal areas. Other vaginal infections such as *Trichomonas* and *Gardnerella* vaginosis that are common in women of reproductive age are less common in older women, likely because of the higher vaginal pH. A wet preparation revealing sheets of inflammatory cells without bacterial forms can represent advanced atrophy rather than an infectious cause. In women with inflammatory atrophy, the vagina will look inflamed (ie, petechia) with serous exudate, rather than thin, pale, and dry as is typical in advanced atrophy. Local estrogen cream may thus need to be considered as well. A clinician should not be hesitant to inquire about sexual practices when a woman presents with recurrent vaginal infections, vesicular lesions, or other changes suggestive of a sexually transmitted disease.

DISORDERS OF THE VULVA

With aging, the skin of the vulva loses elasticity, and the underlying fat and connective tissues undergo degeneration, with loss of collagen and thinning of the epithelial layer. Consequently, postmenopausal women not on estrogen are predisposed to a variety of dermatologic disorders. The assessment of vulvar complaints must include direct examination. Any pigmented lesion that does not respond to topical corticosteroid or estrogen treatment should be promptly biopsied if consistent with individual treatment goals of the patient.

Vulvar skin irritation can result from a variety of agents and causes burning, itching, and edema. Hygienic products used for urinary or fecal incontinence can lead to chemical dermatitis, as can urine itself. Treatment of incontinence is important to solve this problem. Vulvar burning or pain is rarely due to estrogen deficiency, and this complaint should be investigated rather than treated with ever-increasing dosages of estrogen.

Vulvodynia, a chronic vulvar pain syndrome, is seen in both pre- and postmenopausal women. The International Society for the Study of Vulvovaginal Diseases (ISSVD) categorizes vulvodynia as either generalized or localized. The condition is further divided into provoked (sexual, nonsexual), unprovoked, or mixed. Treatment of vulvodynia can be challenging and should be approached at multiple levels, including local anesthetic agents, antidepressant therapy and/or other pain modulating agents, pelvic floor rehabilitation, etc.

Vulvar excoriation can result from scratching of an inflamed vulva. Local corticosteroids such as hydrocortisone 1% ointment applied daily, sitz baths, or use of a bidet can help alleviate vulvar irritation. Any chronically irritated area should be biopsied to exclude a malignancy.

The term "vulvar dystrophy" has been abandoned, and the ISSVD now uses a classification based on common histologic patterns. The classification system excludes histologically well-defined neoplasias and easily categorizable infections. For categorization of vulvar intraepithelial neoplasia (VIN), the older terms VIN 1, 2, or 3 have been replaced by VIN usual type versus VIN well differentiated. While VIN usual type appears to be related to the human papilloma virus and includes warty, baseloid, and mixed types, VIN well differentiated does not appear to be related to human papilloma virus, and it has a 95% association with vulvar cancer seen primarily in postmenopausal women. Because VIN has a varied clinical presentation, a biopsy of any vulvar lesion should be considered.

Nonneoplastic Vulvar Lesions

Lichen sclerosus causes over one-third of all vulvar dystrophies and can extend beyond the vulva to the perirectal areas. It is rarely precancerous. There is epithelial thinning with edema and fibrosis of the dermis. It can progress to shrinkage and adherence of the labia minora with reduction in introital caliber. Lesions are typically shiny, white or pink, and parchment-like; they can be asymptomatic or cause itching, vaginal soreness, and dyspareunia. Diagnosis is confirmed on biopsy of the involved vulvar areas. Recommended treatment involves daily application of a potent topical corticosteroid, clobetasol propionate 0.05%. Treatment should be continued for at least 3 mo. Testosterone, the mainstay of therapy until recently, is significantly less effective than clobetasol (SOE=A). Further measures include wearing cotton underwear and avoiding irritant soaps. Topical emollient agents including lanolin can be helpful, but petroleum jelly should be avoided.

Squamous hyperplasia appears as thickened, hyperplastic, elevated white keratinized lesions that can be difficult to distinguish clinically from VIN or condylomata. However, it is benign. Biopsy should precede treatment. Topical mid-potency corticosteroids such as triamcinolone 0.1% twice daily for a few weeks (or longer with thick lesions) typically resolve the lesions; intermittent therapy may be necessary.

Other vulvar lesions include lichen simplex chronicus, which presents with vulvar pruritus, and lichen planus, which presents as erosive, ulcerative lesions of the vulva or vagina that can result in significant discomfort and scarring. Mid-potency corticosteroids applied topically or intravaginally are recommended. In lichen planus that involves the vagina, daily local estrogen cream should also be used.

Vulvar Neoplasia

Patients with suspicious, unusual, or symptomatic vulvar lesions should be referred for biopsy. VIN lesions are not usually precancerous. VIN is most often seen in postmenopausal women, but the incidence of VIN does not increase with age. Over half of cases are asymptomatic. The most common complaint in symptomatic cases is pruritus. The clinical appearance is the same as squamous hyperplasia or may be simply pigmentation. Lesions are often multifocal.

Invasive cancer of the vulva is an age-related malignancy; half of all cases occur after age 70. The vast majority are squamous cell carcinomas. Malignant melanoma, sarcoma, basal cell carcinoma, and adenocarcinoma account for <20% of cases. Treatment involves surgery (radical vulvectomy), occasionally accompanied by radiation.

DISORDERS OF PELVIC FLOOR SUPPORT

Childbearing and other activities that increase intra-

Table 51.1—Classification of Pelvic Organ Prolapse

Class	Description
1st degree	Extension to the mid-vagina
2nd degree	Approaching the hymenal ring
3rd degree	At the hymenal ring
4th degree	Beyond the hymenal ring

SOURCE: Data from American College of Obstetricians and Gynecologists. *Pelvic Organ Prolapse*. Washington, DC: American College of Obstetricians and Gynecologists. Technical Bulletin No. 214; 1995.

abdominal pressure cause progressive weakening of the connective tissue and muscular supports of the genital organs and can lead to genital prolapse. Constipation, chronic coughing, and heavy lifting commonly increase intra-abdominal pressure. Common symptoms of prolapse include pelvic pressure, lower back pain, urinary or fecal incontinence, difficulty with rectal emptying, or a palpable mass. Traditional classification of vaginal prolapse includes differentiated protrusion of the posterior vaginal wall (enterocele or rectocele), descent of the anterior vaginal wall (cystocele), and prolapse of the vaginal apex. These conditions are demonstrated by having the patient bear down or cough while in the dorsal lithotomy position, but the full extent of prolapse is better appreciated with a standing Valsalva maneuver. Vaginal prolapse is a pelvic organ hernia through the vaginal hiatus.

For the 1995 American College of Obstetrics and Gynecology classification of pelvic organ prolapse, see Table 51.1. The International Continence Society and the American Urogynecologic Association adopted a subsequent, rather complex prolapse classification system (Pelvic Organ Prolapse Quantification [POPQ]) that is based on measurement of the distance between vaginal anatomic sites and the hymenal ring, as well as on vaginal length and perineal dimensions. The purpose of this classification, which is used by specialty societies, is to more objectively and reproducibly describe the degree of prolapse.

Mild prolapse (first or second degree [Table 51.1]) can be retarded with adequate estrogenization and Kegel exercises to strengthen the pelvic floor musculature (SOE=C). Genital prolapse does not always lead to bladder dysfunction and should not be assumed to be the cause of incontinence (see "Urinary Incontinence," p 207). Correcting advanced prolapse can cause or exacerbate urinary incontinence by "unkinking" the urethra or bladder neck. However, large cystoceles or rectoceles can produce urinary retention, and reduction of the cystocele can restore normal bladder function.

Pessaries

Pessaries are commonly used in an effort to delay or avoid surgery. Their use in older women may be indicated to provide comfort and restore bladder function when comorbid illness makes surgery undesirable (SOE=C). Such women may elect long-term pessary use with ongoing oversight by their primary health care provider and gynecologist. Available pessaries are made from rubber, plastic, or silicone. A variety of shapes and sizes are available: doughnuts, rings, cubes, inflatable balls, and foldable models.

The choice of pessary is influenced by the degree of prolapse, presence of incontinence, type of accompanying tissue relaxation, and ease of care. Patients with prolapse and no incontinence require only space-occupying types (ie, doughnut). Those with stress incontinence benefit from a foldable lever-type, which restores bladder neck support. Ring pessaries are easier to insert and remove and may be preferred by older women, especially those who used a contraceptive diaphragm in their youth. For those with advanced degrees of apical or anterior wall prolapse, a more rigid pessary, such as Gellhorn with a stem, may be needed. Although more difficult to insert and remove, this pessary type is very popular because of its high degree of efficacy. Self-care can be more challenging. Cube pessaries should be used with caution because they can adhere to the vaginal walls because of the suction effect and result in mucosal ulcerations when removed.

Pessary selection often proceeds by trial and error; the optimal pessary fits snugly but comfortably and allows voiding and defecating without difficulty. After pessary selection and insertion, clinical follow-up within a few days is essential to ascertain satisfactory usage. After initial fitting and recheck, pessaries should be removed, cleaned, and the vaginal walls inspected.

Pessary care requirements often influence the selection of a device and the amount of follow-up required. If an older woman's mobility or manual dexterity permits, she should remove the pessary two nights per week, wash it with soap and water, and reinsert it with a water-soluble lubricant after arising in the morning. She should use 1 g vaginal estrogen cream the two nights the pessary is out. Women who cannot perform this level of self-care should be assisted at periodic office or home care visits if needed (ie, every 6–12 weeks) by a nurse practitioner. All women with pessaries should be instructed to report any unusual discharge, bleeding, or discomfort, and any changes in bladder or bowel function, and all should have a pelvic examination once or twice a year. If discomfort is present or the device becomes uncomfortable, a different size or type should be tried. Pessaries do not work as well with marked vaginal outlet relaxation. If a pessary is left in place for long periods without monitoring, fistulation can

develop, or fibrous tissue can form around the pessary, and removal under anesthesia may be necessary.

Surgery for Prolapse

Surgical treatment of vaginal prolapse can be classified as either reconstructive or obliterative. Reconstructive procedures are designed to restore normal anatomy, whereas obliterative procedures result in total or partial closure of the vaginal canal. Vaginal reconstructive procedures include sacrospinous fixation (for apical prolapse), anterior repairs (for a cystocele), and posterior repairs (for a rectocele). These can safely be done under regional anesthesia, which minimizes anesthetic risks. Abdominal reconstructive procedures include sacrocolpopexy (for apical prolapse) and paravaginal repairs (for a cystocele); they typically require general anesthesia. Urinary and fecal incontinence procedures can also be performed at the time of the prolapse surgery. See also "Urinary Incontinence," p 207.

POSTMENOPAUSAL VAGINAL BLEEDING

Postmenopausal bleeding (defined as bleeding after 1 yr of amenorrhea) occurs in a significant number of older women. A referral to gynecology is needed to establish diagnosis. The challenge is not only to exclude gynecologic malignancies but also to alleviate the symptoms and eliminate the cause of benign conditions. Causes of bleeding can be grouped according to anatomic areas and endocrine dysfunction (Table 51.2). Not all complaints of postmenopausal bleeding are related to the reproductive organs;

Table 51.2—Causes of Postmenopausal Vaginal Bleeding

Cervical	Carcinoma Cervicitis Polyp
Endocrinologic	Exogenous hormones Perimenopausal ovarian function
Ovarian	Functioning ovarian tumor
Uterine	Endometrial atrophy Hyperplasia Neoplasia Polyp Submucosal leiomyoma
Vaginal	Atrophy Inflammation Tumor Ulceration
Vulvar	Carcinoma Laceration or ulceration Urethral caruncle
Other	Coagulation disorder Rectal lesion Urinary tract infection

Chapter 51: Gynecologic Diseases and Disorders **419**

patients may be confused as to the origin of the bleeding. Proper evaluation involves complete pelvic examination looking for any vaginal, cervical, or uterine source and directed diagnostic studies. Endometrial hyperplasia and cancer can be evaluated by taking an endometrial biopsy or by measuring the endometrial thickness on vaginal probe ultrasound. Although neither ultrasound nor biopsy is 100% specific, an endometrial thickness of <5 mm on ultrasound essentially excludes hyperplasia and malignancy. Dilation and curettage is reserved for cases in which tissue cannot otherwise be adequately sampled or when bleeding persists. The use of direct visualization (hysteroscopy) during the procedure is the most accurate method for tissue sampling. New techniques to destroy the endometrial lining (ablation) by heat, cold, radiotherapy, or excision can be helpful in women whose bleeding is proved to be due to nonmalignant conditions.

Exogenous hormone replacement is a common cause of postmenopausal bleeding. Women on continuous combined estrogen-progesterone replacement who continue to have bleeding after 1 yr should be evaluated. Some specialists recommend biopsy if bleeding persists beyond 6 mo. Women on cyclic hormone therapy who bleed at an unexpected time during the cycle should also be evaluated. See also estrogen therapy in "Endocrine and Metabolic Disorders," p 501.

REFERENCES

- DeLancey JO. The hidden epidemic of pelvic floor dysfunction: Achievable goals for improved prevention and treatment. *Am J Obstet Gynecol.* 2005;192(5):1488−1495.

- Haefner HK, Collins ME, Davis GD, et al. The vulvodynia guideline. *J Low Genit Tract Dis.* 2005;(1):40–51.

- Shah SM, Sultan AH, Thakar R. The history and evolution of pessaries for pelvic organ prolapse. *Int Urogynecol J Pelvic Floor Dysfunct.* 2006;17(2):170−175.

CHAPTER 52—PROSTATE DISEASE

KEY POINTS

- A number of treatment options exist for benign prostatic hyperplasia (BPH), including watchful waiting, medications, minimally invasive procedures, and more extensive operations. The choice is influenced by the extent of symptoms, the presence of complications from outflow obstruction, and patient preferences.

- The use of 5α-reductase inhibitors for BPH is especially indicated when the prostate gland is large.

- Two trials of prostate cancer screening using serial prostate-specific antigen (PSA) measurement in men 55−74 yr old indicate that screening leads to significant overdiagnosis and overtreatment of clinically insignificant tumors. The trials show somewhat conflicting results on mortality after a decade of screening, one showing no mortality benefit and the other observing a very modest benefit. Men should be well informed about the risks and benefits of PSA screening before making a decision whether or not to be screened.

- Several treatment options exist for men with localized prostate cancer, including watchful waiting, resection of the gland and seminal vesicles, and radiation therapy. How the patient balances the potential benefits and burdens of the various options will influence the choice of therapy.

- For patients with chronic prostatitis, efforts should be made to identify the causative organism, and even with a prolonged course of appropriate antibiotics, a cure can be expected in fewer than half the patients.

With advancing age, the prevalence of prostate diseases increases dramatically. The three most common conditions are BPH, prostate cancer, and prostatitis. Self-reported prostate disease affects about 3 million American men. BPH develops in over half of men ≥65 yr old and affects the overwhelming majority of men >85 yr old. Prostate cancer is the second leading cause of cancer death in men, and many men have asymptomatic or low-grade tumors that cause few or no health problems. The prevalence of prostatitis is similar to that of ischemic heart disease or diabetes mellitus.

BENIGN PROSTATIC HYPERPLASIA

Epidemiology

BPH is a noncancerous enlargement of the epithelial and fibromuscular components of the prostate gland. The epithelial component normally makes up 20%–30% of prostate volume and contributes to the seminal fluid. The fibromuscular component comprises 70%–80% of the prostate and is responsible for expressing prostatic fluid during ejaculation. Age and long-term androgen stimulation induce development of BPH. Microscopic appearance of BPH can be seen as early as age 30, is present in 50% of men by age 60, and is present in 90% of men by age 85. In half of these cases, microscopic BPH develops into palpable macroscopic BPH. Of those with macroscopic BPH, only half develop into clinically significant disease brought to medical attention. BPH is one of the most common conditions in aging men; in the United States annually it accounts for more than 1.7 million office visits and 250,000 surgical procedures.

Prostatism, or Lower Urinary Tract Symptoms

The symptoms of BPH are nonspecific; other diseases can result in identical symptoms. The pathophysiology of BPH symptoms is not completely understood, but presumably it involves the periurethral zone of the prostate gland, which results in obstructed urine flow and compensatory responses of the bladder, such as hypertrophy and decreased capacity. The urethral obstruction has both mechanical (obstructing mass) and dynamic (smooth muscle contractions) components. The resulting lower urinary tract symptoms are divided into irritative (eg, frequency, urgency, nocturia) and obstructive (eg, hesitancy, intermittency, weak stream, incomplete emptying) manifestations. A quantitative symptom index for severity assessment and treatment response monitoring, which was developed by the American Urological Association and adopted by the World Health Organization, is known as the International Prostate Symptom Score. Although tracking symptom severity is useful in the longitudinal management of patients, symptom severity has not been found to correlate with prostate size, urine flow rates, or postvoid residual volume. BPH primarily affects quality of life, although complications such as recurrent urinary tract infection, bladder stones, urinary retention, chronic renal insufficiency, and hematuria can develop.

Diagnosis

Differential diagnosis of lower urinary tract symptoms includes endocrine disorders (especially diabetes mellitus), neurologic disorders, urinary tract infections,

---

STRENGTH-OF-EVIDENCE (SOE) RATING DEFINITIONS

A = consistent and good quality patient-oriented evidence
B = somewhat inconsistent or limited quality patient-oriented evidence
C = very inconsistent or very limited patient-oriented evidence, disease-oriented evidence, and/or consensus from professional organizations
D = unstudied common practice or opinion

See inside front cover for detailed information regarding the SOE classification.

---

sexually transmitted diseases, kidney or bladder stones, and medications (especially medications with anticholinergic and diuretic effects). Digital rectal examination (DRE) can be unremarkable or reveal an enlarged, smooth, rubbery, symmetrical gland. Urinalysis is routinely performed to evaluate for urinary tract infection, hematuria, and glycosuria. A baseline serum creatinine measurement assesses kidney function and the possibility of obstructive uropathy or intrinsic renal disease, or both. Additional optional tests include postvoid residual urine volume (often done by office or bedside bladder scan), urine flow rates, and pressure flow studies. These tests can be considered when the diagnosis is uncertain or an invasive treatment is being planned.

Treatment Approaches

BPH therapy depends on the patient and is driven by the impact of symptoms on the patient's quality of life (Table 52.1). All patients should be educated regarding lifestyle modification by adjusting fluid intake (eg, avoiding caffeine) and avoiding medications (especially anticholinergics) that aggravate symptoms. Men with mild to moderate symptoms may be satisfied with lifestyle modification only. Both medical and surgical treatments are also available, with medication the usual first approach. Indications for surgical treatment include patient preference, dissatisfaction with medication, and refractory urinary retention, as well as renal dysfunction, bladder stones, recurrent urinary tract infections, or hematuria if these are clearly due to prostatic obstruction.

Medical Treatment

The two main pharmacologic approaches are α-adrenergic antagonist and 5α-reductase inhibitor therapy (SOE=A).

α-Adrenergic antagonists, or α-blockers, are directed at the dynamic component of urethral obstruction. Smooth muscle of the prostate and bladder neck has a resting tone mediated by α-adrenergic innervation. α-Blockers relax the smooth muscle in the hyperplastic prostate tissue, prostate capsule, and bladder neck, thus decreasing resistance to urinary flow. Of the two major α-adrenergic receptors, α_1 receptors predominate in the prostate, with the α_{1a} subtype comprising 70% of these receptors. α-Blockade development for BPH therapy has progressed from selective α_1 agents (prazosin, alfuzosin) to long-acting selective α_1 agents (terazosin, doxazosin) and then to long-acting α_{1a} subtype selective agents (tamsulosin, silodosin, alfuzosin). The most common adverse events of α_1 agents are dizziness, mild asthenia (fatigue or weakness), and headaches. Postural hypotension occurs infrequently and can be minimized by careful dosage titration.

Table 52.1—Management Options for Benign Prostatic Hyperplasia

Category	Interventions	Rationale	Comments
Lifestyle modification	Reduce nighttime fluids to manage nocturia; eliminate bladder irritants (eg, caffeine, alcohol, nicotine)	Factors outside the urinary tract contribute to urinary symptoms	Often sufficient management for mild symptoms; complements management for moderate to severe symptoms

Pharmacologic management	α-*Adrenergic antagonists*
	  ▪ Selective α_1: prazosin[OL], alfuzosin
	  ▪ Long-acting selective α_1: terazosin, doxazosin
	  ▪ Long-acting selective α_{1a} subtype selective: tamsulosin, silodosin, alfuzosin
		Relaxation of smooth muscle in hyperplastic prostate tissue, prostate capsule, and bladder neck decreases resistance to urinary flow	Adverse events: dizziness, mild asthenia, headaches, postural hypotension (reduced with careful dosage titration, not present with selective α_{1a} subtypes), abnormal ejaculation, rhinitis

	5α-Reductase inhibitors: finasteride, dutasteride	Reduced tissue levels of dihydrotestosterone result in prostate gland size reduction	Most effective for men with larger prostates (>40 g); results may not be evident for up to 6 mo
Surgery	Transurethral resection of the prostate; transurethral incision of the prostate; open prostatectomy; transurethral vaporization of the prostate; stent placement	Removal or expansion of periurethral prostate tissue reduces obstruction to urinary flow	Indicated for recurrent urinary tract infection induced by benign prostatic hypertrophy, recurrent or persistent gross hematuria, bladder stones, renal insufficiency

The enzyme 5α-reductase is required for the conversion of testosterone to the more active dihydrotestosterone. Finasteride and dutasteride are inhibitors of 5α-reductase and reduce tissue levels of dihydrotestosterone, thus reducing prostate gland size. Improvements in symptom scores and urine flow rates may not be evident for up to 6 mo. The 5α-reductase inhibitors are most effective in men with larger prostates (>40 g, about the size of a plum) (SOE=A). Because 5α-reductase inhibitors reduce serum PSA levels by an average of 50%, baseline serum PSA determination is recommended for men in whom prostate cancer surveillance is planned. Subsequently, after a 6-mo trial if continued 5α-reductase inhibitor use is desired, a new baseline PSA level is obtained on medication treatment and then every year for cancer surveillance.

When used together over years, the combination of α-adrenergic antagonists with 5α-reductase inhibitors has been shown to be safe and to reduce clinical progression of BPH better than either agent alone (SOE=A). In particular, a lower risk of urinary retention, urinary incontinence, renal insufficiency, and recurrent bladder infections is associated with combination therapy. Trials of BPH therapy with the herbal preparation *Serenoa repens,* or saw palmetto, show conflicting results. Limited data from smaller studies suggested that it improves urinary symptoms and flow measures in men with BPH, while a more recent trial of a specific saw palmetto extract showed benefit no greater than that of placebo. Saw palmetto is a very popular treatment and its risks appear limited, but its benefits are uncertain. See also "Complementary and Alternative Medicine," p 81.

Surgical Treatment

Surgical management includes transurethral resection of the prostate, transurethral incision of the prostate, open prostatectomy, transurethral vaporization of the prostate, and device insertion such as stent placement. Surgical approaches offer the best chance for symptom improvement but also have the highest rates of complications. The benefits of various surgical treatments are generally considered equivalent, but complication rates differ. Transurethral resection of the prostate is the standard of care to which other BPH treatments are compared, and it has an 80% likelihood of successful outcome in properly selected patients (SOE=A). Usually performed under spinal anesthesia, a transurethral resection of the prostate involves the passage of an endoscope through the urethra to surgically remove the inner portion of the prostate. Long-term complications can include retrograde ejaculation, urethral stricture, bladder neck contracture, incontinence, and impotence. Transurethral incision of the prostate is an endoscopic procedure via the urethra to make one or two cuts in the prostate and prostate capsule, relieving urethral constriction. Limited to small prostate glands (<30 g), transurethral incision of the prostate offers lower rates of retrograde ejaculation, bleeding, and contractures. Open prostatectomy involves removal of the inner portion of the prostate through a retropubic or suprapubic incision. It is best used for patients with larger prostates or with complicating conditions such as bladder stones or urethral strictures. Open prostatectomy is associated with incisional morbidity, longer hospitalization, and greater risk of impotence.

Transurethral vaporization of the prostate uses a high-energy electrode inserted via the urethra to vaporize the prostate. This approach has little bleeding but creates more prolonged irritative voiding. Prostatic stents are used to maintain expansion of the prostatic urethra and have both temporary and permanent uses.

PROSTATE CANCER

Incidence and Epidemiology

Prostate cancer is the most common noncutaneous cancer and the second leading cause of cancer deaths among men in the United States. It was estimated that in 2008, 186,320 men would be diagnosed with and 28,660 men would die from prostate cancer. The incidence increases with age and is rare in men <40 yr old. A prevalence study of 340 healthy men scheduled for organ donation, reported in 2008, found the prevalence of prostate cancer was 0.5% in men <50 yr old, 23.4% in men 50–59 yr old, 35% in men 60–69 yr old, and 45.5% in men >70 yr old. Earlier autopsy studies that included debilitated men have found prevalence rates as high as 80% in men >80 yr old. The incidence of disease varies according to race, with black Americans having the highest risk in the world. Among black men, prostate cancer occurs at an earlier age, has a higher mortality rate, and tends to be at a more advanced stage at diagnosis. Family history is a contributing factor. Men with one first-degree relative affected have more than a 2-fold increased risk (SOE=B). Androgens are necessary for prostate cancer pathogenesis; the disease does not occur in men castrated before puberty. History of sexually transmitted disease can be associated with an increased risk of prostate cancer (SOE=B). The association between prostate cancer and omega-3 fatty acid intake, alcohol intake, or vasectomy is inconclusive.

Symptoms

Cancer usually arises in the peripheral zone of the prostate. Most men, especially those with early-stage, potentially curable disease, are asymptomatic. Prostate cancer spreads by three routes: direct extension, the lymphatics, and the bloodstream. Direct invasion of the urethra and bladder can lead to irritative voiding symptoms, urinary incontinence, and hematuria. Extension of disease to adjacent nerves can cause impotence and pelvic pain. Nodal metastasis can cause extrinsic ureteral obstruction. Leg edema can develop from lymphatic obstruction. Hematogenous metastasis to bone can cause severe local pain, normochromic normocytic anemia, pathologic fractures, and spinal cord compression. Less commonly, hematogenous metastasis involves viscera, namely the lung, liver, and adrenal glands.

Screening Controversy

The benefit of early detection and the best approach to treatment of prostate cancer are controversial. There is a large reservoir of prostate cancer that does not need to be diagnosed because most men with prostate cancer die with the disease, not from it. However, the well-recognized burden of progressive prostate cancer is a potential impetus for early detection and management.

Initial results of two prospective, randomized controlled trials of prostate cancer screening were published in 2009, reporting somewhat conflicting findings. The Prostate, Lung, Colorectal, and Ovarian Cancer Screening Trial found no significant difference in prostate cancer mortality between screened and unscreened groups after 7–10 yr of follow-up. The European Randomized Study of Screening for Prostate Cancer, which was actually a collection of smaller trials in different European countries, found a 20% decrease in prostate cancer mortality in the screened group over a mean of 8.8 yr of follow-up; the absolute risk difference associated with screening was 0.071%, meaning that 1,410 men would need to be screened and 48 additional cases of prostate cancer would be treated for every prostate cancer death prevented. Both trials documented significantly increased prostate cancer incidence associated with screening. Men who were >74 yr old at baseline were not enrolled in either trial. The two trials had significant methodologic differences, particularly for inclusion criteria, enrollment size, frequency and mode of screening, definition of a positive PSA level, and follow-up.

Screening for prostate cancer remains a controversial topic with different recommendations and guidelines from various task forces and specialty societies. In 2008, the U.S. Preventive Services Task Force issued updated recommendations, concluding that there is insufficient evidence to assess the balance of benefits and harms of screening for prostate cancer in men <75 yr old, and specifically recommending *against* screening in men ≥75 yr old. Other societies, including the American Cancer Society and the American Urological Association, recommend offering PSA measurement and DRE to men annually starting at age 50 for men with at least a 10-yr remaining life expectancy and earlier (age 40) for men at high risk (black men, first-degree relative affected). Because screening for prostate cancer may lead to harm, including psychologic stress and adverse effects of further diagnostic testing, or adverse effects of treatment if prostate cancer is detected, clinicians should carefully discuss options and consequences with patients before proceeding with screening in asymptomatic men.

Screening and Diagnostic Tests

DRE allows palpation of the posterior surfaces of the lateral lobes of the prostate, where cancer most often begins. Cancer characteristically is hard, nodular, and irregular. Although DRE is less sensitive than PSA in detecting prostate cancer, it can sometimes detect cancers in men who have a normal PSA level. Its use as a single screening test is greatly limited, however, because parts of the prostate gland cannot be palpated. About half of the cancers thought to be limited to the prostate on the basis of DRE are found during surgery to have already spread. DRE has many false-positive results; about one-third of men with positive DRE tests have prostate cancer on biopsy. Local extension of prostate cancer into the seminal vesicles can often be detected by DRE, which may be valuable in staging of disease. Thus, despite its limitations, DRE has a role in prostate cancer staging and in screening asymptomatic patients who choose to be screened.

The serum PSA test is not specific for prostate cancer. PSA increases in benign conditions of the prostate, namely, hypertrophy and prostatitis, and in transient response to conditions such as ejaculation and prostatic massage. The sensitivity of the PSA test is also imperfect. Decreased PSA values have been associated with acute hospitalization and use of medications such as 5α-reductase inhibitors and saw palmetto. PSA levels are normal in 30%–40% of men with cancer confined to the prostate (ie, false-negative tests). The reported positive predictive value of PSA in screening studies is 28%–35%: about one-third of men with increased PSA levels have prostate cancer demonstrated by fine-needle biopsy.

Several approaches to improve the accuracy of PSA testing have been developed. PSA density is derived from the PSA concentration divided by the volume of the prostate gland (measured by ultrasound). Prostate cancer results in higher PSA levels per unit volume than BPH and should therefore yield a higher PSA density. The PSA rate of change or velocity is more specific for prostate cancer than a single PSA measurement. Using a PSA velocity value of ≥ 0.75 ng/mL/yr achieves 90% specificity, whereas using a single PSA level >4 ng/mL achieves 60% specificity. This high specificity for PSA velocity is realized even in normal-range serum PSA levels (<4 ng/mL). Another approach involves age-adjusted PSA reference ranges because PSA values increase with age. Finally, the ratio of free to complexed PSA can be measured, recognizing that PSA bound to α_1-antichymotrypsin accounts for a larger proportion of total PSA with prostate cancer than with BPH.

Abnormal DRE or PSA tests lead to transrectal ultrasound-guided biopsy of the prostate for patho-

Table 52.2—Staging Systems for Prostate Cancer

TNM Stage	Jewett-Whitmore Stage	Description
T1	A1, A2	Tumor is an incidental finding.
T1c		Tumor is identified by needle biopsy as a follow-up to screening that detected increased PSA.
T2	B1, B2	Tumor is palpable, confined to prostate.
T3	C1, C2	Tumor extends beyond the prostate capsule, may involve seminal vesicles.
T4	C2	Tumor invades adjacent structures (eg, bladder neck, rectum, pelvic wall).
N	D1	Lymph node metastasis present.
M	D2	Distant metastasis present.

NOTE: TNM = tumor, regional node, metastasis
SOURCE: For further details, see AUA Prostate Cancer Clinical Guidelines Panel. *Report on the Management of Clinically Localized Prostate Cancer.* Baltimore, MD: American Urological Association; 1995.

logic diagnosis. Cancer can appear as a hypoechoic density, but ultrasonography is not specific enough to be used as a screening tool. Any suspicious areas (by DRE or ultrasound) are biopsied. In addition to, or in the absence of suspicious areas, spring-loaded core needle biopsies are routinely taken from the base, middle, and apex of each lobe (six samples total, termed sextant biopsy). Sextant biopsy can be enhanced by extended biopsy schemes that sample more gland areas, particularly the lateral aspects. In a systematic review, prostate biopsy schemes that consist of 12 cores (standard sextant biopsy plus laterally directed cores) achieved a reasonable balance between cancer detection rates and adverse events.

Grading

The Gleason grading system is the most commonly used system that is based on the histologic appearance of prostate cancer. The Gleason grade ranges from 1, or well differentiated, to 5, or poorly differentiated. The Gleason score is the sum of the most common Gleason grade observed plus the next most common Gleason grade seen. The Gleason score ranges from 2 to 10. Gleason scores are sometimes grouped as 2–4, well differentiated; 5–7, moderately differentiated; 8–10, poorly differentiated. Well-differentiated tumors have a favorable prognosis; poorly differentiated tumors, an unfavorable prognosis (SOE=A). Most clinically detected tumors are moderately differentiated.

Staging

Staging of prostate cancer is necessary for planning disease management. Two classification systems are used: the tumor, regional node, metastasis (TNM) system and the Jewett-Whitmore (ABCD) system (Table 52.2). Usually detected by transurethral resection of the prostate, incidentally discovered cancers are staged according to the amount of tissue involved (T1 or A). Stage T1c reflects the growing number of tumors detected because of an increased PSA level. Tumors detectable by DRE and confined to the prostate (T2 or B) are subdivided on the basis of the amount of tumor that is palpable. Staging is also based on the degree of extension and invasion of surrounding structures in tumors that extend beyond the prostatic capsule (T3 to T4 or C), and on presence of metastasis (M1 or D).

The initial staging evaluation includes PSA level, DRE findings, transrectal ultrasonography results, and Gleason score. Bone scans may be performed on patients with PSA values >10 ng/mL, Gleason score >6, or complaints of bone pain (SOE=D). For patients electing active treatment, surgical assessment of lymph node involvement (pelvic lymphadenectomy) is performed by itself or in conjunction with prostate surgery or implantation of radioactive seeds. CT scans are often used for active treatment planning.

In the past, CT scans, MRI scans, pedal lymphangiography, and pelvic lymph node dissection were routinely used in various combinations to evaluate the extent of prostate cancer. In the initial staging evaluation of patients with prostate cancer, these tests should be eliminated because they have been associated with unacceptably high false-negative and false-positive results. A subset of patients appear to benefit from CT scans combined with fine-needle aspiration. Patients who have a PSA >25 ng/mL, a Gleason score >6, and a palpable abnormality on DRE are recommended to undergo a CT scan with fine-needle aspiration if a lymph node >6 mm is present (SOE=D). Many of these patients will be diagnosed with nodal metastasis and are thus spared the need for bilateral pelvic lymph-node dissection and its associated morbidity.

The serum PSA level should be used to eliminate the staging radionuclide bone scan (SOE=C). In the asymptomatic, newly diagnosed, previously untreated prostate cancer patient, a PSA concentration ≤10 ng/mL has been associated with rare (0–0.8%) findings of skeletal metastases. Adopting recommendations to eliminate the staging radionuclide bone scan in this population will substantially reduce testing, because 50%–60% of men with newly diagnosed prostate cancer have a serum PSA concentration in this range.

Management of Localized Disease

Localized cancer lends itself to cure, but the prevalence of men dying with prostate cancer (often asymptomatic) but not from the disease questions the necessity of treatment. There remains a lack of evidence that treatment prolongs life when treatment is compared with watchful waiting. Thus, three approaches to localized prostate cancer are routinely advocated: watchful waiting, radical prostatectomy, and radiation therapy (Table 52.3).

Watchful waiting (also called *expectant* or *conservative management; surveillance*) is the approach offered most commonly to men with <10 yr of remaining life expectancy, who have significant medical comorbidities, or whose tumor is small and well to moderately differentiated. Conservative management studies have shown that 10 yr disease-specific survival is 89%–96% for men with Gleason score 2–5 tumors, 70%–82% for men with Gleason score 6 tumors, 30%–58% for men with Gleason score 7 tumors, and 13%–40% for men with Gleason score 8–10 tumors. Because most men with prostate cancer are asymptomatic, watchful waiting attempts to spare men the burden of unnecessary treatment. However, waiting for symptoms in men with prostate cancer before starting treatment means sacrificing the opportunity for cure. Patients are offered palliation if and when symptoms develop. A newer approach, active surveillance, combines the concept of expectant management with the option for deferred curative intent treatment. The optimal selection criteria and surveillance strategy for active surveillance have not been defined. Active surveillance selection criteria include cases detected by PSA screening with Gleason scores <7 and small volume involvement (<3 of 6 biopsy cores, <50% malignant involvement within each core). The National Comprehensive Cancer Network guidelines for active surveillance suggest serum PSA measurement as often as every 3 mo, DRE as often as every 6 mo, and repeat prostate biopsy as often as annually (SOE=C).

Radical prostatectomy involves the surgical removal of the entire prostate gland and the seminal vesicles. It can be performed through a perineal (incision near the rectum) or retropubic (lower abdominal incision) approach. The perineal approach allows an easier vesicourethral anastomosis and less bleeding, whereas the retropubic approach allows access to the pelvic lymph nodes and spares the neurovascular supply to the corpora cavernosa (with improved potency). The major complications of radical prostatectomy are urinary incontinence and erectile dysfunction. Surgery is thought to have the highest incidence of posttreatment sexual dysfunction. In a population-based study of 1,291 men undergoing radical prostatectomy for clinically localized prostate cancer, 59.9% reported erections not firm enough for sexual intercourse and 8.4% were incontinent 18 mo later (SOE=C). After radical prostatectomy, men are more likely to experience stress incontinence, with

Table 52.3—Management Approaches for Prostate Cancer

Management	Description	Comments	Selected Adverse Effects
Localized			
Watchful waiting	Prostate cancer is not treated until symptoms develop	Offered to men with <10 yr of remaining life expectancy; significant medical comorbidities; small, well-differentiated tumors; or unwillingness to bear treatment burdens Awaiting symptoms sacrifices opportunity for cure	Anxiety
Radical prostatectomy	Surgical removal of the entire prostate gland and seminal vesicles	Offered to men who have no surgical contraindications Adverse effects realized immediately	Erectile dysfunction, urinary incontinence
External beam radiation therapy	Standard regimen delivers 6,000–7,000 rads of pelvic radiation over 5-8 wk period	Radiation reaches tissues outside the prostate, including pelvic lymph nodes Adverse effects occur initially from radiation-induced inflammation, then develop over time as scar tissue develops	*Acute*: proctitis, urethritis *Chronic*: erectile dysfunction, urinary incontinence, bowel dysfunction
Brachytherapy	Radioactive seeds (eg, iridium, palladium) are implanted into the prostate gland using CT scan guidance	Improvements in prostate imaging allow uniform distribution of seed, overcoming past limitations Adverse effects occur initially from radiation-induced inflammation, then develop over time as scar tissue develops	*Acute*: prostatitis, urinary retention, hematuria *Chronic*: erectile dysfunction, urinary incontinence, bowel dysfunction
Locally Advanced			
Radiation therapy	See external beam radiation (above)	Offered to men with prostate cancer extending beyond capsule or into seminal vesicles Asymptomatic cancer period may be prolonged	See external beam radiation (above)
Androgen deprivation	Hormone therapy can be combined with radiation therapy	Neoadjuvant androgen deprivation provides additional benefit toward increased survival and freedom from metastases; due to adverse effects, controversy exists regarding early versus delayed use of androgen deprivation	Erectile dysfunction, loss of libido, loss of stamina, increased fatigue, hot flashes, diminished muscle mass, premature osteoporosis
Advanced/Metastatic			
Complete androgen ablation	Combined approach of reducing androgens to castration levels and inhibiting binding of androgen to its receptor	Includes orchiectomy or LHRH agonists with antiandrogens	Erectile dysfunction, loss of libido, loss of stamina, increased fatigue, hot flashes, diminished muscle mass, premature osteoporosis
Orchiectomy	Surgical castration	Oldest, safest, least expensive approach; rejected by half of American men	Erectile dysfunction, loss of libido, loss of stamina, increased fatigue, hot flashes, diminished muscle mass, premature osteoporosis
LHRH agonists	Chemical castration	Alternative to surgical castration, equally effective Causes initial increase in serum testosterone levels	Erectile dysfunction, loss of libido, hot flashes, gynecomastia, insomnia, GI upset, dizziness

Table 52.3—Management Approaches for Prostate Cancer (continued)

Management	Description	Comments	Selected Adverse Effects
Antiandrogens	Inhibit binding of androgen to its receptor	Used at initiation of LHRH agonists to block effect of increased testosterone levels Used after castration to block effect of residual small amount of androgen being produced by adrenal glands	Erectile dysfunction, loss of libido, gynecomastia, insomnia, GI upset, dizziness
Other	Symptom-specific approaches are used as indicated	For example, focal radiation therapy can be provided to the site of a bony metastasis to reduce both pain and risk of fracture	Intervention specific

NOTE: LHRH = luteinizing hormone-releasing hormone

symptoms ranging from occasional leakage to no urinary control. Bladder neck contractures also occur, resulting in obstructive voiding symptoms and urinary retention. The relationship between these symptoms and sense of bother is not direct; for example, those with the most leakage may have little bother while those with minimal leakage may report substantial bother.

Data regarding the benefits of radical prostatectomy are still lacking. Two randomized controlled trials have compared radical prostatectomy to watchful waiting. In one study of 695 men with 10-yr follow up, prostatectomy compared with watchful waiting reduced both death from prostate cancer (10% versus 15%) and distant metastases (15.2% versus 25.4%). In the second study of 142 men, no statistically significant differences in survival were found; however the study lacked sufficient power to detect moderate treatment differences. Both studies were conducted before prostate cancer detection with PSA testing was available. Two surgical improvements currently under investigation to reduce morbidity include the laparoscopic approach and robotic assistance. The laparoscopic approach has raised concerns of poorer results related to positive surgical margins, return of continence, and preservation of potency. Robotic approaches have not shown advantage in hospital length of stay, postoperative pain, or blood replacement (SOE=C). Long-term outcomes are not yet known for either the laparoscopic or robotic approach. Thus, radical prostatectomy can be offered to men with locally confined disease, with >10 yr of remaining life expectancy, and without contraindications to undergoing surgery (SOE=B).

Radiation therapy is provided through external beam radiation or through implantation of radioactive sources (known as *brachytherapy*). The standard regimen of external beam radiation delivers a total of about 6,000–7,000 rads over 5–8 weeks. Hypofractionated schemes use higher doses per fraction that achieve biologically similar doses over 4–5 weeks. Pelvic lymph nodes can be radiated as well. Proctitis and urethritis are common acute adverse events. Chronic complications include erectile dysfunction, urinary incontinence, and chronic proctitis. The incidence of urinary stress incontinence after radiation therapy is significantly less than with surgery but that of irritative voiding dysfunction is greater. Bowel dysfunction, uncommon after surgery, affects more than half of patients after radiation. Bowel symptoms include diarrhea, rectal urgency, and fecal soiling. Most patients classify these bowel symptoms as minor with little to no effect on quality of life. Conformal radiation therapy is a mode of high-precision external-beam radiation that uses high-resolution CT scan data and advanced computer technology to conform the radiation dose to the three-dimensional configuration of the tumor. This newer technology shows promise in reducing complications and adverse events. Local control and cancer survival rates appear to be comparable to those of radical prostatectomy, at least for the first 5–8 yr (SOE=C). Comparisons between treatments are difficult because men undergoing radiation treatment tend to be older, less medically fit, and usually have not been pathologically staged.

Brachytherapy involves retropubic or perineal implantation of radioactive seeds, usually iridium or palladium. Improvements in three-dimensional imaging of the prostate through CT scan or ultrasound guidance have allowed more uniform distribution of seeds throughout the prostate and overcome many of the past limitations of brachytherapy. Potency is better preserved with seed implants. Urinary symptoms include frequency, dysuria, and urge incontinence. Bowel symptoms include rectal urgency and rectal bleeding. The morbidity of seed implants appears to improve over time after the initial seed placement and associated prostate inflammation and swelling. In retrospective series, it appears that brachytherapy is comparable to radical prostatectomy and external beam radiation for low-risk disease. However, brachytherapy outcomes appear less favorable for tumors with higher Gleason score or higher pretreatment PSA levels (SOE=C).

Management of Locally Advanced Prostate Cancer

Locally advanced prostate cancer extends beyond the capsule or invades the seminal vesicle, without evidence of distant or nodal metastasis. Radiation therapy is the recommended treatment, and neoadjuvant androgen deprivation provides additional benefit toward increased survival and freedom from metastases (SOE=B). However, controversy exists as to when androgen deprivation should be started. Patients may have a prolonged asymptomatic cancer period, while significant negative quality-of-life changes from long-term androgen deprivation occur, including loss of stamina, increased fatigue, hot flashes, diminished muscle mass, and premature osteoporosis. While radiation therapy with neoadjuvant androgen deprivation is a standard approach for locally advanced disease, some advocate that patients should be given the choice of early versus delayed androgen deprivation.

Management of Advanced Disease

Advanced disease is treated with androgen ablation and symptom-specific approaches, such as focal radiation therapy to painful bone metastasis. Androgen ablation aims to eliminate prostate cancer growth stimulation and includes orchiectomy or luteinizing hormone-releasing hormone (LHRH) agonists with antiandrogens. Orchiectomy and LHRH agonists are equally effective at reducing androgens to castration levels. Orchiectomy is the oldest, safest, least expensive approach but is rejected by nearly half of American men. LHRH agonists such as leuprolide and goserelin result in castration levels about 1 mo after an initial increase in serum testosterone levels. Antiandrogens (eg, flutamide) are often given before starting LHRH agonists to blunt the effects of the initial testosterone increase. Antiandrogens inhibit the binding of androgen to its receptor. After castration, a small amount of adrenal androgen exists and may allow continued stimulation of prostate cancer growth. Antiandrogens can be combined with chemical or surgical castration, a practice called *complete androgen ablation*. Survival rates for antiandrogens alone are inferior to those for chemical or surgical castration alone; complete androgen ablation offers slight improvement in survival over that offered by castration only (SOE=B).

Radiation therapy is useful for relieving the pain of isolated bone metastasis and reducing the risk of fracture of bones with significant destruction. Diffuse bone metastases require alternative approaches. Bone-seeking radiopharmaceuticals such as strontium or radium can be beneficial for pain control (SOE=B). Androgen deprivation decreases bone pain in two-thirds of symptomatic patients (SOE=B). Bisphosphonates also decrease bone pain (SOE=B).

PROSTATITIS

Etiology

Prostatitis is an inflammatory condition of the prostate that can result from acute bacterial, chronic bacterial, or nonbacterial causes. The most common sources of acute or chronic infection are ascending urethral infection or reflux of infected urine into the prostatic ducts, or both. Direct extension or lymphatic spread from the rectum or hematogenous spread also occurs. Acute prostatitis is an infectious process that is more common in young men. Pathogens in men ≤35 yr old often include *Neisseria gonorrhea* and *Chlamydia trachomatis*. In older men, acute prostatitis is associated with indwelling urethral catheter use, and coliforms are the suspected bacterial cause. In >80% of patients with prostatitis, no infectious agent is identified.

Diagnosis

Acute bacterial prostatitis is characterized by fever, chills, dysuria, and a tense or boggy, extremely tender prostate. Because bacteremia can result from manipulation of the inflamed gland, minimal rectal examination is indicated. Gram's stain and culture of the urine can identify the causative agent.

Chronic bacterial prostatitis presents classically as recurrent bacteriuria caused by the same organism, although most patients do not have this presentation. Patients have varying degrees of obstructive or irritative voiding symptoms and perineal pain. The prostate often feels normal. First-void or midstream urine is compared with expressed prostatic secretion or urine collected after prostatic massage. The expressed sample should reveal leukocytosis and the causative agent. Sterile expressant with leukocytosis suggests nonbacterial prostatitis.

Treatment

Acute bacterial prostatitis is treated with antibiotics and can require hospitalization. The severe inflammation allows antibiotics to penetrate the prostate, and prompt response to empiric therapy is expected. CT or MRI should be considered to evaluate for an abscess if recovery is delayed. Antibiotic selection should be based initially on results of a urine Gram's stain, with subsequent consideration of sensitivity profiles. Fluoroquinolones are highly effective in most cases.

Antibiotics are less effective for chronic bacterial prostatitis because of their poor penetration of the prostate. Prolonged therapy (6–16 weeks) offers a cure rate of 30%–40%. Continuous low-dose antibiotic suppression therapy can be offered for those with frequent symptomatic relapse. Total prostatectomy offers cure but at a high risk-to-benefit ratio. Transurethral resection of the prostate is safer but cures only one-third of patients.

Nonbacterial prostatitis is treated symptomatically. A small percentage of cases can involve occult infections, and empiric antibiotic therapy is often used. Efforts to reduce pain and discomfort include anti-inflammatory agents, sitz baths, fluid adjustments (avoid caffeine), anticholinergic agents, and α-adrenergic antagonists.

ACOVE-3* QUALITY INDICATORS PERTAINING TO PROSTATE DISEASE

Benign prostatic hyperplasia (BPH) history

- If a male vulnerable older adult complains of new or worsening urinary frequency, urgency, urinary incontinence, nocturia, decreased force of stream, feeling of incomplete bladder emptying, or postvoid dribbling (lower urinary tract symptoms [LUTS]), then a history should document the following:
  ○ Medications associated with symptoms
  ○ Neurologic conditions that can affect the urologic system
  ○ Prior urologic, neurosurgical, orthopedic, or general surgery procedures
  ○ Whether symptoms are bothersome
  ○ Prior treatment

BPH examination

- If a male vulnerable older adult complains of new LUTS, then a rectal examination (including prostate size, degree of tenderness, and nodularity) and abdominal examination should be performed.

Urine evaluation

- If a male vulnerable older adult complains of new or worsening LUTS, then a urinalysis (microscopic examination or dipstick) should be performed, as well as a urine culture if the urinalysis demonstrates pyuria or hematuria.

Postvoid residual

- If a male vulnerable older adult presenting with new or worsening urinary incontinence or complaints of incomplete emptying or LUTS and has neurologic disease (eg, spinal cord injury, multiple sclerosis) or has had a procedure that can affect innervation of the bladder or urethral sphincter mechanism (eg, spinal surgery), then he should have a postvoid residual measurement.

Urologic trauma

- If a male vulnerable older adult presenting with new or worsening LUTS has a history of lower tract urologic surgery or urethral trauma (including traumatic catheterizations), then he should be referred to a urologist within 2 mo.

Hematuria

- If a male vulnerable older adult has new microhematuria (>3 RBCs/high-power field) and a negative urine culture (or has 1 positive and 1 negative urinalysis), then a repeat urinalysis should be performed within 1 mo.
- If a male vulnerable older adult has unexplained gross hematuria or microhematuria (>3 RBCs/high-power field on 2 of 3 urinalyses) and a negative urine culture, then he should have the following within 3 mo:
  ○ Serum creatinine
  ○ Upper urologic tract imaging
  ○ Referral to a urologist or nephrologist

Prostate-specific antigen (PSA) testing

- If a male vulnerable older adult receives a screening PSA test, then the chart should document a discussion of the pros and cons of the test.

Referral indications

- If a male vulnerable older adult with presumed BPH has bladder stones, urinary retention (>1 episode), urinary tract infection, or renal failure with hydronephrosis, then the patient should be referred to a urologist.

BPH treatment

- If a male vulnerable older adult with BPH has an American Urological Association Symptom Index (AUA SI) score of ≤7, the symptoms are not bothersome, and the patient is not known to have bilateral hydronephrosis, bladder stones, hematuria attributable to the prostate, or urinary tract infection, then he should not be prescribed medications or surgery for BPH.
- If a male vulnerable older adult with BPH has moderate to severe symptoms (or an AUA SI score >7) that are bothersome, then the medical record should document that treatment options were discussed (eg, medical, surgical, watchful waiting).

Preoperative urine evaluation

- If a male vulnerable older adult has surgery for BPH, then a urinalysis or a urine culture should have been done within 6 weeks before surgery and treated, if necessary.

REFERENCES

■ Issa MM, Kraft KH. 5alpha-reductase inhibition for men with enlarged prostate. *J Am Acad Nurse Pract.* 2007;19(8):398–407.

■ Propert KJ, McNaughton-Collins M, Leiby BE, et al. A prospective study of symptoms and quality of life in men with chronic prostatitis/chronic pelvic pain syndrome: the National Institutes of Health chronic prostatitis cohort study. *J Urol.* 2006;175(2):619–623.

■ Wilt TJ, MacDonald R, Rutks I, et al. Systematic review: comparative effectiveness and harms of treatments for clinically localized prostate cancer. *Ann Intern Med.* 2008;148(6):435–448.

CHAPTER 53—DISORDERS OF SEXUAL FUNCTION

KEY POINTS

■ Normal age-associated changes lead to a decline in sexual interest and decreased ability; however, complete sexual dysfunction is not a part of healthy aging.

■ Physiologic changes in sexual response occur in both men and women. It is important to distinguish between normal age-associated changes and pathologic conditions that can be related to medications or medical disorders.

■ Many older women have sexual dysfunction but do not report it to their primary care practitioners unless asked.

■ Multiple options are available to treat male and female sexual dysfunction.

■ Sexuality is an important part of quality of life for many older adults; treatment of sexual dysfunction can lead to improvements in quality of life.

Our understanding of sexual function and dysfunction in older men has increased significantly in recent years. There is less scientific information on the sexuality of older women, possibly because of the difficulty of measuring the female sexual response. However, the 2007 National Social Life, Health, and Aging Project (NSLHAP) provides insights into the sexual activity, behavior, and problems of older men and women in America.

FEMALE SEXUALITY

Age-Associated Changes

Many factors play an important role in the sexual response of older women, including changes that occur with menopause, cultural expectations, relationship problems, previous sexual experiences, chronic illnesses, and depression. American women live about 29 yr after menopause and outlive their spouses an average of 8 yr. Although the frequency of intercourse decreases with aging, sexuality remains important for older women. Among 513 women 75–85 yr old in the NSLHAP, 37.2% were married, 1.2% were living with a partner, and 16.7% reported sexual activity with their spouse or other partner in the previous year. Of those who were sexually active with a partner, 54.1% reported sexual activity at least 2 or 3 times per month. Among those women who had a spouse or other partner but had been sexually inactive in the previous 3 mo, 64.8% attributed the inactivity to the partner's physical health problems or limitations and 24.8% to their own health problems.

The female sexual response cycle changes with aging. During the excitement phase, the clitoris may require longer direct stimulation, and genital engorgement is decreased. Vaginal lubrication is reduced, although with increased foreplay and gentle stimulation, lubrication is usually adequate for intercourse. During the plateau phase, there is less expansion and vasocongestion of the vagina. During orgasm, fewer and weaker contractions occur, although older women can still achieve multiple orgasms. Occasionally during orgasm, older women experience spastic and painful contractions of the uterine musculature. During the resolution phase, vasocongestion is lost more rapidly. Most of these changes are thought to be due to a decline in serum estrogen concentration after menopause, but a vasculogenic component can contribute to postmenopausal sexual dysfunction.

Female Sexual Dysfunction

For the most part, menopause is accompanied by decreased sexual function, with decreased sexual interest, responsiveness, and coital frequency. In addition, there is an increase in urogenital symptoms, often not discussed with the clinician. For example, in the NSLHAP, among women 75–85 yr old who were sexually active, the most common sexual problem was lack of interest (49.3%), followed by difficulty with lubrication (43.6%), inability to climax (38.2%), sex not pleasurable (24.9%), and pain during intercourse (11.8%).

Dyspareunia, defined as pain with intercourse, can be due to organic or psychologic factors, or a combination. For example, a woman can experience an episode of dyspareunia because of postmenopausal vaginal atrophy. With each subsequent sexual encounter, she anticipates pain, causing inadequate arousal with decreased lubrication. Because of this cycle, the woman continues to experience dyspareunia, even after the vaginal atrophy has been treated. The most common organic cause of dyspareunia is atrophic vaginitis due to estrogen deficiency. Other causes include inadequate lubrication, localized vaginal infections, cystitis, Bartholin cyst, retroverted uterus, marked uterine prolapse, endometriosis, pelvic tumors, excessive penile thrusting, or vaginismus (involuntary muscle spasms).

Estrogen replacement can improve symptoms of vulvovaginal atrophy, but it has little effect on libido or sexual satisfaction (SOE=B). Libido is thought to depend on testosterone (even in women), rather than on estrogen. The ovaries and adrenals are the main sources of androgens in women. The effects of female androgen deficiency were originally identified in women treated for advanced breast cancer with oophorectomy and adrenalectomy. When deprived of androgens, these women reported loss of libido. Because there are no normative data on plasma total and free testosterone in women and no well-defined clinical syndrome of androgen deficiency, The Endocrine Society has not recommended making a diagnosis of androgen deficiency in women.

Older women commonly have multiple medical conditions, some of which affect sexuality. However, scientific studies on the effect of chronic diseases and medications on the sexuality of older women are limited. Women with diabetes mellitus are less likely to be sexually active, and report decreased libido and lubrication and longer time to reach orgasm. Rheumatic diseases affect sexuality via functional disability. After mastectomy for breast cancer, 20%–40% of women experience sexual dysfunction, possibly because of disruption of body image, marital and family problems, spousal reaction, adjuvant therapy, or the psychologic impact of a breast cancer diagnosis. Several drugs can adversely affect sexual function, including antihistamines, antihypertensives, antidepressants, antipsychotics, antiestrogens, CNS stimulants, narcotics, alcohol, and anticholinergic drugs.

Psychosocial factors have an important role in sexual dysfunction. Women commonly marry men older than themselves and live longer than men. Consequently, heterosexual older women are likely to spend the last years of their lives alone. Even when a partner is available, he might have erectile dysfunction. Finally, lack of privacy can be a problem when an older couple lives with their children or in a nursing home.

Evaluation and Treatment

The history is the most important part of the evaluation of sexual function. Careful and sensitive questioning can detect problems that a woman might not otherwise volunteer. Clinicians should ask about dyspareunia, lack of vaginal lubrication, and previous negative experiences, such as rape, child abuse, or domestic violence. Medications should be carefully reviewed. A woman with dyspareunia should undergo a pelvic examination to exclude organic causes.

Dyspareunia due to atrophic vaginitis and decreased lubrication responds well to topical or systemic estrogen therapy. However, it is important to explain to the patient that complete restoration of vaginal tissue function can take up to 2 yr. A vaginal estradiol ring or tablet delivers low-dose estrogen locally with lower systemic absorption and risks of systemic adverse events than does vaginal estrogen. If the patient is not a candidate for or does not want to use estrogen, water-soluble vaginal lubricants (eg, Replens, Astroglide, K-Y jelly) are beneficial. Importantly, local stimulation through regular intercourse helps maintain a healthy vaginal mucosa. Longer foreplay allows more time for vaginal lubrication, just as older men often need longer and more direct stimulation to achieve an adequate erection.

Decreased libido may respond to testosterone, but no androgen preparation is approved by the FDA for sexual desire disorders in women. In four placebo-controlled, randomized trials of low-dose testosterone patch in surgical menopausal women with low sexual desire published in 2005 and 2006, all women were on systemic estrogens. A testosterone

Table 53.1—Treatment Options for Sexual Dysfunction in Older Women

Symptom	Possible Cause	Therapy
Decreased desire	Low testosterone from natural or surgical menopause	Testosterone[OL] is not recommended by The Endocrine Society
	Chronic illness	Treatment of underlying illness
	Depression	Antidepressant medication
	Relationship problems	Marital therapy
	Medications	Review of drugs ingested
Decreased lubrication	Vaginal dryness or atrophy from postmenopausal status	Longer foreplay, regular intercourse, lubricants, topical estrogens
	Anticholinergic medications	Review of medications, including OTC drugs
Delayed or absent orgasm	Neurologic disorders, diabetes	Treatment of underlying illness
	Psychologic problems	Cognitive-behavioral therapy, masturbation, Kegel exercises
Pain with intercourse	Organic cause	Treatment of underlying physical condition
	Vaginal dryness, atrophy	Longer foreplay, regular intercourse, lubricants, topical estrogens
	Vaginismus (involuntary vaginal contractions)	Psychotherapy, cognitive-behavioral therapy

patch delivering 300 mcg/d dosed twice weekly or daily improved sexual desire and other sexual function domains. Androgenic adverse events such as acne and hirsutism were uncommon, and concentrations of high-density lipoprotein cholesterol did not decrease as in studies with oral methyltestosterone.

In 2007 data from the Phase III studies known as the Investigation of Natural Testosterone in Menopausal Women Also Taking Estrogen in Surgically Menopausal Women (INTIMATE SM), total satisfying sexual activity was significantly increased in women who received the testosterone patch than in those who received placebo. There are less data in naturally menopausal women, but the results of a similar study (INTIMATE NM, in which NM stands for natural menopause) showed that the testosterone patch improved sexual interest and response in women who have undergone natural menopause and have decreased sexual desire. In 2008, the APHRODITE trial demonstrated that the testosterone patch is also effective in women with natural or surgically induced menopause and decreased libido who are not taking estrogens. Although the testosterone patch seems effective (SOE=B), the trials discussed above were only 6 mo long, and there are no data about the long-term safety of the testosterone patch in women. The Endocrine Society clinical practice guideline on androgen therapy in women recommends against the generalized use of testosterone by women because of the above concerns. Testosterone for women is available only as oral methyltestosterone in combination with esterified estrogens and is approved by the FDA for moderate to severe vasomotor symptoms that are not improved with estrogens alone. The testosterone patch is not FDA approved for women. Further studies of the best dosage, delivery system, long-term efficacy, and safety of testosterone are needed.

Randomized trials of sildenafil for female sexual dysfunction yielded conflicting results (SOE=C). The manufacturer has therefore decided not to apply for use of sildenafil in women for this indication. Finally, older women should receive education about male sexual aging in addition to female sexual aging. Otherwise, an older woman might mistakenly attribute her partner's diminished erection and need for more genital stimulation to her own inability to arouse her partner. Other psychologic issues, including depression, history of sexual abuse, and relationship problems, should be addressed and treated with antidepressants, psychotherapy, and marital therapy, as necessary (SOE=C). For a summary of treatments for female sexual dysfunction, see Table 53.1.

MALE SEXUALITY

Age-Associated Changes

As men age, their sexuality changes. The frequency of sexual intercourse and the prevalence of engaging in any sexual activity decrease. Young men report having intercourse 3 to 4 times per week, whereas only 7% of men 60–69 yr old and 2% of those ≥70 yr old report the same frequency. Among men 60–70 yr old, 50%–80% engage in any sexual activity, a prevalence rate that declines to 15%–25% among men ≥80 yr old (SOE=A). However, sexual interest often persists despite decreased activity. The man's level of sexual activity, interest, and enjoyment in his younger years often determines his sexual behavior with aging. Factors contributing to a man's decreased sexual activity include poor health, social issues, partner availability, decreased libido, and erectile dysfunction. Although men 75–85 yr old continue to prefer vaginal intercourse, approximately 50% report difficulty with erectile function.

Table 53.2—Causes of Sexual Dysfunction in Older Men

Causes (in order of prevalence)	Characteristics
Vascular disease	▪ Gradual onset Vascular risk factors: diabetes mellitus, hypertension, hyperlipidemia, tobacco use
Neurologic disease, eg, radiation therapy, spinal cord injury, autonomic dysfunction, surgical procedures	▪ Gradual onset Neurologic risk factors: diabetes mellitus; history of pelvic injury, surgery, or irradiation; spinal injury or surgery; Parkinson's disease; multiple sclerosis; alcoholism Loss of bulbocavernosus reflex
Medications, eg, anticholinergics, antihypertensives, cimetidine, antidepressants	▪ Sudden onset Lack of sleep-associated erections or lack of erections with masturbation Temporal association with a new medication
Psychogenic, eg, relationship conflicts, performance anxiety, childhood sexual abuse, fear of sexually transmitted diseases, "widower's syndrome"	▪ Sudden onset Sleep-associated erections or erections with masturbation are preserved
Hypogonadism	▪ Gradual onset Decreased libido more than erectile dysfunction Small testes, gynecomastia Low serum testosterone concentration
Endocrine, eg, hypothyroidism, hyperthyroidism, hyperprolactinemia	▪ Rare, <5% of cases of erectile dysfunction

Aging is associated not only with changes in sexual behavior but also with changes in the stages of sexual response. During the excitement phase, there is a delay in erection, decreased tensing of the scrotal sac, and loss of testicular elevation. The duration of the plateau stage is prolonged, and pre-ejaculatory secretion is decreased. Orgasm is diminished in duration and intensity, with decreased quantity and force of seminal emission. During the resolution phase, detumescence and testicular descent are rapid. The refractory period between erections is also longer. However, erectile failure is not a part of healthy aging but rather is frequently caused by age-associated disease or its treatment (eg, radical prostatectomy for prostate cancer) (SOE=B).

Erectile Dysfunction

Erectile dysfunction (ED) is the most common sexual problem of older men. ED is the inability to achieve or maintain an erection adequate for sexual intercourse. The prevalence of ED increases with age; by age 70 yr, 67% of men have ED. This high prevalence is important; in a study comparing affected and unaffected men, men with sexual dysfunction reported impaired quality of life. For a summary of the causes of sexual dysfunction in men, see Table 53.2.

The most common cause (30%–50%) of ED in older men is vascular disease (SOE=A). Risk of vascular ED increases with traditional vascular risk factors, eg, diabetes mellitus, hypertension, hyperlipidemia, and smoking. In fact, ED is a predictor of future major atherosclerotic vascular disease (ie, myocardial infarction and stroke).

Obstruction from atherosclerotic arterial occlusive disease likely impedes the intracavernosal blood flow and pressure needed to achieve a rigid erection. In addition, atherosclerotic disease can cause ischemia of trabecular smooth muscle and result in fibrotic changes leading to failure of venous closure mechanisms. Venous leakage leading to vascular ED can also result from Peyronie's disease, arteriovenous fistula, or trauma-induced communication between the glans and the corpora. In anxious men who have excessive adrenergic-constrictor tone and in men with injured parasympathetic dilator nerves, ED can result from insufficient relaxation of trabecular smooth muscle.

The second most common cause of ED in older men is neurologic disease (17%–37%). Disorders that affect the parasympathetic sacral spinal cord or the peripheral efferent autonomic fibers to the penis impair penile smooth muscle relaxation and prevent the vasodilation necessary for erection. In patients with prostate cancer, all forms of (curative) treatment frequently cause neurogenic erectile failure (brachytherapy or external radiation, 50%; radical prostatectomy with nerve sparing, 45%–80%) and pain on orgasm (SOE=B). Common health problems such as diabetes mellitus, stroke, and Parkinson's disease can cause autonomic dysfunction that result in erectile failure. Finally, surgical procedures such as cystectomy and proctocolectomy commonly disrupt the autonomic nerve supply to the penis, resulting in postoperative ED.

Numerous commonly used medications have been associated with ED for which the mechanism, for the most part, is unknown. In approximately 5% of men with ED, the ED is drug-induced. Those medications with anticholinergic effects, such as antidepressants, antipsychotics, and antihistamines, can cause ED by blocking parasympathetic-mediated penile artery vasodilatation and trabecular smooth muscle relaxation. Almost all antihypertensive agents have been associated with ED; of these, β-blockers, clonidine, and thiazide diuretics have higher incidence rates, whereas ACE inhibitors and angiotensin-receptor blockers have lower incidence rates (SOE=B). One mechanism by which antihypertensives can cause ED is lowering blood pressure below the threshold needed to maintain sufficient blood flow for penile erection, especially in those men who already have penile arterial disease. OTC medications such as cimetidine and ranitidine can also cause ED. Cimetidine, an H_2-receptor antagonist, acts as an antiandrogen and increases prolactin secretion; thus, it has been associated with loss of libido and erectile failure. Ranitidine can also increase prolactin secretion, although less commonly than does cimetidine.

The prevalence of psychogenic ED correlates inversely with age. In approximately 9% of men ≥65 yr old with ED, the ED is psychogenic. Psychogenic ED can develop via increased sympathetic stimuli to the sacral cord, inhibiting the parasympathetic dilator nerves and thus inhibiting erection. Common causes of psychogenic ED include relationship conflicts, performance anxiety, childhood sexual abuse, and fear of sexually transmitted diseases. Older men may have "widower's syndrome," in which the man involved in a new relationship feels guilt as a defense against subconscious unfaithfulness to his deceased spouse.

Hyperthyroidism, hypothyroidism, and hyperprolactinemia have been associated with ED. However, <5% of ED is caused by endocrine abnormalities. Thus, endocrine evaluation of men with ED but intact libido is of limited value (SOE=B).

The role of androgens in erection is unclear. Hypogonadal men show smaller and slower developing erections in response to fantasy, which is improved with androgen replacement. However, even men with castrate levels of testosterone can attain erections in response to direct penile stimulation. Thus, it may be that erection from direct penile stimulation is androgen independent, whereas erection from fantasy is androgen dependent. Overall, testosterone appears to play a larger role in libido. Hypogonadal men respond better to phosphodiesterase inhibitors after testosterone replacement therapy.

Evaluation of Erectile Dysfunction

The initial step is to obtain a sexual, medical, and psychosocial history. Sexual history should clarify whether the problem consists of inadequate erections, decreased libido, or orgasmic failure. The onset and duration of ED, the presence or absence of sleep-associated erections, and the associated decline in libido are clues to the likely cause.

Sudden onset suggests psychogenic or drug-induced ED. A psychogenic cause is likely if there is a sudden onset but retention of sleep-associated erections or if erections with masturbation or a partner are intact (SOE=A). If sudden-onset erectile failure is accompanied by lack of sleep-associated erections and lack of erection with masturbation, temporal association with new medication should be investigated. A gradual onset of ED associated with loss of libido suggests hypogonadism. Gradual onset associated with intact libido (most common presentation) suggests vascular, neurogenic, or other organic causes.

Medical history is directed at discerning those factors likely to be contributing to ED. Vascular risk factors include diabetes mellitus, hypertension, coronary artery disease, peripheral arterial disease, hyperlipidemia, and smoking. Neurogenic risk factors include diabetes mellitus; history of pelvic injury, surgery, or radiation; spinal injury or surgery; Parkinson's disease; multiple sclerosis; or alcoholism. An extensive medication review, including OTC medications, is essential. Finally, the psychosocial history should assess the patient's relationship with the sexual partner, the partner's health and attitude toward sex, economic or social stresses, living situation, alcohol use, and affective disorders.

On physical examination, attention should be paid to signs of vascular or neurologic diseases. Peripheral pulses should be palpated. Signs of autonomic neuropathy (eg, orthostatic hypotension and absent heart rate response to standing) and loss of the bulbocavernosus reflex suggest neurologic dysfunction. The genital examination includes palpating the penis for Peyronie's plaques and assessing for testicular atrophy. A femoral bruit and diminished (or absent) pedal pulses suggests arterial insufficiency. An absent bulbocavernosus reflex suggests penile neuropathy. A loss of secondary sexual characteristics, small testes, and gynecomastia suggest hypogonadism or hyperprolactinemia.

Appropriate laboratory evaluations are those that target relevant comorbid conditions such as diabetes mellitus and vascular disease or that evaluate neurologic disorders if suggested by the physical examination. The measurement of serum testosterone should be considered in the setting of other symptoms of androgen deficiency. For specific recommendations regarding testing, see "Endocrine and Metabolic Disorders," p 491.

An at-home therapeutic trial of a phosphodiesterase inhibitor (sildenafil or vardenafil) is easier

Table 53.3—Treatment Options for Erectile Dysfunction

Treatment	Route/ Administration	Applicable Conditions	Onset	Duration of Action	Dosage	Selected Adverse Events
Sildenafil	Oral	N, A?, V?	60 min	4 h	25–100 mg	Headache, flushing, rhinitis, dyspepsia, transient color blindness; contraindicated with nitrate use and α-blockers
Vardenafil	Oral	N, A?, V?	45 min	4 h	5–20 mg	Headache, flushing, rhinitis, dyspepsia; contraindicated with nitrate use and α-blockers
Tadalafil	Oral	N, A?, V?	45–60 min	24–36 h	5–20 mg	Headache, dyspepsia, flushing, rhinitis; contraindicated with nitrate use and α-blockers
Vacuum device	External	P, N, V, A?	<5 min	30 min	—	Petechiae, bruising, painful ejaculation
Papaverine[OL]	Intracavernosal	N, A?, V?	10 min	30–60 min	15–60 mg	Prolonged erection, fibrosis, ecchymosis
Alprostadil	Intracavernosal	N, A?, V?	10 min	40–60 min	5–20 mcg	Prolonged erection, pain, fibrosis
Phentolamine[OL]	Intracavernosal	N, A?, V?	10 min	30–60 min	0.5–1 mg	Prolonged erection, fibrosis, headache, facial flushing
Medicated urethral system for erection (MUSE)	Intraurethral	N, A?, V?	10–15 min	60–80 min	250–1000 mcg	Penile pain or burning, hypotension
Penile prosthesis	Surgical	N, A, V		replacement in 5–10 yr		Infection, erosion, mechanical failure
Sex therapy	Counseling	P	weeks	years	weekly	Anxiety

NOTE: A = arteriogenic; N = neurogenic; P = psychogenic; V = venogenic; ? = possibly

than an in-office diagnostic penile injection of a vasodilator. The initial dose should be low (sildenafil 25–50 mg or vardenafil 5–10 mg) in men suspected of having neurogenic ED. A poor response suggests vasculogenic ED. Further therapeutic trial with sildenafil at 100 mg or vardenafil at 20 mg may prove to be effective. An at-home therapeutic trial using tadalafil (5–10 mg) can be considered, but the long half-life complicates matters if an adverse event occurs with the first dose.

More extensive diagnostic tools are available but not commonly used. Nocturnal penile tumescence testing is of little value, except to confirm a psychogenic cause. The penile-brachial pressure index can be helpful in assessing arteriogenic ED. This index measures the loss of systolic pressure between the arm and the penis. When measured before and after exercise, it can be used to assess for a pelvic steal syndrome, which is the loss of erection associated with initiation of active pelvic thrusting, presumably due to the transfer of blood flow from the penis to the pelvic musculature. More invasive and expensive tests such as Doppler ultrasound to assess penile arterial function, dynamic infusion cavernosometry to assess venous leakage syndrome, and penile arteriography are generally reserved for research or penile vascular surgery candidates.

Treatment of Erectile Dysfunction

Multiple effective therapeutic options are available for the treatment of ED. Treatment should be individualized and based on cause, personal preference, partner issues, cost, and practicality (Table 53.3).

Oral therapy for ED with sildenafil, vardenafil, or tadalafil has revolutionized treatment of male sexual dysfunction. Sildenafil is a type-5 phosphodiesterase inhibitor that potentiates the penile response to sexual stimulation. It improves the rigidity and duration of erection. It is taken 1 hour before sexual activity and has no effect until sexual stimulation occurs. Because absorption is attenuated when sildenafil is ingested with a fatty meal, patients need to be educated about this issue. Vardenafil is a more potent and specific phosphodiesterase inhibitor. A lower effective dose and better adverse-event profile (no effect on color vision) make vardenafil a reasonable option. Tadalafil is a longer-acting phosphodiesterase inhibitor with an adverse-event profile similar to that of vardenafil but with the added potential problem of muscle pain. All three of these agents are contraindicated for concomitant use with nitrate medications, because the combination can produce profound and fatal hypotension. Choosing between the three currently available phosphodiesterase inhibitors should likely be based on price and patient preference. Because of the longer duration of action of tadalafil, men tend to select it when given the choice (SOE=B).

Vacuum tumescence devices are another option. The apparatus consists of a plastic cylinder with an open end into which the penis is inserted. A vacuum device attached to the cylinder creates negative pressure within the cylinder, and blood flows into the penis to produce penile rigidity. A penile constriction ring placed at the base of the penis then traps the blood in the corpora cavernosa to maintain an erection for about 30 minutes. The vacuum device is effective for psychogenic, neurogenic, and venogenic ED, but it requires a lot of manual dexterity. Local pain, swelling, bruising, coolness of penile tip, and painful ejaculation are potential adverse events. It is important to remove the constriction ring after 30 minutes.

Intracavernous injection of vasoactive drugs such as papaverine, phentolamine, and alprostadil are effective in producing erections adequate for sexual activity (SOE=A) but are used much less frequently since oral therapy has become available. Alprostadil, which is the only agent approved by the FDA for intracavernous injection, produces erections that last 40–60 minutes. Phentolamine[OL] is mainly used in combination therapy with papaverine[OL] or alprostadil, or both. Potential adverse events are bruising, ecchymoses or hematoma, local pain, fibrosis from repeated injections, and priapism. Alprostadil appears to cause less scarring and priapism than papaverine. If an erection lasts >4 hours, detumescence is necessary by aspiration of blood from the corpora cavernosa or injection of phenylephrine, because there is the potential for intracavernous hypoxia and fibrosis of trabecular smooth muscle, which can prevent future erections. In general, intracavernosal therapy should probably be reserved for patients in whom oral therapy with a phosphodiesterase inhibitor is not effective. Alprostadil can also be administered intraurethrally using medicated urethral system for erection (MUSE). This system contains a small pellet of alprostadil that is placed within the urethra and is rapidly absorbed through the urethral mucosa to produce an erection within 10–15 minutes. Possible adverse events are penile pain, urethral burning, and a throbbing sensation in the perineum.

Testosterone supplementation increases libido and can improve ED in men with true hypogonadism (SOE=B). It is available as an intramuscular injection (testosterone enanthate or cypionate) or topical transdermal patch and gel. Possible adverse events associated with testosterone include polycythemia, prostate enlargement, gynecomastia, and fluid retention. It is important to perform a digital rectal examination to assess the prostate and obtain a baseline prostate-specific antigen level before beginning therapy. If prostate-specific antigen or hematocrit increases with testosterone therapy, it usually does so within 6 mo. Therefore, these levels should be checked every 3 mo during the first year of therapy, then every 12 mo thereafter.

Surgical implantation of a penile prosthesis is another therapeutic option. Mechanical failure, infection, device erosion, and fibrosis are possible complications. However, since the availability of alprostadil and, more recently, phosphodiesterase inhibitors, surgical implantation of a penile prosthesis is rarely done (ie, men with severe arterial occlusive disease). Nevertheless, long-term patient satisfaction with penile prosthesis is actually higher than with oral therapy (SOE=B). Penile revascularization surgery has limited success.

Men with psychogenic ED should be referred to a mental health or other professional specializing in treatment of sexual disorders for further evaluation and treatment.

REFERENCES

■ Lindau ST, Schumm LP, Laumann EO, et al. A study of sexuality and health among older adults in the United States. *N Engl J Med.* 2007;357:22–34.

■ Rheaume C, Mitty E. Sexuality and intimacy in older adults. *Geriatr Nurs.* 2008;29(5):342–349.

■ Tolra JR, Campana JM, Ciutat LF, et al. Prospective, randomized, open-label, fixed-dose, crossover study to establish preference of patients with erectile dysfunction after taking the three PDE-5 inhibitors. *J Sex Med.* 2006;3(5):901–909.

■ Wallace M. Sexuality Assessment for Older Adults. *Try This: Best Practices in Nursing Care to Older Adults.* 2007;(10). Available at http://consultgerirn.org/uploads/File/trythis/try_this_10.pdf

CHAPTER 54—MUSCULOSKELETAL DISEASES AND DISORDERS

KEY POINTS

- In addition to arthritis, musculoskeletal complaints in older adults can result from other disorders, including derangement of tendons, bursae, muscles, connective tissue, and nerves.

- Imaging and laboratory studies should be used to confirm clinical impressions rather than to search for a diagnosis. Older adults often exhibit incidental abnormalities on imaging and laboratory testing.

- Comorbid medical conditions and treatments should be considered, and potential toxicities weighed against potential treatment benefits.

- Exercise and other nondrug treatments should be considered in management of all articular and regional musculoskeletal problems.

DIAGNOSTIC APPROACH TO MUSCULOSKELETAL COMPLAINTS IN OLDER ADULTS

The following 3 questions yield information critical to the diagnosis of musculoskeletal complaints:

1. Do the symptoms arise from the joint or elsewhere?

2. Is the process inflammatory?

3. How many joints are involved?

Do the symptoms arise from the joint or elsewhere? Arthritis symptoms or pain and stiffness are usually accompanied by physical findings of warmth, swelling, tenderness at the joint line, and painful passive motion (with the patient relaxed). Pain on active but not passive motion, and tenderness elicited on palpation of structures around the joint suggest a periarticular source and resulting bursitis, tendinitis, etc, rather than arthritis.

Arthritis—reproducible on active and passive joint range of motion; joint line is painful or tender on palpation; range of motion may or may not be limited. Inflammatory signs, including warmth, erythema, swelling, or effusion may be present.

Tendinitis—reproducible on active but not passive range of motion; inflammatory signs may be present. Range of motion is preserved unless limited because of contracture. Maneuvers that are specific to the region are helpful when pain is elicited (eg, forced supination against resistance results in anterior shoulder pain due to bicipital tendinitis).

Bursitis—tenderness on palpation over the bursa. Active range of motion may be painful, but passive range of motion is neither painful nor limited unless there is an underlying arthritis. Inflammatory findings may be present.

Bone—present and not reproducible with range of motion. Localized tenderness may be present, and the source may be distinct from the joint.

Is the process inflammatory? Older adults with arthritis should be assessed for inflammatory signs and symptoms. Stiffness that is present on awakening and that persists for hours is a prominent feature of inflammatory arthritis. In contrast, noninflammatory stiffness generally resolves within an hour after awakening or recurs after periods of inactivity. Unintentional weight loss, fever, loss of appetite, or a general feeling of poor health are features of a systemic illness and can accompany an inflammatory arthritis. The presence of rash, fever, stomatitis, dysphagia, Raynaud phenomenon, or true muscle weakness suggests an autoimmune rheumatologic disorder. Inflammatory features of arthritis should also be sought out during the physical examination. Joints that are palpably warmer than surrounding tissues, visibly red, or swollen are inflamed. Effusions may occasionally be palpated.

How many joints are involved? Identifying the number of involved joints can often be helpful in guiding diagnosis (Table 54.1). A monoarthritis can be infectious (eg, bacterial, fungal), crystal-mediated, traumatic, or degenerative. Arthrocentesis should be performed to evaluate the cause of an undiagnosed monoarthritis to exclude an infection and to evaluate for crystals. Arthritis involving 2 or 3 joints (pauciarthritis) can also be crystal mediated or degenerative, but it can also be due to reactive arthritis (Reiter's syndrome), spondyloarthritis, or related to inflammatory bowel. Finally, the differential diagnosis of arthritis involving ≥4 joints (polyarticular arthritis) includes crystal-mediated arthritis, degenerative arthritis, rheumatoid arthritis, systemic lupus erythematosus, and viral arthritis (eg, hepatitis, parvovirus B19, etc).

STRENGTH-OF-EVIDENCE (SOE) RATING DEFINITIONS

A = consistent and good quality patient-oriented evidence
B = somewhat inconsistent or limited quality patient-oriented evidence
C = very inconsistent or very limited patient-oriented evidence, disease-oriented evidence, and/or consensus from professional organizations
D = unstudied common practice or opinion

See inside front cover for detailed information regarding the SOE classification.

Table 54.1—Differential Diagnosis of Arthritis

Monoarthritis (1 joint)	Pauci-arthritis (2 or 3 joints)	Polyarthritis (≥4 joints)
Infection related (eg, bacterial, fungal, TB, Lyme disease)	Crystal-mediated	Crystal-mediated
Crystal-mediated	Enteropathic (eg, inflammatory bowel disease)	Immune complex (eg, lupus, serum sickness)
Trauma	Infection related (eg, Lyme disease, rheumatic fever, endocarditis)	Infection related (eg, Lyme disease, viral arthritis, rheumatic fever, endocarditis)
Hemarthrosis	Psoriatic arthritis	Psoriatic arthritis
Osteoarthritis	Reactive (Reiter's syndrome)	Reactive (Reiter's syndrome)
	Sarcoid (knees, ankles)	Rheumatoid arthritis
	Spondyloarthritis	Osteoarthritis
	Osteoarthritis	
	Amyloid (large, upper)	

Diagnostic Testing

Laboratory testing should be pursued with the caveat that many tests are neither sensitive nor specific, but they can play a confirmatory role when interpreted in the appropriate clinical context. The Westergren erythrocyte sedimentation rate (ESR), rheumatoid factor, and antinuclear antibodies are three laboratory tests used to evaluate rheumatic disease. Although these laboratory studies are of great value to confirm a diagnosis in older adults with clinically apparent disease, the abnormal values should be interpreted cautiously due to reduced specificity of these tests with aging, ie, the tests may be abnormal in healthy older adults.

The ESR can be increased in older adults even in absence of identifiable illness, and it increases normally with aging according to the following formula: men: 17.3 + 0.18 (age); women: 22.1 + 0.18 (age). The ESR is useful in evaluating patients with headache, fever of unknown origin, or unintentional weight loss if temporal/giant cell arteritis is suspected; however, diagnosis requires biopsy of the temporal arteries. ESR increases can also accompany nonrheumatic systemic illness and therefore cannot distinguish giant cell arteritis from systemic infection, myeloma, or other advanced malignancy.

Rheumatoid factor is an antibody (usually IgG) that reacts with the Fc portion of IgG. It can be detected in 70%–80% of patients with rheumatoid arthritis but is not specific to this disease. It can also be detected in up to 30% of apparently healthy older adults, but when present is usually at a titer of 1:80 or less. This test may be most useful in evaluation of older adults with symmetric inflammatory polyarthritis that is characteristic of rheumatoid arthritis. More recent studies suggest that using anti-citrullinated peptide antibodies (anti-CCP) together with the rheumatoid factor latex assay enhances specificity in diagnosis of rheumatoid arthritis. Neither test should be used to evaluate older adults with diffuse and vague musculoskeletal complaints in the absence of symmetric inflammatory small-joint findings on examination.

Antinuclear antibodies (ANAs) are immunoglobulins directed against DNA, RNA, and other nuclear or cytoplasmic proteins. Both the pattern of immunofluorescence (rim, speckled, nucleolar, or diffuse) and titer provide useful clinical information. ANAs can be found in healthy older adults but usually are in a diffuse pattern at a low titer in absence of rheumatic disease. The ANA test is highly sensitive for systemic lupus erythematosus in that a negative test essentially excludes it. ANAs can be present in high titers in older adults with systemic or medication-induced lupus, inflammatory muscle disease, or scleroderma.

Arthrocentesis should be performed when infection or crystalline-mediated inflammatory joint disease is suspected. Fluid should be sent for cell count, Gram's stain, culture, and crystal analysis. Bloody effusions may be due to joint trauma or crystalline disease and may signal a coagulopathy or periarticular fracture.

Radiographs

Radiographs should be obtained to confirm a diagnosis of arthritis and distinguish inflammatory (eg, rheumatoid arthritis) or destructive (eg, septic, psoriatic) arthritis from noninflammatory (eg, osteoarthritis) forms of arthritis. Inflammatory joint findings are symmetric joint space narrowing, juxta-articular or generalized osteopenia, and erosions at or next to the joint. In contrast, degenerative arthritis or osteoarthritis is characterized by asymmetric joint space narrowing, osteophytes, sclerosis, and cysts. Presence of radiographic osteoarthritis does not exclude the possibility that a periarticular or inflammatory condition coexists. Radiographs can also help distinguish arthritis from a periarticular or bony process (eg, osteomyelitis, periostitis, fracture).

MRI provides high-resolution imaging of articular (cartilage, synovium, meniscus, ligaments) and periarticular structures (bone, tendon, bursae) and should be performed when joint instability is suspected (eg, internal derangement of the knee after trauma, cervical spine in rheumatoid arthritis patients before elective surgery). MRI is also the imaging modality of choice to evaluate back pain with neurologic deficits and to assess spinal cord integrity at any level. MRI can detect intraosseous processes, including infection, occult fracture, and avascular necrosis. It is significantly more expensive and not superior to plain radiographs for imaging the wrist, hand, and foot.

Despite the high level of resolution achievable with MRI, CT scanning remains the imaging modality of choice to evaluate cortical abnormalities of axial bone (eg, spine, sacroiliac joint) and of intermediate to large joints.

EVALUATION OF REGIONAL MUSCULOSKELETAL COMPLAINTS

The Painful Shoulder

Shoulder pain is a common problem in older adults. Pain in the shoulder can be referred (from the cervical spine, heart, or subdiaphragm), occur as a local manifestation of a systemic process (eg, rheumatoid arthritis, polymyalgia rheumatica, or amyloidosis), or arise from the shoulder itself (eg, bursitis, tendinitis, capsulitis, and arthritis).

Subacromial bursitis causes a dull ache that precludes sleeping on the affected side with tenderness to palpation diffusely along the shoulder. Bicipital tendinitis causes pain in the anterior-lateral aspect of the humeral head. Forced supination of the forearm against resistance with the elbow flexed at 90 degrees reproduces the pain (Yergason sign). In contrast, rotator cuff tendinitis results in shoulder pain that is worse between 60 and 120 degrees of abduction. Patients may have mild to no symptoms on passive abduction but often "drop" their arm when asked to abduct against gravity. This is difficult to distinguish clinically from an incomplete tear of the rotator cuff. However, patients with a complete rotator cuff tear are unable to sustain the weight of their arm against gravity at all. Older adults are susceptible to rotator cuff injuries with even minor trauma (eg, lifting groceries, catching their fall). Adhesive capsulitis (ie, "frozen" shoulder) is a painful loss of range of motion in all directions; it can result from stroke, trauma, untreated arthritis, or relatively minor injury. Patients with diabetes can develop adhesive capsulitis without any inciting event. Osteoarthritis, rheumatoid arthritis, and calcium pyrophosphate dehydrate deposition disease (CPPD) can all contribute to shoulder pain. Plain radiographs are most useful in assessing the shoulder for evidence of joint degeneration and can demonstrate calcification of the tendons or superior migration of the humeral head in the case of a complete rotator cuff tear. Shoulder pain often responds to local steroid injections administered in conjunction with physical therapy. Surgical intervention is rarely pursued for these conditions in older adults.

The Painful Elbow

Bursitis and arthritis most commonly cause elbow pain, although tendinitis can contribute in overuse syndromes. Olecranon bursitis, with swelling of the bursa and pain only at the extremes of range of movement, is commonly associated with rheumatoid arthritis and gout, both of which also result in palpable nodules or tophi. Olecranon bursitis can be managed conservatively by using padding and avoiding pressure on the elbow. Excessive redness, warmth, or exquisite tenderness prompts evaluation for infection. Unlike bursitis, arthritis results in painful passive motion (supination or flexion) and tenderness on palpation over the joint line. Arthritis of the elbow can be part of an inflammatory arthritis (eg, rheumatoid arthritis, spondyloarthropathy, gout) but should be evaluated for an infectious cause if it presents as a monoarthritis. Overlying cellulitis does not preclude joint aspiration for culture and cell count, but empiric antibiotic coverage is warranted.

The Painful Wrist

Few conditions cause wrist pain. Arthritis of the wrist results in painful passive motion that is usually accompanied by fullness and tenderness on palpation that can be due to either synovial tissue inflammation or joint effusion. Inflammatory arthritis that affects the wrist also results in other joint involvement that can be appreciated on examination (rheumatoid arthritis, gout, CPPD). Monoarthritis should be evaluated for the possibility of septic arthritis or gout. Radiographs are useful in distinguishing between these different types of arthritis. MRI should be pursued in patients with tenderness over the ulnar styloid process to detect impending extension tendon rupture that requires tendon transfer surgery. Occasionally, wrist pain can be a manifestation of periostitis. Examination reveals tenderness on compression of the distal radius or ulna that can be confirmed on radiograph or bone scan.

In carpal tunnel syndrome, the impingement of the median nerve causes pain and paresthesia of the hand that are prominent at night. Paresthesia can be reproduced by tapping over the flexor retinaculum (Tinel's sign) or by forced flexion of the wrist (Phalen's sign). Carpal tunnel syndrome can be the result of overuse or arthritis of the wrist joint, or a manifestation of a systemic disease (eg, diabetes, hypothyroidism, amyloidosis). The diagnosis is confirmed by demonstrating nerve conduction delay at the wrist. Older adults with cervical spine arthritis can manifest a "double crush" phenomenon that can be detected on electrodiagnostic testing. Management options include the consistent use of neutral wrist splints (SOE=B) and judicious glucocorticoid injections (SOE=B) into the carpal tunnel, taking care not to inject the median nerve. Surgical decompression should be pursued if conservative measures fail or if thumb apposition weakness or thenar muscle atrophy is apparent.

The Painful Hip

Hip pain in older adults can be referred from the spine, retroperitoneal area, or knee, or can arise in the joint and surrounding area. Trochanteric bursitis results in pain that is localized over the lateral proximal thigh and that can be reproduced on palpation over the trochanter. Patients often complain of difficulty sleeping on the affected side. Response is good to glucocorticoid injection. Iliotibial band syndrome also causes lateral thigh pain that is worse with walking and can be reproduced by having the patient bend forward at the waist while crossing the legs. Although responsive to steroid injection, iliotibial band syndrome should also be managed with stretching exercises and massage. Arthritis is suggested by hip pain that is reproduced on passive motion, often accompanied by reduced range of motion, especially internal rotation. Weakness of the hip muscles may be notable with a positive Trendelenburg sign or lurch during walking. Pain that is diffuse and bilateral and accompanied by prolonged morning stiffness should raise the possibility of polymyalgia rheumatica. Plain radiographs are useful to evaluate for osteoarthritis, rheumatoid arthritis, Paget's disease of the bone, and fractures, while avascular necrosis is best demonstrated by MRI. Patients with hemoglobinopathy, traumatic injury to the hip, or malignancy who are receiving chronic steroid therapy and who report hip pain that is not reproduced on passive motion should be evaluated with a radiograph or MRI for avascular necrosis, osteomyelitis, or bone metastasis. Therapies are aimed at the underlying cause but usually include devices to reduce weightbearing on the affected hip (eg, cane, orthotics), weight loss and exercise, medications, and surgery.

The Painful Knee

According to data from the third National Health and Nutrition Examination Survey (NHANES III), knee pain affects >20% of adults ≥60 yr old, with an incidence approaching 30% for those ≥80 yr old.

The anserine bursa is located inferomedially to the knee joint, and when inflamed causes knee pain

that is most notable at night. There is exquisite tenderness to palpation over the area, with occasional swelling and erythema. Injection with a small amount of glucocorticoid mixed with anesthetic can be both diagnostic and therapeutic (SOE=C). In contrast, knee pain with visible fluid or swelling at the superior aspect of the knee is more consistent with suprapatellar bursitis. This is commonly exacerbated by frequent kneeling and is common in gardeners and painters. Because mechanical irritation with prolonged kneeling aggravates the suprapatellar bursa, avoidance of kneeling is recommended rather than injections or NSAIDs. Adequate padding between the knees while sleeping (for anserine bursitis) and thick padding while kneeling (for suprapatellar bursitis) can alleviate symptoms as well as prevent recurrence (SOE=C).

Arthritis should be suspected with a history of knee pain that is aggravated by activity (eg, bending, stooping, walking) and alleviated with rest. The skin may or may not be warm. Passive motion and palpation of the joint line reproduces the pain. Usually there is no joint effusion, but occasionally there may be a small effusion. Patients with posterior knee pain should be examined for a popliteal cyst. Inspection of both popliteal fossae with the patient standing can reveal asymmetric fullness on one side and can be confirmed by ultrasound. The knee should be assessed for ligamentous instability (medial and lateral collateral and cruciate) by gently stressing the joint in all directions. Patients should be asked about symptoms of locking or instability. Rotational extension can elicit pain localized to the site of meniscal disease, and MRI is needed to assess the extent of damage. Other causes of knee pain include crystalline-mediated (gout, CPPD), rheumatoid, psoriatic, and reactive arthritis, as well as avascular necrosis of the tibia, referred pain from hip disease, and septic arthritis.

The Patient with Diffuse Pain

Patients complaining of pain that is diffuse and does not respect articular boundaries, or of persistent symptoms despite maximal medical and adjunctive therapy should be evaluated further. Persistent pain with diffuse tenderness of periarticular regions warrants evaluation for metabolic disturbances that affect bone such as vitamin D deficiency, hyperparathyroidism, or hypothyroidism. Systemic infection of any source can manifest with diffuse pain. Chronic somatic pain can be a manifestation of depression as well.

Fibromyalgia is a chronic disorder characterized by chronic, widespread muscle pain and tenderness that is associated with nonrestorative sleep and fatigue. It is frequently accompanied by fatigue, insomnia, depression, and anxiety. Although the average age of fibromyalgia patients is reported to be in the 40s, older adults are not spared from the development or persistence of this condition. The precise cause of fibromyalgia is not known, but research suggests it is related to a problem with the processing of pain in the CNS. No clinical laboratory tests or imaging studies are available to confirm a diagnosis. Commonly requested laboratory (eg, thyroid, vitamin D, antinuclear antibody, sedimentation rate, C-reactive protein) and imaging studies are usually negative or normal.

Aerobic exercise and stretching is recommended for all but should be initiated slowly and progressed patiently to avoid overuse and strain injuries. Tricyclic antidepressants[OL] can be helpful (SOE=B) but should be started at low dosages and increased slowly with caution because of anticholinergic adverse events. Duloxetine, pregabalin, and gabapentin[OL] have been studied in treatment of fibromyalgia and may have modest benefit for some patients (SOE=B). Muscle relaxants have also been used.

For an approach to complaints of back or neck pain, see "Back and Neck Pain," p 450.

GENERAL MANAGEMENT STRATEGIES

Comorbid Conditions

Thorough assessment of comorbid illnesses is a necessary part of caring for older adults with musculoskeletal disorders. Diseases and their treatments often compete and complicate medical management, while increasing risk of functional limitations. In addition, specific diseases in combination are of clinical importance. For example, comorbid heart disease with rheumatoid arthritis can present a significant clinical challenge, due to potential effects of anti-inflammatory therapy or joint replacement on risk of significant cardiovascular complications.

Arthritis and pain contribute to functional limitations in late life, and the accompanying muscle weakness increases risk of further functional decline and disability. Being overweight or obese contributes to mobility limitations that are compounded by arthritis of weight-bearing joints. Rehabilitative interventions targeting muscle weakness and obesity are recommended for maintaining function despite the ongoing presence of articular and nonarticular diseases. See "Frailty," p 161; and "Malnutrition," p 195.

Older adults with arthritis of weight-bearing joints are at increased risk of injurious falls and fracture, attributed in part to proprioceptive deficits. Studies suggest that pain may increase the propensity to trip on an obstacle. These factors suggest that alleviating painful symptoms along with muscle and proprioception training should be implemented along with other strategies for falls prevention. See "Falls," p 224.

Nonpharmacologic Strategies

As with any chronic disease treatment, patient education should be considered the first step in management of musculoskeletal disorders. Involvement of family and other caregivers can be helpful. Educational groups or classes have been shown to reduce pain severity, medical visits, and reliance on medications, while improving self-efficacy and promoting physical activity (SOE=B).

Several well-designed studies have demonstrated the integral value of exercise in managing rheumatoid arthritis, osteoarthritis, polymyositis, and systemic lupus erythematosus (SOE=A). Patients should be provided with an exercise "prescription" that details warm-up activities, followed by instructions for the type of exercise (eg, strengthening, flexibility, and endurance), intensity, duration, and frequency during a given week. Patients should be advised to watch for signs of excessive joint strain, including swelling, fatigue, weakness, or pain during activity or that lasts >1–2 hours after exercise.

Therapeutic ultrasound is widely prescribed for pain and loss of function due to osteoarthritis. Ultrasound uses high-frequency (0.8–1 MHz) sound waves to reduce painful symptoms by pulsed delivery for acute pain and inflammation, or by continuous delivery for patients with chronic symptoms that have resulted in joint limitations (SOE=C).

Cold and heat are useful adjuncts that can decrease both pain and muscle spasms (SOE=C). Use of ice or cold packs should be limited to 20 minutes or when the area becomes numb. Cautious use of heat can reduce pain and muscle spasm but should be limited to 20-minute intervals using a heating modality that is unlikely to cause skin scalding. Contrast therapy, which alternates between hot and cold treatment modalities, can provide additional therapeutic benefits than either alone (SOE=C).

Massage can alleviate painful symptoms. Acupuncture has been included as a potentially useful adjunct for patients with back pain (SOE=A). Transcutaneous electrical nerve stimulation (TENS) is yet another alternative that delivers electrical stimulation that can be combined with acupuncture (SOE=B). Finally, neuromuscular electrical stimulation (NMES) delivers low-voltage electrical impulses through surface electrodes placed over motor points of the targeted muscle, inducing muscle contraction. NMES may be an alternative for patients who are unable to participate in exercise because of severe pain or contraindications (SOE=D).

Occupational and physical therapists can recommend devices that serve to alleviate painful symptoms, stabilize lax joints, lessen joint strain, improve gait mechanics and stability, and lessen risk of falling (SOE=C). Involvement of therapy services early in the management plan is highly advisable.

Pharmacologic Therapies for Pain

Selection of medications requires particularly careful attention to potential for adverse drug events in the geriatric population. Medications generally are indicated only for significant symptoms or when nonpharmacologic approaches have failed. Topical balms and creams, applied 2 or 3 times daily, can help control arthritis symptoms in small and intermediate joints (SOE=C). Capsaicin cream is effective for osteoarthritis of the hand(s) but must be used carefully to avoid contact with mucous membranes (SOE=B).

Acetaminophen (500–1,000 mg q8h) remains the preferred simple analgesic for older adults (SOE=A). The risk of nephropathy from acetaminophen remains low when it is used in modest dosages in patients without preexisting kidney disease and with cautious supervision in patients with renal insufficiency. However, excessive dosages can result in hepatotoxicity.

NSAIDs can be prescribed at either analgesic (lower) or anti-inflammatory dosages, but because of their toxicity in older adults, they are recommended only in suitable candidates for short periods. Analgesic medications include choline magnesium trisalicylate (750 mg q8h), ibuprofen (200–800 mg q8h), and etodolac (200–300 mg q8h). Nonacetylated salicylates such as salsalate or magnesium choline salicylate and COX-2 agents are thought to have lower GI toxicity when used short term but equivalent GI toxicity when used long term, and they are far more expensive than generic ibuprofen. All agents in this class are equally effective at their recommended dosages. Patients with a high risk of GI bleeding and ulceration should either avoid NSAIDs or be given prophylaxis concurrent with NSAID use (ie, prostaglandin analogs or proton-pump inhibitors). Patients prescribed NSAIDs should be monitored for renal insufficiency and fluid retention, which can be particularly severe in patients who have heart failure or are taking ACE inhibitors. Delirium is common in older adults with NSAID use. COX-2 inhibitors have been associated with higher rates of stroke and myocardial infarction, leading to the withdrawal of rofecoxib from the market, followed by manufacturers' withdrawal of valdecoxib. Some relatively selective COX-2 inhibitors remain available (ie, nabumetone, etodolac, and meloxicam).

Because of their adverse events, prednisone and other glucocorticoids should not be used indiscriminately. Consultation with a rheumatologist can be helpful when considering immunosuppressive treat-ments. Dosages used depend on the particular disease being treated, with benefits usually realized within 5–10 days. Toxicities of glucocorticoids include cataracts, poor wound healing, gastric ulcers, mental status change, hyperglycemia, hypertension, osteoorosis, and immunosuppression. Full recovery of the hypothalamic-pituitary axis can require up to a year after chronic steroid use. Individuals on chronic steroid therapy should also receive therapy to prevent osteoporosis, usually with calcium, vitamin D, and bisphosphonates.

Finally, narcotic medications, started in low dosages and titrated slowly, are often useful in managing acute or chronic musculoskeletal pain that is unresponsive to exercise, use of assistive devices, hot and cold therapies, or acetaminophen. See also "Persistent Pain," p 109.

APPROACH TO SPECIFIC RHEUMATOLOGIC DISEASES

Osteoarthritis

Depending on the source of data and which joint is involved, osteoarthritis (OA) is present in 50%–90% of older adults. It is the major cause of knee, hip, and back pain in older adults, and it will increase in both incidence and prevalence with the aging of the population and increasing rates of obesity.

Cartilage degeneration is the hallmark of OA, with fibrillation and ulceration that begins superficially and eventually extends into deeper layers. However, evidence indicates that OA is not a purely degenerative disease restricted to the cartilage; subchondral bone abnormalities and focal synovial inflammation have also been seen in pathologic specimens. These pathologic characteristics are thought to arise as a result of repetitive cycles of degradation and repair responses that eventually become inadequate to maintain joint health. Inflammatory cytokines, matrix-degrading metalloproteinase enzymes, and chondrocyte apoptosis are likely contributors to this process.

OA commonly affects the hands, knees, hips, and cervical and lumbar spine, but it can develop in any joint that has suffered injury or other disease. For the American College of Rheumatology diagnostic criteria for OA of the hand, knee, and hip, see Table 54.2. On examination, bony enlargement and crepitus suggest OA. In the fingers, this enlargement is called Heberden's nodes when it occurs in the distal interphalangeal joints and Bouchard's nodes in the proximal interphalangeal joints. Joint tenderness and warmth may appear, but intense inflammation suggests an alternative or concomitant diagnosis.

Table 54.2—American College of Rheumatology Criteria for Osteoarthritis

Hand	Knee	Hip
Hand pain, aching, or stiffness	Knee pain	Hip pain
and	*and*	*and*
Hard tissue enlargement of two or more joints of the DIP, PIP, or CMC	Radiographic osteophytes	Two or more of the following:
and	*and*	▪ ESR <10 mm/h
Two or more DIP joints with hard tissue enlargement	One or more of the following:	▪ Radiographic femoral or acetabular osteophytes
and	▪ Age ≥50 yr	▪ Radiographic joint space narrowing
Fewer than three swollen MCP joints	▪ Morning stiffness <30 min	
or	▪ Crepitus on motion	
Deformity in two or more signal joints (DIP, PIP, first CMC)		

NOTE: DIP=distal interphalangeal, PIP=proximal interphalangeal, CMC=carpometacarpal (thumb base), MCP=metacarpophalangeal, ESR = erythrocyte sedimentation rate (Westergren)

SOURCES: Data from Altman R, Alarcon G, Appelrouth D, et al. The American College of Rheumatology criteria of the classification and reporting of osteoarthritis of the hand. *Arthritis Rheum.* 1990;33(11):1601–1610; Altman R, Asch E, Bloch D, et al. Development of criteria for the classification and reporting of osteoarthritis. Classification of osteoarthritis of the knee. Diagnostic and Therapeutic Committee of The American College of Rheumatology *Arthritis Rheum.* 1986;29(8):1039–1049; and Altman R, Alarcon G, Appelrouth D, et al. The American College of Rheumatology criteria for the classification and reporting of osteoarthritis of the hip. *Arthritis Rheum.* 1991;34(5):505–514.

Osteophytes are the radiographic counterpart of this enlargement, and asymmetric joint space narrowing is also common (Figure 54.1). MRI can help evaluate back and neck symptoms that may require surgical intervention.

The objectives of OA management are to alleviate painful symptoms, prevent disease progression, maximize function, and minimize disease-related complications. Weight reduction can help reduce pain and improve function in patients with OA of the knee, hip, or spine. In knee OA, neoprene braces can alleviate patellofemoral symptoms by improving patellar tracking, and can provide a greater sense of joint stability by improving joint proprioception. Specific orthoses designed to reduce medial knee pain by unloading the medial compartment of the knee include a valgus unloader brace and a lateral wedge insole. A simpler investment in a well-designed running shoe can also lessen pain and damage by decreasing the impact transmitted during ambulation. Finally, a properly fitted and used cane can provide stability as well as unloading the symptomatic knee or hip.

Topical therapies (eg, analgesic balms, capsaicin, topical NSAIDs) can be useful in hand or knee OA (SOE=C). Regular and consistently prescribed acetaminophen is the initial pharmacologic recommendation (SOE=A), followed by low-dose narcotic medications, or in cases of narcotic intolerance, NSAIDs. Studies evaluating glucosamine and chondroitin sulfate for pain have conflicting results, with more recent higher quality studies showing no superiority over placebo for patients with knee OA (SOE=A).

Glucocorticoid injections can be used for knee pain, although whether they are more effective than placebo injection is unclear (SOE= B). Hyaluronic acid and hyaluronan polymers given in a series of weekly injections in the knee are approved for intra-articular viscosupplementation therapy. The benefits of these preparations vary substantially between patients but last longer than benefits of corticosteroid injections in those who respond (SOE=B).

Several surgical procedures and joint replacement can be considered for patients with large-joint OA. Arthroscopic debridement for knee OA is usually reserved for patients who report mechanical symptoms (eg, locking, "giveway" weakness), but effectiveness has not been proved (SOE=C). Joint-"sparing" high tibial osteotomy can realign the knee but requires considerable rehabilitation. Unicompartment joint replacement can be done in patients whose disease is limited to one compartment (eg, isolated medial, lateral, or patellofemoral knee OA) (SOE=B). Total joint arthroplasty can be considered in patients with more extensive, disabling disease of the knee or hip. Although surgery remains the definitive intervention, it should be performed when the patient is likely to be able to withstand both the surgery and the ensuing rehabilitation and is debilitated enough from the OA that the benefits of surgery outweigh the risks.

Rheumatoid Arthritis

Although significantly less prevalent than osteoarthritis, rheumatoid arthritis (RA) is an important disease of older adults. Up to 40% of patients with RA are >60 yr old; some of these individuals have aged with the disease, while 20%–55% develop RA late in life.

Older adults with late-onset RA may present similarly to young adults with acute inflammatory polyarthritis that involves the small joints of the hands and feet and that is accompanied by a positive

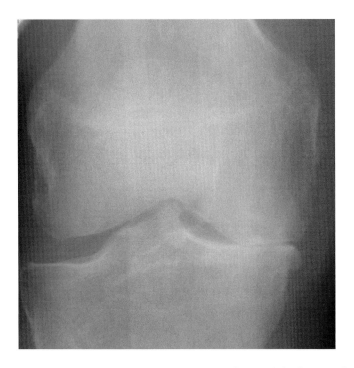
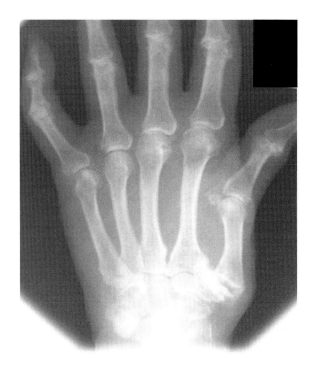

Figure 54.1—*Left*: Radiograpic osteoarthritis of the knee with medical compartment osteophytes, joint space narrowing, and sclerosis. *Right*: Radiographic osteoarthritis of the hand with osteophytes, asymmetric joint space narrowing, and sclerosis of varying degrees of the thumb base (carpometacarpal joint) and interphalangeal joints.

rheumatoid factor. Seronegative presentations that are unique to older adults include the "RS3PE" syndrome of remitting symmetric seronegative synovitis with peripheral edema, and an inflammatory arthritis of the shoulder and hips similar to polymyalgia rheumatica (PMR). In fact, descriptive studies suggest that late-onset RA should be considered in the differential diagnosis of PMR and vice versa. Other diseases that mimic RA include CPPD and carcinoma polyarthritis.

As with young adults, the diagnosis of RA relies on clinical, radiologic, and laboratory criteria as set forth by the American College of Rheumatology (Table 54.3). In contrast to young adults with RA, older adults with RA are more likely to have a higher initial ESR.

Descriptive studies suggest that patients with seropositive RA, even if of late onset, should be managed aggressively, including use of disease-modifying anti-inflammatory drugs (DMARDs) (SOE=B). Methotrexate is well tolerated, but older adults may require a lower dose; it should be given with daily folic acid. Cases of lymphoproliferative disease have been reported with long-term methotrexate treatment. Hydroxychloroquine is also well tolerated, but patients must be monitored for macular toxicity. Leflunomide has been demonstrated to prevent radiographic progression in younger adults, but experience is minimal in older adults (SOE=B). It has a relatively fast onset of action (about 4 weeks)

compared with other DMARDs. Older agents, such as penicillamine, sulfasalazine, gold, and cyclophosphamide, are less well tolerated by older adults, and are rarely used.

Several biologic agents for RA are available, but experience with these agents in older adults is limited, so their use is generally limited to those in whom conventional DMARD therapy has not been effective. These agents work by inhibiting tumor necrosis factor α (etanercept, infliximab, and adalimumab), antagonizing the interleukin receptor (anakinra), serving as a fusion protein (abatacept), or binding B cells (rituximab); they are given via injection or infusion. Rituximab, infliximab, and adalimumab all increase the risk of granulomatous infections with organisms such as *Mycobacterium tuberculosis*, atypical mycobacteria, yeast, *Listeria*, and *Nocardia*. Infliximab can also cause postinfusion fever, chills, headache, chest pain, and dyspnea. Anakinra is associated with bacterial respiratory tract infections.

Low-dose prednisone (10–15 mg/d) may be used as the primary treatment for seronegative PMR-like disease and the "RS3PE" syndrome. However, in contrast to classic PMR, late-onset RA may not respond promptly to low-dose prednisone. Prednisone alone is often not sufficient in managing seropositive RA but may be useful as an adjunctive agent. Its use is associated with increased risk of infectious complications, fluid retention, and osteoporosis.

Table 54.3—American College of Rheumatology Criteria for Rheumatoid Arthritis

Presence of at least four of the following signs and symptoms:

- Morning stiffness for at least 6 weeks
- Arthritis of three or more joint areas for at least 6 weeks
- Arthritis of the hand joints for at least 6 weeks
- Symmetric arthritis for at least 6 weeks
- Subcutaneous rheumatoid nodules
- Increased serum rheumatoid factor (and anti-CCP antibodies)
- Radiographic changes that include erosions or unequivocal bony calcification in periarticular bone

SOURCE: Data from Arnett FC, Edworthy SM, Bloch DA, et al. The American Rheumatism Association 1987 revised criteria for the classification of rheumatoid arthritis. *Arthritis Rheum.* 1988;31(3):315–324.

Gout

Gout can cause both severe pain and debility. Women generally do not develop gout until menopause, at which time the rate in women matches that in men. Diuretic use is an important predisposing factor. The clinical characteristics of gout can differ appreciably in older adults. Gout can present as a subacute smoldering oligoarthritis rather than as an acute, monarticular, and incapacitating attack, as in classic podagra. Tophaceous deposits in the distal and proximal interphalangeal joints can be mistaken for or coexist with osteoarthritis. Similarly, tophi at the extensor surfaces can be confused with rheumatoid nodules. Acute attacks can be precipitated by trauma, acute nonarticular illness requiring hospitalization, dehydration (acute gout is particularly common after surgery), and abrupt changes in uric acid concentration.

For a diagnosis of gout to be established, the presence of sodium urate crystals from synovial fluid or an aspirate of a tophus must be demonstrated. Sodium urate crystals are strongly birefringent and needle shaped and can be demonstrated in synovial fluid obtained in the intercritical phase, as well as during an acute flare. Radiographs show juxta-articular erosions of the involved joints. An overhanging edge (ie, Martel's sign) can be seen and is helpful in distinguishing gout from rheumatoid arthritis. With rare exception, asymptomatic hyperuricemia precedes the development of gouty arthritis. However, hyperuricemia is not uniformly present at the time of an acute gout attack, nor does the presence of hyperuricemia confirm a diagnosis of gout.

An acute gout attack is best managed with a short-acting NSAID in those who can tolerate it, although narcotic medications or oral, intramuscular, or intra-articular glucocorticoids can be used. Intramuscular or short-term oral glucocorticoids (prednisone 30 mg/d for 5 days) are preferred in managing a polyarticular gouty flare. Colchicine can also be used to treat an acute gouty attack. The approved dose for an acute attack is 1.2 mg at the onset of the attack and then 0.6 mg 1 hour later (total dose 1.8 mg). For patients who have recurrent episodes of gout, colchicine can be added to reduce the frequency of gouty attacks. Conventional dosing is 0.6 mg q12h; the dosage should be reduced to 0.6 mg/d to three times weekly in patients with renal insufficiency, and colchicine should not be used at all in patients with hepatic insufficiency. Medications such as allopurinol, febuxostat, or probenecid, which can acutely lower uric acid levels, should not be used in the management of acute gout, because premature lowering of uric acid level will paradoxically intensify and prolong an acute gout attack. Probenecid works as an uricosuric agent but is ineffective if creatinine clearance is <30–40 mL/min. Allopurinol and febuxostat inhibit uric acid formation and are useful in management of chronic gout, particularly for those with tophi, renal stones, or for whom colchicine is ineffective; the dosage should be adjusted for renal or hepatic impairment.

Calcium Pyrophosphate Dihydrate Deposition Disease

CPPD, also known as "pseudogout," has many manifestations. Depending on the joint affected, it can mimic rheumatoid arthritis, inflammatory osteoarthritis, gout, or septic arthritis. It is most commonly diagnosed by finding *chondrocalcinosis* on plain radiographs (Figure 54.2). CPPD is associated with disorders of calcium metabolism (eg, hypomagnesemia, hypophosphatemia, hyperparathyroidism), hypothyroidism, and hemochromatosis. CPPD of the wrist can mimic rheumatoid arthritis but can be distinguished by prominent synovitis and chondrocalcinosis of the wrist and metacarpophalangeal joints; it is rheumatoid factor and anti-CCP antibody negative. CPPD can also mimic inflammatory osteoarthritis with rapid joint destruction of the wrist, patellofemoral knee compartment, and hip joint.

CPPD can also cause an acute, intermittently inflammatory arthritis of the knee, hip, wrist, and metacarpophalangeal joints, with elbow, shoulder, and ankle involvement less common. CPPD can mimic an acute gout attack with sudden onset of pain and swelling that coincide with or immediately follow an acute illness or traumatic event such as surgery. When fever is present, distinguishing CPPD from septic arthritis is imperative.

Arthrocentesis with crystal analysis is diagnostic and useful to distinguish CPPD from gout and infection. CPPD crystals are weakly positive birefringent rhomboids or squares. Chondrocalcinosis is

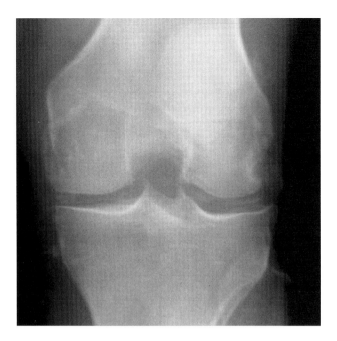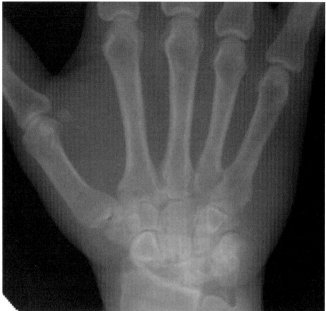

Figure 54.2—*Left*: Chondrocalcinosis of the meniscus. *Right*: Chondrocalcinosis of the triangular cartilage of the wrist.

apparent on plain radiographs (Figure 54.2), appearing as a stippled or linear calcification of the articular cartilage of the knee, wrist, hip, shoulder, and pubic symphysis.

Arthrocentesis can result in significant relief of painful symptoms with CPPD. Short-acting NSAIDs and steroidal agents are also useful in management of CPPD in patients who can tolerate them (SOE=C). Intra-articular and parenteral corticosteroids are recommended for patients who cannot tolerate NSAIDs. Given once and possibly repeated in 1–2 days, triamcinolone acetonide (60 mg IM), betamethasone (7 mg IM), or methylprednisolone (125 mg IV) are all safe and effective. Use of colchicine to prevent future acute episodes of CPPD has not been substantiated in clinical trials.

Polymyalgia Rheumatica

Polymyalgia rheumatica (PMR) is a condition unique to older adults. Approximately 53 new cases develop per 100,000 persons per year, with an estimated prevalence of 600 cases per 100,000 and higher prevalence with increasing age.

PMR should be suspected in patients ≥50 yr old with persistent pain or stiffness of the upper arms, shoulders, hips, or thighs that is accompanied by constitutional symptoms of fatigue, low-grade fever, and weight loss. Patients lack physical evidence of an inflammatory arthritis of the small hand joints, distinguishing PMR from rheumatoid arthritis, and they also have normal muscle bulk and strength.

Diagnostic criteria include limb-girdle stiffness, an ESR often >50 mm/h, and normal levels of muscle enzymes. Recent studies of PMR have confirmed the presence of synovitis identical to that seen in rheumatoid arthritis, with synovial thickening, effusions, and lymphocytic synovial infiltration. PMR can progress to chronic polyarthritis that fulfills criteria for rheumatoid arthritis.

Mild symptoms of PMR can respond to NSAIDs. However, most patients require prednisone (10–20 mg/d as a single dose given in the early morning) (SOE=B). Symptoms should abate within 7 days, but the starting dosage should be maintained for 4–6 weeks before tapering is attempted. Dosage reduction should be gradual (eg, by 1 mg/mo) with monitoring for symptom recurrence and laboratory studies (C-reactive protein, ESR) suggesting reactivation. Short-acting NSAIDs can be added to assist with controlling symptoms during the taper. Concomitant giant cell arteritis or an alternative diagnosis of rheumatoid arthritis should be considered in patients whose response to therapy is incomplete or not sustained. The duration of treatment required varies considerably, from 3 mo to several years. Osteoporosis prophylaxis is recommended for all patients on systemic steroids for >2 mo.

Giant Cell Arteritis and Temporal Arteritis

Giant cell arteritis (GCA) is a granulomatous vasculitis that involves large and medium-sized arteries. The overlap between arteritis and polymyalgia rheumatica (PMR) is notable. Approximately 10%–20% of patients with PMR will also have GCA, and 66% of patients with GCA also have PMR symptoms. Therefore, all patients with PMR with any symptoms above the neck should have a temporal artery biopsy to evaluate for GCA.

Head and neck manifestations of temporal arteritis include headache, jaw and tongue claudication with tenderness, erythema, or nodularity occasionally palpable along the temporal artery. Optic nerve pallor or swelling portends ischemia with impending blindness that warrants immediate glucocorticoid therapy. GCA can also appear as sudden blindness with no prior systemic illness or with claudication in the arms. Other manifestations can include stroke, ischemic necrosis of tongue or scalp, or rarely myocardial infarction. Aortic aneurysm, predominantly thoracic, is a late manifestation of GCA even when previously appropriately treated. The incidence of aneurysm in GCA is about 10%, with discovery of thoracic and abdominal aneurysm 5.9 and 2.5 yr, respectively, after GCA diagnosis. Constitutional symptoms of weight loss, malaise, fever, and depression may be the only manifestations of GCA.

Temporal artery biopsy is the gold standard for diagnosis; a specimen several centimeters in length should be obtained from the symptomatic side and immediately processed by frozen section staining of multiple cross- and longitudinal sections; a section of the contralateral side can be obtained if the initial specimens are negative. Evidence of vasculitis without giant cells suggests other diagnoses (eg, polyarteritis nodosa) that may require cytotoxic therapy. Ultrasound, angiography, MRI with gadolinium, and positron emission tomography have been investigated as diagnostic modalities for demonstrating vascular inflammation; however, none has replaced biopsy as the gold standard diagnostic test.

Patients suspected of having GCA should begin prednisone treatment while awaiting biopsy to reduce the risk of sudden blindness. Fortunately for diagnostic purposes, pathologic evidence of GCA persists for up to 2 weeks of prednisone therapy. Prednisone is given at a dosage of 40–60 mg/d and should be maintained for at least 1 mo before considering dosage reduction. Intravenous glucocorticoids (prednisolone or methylprednisolone 80–100 mg) are occasionally recommended for patients at high risk of blindness or impending ischemic events of other organs. Treatment should continue for approximately 2 yr. Long-term glucocorticoid therapy warrants prophylaxis for osteoporosis. Published studies of methotrexate as a steroid-sparing agent have not consistently proved it to be effective. Monitoring for return of symptoms of PMR or temporal arteritis and increase of inflammatory markers should continue lifelong after ceasing immunosuppressive therapy.

Systemic Lupus Erythematosus

Systemic lupus erythematosus is an autoimmune multisystemic disease that most commonly affects women of child-bearing age, yet up to 20% of cases are seen in older adults. When onset is after 50 yr of age, the condition is referred to as "elderly onset lupus."

Elderly onset lupus should be considered in the differential diagnosis of rash (need not be malar in distribution), nonerosive arthritis, serositis (pleuritis, pericarditis), cytopenias (leukopenia, hemolytic anemia, or thrombocytopenia), neuropsychiatric symptoms (cognitive, seizures), symptoms of sicca (in the absence of medication-induced dry mouth), and Raynaud's phenomenon. Renal involvement (eg, urinary casts, proteinuria) is less common in older lupus patients than in younger lupus patients. Additional physical findings can include periungual or palmar erythema, asymptomatic oral or nasal ulcers and livedo reticularis—when present, these should raise suspicion of anticardiolipin antibody syndrome (venous or arterial thromboembolic phenomena). Vague manifestations for which lupus should be considered include fever, Raynaud's phenomenon, and thromboembolic phenomena (including stroke).

The diagnosis rests on a constellation of clinical criteria along with serologic evidence of autoimmunity (positive antinuclear antibody, anti-double-stranded DNA, anti-Sm, or false-positive test for syphilis). Rheumatoid factor, anti-Ro/Sjögren's syndrome (SS) A and anti-La/SSB are more often positive in patients with elderly onset lupus.

Distinguishing elderly onset lupus from drug-induced lupus erythematosis is often clinically difficult. Both have a positive antinuclear antibody test, although drug-induced lupus erythematosis is associated with a speckled pattern with antihistone antibodies. Anti-double-stranded DNA and hypocomplementemia, both useful in monitoring disease activity in younger patients, are less frequently found in older patients. Renal biopsy should be pursued to evaluate patients with proteinuria or an active urine sediment to determine the underlying pathophysiology before starting treatment. Serologic evaluation for thromboembolic phenomena includes IgG and IgM anticardiolipin antibody levels and lupus anticoagulant testing, with mixing studies for a circulating anticoagulant to explain prolonged partial thromboplastin times.

Treatment recommendations are based entirely on extrapolation from younger adults; no studies of these therapies have been done in older adults with lupus (SOE=D). Short-acting NSAIDs can be used to treat arthritis and serositis in older adults who can tolerate them. Hydroxychloroquine is effective in managing skin and joint manifestations (begun at 200 mg/d for a week, then increased to 400 mg/d). However, older adults should be evaluated for age-associated macular degeneration and monitored for visual field deficits while receiving hydroxychloroquine treatment. Patients who are cardiolipin and lupus anticoagulant positive should receive preventive anticoagulant therapy. Intravenous methylprednisolone and monthly intravenous pulse cyclophosphamide is reserved for severe or renal (with an active urine sediment) or CNS disease. Methotrexate[OL], azathioprine[OL], or cyclosporine[OL] can be of benefit as corticosteroid-sparing agents.

Polymyositis and Dermatomyositis

Inflammatory muscle diseases, including polymyositis and dermatomyositis, form a heterogeneous and uncommon group of skeletal muscle diseases. Incidence of these diseases peaks in adults in their 50s, but they can occur at any age.

Muscle weakness is the central feature of myositis, and it is most prominent in the proximal muscle groups. Patients report difficulty with tasks such as standing from a chair, ascending stairs, or lifting a light package above the head. Muscle tenderness is usually not a manifestation and should raise suspicion of other conditions. Arthritis, when present, is inflammatory and occasionally erosive, suggesting overlap with rheumatoid arthritis. Esophageal dysmotility can cause dysphagia, hoarseness, and aspiration. Arrhythmia, symptoms of congestive heart disease, dyspnea on exertion, or persistent cough can also be present and suggest cardiac or interstitial lung disease. Raynaud's phenomenon or Sjögren's syndrome can also be present. Dermatomyositis is characterized by a facial rash that can involve the eyelids (heliotrope) or the nose and malar areas, or be more generalized. Rash can also be apparent over the neck and upper torso in sun-exposed areas. Gottron's papules (skin thickening over the interphalangeal joints) can also be seen.

Initial diagnostic efforts should focus on excluding conditions that can result in muscle weakness, such as medication (eg, steroids, HMG-CoA reductase inhibitors), and metabolic derangements (eg, thyroid disorders, diabetes, vitamin D deficiency, electrolyte abnormalities) before muscle biopsy is pursued. Serum levels of muscle enzymes (creatine kinase, aldolase) are usually markedly increased. Electromyographic testing is used to exclude neuropathy. MRI using fat-suppression sequences can help to select which muscle to biopsy. Muscle biopsy remains the gold standard to confirm the diagnosis and also to distinguish among the subtypes of myosites. A diagnosis of polymyositis warrants an evaluation for cardiac and pulmonary disease; a diagnosis of dermatomyositis, and less so with polymyositis, warrants a search for underlying malignancy. Associations with colon, lung, breast, prostate, ovarian, and uterine tumors have been reported, as have remission of polymyositis and dermatomyositis after treatment of the underlying malignancy.

Glucocorticoids are the initial therapy for polymyositis and dermatomyositis. Prednisone at 1 mg/kg/d is a typical starting dosage; for severe disease, an initial dose of methylprednisolone 1,000 mg IV is often used. Prednisone can be tapered after an initial phase of improved muscle strength and normalized muscle enzyme concentrations. However, prolonged glucocorticoid use at high dosages can result in a myopathy with resultant proximal muscle weakness. Therefore, tapering the total dose by 10%–20% per month should be attempted. Methotrexate[OL], given parenterally, in a weekly pulse regimen can be combined with corticosteroids and can also have a steroid-sparing effect in long-term therapy. Weekly oral methotrexate[OL] is effective in managing refractory skin manifestations of dermatomyositis.

Supervised exercise over 6-week and 6-month study periods has proved beneficial in polymyositis (SOE=B), improving function without aggravating underlying disease.

Sjögren's Syndrome and Sjögren's Disease

Sjögren's disease is a systemic, multiorgan chronic disease with lymphocytic infiltration of exocrine glands. It should be considered in patients with interstitial lung disease; malabsorption; CNS disease that mimics multiple sclerosis; unexplained renal, liver, or thyroid disease; or rash. Sicca symptoms (dry mouth and dry eyes) are common but are frequently caused by medications and other connective tissue syndromes.

An ophthalmologic examination that includes a Schirmer test and slit-lamp examination (to assess corneal damage) can confirm the presence of keratoconjunctivitis. Antinuclear, anti-SSA, and anti-SSB antibodies are usually present. Rheumatoid factor and a variety of autoantibodies are often seen. Biopsy of a skin rash can verify the presence of cutaneous vasculitis. Biopsies of a salivary or lacrimal gland can confirm the presence of characteristic lymphocytic infiltration.

Sugar-free candies and artificial saliva can alleviate symptoms of xerostomia. Symptomatic treatment of xerophthalmia consists of lubricating ointments and artificial tears. Punctal plugs can be tried to retain tears. Ophthalmic cyclosporine can be used to treat inflammatory eye disease. Treatment of an underlying inflammatory disease (eg, rheumatoid arthritis, systemic lupus erythematosus, myositis, scleroderma) can improve symptoms as well.

ACOVE-3* Quality Indicators Pertaining to Musculoskeletal Diseases and Disorders

Assess pain and function

- If a vulnerable older adult has symptomatic osteoarthritis (OA) of the knee or hip, then pain should be assessed when new to a primary care or musculoskeletal disease practice and annually.
- If a vulnerable older adult has symptomatic OA of the knee or hip, then functional status should be assessed when new to a primary care or musculoskeletal disease practice and annually.

Exercise therapy

- If an ambulatory vulnerable older adult has symptomatic OA of the knee or hip for >3 mo and is able to exercise, then a directed or supervised muscle strengthening or aerobic exercise program should be recommended and activity reviewed annually.

Ambulatory assistive device

- If a vulnerable older adult has symptomatic OA of the hip or knee and has difficulty walking that makes ADLs difficult for >3 mo, then the need for ambulatory assistive devices should be assessed.

Nonambulatory assistive device

- If a vulnerable older adult has symptomatic OA and has difficulty with nonambulatory ADLs, then the need for assistive devices for ADLs should be assessed.

First-line pharmacologic therapy

- If a vulnerable older adult is started on pharmacologic therapy to treat OA, then acetaminophen should be tried first.

Total joint replacement

- If a vulnerable older adult has severe symptomatic OA of the knee or hip despite nonsurgical therapy, then a referral to an orthopedic surgeon should be made.

Related quality indicators for Musculoskeletal Diseases and Disorders

- Use of acetaminophen, NSAIDs, and aspirin (see "Persistent Pain," p 109)

***Assessing Care of Vulnerable Elders – 3rd Set. See page inside front cover for explanation.**

REFERENCES

- Antall GF. The use of guided imagery to manage pain in an elderly orthopaedic population. *Orthop Nurs.* 2004;23(5):335–340.

- Jackson CE. A clinical approach to muscle diseases. *Semin Neurol.* 2008;28(2):228–240.

- Singh H, Torralba KD. Therapeutic challenges in the management of gout in the elderly. *Geriatrics.* 2008;63(7):13–18, 20.

- Zhang W, Moskowitz RW, Nuki G, et al. OARSI recommendations for the management of hip and knee osteoarthritis, Part II: OARSI evidence-based, expert consensus guidelines. *Osteoarthritis Cartilage.* 2008;16(2):137–162.

CHAPTER 55—BACK AND NECK PAIN

KEY POINTS

- Back problems are the third most common reason for physician visits by older adults, and degenerative conditions of the spine are the most common cause of these problems.

- Pain that is insidious in onset, progressive in its course, and nonpositional; that is associated with night pain and systemic symptoms or signs; and that persists for >1 mo should raise concerns about tumor or infection. Nonsystemic causes of pain are characterized by intermittent, often positional pain that is worse at onset and usually improves with time.

- The physical examination of the back, hips, and legs is essential in the assessment of older adults with back pain. Plain radiographs remain the most useful starting point in the diagnostic evaluation of back pain.

- Management requires a therapeutic approach that addresses the structural problems most likely to be causing the pain.

- Neck pain is most often due to mechanical disease of the cervical spine and is best diagnosed on physical examination.

Back problems are the third most common reason for physician visits by older adults. In the Framingham study, 22% of patients ≥68 yr old had back pain on most days. The causes, natural history, and prognosis of back pain are different in older individuals than in younger ones. Herniated discs are rare in older adults, while lumbar spinal stenosis, mechanical instability of the lumbar spine, and osteoporotic fractures are common causes of back pain.

Systemic conditions such as tumors and infections, although a rare cause of back pain, are more common in older adults. Diagnostic imaging studies can complicate the evaluation of pain in older adults, because the incidence of anatomic abnormalities that may or may not be the cause of the pain is very high. The natural history of mechanical low back pain has been well defined in younger individuals but not in older adults.

A systematic approach to the diagnosis of lower back pain in older adults requires knowledge of the typical presentation of common back conditions of older adults, an understanding of the anatomy of the lumbar spine, the identification of physical findings associated with common abnormalities, and the judicious use of diagnostic imaging studies (Table 55.1). The lack of specificity of diagnostic imaging tests heightens the importance of the history and physical examination in evaluation. The CBC and sedimentation rate are very helpful tests in the evaluation of possible infection or tumor.

SYSTEMIC CAUSES

The history and physical examination can usually distinguish systemic from mechanical causes of back pain. Systemic conditions such as tumors or infections of the spine usually have an insidious onset of pain that becomes more and more persistent over time. This pain is usually nonpositional, can occur at night, and can be associated with systemic systems and signs. The pain of mechanical disease is usually intermittent, positional, and often worse at onset. The absence of the typical physical examination findings of motor weakness of the L4 through S1 innervated muscles of the hip and foot may also indicate systemic disease. The likelihood of cancer as a cause of back pain increases in adults ≥50 yr old, those with a previous history of cancer, and those with pain that persists >1 mo.

Fever, discrete local vertebral tenderness, upper lumbar or thoracic pain, and nonpositional pain can indicate vertebral infection. Approximately 10% of older adults with endocarditis have back pain. Infection can produce back pain in individuals at risk of endovascular infections, such as those on hemodialysis, with chronic indwelling venous access catheters, with a history of recent or chronic urinary tract infections, or with a history of intravenous drug abuse.

A number of visceral problems, such as abdominal aortic aneurysms, bladder distention secondary to urinary retention, large uterine fibroids, and intra-abdominal infections or tumors, can present with back pain. Referred pain from these conditions should be suggested by the historical pattern of the pain, the absence of positional changes, and a normal physical examination of the lumbosacral spine.

NONSYSTEMIC CAUSES

Lumbar Spinal Stenosis

Lumbar spinal stenosis results from a narrowing of either the central or lateral aspect of the lumbar spine canal. The characteristic symptom of lumbar spinal

Table 55.1—Conditions Causing Back Pain in Older Adults

Condition	History	Examination	Laboratory Tests, Imaging
Tumor	Persistent, progressive pain at rest; systemic symptoms	No focal abnormalities	Anemia, increased ESR, abnormal bone scan or MRI
Infection	Persistent pain, fever; at-risk patient (eg, indwelling catheter)	Tender spine	Increased ESR, WBC; positive bone scan or MRI
Unstable lumbar spine	Recurring episodes of pain on change of position	Pain going from flexed to extended position	One disc space narrowed and sclerotic spondylolisthesis
Lumbar spinal stenosis	Pain on standing and walking relieved by sitting and lying	Immobile spine; L4, L5, S1 weakness	MRI or CT scan showing stenosis
Sciatica	Pain in the posterior aspect of leg; may be incomplete	Often positive straight leg raise; L4, L5, S1 weakness	Variable diagnostic imaging findings
Vertebral compression fracture	Sudden onset of severe pain; resolves in 4–6 weeks	Pain on any movement of spine; no neurologic deficits	Vertebral end-plate collapse; compression fracture seen on plain film
Osteoporotic sacral fracture	Sudden lower back, buttock, or hip pain	Sacral tenderness	H-shaped uptake on bone scan

NOTE: ESR = erythrocyte sedimentation rare

stenosis is pain in the back radiating into the buttock or leg that is worse on standing and walking and relieved with sitting. The presence of lumbar spinal stenosis on diagnostic imaging studies in up to 20% of people without the clinical syndrome heightens the importance of the history and physical examination in this diagnosis.

Flexion of the lumbar spine results in an increase in spinal canal volume and a decrease in nerve root bulk. Extension of the lumbar spine results in a decrease in spinal canal volume and an increase in nerve root bulk. Therefore, positions that flex the spine, such as sitting, bending forward, walking uphill, and lying in a flexed position, all relieve symptoms, while positions that extend the lumbar spine, such as prolonged standing, walking, and walking downhill, all exacerbate symptoms.

Lumbar spinal stenosis causes pain either in the back or in the legs, made worse by standing or walking. Pain in the calf when walking can often mimic the claudication of arterial insufficiency and is referred to as *pseudoclaudication*. Continued walking after this point can result in combinations of paresthesia, numbness, and weakness in one or both legs. Walking uphill is easier than walking downhill, and walking with an assistive device, such as a shopping cart, which allows some flexion of the lumbar spine, is usually better tolerated. These symptoms are usually progressive and consistent, not intermittent. There is often subtle weakness in the muscles innervated by the L4, L5, and S1 nerve roots. (See Table 55.2 and the assessment section, below.)

Sciatica

Sciatica describes a lancinating pain, usually felt from the buttock down the posterior aspect of the leg to the foot; it may occur only in isolated regions of the distribution of the sciatic nerve. In older adults, there are two common patterns of sciatica. Sciatic pain that comes on only with standing and walking and that limits the person's ability to walk is usually a result of lumbar spinal stenosis. In other cases, sciatic pain can have a relatively sudden onset, be present at rest, and be exacerbated by sudden maneuvers, such as getting out of a bed or chair. This abrupt and persistent pain, not necessarily related to the erect position, usually resolves spontaneously in several weeks. The diagnosis of sciatica can be confirmed by demonstrating weakness of the L4, L5, and S1 innervated muscles of the foot, ankle, and hip. (See Table 55.2 and the assessment section, below.)

Unstable Lumbar Spine

Lumbar degenerative disc disease may produce a *relatively* unstable lumbar spine. Individuals with this condition often have episodes of severe pain in the back or in the distribution of the sciatic nerve. This pain usually comes on suddenly, often after abrupt movements. It usually lasts only minutes to hours but recurs frequently. This pain also comes on with significant flexion or extension of the lumbar spine. On physical examination, the patient often has guarded movements of the lumbar spine and pain when moving from the flexed to the extended position. Significant disc space narrowing, vertebral end-plate sclerosis, and osteophytosis at one disc space, out of proportion to the other spaces, is often seen in patients with lumbar spine instability.

Osteoporotic Vertebral Compression Fractures

Although only one-third of vertebral compression fractures are symptomatic, the symptoms can be quite

Table 55.2—Innervation of Lower Extremities

Function	Muscle	Peripheral Nerve	Nerve Root
Great toe dorsiflexion	Extensor hallucis longus	Deep peroneal	L5
Ankle dorsiflexion	Tibialis anterior	Deep peroneal	L4, L5
Ankle eversion	Peroneus longus, brevis	Superficial peroneal	L5, S1
Ankle plantar flexion	Gastrocnemius, soleus	Tibial	S1, S2
Knee extension	Quadriceps	Femoral	L3, L4
Hip flexion	Iliopsoas	Femoral	L2, L3
Hip adduction	Adductor magnus, brevis, longus	Obturator	L3, L4
Hip abduction	Gluteus medius	Superior gluteal	L4, L5
Hip extension	Gluteus maximus	Inferior gluteal	L5, S1

Table 55.3—Assessment of Lower Back Pain in Older Adults

Symptoms	Conditions
Acute pain	Vertebral compression fracture Disc displacement Osteoporotic sacral fracture Visceral pain (eg, aortic aneurysm)
Positional pain	
Increased with standing and walking and relieved with sitting	Lumbar spinal stenosis
Brought on by bending, lifting, or unguarded movements	Unstable lumbar spine
Persistent pain (gradually increasing, nonpositional)	Tumor Infection

severe. The pain from an acute vertebral fracture usually lasts from 2 wk to 2 mo. The onset of pain is abrupt, and intense pain is felt deep at the site of the fracture. Tenderness is often marked over the involved vertebra. The pain is usually worse on standing and walking, and relieved with lying down. Although the pain commonly radiates to the flank, abdomen, and legs, neurologic sequelae should not occur in patients with spontaneous osteopenic fractures. Symptomatic fractures most often affect the lower thoracic and lumbar vertebrae.

The acute pain resolves slowly. In one study, analgesic use decreased by 16% at day 5 and by 33% at day 14. Patients often have trouble walking for 2 weeks and restrict their activity for approximately 1 mo.

The impact of these fractures, and osteoporosis in general, on chronic back pain and the function of older adults is unclear. Patients with these fractures are more apt to have further fractures, are more disabled, and have a higher mortality than those without fractures. An increase in chronic back pain, however, is seen only in patients with extensive fractures.

Osteoporotic Sacral Fractures

Lower back pain in older women may be due to osteoporotic sacral fractures. This pain often occurs spontaneously, usually involving the lower back. Pain can also be felt in the buttock or hip area. Sacral tenderness on physical examination is usually present. The incidence of associated additional osteoporotic fractures is high.

Plain radiographs are usually negative. Technetium bone scans show a characteristic H-shaped uptake over the sacrum. A CT scan shows displacement of the anterior border of the sacrum. Prognosis for recovery is excellent, with no neurologic deficits. The pain usually resolves in 4–6 weeks.

ASSESSMENT

See Table 55.3.

History

Pain that is insidious in onset, progressive in its course, nonpositional, associated with night pain and systemic symptoms or signs, and that persists for >1 mo should raise concerns about tumor or infection. Nonsystemic causes of pain are characterized by intermittent, often positional pain that is worse at onset and that usually improves over time.

Diseases of the hip often result in pain in the back and leg in a distribution that resembles that of back disease. Back disease is more apt to cause pain when an individual goes from the supine to the sitting position. The hip is more apt to be the cause of the pain if the individual has pain in the groin, a limp, or limited range of motion of the hip.

Table 55.4—Physical Examination of Older Adults with Lower Back Pain

Sign	Condition
Paravertebral muscle spasm	Mechanical disease
Asymmetric range of motion of the lumbar spine	Mechanical disc disease Unstable lumbar spine
Spinal tenderness	Vertebral compression fracture Infection
Weakness of L4–L5 and L5–S1 muscles	Mechanical disc disease Lumbar spinal stenosis
Normal examination of lumbar spine	Osteoporotic sacral fracture Hip disease Tumor Referred visceral pain

Table 55.5—Lumbosacral Nerve Root Compression

Root	Motor	Sensory	Reflex
L4	Quadriceps	Medial foot	Knee jerk
	Dorsiflexors	Dorsum of foot	Medial hamstring
L5	Dorsiflexors	Dorsum of foot	Medial hamstring
S1	Plantar flexors	Lateral foot	Ankle jerk

SOURCE: Reuben DB, Herr KA, Pacala JT, et al. *Geriatrics At Your Fingertips*, 12th ed. New York: American Geriatrics Society; 2010. Reprinted with permission.

Physical Examination

The physical examination of the back, hips, and legs is essential in the assessment of an older adult with back pain (Table 55.4). The finding of subtle but asymmetric weakness of the hip, ankle, and foot muscles innervated by the lumbar and sacral nerves can help elucidate the cause of back and leg pain.

A thorough back examination begins with the patient in the upright position. The back should be moved through all four planes of movement of the lumbar spine: side flexion to the right, side flexion to the left, forward flexion, and extension. Asymmetric limitation of the range of motion of the lumbar spine, or reproduction of the pain with these maneuvers, often indicates mechanical disease of the lumbar spine. The pain of lumbar spinal stenosis is often produced by spinal extension.

The remainder of the examination is performed with the patient in the supine position. A straight leg raise test can be informative if positive, but a negative test does not exclude any condition. Each patient with a back complaint should have a complete examination of the hips, focusing on the passive range of motion. The examiner should be able to abduct the hip to 40 degrees before the pelvis starts to tilt. The hip should flex beyond 110 degrees, externally rotate 50–60 degrees, and internally rotate 15–20 degrees.

Manual examination of the leg muscles can be helpful. Nerve root irritation from a spinal process should affect all the muscles innervated by these nerve roots. Thus, an individual with lumbar spine disease at the L4–L5 and the L5–S1 level should have weakness of the hip abductor and hip extensor, as well as of the ankle dorsiflexor, great toe dorsiflexor, and ankle evertor. A patient with a peroneal palsy should have weakness of the great toe extensor, ankle dorsiflexor, and ankle evertors, but no involvement of the hip abductors and hip extensors. See Table 55.5.

Observation of the patient can be very helpful. Patients with lumbar spinal stenosis often bend forward more and more as they walk, while patients with hip disease are apt to limp.

Laboratory Tests and Imaging

Although not recommended in the evaluation of younger patients in the routine evaluation of low back pain, a plain lumbar spine radiograph can be a helpful test in evaluating back pain in older adults, particularly if there is suspicion of an underlying systemic condition. This single diagnostic tool can demonstrate degenerative disc and joint disease, vertebral compression fractures, deformities such as spondylolisthesis and scoliosis, and systemic disorders such as osteoporosis and Paget's disease. A CBC with an erythrocyte sedimentation rate is perhaps the most useful screening laboratory test for an underlying systemic disease.

A technetium bone scan is useful in evaluating a suspected infection or neoplasm. CT and MRI have replaced myelography in assessing the neural canal. CT imaging is, in many cases, slightly superior in demonstrating the bony architecture of the spine, whereas the MRI is more sensitive to morphology of soft tissue, including disc, ligamentum flavum, neoplasm, and infection. Either CT or MRI studies are necessary to document spinal stenosis if surgical treatment is contemplated.

The use of diagnostic imaging studies is tempered by the high false-positive rates of these studies in older adults. A diagnostic imaging study simply identifies an anatomic abnormality—it does not demonstrate that this abnormality is the cause of the pain. In one study, 57% of adults ≥60 yr old, with no history of lower back pain or sciatica, had abnormal lumbar spine MRIs. Of these individuals, 36% had a herniated nucleus pulposus, and 21% had lumbar spinal stenosis. In another study, only 36% of asymptomatic individuals had normal discs at all levels; the prevalence of disc abnormalities increased in older adults. Other studies have shown similarly high rates of abnormal findings in asymptomatic individuals. These studies reinforce the need to correlate carefully the history and physical examination with the findings on diagnostic imaging studies.

MANAGEMENT

Management of back pain is hampered by the common difficulty of making a definitive diagnosis. Patients can do well, however, with a therapeutic approach that addresses the structural problems most likely to be causing their pain.

Treatment of an unstable lumbar spine is symptomatic. Nonopioid analgesics are often helpful in the early stages. As soon as the acute symptoms subside, a gentle, progressive exercise program should be started that is designed to strengthen and improve the efficiency of the spinal and abdominal musculature. An aquatic program offers the dual benefits of rapid rehabilitation with a low incidence of reinjury. Walking in chest-high water against resistance and performing the flutter kick are two simple aquatic exercises (SOE=D).

Chronic mechanical pain is often caused by excessive vertebral motion that is more pronounced and repetitive. Management is aimed at eliminating or reducing motion. This can be done internally by strengthening the paraspinous and abdominal muscles, thus providing an internal "brace" for the lumbar spine. It must be stressed that this exercise should be a lifetime commitment. Lumbar sacral corsets and braces provide an external method of immobilizing the lumbar spine. In severe cases that have not responded to conservative therapy, surgical fusion can be considered (SOE=D).

Analgesia is the most important goal of treatment of vertebral compression fractures, while trying to avoid the complications of the bed rest required by the patient's pain. Spinal extension exercises also may be helpful. Calcitonin[OL] has been demonstrated to decrease the pain associated with acute vertebral fractures.

Vertebroplasty is the percutaneous injection of bone cement into a collapsed vertebra. Two randomized trials demonstrated no difference in pain relief between vertebroplasty and placebo subjects who had fracture pain for a median of 9 weeks in one trial and 18 weeks in the other (range 1−52 weeks) (SOE=A). The role of this procedure in the management of an acute vertebral compression fracture is still unclear and unproved. Given the good natural history of the pain in most patients with vertebral compression fractures, however, this procedure should not be considered first-line therapy for these fractures (SOE=D).

Because mechanical encroachment on lumbar nerve roots causes lumbar spinal stenosis, conservative therapy is limited. Epidural corticosteroid injections have been used extensively for the sciatica associated with lumbar spinal stenosis, but a review of controlled trials of this therapy did not demonstrate efficacy of injection over controls.

Lumbar spinal stenosis is the most common indication for spinal surgery in older adults. In a prospective study of surgery for spinal stenosis, the ideal candidates for surgery were found to be those patients with severe narrowing of the spinal canal, minimal associated back pain, no coexisting conditions that affect walking, and symptom duration of <4 yr. In two randomized, controlled trials and a high-quality observational study, surgery provided earlier and greater pain relief and improvement in functional status, but those gains narrowed over the course of follow-up (SOE=A).

NECK PAIN

Causes

Although neck pain can be due to inflammatory and systemic conditions, it is most often due to mechanical disease of the cervical spine. Inflammatory conditions such as polymyalgia rheumatica and rheumatoid arthritis are characterized by morning stiffness, systemic complaints such as fatigue, fever, and weight loss, and other muscle and joint complaints.

Mechanical disease of the cervical spine can cause neck and occiput pain, scapula and trapezius pain, radicular pain down the arm, as well as spastic paraparesis due to cervical myelopathy.

The referral pain pattern of cervical spine disease has been demonstrated by a number of injection studies. C2–C3 disease is felt in the occiput; C3–C4 and C4–C5 problems are referred into the posterior and lateral aspects of the neck; C5–C6 lesions are referred into the trapezius and upper cervical region;

C6–C7 disease is felt in the retroscapular region, often as far down as the mid to lower thoracic region. This referral process produces not only pain in these regions but also local muscle spasm and tenderness, often mistaken for "trigger points."

Irritation of a cervical nerve root produces lancinating pain and numbness in the neck and upper scapular region, radiating into the arm in a dermatomal distribution. Characteristic weakness of the arm muscles (see below) confirms the specific nerve root involved.

Narrowing of the cervical canal can produce the syndrome of cervical myelopathy, which is characterized by clumsiness, weakness, and spasticity of the legs, bladder spasticity, and upper motor neuron signs of the legs (clonus, hyperreflexia, and Babinski signs). Although progressive signs and symptoms call for an aggressive diagnostic and therapeutic approach, the natural history of this problem can be quite variable, and surgical intervention is not always necessary.

Assessment

Mechanical disease of the cervical spine is best diagnosed on physical examination. The cervical spine has four planes of movement: rotation to the right, rotation to the left, flexion, and extension. Asymmetric limitation of the range of motion of the cervical spine in some but not all of these movements, and weakness of the arm muscles innervated by the cervical nerve root, indicate mechanical disease of the cervical spine. The shoulder abductor and elbow flexor muscles are innervated by C5 and C6 nerve roots, the wrist extensor and thumb opponens muscles by C6 and C7, and the elbow extensor and finger abductors muscles by C7 and C8. Weakness of the C7- and C8-innervated muscles is most common with cervical disc disease, because the

C7–T1 interspace is the most common site of cervical spine lesions. Individuals with mechanical disease of the cervical spine often awake in the morning with pain in the trapezius and scapular region, do not have full rotation of the cervical spine, and have difficulty with such activities as backing a car out of a driveway.

Diagnostic Imaging

The role of diagnostic imaging tests in the diagnosis and management of neck pain is unclear. A plain radiograph of the cervical spine has limited value, in that 80% of adults ≥55 yr old have signs of degenerative cervical disc disease on these films. MRIs of the cervical spine also show degeneration in at least one level in almost 60% of adults ≥40 yr old. These anatomic abnormalities call for interventions only if they are consistent with significant historical and physical features of the patient's condition.

Management

There is much controversy about the therapy of mechanical disease of the cervical spine. Two studies from the Netherlands and Finland, done on younger individuals, have had promising results for manual therapy and active neck muscle training in the treatment of neck pain. In a Cochrane review of the management of neck disorders, the combination of mobilization and/or manipulation along with active exercises was beneficial for persistent mechanical neck disorders. Mobilization and/or manipulation done alone or combined with other treatments such as heat were not effective. These therapies were effective only when combined with an exercise program.

ACOVE-3* Quality Indicators Pertaining to Back and Neck Pain

- See "Persistent Pain," p 123; and "Musculoskeletal Diseases and Disorders," p 437.

References

- Katz JN, Harris MB. Lumbar spinal stenosis. *N Engl J Med.* 2008;358(8):818–825.
- Peloso P, Gross A, Haines T, et al. Medicinal and injection therapies for mechanical neck disorders. *Cochrane Database Syst Rev.* 2007;(3):CD000319.
- van der Veld G, Hogg-Johnson S, Bayoumi AM, et al. Identifying the best treatment among common nonsurgical neck pain treatments: a decision analysis. *Spine.* 2008;33(4 Suppl):S184–S191.
- Wollman S. Low back pain. *Nursing.* 2003;33(10):49.

CHAPTER 56—DISEASES AND DISORDERS OF THE FOOT

KEY POINTS

- Foot and ankle problems are common in older adults. Efficient diagnosis and treatment are critical to maintain function and quality of life.

- Long-term effects of common structural foot deformities, including collapsing pes plano valgus, cavus foot, and equinus deformity, cause significant disability in older adults.

- Skin disorders of the foot are common in older adults. Complete assessment of the skin of the foot is necessary to identify skin conditions and potential malignancies.

- Surgical intervention for treatment of foot deformities can alleviate pain and improve function in older adults who are appropriate surgical candidates. Most surgical interventions in older adults can be performed under local anesthesia.

- Systemic diseases can create long-term effects on the foot and ankle.

Foot problems can have a deleterious effect on the functional capacity and quality of life of older adults. These problems can affect the daily lives of older adults and lead to inactivity and overall morbidity. Foot problems vary in severity from dry xerotic skin on the plantar surface of the foot to an infected limb-threatening diabetic foot ulcer in a patient with peripheral arterial disease. In general, foot problems are musculoskeletal and/or dermatologic, although vascular, neurologic, and a variety of systemic diseases can also affect the foot. The clinician needs to identify these specific problems for either treatment or referral to the appropriate specialist depending on the preliminary diagnosis or presentation.

The prevalence of foot problems in older adults varies by level of disability and site of care. Studies to determine prevalence have looked at nursing-home (long-term rehabilitation), inpatient, and outpatient settings, and at age- and morbidity-specific populations, all of which confirm that the prevalence of foot pathology increases with a person's age. The more common problems identified by these studies are nail disorders, corns/calluses, hammertoes, hallux valgus, plantar fasciitis, and flat feet. Studies of the geriatric population demonstrate that foot complaints can inhibit daily activities such as getting out of a chair, walking, and stair climbing. Foot complaints are also associated with increased fall risk in the aging population. Approximately one-third of the geriatric population has some foot pathology, with a higher incidence in patients who are within a medical facility such as a nursing home or hospital.

THE ROLE OF THE PRIMARY CLINICIAN IN FOOT CARE

Regular assessment of the feet is recommended. Practitioners should be aware of their patients' foot conditions and the complications of systemic diseases, such as diabetes mellitus, peripheral arterial disease, arthritic changes, neurologic disorders, and mental health symptoms that manifest as foot symptoms and signs. Primary practitioners should recognize common foot problems and refer patients for podiatric care and management in a timely and appropriate manner. Quality of life and the functional capacity of older adults can be significantly improved by early detection and comprehensive management of foot problems (SOE=D).

COMMON DEFORMITIES OF THE FOOT

See Table 56.1.

Collapsing Pes Plano Valgus Foot (Pes Planus), Cavus Foot, Equinus Deformity

Long-term effects of foot deformities can cause significant disability in older adults. In general, these deformities have derived from the longstanding effects of a pathologic foot. A pathologic foot is one that abnormally distributes weight during gait and creates stress on the musculoskeletal structure of the foot, resulting in pain. This physical stress of the foot over a lifetime can result in tissue atrophy, arthritis, and subluxation of joints in the foot. Two generalized pathologic foot types create this disability: collapsing pes plano valgus (low arch morphology) and cavus foot (high arch morphology). Equinus, the effect of a tight heel cord (Achilles tendon), is a deforming force on the foot that can be identified in both pes planus and pes cavus foot types.

Table 56.1—Common Disorders of the Foot

Disorder	Definition or Description
Bunion	Prominent and dorsal medial eminence of the first metatarsal; associated with hallux valgus
Calcaneal spur/heel spur	A calcification of the attachment of the plantar fascia, usually at the medial plantar tuberosity of the calcaneus. The spur projects anteriorly and is the consequence of chronic repetitive trauma or stress resulting from biomechanical and pathomechanical change. When ligamentous calcification occurs, inflammation and associated pain at the attachment result. This may be referred to as heel pain syndrome and may be related to plantar fasciitis.
Cystic erosion	Areas of radiolucency usually noted with arthritic changes, such as rheumatoid arthritis, and usually occurring in the metatarsal heads with associated joint changes
Digiti flexus	Fixed or flexible flexion at the metatarsal phalangeal joints, ie, hammertoe
Digiti quinti varus	Valgus displacement or splaying of the fifth metatarsal, with a resulting varus or inward deviation of the fifth toe
Dislocation of lesser metatarsal phalangeal joint	Toe joint is out of its socket
Entrapment syndrome	Occurs when a nerve is compressed by ligamentous or other soft-tissue inflammation, resulting in pain and possibly numbness and neuropathic symptoms. The most common sites are the posterior tibial nerve and the intermetatarsal nerves, plantarly.
Equinus	Tight Achilles tendon
Haglund's deformity	A hyperostosis of the posterior and superior portion of the calcaneus, enlarging the calcaneus, which can in turn place pressure on the attachment of the Achilles tendon. The presence of the deformity also can produce a pressure area for the heel counter of the shoe. It is easily demonstrated on a lateral radiograph of the foot and can be associated with tendinitis or bursitis, usually resulting from an incompatibility of foot to shoe last.
Hallux abducto valgus	An alternative clinical diagnosis for hallux valgus, or bunion. There is a varus splaying of the first metatarsal with a valgus and rotational deformity of the phalanges of the great toe.
Hallux limitus and rigidus	A degenerative joint change involving the first metatarsal phalangeal joint, resulting from dorsal spurs, with a marked limitation or absence of any range of motion. The difference between hallux limitus and rigidus is based on the radiographic interpretation and difference in function.
Hallux valgus	Deviation of the tip of the great toe, or main axis of the toe, toward the outer or lateral side of the foot, ie, bunion
Hammertoe	Muscle tendon imbalance causing contraction of the proximal or distal interphalangeal joint, or both
Metatarsalgia	Pain in the forefoot near the heads of the metatarsals
Morton's neuroma/Morton's syndrome	A congenital shortening of the first metatarsal shaft, which creates an abnormal metatarsal arc. Excessive weight is placed on the second metatarsal head during gait and stance. The dynamics and pathomechanics of the foot are modified and can lead to hallux valgus, abducto valgus, or rotational deformity of the hallux.
Periostitis	Inflammation of the periosteum
Pes cavus	Higher than normal arch that is commonly associated with neurologic change. In older adults, excessive pressure is usually placed on the metatarsal heads. With atrophy of the plantar fat pad and displacement, pressure is increased, which can serve as a predisposing cause for pain and ulceration.
Pes planus	A flattening of the medial longitudinal arch, in which the calcaneal pitch on a radiograph is usually below 15 degrees (ie, flat feet)
Pes valgo planus	Clinical picture same as that of pes planus, with an addition of pronation, demonstrated by a lateral deviation of the Achilles tendon and an outward and rotational deformity of the foot.
Plantar fasciitis	Inflammation and pain involving repetitive microtrauma to the plantar fascia, particularly at its posterior calcaneal attachment; associated with biomechanical and pathomechanical changes in the function of the foot. It is related to calcaneal spurs, ligamentous calcification, and tissue atrophy.
Subluxation	Deviation of a joint's position
Tailor's bunion	Prominence of the dorsal lateral aspect of the fifth metatarsal head
Tarsal tunnel syndrome	An entrapment neuropathy of the posterior tibial nerve
Tenosynovitis	Inflammation of the synovial sheath of a tendon complex; sometimes associated with a tendon tear
Tibialis posterior dysfunction	Chronic rupture or weakening of the tibialis posterior tendon secondary to long-term pes planus
Valgus position	Frontal plane position in which pressure is inwardly directed in the foot
Varus position	Frontal plane position in which pressure is outwardly directed in the foot

Collapsing pes plano valgus is a foot type with an unstable medial longitudinal arch leading to a "flat foot." The instability can occur in the talonavicular joint, the navicular cuneiform joint, and/or the first metatarsal cuneiform joint. This instability causes the forefoot to abduct on the rear-foot, and the rear-foot to go into valgus attitude in respect to the ankle joint. Essentially, the longitudinal arch collapses on the weight-bearing surface during stance, resulting in the subluxation of joints leading to arthrosis. Early in life, this deformity is usually quite flexible and can be treated with functional orthoses to help support the arch during stance. However, later in life, the foot becomes more rigid and is treated with an accommodative orthoses that absorbs the abnormally high pressure on the pes planus foot type. The deformity can be congenital or acquired, but the extent of the deformity depends on activity level, body type, shoeing, etc. Patients with this type of foot have a number of other associated deformities. These include posterior tibial tendon dysfunction, hallux valgus (bunion deformity), lesser metatarsal phalangeal joint dislocations (chronic dislocation of the toe joints), hammertoes, and neuromas.

The cavus foot type is generally rigid and a very poor shock absorber. It also can be congenital, or if acquired later in life, it usually has a neurologic origin. Cavus foot frequently has a metatarsus adductus (inward orientation of the metatarsal bones) component. Older adults with this foot type generally have loss of the fat pad in the heel as well as in the submetatarsal head region (ball of the foot). Associated deformities include cocked hallux (hammertoe of the great toe), sagittal dislocation of the metatarsal phalangeal joints, metatarsalgia, mid-foot dorsal exostoses (bone spurs), and rigid hammertoe deformities.

Equinus is the effect of a tight Achilles tendon on the foot. This is frequently a component of a pes planus or cavus foot, but it can be seen in a foot that appears grossly normal as well. It is a tightness of either the gastrosoleal complex or the gastrocnemius muscle complex. Equinus can cause various symptomatology, including Achilles tendinitis, plantar fasciitis, metatarsalgia, and hammertoe deformities.

Associated Common Deformities

Specific associated deformities can develop due to the pathomechanics of the general deformities.

Posterior Tibial Tendon Dysfunction

Posterior tibial tendon dysfunction is a foot deformity that is defined as the gradual tearing and/or rupturing of the tibialis posterior tendon. The tibialis posterior muscle arises from the posterior aspect of the leg, and its tendon courses posteromedially across the ankle

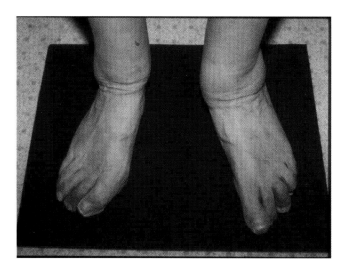

Figure 56.1—Stage 3 tibialis posterior dysfunction

joint and inserts primarily into the navicular joint. It also has small connections to remaining tarsal bones. The muscle serves as a powerful inverter and plantar flexor of the foot. The loss of this muscle's function creates significant disability, especially in obese patients. It causes collapse of the longitudinal arch, which causes subluxation of the rear-foot tarsal joints and eventually the ankle joint. The dysfunction is divided into four stages. Stage I is a tendinitis of the tibialis posterior tendon without foot deformity. Stage II is tearing or rupturing of the tibialis posterior tendon, which creates a flexible (fully reducible) deformity. Stage III is a Stage II deformity that has become arthritic and rigid (Figure 56.1). Stage IV occurs when the pronatory forces weaken the deltoid ligament, resulting in a valgus ankle deformity. This can be crippling in older patients.

Conservative treatment ranges from orthoses built to place the foot in a supinatory position to bracing with either an ankle-foot orthoses or a Richie brace®, a custom brace that provides increased foot control. Surgical treatment varies depending on the stage of deformity. Stage I deformity is treated with synovectomy and repair of the tendon, Stage II requires calcaneal osteotomies and tendon transfers to reconstruct the foot, Stage III requires arthrodesis of the rear foot, and Stage IV requires a plantar arthrodesis. Studies have demonstrated that Stage I and II repairs can improve function and reduce symptoms (SOE=B).

Hallux Valgus

One-third of people >65 yr old have a hallux valgus deformity (bunion). The hallux valgus deformity is a subluxation of the first metatarsal phalangeal joint, resulting from the adduction of the first metatarsal and the abduction of the hallux. This deformity

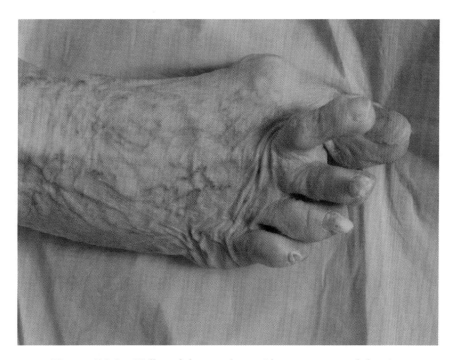

Figure 56.2—Hallux abducto valgus with crossover toe deformity

essentially progresses during a person's lifetime. There is usually hypermobility of the first metatarsal cuneiform joint. The prominence and subluxation can be painful, especially when the person is wearing shoes because of pressure at the bunion deformity. Hallux valgus deformities that have been present for a lifetime frequently are arthritic. These deformities are treated conservatively by adapting the patient's shoe to the deformity, ie, wider shoes/toe box and various padding techniques. Surgery is considered if the deformity is symptomatic and unresponsive to conservative care. Specific procedures depend on the severity of the deformity and on the patient's health and activity level. Studies evaluating orthopedic quality of life indicators and Short Form-36 after repair demonstrated reduction of symptoms and a return to shoe gear usually independent of the procedure. These findings were consistent over all age ranges (SOE=B).

Hallux Limitus

Hallux limitus is an arthritic condition occurring at the first metatarsal phalangeal joint. Normal motion of the first metatarsal phalangeal joint has been reported from 75 degrees to 35 degrees. Hallux limitus occurs when there are clinical findings of arthritis, including crepitus and a decrease of normal motion. Hallux rigidus is present when there is very little motion and the joint is essentially functioning as if fused. The cause of hallux limitus is thought to be from sagittal plane instability (the first metatarsal has increased dorsi and plantarflexion) of the first toe, resulting in hypermobility. This causes elevation of the first toe and thus impingement of the joint. Over time, this

process results in an arthritic joint. Traditional treatment consists of orthoses that attempt to prevent motion at the first metatarsal phalangeal joint and thereby relieve pain. A study examining >700 patients revealed more than half of the patients were successfully treated with conservative orthotic therapy, making it a viable approach as an initial treatment (SOE=B). An alternative approach in patients who still have some motion at the joint is to construct an orthoses with a first ray cut out, thereby plantarflexing the first metatarsal and placing the joint in a mechanically better position as the patient shifts weight from heel to ball of the foot when walking. The surgical approach of hallux limitus can vary from removal of bone spurs (cheilectomy) to osteotomies, joint implants, and arthrodesis of the joint. When surgery is required, it can successfully reduce symptoms and increase function (SOE=B).

Hammertoe Deformities

Hammertoes are caused by a muscle tendon imbalance that occurs around the metatarsal phalangeal joint. Hammertoes are a buckling (contraction) at the proximal interphalageal joint (PIPJ) or the distal interphalangeal joint (DIPJ) of the lesser toes. In a "classic" hammertoe, there is a flexor contracture at the PIPJ. A mallet toe is a hammertoe that contracts at the DIPJ, and a claw toe is a hammertoe that contracts at the PIPJ and the DIPJ. Hammertoes can be flexible and easily reducible, or they can be rigid and nonreducible. The rigid hammertoes are generally more painful and create problems when wearing shoes. When hammertoes press against the shoe, a

Table 56.2—Shoe Terms

Term	Definition or Description
Custom-made molded shoes	Made from an impression of the foot either by a plaster cast or foam imprint
Extra depth shoe	Provides additional space in the toe box
Heel counter	Back of the shoe that the heel fits in; shoes with a stiffer and higher heel counter have more stability
Rocker bottom sole	Modification of the sole
Shock-absorbing heel	Hard but absorbent material that provides shock absorption; good for patients with a cavus foot and obese patients
Thomas heel modification	A distal medial extension of the heel that provides stability of the arch
Toe box	Part of the shoe that contains the toes
Velcro lacing	Hook and loop tape used to secure the shoe closed, rather than conventional laces

callus or corn is created. This can cause pain and require periodic debridement. Treatment of hammertoes can consist of digital padding, wide toe box in shoes or custom shoes, debridement of callus, or surgical correction of the deformity (SOE=C).

Chronic Dislocated Metatarsal Phalangeal Joint

The end-stage of a hammertoe deformity is a chronically dislocated joint. This is not uncommon in older adults and is caused by long-term biomechanical pathology occurring in the forefoot. This is also seen sometimes at an earlier age in patients with rheumatoid arthritis. The toe generally dislocates on top of the metatarsal head, which places pressure on the ball of the foot. When this occurs on the second toe, it is usually associated with a hallux valgus deformity and can result in a cross-over deformity (Figure 56.2). Metatarsal phalangeal joint dislocations are a source of chronic pain and can cause plantar ulcerations, especially in those who suffer from neuropathy. Patients developing metatarsal phalangeal joint dislocations usually require accommodative shoes with increased toe box height to reduce dorsal pressure. When shoes can no longer control symptoms and skin breakdown, surgical reconstruction may be necessary (SOE=A).

Neuroma

Neuromas are commonly seen in the foot between the third and fourth metatarsal heads, where they are referred to as Morton's neuromas. A neuroma is a benign growth of a peripheral nerve caused by chronic entrapment. It is theorized that the common metatarsal nerve is entrapped by the deep intermetatarsal ligament as it courses underneath the ligament and forms the digital nerve branches. Conservative treatment of neuroma is metatarsal pads, orthoses, corticosteroid injections, cryotherapy, and alcohol injections. Surgical treatment is release of the intermetatarsal ligament or primary excision of the neuroma. A comparative review of surgical intervention consistently demonstrated favorable results with 80% of patients reporting a high level of satisfaction (SOE=B).

General Treatment Strategies

Orthoses and Shoewear for Older Adults

Orthoses are external devices that are placed either on the foot or into the shoe to accommodate for a foot deformity or to alter the function of the foot to relieve physical stress on a certain portion of the foot. Orthoses placed on the foot would include temporary felt padding or silicone/putty spacers to accommodate for structural deformities (ie, hallux valgus, hammer toes, tailor's bunion, etc). Orthoses placed in the shoe are either OTC devices or custom made. The OTC devices are generally made of lightweight polyethylene foam, soft plastics, or silicone, and are produced for a certain size of foot. A custom-made device is constructed from an impression of a person's foot. Impressions historically have been made by plaster casting of the foot in a subtalar joint neutral position. More recently, impressions have been made through computerized assessment or through a foam box. The devices are then made to the impression, taking into account the structural deformities. These devices are generally made from a variety of flexible and rigid plastics and fit into the shoe.

Shoewear is commonly ill-fitting in older adults and can be a source of foot pain. Studies have indicated that approximately 75% of people >65 yr old wear shoes that are too small. Appropriate shoewear can alleviate foot pain as well as protect the foot from injury. Older adults should be advised to purchase a shoe that fits well, has a sturdy heel counter, a firm beveled sole, and good traction. Narrow high heels should be avoided. A wide heel <6 cm in height can be appropriate for women who have tight heel cords and have been wearing high-heeled shoes all their lives. Older adults wearing heels >6 cm high are at a greater risk of falls. Proper

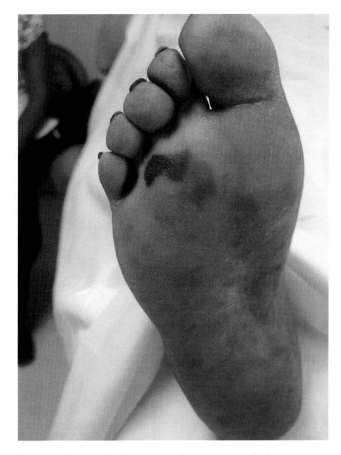

Figure 56.3—Malignant melanoma, acral lentiginous type, located on the plantar aspect of the forefoot

shoes and inserts that reduce pressure can decrease pain and improve function in older adults (SOE=B). See Table 56.2.

Surgical Considerations of Foot Deformities

Foot surgery in older adults has increased substantially in the past 30 yr largely because of the growth of this segment of the population. Studies have indicated that poor outcomes in surgery are generally the result of the overall health of an individual and not the chronologic age. Foot problems that are not alleviated by conservative methods are amenable to surgical solutions when relief of pain and restoration of function are the goals. Most podiatric surgical procedures for older adults can be performed under local anesthesia with monitored sedation, thereby minimizing surgical risk.

SKIN AND NAIL DISORDERS

Skin Neoplasms

Skin neoplasms on the foot are common in older adults and are rarely malignant. The true incidence of skin lesions in the older population is unknown but is likely quite high. Suspicious lesions require biopsy. Common benign lesions include the following:

- Keratotic lesions – calluses or corns seen commonly over sites of pressure; common terms are heloma durum (hard corn), heloma molle (soft corn), and tyloma (wide spread callus).
- Plantar verruca – The most common skin disorder of the foot, this viral infection of the plantar aspect is caused by a strain of the papilloma virus. Lesions are circular, punctate, and flat. A cluster of the lesions is referred to as a mosaic wart. The lesions commonly contain thrombosed vessels. Skin lines are interrupted. Treatments include topical salicylic acid, bleomycin injections, cryotherapy, CO$_2$ laser treatment, and surgical excision. These must be used with caution in older adults with reduced circulation and impaired healing. Treatment of verrucoid lesions in older adults may require mixing approaches and treating associated complications (eg, treating hyperkeratosis with keralytic agents such as urea) (SOE=B).
- Epidermal inclusion cysts – created by a portion of epidermis proliferating in the dermis.
- Dermatofibromas – flat-topped, raised, and firm lesions; generally not treated unless located across a joint or irritated by shoewear. A high recurrence rate is noted after excision.
- Hemangioma – These common vascular tumors contain abundant capillaries and are flat-topped, red lesions typically seen on the plantar aspect of the foot.

Malignant lesions are uncommon in the foot but can easily go undiagnosed and generally have a poor outcome. It is important to fully evaluate pigmented lesions of the foot and perform biopsies of any suspicious lesions. Characteristics of a potentially malignant lesion are new lesions in a patient ≥60 yr old or lesions that change shape, color, or diameter. Lesions not responding to conservative therapy and slow or nonhealing ulceration of the foot should be biopsied to exclude a potential underlying neoplasm. Morbidity associated with these lesions increases at age 60 and over. Malignant lesions identified in the foot include basal cell carcinoma, Bowen's disease, squamous cell carcinoma, and malignant acral lentiginous melanoma (Figure 56.3).

Xerosis

Excessive dryness, or xerosis, is associated with a lack of hydration and lubrication. The number of sebaceous and sweat glands decrease in older adults. Plantar skin lacks sebaceous glands. It is therefore common for fissures to develop on the heel resulting in dryness and increased stress on the heel. Management aims to prevent infection and other complications. Urea cream or solution (10%, 20%, or 40%) or ammonium lactate (12%) may be helpful as a mild and safe keratolytic. A heel sleeve or pad made with mineral oil or a heel cup can help minimize trauma to the heel, thus reducing the potential for complications. Urea and/or lactic acid–based emollients have been shown to be effective but must be used daily and applied after bathing (SOE=C).

Eczema

Eczema is inflamed skin that is not infected. The most common types in older adults are xerotic eczema, venous stasis eczema, and drug-induced eczema. Treatment is generally a combination of emollients and steroid creams, with or without occlusive dressings.

Nail Disorders

Ingrown Nails and Paronychia

Nail disorders are the most common disorders of the foot. Onychocryptosis is the incurvation of the edge of the nail plate into the nail groove. It generally occurs in the distal portion of the nail groove and is secondary to long-term improper nail cutting, narrow shoes, and/or genetically incurvated nail matrixes. A chronically ingrown nail is best treated either with a partial nail avulsion or a permanent matricectomy.

Paronychia is a localized infection caused by the nail embedding into the nail groove. A paronychia may require incision and drainage of the abscess with removal of the nail spicule. All infected granulation tissue is resected and depending on the presence of cellulitis or comorbidities, antibiotic treatment may be needed. Toes with chronic paronychias should be radiographed to exclude underlying osteomyelitis, especially in patients with diabetes or peripheral arterial disease.

Onychomycosis

Onychomycosis is a fungal infection of the nail plate. Approximately one-third of the older population has onychomycosis, with an increased incidence in older adults with obesity, immunodeficiency, diabetes, peripheral arterial disease, chronic tinea pedis, or psoriasis. Dermatophytes account for 80% of infections, with the remainder caused by saprophytes or yeast.

Onychomycosis causes thickening of the nail plate and can create pain (Figure 56.4). In patients

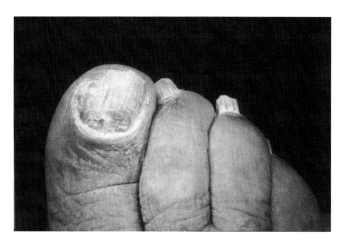

Figure 56.4—Onychomycosis. Nails infected by fungi are often yellow, thickened, and friable, with yellow-brown debris under the nail plate.

with neuropathy, onychomycosis can be a source of nail bed ulcerations. Treatment includes topical and oral antifungal medications, as well as permanent excision of the nail plate. A decision to treat is usually made because of the cosmetic concern of a yellow friable nail, other comorbidities (particularly diabetes mellitus, in which the break in the epidermal barrier due to the fungal infection can serve as a route for bacterial infections), and occasionally pain. No topical antifungal agents are effective against onychomycosis (SOE=A). A topical nail lacquer, ciclopirox (applied daily for 1 yr), is available to treat onychomycosis, but <12% of patients in clinical studies achieve clear or almost clear toenails with its use. Oral antifungals such as terbinafine, fluconazole, and itraconazole are effective for onychomycosis, but their duration of treatment, adverse event profile, and high rate of relapse after discontinuation warrant careful consideration for use in older adults. These agents are primarily metabolized by the liver and can interact with many medications that are commonly administered to older adults. Treatment can take 3–4 mo, and the rate of relapse of onychomycosis is high. Comorbities such as diabetes, secondary fungal infections, and quality of life should be considered before initiating treatment.

SYSTEMIC DISEASES AFFECTING THE FOOT AND ANKLE

Diabetes Mellitus

Diabetes is the most important disease affecting foot health in older adults. Complications of diabetes can cause the loss of limbs and significant disability. See also "Diabetes Mellitus," p 504. It has been estimated that 50%–75% of all amputations in patients with diabetes could be prevented by foot health education, periodic clinician assessment, and early intervention. The ocular complications of diabetes can affect the ability of patients to see ingrown toenails, corns, and ulcers. Other complications of diabetes that contribute to poor foot health include neuropathy, vascular insufficiency, dermopathy, atrophy of the muscles and soft tissues, and deformity. Neuropathy, especially sensory impairment, is a precursor to ulcers. Paresthesias, decreased vibratory sense, and loss of sensation are among the most important neuropathic changes that contribute to ulcer formation in older diabetic patients.

Arterial insufficiency causes pallor, a loss or decrease in the posterior tibial and dorsalis pedis pulse, dependent rubor, and decreased capillary filling time in the toes. Severe vascular disease can result in rest pain that typically occurs at night. A loss of the plantar metatarsal fat pad is associated with vascular insufficiency and predisposes to ulcerations at the site of bony prominences or deformities of the foot.

Foot ulcers are a common result of the multiple pathologies found in patients with diabetes. Prevention and early recognition are the most important strategies in managing foot ulcers. Clinicians should ensure that older diabetic patients have their feet examined a least annually. Diabetic patients are often instructed to remove their shoes at all visits to make a quick visual inspection of the feet and between the toes to ensure no skin breakdown. Patients and caregivers should be instructed in the importance of daily foot inspections. Preventive strategies include optimizing glycemic control, and monitoring and treating peripheral neuropathy, arterial disease, limited joint mobility, bony deformities, hyperkeratosis, and onychodystrophy (SOE=C). Diabetic foot prevention has been shown to be both cost-effective and limb saving in this high-risk population (SOE=A). Assessing sensation using the Semmes-Weinstein monofilament and monitoring reflex changes help the clinician to assess the risk of development of ulcers and to help prevent ulcers in patients with diabetes. Reducing excessive pressure, shock, and shear by accommodating, stabilizing, and supporting deformities by weight diffusion and dispersion is also important in ulcer prevention (SOE=C). Early intervention of high-risk feet with proper shoes and foot care reduces complications as demonstrated in the LEAP (Lower Extremity Amputation Prevention) program and Medicare LOPS (Loss of Protective Sensation) program.

When prevention fails and an ulcer develops, the history should focus on duration, inciting event or trauma, prior ulcerations, previous attempts at wound care, and use of pressure off-loading procedures. The examination should include an assessment of the location and depth of the ulcer, the presence of infection, ischemic or neuropathic changes, edema,

and the presence of a Charcot joint. Imaging should be performed to exclude osteomyelitis (SOE=B) and may include plain radiography, CT, technetium bone scans, indium scans, and MRI. Noninvasive vascular studies include Doppler and transcutaneous oxygen tension. Consultation with a vascular specialist may be needed when vascular insufficiency is severe or the wounds are nonhealing. See "Pressure Ulcers and Wound Care," p 283.

The general principles of management include debridement, pressure relief, off-loading, avoidance or limitation of weight bearing, proper dressings, management of infection with antibiotics, management of ischemia, medical management of comorbidities, and hospitalization and surgical management when necessary. Weight bearing can be modified by the use of crutches and wheelchairs as well as contact casts, walkers, boots, braces, total contact orthotics, modified surgical shoes and boots, and appropriate dressings. A wide variety of dressings and topical agents are available; selection is guided by the nature of the ulcer and its complications. Topical agents include saline, antiseptics, topical antibiotics, enzymes, growth factors, and dermal skin substitutes. Vacuum-assisted closure and hyperbaric oxygen chambers can also aid in the closure of difficult-to-heal wounds in patients with diabetes (SOE=B). Empiric antibiotic therapy should be started early when there is a suspicion of infection. With osteomyelitis or limb-threatening infection, hospitalization is usually indicated. The choice of antibiotic is based on the clinical symptoms, culture and sensitivity, and the presence of deep infection, bone exposure, or sepsis, as well as whether soft tissue or bone is infected (SOE=B).

Peripheral Arterial Disease

Older adults with peripheral arterial disease demonstrate many of the same signs and symptoms as those with diabetes mellitus. In contrast to neuropathic ulcers, vascular ulcers are extremely painful. See "Cardiovascular Diseases and Disorders," p 360.

Arthritis

Osteoarthritis is common in older adults. It occurs in weight-bearing joints and causes pain, swelling, stiffness, limitation of movement, and deformity. It may be worsened by chronic trauma, strain, or obesity. Gouty arthritis is monoarticular and is most common in the first metatarsal phalangeal joint. It results early in intense pain and erythema and later in joint damage.

Rheumatoid arthritis affects the hands and feet equally and is usually symmetric in its presentation.

It can also result in muscle wasting and marked deformity. The metatarsal phalangeal joints become dislocated or subluxed; there is increased protrusion of the metatarsal heads, and walking becomes painful.

If conservative treatment with orthotics and special shoes do not relieve the pain, surgery may help to allow less painful ambulation. See "Musculoskeletal Diseases and Disorders," p 443.

ACOVE-3* QUALITY INDICATORS PERTAINING TO DISEASES AND DISORDERS OF THE FOOT

Diabetic foot examination

■ If a vulnerable older adult has diabetes mellitus, then a foot examination should be performed annually.

*Assessing Care of Vulnerable Elders – 3ʳᵈ Set. See inside front cover for explanation.

REFERENCES

■ Bowker JH, Pfeifer MA. *Levin and O'Neal's The Diabetic Foot.* 7th ed. St. Louis, MO: Mosby; 2007.

■ Menz HB. *Foot Problems in Older People: Assessment and Management.* Philadelphia, PA: Churchhill Livingstone; 2008.

CHAPTER 57—NEUROLOGIC DISEASES AND DISORDERS

KEY POINTS

■ Cerebrovascular disease is a leading cause of disability and death among older adults.

■ Control of systolic hypertension is the most important factor in preventing stroke.

■ Common causes of late-life seizures include vascular disease, new mass lesions, and withdrawal of alcohol or medications.

■ Parkinson's disease may be recognized by an insidious onset of asymmetric tremor or muscular rigidity.

The number of disorders that affect the nervous system increases rapidly with advancing age. Subtle neurologic abnormalities often are detected on examination. In one study of nearly 500 older adults, the following signs were found that could not be attributed directly to any specific medical or neurologic disease: diminished arm swing (present in 29% of those examined), diminished toe vibration sense (21%), hyperreflexia in arms (10%), unequal nasolabial folds (9%), absent pupillary response (9%), Babinski sign (7%), diminished toe position sense (7%), and decreased arm strength (5%). False findings imply that the diagnosis of significant neurologic disease may be more difficult in the setting of these "normal" signs. Still, a large percentage of older adults have neurologic disease, which causes a variety of impairments. The goal is to determine the significance of these abnormalities, to make an accurate diagnosis, and to implement appropriate treatment.

CEREBROVASCULAR DISEASES

Stroke is a leading cause of disability and death among older adults. A stroke occurs approximately every 40 seconds in the United States. The incidence of stroke increases with advancing age, approximately doubling with each decade. The incidence of stroke for men is 2.1 per 1,000 person-years at ages 55–64 yr, 4.5 per 1,000 person-years at ages 65–74 yr, and 9.3 per 1,000 person-years at ages 75–84 yr. The incidence of stroke for women is 25%–30% lower than that for men in comparable age groups, but it surpasses that of men ≥85 yr old.

Throughout the latter half of the 20th century, the incidence of stroke declined in the United States, Canada, and Western Europe. This drop may be attributable to better control of modifiable risk factors, including hypertension, heart disease, diabetes mellitus, cigarette smoking, increased blood lipids, and alcohol use. Hypertension is the most prevalent risk factor for stroke, and its treatment results in a substantially reduced risk of stroke. Treatment of isolated systolic hypertension in older adults reduces the risk of stroke by nearly 40% (SOE=A). (See "Hypertension," p 384.) Another important risk factor is heart disease, including atherosclerotic coronary heart disease, left ventricular hypertrophy, valvular heart disease, valve replacement, and valvular and nonvalvular atrial fibrillation. (See "Cardiovascular Diseases and Disorders," p 360.) Several studies have confirmed a 2- to 4-fold increased risk of stroke in individuals with diabetes mellitus (SOE=A). Studies suggest that tight control of blood-glucose levels might reduce the risk of stroke in individuals with diabetes mellitus, although the evidence for reduction of other vascular complications (eg, retinopathy, nephropathy) is somewhat more compelling. (See "Diabetes Mellius," p 504.) Additionally, aggressive treatment of hypertension and hyperlipidemia in this patient population is a crucial component in lowering the risk of stroke. Cigarette smoking independently increases the risk of stroke as much as 3-fold (SOE=A). The incidence of stroke declines significantly even after 2 yr of smoking cessation, and after 5 yr the level of risk returns to that of nonsmokers. Increased blood lipids and excessive alcohol use are other important risk factors for stroke.

Besides being the most common acute, serious neurologic disease, stroke is also a leading cause of death. Intracerebral hemorrhage carries a higher rate of morbidity and mortality than ischemic stroke. The fatality rate within 1 mo of an acute stroke is 20%–30% across all age groups; mortality is highest among older adults. Survival in part depends on the location and severity of the stroke. In ischemic stroke, the most important predictor is the severity of neurologic signs, which can be quantified after stroke by use of an instrument such as the NIH Stroke Scale (http://www.nihstrokescale.org). This severity scale has become widely used by physicians, nurses, and paramedics to describe the degree of impairment after stroke. In general, a score of <5 in this scale, which ranges from 0 to 42, is associated with a very good prognosis. Individuals with a score >20 have a very poor prognosis and a high likelihood of major complications. See "Rehabilitation," p 130.

Neurologic causes of death include the brain injury itself or resultant brain edema. Common medical causes of death are myocardial infarction, arrhythmia, heart failure, aspiration pneumonia, and pulmonary embolism. Age in itself does not influence the gross neurologic aspects of stroke, but older age is associated with lesser recovery in ADLs. Older stroke patients can benefit from formal rehabilitation.

STRENGTH-OF-EVIDENCE (SOE) RATING DEFINITIONS

A = consistent and good quality patient-oriented evidence
B = somewhat inconsistent or limited quality patient-oriented evidence
C = very inconsistent or very limited patient-oriented evidence, disease-oriented evidence, and/or consensus from professional organizations
D = unstudied common practice or opinion

See inside front cover for detailed information regarding the SOE classification.

Special consideration should be given to those suffering a transient ischemic attack (TIA). TIA is defined as a transient neurologic deficit lasting <24 hours due to focal brain or retinal ischemia. This definition is undergoing revision largely because of new imaging techniques and new insights into the pathophysiology of TIA. TIA is a medical emergency. This cohort of individuals represents those at highest risk of going on to develop acute stroke. Individuals with TIA have approximately 3 times the risk of developing ischemic stroke than those who have already suffered a stroke. In addition, nearly 50% of this risk occurs in the first 48 hours. These data emphasize the importance of careful monitoring of those suffering a TIA. Factors predictive of development of stroke after TIA are age, duration of symptoms, motor or speech symptoms, and presence of hypertension and/or diabetes. Treatment for patients with TIA is essentially the same as for patients with acute ischemic stroke, and treatment is specific to what is found during the evaluation. See treatment of acute ischemic stroke, p 466.

Internal Carotid Artery Disease

A lesion at the origin of the internal carotid artery, most commonly secondary to atherosclerosis, can lead to transient monocular blindness (ie, amaurosis fugax) or a cerebral hemispheric deficit (eg, focal motor, sensory, or cognitive symptoms or signs), because both the retina and cerebral hemispheres derive their blood supply from the internal carotid artery. Hemispheric deficits include hemiparesis or hemisensory loss, homonomous hemianopia, aphasia, or apraxia. The initial evaluation of patients with these symptoms or signs usually includes a neuroimaging study (CT or MRI) and noninvasive imaging of the carotid arteries (B-mode ultrasonography and Doppler ultrasonography or magnetic resonance angiography). For patients with ≥70% symptomatic stenosis, carotid endarterectomy significantly reduces subsequent stroke risk (number needed to treat [NNT]=15 over 2–6 yr of follow-up), provided that the patient has few comorbidities and that many endarterectomies are performed at the institution (SOE=A). Under these conditions, the surgery can be performed with reasonable safety in older adults provided that medical comorbidity is relatively low. Endovascular treatment with carotid artery angioplasty, stenting, and use of an emboli-protection device has been shown to demonstrate similar efficacy and safety, with less procedural morbidity, than endarterectomy for significant stenosis (SOE=B), making this procedure an attractive option in patients with significant comorbities (especially those at high risk of general anesthesia or with prior neck radiation exposure, prior carotid endarterectomy, or contralateral carotid occlusion). The optimal treatment for symptomatic carotid stenosis of <70% or of asymptomatic carotid stenosis is still not clear; treatment options include carotid endarterectomy, endovascular treatment, or medical management. Medical management should seek to optimize blood pressure, lipid status, and antiplatelet agents.

Aspirin is the mainstay of antiplatelet therapy for secondary atherosclerotic stroke prevention (SOE=A; relative risk reduction 15%–20%; NNT approximately 60 for prevention of one stroke over 1 yr of therapy). Studies on the use of aspirin in stroke prevention suggest that dosages >325 mg/d do not add therapeutic benefit, but the minimal necessary dosage has not been fully investigated. Many clinicians routinely prescribe 81–325 mg/d, although even the lower dosage can cause GI irritation and blood loss. When aspirin monotherapy is not sufficient, other platelet-inhibiting medications are widely prescribed. These can include sustained-release dipyridamole combined with aspirin. Clopidogrel 75 mg/d is an alternative for patients who cannot tolerate aspirin.

The only clear role for warfarin in primary or secondary stroke prevention is in the setting of cardioembolic disease. Two large trials (Warfarin-Aspirin Recurrent Stroke Study and Warfarin-Aspirin in Symptomatic Intracranial Disease) found no benefit in the use of warfarin over aspirin for secondary stroke prevention (SOE=A). Specific indications for warfarin include atrial fibrillation, severe valvular disease, and known intracardiac clot secondary to myocardial infarction.

Vertebrobasilar Arterial Disease

Syndromes associated with vascular lesions in the posterior circulation (ie, vertebral and basilar arteries) result in impairment of the cranial nerves, or dysfunction of the descending motor or ascending sensory tracks within the brain stem. Because of the large number of pathways passing through the brain stem, vertebrobasilar occlusion results in myriad signs, including abnormal eye movements; Horner's syndrome; unilateral or bilateral or crossed motor and sensory abnormalities in the face, arm, or leg; ataxia; dysarthria; dysphagia; and even stupor or coma. Because the thalamus and posterior portions of the cerebral hemispheres also are supplied by the vertebrobasilar system, behavioral and visual symptoms also can occur. Treatment of posterior circulation cerebrovascular disease is typically medical, but as new technology emerges endovascular therapies are a potential option (SOE=D).

Lacunar Disease

Lacunar disease secondary to occlusion of small penetrating vessels is presumably the consequence of lipohyalinosis (lipid deposition and hyalinization) or local arteriolosclerosis. Lacunar strokes can result in several well-defined syndromes, including pure motor hemiplegia, pure hemisensory stroke, ataxic hemiparesis, and dysarthria-clumsy hand syndrome. Risk factors include hypertension and diabetes mellitus. The most effective means of managing lacunar disease is aggressive treatment of these risk factors (SOE=B). Although aspirin is prescribed for stroke prevention in patients who have suffered lacunar strokes, it has not been shown to prevent lacunar strokes specifically. A large multicenter randomized controlled trial addressing this issue is ongoing as of Jan 2010. Lacunar strokes can occur independently or concurrently with large-vessel cerebrovascular disease.

Treatment of Acute Ischemic Stroke

The current protocol for care of the older stroke patient includes optimizing hydration status; controlling blood pressure while avoiding acute hypotension; preventing deep-vein thrombosis; detecting and treating coronary ischemia, heart failure, and cardiac arrhythmias; and starting long-term treatment with antiplatelet agents or oral anticoagulation to prevent recurrent stroke, depending on the presumed cause. Dehydration on presentation is common, but rehydration is usually gradual to reduce the risk of cerebral edema. In patients with clinically evident cerebrovascular disease immediately after an ischemic cerebral infarction, treatment of hypertension should be delayed (unless blood pressure is very high, eg, >220/120 mmHg) until the situation stabilizes. Even when treatment has been delayed temporarily, the eventual goal is to reduce blood pressure gradually (eg, a goal of 15% reduction over the first 24 hours) while avoiding orthostatic hypotension. The target systolic blood pressure should be 10–20 points higher than the baseline pressure; if the baseline is unknown, systolic pressure should not be lowered beyond 160 mmHg. Patients with acute ischemic stroke who are treated with thrombolytic agents require careful blood-pressure monitoring, especially during the first 24 hours of treatment. Patients with a history of ischemic heart disease or arrhythmia, and patients with large strokes should be monitored by electrocardiography for 48 hours. For large cardioembolic strokes (eg, involving most of the middle cerebral artery territory or involving both middle and anterior cerebral artery territories), anticoagulation therapy is usually not initiated until at least 48 hours after onset. Earlier anticoagulation does not improve outcome. Early initiation of aspirin[OL] therapy has a low risk of hemorrhagic adverse events and might modestly improve outcome.

The only medication approved by the FDA for ischemic stroke is recombinant tissue-plasminogen activator (rt-PA [alteplase]). Infusion of this medication within 3 hours of stroke onset approximately doubles the chances of a favorable outcome at 3 mo (SOE=A; very limited data in older adults). However, the benefits of rt-PA must be weighed against the increased risk of intracranial hemorrhage, which can be fatal or result in worsened neurologic status. Most hemorrhagic events occur among patients with severe strokes, and outcomes among patients with severe strokes are very poor without treatment. Use of rt-PA requires careful assessment by a physician experienced in the treatment of stroke. rt-PA should be considered in all patients who present within 3 hours of onset of neurologic deficit and in whom CT confirms the absence of intracranial hemorrhage. Major contraindications include major surgery within the previous 2 weeks, previous intracranial hemorrhage, sustained systolic blood pressure >185 mmHg or diastolic >110 mmHg, symptoms of subarachnoid hemorrhage, recent urinary or GI tract bleeding, coagulopathy, thrombocytopenia, or INR >1.7. The NIH Stroke Scale is helpful for stratifying ischemic stroke patients according to risk and benefit for rt-PA. Patients with scores <5 generally have a favorable outcome regardless of treatment; patients with scores >20 have a substantially increased rate of hemorrhagic complications. Although older adults experience higher rates of bleeding complications than those <65 yr old (SOE=A), the increased risk does not automatically preclude treatment. See also stroke rehabilitation in "Rehabilitation," p 136.

Intracerebral Hemorrhage

Intracerebral hemorrhage accounts for 15%–20% of all strokes. Approximately 80% occur between the ages of 40 and 70 yr. A racial distribution suggests that black Americans and Asian Americans may be at slightly higher risk than white Americans.

The most common risk factor for intracerebral hemorrhage is hypertension, which is present in 75%–80% of cases. Excessive use of alcohol is also associated with a higher incidence. Common locations for hypertensive bleeds are the putamen, thalamus, cerebellar hemisphere, pons, and cerebrum. In older adults, a common cause of cerebral lobar hemorrhage is cerebral amyloid angiopathy, which usually occurs without systemic amyloidosis. In these cases, intracranial bleeds tend to be recurrent. Hemorrhage can be complicated by the use of antiplatelet agents and anticoagulants. Other secondary causes of intracerebral hemorrhage should not be overlooked; these include trauma, arteriovenous malformations, and aneurysms. Acute treatment is supportive, with interim control of severe hypertension and discontinuation of antithrombotic medication. Large lobar or

intraventricular hemorrhages can be considered for neurosurgical drainage.

The decision to restart anticoagulation or antiplatelet medications after intracerebral hemorrhage can be difficult. It depends on many factors, including but not limited to, the reason the medications were started, the cause of the hemorrhage, the risk of future ischemic events, and the neurologic state of the patient. In those at high risk of future ischemic cerebrovascular events, such as those with mechanical valve replacement and those with atrial fibrillation and prior stroke, restarting anticoagulation 7–10 days after hemorrhage appears to be safe (SOE=B).

SUBDURAL HEMATOMA

A subdural hematoma is a collection of blood between the dura and the arachnoid. It is usually due to head trauma, although the trauma may be mild, particularly in older adults. In approximately 15% of cases, the hematomas are bilateral.

Perhaps most relevant in older adults is the chronic subdural hematoma. The incidence of chronic subdural hematoma increases with age, from 0.13 per 100,000 person-years for those in their 20s to 7.4 per 100,000 person-years for those in their 70s. In 50% of chronic subdural hematomas, there is no history of head injury, although other risk factors include clotting disorders, shunting procedures (eg, ventriculoperitoneal shunting for normal-pressure hydrocephalus separating the blood vessels from the dura, resulting in tears), and seizures.

The symptoms of chronic subdural hematoma are headache, slight or severe cognitive impairment, and hemiparesis. Some individuals may have seizures. Focal neurologic signs (eg, weakness, sensory loss, and change in sensation) can be present. Neuroimaging studies reveal an extra-axial collection of blood.

Treatment varies depending on whether the hematoma is symptomatic or an incidental finding on a neuroimaging study. If symptomatic and the patient's condition is worsening, then removal of the clot may be attempted. If asymptomatic or if the patient's condition is improving, then clinical monitoring is appropriate, because the hematoma may resolve without surgery.

HEADACHES

There is evidence to suggest that the prevalence of headaches diminishes with age. One study demonstrated that although 74% of men and 92% of women between the ages of 21 and 34 yr have headaches, these proportions drop to 22% and 55% after the age of 75 yr. Headache is one of the most common medical complaints in young persons, and yet one study suggests that it is the tenth most common symptom in older women and the fourteenth most common symptom in older men. Headache incidence also declines with age; only 2% of all sufferers of an initial migraine are >50 yr old.

Persistent headaches are more likely to represent systemic or intracranial lesions (ie, nonbenign conditions) in older adults than in younger adults. In one study, 10% of headaches among younger patients represented systemic or intracranial lesions; in older adults, this proportion was 34%. These nonbenign conditions include intracranial masses (eg, primary or secondary tumors, subdural hematomas), cervical spondylosis, COPD, carbon monoxide poisoning, and giant cell arteritis. In addition, many commonly used medications can cause headaches that are dull, diffuse, and nondescript, including vasodilators (eg, nitrates), antihypertensives (eg, reserpine, atenolol, and methyldopa), antiparkinsonian agents, and stimulants.

One secondary cause of headache specific to older adults is giant cell (temporal) arteritis. This disease does not appear to develop in those <50 yr old and peaks in incidence between the ages of 70 and 80. Women are affected twice as often as men. Pain may be centered at the temporal or occipital arteries. Palpation of the scalp arteries may reveal focal tenderness and nodularity. Complaints of visual changes, low-grade fever, polymyalgia, and constitutional symptoms further suggest the diagnosis. See giant cell arteritis and temporal arteritis in "Musculoskeletal Diseases and Disorders," p 446, for information regarding diagnosis and treatment of this condition.

The common primary headache disorders can be classified into migraines (with or without aura) and tension-type headaches. Migraines are often unilateral, pulsating headaches of moderate or severe intensity associated with nausea, vomiting, or photophobia. Auras, when they occur, usually precede the headache and are manifested by transient neurologic symptoms that can be localized to the cerebral cortex or brain stem. Visual phenomena are among the most common types of auras. In contrast to migraines, tension-type headaches are often more diffuse, have a pressing or a tight quality, and are much less associated with nausea or vomiting.

Headaches in older adults can present as they do in younger people, as described above, or in atypical ways. With migraines in particular, auras tend to disappear with age, and in some individuals the headaches disappear while auras remain. The occurrence of an isolated visual or sensory aura in the absence of a headache can be diagnostically challenging in the sense that these symptoms can be signs of transient ischemic attacks as well.

The treatment of headaches can be categorized as either abortive (ie, treating an attack that has already begun) or preventive. Apart from various OTC preparations, abortive therapies include ergotamines or triptans (eg, sumatriptan), which act by central serotonergic mechanisms. These medications are mild vasoconstrictors and contraindicated in patients with uncontrolled hypertension, stroke, or coronary artery disease. Generally, safety data in geriatric populations are lacking. Preventive therapies include β-blockers (eg, propranolol, atenolol^{OL}), valproic acid, topiramate, tricyclic antidepressants^{OL}, and calcium channel blockers^{OL}. The choice of an agent should be guided by an effort to avoid adverse events and drug interactions.

Older adults may not tolerate headache medications as well as younger patients; moreover, a medication may be contraindicated by comorbidities or existing medication regimens. For example, β-blockers and tricyclic antidepressants, which are often used as preventive therapy, can be associated with lethargy or sedation.

MOVEMENT DISORDERS

A movement disorder can be defined simply as abnormal involuntary movements. These movements are not the result of weakness or sensory deficits; they are the result of dysfunction of the basal ganglia or the extrapyramidal motor system. Movement disorders can be classified as hyperkinesias (excessive movement) or hypokinesias (paucity of movement). A particular movement disorder (eg, Parkinson's disease) can be characterized by several types of involuntary movements (eg, tremor, bradykinesia). Several movement disorders are especially common among older adults.

Parkinson's Disease

Parkinson's disease is a progressive neurodegenerative disease in which cell death in the substantia nigra and consequent reduction in brain dopamine levels results in a constellation of signs, including tremor at rest, bradykinesia, rigidity, and postural instability. The pathologic hallmark of the disease is the Lewy body, an intracellular inclusion body found in the substantia nigra.

The incidence increases dramatically with age, and the prevalence among people in their 70s and 80s in the United States is approximately 200 cases per 100,000 (0.2%). The prevalence among those in their 70s and 80s in other countries (Iceland, India, Scotland, Australia) has been estimated to be even higher, approaching 1,000 to 2,000 per 100,000 (1% to 2%). The disease most commonly appears between the ages of 50 and 79 yr. In a small proportion of cases, the disease clusters within families and has a genetic basis. In a small number of these families, the disease has been linked to a region on the long arm of chromosome 4 that encodes the neuronal protein α-synuclein. In addition, environmental toxins (eg, manganese and pesticides) have been associated with some forms of the disease.

The disease begins insidiously and asymmetrically. The clinical manifestations include tremor, usually in one hand or sometimes in both, classically involving the fingers in a pill-rolling motion. The tremor (slow frequency, usually 3–5 Hz) is present at rest and usually decreases with active, purposeful movement. Muscular rigidity is usually readily evident on passive movement of a limb. Passive movement may demonstrate a smooth resistance or superimposed ratchet-like jerks (ie, cogwheel phenomenon). The term *bradykinesia* is often used to describe either a slowness in initiating movement (ie, a paucity of spontaneous movements) or movements themselves that are slow, and the term *freezing* is used to describe sudden interruption of movement. Other clinical features of Parkinson's disease may include the following:

- tachykinesia: the tendency for movements to become smaller and faster

- tachyphemia: the tendency to speak more and more rapidly until all the words run together into a mumble

- micrographia: the tendency to make loops that become smaller and tighter when drawing loops across a page, to exhibit handwriting that is very small

- festinating gait: taking steps that inadvertently quicken and become smaller

- impaired finger tapping: the amplitude of the tapping lessens and the movements become more rapid until the fingers seem stuck together

Postural abnormalities are evident in the standing and sitting positions, and an erect posture is not readily assumed or maintained. The head tends to fall forward on the trunk. The tendency to fall forward (propulsion) or backward (retropulsion) results from the loss of postural reflexes. Bradykinesia prevents the patient from stopping the fall, either by taking a step or moving the arms. The face can become mask-like, with lack of expression and diminished eye blinking.

Mood abnormalities, usually depression or anxiety, are common, as are cognitive impairment and dementia. These may severely restrict the medications that might be used to relieve the tremor, bradykinesia, and rigidity.

Patients with parkinsonism can present for a multitude of reasons, but the most common are tremor and gait instability. Distinguishing between the parkinsonian resting tremor and other types of tremor

such as essential tremor can be at the crux of making the diagnosis. Another early diagnostic challenge may be distinguishing mild early parkinsonism from the changes that can accompany aging (eg, slowing down, loss of balance, stiffness, difficulty walking, stooped posture). However, the bradykinesia and rigidity of Parkinson's disease are usually asymmetric at onset, with one side slightly affected and the other remaining normal. In addition, tremor at rest is not a feature of normal aging, and although older adults may complain of stiffness, true extrapyramidal rigidity is otherwise uncommon.

The diagnosis is made clinically by demonstrating the classic features described above and excluding other possible causes. Neuroimaging should be considered in atypical presentations such as the abrupt onset of tremor, focal weakness, sensory disturbances, or reflex abnormalities not attributed to muscle tone asymmetry. Falls early in the course of the disease may alert the physician to one of the Parkinson's plus syndromes (see multiple system atrophy, below), as opposed to idiopathic Parkinson's disease.

Once the diagnosis is made, treatment programs are multifactorial and must be individualized. Treatment of Parkinson's disease is truly an art. Nonpharmacologic therapy includes a regular exercise program. Many older adults benefit from a course of physical therapy aimed at restoring their confidence in walking and maintaining balance, as well as being taught simple tips to help manage unpredictable and disabling freezing episodes, and when needed, how to select a cane or walker of the appropriate size and weight. A home visit by an occupational therapist can help to plan the appropriate placement of wall rails, grab bars, and other such assistive devices that reduce the possibility of falling. Across all settings, a function-focused care approach is needed to help patients with Parkinson's disease maintain and optimize their function and avoid the tendency caregivers have to take over care.

For patients with milder disease and no signs of dementia, dopamine agonists may be used initially as monotherapy. A cautious induction period with each is required, because nausea, orthostatic hypotension, and confusion are common adverse events. Dopamine agonists include ropinirole (given in starting dosages of 0.25 mg/d and increased as needed to dosages of 3 mg/d) and pramipexole (given in starting dosages of 0.125 mg/d and increased as needed to dosages of 4.5 mg/d).

Selegiline is another agent that has been used as early monotherapy. It acts to inhibit monoamine oxidase B (MAO-B), one of the enzymes responsible for dopamine breakdown. Selegiline in dosages of 5 mg twice a day (8 am and noon) can delay the need for additional antiparkinsonian agents (SOE=B). However, whether selegiline slows the disease progression or just suppresses symptoms is controversial. Selegiline is generally well tolerated, although some patients can experience adverse events, including nausea, insomnia, confusion, anxiety, and feeling "revved up." Although chemically related to other monoamine oxidase inhibitors, selegiline does not require dietary restrictions. Rasagiline is a newer selective MAO-B inhibitor that has been approved by the FDA as early monotherapy or as adjunct therapy (SOE=A). In early safety trials, a larger incidence of melanoma was seen in the rasagiline group compared with that in the placebo group. It is unclear whether this is secondary to the drug or the disorder, given there is a higher incidence of melanoma in the idiopathic Parkinson's disease population. Routine dermatologic evaluations are recommended for all patients with idiopathic Parkinson's disease.

Amantadine, a medication particularly useful for treating tremor, is generally prescribed at 100 mg q8–12h. Its mild anticholinergic action appears to play a role in its antiparkinsonian effects. It also promotes dopamine release in the corpus striatum. Older adults taking amantadine can develop cognitive adverse events, including hallucinations.

The most effective treatment, considered the gold standard, of patients with Parkinson's disease is levodopa combined with carbidopa. Levodopa is converted to dopamine in both the CNS and the periphery via dopa decarboxylase. Peripheral conversion is reduced by combining levodopa with carbidopa (a dopa decarboxylase inhibitor), which does not cross the blood-brain barrier. This formulation decreases peripheral adverse events. Treatment usually begins with a half tablet of the 25/100 combination (ie, 25 mg carbidopa to 100 mg levodopa) q12–24h. Every 1–2 weeks, the dose can be increased by one-half to one tablet, to reach a dosage of one full tablet q8h, if needed and if adverse events are tolerable. If disabling bradykinesia, rigidity, postural instability, or tremor is still present, the dosage can be gradually increased further, with cautious observation of adverse events. Older adults, particularly if cognitively impaired, rarely tolerate levodopa at more than 1,000 mg/d. The controlled-release form (25/100 and 50/200) generally requires a slightly higher total daily dose.

Common adverse events of levodopa-carbidopa include nausea, abdominal cramping, orthostatic hypotension, and confusion. Treatment of the motor manifestations of parkinsonism is important, but many older adults also complain of difficulty with constipation and insomnia. Constipation is particularly bothersome to older patients taking levodopa, which tends to exacerbate the constipation associated with reduced levels of physical activity. Treatment includes a diet rich in fruit and fiber, prune and other juices, frequent consumption of liquids, and use of osmotic laxatives. Older Parkinson's disease patients with insomnia should also be given individualized treatment. Some patients wake up at night because of severe feelings of stiffness and malaise caused by low dopamine levels. Higher bedtime doses, or even sustained-release forms, of levodopa are appropriate. Patients can also experience insomnia because they are sleeping too much during the day, which can be an adverse event of levodopa therapy. In these cases, it may be important to reduce the dosage of levodopa and to correct the reversed sleep-wake cycle. Urinary urgency may be a feature of Parkinson's disease that can also cause frequent nighttime awakenings.

By approximately 5 yr of levodopa therapy, half of patients develop dyskinesias from the drug. The "on" phenomenon refers to periods of good function, albeit frequently accompanied by these dyskinesias. Also at this stage, levodopa will begin to lose efficacy over a shorter time period, requiring an increase in dosage frequency, referred to as the "off" phenomenon. This can result in frank freezing episodes. It is not clear whether this represents progression of the underlying disease process or loss of drug efficacy. However, because of this "on-off" phenomenon, other alternatives should be considered for initial therapy when the patient's remaining life expectancy is projected to be significantly >5 yr in an attempt to maximize drug efficacy.

When the "off" phenomenon becomes an issue, there are several potential solutions. Adjustments can be made to the dosing strength and frequency of levodopa-carbidopa therapy. Selegiline can be added if not already in use. Catechol-O-methyl-transferase (COMT) inhibitors can also be used as an adjunct to levodopa-carbidopa therapy. COMT inhibitors block peripheral breakdown of levodopa, thereby increasing bioavailability. Adverse events of these medications are similar to those of levodopa. Of note, tolcapone has a black box warning for fatal hepatotoxicity and requires monitoring of liver function tests every 2–4 weeks for the first 6 mo of therapy. This hepatotoxicity has not been observed with entacapone and, therefore, its use does not require monitoring.

Surgical options can be considered for Parkinson's disease patients who have symptoms that cannot be controlled by medical therapies. Deep brain stimulation (DBS) of the globus pallidus or subthalamic nucleus is most effective for patients who have fluctuating tremor and dyskinesias, despite medical therapy, and who have few comorbidities. DBS significantly increases "on" time and decreases troubling dyskinesias (SOE=B). Complications of DBS include surgical site infection, intracranial hemorrhage, death (about 1%), cognitive and speech problems, and an increased risk of falls (SOE=B).

A major factor influencing the treatment of older adults with Parkinson's disease is their propensity to develop confusion and psychosis on antiparkinsonian medications. In general, the therapeutic regimen should be kept simple. Rather than small dosages of multiple medications, higher dosages of one or two medications is less likely to result in toxic adverse events. Levodopa provides the most improvement in the motor manifestations of Parkinson's disease relative to its toxic effects on the CNS, whereas medications with anticholinergic properties (eg, trihexyphenidyl, amantadine) provide the least benefit. The dopamine agonists (bromocriptine, ropinirole, pramipexole) fall in between. Although psychosis can be treated effectively with clozapine or quetiapine, which have fewer extrapyramidal adverse events than other antipsychotic agents, confusion and disorientation can be treated more simply by lowering the dosages of antiparkinsonian medications. In this setting, anticholinergic medications should be the first to be discontinued, followed by selegiline, dopamine agonists, and finally levodopa.

All dopamine agonists, and to a lesser extent levodopa, have been associated with sudden sleep attacks in which patients may fall asleep abruptly while driving. Additionally, all these medications have been associated with compulsive behaviors such as gambling. Patients should be warned of these rare but potentially serious adverse events related to therapy, and clinicians should ask about these behaviors during routine follow-up visits.

Multiple System Atrophy

A histopathologic understanding of three parkinsonian syndromes—olivopontocerebellar atrophy, Shy-Drager syndrome, and striatonigral degeneration—has permitted these overlapping syndromes to be included within the rubric of multiple system atrophy (MSA). Sometimes called a *Parkinson's plus disease*, MSA is characterized by parkinsonism (ie, rigidity, tremor, bradykinesia, and postural instability) plus autonomic symptoms, cerebellar signs, and sometimes myoclonus. Other features that can accompany MSA are upper motor signs, severe dysarthria, stridor, dystonia, and an amyotrophic lateral sclerosis (ALS)–like condition. The diagnosis is clinical, and MSA can initially be indistinguishable from idiopathic Parkinson's disease. A key feature, however, that can help differentiate between MSA and idiopathic Parkinson's disease is a limited, less robust response in MSA patients to levodopa-carbidopa therapy, especially in terms of the tremor. The mean age of onset for MSA is 55 yr; it is slightly more common in men, and it progresses to death in approximately 7 yr on average.

Autonomic symptoms are often the first to allow MSA to be differentiated from Parkinson's disease. Patients complain of dizziness, lightheadedness, or syncope on standing, and of postexertional weakness, gait unsteadiness, and dimming of vision. Impaired temperature control, reduced sweating, sphincter disturbance with urinary or fecal incontinence, diarrhea, constipation, impotence, iridic atrophy, impaired eye movements, Horner's syndrome, and anisocoria can also be seen.

Orthostatic hypotension is often the most disabling symptom. Nonpharmacologic treatment of the autonomic dysfunction includes eating small meals, getting up slowly, and avoiding excessive straining during bowel movements. Compressive clothing and elastic stockings, increased salt and fluid intake, and sleeping in a reverse Trendelenburg position can ameliorate some of the orthostatic symptoms. Medications that are sometimes useful in treating the orthostatic hypotension include midodrine and fludrocortisone[OL]. Use of these medications occasionally results in supine hypertension, which requires close blood-pressure monitoring. Levodopa can initially help the rigidity, bradykinesia, and postural instability. Unfortunately, dopamine replacement often worsens the orthostatic hypotension. Falls, another common problem for these patients, are exacerbated by orthostatic hypotension. A plan of care to optimize function and prevent falls is critical.

Progressive Supranuclear Palsy

Progressive supranuclear palsy accounts for approximately 4% of cases of parkinsonism. It is marked by supranuclear gaze palsy, square wave jerks (defined below), and cognitive impairment. Onset is usually during the late 50s or early 60s. The pathogenesis is unknown. The disease usually progresses rapidly, with marked incapacity occurring within 3–5 yr and death within 10 yr, generally as a result of intercurrent infection or other complications of immobility.

Progressive supranuclear palsy derives its name from progressive impairments of voluntary gaze. Most patients develop eye movement restrictions at approximately year 4 of the disease course. Patients are unable to voluntarily look downward or upward (upward gaze is less severely involved). Limitation of voluntary gaze is termed *supranuclear*. Because the vestibular nuclei are still able to direct eye movements, when the examiner abruptly tips the head, the eyes can be driven to look downward or upward. In addition to gaze palsy, patients with progressive supranuclear palsy often exhibit macro-square wave jerks. During fixation, small brief saccadic-appearing eye movements occur every few seconds. These eye movements are involuntary and give the appearance of scanning eye movements around a small target.

As the disease progresses, its appearance differentiates from that of idiopathic Parkinson's disease. Resting tremor is usually mild, and the rigidity is more pronounced at the neck and trunk. Axial rigidity is often striking, so that the neck is hyperextended and contracted facial muscles bear an expression of sustained surprise. Gait is disturbed early in the course, and falls are frequent in most patients. Cognition is often affected, with personality changes, impaired judgment, and sometimes inappropriate laughing and crying. Unlike in MSA, other than urinary incontinence, autonomic dysfunction is atypical.

No fully effective treatment is available. Treatment with levodopa may partially reduce the rigidity, although the dramatic response to levodopa that is experienced by patients with Parkinson's disease is usually lacking. Generally, any improvement is transient.

Chorea

Chorea is a flowing, continuous, random movement that flits from one part of the body to another. A variety of conditions are associated with chorea in older adults. The pathologic basis for chorea is dysfunction of the striatum.

Choreiform movements that sometimes occur as an isolated symptom in adults ≥60 yr old are termed *senile chorea*. Involuntary complex movements of the face, mouth, and tongue can occur alone or with unilateral or bilateral limb movements. Neither mental disturbance nor family history of Huntington's chorea is associated with senile chorea. Pathologic findings often include degeneration of the putamen or caudate nucleus, or both.

Chorea can be treated with dopamine-receptor blocking medications (eg, haloperidol^{OL}), but a potential adverse effect is tardive dyskinesia. Agents that block the release of dopamine presynaptically (eg, reserpine^{OL}) are another option, and they are not associated with tardive dyskinesias; however, reserpine can be associated with depression and orthostatic hypotension. Metyrosine^{OL} inhibits the enzyme tyrosine hydroxylase, which catalyzes the conversion of tyrosine to dihydroxyphenylalanine. Therefore, metyrosine blocks the formation of dopamine and can be effective in treating chorea. Although not associated with tardive phenomena, metyrosine^{OL} can cause somnolence. All of these medications can produce parkinsonism as an adverse event, which is usually dose dependent and reversible when the medication is discontinued.

Drug-Induced Movement Disorders

Several different types of involuntary movements can arise as a result of the use of medications. It is important to distinguish among effects of medications that are acute, chronic but reversible, and chronic and irreversible. One acute effect that can occur with antipsychotic medications is an acute dystonic reaction resulting in oral, lingual, or nuchal dystonia. If the dystonia is severe enough, treatment with intravenous diphenhydramine or lorazepam may be required, although this approach in older adults should be exercised with caution, given the propensity of these agents to produce somnolence or confusion. Fortunately, acute dystonia occurs less frequently in older than in younger adults. Chronic reversible drug effects (effects that resolve when the causative medication is discontinued) include action tremor (eg, lithium, theophylline, valproic acid), parkinsonism (eg, antipsychotic, antiemetic medications), chorea (eg, estrogen, antiepileptic medications), or dystonia (dopamine replacement therapy in Parkinson's disease). Chronic irreversible drug effects or tardive phenomena often begin after the medication (usually an antipsychotic medication) has been used for weeks to months. Movements can include orobuccal dyskinesias, dystonia, akathisia (sensation of needing to move), myoclonus, and tics. Advanced age and duration of treatment with antipsychotic medications are the only well-established risk factors for developing tardive movement disorders. Once the diagnosis of a tardive phenomenon is established, the dosage of medication should be reduced or the medication should be discontinued. Treatment for tardive dyskinesia or tardive dystonia includes anticholinergic agents (eg, trihexyphenidyl), baclofen^{OL}, reserpine^{OL}, or clozapine^{OL}, each of which must be used with caution in older adults. In cases of severe tardive dystonia in which there is neck jerking or sustained eye closure, intramuscular injections of botulinum toxin^{OL} can reduce the frequency and severity of movements.

Essential Tremor

Essential tremor is the most common form of abnormal tremor. The tremor is an action tremor, which is present when the limbs are in active use (eg, while writing or holding a cup). The tremor most commonly involves the arms, although the head and voice are often involved also. Other areas of the body that can be affected include the chin, tongue, and legs. The tremor is often slightly worse in one arm than in the other. One of the striking features of the tremor is that it has a varying amplitude so that during some moments, the tremor is mild or even absent and during others it is severe. The tremor disappears when the arms are relaxed, ie, when the person is sitting with hands in the lap or when standing or walking with arms held at the sides. Functionally, the tremor can interfere with many daily activities, such as eating, writing, or fastening buttons. Stress or anxiety can exacerbate the tremor. The frequency of the tremor is in the 4–12 Hz range; because age is inversely related to the frequency of the tremor, older adults have slower tremor, often in the range of 4–8 Hz.

The prevalence of the disorder increases with advancing age, with as many as 1%–5% of adults ≥60 yr old affected. The age of onset seems to have a bimodal distribution, with peaks in the teens and 20s and in the 50s through the 70s. The prevalence rates among men and women are similar, although head tremor may be more common among women.

Between 17% and 100% of affected individuals report having an affected relative, which suggests that there is a familial form of the tremor. In some families, many individuals are affected over several generations. Familial forms of the tremor have been linked to regions on chromosomes 2p and 3q. The familial and sporadic forms of essential tremor have no apparent clinical differences. The cause of the sporadic form of the illness is not known; age is the only known risk factor for essential tremor.

Distinguishing essential tremor from several other conditions can be difficult. Physiologic tremor, which is present in all people, varies in amplitude, and it may be more noticeable in some individuals. It can also be enhanced by anxiety, stimulants, hypoglycemia, medications, or certain illnesses (eg, hyperthyroidism). The tremor is often faster than that of essential tremor (8–12 Hz), and the amplitude lower. Although those with Parkinson's disease most typically have a tremor at rest, they may also have an action tremor. In addition, if essential tremor is severe enough, it may even be present at rest. However, other features of Parkinson's disease (eg, bradykinesia and rigidity) should not be present in individuals with essential tremor.

The main indications for treatment of essential tremor are embarrassment and disability. The latter can manifest itself either as difficulty performing certain tasks (eg, eating and writing), modifying the way the task is performed (eg, drinking only with a straw out of closed cups), and even avoiding certain tasks. It is important to educate the patient on exacerbating factors such as caffeine and other stimulants, as well as on stress and fatigue. Initial pharmacologic therapy includes β-blocking agents (eg, propranolol, atenolol[OL]), primidone[OL], phenobarbital[OL], diazepam[OL], and newer agents, including gabapentin[OL] and topiramate[OL]. The response to these agents is variable (ie, some patients experience moderate improvement, whereas others experience none), and the tremor is rarely reduced to asymptomatic levels. Among these agents, a β-blocker or primidone would be considered first-line treatment in older adults (SOE=D). Some patients with severe, medically refractory tremor may undergo DBS. As previously stated, DBS in patients with Parkinson's disease has been shown to be effective in improving tremor, motor functioning, and quality of life but with an increased risk of serious adverse events (SOE=B).

EPILEPSY

A seizure is a paroxysmal excessive or a hypersynchronous cerebral neuronal discharge, or both, that results in a transient change in motor function, sensation, or mental state. Recurrent seizures are the defining feature of epilepsy. Depending on whether the seizure discharges involve only a portion of the cortex or the entire cortex, seizures are broadly classified as partial or generalized. Partial seizures are subdivided on the basis of whether or not the seizure is associated with impaired consciousness. Simple partial seizures do not impair consciousness and most often are associated with focal rhythmic motor twitching. Complex partial seizures are associated with altered consciousness and commonly amnesia for the event. Automatisms and other motor manifestations can occur with complex partial seizures. Generalized seizures in older adults are almost invariably convulsive ("grand mal").

New-onset seizures are seen in a bimodal pattern with respect to age, with an initial peak in incidence within the first year of life and a second peak after the age of 60 yr. Disease-specific causes of seizures are more common in older adults, and one-half or more of older adult patients with new-onset seizures have an underlying cause. Common causes include cerebrovascular disease, space-occupying lesions, brain trauma, alcohol withdrawal, and neurodegenerative diseases. Related to this is the observation that the incidence of partial seizures (which frequently have an underlying cause) increases in older adults, whereas the incidence of generalized tonic-clonic seizures (which are more often idiopathic) remains constant with respect to age. Beyond the age of 65 yr, approximately one-half of new-onset cases of seizures have a complex partial pattern. This pattern can be explained by the greater incidence of underlying focal lesions in older age groups.

Because of this propensity for new-onset cases of seizures to be harbingers of focal lesions, the diagnostic evaluation of older adults to exclude an underlying treatable cause is particularly important. The neurologic history and examination should aim to clinically characterize the seizure and localize its source, as well as elicit other signs of a focal lesion or a metabolic disturbance (eg, uremia, hepatic failure). Blood studies (BUN; serum concentrations of sodium, glucose, magnesium, calcium; and liver function tests), MRI, and electroencephalography play important roles.

Once the appropriate evaluation is done, the decision to begin an anticonvulsant should not be taken lightly. More than 50% of people with a single unprovoked seizure do not have another. The presence of a focal brain abnormality, changes on an electroencephalogram (EEG), or a family history of epilepsy raises the likelihood of recurrence and should prompt consideration of pharmacologic therapy.

The treatment of epilepsy in older adults is particularly challenging. The prevalence of adverse drug-disease and drug-drug interactions increases with age. One example of a drug-disease interaction is that between anticonvulsants such as divalproex sodium and hepatic disease, given the tendency of divalproex and other anticonvulsants such as carbamazepine to exacerbate preexisting liver dysfunction, particularly in older adults. Caution should also be taken with the newer anticonvulsants levetiracetam and gabapentin in patients with renal failure.

In terms of drug-drug interactions, many of the anticonvulsant medications are metabolized via the cytochrome P450 system, especially the older agents phenytoin and carbamazepine. Before starting any new medication in patients taking anticonvulsant agents, the possibility of an interaction should be investigated. Further, age-related changes in renal and hepatic function can alter drug metabolism significantly, so that older adults often need lower dosages of anticonvulsant medications. A sizable fraction of many anticonvulsant medications is bound to plasma proteins. Because aging decreases albumin synthesis, free (unbound) levels of anticonvulsant medications (eg, phenytoin) may need to be monitored. Older adults can be particularly sensitive to adverse events of medications. For example, anticonvulsant medications can intensify an underlying dementia or exacerbate mild cognitive decline. A clinical pharmacist can help resolve complex issues of drug interactions, dosages, and adverse events. Finally, older adults may have difficulty with adherence for a variety of reasons. It is particularly important when treating older adults to involve caregivers so that the goals of the treatment, adverse events, and monitoring of progress are understood.

Most anticonvulsant medications are started slowly and the dosages increased gradually (Table 57.1). Reduction in seizure frequency and severity and the onset of adverse events, and not the serum concentration of the medication, should be used to gauge the effects of the medication. If monotherapy has not adequately controlled the seizures and the dosage has been maximized, then monotherapy with another agent should be tried before resorting to combination therapy. The common causes of breakthrough seizures in individuals known to be epileptic are infections, metabolic disturbances, sleep deprivation, and medication noncompliance. Rarely, partial seizures can present in nonconvulsive status epilepticus (NCSE). This is defined as continuous electrical seizure activity without outward convulsion. After a seizure, it is important to distinguish between NCSE and a postictal state. If a patient is not improving gradually or is demonstrating focal neurologic signs such as eye deviation or nystagmus, evaluation with an EEG to exclude NCSE is warranted. An EEG is also warranted in the routine evaluation of a delirious patient with no obvious cause or who does not improve after the proposed underlying cause has been treated.

Surgery for epilepsy has become an increasingly common choice of patients whose seizures have proved refractory to pharmacologic management. The utility of surgery in older adults is not known. Discontinuing anticonvulsant medications should be considered if the patient has not had a seizure for several years, particularly if the original seizure activity was a single or poorly characterized event.

MOTOR NEURON DISEASE

Amyotrophic lateral sclerosis (ALS) is a neurodegenerative condition involving the cell bodies of both upper and lower motor neurons; it is characterized clinically by a progressive weakness and wasting of skeletal muscles, often in combination with bulbar palsy and respiratory failure. The incidence increases with age but reaches a plateau in the 60s. To date, age remains the single most clearly identifiable risk factor for this progressive and fatal disorder.

Patients commonly present with gait disturbance, falls, foot drop, weakness in grip, dysphagia, or dysarthria. On neurologic examination, patients may have a combination of upper motor neuron signs (eg, hyperreflexia, clonus, extensor plantar responses) and lower motor neuron signs (eg, weakness, atrophy, fasciculations). Although cranial nerves can be involved, with weakness of the face, tongue, and palate, the extraocular muscles are usually spared. The electromyogram demonstrates findings consistent with diffuse denervation (ie, diffuse fibrillation potentials, positive sharp waves) and poor recruitment of motor units. The differential diagnosis includes lesions at the level of the foramen magnum or the high cervical cord and vitamin B_{12} deficiency. The prognosis is poor, with survival time averaging 2–3 yr. The presence of bulbar signs carries a poorer prognosis.

Although most new cases of ALS are in older adults, the incidence and prevalence of ALS relative to other more common neurologic disorders is low. Therefore, gait disturbance and focal motor weakness may be attributed to the more common cerebrovascular diseases or to cervical radiculomyelopathy rather than to ALS. Older adults are also more likely to have coexisting neuropathology, adding to the challenge of and delay in diagnosing ALS. In one

Table 57.1—Anticonvulsant Therapy in Older Adults

Medication	Dosage (mg)	Target Blood Level (mcg/mL)	Comments (Metabolism, Excretion)
Carbamazepine	200–600 q12h	4–12	Many drug interactions, mood stabilizer, may cause SIADH, thrombocytopenia, leukopenia (L, K)
Gabapentin	300–600 q8h	NA	Used as adjunct to other agents, adjust dosage on basis of CrCl (K)
Lamotrigine	100–300 q12h	2–4	Prolongs PR interval; risk of severe, potentially fatal rash that depends on speed of titration (risk vitually disappears with slow titration); when used with valproic acid, begin at 25 mg q48h, titrate to 25–100 mg q12h (L, K)
Levetiracetam	500–1,500 q12h	NA	Reduce dosage in renal impairment: CrCl 30–50 mL/min: 250–750 q12h CrCl 10–29 mL/min: 250–500 q12h CrCl <10 mL/min: 500–1,000 q24h
Oxcarbazepine	300–1,200 q12h	NA	Can cause hyponatremia, leukopenia (L)
Phenobarbital	30–60 q8–12h	20–40	Many drug interactions; not recommended for use in older adults (L)
Phenytoin	200–300 q24h	5–20*	Many drug interactions; exhibits nonlinear pharmacokinetics (L)
Pregabalin	50–200 q8–12h	NA	Indicated as adjunct therapy for partial-onset seizures only; not well studied in older adults (K)
Tiagabine	2–12 q8–12h	NA	Adverse-event profile in older adults less well described (L)
Topiramate	25–100 q12–24h	NA	Can affect cognitive functioning at high dosages (L, K)
Valproic acid	250–750 q8–12h	50–100	Can cause weight gain, tremor, hair loss; several drug interactions; mood stabilizer; monitor liver function tests and platelets (L)
Zonisamide	100–400 q24h	NA	Anorexia; contraindicated in patients with sulfonamide allergy (K)

NOTE: SIADH = syndrome of inappropriate secretion of antidiuretic hormone; L = metabolized via liver; K = metabolized via kidneys; NA = not available; CrCl = creatinine clearance

*Phenytoin is extensively bound to plasma albumin. In cases of hypoalbuminemia or marked renal insufficiency, calculate adjusted phenytoin concentration (C):

$$C_{adjusted} = \frac{C_{observed} \text{ (mcg/mL)}}{0.2 \times \text{albumin (g/dL)} + 0.1}$$

If creatinine clearance <10 mL/min, use:

$$C_{adjusted} = \frac{C_{observed} \text{ (mcg/mL)}}{0.1 \times \text{albumin (g/dL)} + 0.1}$$

Obtaining a free phenytoin level is an alternative method of monitoring phenytoin in cases of hypoalbuminemia or marked renal insufficiency.

SOURCE: Adapted with permission from Reuben DB, Herr K, Pacala JT, et al. *Geriatrics At Your Fingertips*, 12th ed. New York: American Geriatrics Society; 2010.

study, those 65 yr old were diagnosed after 19 mo, while those <65 yr old were diagnosed after 3 mo.

Treatment is mostly supportive. Riluzole, which has demonstrated modest effects on survival or time to tracheostomy (SOE=A), is in widespread use. Riluzole is thought to protect against glutamate toxicity, which may be involved in the pathogenesis of ALS. Follow-up in a dedicated multidisciplinary ALS or muscular dystrophy clinic has also been shown to improve quality of life of ALS patients. In these settings, patients can receive multidisciplinary care from a team, including a neuromuscular subspecialist; a chaplain; and physical, occupational, and speech therapists.

MYELOPATHY

In older adults, myelopathy or spinal cord dysfunction is most often the result of compression of the spinal cord. The cervical region is affected most commonly. Intrinsic spinal cord lesions are often the result of

spinal cord tumors or vascular events (eg, infarcts or hemorrhages). Extrinsic compressive lesions are more prevalent; common causes among older adults are cervical spondylosis (with resultant osteophyte formation and degenerative disc disease), disc prolapse or herniation, rheumatoid arthritis resulting in vertebral body subluxation, or spinal metastases. Nearly 80% of adults ≥70 yr old have radiographic evidence of osteophyte formation with significant narrowing of the spinal canal; most are asymptomatic. Spinal stenosis is a congenital abnormally narrow spinal canal. When disc protrusion occurs in an individual with spinal stenosis, it further compromises the ability of a spinal canal that is already limited. Narrowing of the cervical canal can lead to neck stiffness and pain; radicular pain, sensory loss, or weakness in the arms; and weakness and upper motor neuron signs (eg, hyperreflexia, spasticity, Babinski sign) in the legs. Narrowing of the lumbar canal can lead to lower back pain; radicular pain, sensory loss, or weakness in the legs; and upper motor neuron signs in the legs. Other symptoms of spinal cord compression include gait disturbance, falls, or complaints of "numb, clumsy hands." On examination, the patient may exhibit spastic paraparesis (symmetric or asymmetric), sensory loss at a particular cord level, or problems with micturition.

MRI can be helpful for diagnosis, but results must be viewed with caution because abnormal MRI findings are common in asymptomatic older adults. If the patient cannot tolerate MRI due to the presence of metallic objects, a pacemaker, or severe claustrophobia, then spinal CT with intrathecal contrast can be performed.

Conservative management, particularly if neck pain is present, includes activity modification, neck immobilization with a cervical collar, massage, heat treatment, physical therapy, and medications (eg, muscle relaxants and pain medications, including NSAIDs). Decompressive surgery is recommended for persistent pain or a progressive neurologic deficit. Older adults are more prone to have multiple levels of involvement, and some studies have suggested the prognosis after surgery of older adults is poorer than that of younger patients. See also "Back and Neck Pain," p 450.

RADICULOPATHY

Radiculopathy results from compression of a spinal root as it exits the spinal cord. Among older adults, this can be the result of herniated discs or osteophyte formation. Symptomatic nerve root compression may result in complaints of pain radiating down the neck, back, arm, or leg, and on neurologic examination, this can be accompanied by motor and sensory deficits as well as by diminution of reflexes in the distribution of a particular spinal root or roots. See also "Back and Neck Pain," p 450.

PERIPHERAL NEUROPATHY

The prevalence of peripheral neuropathy in older adults has been estimated to be as high as 20%, and some degree of subclinical decrease in peripheral nerve function on electromyography is probably universal in healthy older adults. Peripheral neuropathy can be particularly devastating in older adults because of gait impairment due to sensory and motor deficits and thus a propensity to fall. In developed countries, diabetic neuropathy is the most common form of neuropathy; up to 60% of individuals who have diabetes mellitus and who are ≥60 yr old have a peripheral neuropathy. Several types of neuropathy are associated with diabetes mellitus, including a distal symmetric neuropathy; asymmetric neuropathies that may involve cranial nerves, roots, or plexus; and mononeuropathy multiplex. Other common causes of peripheral neuropathy in older adults are medications (eg, amiodarone, colchicine, phenytoin, lithium, vincristine, isoniazid), alcohol abuse, nutritional deficiencies (eg, vitamins B_6 and B_{12} deficiency, as well as deficiencies of thiamine, folate, and niacin), renal disease (ie, uremia), monoclonal gammopathy (eg, multiple myeloma), and neoplasia (eg, infiltration of peripheral nerves by malignant cells, paraneoplastic syndromes associated with small-cell carcinoma of the lung, breast cancer, ovarian cancer, renal cell carcinoma, and prostate cancer).

The history and physical examination are the most important tools in diagnosis of a peripheral neuropathy. Questions should be geared toward identifying possible causes and risk factors of the individual patient. If the patient is not overtly diabetic, risk factors for diabetes and possible insulin resistance should be assessed. The past history and review of systems can give clues to a systemic disease that could contribute to a peripheral nerve disorder. A history of gastric bypass, eating disorder, or hemodialysis could indicate a possible nutritional deficiency. A thorough medication history, including current medications, should be taken to look for possible causes. A social history can provide evidence of a possible toxic exposure, such as alcohol or an occupational exposure.

Electrodiagnostic studies are considered an extension of the neurologic examination. They can yield valuable information in classifying the neuropathy to help narrow a complicated differential diagnosis. First, they can differentiate between a single or multiple mononeuropathy or a polyneuropathy. Next, they can help classify a polyneuropathy as either axonal or demyelinating. This is important because certain neuropathies affect nerves in different ways. For instance, a diabetic neuropathy is predominantly an axonal neuropathy, as are many of the toxic neuropathies such as alcohol and heavy metal exposure. On the contrary, the hereditary neuropathies more commonly cause peripheral demyelination.

Treatment of the neuropathy depends on the underlying cause and ranges from withdrawal of the causative agent (eg, alcohol, medications) to nutritional supplementation (eg, in nutritional deficiency), or to treatment of the primary cancer (eg, neoplastic neuropathy). There is some evidence that optimizing glucose control can lessen the severity of diabetic neuropathy (SOE=C). Treatment of neuropathic pain includes the use of tricyclic antidepressants and anticonvulsant medications such as carbamazepine[OL], gabapentin[OL], and pregabalin[OL]. Gabapentin and pregabalin are approved for use in treatment of post-herpetic neuralgia, and pregabalin is also approved for use in diabetic neuropathy and fibromyalgia (SOE=A). Topical agents include capsaicin cream and local anesthetic medications.

Another option approved for use in diabetic neuropathy is the antidepressant duloxetine. Duloxetine is a serotonin-norepinephrine reuptake inhibitor in the same class as the antidepressant venlafaxine.

MYOPATHY

Myopathies are characterized by proximal muscle weakness, wasting, and diminished or absent reflexes. They can be accompanied by increases in serum enzymes (eg, creatine kinase) and a myopathic pattern on electromyogram and on muscle biopsy (ie, fiber degeneration that follows a random pattern). Older adults may attribute mild or moderate muscle weakness to aging and therefore may not immediately consult a physician. Proximal muscle weakness, which results in difficulty rising from a chair, climbing stairs, or washing hair, is particularly likely to be falsely attributed to aging or arthritis.

The most common myopathies in older adults are polymyositis, endocrine myopathies, toxic myopathies, and myopathies associated with carcinoma. Polymyositis, a disorder of skeletal muscle with diverse causes, is characterized by lymphocytic infil-tration of the muscles. Muscle biopsy usually shows signs of degeneration, regeneration, and infiltration by lymphocytes. Prednisone treatment should be used with caution in older adults because of its propensity to produce psychosis. In thyrotoxic myopathy, weakness and wasting are greatest in the pelvic girdle muscles and to some extent in the muscles of the shoulder region. Reflexes can be normal, and the diagnosis is based on the distribution of muscle weakness in an individual with thyrotoxicosis. The myopathy improves after the underlying endocrine disorder is treated. Hypothyroidism can also cause a myopathy that improves with thyroid replacement therapy. Myopathy can occasionally be the result of a remote effect of a cancer (ie, a paraneoplastic disorder), with complaints of weakness often preceding the establishment of the cancer diagnosis. Several medications cause myopathy, including corticosteroids, lipid-lowering agents, colchicine, procainamide, and diuretics that produce hypokalemia.

RESTLESS LEGS SYNDROME

See "Sleep Problems," p 276.

ACOVE-3* QUALITY INDICATORS PERTAINING TO NEUROLOGIC DISEASES AND DISORDERS

Carotid artery imaging
- If a vulnerable older adult has a new transient ischemic attack (TIA) or ischemic stroke in the vascular territory of the carotid artery, then a carotid artery imaging study should be done, or it should be documented that the patient is not a carotid procedure candidate.

Carotid endarterectomy
- If a vulnerable older adult has symptomatic carotid stenosis >70%, then the medical record should document a discussion of risks and benefits of carotid procedures or that the patient is not a candidate for a carotid procedure or that a carotid endarterectomy cannot be done with a less than 6%, 30-day morbidity and mortality rate.

Anticoagulate atrial fibrillation
- If a vulnerable older adult has chronic atrial fibrillation and is at medium to high risk of stroke, then anticoagulation should be offered.
- If a vulnerable older adult has chronic atrial fibrillation, medium to high risk of stroke, and has a contraindication to anticoagulation, then antiplatelet therapy should be prescribed.
- If a vulnerable older adult is prescribed anticoagulants for atrial fibrillation, then there should be documentation that the goal for the INR is 2–3 or reason for other goal.

Ischemic stroke prophylaxis
- If a vulnerable older adult has had a TIA or ischemic stroke, then outpatient antiplatelet or anticoagulant therapy should be prescribed within 3 mo after the stroke or TIA or entering a new practice.

Hyperlipidemia and stroke
- If a vulnerable older adult has a new TIA or ischemic stroke, then there should be documentation of a fasting low-density lipoprotein level.

Smoking cessation
- If a vulnerable older adult has a new TIA or stroke, then smoking status should be documented.
- If a vulnerable older adult has a TIA or stroke and is a current smoker, then smoking cessation counseling should be documented annually.

Exercise prescription
- If an ambulatory vulnerable older adult has had a TIA or stroke and is not physically active, then counseling to increase physical activity should be documented annually.

Alcohol misuse

- If a vulnerable older adult has a new TIA or stroke, then assessment of alcohol intake should be documented, and if positive for alcohol intake, alcohol intake should be reassessed annually.
- If a vulnerable older adult has a new TIA or stroke and consumes ≥5 drinks of alcohol per day, then he or she should be counseled to decrease consumption to <2 drinks per day, and this should be documented annually.

Hormone replacement therapy

- If a female vulnerable older adult has had a TIA or stroke and is taking hormone replacement therapy, then hormone replacement therapy should be discontinued or a reason (other than stroke prevention) documented.

Education about stroke

- If a vulnerable older adult presents with a new TIA or stroke, then education of the patient (or caregiver) about stroke symptoms and risk factors should be documented within 6 mo.

Early aspirin therapy

- If a vulnerable older adult is hospitalized with a new acute ischemic stroke, then aspirin should be given within 48 hours (if not already on anticoagulant therapy).

Thrombolytic therapy

- If a vulnerable older adult is hospitalized with an acute stroke and inclusion and exclusion criteria are met, then thrombolytic therapy should be offered.
- If a vulnerable older adult with a new stroke is started on intravenous tissue plasminogen activator for thrombolysis, then inclusion and exclusion criteria should be met.
  - *Inclusion criteria*
    - Clinical diagnosis of stroke with meaningful deficit
    - Baseline CT scan with no intracranial hemorrhage
    - Stroke onset <180 minutes before treatment
  - *Exclusion criteria*
    - Minor or rapidly improving symptoms
    - CT signs of intracranial hemorrhage
    - History of intracranial hemorrhage, seizure at stroke onset, arterial puncture at noncompressible site or lumbar puncture within 1 week, major surgery or serious trauma within 2 weeks, GI or urinary tract hemorrhage within 3 weeks
    - Systolic blood pressure >185 mmHg, diastolic blood pressure >110 mmHg, or aggressive treatment required to lower blood pressure
    - Laboratory values: glucose <50 mg/dL or >400 mg/dL; platelet count <100,000/uL, heparin therapy within 48 hours with associated increased partial thromboplastin time, current anticoagulant therapy with INR >1.7
    - Clinical presentation suggesting postmyocardial infarction pericarditis

Depression evaluation

- If a vulnerable older adult presents with a new stroke, then presence or absence of depression should be documented within 3 mo.

Speech therapy

- If a vulnerable older adult presents with a new stroke and has resulting language difficulties, then a referral for speech therapy should be made within 1 mo.

Dysphagia documentation

- If a vulnerable older adult presents with a new stroke, then presence or absence of dysphagia should be documented in the hospital record.

Rehabilitation for functional deficits

- If a vulnerable older adult presents with a new stroke, then on discharge the patient should have a rehabilitation plan or documentation of no residual functional deficit from the new stroke.

Related quality indicators for Neurologic Diseases and Disorders

- Alimentation for patients who cannot eat, approach to dysphagia (see "Eating and Feeding Problems," p 203)
- Nutrition for malnourished patients (see "Malnutrition," p 195)
- Stroke prophylaxis for vascular dementia (see "Dementia," p 245)
- Antiplatelet therapy for patients with coronary artery disease, warfarin education, and monitoring (see "Cardiovascular Diseases and Disorders," p 360)

*Assessing Care of Vulnerable Elders – 3rd Set. See inside front cover for explanation.

REFERENCES

■ Adams HP, del Zoppo G, Alberts MJ, et al. Guidelines for the Early Management of Adults With Ischemic Stroke: A Guideline From the American Heart Association/American Stroke Association Stroke Council, Clinical Cardiology Council, Cardiovascular Radiology and Intervention Council, and the Atherosclerotic Peripheral Vascular Disease and Quality of Care Outcomes in Research Interdisciplinary Working Groups: The American Academy of Neurology affirms the value of this guideline as an educational tool for neurologists. *Stroke.* 2007;38(5):1655–1711.

■ England JD, Gronseth GS, Franklin G, et al. Practice Parameter: evaluation of distal symmetric polyneuropathy: role of laboratory and genetic testing (an evidence-based review). Report of the American Academy of Neurology, American Association of Neuromuscular and Electrodiagnostic Medicine, and American Academy of Physical Medicine and Rehabilitation. *Neurology.* 2009:72(2):177–184.

■ Weaver FM, Follett K, Stern M, et al. Bilateral deep brain stimulation vs best medical therapy for patients with advanced Parkinson's disease: a randomized controlled trial. *JAMA.* 2009;301(1):63–73.

CHAPTER 58—INFECTIOUS DISEASES

KEY POINTS

■ Immune function wanes with age, and resistance is compromised in older adults not only as a consequence of age-related declines in immunity (ie, immune senescence) but also more importantly because of comorbid disease.

■ Accepted thresholds for "fever" generally do not apply in infected older adults because of their altered febrile response to infection. Fever can be redefined in frail older patients (temperature >2°F over baseline or oral temperature >99°F) to enhance its diagnostic utility.

■ Applying minimal criteria for starting antibiotic therapy in residents of long-term care facilities is likely to reduce inappropriate antibiotic use without jeopardizing patient safety.

■ First-line therapy should be selected carefully in older patients with pneumonia because of the associated high mortality rates and because the causes of pneumonia differ in older versus younger patients.

■ The response to aggressive, highly active antiretroviral therapy is similar in younger and older adults with HIV infection, but diseases associated with advancing age develop earlier in HIV-infected adults, even those with prolonged suppression of HIV replication.

Infection is the major cause of mortality in 40% of those ≥65 yr old, and it contributes to death in many others. Infection is also a significant cause of morbidity in older adults, often exacerbating underlying illness or leading to hospitalization. Pneumonia and other respiratory tract infections, urinary tract infection, and sepsis are all in the top 20 diagnosis-related groups paid by Medicare. Further, older adults are often a "sentinel" population in which new infections (eg, West Nile virus), newly more virulent strains (*Clostridium difficile* colitis), or the return of annual epidemics (eg, influenza) are first noted. Associations of infection and inflammation with age-related chronic diseases suggest that infectious diseases may play an even larger role in the morbidity and mortality of the older adult population than previously realized. This chapter explores the biologic, cultural, and societal factors that influence susceptibility to infection, the presentation of disease, and management suggestions for several common infectious disease syndromes in older adults.

PREDISPOSITION TO INFECTION

Fundamental changes in the immune response occur with aging in large measure not only because of comorbidities but also because of age-related declines in immunity, a phenomenon known as *immune senescence* (Table 58.1). The main features of immune senescence are depressed T-cell responses and T-cell–macrophage interactions (clinically reflected as delayed-type hypersensitivity responses), but deficits of innate immunity are increasingly being recognized, particularly in frail older patients.

Although age itself influences immune function, nonspecific host-resistance factors that change with age also increase the risk of infection in older adults. For example, poor skin integrity predisposes to skin and soft-tissue infection, impaired cough or gag reflexes increase the risk of pneumonia, and increased gastric pH and decreased GI motility predispose to diarrheal illnesses. However, all these changes associated with aging have far less influence on infection risk than comorbid diseases. Diabetes mellitus, chronic renal insufficiency, heart failure, chronic edema due to venous insufficiency, COPD, and stroke are but a few examples of age-related

Table 58.1—Changes in Immune Function Associated with Aging

Type of Immunity	Change With Age	Comment
Innate immunity		
Skin, mucous membranes	↓↓↓	Skin thins and dries with aging
Polymorphonuclear neutrophils		
Adherence, chemotaxis	—	
Ingestion	—	
Intracellular killing	↓	Most changes are due to comorbidity
Adaptive immunity		
Thymic hormones	↓↓↓	
Lymphocyte subsets		
T cells	↓↓↓	Shift from naive to memory subtypes
Natural killer cells	↓↓	Number increases but function declines
Lymphocyte functions		
Proliferative responses	↓↓	
Senescent phenotype	↑↑↑	This refers to oligoclonal expansion of CD8 cells that have replicative senescence, are CD28 negative, and secrete high quantities of proinflammatory cytokines
Cytokine production, secretion		
IL-2, IL-2 receptor	↓↓↓	After stimulation
Interferon-γ	↑	Primarily basal secretion
Prostaglandin E$_2$	↑↑	Basal and stimulated
Delayed-type hypersensitivity	↓↓	
Autoimmunity	↑↑	Autoantibodies common but of unclear significance

NOTE: — = no age-related changes; ↑ = mild increase; ↑↑ = moderate increase; ↑↑↑ = marked increase; ↓ = mild decrease; ↓↓ = moderate decrease; ↓↓↓ = marked decrease; IL=interleukin

comorbid illnesses that increase risk of infection. Comorbidity further influences the outcomes and management strategies for infection in older adults. For example, community-acquired pneumonia in otherwise healthy adults <50 yr old is typically treated on an outpatient basis and rarely causes mortality; however, in older adults with community-acquired pneumonia and multiple comorbid conditions, the greatly increased risk of morbidity and mortality often necessitates hospitalization. In addition, cognitive impairment and other barriers to adherence may increase the difficulty of treating older patients, increasing complications and costs.

A major influence on immune function in older adults is nutritional status. Protein and calorie undernutrition is present in 30%–60% of adults ≥65 yr old on admission to the hospital. Among outpatients, 11% of older adults are malnourished, 90% of which is due to reversible underlying conditions such as depression, poorly controlled diabetes mellitus,

and medication adverse events (SOE=B). Delayed wound healing, increased risk of nosocomial infection, extended lengths of hospital stay, and increased mortality are all associated with malnutrition. Even mildly undernourished older adults (ie, those with a serum albumin of 3–3.5 g/dL) have evidence of immune compromise, poor vaccine responses, and diminished cytokine responses to specific challenges. Nutritional interventions may boost immune function in some older adults, but this remains controversial. Some studies suggest a clinical benefit, particularly in older adults with subclinical nutritional deficiencies, whereas others do not. Differences in study design, population enrolled, duration of follow-up, and definitions of infection (self-reported versus clinician diagnosed) may account for many of these differences. See "Malnutrition," p 200.

Residing in long-term care or nursing facilities also places older adults at increased risk of epidemic disease such as influenza. Widespread antibiotic use in these settings increases the likelihood of acquiring diseases caused by antibiotic-resistant organisms; methicillin-resistant *Staphylococcus aureus*, vancomycin-resistant enterococci, and multiply resistant gram-negative rods are more common causes of infection in institutionalized than in community-dwelling older adults. Resistance issues are aug-

---

STRENGTH-OF-EVIDENCE (SOE) RATING DEFINITIONS

A = consistent and good quality patient-oriented evidence
B = somewhat inconsistent or limited quality patient-oriented evidence
C = very inconsistent or very limited patient-oriented evidence, disease-oriented evidence, and/or consensus from professional organizations
D = unstudied common practice or opinion

See inside front cover for detailed information regarding the SOE classification.

mented in the nursing home by debilitated hosts, close proximity of residents, poor staff compliance with prevention strategies (eg, influenza immunization), and difficulties in implementing infection-control measures in long-term care.

DIAGNOSIS AND MANAGEMENT OF INFECTIONS

Presentation

Older adults often present without typical signs and symptoms, even in severe infection. Fever, the most readily recognized feature of infection, may be absent in 30%–50% of frail older adults with serious infections, even pneumonia or endocarditis. The cause of impaired febrile responses in older adults is incompletely understood, but diverse mechanisms of thermoregulation are involved, including a reduced basal body temperature in many older adults and blunted thermogenesis by brown adipose tissue.

Because of the altered febrile response to infection, many authors have suggested a redefinition of *fever* in older adults. Given the sensitivity, specificity, and positive and negative predictive values, fever in older nursing-home residents can be redefined appropriately as a temperature >2°F (1.1°C) over baseline (if a baseline is available) or, perhaps more practically, an oral temperature >99°F (37.2°C) or a rectal temperature >99.5°F (37.5°C) on repeated measures (SOE=B). This definition of fever has a sensitivity of 82.5% in nursing-home residents, and the specificity remains high at 89.9% (Table 58.2). These data were generated in a cohort of frail, older, veteran men in a nursing home. It would seem reasonable to apply the same definitions to frail, older adults of either sex in the community, although the performance characteristics of this definition of fever in otherwise healthy older adults have not been validated.

The absence of fever is only one way that infectious diseases can present atypically in older adults. For example, pneumonia can be signaled by a nonspecific decline in baseline functional status, such as confusion or falling, without cough, sputum production, or shortness of breath. Anorexia and decreased oral intake may be the primary manifestation of infection, or exacerbation of an underlying illness (eg, atrial fibrillation) may become the predominant feature. Cognitive impairment, when present, further contributes to the often confusing presentation of infections in older adults. Many cognitively impaired older adults are unable to communicate symptoms accurately, and clinicians must be ready to pursue objective assessments such as laboratory and radiologic evaluations at a lower threshold, unless advance directives indicate otherwise.

Table 58.2—Defining Fever in Frail, Older Residents of Long-Term Care Facilities

Definition	Sensitivity	Specificity	(+) Likelihood Ratio	(−) Likelihood Ratio
T >101°F (38.3°C)	40.0%	99.7%	133	0.6
T >100°F (37.7°C)	70.0%	98.3%	41	0.3
T >99°F (37.2°C)	82.5%	89.9%	8	0.2

NOTE: (+) Likelihood ratio = sensitivity / (1− specificity); (−) Likelihood ratio = (1− sensitivity) / specificity; T = temperature
SOURCE: Data from Castle SC, Yeh M, Toledo S, et al. Lowering the temperature criterion improves detection of infections in nursing home residents. *Aging Immunol Infect Dis.* 1993;4(2):67–76.

Antimicrobial Management

Drug distribution, metabolism, excretion, and interactions can be altered with age. Aging in the absence of any comorbid disease is associated with decreased renal function, and antibiotic dosages may need to be reduced in older adults. (See "Pharmacotherapy," p 72.) Furthermore, antibiotics interact with many other medications commonly prescribed for older adults. Digoxin, warfarin, oral hypoglycemic agents, theophylline, antacids, lipid-lowering agents, antihypertensive medications, and H_2-receptor antagonists all have significant interactions with commonly prescribed antimicrobials. Drug concentrations can increase (eg, enhanced digoxin toxicity associated with macrolides, tetracyclines, and trimethoprim) or decrease (eg, reduced absorption of some fluoroquinolones with antacids) with concomitant medication administration. Atrophic gastritis, a common problem in older adults, and H_2 blockers or proton-pump inhibitors can reduce the absorption of some antimicrobials, such as ketoconazole or itraconazole. Finally, adherence to prescribed regimens may be limited as a consequence of poor cognitive function, impaired hearing or vision, multiple medications, and financial constraints.

The choice and timing of antibiotics may also be important. In sepsis, pneumonia, and other severe infections, an increasing body of evidence suggests that broad coverage is warranted initially because outcomes (ie, mortality, length of stay in intensive care) are improved when the offending organism is covered by the *initial* antibiotic regimen. In older adults with pneumonia, data suggest that delaying the start of therapy for ≥4 hours after admission to the hospital is associated with an increased risk of mortality (SOE=B). "De-escalation," a narrowing of antibiotic choice to specific therapy if the offending organism is identified by culture or other diagnostic studies, is essential for antibiotic stewardship and should be done whenever possible. Unfortunately, diagnostic studies (eg, obtaining sputum) are often

Table 58.3—Suggested Minimal Criteria for Initiation of Antibiotic Therapy in the Long-Term Care Setting

Condition	Minimal Criteria
Urinary tract infection, without catheter	Fever *and* one of the following: new or worsening urgency, frequency, suprapubic pain, gross hematuria, CVA tenderness, incontinence
Urinary tract infection, with catheter	Fever or one of the following: new CVA tenderness, rigors, or new-onset delirium
Skin and soft-tissue infection	Fever or one of the following: redness, tenderness, warmth, new or increasing swelling of affected site
Respiratory infection	Fever ≥102°F (38.9°C) *and* one of the following: RR >25, productive cough Fever >100°F <102°F *and* one of the following: RR >25, pulse >100, rigors, new-onset delirium Afebrile with COPD *and* new or increased cough with purulent sputum Afebrile without COPD *and* new or increased cough *and* either RR >25 or new-onset delirium
Fever without source of infection	At least one of the following: new-onset delirium, rigors If these are not present, evaluate without initiating antibiotics Antibiotics probably should not be instituted as a diagnostic test, but if initiated as such, discontinue in 3–5 days if no improvement and evaluation negative

NOTE: CVA = costovertebral angle; RR = respiratory rate (per minute)
SOURCE: Data from Loeb M, Bentley DW, Bradley S, et al. Development of minimum criteria for the initiation of antibiotics in residents of long-term care facilities: results of a consensus conference. *Infect Control Hosp Epidemiol.* 2001;22:120–124.

difficult in older adults or are unavailable in long-term care settings. These factors and the atypical presentation of infection noted above often lead to early initiation of antimicrobials in older adults, particularly in long-term care. However, this practice results in inappropriate use of antibiotics in up to 75% of cases in long-term care. The use of strict, minimal criteria for initiation of antimicrobials in long-term care is most likely to reduce inappropriate antibiotic use without jeopardizing patient safety (Table 58.3) (SOE=C).

INFECTIOUS SYNDROMES

Bacteremia and Sepsis

Bacteremia is a common cause of hospitalization in older adults. Older patients with bacteremia are less likely than their younger counterparts to have chills or sweating, and fever is often absent. Gastrointestinal and genitourinary sources of bacteremia are more common; thus, the causative bacteria are more likely to be gram-negative rods or enterococci in older adults versus younger patients.

Bacteremia carries a poor prognosis in older adults. For example, nosocomial gram-negative bacteremia carries a mortality rate of 5%–35% in young adults, but 37%–50% in older adults. Major contributing factors include coexisting diseases that reduce physiologic reserve and the more common use of invasive devices (eg, intravenous or urinary catheters) that make eradication of organisms difficult.

The management of bacteremia and sepsis in older and younger patients is similar. Rapid administration of appropriate antibiotics aimed at the most likely sources is essential, and early "goal-directed"

therapy for volume resuscitation has proven benefit in populations of all ages with sepsis (SOE=B). The use of activated protein C as adjunctive therapy in older adults with sepsis has raised concern about increased bleeding. However, in a randomized trial of activated protein C in patients ≥75 yr old with sepsis, the survival benefit was preserved despite a slightly increased risk of serious bleeding (SOE=B).

Pneumonia

Patients aged ≥65 yr old account for >50% of all pneumonia cases, and annual hospitalization rates for pneumonia range from 12 per 1,000 among community-dwelling adults ≥75 yr old to 32 per 1,000 among nursing-home residents. In fact, the cumulative 2-yr risk of pneumonia for long-term care residents is approximately 30%. Mortality caused by pneumonia in older adults is three to five times that in young adults, but the rate is profoundly influenced by comorbidity. Comorbidity, defined in one study as cancer, collagen vascular disease, or advanced liver disease, was the strongest independent predictor of mortality in community-acquired pneumonia in older adults, with a relative risk (RR) of 4.1. Other independent risk factors for pneumonia-related mortality include age ≥85 yr old; debility (decreased motor function); serum creatinine >1.5 mg/dL; and the presence of hypothermia (<36.1°F), hypotension (<90 mmHg systolic), or tachycardia (>110 beats per minute) on admission (SOE=A). Long-term follow-up data also suggest that community-acquired pneumonia in older adults indicates a higher risk of subsequent all-cause mortality over the next 12 yr, as a consequence of both recurrent pneumonia (RR 2.1 [1.3–3.4]) but also cardiovascular disease (RR 1.4 [1.0–1.9]) (SOE=A).

The causes of pneumonia in younger and older adults differ. In older patients, *Streptococcus pneumoniae* is still the predominant organism, but gram-negative bacilli (eg, *Haemophilus influenzae, Moraxella catarrhalis, Klebsiella* spp) are much more common than in younger adults, particularly in patients with COPD or who reside in long-term care facilities. *Staphylococcus aureus* and respiratory viruses are also common causes of community-acquired pneumonia in nursing-home residents. Obtaining a microbiologic diagnosis is often difficult in older adults who rarely produce sputum. Blood cultures should be obtained before antimicrobial therapy but are positive in only 10%–15% of patients. An often overlooked diagnostic test for pneumonia is that of urinary antigen testing for *Strep pneumoniae* (sensitivity 70%–80%; specificity 77%–97%) or *Legionella pneumophila* (sensitivity 70%–80%; specificity 77–97%). Importantly, the sensitivity of these tests is not affected for some time (up to 24 hours) after the initiation of antimicrobial therapy. The test for legionellosis detects only serogroup 1, which causes 80% of all legionella infection.

Guidelines for pneumonia therapy have evolved to account for the emergence of resistant bacteria, particularly drug-resistant *Strep pneumoniae*, and the recognition of comorbidities, healthcare setting versus community-acquired illness, and specific pathogens of interest in certain settings (eg, *Staph aureus* after viral influenza infection). Because of their ease of administration and broad activity against respiratory pathogens, respiratory fluoroquinolones are used often in older adults, and they are one of the first-line therapies suggested by more recent guidelines. Guidelines of the Infectious Diseases Society of America for treatment of community-acquired pneumonia suggest the following as first-line therapy in adults ≥60 yr old with or without comorbidity: a β-lactam/β-lactamase combination or advanced-generation cephalosporin (eg, ceftriaxone or cefotaxime) with or without a macrolide. Alternatively, one of the newer fluoroquinolones with enhanced activity against *Strep pneumoniae* (eg, levofloxacin, moxifloxacin, gemifloxacin) may be used. However, several notes of caution are needed regarding fluoroquinolone use in older adults: first, fluoroquinolones kill bacteria better at higher concentrations, and outcomes are better in older adults when high drug concentrations are present (SOE=B). Thus, full-dosage therapy should be provided (ie, the adage of "start low, go slow" often invoked for drug therapy in older adults is *not* appropriate for this class of drugs). Second, if tuberculosis is a realistic possibility, fluoroquinolone use should be reserved. Use of fluoroquinolones to treat community-acquired pneumonia can lead to delayed diagnosis of tuberculosis (by an average of >40 days) and to fluoroquinolone resistance in the organism.

Finally, significant adverse events, including dizziness and cardiac conduction abnormalities (QT prolongation), may limit the use of fluoroquinolones in certain older adults; however, the overall safety of fluoroquinolones in older adults without underlying conduction abnormalities or specific contraindications is quite good (SOE=B).

Nursing-home–acquired pneumonia or hospital-acquired pneumonia in older adults requires broader initial therapy than does community-acquired pneumonia because of the broader spectrum of organisms causing infection. In the nursing-home setting, polymicrobial infection, often due to aspiration, and *Staph aureus* are much more common than in the community setting. In the hospital setting, gram-negative bacilli predominate, but *Staph aureus* is more common as well and is more likely to affect specific antibiotic choices because of resistance. Outcomes data suggest that response to therapy is greater when the initial antibiotic regimen covers the offending agent. Thus, initial regimens should be broadly inclusive, followed by step-down therapy to more narrow coverage if the causative agent is identified. Importantly, if patients are known to be colonized with methicillin-resistant *Staph aureus* (MRSA), initial regimens should include vancomycin or linezolid until MRSA is excluded as the causative agent. Further, data suggest that patients with clinically improving hospital-acquired pneumonia not caused by nonfermenting gram-negative bacilli (eg, *Pseudomonas, Stenotrophomonas*) can be treated with shorter courses of antibiotics (7 or 8 days, rather than the 2 weeks commonly used in the past). Shorter courses (8 days versus 15 days) of antibiotics are associated with equivalent efficacy and less antibiotic resistance (SOE=A).

The prevention of pneumonia in older adults is a complex issue, and a multipronged approach is most likely to be effective. Immunization of at-risk individuals is by far the most well-studied measure. Annual influenza vaccine and pneumococcal vaccine should be administered to all older adults (see "Prevention," p 61). In addition to vaccines, smoking cessation and aggressive treatment of comorbidities (eg, minimizing aspiration risk in patients after stroke, limiting use of sedative hypnotics) can reduce the risk of infection. Finally, system changes with attention to infection control (isolation, cohorting, skin testing for tuberculosis with purified protein derivative, and immunization policies for staff/visitors) can be particularly effective in the nursing home.

Influenza

Influenza results in approximately 40,000 deaths annually in the United States, nearly all of which are in the older adult population. The clinical syndrome of influenza is easily recognized by most clinicians, particularly in the setting of local activity or outbreak settings frequently seen in the nursing home. Although some controversy exists with regard to the effectiveness of influenza vaccine in frail older adults, the bulk of the data suggests the vaccine is 60%–80% efficacious in older adults for preventing severe disease, hospitalization, and death. Therefore, annual immunization is recommended for all adults >50 yr old, and for anyone of any age who wishes to reduce the risk of serious influenza (SOE=A).

Several medications are available for treatment and prophylaxis of influenza. M2 inhibitors (amantadine and rimantadine) block the M2 ion channel of influenza and are effective only against influenza A; their use is limited by widespread resistance (>90% of the most virulent strains). Further, amantadine is particularly difficult to use in older adults because of the extensive dosage adjustments required for small changes in kidney function and marked adverse events, particularly CNS symptoms. In contrast, neuraminidase inhibitors (zanamivir and oseltamivir) are effective against both influenza A and B; they inhibit the virus by interfering with an essential enzyme, neuraminidase, that cleaves sialic acid to expose host cell receptors for the virus. Oseltamivir, a capsule, is preferred over zanamivir in older adults because zanamivir must be inhaled, and it is difficult for many older adults to properly use the product. Treatment of influenza is effective if started in the first 48 hours, but it is most effective if started within 24 hours of symptom onset (SOE=A). Oseltamivir and zanamivir can also be used for prevention in outbreak situations (eg, in long-term care) when combined with appropriate vaccination strategies (SOE=A).

Urinary Tract Infection

Urinary tract infection (UTI) is among the most common of clinical illnesses in older adults, with an incidence of 10.9 per 100-person years in men and 14 per 100 person-years in women ≥65 yr old. Gram-negative bacilli (eg, *Escherichia coli*, *Enterobacter* spp, *Klebsiella* spp, *Proteus* spp) are most common, but there is an increase in more resistant isolates, such as *Pseudomonas aeruginosa*, and in gram-positive organisms, including enterococci, coagulase-negative staphylococci, and *Streptococcus agalactiae* (group B strep). In patients with indwelling catheters, the microbes listed still predominate, but it is also common to encounter additional organisms, including enterococci, *Staph aureus*, and fungi, particularly *Candida* spp. The organisms colonizing urinary catheters commonly develop biofilms and are difficult to resolve with the same urinary catheter in place.

Asymptomatic Bacteriuria Versus Urinary Tract Infection

Up to 15% of women in the community and 40% of women in nursing homes have asymptomatic bacteriuria; the incidence in men is approximately half that in women. Rates are even higher with the use of condom catheters (87%) or Foley catheters (nearly 100%). Numerous studies have suggested that there is no clinical benefit from the treatment of asymptomatic bacteriuria, and that treatment is associated with significant adverse events, expense, and the potential for selection of resistant organisms. Thus, no treatment is recommended (SOE=A). The clinical difficulty is deciding what is symptomatic and, thus, when a urine culture should be ordered, particularly in the nursing-home setting. The presentation of infection can be quite subtle in older adults, and a change in functional status often prompts the collection of a urine specimen even in the absence of fever, dysuria, or other typical clinical features. Similarly, empiric antimicrobial therapy should be started only when infection is documented or highly suspected.

Urinary Tract Infection in Women

In contrast to asymptomatic bacteriuria, symptomatic UTI requires therapy. Therapy is based on the location of infection (upper versus lower tract disease) and the likely causative agent. Lower tract UTI (ie, cystitis), characterized by dysuria, frequency, and urgency (not fever, which generally indicates upper tract disease), is often treated in young women for 1–3 days, and 3–7 days of therapy is probably sufficient for uncomplicated cystitis in older women (SOE=B). Randomized trials in older women indicate that fluoroquinolones are more efficacious than trimethoprim-sulfamethoxazole (TMP-SMX), likely because resistance rates of *E coli* to TMP-SMX are 10%–20% in most areas of the United States; however, with wider use of fluoroquinolones, resistance to these agents is also increasing. Other reasonable choices in some settings include amoxicillin (particularly for enterococcal infection) and first-generation cephalosporins in patients with multiple antibiotic intolerances. Culture is not required unless first-line therapy is not effective (SOE=A).

Upper UTI (ie, pyelonephritis), characterized by fever, chills, nausea, and flank pain, is commonly accompanied by lower tract symptoms and requires a longer period of therapy (7–21 days). Because of the excellent bioavailability of many antibiotics, particularly the fluoroquinolones, intravenous therapy is not essential if the patient can tolerate oral medications. In a study comparing fluoroquinolones with TMP-SMX for upper tract UTI in younger women (18–58 yr old), fluoroquinolones were more effective (microbiologic cure rate 99% versus 89% for

TMP-SMX; clinical cure rate 96% versus 83% for TMP-SMX) because of the presence of organisms resistant to TMP-SMX. This is likely to be true in older adults as well. Intravenous administration of antibiotics remains the standard of care for patients with suspected urosepsis, those with upper tract disease due to relatively resistant bacteria such as enterococci, or those unable to tolerate oral medications. Culture and sensitivity data are more useful in guiding antimicrobial therapy in upper tract UTIs than in lower tract disease and should be obtained in most cases (SOE=A).

Prophylactic antibiotics intended to prevent frequently recurrent UTIs in older women are not recommended because of the high incidence of the development of resistant organisms. Several measures may decrease the frequency of recurrence, including intravaginal or systemic estrogen replacement that changes the vaginal flora, thus reducing the risk of UTI, or perhaps ingestion of cranberry juice ($\geq$300 mL/d).

Urinary Tract Infection in Men

Prostatic disease (primarily hyperplasia) or functional disability, such as autonomic neuropathy from diabetes mellitus with incomplete bladder emptying, account for most lower and upper UTIs in older men. Thus, short-course therapy for UTIs in older men is inappropriate. Therapy should last at least 14 days, and if prostatic involvement is suspected (ie, acute or chronic prostatitis), at least 6 weeks (SOE=B). The causative organisms and treatment choices are similar to those outlined above for older women. Fluoroquinolones and TMP-SMX are most widely used when prostatic involvement is suspected and culture data confirm the organism's susceptibility because, of the available agents, these two penetrate the prostate best. Because treatment for all UTIs in men is generally longer than in women and the prostate is a common reservoir for recurrent UTIs, culture and sensitivity data should guide therapy for virtually all UTIs in men (SOE=C).

Tuberculosis

Worldwide, approximately 1.7 billion people are infected with *Mycobacterium tuberculosis*, 16 million in the United States. Adults $\geq$65 yr old account for one-fourth of all active tuberculosis (TB) cases in the United States. The vast majority of active TB in older adults is in community dwellers, but the rate of infection in long-term care residents is much higher: skin-test studies show prevalence rates of skin-test reactivity in the range of 30%–50%. This high prevalence is due to exposure to *M tuberculosis* in the early 1900s, when it was estimated that 80% of all individuals were infected by age 30. Most active cases of TB in older adults are, therefore, due to reactivated disease, but primary infection may account for 10%–20% of cases and is of particular concern in nursing-home outbreaks.

As with most other infections, TB may not present in classic fashion (ie, cough, sputum, fever, night sweats, weight loss) in older adults. Often fatigue, anorexia, decreased functional status, or low-grade fever are presenting manifestations. Most tuberculous disease in older adults occurs with lung involvement (75%), and pneumonic processes in older adults, particularly those that occur in a postacute manner, should raise a high index of suspicion for *M tuberculosis* infection. Older adults are more likely than their younger counterparts to have extrapulmonary disease. Other sites include miliary (disseminated) disease, tuberculous meningitis or osteomyelitis, and urogenital disease, but virtually any body structure or organ system can be involved and can account for the major presenting symptom.

A diagnosis of active disease usually requires isolation of the organism from sputum, urine, or other clinical specimen. Current techniques have improved the speed of diagnosis, particularly for identifying the species of *Mycobacterium* after isolation. This is now typically accomplished within 24 hours of obtaining a positive culture by use of DNA probes. Direct polymerase chain reaction of clinical specimens or other rapid diagnostic techniques are not available or reliable in most local laboratories, but such tests can be available in research settings. They are most likely to be helpful for establishing a diagnosis from cerebrospinal or pleural fluid, which yields positive cultures in only 10%–15% of cases.

The most confusing area of TB diagnostics is typically interpretation of the results of purified-protein derivative (PPD) skin tests. In all populations, induration of $\geq$15 mm 48–72 hours after placement of a 5-tuberculin unit PPD indicates a positive test. Induration $\geq$10 mm is considered a positive test in nursing-home residents, recent converters (previous PPD <5 mm), immigrants from countries with high endemicity of *M tuberculosis* infection, underserved populations in the United States (homeless people, black Americans, Hispanic Americans, and Native Americans), and those with specific risk factors (eg, gastrectomy, >10% below ideal body weight, chronic kidney failure, diabetes mellitus, or immunosuppression, including that caused by corticosteroids or malignancy). In individuals infected with HIV, those with a history of close contact with people with active *M tuberculosis*, and those with chest radiographs consistent with *M tuberculosis* infection, $\geq$5 mm induration is considered a positive PPD test. Anergy panel testing in conjunction with PPD testing is of little value and is not recommended (SOE=C).

Long-term care facilities should use a two-step procedure for PPD testing during the initial evaluation of residents (SOE=C). Two-step testing requires retesting of patients within 2 weeks. If the second skin test results in ≥10 mm of induration or the increase in the size of the induration from the first to the second skin test is ≥6 mm, the patient is considered PPD positive. Further evaluation is then needed.

The treatment of active TB in older adults is similar to that in young adults. Four-drug therapy (usually isoniazid [INH], rifampin, pyrazinamide, and ethambutol or streptomycin) is recommended as initial therapy, with tapering to one of several two- or three-drug regimens once susceptibility testing is available. The most common regimen is INH, rifampin, and pyrazinamide for 2 mo, followed by INH and rifampin for an additional 4 mo.

Prophylaxis with 9 mo of INH for asymptomatic individuals with a positive PPD should be provided *regardless of age* in adults who are recent converters (defined in adults >35 yr old with a PPD that has gone from <10 mm to ≥15 mm within 2 yr), or regardless of duration of PPD positivity if an individual has any of the specific risk factors highlighted above. Patients with a positive PPD of unknown duration should receive INH prophylaxis, even those >35 yr old (as opposed to recommendations in the 1990s). Older adults should be monitored closely for symptoms and signs of peripheral neuropathy (due to INH and preventable by coadministration of pyridoxine) and hepatitis (due to treatment with INH, rifampin, or pyrazinamide). Shorter-course therapy with 2 mo of rifampin and pyrazinamide is effective but has a much higher incidence of hepatotoxicity than INH treatment and thus should be used only in very specific circumstances (SOE=B).

Infective Endocarditis

Since the early part of the 20th century, infective endocarditis has undergone a transformation from a disease of young adults primarily due to rheumatic or congenital valve anomalies to one of older adults associated with degenerative valvular disorders and prosthetic valves. Native-valve endocarditis is typically caused by viridans streptococci and *S aureus*, and occasional infections are due to HACEK organisms (a group of typically nonfermenting gram-negative rods that primarily inhabit the oral cavity and include the genera *Haemophilus*, *Actinobacillus*, *Cardiobacterium*, *Eikenella*, and *Kingella*). Gastrointestinal and genitourinary organisms, such as enterococci and gram-negative rods, are more common in native-valve infective endocarditis in older adults, and coagulase-negative staphylococci are a common cause of prosthetic-valve endocarditis, particularly in the first 60 days after placement of a prosthetic valve.

The diagnosis of endocarditis is often difficult in older adults. Fever is less common in older patients than in younger ones, occurring in 55% versus 80%, respectively, as is leukocytosis, occurring in 25% versus 60%. Rates of positive blood cultures do not vary by age; however, degenerative, calcific valvular lesions and prosthetic valves lower the sensitivity of transthoracic echocardiography to 45% in older patients (versus 75% in younger patients). Transesophageal echocardiography (TEE) improves the diagnostic yield for infective endocarditis, but the lack of positive findings on TEE never excludes it. TEE is of particular value in resolving the clinical problem of *S aureus* bacteremia. Positive findings on TEE support prolonged antibiotic administration (4–6 weeks) versus short-course (2 weeks) therapy. However, TEE is invasive and expensive. Interestingly, age does not appear to play a major role in mortality risk, with a 2-yr survival of 75% for infective endocarditis in all age groups unless major comorbidities are also present.

Antibiotic treatment of infective endocarditis is directed at the identified pathogen or the most likely causes, if blood cultures are negative. Therapy is administered intravenously for 2–6 weeks. Surgical therapy should be considered in cases of severe valvular dysfunction, recurrent emboli, marked heart failure, myocardial abscess formation, fungal endocarditis, or when appropriate antibiotic treatment does not yield negative blood cultures.

Recommendations for endocarditis prophylaxis for dental procedures were revised in 2007, focusing on providing prophylaxis only in the highest-risk patients and eliminating recommendations for prophylaxis for those undergoing gastrointestinal or genitourinary procedures (Table 58.4 and Table 58.5).

Prosthetic Device Infections

Permanent implantable prosthetic devices are common in older adults. Prosthetic joints, cardiac pacemakers, artificial heart valves, intraocular lens implants, vascular grafts, penile prostheses, and a variety of other devices are placed more often in older than in younger adults. A discussion of all prosthetic device infections (PDIs) is beyond the scope of this chapter, but several general concepts can be summarized.

PDIs are usually separated into early versus late infections because the causative agents differ significantly. Early PDIs, most commonly defined as occurring <60 days after device implantation, are primarily due to contamination at the time of implantation or to events associated with the acute hospital-

Table 58.4—Endocarditis Prophylaxis (AHA Guidelines)

Cardiac Conditions Requiring Prophylaxis

Prosthetic cardiac valve
Previous infective endocarditis
Cardiac transplant recipients who develop cardiac valvulopathy
Unrepaired cyanotic congenital heart disease
Repaired congenital heart disease with residual defects at the site or adjacent to the site of a prosthetic patch or device
Congenital heart disease completely repaired with prosthetic material or device (prophylaxis needed for only the first 6 mo after repair procedure)

Cardiac Conditions Not Requiring Prophylaxis

All cardiac conditions or procedures not listed above

Procedures Warranting Prophylaxis (*only* in patients with cardiac conditions listed above)

Dental procedures requiring manipulation of gingival tissue, manipulation of the periapical region of teeth, or perforation of the oral mucosa (includes extractions, implants, reimplants, root canals, teeth cleaning during which bleeding is expected)
Invasive procedures of the respiratory tract involving incision or biopsy of respiratory tract mucosa
Surgical procedures involving infected skin, skin structures, or musculoskeletal tissue

Procedures Not Warranting Prophylaxis

All dental procedures not listed above
All noninvasive respiratory procedures
All gastrointestinal and genitourinary procedures

SOURCE: Reuben DB, Herr KA, Pacala JT, et al. *Geriatrics At Your Fingertips.* 11th ed. New York: American Geriatrics Society; 2009:191. Reprinted with permission.

ization (ie, occult bacteremias caused by intravenous catheters). Thus, coagulase-negative staphylococci predominate, and *S aureus* and diphtheroids are common as well; gram-negative bacilli and fungi are relatively rare causes of early PDI. Late PDIs are usually caused by organisms that commonly cause transient bacteremia (in older adults this is most often skin, respiratory, gastrointestinal, or genitourinary organisms). Staphylococci, including coagulase-negative staphylococci, play a major role in both early and late PDIs, although their relative importance is greater in early PDIs. Thus, empiric staphylococcal therapy should be provided in either early or late PDIs if a specific causative agent is not identified.

In general, hardware removal is required to clear PDIs. However, early antibiotic treatment, in some instances combined with aggressive surgical drainage, can be successful. Small studies in prosthetic joint infection suggest that initial debridement and culture and a brief course (2 weeks) of intravenous antibiotics followed by combination oral two-drug therapy that includes rifampin may obviate the need for device removal. Until more definitive data are available, it is prudent to restrict this approach to patients with a short duration of symptoms (<3 weeks), those who

are likely to have difficulty tolerating another surgical procedure, or those in whom return to full functional status is not a realistic goal because of comorbidities. In those older adults in whom full function is the goal, the best chance for cure is a two-stage procedure in which the device is removed and antibiotics are given for an extended period (6–8 weeks), followed by delayed reimplantation. Of course, for life-saving devices, such as mechanical valves or implantable defibrillators, this is not an option. Infected prosthetic devices are usually surrounded by microbial biofilms, such as microbe-derived glycocalyx. Biofilms reduce antibiotic penetration and thus greatly increase the concentrations of antibiotic needed for bactericidal activity. Furthermore, many conditions associated with infected prostheses are also accompanied by poor blood flow to the area. Therefore, it is preferable to use bactericidal antibiotics, often in combination with a second agent that penetrates biofilms and poorly perfused areas (eg, rifampin for staphylococci).

Bone and Joint Infections

Native bone and joint infections in the absence of prostheses occur in older adults. Septic arthritis is more likely to occur in joints with underlying pathology (eg, rheumatoid changes, gout, osteoarthritis), and early arthrocentesis is indicated in any mono- or oligo-articular syndrome to exclude infection. *Staphylococcus aureus* is the most likely pathogen; infections are only rarely due to gram-negative bacilli and streptococci. Aggressive antibiotic therapy combined with serial arthrocentesis may be as effective as open surgical drainage in uncomplicated septic arthritis, while also preserving better joint function. Surgical drainage is required if this more conservative strategy is not successful.

Osteomyelitis in older adults can be due to hematogenous seeding from a bacteremia or contiguous spread from an adjacent focus. *Staphylococcus aureus* is the predominant organism, but gastrointestinal and genitourinary flora are again more common in older adults, emphasizing the advantage of a specific microbiologic diagnosis to guide therapy. Pressure ulcer infections and diabetic foot infections are very common, particularly in institutionalized older adults, and they commonly require surgical consultation combined with aggressive antimicrobial therapy aimed at mixed aerobic and anaerobic bacteria.

HIV Infection and AIDS

HIV infection in older adults was initially limited to those who had received blood transfusions for surgical

Table 58.5—Endocarditis Prophylaxis Regimens

Situation	Regimen (Single Dose 30–60 Minutes Before Procedure)*
Oral	Amoxicillin 2 g po
Unable to take oral medication	Ampicillin 2 g, cefazolin 1 g, or ceftriaxone 1 g IM or IV
Allergic to penicillins or ampicillin	Cephalexin 2 g, clindamycin 600 mg, azithromycin 500 mg, or clarithromycin 500 mg po
Allergic to penicillins or ampicillin and unable to take oral medication	Cefazolin 1 g, ceftriaxone 1 g, or clindamycin 600 mg IM or IV

* For patients undergoing invasive respiratory tract procedures to treat an infection known to be caused by *Staphylococcus aureus*, or for patients undergoing surgery for infected skin, skin structures, or musculoskeletal tissue, regimen should include an antistaphylococcal penicillin or cephalosporin.

SOURCE: Data from Wilson W, Taubert KA, Gewitz M, et al. Prevention of infective endocarditis. Guidelines from the American Heart Association. A guideline from the American Heart Association Rheumatic Fever, Endocarditis, and Kawasaki Disease Committee, Council on Cardiovascular Disease in the Young, and the Council on Clinical Cardiology, Council on Cardiovascular Surgery and Anesthesia, and the Quality of Care and Outcomes Research Interdisciplinary Working Group. *Circulation* (online) 2007. http://circ.ahajournals.org/cgi/reprint/CIRCULATIONAHA.106.183095 (accessed Jan 2011).

procedures. However, increasing numbers of older Americans with HIV have acquired their infection via sexual activity. In addition, improvements in treatment have resulted in a large population of adults aging with HIV infection. By 2015, >50% of U.S. adults infected with HIV will be ≥50 yr old. Older adults constitute approximately 10% of all new diagnoses of AIDS in the United States, but this group and their clinicians often suffer from a lack of HIV awareness. Nonspecific symptoms such as forgetfulness, anorexia, weight loss, and recurrent pneumonia are often dismissed as age related, delaying HIV testing. Untreated HIV infection in older adults tends to pursue a more rapid downhill course, perhaps because of impaired T-cell replacement mechanisms with advanced age and the impact of additional comorbidities. However, if older adults are treated with aggressive highly active antiretroviral therapy (HAART), the antiviral response is similar to that seen in young adults. In fact, older adults often are more adherent with complicated HAART regimens than young adults. However, despite this response, increasing data suggest immune reconstitution is less robust in older adults with HIV infection.

Treatment regimens and prophylaxis of opportunistic infections with HAART are similar to those used in younger patients. Indications that HIV therapies can accelerate atherosclerosis and glucose intolerance suggest that an aggressive approach to prevention of cardiovascular disease in older HIV-infected adults is warranted and may lead to specific recommendations in older adults if associations of metabolic changes with specific HIV therapies become clearer. Other age-related comorbidities are also more common in HIV-infected individuals, even those with well-controlled viral replication (ie, a peripheral blood viral load <50 copies/mL). Many types of cancer, osteoporosis, and cirrhosis are all more prevalent in this population, and appear to develop about a decade earlier in HIV-infected individuals versus appropriately matched, uninfected controls. Older adults appear to be more susceptible to specific complications associated with HIV infection such as encephalopathy. Finally, older

HIV-infected adults are more likely than uninfected, age-matched adults to have multiple comorbidities, which increases the complexity of their care and the potential for medication interactions.

HIV prevention is rarely discussed in the geriatric community but is important if the trend of increasing sexual acquisition of HIV in older adults is to be reversed. Most older women do not believe that they are at risk of HIV infection, yet heterosexual activity is the primary mode of infection in this group. The concept of HIV-risky behavior is not well known among older adults, because HIV was not a problem during their adolescence or young adulthood. Older adults must be included in educational programs aimed at ensuring safe sexual practices and increasing awareness of the benefits of testing and effective HIV therapy.

Miscellaneous Infectious Syndromes

Bacterial meningitis is most common at the age extremes of life, and most meningitis-associated fatalities are in older adults. *Streptococcus pneumoniae* remains the most common cause in older adults, but gram-negative bacilli (20%–25%), *Listeria* spp (up to 10%), and TB are more common than in young adults. Because many *Strep pneumoniae* are now resistant to β-lactam antibiotics (up to 30% penicillin resistance and 10% ceftriaxone resistance nationwide), ceftriaxone or cefotaxime *plus* vancomycin are recommended as empiric therapy for bacterial meningitis in older adults until a specific isolate can be tested for antimicrobial susceptibility. Ampicillin is the drug of choice for *Listeria* spp, and more resistant gram-negative rods (eg, *Pseudomonas* spp) require ceftazidime or an extended-spectrum penicillin with or without intrathecal aminoglycoside therapy.

Neurosyphilis remains one of the most perplexing diagnoses in medicine. It is often raised as a possible underlying process in stroke or dementia in older adults. Syphilis should also be considered in unilateral deafness, gait disturbances, uveitis, and optic neuritis. In reality, there is no gold-standard test to exclude neurosyphilis. Neurosyphilis can only be

Table 58.6—Fever of Unknown Origin in Older Adults

Causes	Approximate % of Cases	
Infections	35	
Intra-abdominal abscess		12
Infective endocarditis		10
Other		7
Tuberculosis		6
Collagen vascular disorders	28	
Giant cell arteritis, polymyalgia rheumatica		19
Polyarteritis nodosa		6
Other		3
Malignancy	19	
Lymphoma		10
Carcinoma		9
Others (pulmonary emboli, drug fever)	9	
No diagnosis	5–10	

SOURCE: Data pooled from multiple studies: Esposito AL, Gleckman RA. Fever of unknown origin in the elderly. *J Am Geriatr Soc.* 1978;26(11):498; Knockaert DC, Vanneste LJ, Bobbaers HJ. Fever of unknown origin in elderly patients. *J Am Geriatr Soc.* 1993;41(11):1187–1192.

"ruled in" by such tests. However, suspicion is often first raised when a serum rapid plasma reagent or Venereal Disease Research Laboratory test (VDRL) is positive. A reasonable diagnostic evaluation after discovery of such a positive test includes confirmation of nonspecific tests (rapid plasma reagent and VDRL) with a specific test (microhemagglutination-*Treponema pallidum*, or fluorescent treponemal antibody absorption); if tests are confirmed, lumbar puncture should be performed for cell counts, glucose, protein, and cerebrospinal fluid (CSF) VDRL. A positive VDRL on CSF is diagnostic of neurosyphilis, but the sensitivity of this test is approximately 75% in most series. Other diagnostic tests are controversial. The ratio of intrathecal to serum-specific treponemal antibody (standardized to the total IgG in CSF and serum) may also be helpful, with ratios of ≥3 indicating likely infection. In the absence of these tests, it must be the judgment of a skilled clinician as to whether minor abnormalities in CSF (eg, low-level pleocytosis) and the clinical picture support the diagnosis and warrant therapy for neurosyphilis. Optimal treatment of neurosyphilis remains penicillin G, but a study in HIV-infected patients suggests that ceftriaxone may be an acceptable alternative.

Advancing age is the major risk factor for reactivated varicella-zoster virus causing herpes zoster (or "shingles"); the most disabling complication, post-herpetic neuralgia, is common in older adults. See "Dermatologic Diseases and Disorders," p 340, for diagnosis and treatment. Zoster vaccine is recommended for all immunocompetent adults ≥60 yr old, and it reduces the risk of zoster and post-herpetic neuralgia by >50% (SOE=A).

Facial nerve palsy (Bell's palsy) is common in older adults and associated with at least three infectious causes: herpes simplex virus, varicella zoster virus, and *Borrelia burgdorferi* (which causes Lyme disease). There are no strong data, at present, to suggest benefit of antiviral therapy for facial nerve palsies due to herpes simplex virus, but trials are underway. If facial nerve palsy is seen as part of an episode of varicella zoster virus, treatment is indicated. If Lyme disease is suspected clinically, the patient should receive oral amoxicillin 500 mg q6h for 14 days, oral doxycycline 100 mg q12h for 14 days, or intravenous ceftriaxone 2 g/d for 14 days.

Gastrointestinal infections are common among older adults. Diverticulitis, appendicitis, cholecystitis, intra-abdominal abscess, and ischemic bowel can present diagnostic dilemmas in the absence of fever or increased WBC counts. A high index of suspicion is necessary in older adults. CT or labeled WBC studies are most likely to be of value in establishing the diagnosis of intra-abdominal infection, and ultrasonography is an easy, readily available tool to assist in diagnosing cholecystitis, appendicitis, or abscess. Ischemic bowel often requires angiography.

Infectious diarrhea is also common in older adults. Older patients with achlorhydria are at particular risk because a lower bacterial inoculum is necessary to cause disease. Decreased intestinal motility associated with specific medications and advanced age may further increase susceptibility to infection. Epidemics occurring in the long-term care setting are commonly due to *E coli*, viruses, salmonellae, or *Shigella* spp. Frequent use of antimicrobials in older adults also increases the risk of *C difficile* colitis, and the risk of severe disease is greatest in this age group. Recently, *C difficile* infection has increased in incidence and severity, most prominently affecting older adults. The reasons for this are uncertain but likely relate to spread of more virulent strains, widespread use of fluoroquinolone antibiotics, and perhaps proton-pump inhibitors (SOE=B). Data suggest vancomycin is more effective than metronidazole for *C difficile* disease and should be used as first-line therapy when severe disease is present. Metronidazole is still suggested as first-line therapy for mild to moderate disease. Relapse is more common in older adults and may require tapering of vancomycin (to be done over several months). Prevention of *C difficile* disease is mainly accomplished by reducing the unneeded antibiotics and the duration of needed antibiotic use. This is highlighted by data showing that one of every three courses of antibiotics in nursing-home residents results in *C difficile* disease. See "Gastrointestinal Diseases and Disorders," p 391.

FEVER OF UNKNOWN ORIGIN

Fever of unknown origin (FUO) is defined as temperature >38.3°C (101°F) that lasts for at least 3 weeks and is undiagnosed after 1 week of medical evaluation. Several studies have examined this syndrome in older patients and demonstrated differences between older and younger adults. The cause of FUO can be determined in >90% of cases in older adults, and one-third have treatable infections, such as intra-abdominal abscess, bacterial endocarditis, tuberculosis, perinephric abscess, or occult osteomyelitis, with an incidence of infection similar to that in younger patients. In contrast, collagen vascular diseases are more common causes of FUO in older than in younger patients. These are primarily due to giant cell arteritis, polymyalgia rheumatica, and polyarteritis nodosa but rarely to Wegener granulomatosis. In several published series, 28% of all FUOs in older adults were due to collagen vascular diseases (Table 58.6). Neoplastic disease accounts for another 20%, but with rare exceptions, fever due to cancer is primarily caused by hematologic malignancies (eg, lymphoma and leukemia) and not solid tumors. Medications are another cause of FUO in older adults. Rare causes in this age group include deep-vein thrombosis with or without recurrent pulmonary emboli and hyperthyroidism.

For a diagnostic approach to FUO in older adults, see Table 58.7.

Table 58.7—Evaluation of Fever of Unknown Origin in Older Adults

1. Confirm fever; conduct thorough history (include travel, *Mycobacterium tuberculosis* exposure, medications, constitutional symptoms, symptoms of giant cell arteritis) and physical examination. Discontinue nonessential medications.

2. Initial laboratory evaluation: CBC with differential, liver enzymes, erythrocyte sedimentation rate, blood cultures × 3, PPD skin testing, thyrotropin, antinuclear antibody, consider antineutrophilic cytoplasmic antibody or HIV-antibody testing in specific cases.

3. a) Chest or abdomen or pelvic CT scan—if no obvious source *or*

   b) Temporal artery biopsy—if symptoms or signs consistent with giant cell arteritis or polymyalgia rheumatica and increased erythrocyte sedimentation rate *or*

   c) Site-directed evaluation on basis of symptoms or laboratory abnormalities, or both.

4. If 3a is performed and no source is found, then 3b, and vice versa.

5. Bone marrow biopsy—yield best if hemogram abnormal—send for hematoxylin and eosin stain, special stains, cultures, *or* liver biopsy—very poor yield unless abnormal liver enzymes or hepatomegaly

6. Indium-111 labeled WBC or gallium-67 scan—nuclear scans can effectively exclude infectious cause of fever of unknown origin if negative.

7. Laparoscopy or exploratory laparotomy

8. Empiric antibiotic trial—typically reserved for antituberculosis therapy in rapidly declining host or high suspicion of tuberculosis (ie, prior positive PPD)

NOTE: PPD = (tuberculin) purified protein derivative

ACOVE-3* QUALITY INDICATORS PERTAINING TO INFECTIOUS DISEASES

Pneumonia

- If a vulnerable older adult is admitted to the hospital for pneumonia, then antibiotics should be administered within 4 hours of arrival.
- If a vulnerable older adult is admitted to the hospital with community-acquired pneumonia with hypoxia (oxygen saturation <90%), then oxygen should be administered.
- If a vulnerable older adult hospitalized with community-acquired pneumonia is switched from parenteral to oral antimicrobial therapy, then the oral medication should have equivalent or near-equivalent bioavailability, or there should be documentation of the following:
  ○ Signs of clinical improvement
  ○ Ability to tolerate other oral medications, food, and fluids
  ○ Hemodynamic stability (heart rate <100 beats per minute, systolic blood pressure >90 mmHg, respiratory rate <24, temperature ≤37.8°C [100°F], oxygen saturation >90% on room air)
- If a vulnerable older adult with community-acquired pneumonia is discharged home, then he or she should have been hemodynamically stable on the day before and the day of discharge.

*Assessing Care of Vulnerable Elders – 3rd Set. See inside front cover for explanation.

REFERENCES

- High K, Bradley S, Mehr D, et al. Clinical practice guideline for evaluation of fever and infection in long-term care facilities: 2008 update by the Infectious Diseases Society of America. *Clin Infect Dis.* 2009;48(2):149–171.

- Luther VP, Wilkin A.M. HIV infection in older adults. *Clin Geriatr Med.* 2007;23(3):567–583.

CHAPTER 59—ENDOCRINE AND METABOLIC DISORDERS

KEY POINTS

- Thyrotropin (thyroid stimulating hormone) is an adequate screening test for thyroid function in a healthy older adult outpatient population, but both free T_4 and thyrotropin should be used to evaluate thyroid status in sick older adults.

- Chronic adrenal insufficiency presents with nonspecific symptoms such as anorexia, nausea, weight loss, abdominal pain, weakness, hypotension, and impaired function. It should be considered as a cause of unexplained cachexia, mobility disability, and hypotension, even in the absence of hyponatremia and hyperkalemia.

- Vitamin D deficiency is common and not only contributes to bone loss due to osteoporosis and osteomalacia but also has been associated with muscle weakness and falls.

- The most common causes of hypercalcemia are primary hyperparathyroidism in outpatients and malignant hypercalcemia (eg, caused by squamous cell cancers, breast cancer, myeloma, and lymphoma) in the inpatient setting.

- There is little evidence of long-term clinical benefit from supplementation with dehydroepiandrosterone (DHEA), testosterone, and growth hormone in older adults.

Impaired homeostatic regulation, a hallmark of aging, occurs in many endocrine systems but may become manifest only during stress. For example, fasting blood glucose concentrations change little with normal aging, increasing 1–2 mg/dL per decade of life. In contrast, glucose concentrations after glucose challenge increase much more in healthy older adults than in young adults. In some cases, a loss of function in one aspect of endocrine function can result in a compensatory change in endocrine regulation and be associated with changes in catabolism that maintain homeostasis. For example, decreased testosterone production by the testes, which is seen in many older men, may be partially compensated for by an increase in pituitary luteinizing hormone secretion

and offset by a decrease in testosterone metabolism. In other instances, compensatory changes or changes in hormone catabolism do not fully offset age-related impairment in endocrine functions, as illustrated by the age-related decline in basal serum aldosterone concentrations. In this case, a decline in aldosterone clearance fails to offset the decrease in aldosterone secretion.

As with diseases in other organ systems, endocrine disorders in older adults often have nonspecific, muted, or atypical symptoms and signs. Some of these presentations are well-defined syndromes that are seen almost exclusively in older adults, such as apathetic thyrotoxicosis or hyperosmolar nonketotic state in patients with type 2 diabetes mellitus. However, more commonly, endocrine disorders present with subtle, nonspecific symptoms, such as cognitive impairment or reduced functional status, or an absence of any complaints. Indeed, the diagnosis of endocrinopathies such as primary hyperparathyroidism, type 2 diabetes mellitus, hypothyroidism, and hyperthyroidism in older adults is commonly established as a result of abnormalities found on routine laboratory screening.

Laboratory evaluation of older adults for endocrine disorders can be complicated by coexisting medical illnesses and medications. For example, the presence of serious acute or chronic nonthyroidal illness can lead to the mistaken impression of a thyroid disorder because of the reduction or increase in T_4 concentrations and sometimes increased or decreased thyrotropin concentrations in sick but euthyroid older adults. As a result of biological and assay variability, hormone concentrations may vary considerably in the short term. Therefore, abnormal hormone measurements should always be repeated to confirm endocrine dysfunction, and a stimulatory or suppression test may be required to firmly establish a diagnosis of endocrine hypofunction or hyperfunction, respectively. Furthermore, ranges of normal laboratory values for endocrine testing are commonly established in younger adults, and even age-adjusted norms for laboratory tests may be confounded by the inclusion of older adults who are ill. Consequently, normal ranges for healthy older adults are not available for most laboratory tests.

THYROID DISORDERS

With aging, a decrease in T_4 secretion is balanced by a decrease in T_4 clearance, resulting in unchanged circulating T_4 concentrations. T_3 concentrations are unchanged until extreme old age, when they decrease slightly. However, T_3 concentrations are commonly decreased in nonthyroidal illness because of decreased peripheral conversion of T_4 to T_3. Thyrotropin concentrations are unchanged or minimally changed in healthy older adults.

Nonspecific, atypical, or asymptomatic presentations of thyroid disease are common in older adults. Laboratory testing in the stable outpatient using thyrotropin measurements is the most reliable way to identify hypothyroidism or hyperthyroidism in older adults who are not acutely ill. Screening for thyroid disease by measurement of thyrotropin every 2 yr is recommended for older adults (SOE=C). In addition, the prevalence of hypothyroidism or hyperthyroidism is sufficiently high to warrant thyrotropin testing in all older adults with a recent decline in clinical, cognitive, or functional status, or on admission to a nursing home. However, the results of thyroid function testing can be confusing in euthyroid patients with significant concurrent illnesses, as discussed below.

Hypothyroidism

Most prevalence estimates of hypothyroidism in older adults range from 0.5% to 5% for overt disease, and from 5% to 10% for subclinical hypothyroidism, depending on the population studied. As in younger people, most cases of hypothyroidism in older people are due to chronic autoimmune thyroiditis (Hashimoto disease).

Symptoms of hypothyroidism are often atypical in older adults. Some clinical features of hypothyroidism (eg, dry skin, decreased skin turgor, slowed mentation, weakness, constipation, anemia, hyponatremia, arthritis, paresthesias, peripheral neuropathy, gait disturbances, edema, and increased myocardial fraction of creatine kinase) can misleadingly suggest other diseases. Furthermore, these symptoms usually have an insidious onset and a slow rate of progression. As a result, the diagnosis of hypothyroidism is recognized on clinical examination in only 10%–20% of cases in older adults, and laboratory screening is necessary to detect most cases of hypothyroidism in this population. In addition, older adults with mild hypothyroidism who develop serious nonthyroidal illness may rapidly become severely hypothyroid, a situation that increases susceptibility to myxedema coma. Demented older adults with hypothyroidism rarely recover normal cognitive function with thyroid replacement, but cognition, functional status, and mood may improve with treatment of the hypothyroidism.

Subclinical hypothyroidism, characterized by increased serum thyrotropin and normal free T_4 concentrations, is found in up to 15% of people ≥65 yr old, and is more common in women. Subclinical hypothyroidism is associated with increased low-density lipoprotein (LDL) cholesterol levels and subtle defects in left ventricular diastolic and systolic function. Thyroid hormone replacement lowers total and LDL cholesterol levels in patients with mild thyroid failure, but it is unknown whether levothyroxine therapy is preferable to other lipid-lowering strategies in this situation. The relative risk of coronary heart disease and cardiovascular and all-cause mortality is increased among people with subclinical hypothyroidism who are <65 yr old but not in those ≥65 yr old.

It is unclear whether thyroid hormone replacement improves outcomes in people of any age with subclinical hypothyroidism. In a prospective observational study of adults 85–89 yr old, adverse effects associated with increased thyrotropin concentrations were not identified, and participants with higher thyrotropin concentrations appeared to live longer, suggesting that mild hypothyroidism may be protective in this age group. Randomized trials of T_4 supplementation in older adults with subclinical hypothyroidism have not shown a consistent improvement in symptoms, although people with thyrotropin concentrations >10 mIU/L can derive symptomatic benefit. Accordingly, T_4 replacement may be indicated in older adults with progressively increasing thyrotropin concentrations or a thyrotropin concentration persistently >10 mIU/L. Furthermore, the presence of high titer antithyroid peroxidase antibodies (consistent with Hashimoto's disease) is associated with eventual overt hypothyroidism, arguing for thyroid replacement even in asymptomatic patients (SOE=C).

By itself, an increased thyrotropin concentration is usually due to primary hypothyroidism, but thyrotropin concentrations may be transiently increased during recovery from acute illnesses. Therefore, the diagnosis of hypothyroidism should be confirmed by the combination of an increased thyrotropin concentration and a decreased free T_4 or free T_4 index, or by the demonstration of a persistently increased thyrotropin concentration, or both. Other potentially confusing scenarios in the diagnosis of hypothyroidism include the *low T_4 syndrome*, seen in euthyroid patients with severe nonthyroidal illnesses who have a decreased free T_4 index without increased thyrotropin concentrations. Free T_4 concentrations are usually normal in the low T_4 syndrome, with increased concentrations of reverse T_3. Thyroid hormone supplementation has not been shown to be beneficial in these patients. A normal (or low) thyrotropin concentration together with a low free T_4 concentration can also suggest *secondary hypothyroidism*, which is differentiated from the low T_4 syndrome by the presence of hypopituitarism (deficiencies in

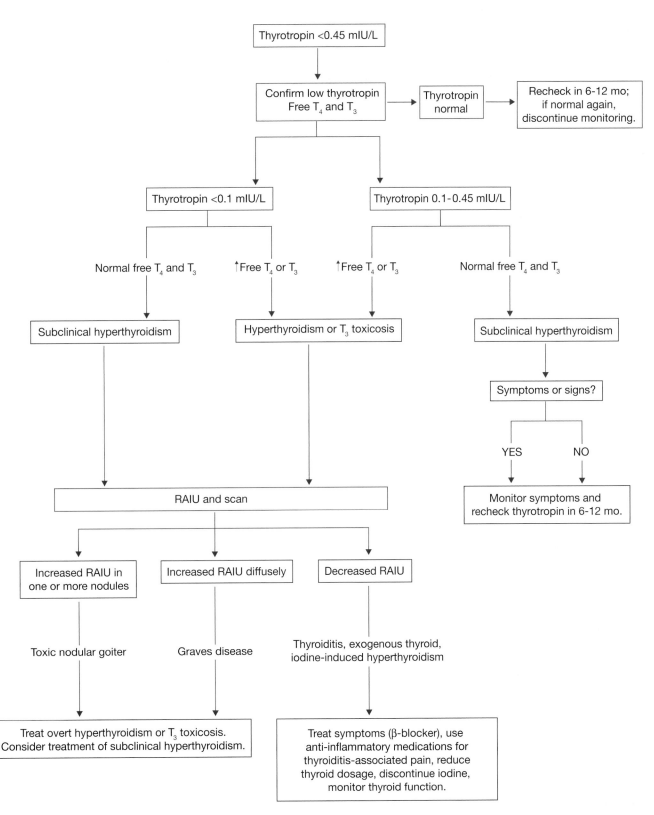

Figure 59.1—Management of low thyrotropin level

NOTE: RAIU = radioactive iodine uptake

other pituitary hormones) and decreased reverse T_3 concentrations. Rarely, older adults with primary hypothyroidism can also have inappropriately normal thyrotropin concentrations resulting from suppression of thyrotropin by fasting, acute illnesses, and medications such as dopamine, phenytoin, or glucocorticoids.

T_4 replacement is usually started at a low dosage (eg, 25 mcg/d) in older adults, increasing the dosage every 4–6 weeks until thyrotropin concentrations reach the normal range. However, in patients with severe cardiac disease, it is sometimes prudent to begin replacement therapy at even lower dosages (eg, 12.5 mcg/d) if patients are asymptomatic or have minimal symptoms of hypothyroidism (SOE=D). In these patients, thyroid replacement should not be withheld for fear of exacerbating cardiac disease; instead, the goal is to reduce or eliminate symptoms of hypothyroidism without causing intolerable exacerbation of cardiac symptoms, such as angina. Older adults who are severely hypothyroid at presentation should receive larger initial T_4 replacement doses of 50–100 mcg, or as high as 400 mcg IV for those with myxedema stupor or coma, even if there is preexisting heart disease (SOE=D). Older adults with severe hypothyroidism or myxedema stupor or coma should also receive testing to exclude concomitant adrenal insufficiency as well as stress doses of glucocorticoids before receiving T_4 to avoid precipitating an adrenal crisis with T_4 replacement.

Thyroid hormone requirements decrease with aging because of a decreased clearance rate, and T_4 replacement dosages are as much as a third lower in older than in younger adults. The average T_4 replacement dosage in older adults is approximately 110 mcg/d. Thyroid hormone is best taken fasting to avoid reduced absorption related to food and other medications (eg, calcium, iron, or soy). Over-replacement of thyroid hormone should be avoided, because osteopenia related to increased bone turnover and exacerbation of heart disease may occur. With correction of the hypothyroid state, the clearance rate of medications such as anticonvulsants, digoxin, and opioid analgesic agents may be affected, necessitating dosage adjustments.

Hyperthyroidism

Hyperthyroidism develops in 0.5%–2.3% of older adults, and 15%–25% of all cases of thyrotoxicosis are in adults ≥60 yr old. In the United States, most cases in older adults are due to Graves disease, but toxic multinodular goiter and autonomously functioning adenomas are more common in older than in young adults, especially in populations with low iodine intake.

Hyperthyroidism often presents with vague, atypical, or nonspecific symptoms in frail older adults. Many findings that are common in younger adults (eg, tremor, hyperkinesis, heat intolerance, tachycardia, frequent bowel movements, ophthalmopathy, increased perspiration, goiter, brisk reflexes) are less common or absent in older adults, whereas other manifestations, such as atrial fibrillation, heart failure, muscle atrophy, and weakness, are more common in older adults. Older adults can present with *apathetic thyrotoxicosis*, a well-known clinical presentation of hyperthyroidism that is rarely seen in younger adults, in which the usual hyperkinetic presentation is replaced by depression, inactivity, lethargy, or withdrawn behavior, often in association with symptoms such as anorexia, weight loss, constipation, muscle weakness, or cardiac symptoms. A low thyrotropin concentration is associated with a 3-fold higher risk of developing atrial fibrillation within 10 yr, and hyperthyroidism is present in 13%–30% of older adults with atrial fibrillation. Hyperthyroidism is a cause of secondary osteoporosis and should be considered in the evaluation of patients with decreased bone mass.

A highly sensitive thyrotropin test is adequate as an initial test for hyperthyroidism in relatively healthy older adults, but the diagnosis should be confirmed with a free T_4 test. For the approach to evaluating and treating a low thyrotropin concentration, see Figure 59.1. Most asymptomatic older adults with low serum thyrotropin concentrations are clinically euthyroid and have normal T_4 and T_3 concentrations, with normal thyrotropin on repeat testing 4–6 weeks later. T_3 *thyrotoxicosis*, with increased T_3 but normal T_4 concentrations, occurs in a minority of hyperthyroid patients, but it is more common with aging, especially in older adults with toxic adenomas or toxic multinodular goiter. However, in contrast to young adults, many older adults with hyperthyroidism do not have increased T_4 or T_3 concentrations, probably because of decreased conversion of T_4 to T_3 associated with aging and nonthyroidal illness. Diagnostic confusion can occasionally occur in euthyroid patients with conditions or medications causing increased T_4 concentrations, called *high T_4 syndrome*. The high T_4 syndrome can develop with medications or illnesses that decrease the conversion of T_4 to T_3 (high-dose glucocorticoids or β-blocking agents, acute fasting) or that increase circulating concentrations of thyroid-binding globulin (estrogens, clofibrate, hepatitis).

Subclinical hyperthyroidism is present in approximately 2% of older adults without known thyroid disease. In patients with a thyrotropin <0.1 mIU/L, 1%–2% per year develop overt hyperthyroidism, whereas overt disease develops uncommonly in those with thyrotropin concentrations between 0.1 and 0.45 mIU/L. Thyrotropin concentrations normalize over time in many of these patients. There is good evidence for an association between subclinical

Table 59.1—Indications for Thyroid Ultrasonography

Screening
- History of head and neck irradiation
- Multiple endocrine neoplasia type 2
- Family history of thyroid cancer

Diagnosis
- Unexplained cervical lymphadenopathy
- Guidance for fine-needle aspiration of single or multiple thyroid nodules
- Identification of nodular characteristics suspicious of cancer

hyperthyroidism and atrial fibrillation for thyrotropin concentrations <0.45 mIU/L (SOE=A). Subclinical hyperthyroidism can increase left ventricular mass and cardiac contractility and can cause delayed diastolic relaxation, but these effects are of uncertain clinical importance. In a meta-analysis of 5 population-based cohort studies, subclinical hyperthyroidism tended to be associated with modestly increased cardiovascular morbidity other than atrial fibrillation, cardiovascular mortality, and all-cause mortality regardless of age, although these findings were not significant. Subclinical hyperthyroidism can accelerate bone mineral density loss, especially in people with a thyrotropin concentration <0.1 mIU/L. In postmenopausal women, ongoing bone losses associated with thyrotropin concentrations <0.1–0.2 mIU/L are stabilized by treating the hyperthyroidism. Large, population-based studies have not found an increase in neuropsychiatric and systemic symptoms in people with subclinical hyperthyroidism. Treatment of hyperthyroidism should be considered in older adults with thyrotropin concentrations <0.1 mIU/L due to Graves or nodular thyroid disease (SOE=C). Evidence is insufficient to recommend treating older adults with thyrotropin concentrations between 0.1 and 0.45 mIU/L, although treatment consideration has been advocated based on increased risk of atrial fibrillation in this group.

Thyroid scanning and measurement of radioactive iodine uptake may be useful in confirming hyperthyroidism and defining the cause. It is important to identify hyperthyroid patients with low radioactive iodine uptake because these patients do not respond to radioactive iodine therapy or antithyroid medications and are treated symptomatically. Radioactive iodine therapy is the treatment of choice for most older adults with hyperthyroidism due to Graves disease or toxic nodular thyroid disease. Radioactive iodine treatment is usually curative in patients with toxic adenoma, but higher or repeated doses are often necessary for patients with toxic multinodular goiter. Antithyroid drugs such as methimazole or propylthiouracil are given before radioactive iodine, to control symptoms and to avoid a worsening of

thyrotoxicosis due to transient release of thyroid hormone after radioactive iodine. β-Blocking agents are helpful to manage symptoms such as tachycardia, tremor, and anxiety[OL], but patients should be monitored for changes in cardiopulmonary function. After radioactive iodine therapy, patients should be monitored by serial measurements of thyrotropin concentration for the eventual development of hypothyroidism or for persistent or recurrent hyperthyroidism. With resolution of hyperthyroidism, the clearance rate of other medications may decrease, necessitating dosage adjustments to avoid excessive drug concentrations.

Nodular Thyroid Disease and Thyroid Cancer

The incidence of multinodular goiter increases with age. Multinodular goiters often have autonomously functioning areas, so that administration of exogenous thyroid hormone to suppress these goiters can cause iatrogenic hyperthyroidism. Older adults with multinodular goiter can develop iodine-induced thyrotoxicosis after receiving radiocontrast or amiodarone.

Approximately 90% of women ≥70 yr old, and 60% of men ≥80 yr old have thyroid nodules. Most of these nodules are nonpalpable. Thyroid nodules are more likely to be malignant in people ≥60 yr old, especially men. The incidence of differentiated thyroid cancers is similar in older and younger adults, whereas thyroid lymphomas are more common and anaplastic thyroid carcinomas are found almost exclusively in older adults. However, even well-differentiated papillary and follicular carcinomas are more aggressive and are associated with increased mortality in older adults.

Ultrasound is the most sensitive test to detect thyroid nodules. Screening ultrasonography of the thyroid is not indicated in the general population. The procedure should be performed when there is unexplained cervical lymphadenopathy or when risk factors for thyroid cancer are present (Table 59.1). Additionally, ultrasound is warranted in patients with normal or high thyrotropin concentrations and one or more palpable thyroid nodules (SOE=B). However, autonomously functioning thyroid nodules are rarely malignant, so no further evaluation for cancer is required in patients with low thyrotropin concentrations and a "hot" nodule on radionuclide thyroid scanning that corresponds to a palpable nodule. Referral to endocrinology is appropriate to establish diagnosis and management.

DISORDERS OF PARATHYROID AND CALCIUM METABOLISM

Important changes occur with aging in several systems that regulate calcium homeostasis that can lead

Table 59.2—Causes of Age-Related Changes in Calcium Homeostasis

Decreased concentrations of 1,25 dihydroxyvitamin D

   Decreased renal 1α-hydroxylase activity, leading to decreased renal parathyroid hormone responsiveness

   Decreased vitamin D synthesis by the skin

   Decreased sunlight exposure (housebound and institutionalized older adults)

Decreased intestinal absorption of dietary calcium

   Inadequate dietary calcium and vitamin D intake

   Decreased intestinal responsiveness to 1,25 dihydroxyvitamin D

   Decreased gastric acid secretion

   Lactase deficiency (avoidance of dairy products)

Increase in serum parathyroid hormone concentrations

   Slight decrease in serum calcium concentrations

   Decreased renal clearance of parathyroid hormone

   Decreased concentrations of 1,25 dihydroxyvitamin D

to decreased bone mass and in some cases osteoporosis in older adults (Table 59.2). The net effect of these changes is to increase circulating concentrations of parathyroid hormone (PTH), which increases 30% between 30 and 80 years of age. Serum calcium concentrations remain normal as a result of the increase in PTH, but the balance between bone resorption and bone formation is changed in favor of resorption, resulting in decreased bone mass and increased risk of osteoporosis with aging.

Vitamin D Deficiency

Vitamin D deficiency is extremely common, affecting approximately 40%–60% of older adults regardless of whether they are community dwellers, hospitalized patients, or nursing-home residents. In addition, dietary calcium intake is inadequate in most older adults. However, as a consequence of factors mentioned in Table 59.2, older adults are less able than younger adults to compensate by increasing their intestinal absorption of ingested calcium. Increased bone turnover and bone loss, especially of cortical bone, is a major consequence of secondary hyperparathyroidism in vitamin D–deficient older adults. Furthermore, vitamin D deficiency is associated with muscle weakness and can contribute to fall risk in some individuals.

25(OH)D, the main form of vitamin D in circulation, is measured in serum to determine vitamin D status; measurements of 1,25(OH)$_2$D$_3$, the active metabolite of vitamin D, are not useful to assess vitamin D status in most individuals (see below) and are mostly used clinically in those with late-stage chronic kidney disease. Although no consensus exists, increasing evidence suggests the optimal concentration of 25(OH)D in older adults for a variety of clinically relevant end points, including bone density, lower extremity function, and fracture risk, is approximately 36–40 ng/mL (SOE=C). Unfortunately, many

older people have 25(OH)D concentrations below these values, and most postmenopausal women taking medication for osteoporosis have 25(OH)D concentrations <30 ng/mL. A recent report on calcium and vitamin D by the Institute of Medicine states that the cut-off point for levels of vitamin D deficiency or insufficiency are not backed up by rigorous scientific studies.

25(OH)D concentrations <30–40 ng/mL are inversely associated with circulating PTH concentrations, reflecting secondary hyperparathyroidism associated with vitamin D deficiency, whereas PTH concentrations approach their nadir at 25(OH)D concentrations above this range. Treating women with vitamin D sufficient to boost 25(OH)D concentrations rom 20 to 32 ng/mL increases intestinal calcium transport. Thus 25(OH)D concentrations between approximately 30 and 60 ng/mL indicate vitamin D sufficiency with little or no associated secondary hyperparathyroidism and increased efficiency of intestinal calcium absorption.

Vitamin D supplementation reduces the risk of adverse health outcomes such as fractures, but only if the supplementation is adequate[OL]. A meta-analysis of 12 randomized controlled trials (RCTs) of fracture risk in older adults reported that supplementation with vitamin D$_3$ (cholecalciferol) at 400 IU/d had little effect on the risk of nonvertebral or hip fractures, whereas 700–800 IU/d reduced the relative risk of hip fracture by 26% (pooled RR: 0.74; confidence interval [CI] 95%, 0.61–0.88), and the relative risk of other nonvertebral fractures by 23% (pooled RR: 0.77; CI 95%, 0.68–0.87), versus calcium alone or placebo (SOE=A). The pooled absolute risk difference for hip fracture was 0.009 (ie, absolute RR of 0.9%), with a number needed to treat (NNT)=111. For nonvertebral fractures, the pooled absolute risk difference was 0.016 (an absolute RR of 1.6%), with an NNT=62.

This protective effect of vitamin D supplementation on fracture risk may be mediated not only by its beneficial effect on bone density, but also by its effect on leg strength and fall risk. In community-dwelling and institutionalized older adults, vitamin D supplementation reduced the incidence of falls by 22% (pooled corrected odds ratio [OR]=0.78; CI 95%, 0.64–0.92) compared with that in those receiving calcium or placebo. The pooled absolute risk difference was 0.07, or a 7% reduction in absolute risk (CI 95%, 2%–12%), with an NNT=15. Subgroup analysis suggested that higher dosages of vitamin D, again in the range of 700–800 IU/d, were needed to reduce fall risk. Of note, these beneficial effects were most apparent in less active older women, whereas community-dwelling older men appeared not to benefit.

Vitamin D supplementation may also be beneficial for prevention of colorectal cancer and adenomas[OL] (SOE=B). Vitamin D is thought to act locally on colonic epithelial cells, decreasing cell proliferation and increasing cell differentiation. Epidemiologic studies have generally observed an inverse relationship between either 25(OH)D concentrations or vitamin D intake and the risk of colorectal cancer and/or adenomas, although data from the Nurses' Health Study suggest that the risk of colorectal cancer was reduced only in those taking vitamin D consistently at dosages above 550 IU/d for >10 yr. More limited data suggest that vitamin D supplementation may have a beneficial effect on other diseases and health outcomes, including periodontal disease, cardiovascular disease, hypertension, multiple sclerosis, glucose intolerance, type 2 diabetes mellitus, tuberculosis, and cancers other than colorectal cancer.

A meta-analysis of 18 RCTs in which 57,311 mostly middle-aged and older participants were enrolled found an association between vitamin D supplementation and decreased risk of death. The RR for death from any cause in treated persons was 0.93 (CI 95%, 0.87–0.99). Although these findings are intriguing, population-based, randomized, placebo-controlled trials are needed to confirm the effect of vitamin D supplementation on overall mortality.

How much vitamin D should be prescribed for older adults? Currently recommended levels of vitamin D supplementation (ie, up to 800 IU/d of cholecalciferol [vitamin D_3]) are inadequate to achieve 25(OH)D concentrations of 30 ng/mL in most older adults without substantial sun exposure. If testing is done, people with 25(OH)D concentrations <30 ng/mL may benefit from higher dose vitamin D supplementation for a short period, eg, ergocalciferol (vitamin D_2) 50,000 IU/wk for 12 wk[OL] (SOE=A). When 25(OH)D concentrations are not known, most older adults should receive cholecalciferol at a dosage of at least 2,000–4,000 IU/d (SOE=A); this should be on the higher end for individuals with minimal sun exposure. Maintaining adequate calcium intake (1,000–1,500 mg/d from the diet and supplements) is also important for bone health and prevention of secondary hyperparathyroidism. High-dose supplementation may cause vitamin D intoxication with hypercalcemia, hypercalciuria, impairment of kidney function, and bone loss, but dosages of 10,000 IU/d do not cause toxicity when taken for up to 5 mo. A few patients who are unable to take daily oral supplements may benefit from oral vitamin D at 100,000 IU every 6 mo with minimal risk of hypercalcemia. See also prevention and treatment of osteoporosis in "Osteoporosis," p 239.

Hypercalcemia

Primary hyperparathyroidism and malignancy are the most common causes of hypercalcemia in older adults. The annual incidence of primary hyperparathyroidism is approximately 1 per 1,000, and the disease is 3-fold more prevalent in women than in men. Most patients with primary hyperparathyroidism are asymptomatic, and the diagnosis is made after an incidental finding of hypercalcemia. When the disease is symptomatic, older adults are more likely than younger adults to present with neuropsychiatric symptoms such as depression and cognitive impairment, neuromuscular symptoms such as proximal muscle weakness, or osteoporosis. For typical laboratory findings in primary hyperparathyroidism and other common causes of hypercalcemia, see Table 59.3. The diagnosis of primary hyperparathyroidism is confirmed with an increased or high normal PTH concentration, by the use of an assay for intact PTH, in the presence of hypercalcemia. Referral to endocrinology should be made for further treatment decisions.

Patients with serum calcium concentrations less than 1 mg/dL above the normal range who are asymptomatic and managed conservatively should avoid lithium carbonate, thiazide diuretics, dehydration, and immobilization. Baseline assessment in these patients should include blood pressure; serum calcium, phosphate, and creatinine; creatinine clearance; and bone densitometry. Follow-up assessments should include serum calcium and creatinine every 12 mo, and bone densitometry (at 3 sites) every 12–24 mo (SOE=C). In addition, these patients should be followed clinically for the development of nephrolithiasis, fractures caused by minimal trauma, and neuropsychiatric or neuromuscular symptoms. At present, no medications are approved specifically for the treatment of primary hyperparathyroidism. Medical management options for hyperparathyroidism in-

Table 59.3—Typical Laboratory Results in the Differential Diagnosis of Hypercalcemia

Laboratory Test	Primary Hyperparathyroidism	Humoral Hypercalcemia of Malignancy	Local Osteolytic Hypercalcemia
Serum calcium	↑	↑ or ↑↑	↑ or ↑↑
Serum phosphate	↓ or low-normal	↓	↑
Urine calcium	↑	↑	↑
Parathyroid hormone	↑	↓↓	↓↓
Parathyroid hormone-related peptide	0	↑	0

NOTE: The diagnosis of malignancy-related hypercalcemia is normally straightforward, and extensive diagnostic testing is rarely required. ↑ = increased; ↑↑ = markedly increased; ↓ = decreased; ↓↓ = markedly decreased; 0 = undetectable

clude β-blocking agents^OL, oral phosphate only in patients with low serum phosphate concentrations and good kidney function^OL, and possibly raloxifene^OL. Alendronate, a bisphosphonate, improves bone mineral density in patients with primary hyperparathyroidism without affecting calcium or PTH concentrations^OL (SOE=B). Cinacalcet, a calcimimetic agent that inhibits parathyroid cell function, reduced or normalized serum calcium concentrations and reduced PTH concentrations without changing bone mineral density in study participants treated for up to 5.5 yr^OL. However, it is unknown whether cinacalcet can prevent fractures and nephrolithiasis or relieve neuropsychiatric symptoms associated with this disorder.

In hospitalized patients, the most common cause of hypercalcemia is a malignancy that produces PTH-related peptide (PTHrp), with hypercalcemia resulting primarily from increased net bone resorption. The presence of an underlying cancer is usually evident on examination and routine diagnostic testing. Squamous cell cancers of the lung or head and neck are common causes of hypercalcemia due to PTHrp production. Other common malignancies associated with hypercalcemia include breast cancer, lymphoma, and myeloma, although the mechanisms of the hypercalcemia associated with these malignancies are usually not PTHrp-mediated and may be responsive to glucocorticoid treatment. Acute treatment for hypercalcemia of malignancy includes volume replacement with intravenous saline, often followed by diuresis with a loop diuretic only when volume repletion is complete. A parenteral bisphosphonate such as pamidronate or zoledronic acid should be given, along with treatment of the underlying malignancy, if possible. In addition to their usefulness in the treatment of hypercalcemia, high-potency bisphosphonates such as zoledronic acid may decrease bone pain and the risk of pathologic fractures in patients with osteolytic bone metastases from a variety of cancers (SOE=A). Nephrotoxicity associated with these agents may be minimized by adhering to recommended dosages and infusion times. However,

these agents should be used cautiously if at all in people with a creatinine clearance of ≤30 mL/min. Cancer patients receiving parenteral bisphosphonates who have had recent dental extractions, dental implants, poorly fitting dentures, or preexisting disease are at risk of osteonecrosis of the jaw.

Paget's Disease of Bone

Paget's disease is characterized by localized areas of increased bone remodeling, resulting in a change in bone architecture and an increased tendency to deformity and fracture. Its prevalence increases with aging, affecting 2%–5% of people ≥50 yr old. Paget's disease is usually asymptomatic and is often diagnosed as an incidental finding on radiographs or during evaluation for an unexplained increase in serum alkaline phosphatase. The most commonly affected sites are the pelvis, spine, femur, tibia, and skull. When Paget's disease is symptomatic, pain is the most common presenting symptom, either localized to the affected bones or resulting from secondary osteoarthritic changes, often in the hips, knees, and vertebrae. When bone deformities occur, the long bones of the legs are usually affected, often with bowing. Skull involvement may result in compression of the eighth cranial nerve and sensorineural hearing loss. The most devastating complication of Paget's disease is malignant transformation of the affected bone, especially the development of osteosarcoma. Treatment is not usually necessary for asymptomatic Paget's disease, unless there is concern of hearing loss from skull involvement, nerve root or spinal cord compression from vertebral involvement, or hip fracture from femoral neck involvement. Bisphosphonates suppress the accelerated bone turnover and bone remodeling that is characteristic of Paget's disease, and they are the treatment of choice (SOE=C). These agents are effective in treating bone pain associated with Paget's disease (SOE=A), and sustained biochemical remissions are achieved with high-potency bisphosphonates in many patients. Calcium and vitamin D should be administered concomitantly with bisphosphonates to prevent hypocalcemia^OL. NSAIDs may be useful in treating secondary osteoarthritis.

During treatment, patients should be monitored clinically for changes in bone pain, joint function, and neurologic status, and with biochemical indices of bone formation (eg, serum osteocalcin or bone-specific alkaline phosphatase), resorption (eg, urinary N-telopeptide), or both.

HORMONAL REGULATION OF WATER AND ELECTROLYTE BALANCE

Unlike young adults, older adults are predisposed to both volume depletion and free water excess. This impairment in regulation of volume status and osmolality is multifactorial, reflecting decreased total body water content as well as changes in antidiuretic hormone (ADH) secretion, osmoreceptor and baroreceptor systems, urine-concentrating capability, renal hormone responsiveness, and thirst sensation. ADH secretion tends to be excessive in older adults, with normal to increased basal ADH concentrations, increased ADH responses to osmoreceptor stimuli such as hypertonic saline infusion, and decreased ethanol-induced inhibition of ADH secretion. This state of relative ADH excess seen with aging, when combined with renal insufficiency, heart failure, hypothyroidism, or diuretic use, predisposes older adults to hyponatremia by impairing free water clearance.

The syndrome of inappropriate antidiuretic hormone (SIADH) is the most common cause of hyponatremia in older adults. Most cases of SIADH are mild and relatively asymptomatic, but even mild chronic hyponatremia (serum sodium of 120–132 mEq/L) may increase the risk of falls, gait impairment, and difficulty sustaining attention in older adults. Medications causing SIADH include the SSRIs, sulfonylureas, carbamazepine, oxcarbazepine, and tricyclic antidepressants.

Older adults are at increased risk of volume depletion. With aging, basal aldosterone secretion declines disproportionately to the decrease in clearance, with a net reduction in circulating aldosterone concentrations of about 30% by the age of 80 yr. At the same time, atrial natriuretic hormone secretion (and renal responsiveness to this hormone) increases with aging. Atrial natriuretic hormone inhibits aldosterone production and causes natriuresis and diuresis through its effects on the kidneys. Taken together, these changes predispose older adults to volume depletion by decreasing the ability of the kidneys to conserve sodium under conditions of fluid deprivation. Baroreceptor ADH responses to hypotension and hypovolemia are decreased in older adults, placing them at additional risk of dehydration. Moreover, renal responsiveness to ADH is decreased with aging, resulting in a decreased ability of the kidneys

to maximally concentrate urine. Finally, even healthy older adults have decreased thirst sensation and may not be aware that they are becoming dehydrated. Demented and immobile older adults are at the highest risk of severe dehydration and hypernatremia.

In addition to predisposing to volume depletion, age-related hyporeninemic hypoaldosteronism also increases the risk of hyperkalemia, especially in older adults with diabetes mellitus or renal insufficiency. The addition of ACE inhibitors, NSAIDs, β-blocking agents, and diuretics with aldosterone-antagonist properties may lead to potentially lethal hyperkalemia in some of these patients. See "Kidney Diseases and Disorders," p 404.

DISORDERS OF THE ADRENAL CORTEX

Basal serum cortisol concentrations do not change with aging, because decreased cortisol secretion is balanced by a decrease in clearance. Stimulation of cortisol production by adrenocorticotropic hormone (ACTH) is unchanged, and cortisol and ACTH responses to stress and secretagogues are unimpaired with aging. Clinically, acute cortisol responses to stress may be higher and more prolonged in older than in younger adults. Accordingly, in nonemergent situations, adrenal function testing should be deferred at least 48 hours after major stressors, such as surgery or trauma. In older adults with a normal ACTH stimulation test in whom adrenal insufficiency is suspected, endocrinology consultation is recommended to assist with further testing.

Hypoadrenocorticoidism

Chronic glucocorticoid therapy is the most common cause of adrenal failure in older adults because of chronic suppression of adrenal function. Recovery of adrenal axis function is variable and may take several months to a year. Autoimmune-mediated adrenal failure is less common in older than in younger adults, but tuberculosis, adrenal metastases, and adrenal hemorrhage in anticoagulated patients are more common causes of adrenal insufficiency in older adults. Additionally, prolonged use of megestrol acetate (eg, as an appetite stimulant) may cause hypoadrenocorticoidism. Older adults with chronic adrenal insufficiency may present with nonspecific symptoms such as anorexia, nausea, weight loss, abdominal pain, weakness, hypotension, or impaired functional status, and hyponatremia and hyperkalemia may not always be present. Accordingly, a high index of suspicion is required to make the diagnosis. Chronic adrenal insufficiency should be considered in patients with unexplained cachexia, mobility impairment, and hypotension. When adrenocortical insufficiency is suspected, the ACTH stimulation test should be performed (SOE=A) and therapy initiated (SOE=D). A normal serum cortisol response 30 or 60 minutes after administration of 250 mcg of ACTH (cosyntropin) is 18–20 mcg/dL. A serum ACTH concentration should be obtained before administration of cosyntropin to distinguish secondary adrenal insufficiency (decreased pituitary ACTH secretion), which is characterized by a low or normal ACTH concentration, from primary adrenal insufficiency, which is associated with a high ACTH concentration. In older adults who are stopping chronic glucocorticoid therapy, the replacement regimen should be tapered gradually (SOE=D), and stress dose coverage should be given for major surgery and other acute physiologic stresses until adrenocortical function has returned to normal (SOE=D). Recovery of hypothalamic-pituitary-adrenal axis may take >9 mo.

Hyperadrenocorticoidism

Exogenous glucocorticoids are the most common cause of Cushing's syndrome in older adults, often causing adverse events, including psychiatric and cognitive symptoms, osteoporosis, myopathy, and glucose intolerance. For patients beginning long-term glucocorticoid therapy, baseline and follow-up bone densitometry measurements are indicated, and calcium, vitamin D, and antiresorptive treatments such as alendronate, risedronate, or zoledronic acid should be started as appropriate for prevention of glucocorticoid-induced osteoporosis. Management of subclinical glucocorticoid hypersecretion is discussed below.

Adrenal Androgens

In contrast to the changes seen in cortisol concentrations with aging, circulating concentrations of the principal adrenal androgen, dehydroepiandrosterone (DHEA), decline progressively with aging, and in octogenarians are only 10%–20% of concentrations in young adults. Low DHEA concentrations are associated with poor health, whereas DHEA concentrations are positively correlated with some measures of longevity and functional status. Given these associations, there has been interest in the potential therapeutic effects of DHEA administration in older adults.

Most studies involving physiologic to mildly supraphysiologic DHEA supplementation in middle-aged and older adults have not found clinically meaningful beneficial effects on body composition. Although DHEA may increase bone mineral density in postmenopausal women (and not in older men), these effects are minimal in comparison with established treatments for osteoporosis. In RCTs of DHEA supplementation for up to 2 yr in older adults

with low DHEA concentrations, improvements were not detected in measures of physical performance, well-being, mood, quality of life, and cognition. Potential risks of DHEA treatment include decreased circulating high-density lipoprotein cholesterol levels in older women, raising the possibility of potential long-term atherogenic effects. Furthermore, DHEA is metabolized to estrogens and to androgens such as testosterone and dihydrotestosterone, and its effects on the risk of breast cancer in women and prostate cancer in men are unknown. Finally, higher dosages of DHEA can cause androgenization in some women and gynecomastia in men. Thus, the safety and efficacy of DHEA supplementation in older adults have not been established, and its use is inappropriate other than in clinical studies.

Women with adrenal insufficiency or who are surgically menopausal develop severe androgen deficiency and may present with symptoms of decreased libido, energy, and well-being. Androgen replacement therapy (eg, with DHEA or testosterone) may be justifiable in these women to treat severe, symptomatic androgen deficiency. However, current guidelines recommend against widespread use of testosterone in women, based on inadequate evidence of appropriate indications and safety in long-term studies.

Testosterone treatment for the indication of hypoactive sexual desire in nonsurgical postmenopausal women is not recommended by The Endocrine Society's 2006 guideline on the topic. Although testosterone appears to improve measures of sexual desire and function in estrogen-replete postmenopausal women, the long-term safety of testosterone therapy and concerns about concomitant long-term estrogen therapy preclude recommendation. There is a lack of data in non-estrogen-replete women, precluding a recommendation for treatment in these women. Additionally, it was felt that a clear definition of hypoactive sexual desire disorder is lacking. See "Disorders of Sexual Function," p 430.

TESTOSTERONE

Despite former controversy, there is now general agreement that total and free testosterone levels and testosterone secretion are lower in healthy older men than in younger men. Many healthy older men exhibit moderate primary testicular failure, with decreased sperm production, testosterone levels, and testosterone secretory responses to gonadotropin administration. In addition, many of these men also have inappropriately normal (ie, not increased) gonadotropin levels in the presence of low testosterone levels, suggesting secondary (hypothalamic or pituitary) testicular failure. Overt testicular failure is common in chronically ill and debilitated older men or in men receiving chronic glucocorticoids or opioids, manifested by testosterone levels well below the normal range and symptoms suggesting androgen deficiency, including decreased libido and impotence, gynecomastia, and hot flushes. Testosterone replacement therapy may generally be warranted in these severely clinically and biochemically androgen-deficient patients, as it would be in hypogonadal young men. However, it is more common to encounter older men with low-normal or mildly decreased serum testosterone levels and nonspecific manifestations, such as decreased libido and potency, reduced energy, depressed mood, weakness, decreased muscle mass, osteopenia, metabolic syndrome, and memory loss. In most cases, these manifestations have multiple causes, but it has been hypothesized that declining testosterone levels with aging contribute to their development, and that testosterone supplementation can help to prevent or treat these disorders.

Male hypogonadism should be diagnosed only in men with signs and symptoms suggesting androgen deficiency, as well as unequivocally low serum testosterone levels. Men with suspected hypogonadism should be evaluated with a serum total testosterone level or preferably, if available, a serum free or bioavailable (non–sex hormone–binding globulin-bound) testosterone level either measured by equilibrium dialysis or calculated from measurements of total testosterone and sex hormone–binding globulin (SHBG), preferably in the morning (SOE=C).

The potential short-term benefits and risks of testosterone supplementation in older men with low-normal or mildly decreased serum testosterone levels in controlled studies of up to 3 years' duration are summarized in Table 59.4. However, it is unknown whether these potential benefits and risks are clinically important or whether longer-term potential benefits outweigh risks. Bearing these uncertainties in mind, a trial of testosterone supplementation may be appropriate in older men with unequivocally low serum total testosterone levels (eg, <2.8 ng/mL) or decreased free or bioavailable testosterone levels, and clinical features suggesting hypogonadism (eg, osteoporosis, muscle wasting or weakness, mild anemia of unclear cause, loss of libido)[OL] (SOE=D). Androgen replacement therapy is inappropriate in asymptomatic older men with low-normal total or free testosterone levels who do not have clinical manifestations consistent with androgen deficiency. Notably, bisphosphonates are clearly efficacious in treating older men with low testosterone and osteoporosis, so testosterone therapy is not appropriate in older men who have no manifestations of hypogonadism other than osteoporosis. Furthermore, testosterone administration is contraindicated in patients with prostate cancer and breast cancer, and should be avoided in

men with an undiagnosed prostate nodule or induration on digital rectal examination, consistently increased PSA, erythrocytosis, and probably in men with severe lower urinary tract symptoms due to benign prostatic hyperplasia or uncontrolled severe heart failure (SOE=C). For available preparations of testosterone, see Table 59.5.

Men should be monitored closely for efficacy as well as adverse events of testosterone treatment, including new or worsening snoring, observed apnea during sleep, or excessive daytime sleepiness that may suggest obstructive sleep apnea syndrome. Routine monitoring for potential adverse effects of testosterone should be performed before initiation of therapy, 3–6 mo after initiation, and then at least annually thereafter (SOE=C); monitoring should include measurement of serum hematocrit (to check for erythrocytosis), serum PSA and digital rectal examination (to assess for prostatic disease), and inquiry into lower urinary tract symptoms. Serum testosterone levels should also be monitored to assess the adequacy of delivery, especially in men receiving transdermal testosterone formulations (patch or gel). An increase in the PSA concentration of >1 ng/mL within 3–6 mo after starting testosterone therapy can indicate the presence of previously undetected prostate cancer, and testosterone should be discontinued until the prostate has been fully evaluated (SOE=C). However, there is no direct evidence that testosterone therapy increases the risk of prostate cancer or symptomatic benign prostatic hyperplasia. See also "Disorders of Sexual Function," p 430.

ESTROGEN THERAPY

Many of the symptoms and signs of hormone deficiency mimic physiologic changes associated with aging. The fact that many hormones also decline with aging has led to an enthusiasm for attempting to reverse unwanted changes associated with aging by the use of hormonal replacement. Based on very compelling epidemiologic data, replacement of estrogen, with or without progesterone, was once standard of care for postmenopausal women, but is no longer because of more recent data from randomized clinical trials demonstrating significant adverse events from such therapy. Estrogen therapy now is largely limited to treatment of menopausal symptoms (see treatment of menopausal symptoms in "Gynecologic Diseases and Disorders," p 416).

Three meta-analyses of observational studies have demonstrated an association of estrogen therapy in women with a reduction in heart disease by half. However, a few long-term prospective studies of secondary prevention demonstrated increased mortality in the first year on therapy, with improved survival in years 2 through 5, leading to no net benefit. In

Table 59.4—Potential Short-Term Benefits and Risks of Testosterone Supplementation in Older Men with Low-Normal or Mildly Decreased Testosterone Concentrations

Study End Point	Effect of Testosterone
Lean body mass	Increased
Fat mass	Decreased
Bone mineral density	Variable (no change or increased)
Strength	Improved grip strength Inconsistent effect on leg muscle strength and performance of functional tasks
Sexual function	Variable; most consistent findings are activation in sexual behavior and increased libido
Mood	Variable; mood and subjective well-being improved in some studies; inconsistent effects on depression
Cognitive	Some cognitive domains improved (eg, verbal memory, visual memory, spatial ability, executive function); worsened effect of practice on verbal fluency
Quality of life	Inconsistent effects; some studies show significant improvement of physical function domain
Lipid profile	Total and low-density lipoprotein cholesterol tend to decrease; high-density lipoprotein cholesterol unchanged
Coronary heart disease	In men with established disease, improved ECG evidence of exercise-induced coronary ischemia (in most studies); variable effect on angina pectoris
Prostate	Prostate-specific antigen (PSA) increased slightly in many patients; can increase risk of prostate biopsy due to rise in PSA concentrations; no effect on voiding symptoms or prostate examination
Hematocrit	Increased 2.5%–5% versus baseline
Long-term clinical outcomes	Unknown

NOTE: This table summarizes results of placebo-controlled studies.

Table 59.5—Testosterone Preparations Available in the United States for Hypogonadal Older Men

Preparation	Initial Treatment Dosage
Testosterone enanthate or cypionate	75 mg IM every week, or 150 mg IM every 2 weeks
Nonscrotal transdermal patch	5 mg transdermal every day
Gel	5–10 g transdermal every day
Buccal tablet	30 mg applied to buccal mucosa q12h
Testosterone pellets	225 mg SC every 4–6 mo

another trial of women with coronary artery disease, no benefit was found from estrogen for angiographic changes of atherosclerosis. The Women's Health Initiative (WHI) is a set of clinical trials to test primary prevention of coronary artery disease with estrogen and estrogen-progesterone combinations. The estrogen-progesterone arm was discontinued early because of the increased risk of coronary disease, breast cancer, stroke, and deep-vein thrombosis (SOE=A); the estrogen-alone arm of the study was discontinued because of increased risk of stroke (SOE=A). Post-hoc analysis of the WHI data suggest that risk of cardiovascular events were increased in older women and with increased years since menopause.

Although observational studies also suggested that estrogen may have a role in preventing dementia, a placebo-controlled trial of estrogen replacement given for 1 yr to 120 women with early to moderate Alzheimer's dementia found no improvement in affective or cognitive outcomes. In the WHI, in a study to assess primary prevention, women in the estrogen arm had clinically important declines in their Mini–Mental State Examination scores or transition to mild cognitive impairment or dementia.

The risks of breast cancer, endometrial cancer, and deep-vein thrombosis/pulmonary emboli associated with the use of estrogen have been well established; these results were confirmed in the WHI trial. A recent study to assess change in risk approximately 3 yr after the WHI trials were discontinued demonstrated continued increased risk with previous estrogen use due to fatal and nonfatal malignancies. The risk of breast cancer was similar to that in the nontreatment arm at the 3-yr follow-up and the previously demonstrated beneficial effects on colon cancer had dissipated, but risk of lung cancer was higher than in the nontreatment arm. Overall mortality was similar in the estrogen and placebo groups. See also estrogen therapy for osteoporosis prevention in "Osteoporosis," p 242.

GROWTH HORMONE

Growth hormone secretion declines with aging, and by 70–80 yr of age, about half of adults have no significant growth hormone secretion over 24 hours. A corresponding decline occurs in concentrations of insulin-like growth factor 1, which mediates most of the effects of growth hormone; it falls to concentrations comparable to those in growth hormone–deficient children in 40% of adults 70–80 yr old.

Adults with growth hormone deficiency due to hypothalamic-pituitary disease exhibit decreased muscle strength, lean body mass, and bone density; increased abdominal obesity; unfavorable lipid profiles; and an increased risk of cardiovascular disease. All improve with growth hormone replacement. Older adults without hypothalamic-pituitary disease have many of the same conditions, which leads to the hypothesis that growth hormone supplementation may have a beneficial effect on these clinically important age-related disorders. Randomized controlled trials of short-term growth hormone supplementation in older adults have reported increased lean body mass (change in lean body mass, 2.1 kg [CI, 1.3 to 2.9]) and decreased fat mass (change in fat mass, –2.1 kg [CI 95%, –2.8 to –1.35]). However, growth hormone was not found to augment improvements in muscle strength achieved with exercise alone, no improvements in functional status were demonstrated, and there were no significant improvements in bone density or lipid levels after adjustment for body composition changes (SOE=A). Furthermore, significant adverse events were common, including carpal tunnel syndrome, arthralgias, edema, and gynecomastia. The long-term efficacy and safety of growth hormone administration in older adults are unknown. Short-term growth hormone supplementation may improve nitrogen balance in older adults with severe illness and catabolic states. However, growth hormone is very expensive, and at present it is not recommended for clinical use in older adults who do not have established hypothalamic-pituitary disease.

MELATONIN

Melatonin, a hormone secreted by the pineal gland, is thought to be involved in the regulation of circadian and seasonal biorhythms. Melatonin secretion is inhibited by exposure to light, resulting in a marked circadian variation in circulating melatonin concentrations. Its sedative effects suggest a role in sleep induction. Most studies show that plasma melatonin concentrations decline throughout life after early childhood, but the physiologic significance of this decline in melatonin secretion is unclear. Numerous claims have been made in the lay press regarding the "antiaging" benefits of melatonin supplementation for various conditions, including insomnia, immune deficiency, cancer, and the aging process itself. Although melatonin may have sleep-inducing properties in older adults with insomnia, the long-term risks and benefits of melatonin supplementation have not been established for insomnia or any other indication.

REFERENCES

- Bhasin S, Cunningham GR, Hayes FJ, et al. Testosterone therapy in adult men with androgen deficiency syndromes: an Endocrine Society clinical practice guideline. *J Clin Endocrinol Metab.* 2006;91(6):1995–2010.

- Gruenewald DA, Matsumoto AM. Aging of the endocrine system and selected endocrine disorders. In: Halter JB, Hazzard WR, Ouslander JG, et al., eds. *Principles of Geriatric Medicine and Gerontology.* 6th ed. New York: McGraw-Hill; 2009:1267–1286.

- Heiss G, Wallace R, Anderson GL, et al for WHI Investigators. Health risks and benefits 3 years after stopping randomized treatment with estrogen and progestin. *JAMA.* 2008;299(9):1036–1045.

CHAPTER 60—DIABETES MELLITUS

KEY POINTS

- Diabetes mellitus, one of the most common chronic conditions in older adults, results in decreased life expectancy, excess complications and comorbidities, a higher risk of other common geriatric conditions (eg, polypharmacy, urinary incontinence, falls, cognitive impairment, depression, and chronic pain), functional impairment, and disability.

- Both diabetes and impaired glucose tolerance are important to identify and address by changes in lifestyle.

- Because of the great heterogeneity in the older population, treatment goals for older diabetic patients must be carefully individualized.

- Although the target blood pressure is debated, attempts to lower blood pressure are important for older hypertensive diabetic patients.

- Diabetes self-management is an important part of diabetes care, and annual self-management training is a covered benefit under Medicare Part B.

Diabetes mellitus is a group of metabolic disorders characterized by hyperglycemia due to abnormalities in insulin secretion, insulin action, or both. It is one of the most common chronic diseases affecting older adults. Estimates of the prevalence among adults ≥65 yr old range between 15% and 20%. Because the general population is aging and rates of obesity are increasing among middle-aged adults, people ≥65 yr old will constitute the majority of diabetic adults in the United States and in other developed countries in the coming decades. In the United States, people ≥65 yr old now account for more than 40% of all people with diabetes. In the coming years, the largest percent increase in diabetes prevalence in any age group will be among those >75 yr old.

The age-adjusted prevalence of diabetes mellitus is higher among black Americans and Hispanic Americans than white Americans. Further, black Americans suffer from complications of diabetes at disproportionately higher rates than white Americans. Research is only starting to decipher the effects of race on diabetes development and outcomes.

Because diabetes may be asymptomatic for many years, it is estimated that up to one-third of older adults with diabetes mellitus are unaware of their condition. Despite the early asymptomatic period, diabetes mellitus is a serious condition associated with significant morbidity and a shortened survival. Older adults with diabetes can expect a 10-yr reduction in life expectancy and a mortality rate nearly twice that of people without this disease. In addition, older adults disproportionately experience the clinical complications and comorbidities associated with diabetes. These complications include atherosclerosis, neuropathies, loss of vision, and renal insufficiency. The rates of myocardial infarction, stroke, and kidney failure are increased approximately 2-fold, and the risk of blindness is increased approximately 40% in older adults with diabetes. Most patients ≥65 yr old who require dialysis have diabetes.

Research is accumulating about important clinical consequences of diabetes that are common in older adults and have serious consequences to health status and quality of life. When diabetes is poorly controlled in older adults, hyperglycemia alone can be the cause of insidious decline characterized by fatigue, weight loss, muscle weakness, and reduced function. Older adults with diabetes are at higher risk than those without diabetes for geriatric syndromes, including incontinence, falls, frailty, cognitive impairment, and depressive symptoms; they also have a higher prevalence of functional impairment and disability. Mobility problems are about 2 to 3 times more likely, and disability in ADLs is about 1.5 times more likely in older adults with diabetes than in those without.

PATHOPHYSIOLOGY

The American Diabetes Association classifies diabetes mellitus affecting older adults into three types. Type 1 is the result of an absolute deficiency in insulin secretion due to autoimmune destruction of the β cells of the pancreas. Type 2 is most commonly due to tissue resistance to insulin action and relative insulin deficiency. A third category is reserved for other specific types of diabetes: injuries to the exocrine pancreas; endocrinopathies characterized by excesses of hormones, such as growth hormone, cortisol, glucagon, and epinephrine, which antagonize insulin action; drug- or chemical-induced diabetes; and infections leading to the destruction of the β cells of the pancreas.

In about 90% of cases, older adults with diabetes have the type 2 form of the disease. Most older adults with type 2 diabetes have had years of glucose intolerance, insulin resistance, and the metabolic syndrome. This "prediabetes" syndrome is also associated with increased risk of atherosclerotic disease, as well as development of type 2 diabetes.

The prevalence of both type 2 diabetes and glucose intolerance increases with age. The reasons for this are not fully known; there appears to be an interaction among several factors, including genetics, lifestyle, and aging influences. Obesity and decreased physical activity, common among older adults, contribute to impairments in insulin action. Glucose intolerance has also been shown to be related to age-associated decline in pancreatic β-cell function and in the insulin-signaling mechanisms that limit the mobilization of glucose transporters needed for insulin-mediated glucose uptake and metabolism in muscle and fat. Changes in body composition that occur with aging, such as increased visceral fat leading to insulin resistance, can also contribute to changes in carbohydrate metabolism. Decreased levels of physical activity in some older adults can exacerbate age-related changes in body composition and increased carbohydrate intolerance. An altered inflammatory environment with aging can also contribute to the higher rates of diabetes in older adults.

In addition to intrinsic physiologic mechanisms, external factors can contribute to glucose intolerance and type 2 diabetes. Some medications commonly used by older adults—diuretics, estrogen, sympathomimetics, glucocorticoids, niacin, and olanzapine—change carbohydrate metabolism and increase glucose concentration. Intercurrent illnesses, such as infections, myocardial infarction, and stroke, as well as other physiologic stresses can lead to worsened hyperglycemia. The heterogeneity in the severity of hyperglycemia among older adults with type 2 diabetes is related to the varying contributions of these factors in each individual.

The pathophysiology of the complications of diabetes is similar in younger and older adults. Prolonged hyperglycemia leads to glycosylation of proteins; the accumulation of these abnormal proteins can cause tissue damage. Also, metabolic products of the aldose-reductase system, such as sorbitol, accumulate in the presence of hyperglycemia. These products can impair cellular energy metabolism and contribute to cell injury and death.

Physiologic changes that develop with diabetes and its complications can interact with physiologic changes associated with aging to further decrease physiologic reserve. Type 2 diabetes and obesity are associated with inflammatory dysregulation, which can also be associated with aging and lead to clinical sequelae such as sarcopenia. Aging is associated with decreased physiologic reserve in multiple organ systems (eg, renal, cardiovascular, CNS), which may interact with end-organ damage due to diabetes, resulting in increased vulnerability to physiologic stressors.

DIAGNOSIS AND EVALUATION

As of 2009, the American Diabetes Association diagnostic criteria for diabetes mellitus do not include any adjustments that are based on age. Three ways to establish the diagnosis of diabetes mellitus are possible, and each must be confirmed, on a subsequent day, by any one of the three methods:

- Symptoms of polyuria, polydipsia, and unexplained weight loss plus a casual plasma glucose concentration of ≥200 mg/dL (11.1 mmol/L). *Casual* is defined as any time of day without regard to time since last meal.

- A plasma glucose concentration after an 8-hour fast of ≥126 mg/dL (7 mmol/L).

- A plasma glucose concentration of ≥200 mg/dL (11.1 mmol/L) measured 2 hours after ingestion of 75 g of glucose in 300 mL of water administered after an overnight fast.

In clinical practice, the presence of two fasting glucose levels of ≥126 mg/dL is the most common method of diagnosis. Older adults with fasting blood glucoses of 110–125 mg/dL are defined as having impaired fasting glucose, a condition associated with increased risk of diabetes development. Some older adults have isolated postchallenge hyperglycemia but do not have high fasting blood glucose concentrations; many of these people would be diagnosed as type 2 diabetes by oral glucose tolerance testing criteria. Isolated postchallenge hyperglycemia does appear to confer increased risk of atherosclerotic complications but not as much as diagnosed type 2 diabetes.

Several diabetes prevention trials demonstrated that in people with glucose intolerance, progression to type 2 diabetes can be prevented by medications and lifestyle changes (SOE=A). Lifestyle changes were found to be slightly more efficacious in older than in younger adults and superior to medications in the older group. These results demonstrate the importance of preventive measures and lifestyle changes in older adults who are at risk of developing type 2 diabetes.

MANAGEMENT

Clinical Evaluation

Older adults with diabetes require a comprehensive evaluation, which in the primary care setting may be done over several patient visits. For patients with significant functional impairments and comorbidities, including those with psychosocial problems and caregiver requirements, a formal, comprehensive geriatric assessment may be needed. Regardless of how the comprehensive evaluation of an older adult with diabetes mellitus is handled, four issues deserve special attention.

First, the history and physical examination must include evaluation of risk factors for atherosclerotic disease and the presence of all comorbid diseases. Diabetes is a well-established risk factor for atherosclerotic cardiovascular disease, so other risk factors such as smoking, family history, hypertension, and hyperlipidemia should also be explored. Diabetes is also associated with multiple vascular complications that may be subclinical or clinical. The presence of coronary artery disease, peripheral vascular disease, neuropathy, foot problems, and medical eye disease must be determined. In many cases, subspecialty consultation (as for retinopathy) and laboratory or diagnostic testing is indicated. In addition, older adults with diabetes are also likely to have prevalent chronic diseases that are not necessarily associated with their diabetes, such as osteoarthritis.

Second, a thorough medication history is important. As previously stated, certain medications can contribute to hyperglycemia. More often, older adults may be on multiple medications for multiple comorbidities and may experience adverse drug events or trouble with medication management or finances, which will affect formulating the treatment plan.

Third, an assessment of functional status is important to help determine whether the patient is able to independently manage his or her diabetes, or whether caregiver input is also needed. Functional assessment will also assist the clinician and the patient in setting diabetes management targets.

Fourth, older adults should be screened for the use of multiple medications, depression, cognitive impairment, urinary incontinence, injurious falls, and pain. Multiple observational studies have shown that these geriatric conditions are more common in older adults with diabetes than without (SOE=B). Finally, each patient's needs for diabetes education and self-management support, including whether to involve a caregiver, should be assessed.

General Principles of Diabetes Management

The clinician develops goals for diabetes management and individualized clinical targets with each older adult with diabetes, involving the caregiver when appropriate. The goals of diabetes management in older adults include the following:

- control of hyperglycemia and its symptoms
- evaluation and treatment of associated risks for atherosclerotic and microvascular disease
- evaluation and treatment of diabetes complications
- support for diabetes self-management and education
- maintenance or improvement of general health status

Although these goals are similar for older and younger people with diabetes, the management of older patients is complicated by the medical and functional heterogeneity of this group. In fact, this heterogeneity is a key consideration in developing individualized diabetes management interventions and clinical targets for older patients with diabetes. Some may have developed diabetes in middle age and have developed multiple related comorbidities. Some may be recently diagnosed but have had undiagnosed diabetes for years and have complications at diagnosis. Others may have just converted from impaired glucose tolerance to diabetes and may have few complications or comorbidities. In addition to medical heterogeneity, older adults with diabetes are heterogeneous in their functional status. Many are active with excellent function. Others may be disabled and frail, with advanced cognitive impairment, multiple comorbidities and complications, and significant functional limitations. Many others are in between, with mild or early functional limitations, several related comorbidities, and multiple risks for worsening morbidity. Several researchers have pointed out the burden that some patients with diabetes complications and other comorbidities experience trying to cope with self-management of multiple chronic diseases.

Another consideration in treating older adults with diabetes is life expectancy and the time needed for clinical benefit from a specific intervention. Clinical trials have demonstrated that approximately 8 yr are needed before the benefits of glycemic control are reflected in a reduction in microvascular complications such as diabetic retinopathy or kidney disease, but that only 2–3 yr are required to see benefits from better control of blood pressure and lipids (SOE=A). It is important to remember that the median remaining life expectancy for a 70-yr-old woman is 14 yr, which is plenty of time for the development of diabetes complications. Therefore, for a person in his or her early 70s who is newly diagnosed or highly functional, diabetes management is no different from that of younger people. However, management must be designed to fit the clinical status of older adults who are significantly functionally impaired or who have multiple comorbidities that limit life expectancy or that significantly increase the risks of hypoglycemia. In all cases, patient preferences and quality of life must be considered.

Solid evidence supports the effectiveness of several components of diabetes care, including control of lipids and blood pressure, control of hyperglycemia, aspirin use, smoking cessation, appropriate eye and foot care, prevention of nephropathy, diabetes education and self-management support for medication adherence, appropriate nutrition, weight loss if indicated, and increased physical activity (SOE=A). Home monitoring of blood glucose has not been found to be cost-effective (SOE=A). Very few of the data supporting these interventions were obtained from research studies of older people. A large, randomized trial of intensive versus moderate control of hyperglycemia showed that very intensive control (targeting HbA$_{1c}$ to <6.5%) is harmful (SOE=A) and that control of hyperglycemia to a target HbA$_{1c}$ <7% in patients with long-standing diabetes reduces microalbuminuria but does not reduce macrovascular events (SOE=A). Thus, the risks and benefits of intensive glycemic control are actively debated, and the most appropriate HbA$_{1c}$ target for people of all ages with type 2 diabetes is unclear. It is likely that many management guidelines can be generalized to many older adults with diabetes, particularly those who are healthy and functional. For some older patients, particularly those with severe comorbidities and disabilities, aggressive management is not likely to provide benefit and may even result in harm, such as hypoglycemia with aggressive glycemic control or hypotension with aggressive blood-pressure control.

Patient preferences regarding management interventions are also important to elicit and consider, because the patient is the one who will ultimately manage his or her diabetes and comorbid conditions. Some patients do not want to follow some management recommendations. Some may fear dependency and the need for assistance more than death. Some may find certain medications or monitoring activities burdensome.

Therefore, it is important to establish individual goals for diabetes management and clinical targets with patients; to reevaluate the clinical, functional, and social status of the patient if these goals and targets are not being met; and to determine if caregiver support or specialty input is needed. A practical clinical method of individualizing and prioritizing diabetes care is to assess goals and preferences, assess patient longevity and functional status, consider the time needed for treatment impact, screen for geriatrics syndromes, and assist patients with decision making and prioritization of treatment strategies.

In 2003, the California Healthcare Foundation and the American Geriatrics Society collaborated to develop one of the first set of guidelines for improving the care of older adults with diabetes mellitus (see the references at the end of the chapter). Many of the specific management interventions outlined below are adapted from this guideline. Since that time, several large trials of diabetes management interventions have included older adults and have added to the evidence base about their management. An excellent review of the evidence, and its gaps, that support management interventions for diabetes among older adults was done by the ACCORD trial investigators (see references at the end of the chapter).

Prevention and Management of Atherosclerotic Complications

Older adults with diabetes are at high risk of atherosclerosis and its complications. In fact, virtually all older adults with diabetes have either clinical or preclinical atherosclerotic disease. Therefore, interventions that reduce the risk of atherosclerotic diseases are extremely important. Smoking cessation counseling and pharmacologic intervention should be offered to any older diabetic adult who smokes. Daily aspirin therapy should be offered to older adults with diabetes if there is not a contraindication to aspirin. Available evidence suggests that dosages from 81 to 325 mg/d are appropriate.

A number of randomized controlled trials (RCTs) provide strong evidence that the management of hypertension in older adults reduces cardiovascular events and mortality; some of these studies included substantial numbers of older adults with diabetes (SOE=A). The best target blood pressure for older diabetic patients is not clear, but experts suggest that in most patients the target blood pressure should be <140/80 mmHg. However, of five major RCTs of blood-pressure control that included people with diabetes, levels <140/80 mmHg were achieved in only one. However, in the ADVANCE trial, with 11,140 people in multiple sites around the world with a mean age of 66 yr, a mean blood pressure of 136/73 mmHg was achieved in the intensive treatment group. The relative risk of cardiovascular death decreased 18% in the intensive group; the relative risk of all-cause death decreased 14% (absolute risk reduction=1.3%, number needed to treat [NNT]=79 for all-cause mortality over 5 yr) (SOE=A). Although observational studies suggest that lowering blood pressure to <130/70 mmHg may provide increased benefit, this target level has not been achieved in any clinical trial of blood pressure management in diabetes. Because some older adults may not be able to tolerate aggressive blood-pressure lowering, hypertension should be treated gradually to avoid complications. Patient preference and adverse events of medication should be considered. See also "Hypertension," p 384.

Evidence for medication choice in older adults with diabetes suggests that most classes chosen (diuretics, ACE inhibitors, β-blockers, and calcium channel blockers) have comparable effectiveness in reducing cardiovascular disease and mortality. Evidence suggests that ACE inhibitors (SOE=A) and angiotensin II receptor blockers (SOE=B) have additional cardiovascular and renal benefit for people with diabetes.

Evidence supports the use of lipid-lowering therapy; RCTs and a meta-analysis have confirmed the benefit of the statin drugs, particularly for secondary prevention of cardiovascular events (SOE=A). In general, most studies with statin management suggest that patients with diabetes benefit more from cholesterol lowering than those without diabetes, and secondary prevention is particularly beneficial. Analyses have calculated NNTs of 14 to 46 for prevention of one major cardiovascular event over 5 yr of lipid-lowering treatment in diabetic patients. However, some controversy still exists regarding the treatment of cholesterol in older adults with diabetes for primary prevention. The one major study (Prospective Study of Pravastatin in the Elderly at Risk, or PROSPER) of statin treatment in older adults, which included some people with diabetes, did not find benefit for primary prevention.

Even with statin therapy, rates of cardiovascular events remain high, and observational and pilot research suggest broader targeting of dyslipidemia. For example, the use of fibrates in patients with low high-density lipoprotein levels may also be of benefit, and this hypothesis is being evaluated in RCTs.

Lipid abnormalities should be corrected in older adults with diabetes when appropriate after considering the individual's overall health status. Evidence suggests that target low-density lipoprotein (LDL) level is <100 mg/dL (SOE=B). Dietary modification can be tried for 6 mo if the LDL level is <100–129 mg/dL. If the LDL level is ≥130 mg/dL, pharmacologic therapy is indicated in addition to lifestyle modifications in diet and activity level. Older adults are always at risk of adverse drug events, so when an older adult with diabetes is prescribed a statin or niacin, or when the dosage is increased, an alanine aminotransferase concentration should be measured within 12 weeks of starting the medication or changing the dosage. Also, some people may develop muscle inflammation with the statins, so symptoms of muscle pain and weakness in the presence of statin therapy must be evaluated. If a fibrate has been started or increased, liver enzymes should be evaluated annually.

Prevention and Management of Microvascular Complications

Microvascular complications of diabetes are major problems among older adults with diabetes and can be important contributors to disability. Diabetic retinopathy can result in decreased vision. Other eye conditions, such as glaucoma and cataracts, are also extremely common in older adults with diabetes. Any older adult with new-onset diabetes should have a screening dilated-eye examination by an eye-care specialist. If there is presence of retinopathy, other eye disease, ocular symptoms, poorly controlled hyperglycemia, or poorly controlled hypertension, a dilated-eye examination should be done every year. If there is no ocular disease or high risk, eye examinations can be performed every other year (SOE=D).

Serious foot problems and amputations are more common among older adults with diabetes. These patients should have a careful foot examination at least annually or more frequently if there is evidence of any problems. To screen for kidney disease, a test for the presence of microalbuminuria should be performed at diagnosis and annually if no abnormalities are detected. Finally, given a higher mortality rate among diabetic patients who develop pneumonia, pneumococcal vaccination is strongly recommended.

Management of Hyperglycemia

Control of hyperglycemia in diabetes is important. Uncontrolled hyperglycemia can lead to symptoms of weight loss, fatigue, sometimes the classic polyuria and polydipsia, and possibly increased infections, so it is important to treat to prevent these symptoms. Treatment of hyperglycemia in type 2 diabetes to prevent vascular complication is more controversial. There is evidence that control of hyperglycemia to near-normal levels may prevent retinal and renal complications, but the effects may be modest and one RCT was stopped early because of an increased mortality rate in the intensively treated group (SOE=A). RCTs of treatment of hyperglycemia to near-normal levels in older adults with diabetes have not confirmed the hypothesis that this would prevent cardiovascular disease, so the target level for hyperglycemia control is not clear. However, management of hyperglycemia to an HbA$_{1c}$ level between 6.5% and 8.5%, depending on the individual patient's management plan and the duration of his or her diabetes, is reasonable (SOE=C). There are many options for drug therapy in older adults with type 2 diabetes, with no clearly preferred algorithm. Few comparisons of the medications are available, and most studies have focused on lowering of hyperglycemia, an intermediate outcome. Little information is available about adverse drug events other than hypoglycemia.

Hyperglycemia-lowering regimens can consist of any of several classes of drugs (Table 60.1 and Table 60.2), used alone or in combination. The regimen should be adjusted over the course of the illness as goals change, the disease progresses, or complications develop. Sulfonylurea preparations have a long record of safety and effectiveness. Hypoglycemia is a serious

Table 60.1—Non-Insulin Agents for Treating Diabetes Mellitus

Medication	Dosage	Formulations	Comments (Metabolism)
Oral Agents			
2nd-Generation Sulfonylureas			Increase insulin secretion; lower HbA$_{1c}$ by 1%–2%
Glimepiride (generic or Amaryl)	4–8 mg once (begin 1–2 mg)	T: 1, 2, 4	Numerous drug interactions, long-acting (L, K)
Glipizide (generic or Glucotrol)	2.5–40 mg once or divided	T: 5, 10	Short-acting (L, K)
(Glucotrol XL)	5–20 mg once	T: ER 2.5, 5, 10	Long-acting (L, K)
Glyburide (generic or Diaβeta, Micronase)	1.25–20 mg once or divided	T: 1.25, 2.5, 5	Long-acting, risk of hypoglycemia (L, K)
Micronized glyburide (Glynase)	1.5–12 mg once	T: 1.5, 3, 4.5, 6	Long-acting, risk of hypoglycemia (L, K)
α-Gucosidase Inhibitors			Delay glucose absorption; lower HbA$_{1c}$ by 0.5%–1%
Acarbose (Precose)	50–100 mg q8h, just before meals; start with 25 mg/d	T: 25, 50, 100	GI adverse events common, avoid if Cr >2 mg/dL, monitor liver enzymes (gut, K)
Miglitol (Glyset)	25–100 mg q8h, with first bite of meal; start with 25 mg/d	T: 25, 50, 100	Same as acarbose but no need to monitor liver enzymes (L, K)
DPP-4 Enzyme Inhibitors			Protect and enhance endogenous incretin hormones; lower HbA$_{1c}$ by 0.5%–1%
Saxagliptin (Onglyza)	5 mg; 2.5 mg if CrCl <50 mL/min	T: 2.5, 5	(K)
Sitagliptin (Januvia)	100 mg once daily as monotherapy or in combination with metformin or a thiazolidinedione; 50 mg/d if CrCl 31–50 mL/min; 25 mg/d if CrCl <30 mL/min	T: 25, 50, 100	(K)
Biguanides			Decrease hepatic glucose production; lower HbA$_{1c}$ by 1%–2%
Metformin (Glucophage)	500–2,550 mg divided	T: 500, 850, 1,000	Avoid in patients >80 yr old (unless CrCl ≥60 mL/min), Cr >1.5 in men, Cr >1.4 in women, heart failure, COPD, increased liver enzymes; hold before contrast radiologic studies; may cause weight loss (K)
(generic or Glucophage XR)	1,500–2,000 mg/d	T: ER 500	Same as above
Meglitinides			Increase insulin secretion; lower HbA$_{1c}$ by 1%–2%
Nateglinide (Starlix)	60–120 mg q8h	T: 60, 120	Give 30 minutes before meals
Repaglinide (Prandin)	0.5 mg q6–12h if HbA$_{1c}$ <8% or previously untreated; 1–2 mg q6–12h if HbA$_{1c}$ ≥8% or previously treated	T: 0.5, 1, 2	Give 30 minutes before meals, adjust dosage at weekly intervals, potential for drug interactions, caution in hepatic or renal insufficiency (L)
Thiazolidinediones			Insulin resistance reducers; lower HbA$_{1c}$ by 0.5%–1.5%; increased risk of heart failure; avoid if NYHA class III or IV cardiac status; discontinue if any decline in cardiac status
Pioglitazone (Actos)	15 or 30 mg/d; maximum 45 mg/d as monotherapy, 30 mg/d in combination therapy	T: 15, 30, 45	Check liver enzymes at start, every 2 mo during first year, then periodically; avoid if clinical evidence of liver disease or if serum ALT levels >2.5 times upper limit of normal; may increase risk of fractures in women (L, K)

Table 60.1—Non-Insulin Agents for Treating Diabetes Mellitus (continued)

Medication	Dosage	Formulations	Comments (Metabolism)
Rosiglitazone (Avandia)*	4 mg q12–24h	T: 2, 4, 8	Probably higher risk of cardiovascular disease than with pioglitazone and other oral hypoglycemic agents; check liver enzymes at start, every 2 mo during first year, then periodically; avoid if clinical evidence of liver disease or if serum ALT levels >2.5 times upper limit of normal; may increase risk of fractures in women (L, K)
Combinations			
Glipizide and metformin (METAGLIP)	2.5/250 mg once; 20/2000 in 2 divided doses	T: 2.5/250, 2.5/500, 5/500	Avoid in patients >80 yr old, Cr >1.5 mg/dL in men, Cr >1.4 mg/dL in women; see individual drugs (L, K)
Glyburide and metformin (Glucovance)	1.25/250 mg initially if previously untreated; 2.5/500 mg or 5/500 mg q12h with meals; maximum 20/2,000/d	T: 1.25/250, 2.5/500, 5/500	Starting dose should not exceed total daily dose of either drug; see individual drugs (L, K)
Liraglutide (Victoza)	0.6–1.8 mg/d SC	3-mL pre-filled pen	Incretin mimetic indicated for type 2 diabetes mellitus; not to be used in combination with insulin; caused dose-dependent and treatment duration–dependent thyroid C-cell tumors in animals (unsure if it does this in people); efficacy: decreased HbA_{1c} by 0.8–1.1%, decreased fasting blood glucose by 15–25 mg/dL, decreased weight by 2.1–2.5 kg.
Pioglitazone and metformin (ACTO plus met)	15/850 mg q12–24h	T: 15/500, 15/850	See individual drugs.
Repaglinide and metformin (PrandiMet)	1/500 mg to 4/1,000 mg twice q12h or q8h before meals; maximum 10/2,500 mg/d	T: 1/500, 2/500	See individual drugs.
Rosiglitazone and glimepiride (Avandaryl)*	1 or 2 tab/d; maximum 8 mg/4 mg	T: 4/1, 4/2, 4/4, 8/2, 8/4	See individual drugs.
Rosiglitazone and metformin (Avandamet)*	4/1,000–8/2,000 in 2 divided doses	T: 1/500, 2/500, 4/500, 2/1,000, 4/1,000	Avoid in patients >80 yr old, Cr >1.5 mg/dL in men, Cr >1.4 mg/dL in women; see individual drugs (L, K)
Pioglitazone and glimepiride (Duetact)	30/2 mg initially; maximum 45/8 mg	T: 30/2, 30/4	See individual drugs.
Sitagliptin and metformin (Janumet)	Begin with current doses; maximum 100/2,000 mg in 2 divided doses	T: 50/500, 50/1,000	See individual drugs.
Injectable Agents			
Exenatide (Byetta)	5–10 mcg SC q12h	1.2-, 2.4-mL pre-filled pen	Incretin mimetic; lowers HbA_{1c} by 0.4%–0.9%; nausea and hypoglycemia common; less weight gain than insulin; avoid if CrCl <30 mL/min (K)
Pramlintide (Symlin)	60 mcg SC immediately before meals	0.6 mg/mL in 5-mL vial	Amylin analog; lowers HbA_{1c} by 0.4%–0.7%; nausea and hypoglycemia common; reduce pre-meal dose of short-acting insulin by 50% (K)

NOTE: ALT = alanine aminotransferase; Cr = creatinine; CrCl = creatinine clearance; ER = extended release; K = renal elimination; L = hepatic elimination; SC = subcutaneously; T = tablet

* FDA has significantly restricted the use of rosiglitazone (*Avandia, Avandaryl, Avandamet*) as of 9/23/10. Due to data suggesting higher cardiovascular risk, such as heart attack and stroke, individuals with Type 2 diabetes who are not currently taking rosiglitazone can be prescribed the medication only if they are unable to achieve glycemic control with an alternative medication. Rosiglitazone will only be available to individuals who are currently taking the medication if they appear to be benefiting from the drug and have been counseled on the risks. For further information, see http://www.fda.gov/Drugs/DrugSafety/PostmarketDrugSafetyInformationforPatientsandProviders/ucm226956.htm.

SOURCE: Reuben DB, Herr KA, Pacala JT, et al. *Geriatrics At Your Fingertips*, 12th ed. New York: American Geriatrics Society; 2010. Reprinted with permission.

Table 60.2—Insulin Preparations

Preparations	Onset	Peak (hours)	Duration (hours)	Number of Injections or Inhalations/day
Rapid-acting				
Insulin glulisine (Apidra)	20 min	0.5–1.5	3–4	3
Insulin lispro (Humalog)	15 min	0.5–1.5	3–4	3
Insulin aspart (NovoLog)	30 min	1–3	3–5	3
Regular (eg, Humulin, Novolin)[a]	0.5–1 h	2–3	8–12	1–3
Intermediate or long-acting				
NPH (eg, Humulin, Novolin)[a]	1–1.5 h	4–12	24	1–2
Insulin detemir (Levemir)	3–4 h	6–8	6–24 depending on dose	1–2
Insulin glargine (Lantus)[b]	1–2 h	—	24	1
Isophane insulin and regular insulin injectable (Novolin 70/30)	30 min	2–12	24	1–2

NOTE: NPH = neutral protamine Hagedorn (insulin)

[a] Also available as mixtures of NPH and regular in 50:50 proportions.

[b] To convert from NPH dosing, give same number of units once a day. For patients taking NPH q12h, decrease the total daily units by 20% and titrate on basis of response. Starting dosage in insulin-naive patients is 10 U once daily at bedtime.

SOURCE: Reuben DB, Herr KA, Pacala JT, et al. *Geriatrics At Your Fingertips*, 12th ed. New York: American Geriatrics Society; 2010. Reprinted with permission.

adverse event, and these medications must be used cautiously in older adults with significant hepatic and renal insufficiency, because the liver is the primary site of metabolism and excretion is via the kidneys. α-Glucosidase inhibitors impair the breakdown of carbohydrates in the gut and limit absorption; the residual carbohydrates in the intestinal lumen are responsible for diarrhea observed in about 25% of older adults who use these drugs. The biguanide preparations also have GI adverse events and can theoretically cause lactic acidosis in older adults with renal insufficiency. However, a Cochrane review of metformin found no significantly increased risk of lactic acidosis. If an older adult is taking metformin, serum creatinine concentration should be measured at least annually and with any increase in dosage. For those ≥80 yr old or those suspected to have reduced muscle mass, renal function should be assessed thoroughly, either through a timed urine collection or application of a formula that corrects serum creatinine for age.

Another class of drugs, the thiazolidinediones, although apparently well tolerated by most patients, carries black box warnings because of a risk of worsening of heart failure and other cardiovascular complications. In a recent meta-analysis of 42 clinical studies, data indicated that one of these drugs, Avandia (rosiglitazone), is associated with an increased risk of myocardial ischemic events, such as heart attack and stroke. As of September 23, 2010 the FDA has restricted the use of Avandia to patients with type 2 diabetes whose diabetes is not controlled on other medications. Restricted access to this drug

will be accomplished through the use of a risk evaluation and mitigation strategy (REMS). Complete details of the FDA safety alert is available at http://www.fda.gov/Safety/MedWatch/SafetyInformation/SafetyAlertsforHumanMedicalProduct s/ucm226994.htm.

Finally, insulin can be used effectively in older adults with type 2 diabetes. Good glycemic control can often be achieved with one or two injections a day of an intermediate-acting insulin preparation. The greatest risk of insulin therapy is hypoglycemia, and some evidence suggests that frail older adults are at higher risk of serious hypoglycemia than are healthier, more functional older adults. The management plan for an older adult with diabetes who experiences severe or frequent hypoglycemia should be evaluated. Referral to subspecialty diabetes care, or more frequent contact with the healthcare team may be needed. Psychosocial reasons for hypoglycemia must be investigated and treated, such as an inability to understand self-management because of cognitive problems, inadequate diabetes knowledge, difficulty in implementing therapy because of disability, or lack of caregiver support.

EDUCATION AND SELF-MANAGEMENT SUPPORT

Because diabetes is a disease for which the patient and/or family/caregivers bear the primary responsibility for management and ultimate control, it is imperative that the patient understands the mechanisms and management of the metabolic derangements and becomes fully involved in diabetes self-management, ie, monitoring and treating the disease and its complications. Therefore, education about diabetes and particularly diabetes self-management are key components of effective care. Often, basic education can be accomplished in the primary care setting. Complex patients with diabetes may need referral to a diabetes educator for one-on-one counseling or group classes, enrollment in a comprehensive diabetes disease management program, or specialty clinician care. Annual diabetes self-management training is a covered benefit under Medicare Part B. Diabetes mellitus education programs may be particularly important in older adults with diabetes who are members of minority groups, particularly black Americans or Hispanic Americans, in whom diabetes is more prevalent than in white Americans. It is extremely important to recognize when caregiver involvement in diabetes self-management activities is required. The caregiver must be highly involved and educated about diabetes and its self-management when the patient is cognitively impaired, is significantly disabled or frail, or has limited proficiency in English.

Diabetes self-management and support must cover several important areas. The older patient, and caregiver if appropriate, must be educated about hypo- and hyperglycemia, including precipitating factors, prevention, symptoms, monitoring, treatment, and indications for notifying the clinician. Although hypoglycemia is unusual in older adults when they are treated with sulfonylurea or insulin, they are still at higher risk than middle-aged diabetics. When appropriate, the patient and caregiver should be taught blood-glucose self-monitoring, and their technique should be reassessed and reinforced periodically.

Diet and physical activity remain important components of the initial and ongoing management of patients with diabetes. Specific dietary recommendations must be tailored for each individual and focus on strategies that improve glycemic control as well as lipids and blood pressure. An individualized meal plan of regular, well-balanced meals consisting of healthy foods in the right amounts with the goal of keeping weight under control is key to diabetes management. Physical activity programs should also be individualized, taking into consideration functional status and presence of diabetic complications . The patient should be assessed regularly for level of physical activity and informed about the benefits of exercise and available resources for becoming more active.

An older adult with diabetes who is prescribed a new medication and any caregiver should be educated on the purpose of the medication, how to take it, and the adverse events that are common or important, with reassessment and reinforcement periodically as needed. Finally, every older adult with diabetes and any caregiver should be educated about risk factors for foot ulcers and amputation and appropriate foot care measures to reduce this risk. Physical ability to provide foot care should be evaluated, with periodic reassessment and reinforcement.

For patient education to be an effective tool in diabetes management, it must take into account the level of adjustment to the disease. In addition, it is critical that the patient and/or family/caregivers understand not only "what" needs to be done but "why" it needs to be done. Self-efficacy strengthening and coping skills training should also be addressed. Support groups, such as those available through the American Diabetes Association, can be extremely helpful for the older patient and/or family/caregivers.

ACOVE-3* QUALITY INDICATORS PERTAINING TO DIABETES MELLITUS

Glycated hemoglobin

■ If a vulnerable older adult has diabetes mellitus, then glycated hemoglobin should be measured annually.

Improving glycemic control

■ If a vulnerable older adult has an increased HbA1c, then a therapeutic intervention should occur:
  ○ HbA_{1c} 9–10.9%: within 3 mo
  ○ HbA_{1c} ≥11%: within 1 mo

Proteinuria

■ If a vulnerable older adult with diabetes mellitus does not have established renal disease and is not receiving an ACE inhibitor or angiotensin-receptor blocker, then a test for proteinuria should be done annually.

■ If a vulnerable older adult with diabetes mellitus has proteinuria, then an ACE inhibitor or angiotensin-receptor blocker should be prescribed.

Foot examination

■ If a vulnerable older adult has diabetes mellitus, then a foot examination should be performed annually.

Periodic retinal examination

■ If a vulnerable older adult with diabetes mellitus has a retinal examination, then the presence and degree of diabetic retinopathy should be documented.

■ If a vulnerable older adult with diabetes mellitus is not blind and did not have retinopathy on a previous examination, then he or she should have a retinal eye examination performed by a specialist every 2 yr.

Blood pressure measurement

- If a vulnerable older adult has diabetes mellitus, then blood pressure should be measured at each primary care and endocrinology visit.

Blood pressure control

- If a vulnerable older adult with diabetes mellitus has a persistent (on 2 consecutive visits) increase in systolic blood pressure (>130 mmHg), then an intervention (eg, pharmacologic, lifestyle, compliance) should occur, or there should be documentation of a reversible cause or other justification for the increase.

Aspirin therapy

- If a vulnerable older adult with diabetes mellitus is not on anticoagulant/antiplatelet therapy, then daily aspirin should be prescribed.

Improving cholesterol

- If a vulnerable older adult with diabetes mellitus has fasting low-density lipoprotein cholesterol >130 mg/dL, then a pharmacologic or lifestyle intervention should be offered within 3 mo.

Related quality indicators for Diabetes Mellitus

- Perioperative assessment and management of diabetes mellitus (see "Perioperative Care," p 92)
- Risks and prophylaxis for aspirin (see "Persistent Pain," p 109)
- Laboratory follow-up of ACE inhibitor (see "Heart Failure," p 376)

*Assessing Care of Vulnerable Elders – 3ʳᵈ Set. See inside front cover for explanation.

REFERENCES

- The American Diabetes Association. Clinical Practice Recommendations 2008. *Diabetes Care.* 2008;31(Supplement 1).
- Brown AF, Mangione CM, Saliba D, et al. Guidelines for improving the care of the older person with diabetes mellitus. *J Am Geriatr Soc.* 2003;51(5 Suppl Guidelines):S265–280.
- Durso SC. Using clinical guidelines designed for older adults with diabetes mellitus and complex health status. *JAMA.* 2006;295(16):1935–1940.
- Morrow AS, Haidet P, Skinner J, et al. Integrating diabetes self-management with the health goals of older adults: a qualitative exploration. *Patient Educ Couns.* 2008;72(3):418–423.

CHAPTER 61—HEMATOLOGIC DISEASES AND DISORDERS

KEY POINTS

- The reserve capacity of hematopoiesis diminishes with advancing age.

- The possibility of a multifactorial cause should be considered when a patient with anemia of chronic disease has a hemoglobin <10 g/dL.

- NHANES III data indicate that about 35% of all anemia among older adults in the United States results from nutrient deficiencies (iron, vitamin B$_{12}$, and/or folate); 45% of all anemia is attributable to chronic disease(s); and in 20% of cases, the anemia is unexplained despite an exhaustive evaluation.

- Coagulation enzyme activity increases with increasing age. This biochemical hypercoagulability can lead to increased thrombotic disease in older adults.

- The incidence of myelodysplasia and acute myeloid leukemia increases with age. Age-related defects in lymphopoiesis are thought to be the basis of the myeloid dominance of adult leukemia.

- Polycythemia vera, essential thrombocythemia, and idiopathic myelofibrosis occur primarily in older adults and have a slow rate of spontaneous transformation to leukemia.

HEMATOPOIESIS

Hematopoietic Stem Cells and Aging

The hematopoietic system derives from a small pool of hematopoietic stem cells (HSCs) that can either self-renew or differentiate along one of several lineages to form mature RBCs, WBCs, or platelets. HSCs differentiate into mature cells through an intermediate set of committed progenitors and precursors, each with decreasing self-renewal potential and increasing lineage commitment. Hematopoiesis is tightly regulated by a complex series of interactions between HSCs, their stromal microenvironment, and diffusible regulatory molecules, the hematopoietic growth factors (HGFs) that effect cellular proliferation. The orderly development of the hematopoietic system in vivo and the maintenance of homeostasis require that a strict balance be maintained between self-renewal, differentiation, maturation, and cell loss. Accumulated DNA damage has been proposed as the principal and unifying mechanism underlying age-dependent HSC decline.

Hematopoietic Response with Aging

Human aging is associated with reduced reserve capacity for hematopoiesis. Abnormalities in function, not evidenced in the basal state, become apparent in the stimulus-driven state. In addition to being lower, the aged response tends to be more variable. Given a comparable stress, hematologic abnormalities are likely to occur earlier and to be of greater severity in older than in younger adults. Thus, the rate of return of the hemoglobin to normal after phlebotomy is blunted, and the ability to mount a granulocyte response to infection is reduced. However, the relative contributions of age per se and age-related comorbidities to this suboptimal response are unclear. Numerous animal studies have shown a reduced ability of the aged hematopoietic system to respond to stimulation. Studies in people have not been as conclusive. See also "Biology," p 8.

Although there is no significant change in basal blood cell counts with aging, the prevalence of anemia tends to increase modestly. This is particularly noted in men ≥75 yr old, who in cross-sectional studies have significantly lower values than their younger counterparts (≤65 yr old). This large effect has not been noted in longitudinal studies. The mechanism for the difference is unclear but is thought to reflect the presence of comorbid illness or reduced erythropoietin (EPO) drive, or both, as a result of declines in androgen concentrations. Older adults do not appear to have an impaired ability to increase hematocrit in response to exogenous EPO or to increase granulocyte count after administration of granulocyte colony-stimulating factor. The severity of neutropenia after chemotherapy in older cancer patients is greater in those who are underweight and malnourished than in those who are not. Age appears to reduce hematopoietic reserve capacity. This, how-

ever, is of clinical relevance only in the presence of other comorbidities (occult or latent).

Aging does not appear to affect the circulating concentrations of EPO and other HGFs; the increase in response to anemia or infection in older adults is equivalent to that in their younger counterparts. However, in response to stress, the blunted hematopoietic response seen with age has been attributed to an impaired ability to release HGFs. This might explain the age-related reduced neutrophil response to infection seen in animal studies and may contribute to increased infection-induced morbidity with aging. The production of certain growth factors, particularly interleukin-6 (IL-6), appears to increase with aging (Table 61.1), leading to the notion that aging is accompanied by dysregulation of growth factor production, with overproduction of some cytokines and underproduction of others.

ANEMIA

Anemia, clearly the most common age-related hematologic abnormality, is seen in both older men and women. According to World Health Organization criteria, anemia is diagnosed if the hemoglobin (Hb) concentration is <13 g/dL in men and <12 g/dL in women. Studies have shown a high prevalence of anemia in older adults who are hospitalized, are seen in geriatric clinics, or are institutionalized. However, if stringent criteria are used to select apparently healthy participants, the prevalence drops. Results from the third National Health and Nutrition Examination Survey (NHANES III) in the United States indicated that the prevalence of anemia was 11% in community-dwelling men and 10.2% in women >65 yr old. In several studies, the prevalence of anemia in the population >80 yr old is reported as being 12%–16% in women and 18%–22% in men.

In the general population, the annual incidence of anemia is estimated to be 1%–2%. In contrast, the incidence of anemia in a well-defined population of people >65 yr old (whites) attending the Mayo Clinic was reported to be 4- to 6-fold higher. In this study, in every age group >65 yr old, the incidence of anemia in men was higher than that in women. This has been attributed to a reduced sensitivity to EPO stemming from declining testosterone concentrations.

Most anemia among NHANES III participants was mild; only 2.8% of women and 1.6% of men had a Hb <11 g/dL. NHANES III also found that of all anemia cases among older adults in the United States, 35% resulted from nutrient deficiencies (iron, vitamin B$_{12}$, and/or folate); 45% was attributable to chronic disease(s); and 20% was unexplained despite an exhaustive evaluation. Several theories have been put forward to explain possible etiologies for these cases of unknown cause, including reduced pluripotent HSC reserve, decreased production of HGFs, reduced

Table 61.1—Physiologic Classification of Anemia

Hypoproliferative	Ineffective	Hemolytic

▪ Iron-deficient erythropoiesis
  Iron deficiency
  Chronic disease
	▪ Macrocytic
	  Vitamin B$_{12}$
	  Folate
	  Myelodysplastic syndrome (refractory anemia)
		▪ Immunologic
		  Idiopathic
		  Secondary

▪ Erythropoietin lack
  Renal
  Endocrine
	▪ Microcytic
	  Thalassemia
	  Sideroblastic
		▪ Intrinsic
		  Abnormal hemoglobin
		  Metabolic

▪ Stem-cell dysfunction	▪ Normocytic
	  Myelodysplastic syndrome
		▪ Extrinsic
		  Mechanical

▪ Aplastic anemia		

SOURCE: Data from Chatta GS, Lipschitz DA. Aging and hematopoiesis. In: Hazzard WR, Blass JP, Ettinger WH Jr., et al., eds. *Principles of Geriatric Medicine and Gerontology.* 5th ed. New York: McGraw-Hill Health Professions Division; 2003:763–770.

sensitivity of HSCs to HGFs, marrow microenvironment abnormalities, unrecognized anemia of chronic disease, occult renal failure, and undiagnosed myelodysplasia. It is also possible that age-associated increases in levels of pro-inflammatory cytokines, such as IL-6, may reduce the responses of stem cells to growth factors, including EPO. Results from the InChianti study examined levels of hemoglobin, EPO, and inflammatory molecules (C-reactive protein, IL-6, IL-1, IL-1b, tumor necrosis factor alpha [TNF α]) in 1,453 older adults. In this population, the inflammatory score increased with age, with a commensurate increase in the EPO level in individuals with a normal hemoglobin and an inappropriately low EPO level in those with anemia.

Evaluation of Anemia

The presence of multiple pathologies in older adults often makes the evaluation of anemia challenging. For practical purposes, 12 g/dL is recommended as a lower limit of normal for hemoglobin for both older men and women. Attempting to define the cause of anemia when the hemoglobin concentration is between 12 and 14 g/dL rarely yields a definitive cause. Even when the hemoglobin concentration is 12 g/dL, a decision as to how aggressively to evaluate a patient with borderline low hematocrit must depend on clinical judgment. Once a decision has been made to investigate low hemoglobin concentration in an older adult, the principles involved in assessment and evaluation are similar to those used in patients of any age.

For a summary of the causes of the various anemias seen in older adults, see Table 61.1. The approach to the patient with anemia should evaluate renal, hepatic, cardiovascular, pulmonary, endocrine, and marrow function. The initial evaluation should include physical examination of these organ systems, medication history, a CBC, a reticulocyte production index, and testing of stool. Microcytosis (mean corpuscular volume [MCV]<84) indicates an impairment of hemoglobin synthesis, and macrocytosis (MCV >100) can be caused by reticulocytosis or more commonly by an abnormality in nuclear maturation. Iron deficiency and vitamin B$_{12}$ deficiency can coexist, resulting in confusing RBC indices. RBC production is estimated from the reticulocyte production index. Hemolytic anemia usually has a reticulocyte index >3, whereas a failure of production is indicated by a reticulocyte index of <2. Decreased production is caused by the hypoproliferative anemias or by ineffective erythropoiesis. An increased lactate dehydrogenase (LDH) concentration and indirect hyperbilirubinemia result from the increased destruction of RBC precursors in the marrow and can be used to distinguish ineffective erythropoiesis from hypoproliferative anemia. For a rational approach to the laboratory evaluation of anemia, see Figure 61.1 and Figure 61.2. A significantly increased reticulocyte count, indirect hyperbilirubinemia, and an increased LDH level are diagnostic of hemolytic anemia. A low reticulocyte count, increased indirect bilirubin, and an increased LDH concentration suggest ineffective erythropoiesis. In older adults with ineffective erythropoiesis, macrocytosis strongly suggests vitamin B$_{12}$ or folate deficiency, and microcytosis should suggest sideroblastic anemia.

The Hypoproliferative Anemias

Iron is the only nutrient that limits the rate of erythropoiesis. Thus, inadequate iron supply for erythropoiesis, the most common cause of anemia in older adults, results in a hypoproliferative anemia. This is diagnosed by the presence of a decreased serum iron and a decreased transferrin saturation (serum iron divided by the total iron binding capacity [TIBC], expressed as a percentage). Absolute iron deficiency (blood loss) is the most common cause of iron-deficient erythropoiesis in younger people. Blood-loss anemia, the anemia of inflammation or chronic disease, and the anemia associated with protein-energy malnutrition are the most prevalent anemias in older populations. Nutritional iron defi-

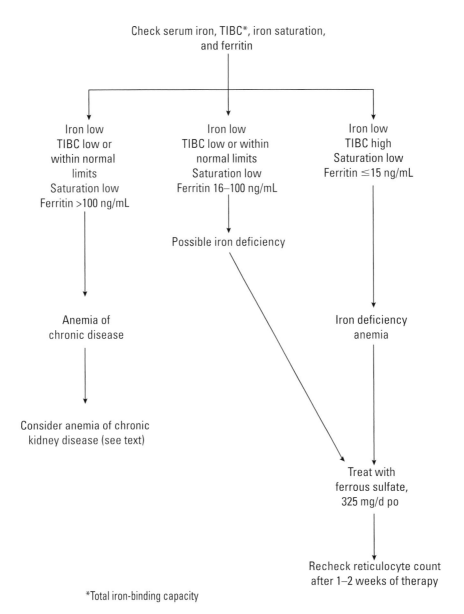

Check serum iron, TIBC*, iron saturation,
and ferritin

Iron low
TIBC low or
within normal
limits
Saturation low
Ferritin >100 ng/mL

Iron low
TIBC low or within
normal limits
Saturation low
Ferritin 16–100 ng/mL

Iron low
TIBC high
Saturation low
Ferritin ≤15 ng/mL

Possible iron deficiency

Anemia of
chronic disease

Iron deficiency
anemia

Consider anemia of chronic
kidney disease (see text)

Treat with
ferrous sulfate,
325 mg/d po

Recheck reticulocyte count
after 1–2 weeks of therapy

*Total iron-binding capacity

Figure 61.1—Evaluation of Hypoproliferative Anemia Due to Possible Iron Deficiency

ciency is very rare in the older age group, despite the prominence of other nutritional problems.

When unexplained iron deficiency does occur, it is almost exclusively due to blood loss from the GI tract. Typical findings in blood-loss anemia are low iron, low serum ferritin, and high TIBC, reflecting absent iron stores. Angiodysplasia of the large bowel and diverticular disease are common causes but should be considered only after a neoplasm has been excluded. Rarely, iron deficiency can result from malabsorption or urinary losses of iron, which occurs in the face of intravascular hemolysis.

The terms *anemia of inflammation* or *anemia of chronic disease* are often used to explain an anemia associated with some other major disease process. Examples include cancer, collagen vascular disorders,

rheumatoid arthritis, and inflammatory bowel disease. Occasionally, the anemia may be the initial manifestation of an occult disease. It is critical that this condition be distinguished from iron-deficiency (blood-loss) anemia, to avoid unnecessary GI tests to identify a cause for blood loss and to prevent the inappropriate prescribing of oral iron therapy

The pathophysiology of the anemia of inflammation or chronic disease is complex and is due to an inability of macrophages to release iron from the breakdown of senescent RBCs. As a consequence, the serum iron decreases and, as with blood-loss anemia, the iron supply is inadequate for erythropoiesis. In contrast to blood-loss anemia with absent iron stores, iron stores are normal or increased in the anemia of inflammation or chronic disease. Laboratory features include a mild anemia, a low serum iron, low

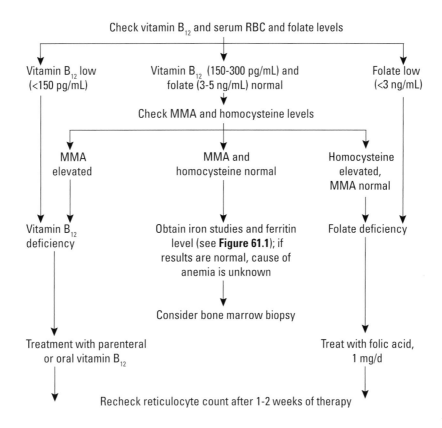

Check vitamin B$_{12}$ and serum RBC and folate levels

- Vitamin B$_{12}$ low (<150 pg/mL) → Vitamin B$_{12}$ deficiency → Treatment with parenteral or oral vitamin B$_{12}$
- Vitamin B$_{12}$ (150-300 pg/mL) and folate (3-5 ng/mL) normal → Check MMA and homocysteine levels
- Folate low (<3 ng/mL)

Check MMA and homocysteine levels:
- MMA elevated → Vitamin B$_{12}$ deficiency
- MMA and homocysteine normal → Obtain iron studies and ferritin level (see **Figure 61.1**); if results are normal, cause of anemia is unknown → Consider bone marrow biopsy
- Homocysteine elevated, MMA normal → Folate deficiency → Treat with folic acid, 1 mg/d

Recheck reticulocyte count after 1-2 weeks of therapy

Figure 61.2—Evaluation of Hypoproliferative Anemia Due to Possible Vitamin B$_{12}$ or Folate Deficiency

transferrin saturation, and normal to increased iron stores (ferritin >50 ng/mL). However, laboratory parameters often can be equivocal, and it may be difficult to distinguish between iron deficiency and defective iron utilization. Hepcidin, a 25 amino acid peptide produced in the liver, has been implicated in the pathogenesis of anemia of chronic disease. Hepcidin functions as a direct mediator of iron homeostasis regulating both intestinal iron absorption as well as release of macrophage iron to erythroid progenitors. Although hepcidin levels have been reported to be increased nearly 100-fold in association with anemia of chronic disease, studies on the clinical utility of hepcidin are limited by the availability of a suitable clinical assay. The possibility of a multifactorial causation, including blood loss, malnutrition, folate deficiency, or hemolysis, should always be considered when the anemia of inflammation or chronic disease is associated with a Hb <10 g/dL. In this circumstance, laboratory investigations commonly have equivocal results; hence, a bone marrow examination may be required. Clinical judgment is critically important in deciding how aggressive the evaluation for anemia ought to be.

Decreased EPO production accounts for the anemia of end-stage renal disease and is implicated in some anemias of cancer and chronic diseases. Many cancer patients have anemia independently of any myelosuppressive therapy. The anemia is characterized by an inability to use iron stores and an inadequate EPO response, indicated by inappropriately low EPO levels. In addition, a component of the erythroid suppression is mediated by cytokines such as IL-1, TNF-α, and transforming growth factor beta (TGF-β). Although the precise incidence of cancer-related anemia is not known, a number of studies have documented a decrease in transfusion frequency after treatment with EPO. Depending on symptoms, erythroid support is recommended for patients with hemoglobin concentrations <10 g/dL. EPO treatment should be started after excluding hemolysis and iron deficiency. Typically, the starting dose of EPO ranges from 20,000 to 40,000 U/week SC. If required, the dosage can be increased to 60,000 U/week. Conversely, some patients require treatment only every 2–3 weeks. Hemoglobin concentrations should be monitored weekly to avoid the vascular sequelae of an iatrogenic polycythemia. A target hemoglobin concentration of 10–12 g/dL is recommended (SOE=B). Most patients respond within 4–6 weeks. Iron should be added to the regimen if ferritin levels fall to <50 ng/mL. If there is no reticulocyte response after 4–6 weeks of EPO treatment, therapy should be discontinued. Although it is difficult to prospectively identify responders, it has been reported that patients with endogenous EPO levels of <200 mU/mL are most likely to respond to treatment with EPO.

Marrow failure due to interference with the proliferation of hematopoietic cells is seen in older adults. The disorder is generally associated with suppression of all marrow elements and is suggested by the presence of peripheral pancytopenia. Common causes include medications, immune damage to the stem-cell population, intrinsic marrow lesions, and marrow replacement by malignant cells or fibrous tissue. The latter is usually associated with a myelophthisic blood picture (nucleated RBCs, giant platelets, and metamyelocytes) as a reflection of the disruption of marrow stromal architecture. The presence of pancytopenia and the absence of iron-deficient erythropoiesis is an indication for bone marrow aspiration and biopsy. Occasionally, isolated suppression of erythropoiesis occurs, which is referred to as *pure red cell aplasia*. This disorder can be related to medication or caused by benign or malignant abnormalities of lymphocytes, including thymoma. These patients have isolated anemia, an increased serum iron, and an absence of erythroid precursors on bone marrow examination.

Ineffective Erythropoiesis

Macrocytic anemias in older adults result from vitamin B_{12} and folate deficiency. The prevalence of pernicious anemia increases with advancing age. Pernicious anemia results from malabsorption of vitamin B_{12} as a consequence of the action of antibodies against gastric parietal cells and intrinsic factor. Atrophic gastritis and decreased secretion of intrinsic factor occur, resulting in failure of vitamin B_{12} absorption. Pernicious anemia is most common in adults >60 yr old and is more common in women. Although cobalamin deficiency is common with aging, anemia secondary to this is rare (see the section on vitamin B_{12}, folate, and homocysteine, below). The presence of pancytopenia, macrocytosis, hypersegmented neutrophils in the peripheral smear, a decreased reticulocyte index, an increased LDH level, and indirect hypobilirubinemia suggests a diagnosis of megaloblastic anemia. The bone marrow classically shows giant metamyelocytes, hypersegmented neutrophils, and enlarged erythroid precursors with more hemoglobin than would be expected from the immaturity of their nuclei (nuclear-cytoplasmic dissociation). Chronic pancreatitis and diseases of the distal ileum (blind loop syndrome) can also cause vitamin B_{12} deficiency. The Schilling test can distinguish a deficiency of intrinsic factor from an abnormality in the ability of the ileum to absorb the vitamin B_{12}–intrinsic factor complex; however, it is no longer commonly done because of expense and inconvenience (versus simply replacing B_{12}). Folate deficiency of sufficient severity to cause anemia in older adults is rare. Alcohol and various drugs also interfere with folate absorption and metabolism. Vulner-

ability to deficiency is significantly greater when folate requirements are increased as a result of inflammation, neoplastic disease, or hemolytic anemia.

The major causes of ineffective erythropoiesis and microcytosis are thalassemia and the sideroblastic anemias. Although thalassemia is generally diagnosed at an earlier age, there are reports of its initial detection in older adults. Mild anemia, a disproportionately low MCV, and the absence of iron deficiency usually point to a diagnosis of thalassemia trait, a condition of little or no clinical consequence. Iron supplements have no role in the treatment of thalassemia trait; on the contrary, they can be detrimental. Acquired sideroblastic anemia, which is primarily a disease of older adults, is a heterogenous group of disorders characterized by the presence of iron deposits in the mitochondria of normoblasts. Referral to a hematologist should be done when these diagnoses are being considered.

Myelodysplastic Syndromes

The *myelodysplastic syndromes* (MDS) are a group of stem-cell disorders characterized by disordered hematopoiesis that occur primarily in the older age group. Refractory anemia and refractory anemia with ringed sideroblasts account for 25%–30% of MDS. Refractory anemia commonly presents as a macrocytic anemia with marrow erythroid hyperplasia and relatively normal myeloid and megakaryocytic lineages. Cytogenetic abnormalities are relatively common in MDS, and one of particular interest in older adults is deletion of the long arm of chromosome 5 (5q−). The median age at presentation is 66 yr, and the 5q− syndrome is characterized by macrocytic anemia, modest leukopenia, normal or increased platelet counts, and marrow erythroid hypoplasia or hyperplasia; it is also more common in women.

Hemolytic Anemias

The causes of hemolytic anemia in older adults are somewhat different than in younger people. Although most patients with congenital disorders will have been previously identified, an occasional older adult with congenital hemolytic anemia can present for the first time with symptoms related to cholelithiasis. Autoimmune hemolytic anemia is the most common cause in the older age group. The diagnosis is made by a positive Coombs' test. In younger people, a cause of the autoimmune hemolysis is only rarely identified. In contrast, in older adults, the anemia is more likely to be associated with a lymphoproliferative disorder (non-Hodgkin's lymphoma or chronic lymphocytic leukemia), collagen vascular disease, or drug ingestion. Corticosteroids and splenectomy are usually effective in patients with red cell antibodies of the IgG type. Patients with red cell antibodies of the IgM variety are more likely to be refractory to such treatment. Microangiopathic hemolytic anemia occurs secondary to either disseminated intravascular coagulation (DIC) or as a manifestation of the syndrome of thrombotic thrombocytopenic purpura (TTP). DIC is usually associated with severe infections or disseminated neoplasm and presents with not only hemolysis but also a consumptive coagulopathy. The presence of red cell fragmentation, thrombocytopenia, a prolonged prothrombin time, a prolonged partial thromboplastin time, and hemosiderinuria suggests this diagnosis. Treatment of DIC entails treating the underlying disorder as well as providing blood product support, including fresh frozen plasma and cryoprecipitate as needed. TTP is characterized by the pentad of fever, intravascular hemolysis, thrombocytopenia, neurologic symptoms, and renal dysfunction. In contrast to DIC, in TTP both the prothrombin time and partial thromboplastin time are normal. Early diagnosis is imperative, because TTP responds very well to treatment with plasmapheresis.

Hemolysis is frequently associated with implantation of prosthetic heart valves. The incidence of hemolysis varies from 5% to 35%, and is affected by a variety of factors, mostly related to the type of valve implanted and to the hemodynamic conditions after implantation. In a report of 278 patients, mild subclinical hemolysis was identified at 12 mo in 26% of patients with a mechanical prosthesis and in 5% with a bioprosthesis. On multivariate analysis, independent predictors of the presence of subclinical hemolysis were mitral valve replacement, use of a mechanical prosthesis, and double valve replacement. Among mechanical valve recipients, double versus single valve replacement and mitral versus aortic valve replacement were correlated with the presence of hemolysis; double valve recipients also showed a more severe degree of hemolysis (SOE=B). Valve-associated anemia is seldom severe. The amount of hemolysis is assessed based on serum levels of LDH and haptoglobin, and on the presence and amount of reticulocytes and schistocytes in the peripheral blood. Treatment of hemolysis includes the supplementation of iron and folate when their deficiency is evident. The use of β-blockers appears to decrease the severity of hemolysis, likely through induction of bradycardia and negative inotropic effects.

VITAMIN B$_{12}$, FOLATE, AND HOMOCYSTEINE

Older adults are more likely than younger ones to have lower concentrations of vitamin B$_{12}$ and folate. In epidemiologic studies, approximately 10% of apparently healthy adults ≥70 yr old were found to have low vitamin B$_{12}$ levels, and 5%–10% were found to have low folate values (SOE=A). Low vitamin B$_{12}$ and folate levels are not necessarily accompanied by macrocytosis or evidence of megaloblastic anemia. Atrophic gastritis leading to vitamin B$_{12}$ malabsorption is the likely cause in most cases of vitamin B$_{12}$ deficiency. Although gastritis can also contribute to low folate levels in older adults, alcohol abuse, drug interactions with folate absorption, and inadequate dietary intake are the most common causes of low folate levels. Some evidence suggests that low vitamin B$_{12}$ levels may contribute to cognitive decline in older adults (SOE=C). There is no question that severe vitamin B$_{12}$ deficiency can result in cognitive loss and significant neurologic deficits. However, most demented patients will not have B$_{12}$ deficiency as the cause of their dementia. Nevertheless, aggressive replacement should always be undertaken when a patient with dementia presents with low levels of vitamin B$_{12}$ or folate.

Even in patients with atrophic gastritis, oral vitamin B$_{12}$ is generally adequate; 10% will be absorbed by mass action alone and not require the presence of intrinsic factor. Thus, a daily dose of 1 mg (1,000 mcg) of vitamin B$_{12}$ will replete a person with concentrations in the low-to-normal range. Parenteral replacement should be used in severe deficiencies with vitamin B$_{12}$, ie, concentrations <100 pg/mL. It has been suggested that in older adults with low normal (<350 pg/mL) B$_{12}$ concentrations, methylmalonic acid (MMA) concentrations be checked to exclude metabolically active B$_{12}$ deficiency. Kidney failure can artificially increase the serum MMA concentration. In those patients with low-normal B$_{12}$ concentrations and macrocytosis (with or without anemia) or neurologic changes, vitamin replacement should be considered, particularly if the MMA concentration is increased. Folic acid can be replaced in dosages ranging from 400 to 500 mg/d. At these dosages, homocysteine concentrations fall (analogous to the fall in MMA when B$_{12}$ is replaced).

Low concentrations of vitamin B$_{12}$ or folate are accompanied by increased concentrations of homocysteine. Epidemiologic studies initially found that B$_{12}$ and folate deficiencies with high levels of homocysteine are associated with cardiovascular disease; however, subsequent trials of homocysteine lowering through vitamin therapy did not reduce end points such as stroke and myocardial infarction (SOE=A), and may increase cancer risk.

PLATELETS AND COAGULATION

Platelet counts do not change with aging, but the concentrations of a large number of coagulation enzymes have been shown to increase with age. These include factors VII, VIII, and fibrinogen. In centenarians, highly significant increases in the concentrations of these factors are noted, as are concentrations of factors IX, X, and thrombin-antithrombin complexes. Fibrin formation is also increased, as evidenced by higher concentrations of fibrinopeptide A. In addition, increased concentrations of D-dimers in older adults would indicate increased hyperfibrinolysis. These observations suggest that aging may be accompanied by increased hypercoagulability. Hyperhomocysteinemia, secondary to low B_{12} concentrations, is also more common in the older age group and may be an additional factor associated with hypercoagulability. However, the very high level of clotting factors and evidence of hypercoagulability in remarkably healthy centenarians have also led to the suggestion that increased coagulation factors may not be markers of increased risks of thrombosis.

Bleeding diatheses are not uncommon in older adults. Unexplained bruises, recurrent nosebleeds, GI losses, or excessive blood loss during surgery or after dental extraction are common presentations. In these patients, screening platelet counts and coagulation studies should be obtained. Tests of platelet aggregation are useful in detecting disorders of platelet function.

Thrombocytopenia is a common cause of bleeding problems in older adults. A platelet count <150,000/mL is considered significant, but bleeding usually occurs at much lower levels. Common causes include decreased production of platelets in the bone marrow, sequestration in enlarged spleens, and increased peripheral destruction. Decreased production of platelets occurs in the leukemias, marrow aplasia, or most commonly in older adults in association with medications that suppress platelet production. The major cause of increased peripheral destruction is immune thrombocytopenia. A lymphoma, collagen vascular disease, or a drug-induced cause is common in older adults with autoimmune thrombocytopenia. Treatment of thrombocytopenia depends on the cause. A referral to a hematologist is warranted to assure accurate diagnosis of the underlying problem.

Platelet function disorders (thrombopathy), though uncommon, can cause significant bleeding in older adults on aspirin therapy. Aspirin irreversibly acetylates cyclooxygenase, affecting arachidonic acid metabolism. The net effect is significant loss of platelet function. In the rare circumstance, spontaneous bleeding can occur or can be precipitated by injury or surgery. Platelet transfusions may be needed.

Bleeding can also occur because of clotting factor deficiencies, which in older adults are usually acquired and caused by the presence of circulating clotting factor inhibitors. The most common is an acquired inhibitor to factor VIII. The onset is often sudden. Titers of anti-factor VIII antibodies can be very high, and presentation is with bleeding into joints and muscle, similar to that in hemophilia A. Treatment involves factor replacement; depending on the severity, prednisone or cyclophosphamide may also be needed. Deficiency of the vitamin K–dependent clotting factors tends to occur in older adults with major illnesses. Disorders of the hepatobiliary tree, antibiotics that neutralize bowel bacteria (a major source of vitamin K), malabsorption, and severe malnutrition are the common causes. The deficits are readily treated with vitamin K.

Liver disease must always be considered in patients who present with excessive bleeding. The prothrombin time is prolonged even in mild to moderate liver disease. The partial thromboplastin time remains normal until liver disease becomes severe. Except for factor VIII (which is produced by endothelial cells), all clotting factors are reduced in liver disease. Liver disease is also associated with DIC; fibrin degradation products are not cleared as well, and platelet function can be affected. The treatment of a bleeding diathesis in liver disease is fresh frozen plasma.

CHRONIC MYELOPROLIFERATIVE DISORDERS

The Philadelphia chromosome–negative chronic myeloproliferative disorders—polycythemia vera (PV), essential thrombocythemia (ET), and idiopathic myelofibrosis (IMF)—have overlapping clinical features but exhibit different natural histories and different therapeutic requirements. All three disorders are seen primarily in the older age group and are characterized by the involvement of a multipotent hematopoietic progenitor cell, marrow hypercellularity, overproduction of one or more marrow lineages, thrombotic and hemorrhagic diatheses, exuberant extramedullary hematopoiesis, and a slow rate of spontaneous transformation to acute leukemia. Referral to a hematologist is warranted if these diseases are suspected.

HEMATOLOGIC MALIGNANCIES, LYMPHOMAS, AND MULTIPLE MYELOMA

See "Oncology," p 521.

REFERENCES

■ Dighiero G, Hamblin TJ. Chronic lymphocytic leukaemia. *Lancet.* 2008;371(9617):1017–1029.

■ Eisenstaedt R, Penninx BW, Woodman RC. Anemia in the elderly: current understanding and emerging concepts. *Blood Rev.* 2006;20(4):213–226.

■ Ferrucci L, Guralnik JM, Bandinelli S, et al. Unexplained anaemia in older persons is characterized by low erythropoietin and low levels of pro-inflammatory markers. *Br J Haematol.* 2007;136(6):849−855.

CHAPTER 62—ONCOLOGY

KEY POINTS

■ Older adults and black Americans of all ages are more likely to develop cancer and present with more advanced disease.

■ Older age has a variable association with the aggressiveness and growth rate of malignant tumors.

■ There has been no demonstrated age-associated resistance to chemotherapy; further, some acute toxicities (eg, nausea, vomiting, and hair loss) are less prominent in older adults.

■ Surgery, radiation, chemotherapy, and biologic therapy are safe and effective treatment interventions for older cancer patients when appropriate precautions are taken based on the patient's comorbidities, vital organ functions, and medications.

Epidemiologic studies indicate that cancer is primarily a burden of geriatric populations. According to the National Cancer Institute's Surveillance, Epidemiology and End Results (SEER) data (collected between 1998 and 2002), 71% of cancer deaths were in people >65 yr old. One in four deaths in the United States is caused by cancer. After age 85, heart disease becomes the number one killer, and the risk of cancer declines for reasons that are not defined. From 2002 to 2004, cancer death rates decreased by 2.6% per year in men and 1.8% per year in women, continuing a trend in improved outcome that began in 1992. Because of the paucity of older adults in clinical trials, it is not clear how much of the improvement in treatment has translated to the benefit of older patients. However, when such data have been evaluated (eg, for colon cancer, breast cancer), it appears that treatment that is effective in younger patients is also effective in older patients (SOE=A). We have much to learn about providing optimal management of cancer in older adults, but emphasizing disease prevention and screening remains an important priority. In fact, the median age for cancer in the United States is 70 yr.

Although cancer has long been recognized as a disease of older people, emphasis on geriatric issues and cancer is a recent development. Experimental data and clinical experience have indicated that tumors are not resistant to treatment by virtue of age alone. However, age is associated with reductions in certain organ functions, and these deficiencies in physiologic reserve might be magnified by comorbid conditions. Cancer treatments can therefore be associated with an increase in adverse events, and treatment should be tailored to the individual, taking into consideration potential increased toxicities and balancing this with expectations of survival in the context of comorbidities.

Three questions form the basis of this new emphasis:

■ Why are tumors more common in older adults?

■ Is there a difference in tumor aggressiveness with advancing age?

■ Should treatment be different for the older patient?

CANCER BIOLOGY AND AGING

Explaining the Increased Prevalence of Cancer with Age

The prevalence of cancer increases with age for at least three reasons. First, cancers, particularly those that occur after menopause, are thought to develop over a long period, perhaps decades. This is best exemplified by the current understanding of colon cancer, which has been shown to develop because of an accumulation of several damaging genetic events occurring in a stochastic manner over time. Thus, if mutations are acquired at a constant rate, older people are more likely to have lived long enough to develop the 8 to 10 genetic lesions it takes to develop a malignancy. In contrast, lymphomas are just as likely to occur in young as in old people. Lymphocytes normally undergo gene rearrangements and mutations to generate antigen receptors, and these processes appear to be particularly vulnerable to errors that can lead to lymphoma at any age.

A second reason for the greater prevalence of cancer with advancing age is that DNA repair mechanisms are thought to decline with age. As a consequence, cells can accumulate damage. Normally, a dividing cell pauses in G1 (the gap after mitosis [M] and before DNA replication [S]) and in G2 (the gap after S and before M) to take inventory and repair any damage before proceeding to the next phase. These are the G1 and G2 checkpoints. Older cells may fail to detect or repair damage and fail to accurately control DNA replication. This leads to aneuploidy and uncontrolled proliferation. In younger people, these aberrations can trigger the death of the cell; in older people, the errors may be tolerated and fail to signal cell death. Cells without functioning checkpoints are vulnerable to loss of growth control.

A third contribution to increased cancer incidence in older people may be a decline in the function of the immune system, particularly in cellular immunity. A number of findings suggest that the immune system can recognize and control certain cancers. A decline in immune function may lead to the emergence of a cancer in an older person that was controlled when that person was younger.

STRENGTH-OF-EVIDENCE (SOE) RATING DEFINITIONS

A = consistent and good quality patient-oriented evidence
B = somewhat inconsistent or limited quality patient-oriented evidence
C = very inconsistent or very limited patient-oriented evidence, disease-oriented evidence, and/or consensus from professional organizations
D = unstudied common practice or opinion

See inside front cover for detailed information regarding the SOE classification.

The Different Characteristics of Cancer with Age

A long-held but incompletely documented clinical dogma that cancers in older people are less aggressive or slower growing has not been consistently supported by epidemiologic data from tumor registries or large clinical trials. Such data can be confounded by geriatric problems that shorten survival independently of the cancer (eg, comorbidity, multiple medications, clinician or family bias regarding diagnosis and treatment in older adults, and age-associated life stresses). These factors may counter any primary influence that aging might have on tumor aggressiveness. Despite these uncertainties, however, there is experimental support for the contention that tumor aggressiveness declines with age. Data obtained from laboratory animals with a wide range of tumors under highly controlled circumstances demonstrate slower tumor growth, fewer experimental metastases, and longer survival in old mice. Tumor growth involves several levels of interaction between the tumor and the host. It may be that tumor angiogenesis is impaired in older people, thereby controlling the rate of tumor growth. The clinical importance of this work is limited, inasmuch as it is difficult to know in any given individual whether the course of the disease will be characterized by an indolent or aggressive pattern of growth.

Breast cancer is the most notable clinical example of an age-associated decline in tumor aggressiveness. Older patients are more likely to have more favorable histologic types, higher levels of estrogen and progesterone receptor expression, lower growth fraction, and less frequent metastases. In a published series on breast cancer patients with primary tumors of ≤1 cm in diameter, the single most important predictor of metastasis to axillary nodes has consistently been found to be patient age: patients <50 yr old have the highest likelihood of spread, whereas those >70 yr old have the lowest likelihood of spread. Stage for stage in breast cancer, older patients seem to have longer survival than younger patients (SOE=A).

By contrast, Hodgkin's disease seems to be a more aggressive disease in older patients. The most likely reason for the age-associated differences in prognosis is that Hodgkin's disease is a different disease in patients ≥45 yr old than in younger patients. Incidence data demonstrate two distinct peak incidence rates, one at age 32 yr and one at age 84 yr. The frequency of particular histologic subtypes of Hodgkin's disease is different in younger and older patients: nodular sclerosis is the most common subtype in younger patients; mixed cellularity is the most common in older patients. In all reported treatment series, older age is an independent prognostic factor.

Table 62.1—Ethnic and Racial Differences in Annual Cancer Incidence, United States, 2000–2004 (per 100,000 population)

Site	White Americans		Black Americans		Hispanic Americans		Asian Americans	
	Male	*Female*	*Male*	*Female*	*Male*	*Female*	*Male*	*Female*
All	556.7	423.9	663.7	396.9	421.3	314.2	359.9	285.8
Breast	—	132.5	—	118.3	—	89.3	—	89.0
Colon	60.4	44.0	72.6	55.0	47.5	32.9	49.7	35.3
Lung	81.0	54.6	110.6	53.7	44.7	25.2	55.1	27.7
Prostate	161.4	—	255.5	—	140.8	—	96.5	—

SOURCE: Data from Jemal A, Siegel R, Ward E, et al. Cancer statistics, 2008. *CA Cancer J Clin.* 2008;58(2):71–96.

Table 62.2—Racial Differences in Cancer Diagnosis and Survival, 1996–2003

Site	Advanced Disease at Diagnosis (%)		5-Yr Survival (%)	
	White Americans	*Black Americans*	*White Americans*	*Black Americans*
Breast	36	46	90	77
Colon	19	24	65	55
Lung	41	43	15	12
Head and neck	59	74	61	40
Bladder	21	34	80	64
Endometrial	25	39	85	61

SOURCE: Data from Jemal A, Siegel R, Ward E, et al. Cancer statistics, 2008. *CA Cancer J Clin.* 2008;58(2):71–96.

Additional study is necessary to document age-associated differences in tumor cell biology.

Acute leukemia, like Hodgkin's disease, appears to be a different disease in older people; the MDR1 drug resistance pump (which eliminates toxins, including certain cancer chemotherapy agents, from the cell) is more commonly expressed, response to treatment is less, and survival is shorter than in younger patients. However, for most cancer types, the molecular biology and clinical behavior of the tumor is similar across the age span.

Ethnic Differences in Cancer Incidence and Mortality

As the demographics of the U.S. population changes, additional information is needed on incidence and on natural history differences in cancers that develop in different ethnic and racial groups. The U.S. Census Bureau estimates that by 2050, Hispanic Americans will account for nearly 25% of the population, and black Americans, Asian Americans, and Native Americans will combine to total another 25%. Overall, black Americans have the highest cancer incidence and mortality rates. Cancer incidence among black Americans is 10% higher than among white Americans, 50%–60% higher than among Hispanic Americans and Asian Americans, and more than twice as high as among Native Americans. The cancer death rate for black Americans is about 30% higher than for white Americans and more than twice as

high as for Hispanic Americans, Asian Americans, and Native Americans. From 1996 to 2003, the 5-yr survival for all cancers was 67% for white Americans and 57% for black Americans.

The factors contributing to the ethnic differences are not defined. However, certain data suggest that when the quality of the health care delivered to white and black Americans is similar, disease outcomes in the two groups are comparable (SOE=B). For specific incidence, diagnosis, and survival data for common cancers in different ethnic groups, see Table 62.1 and Table 62.2.

PRINCIPLES OF CANCER MANAGEMENT

Current forms of cancer treatment include surgery, radiation, chemotherapy, hormone manipulation, and biologic therapy. Age alone does not preclude any of these approaches, but because of normal changes with age in certain organs and also age-associated conditions (comorbidities), special considerations are warranted.

Randomized clinical trials are the most reliable method of studying medical intervention, and treatment decisions are best founded on their results. However, despite efforts from the cooperative oncology groups, patients entered into trials are by and large younger and presumably healthier than the typical geriatric patient with the same disorder.

Furthermore, common end points of these trials are length of survival (for therapeutic interventions) or disease-specific deaths (for prevention studies), and these end points are not always the most appropriate outcomes for older patients (because of their inherently limited life expectancies on the basis of age alone).

More and more, clinical researchers are addressing issues of geriatric oncology. New, geriatrics-oriented trials are focusing more on symptom reduction and quality-of-life outcomes than on life expectancy. Surveys have indicated that older adults, when fully informed, most often choose life-extending treatments, even at the risk of toxicity; it is the clinician and the patient's family that are most focused on quality-of-life issues. Furthermore, for the most part, tumors are not more resistant to treatment in older adults (SOE=B), and acute toxicities (eg, nausea, vomiting, hair loss) may be less prominent in older adults (SOE=B). Thus, although quality of life remains a primary treatment consideration, efforts at extending life should not be denied older adults on the basis of age alone.

The application of the geriatric assessment to patients with cancer and the use of it to determine the capacity of patients to tolerate treatment are in their infancy. Several abbreviated versions of geriatric assessment are being evaluated for their ability to predict treatment tolerability. Even these sophisticated tools need to be applied and interpreted with good clinical judgment. An 85-yr-old man who was mowing his lawn last month but now presents with a tumor-related decline in function is much more likely to tolerate therapy than a person whose baseline level of activity was poor. See "Assessment," p 43.

Cancer Screening

Studies that have contributed to the evidence on which the recommendations are based have included younger individuals, which make it difficult to generalize the findings to the oldest old. Thus, there are no clear guidelines for how to proceed with cancer screening in those over 85 years of age. Older adults, particularly those 85 years and older, are underrepresented in most of the studies that contribute to the body of evidence used to establish cancer screening guidelines. There is no consensus about the value of cancer screening tests in the oldest old. Especially since old age, with its increased prevalence of co-morbid diseases, may reduce the chance that the benefits of screening will be exceeded by the harms of screening. Thus a paradox exists. The USPSTF evidence-based guidelines are based on the premise that screening will improve patient outcomes. However, screening for those 85 years and older seems contradictory since there is very little data that

provide evidence that cancer screening tests are of any benefit for this age group. Many national organizations who publish screening guidelines do not address old age at all and do not have any upper age limits for the PSA, mammography, Pap test, and most recently, colorectal cancer screening. (United States Preventive Services Task Force Screening Guidelines at http://www.ahrq.gov/clinic/uspstfix.htm)

For a complete discussion of issues in cancer screening, along with recommendations for older adult populations, see "Prevention," p 61.

Chemotherapy

Aging can be associated with changes in key pharmacologic parameters of antineoplastic agents and in the susceptibility to end-organ toxicity (Table 62.3).

The most consistent pharmacokinetic change of aging is a progressive delay in the elimination of renally excretable medications because of a reduced glomerular filtration rate. The prolonged half-life of these agents can account in part for more severe toxicity. In a study of women $\geq$65 yr old with metastatic breast cancer, dosages of methotrexate and cyclophosphamide were modified according to the creatinine clearance. As a consequence, myelotoxicity was markedly reduced without compromise of the therapeutic effect.

Owing to differences in their pharmacokinetics and pharmacodynamics, certain medications can be particularly suitable for treating older patients. Oral etoposide provides valuable palliation for small-cell cancer of the lung and large-cell lymphoma, with minimal risk of complications. Fludarabine, which is very active in lymphoproliferative neoplasms, induces apoptosis of cancer cells, a process that can be altered in malignancies occurring in older adults. Vinorelbine and gemcitabine are two newer agents that are active against lung and breast cancer and are well tolerated and effective in older adults.

Hormonal Therapy

Hormonal treatment is effective in cancers of the breast, prostate, and endometrium. Tamoxifen, a selective estrogen-receptor modulator, has antagonistic and partial agonistic effects. It is a useful therapy in adjuvant treatment of breast cancer and also has estrogen-like positive effects on cardiovascular risk factors and bone disease. Other more selective drugs in this category, such as raloxifene, are in clinical testing. Although inactive as a single agent, tamoxifen[OL] is synergistic with chemotherapy in the management of malignant melanoma. For currently used hormonal agents, see Table 62.4. Most of these are well tolerated by older adults and commonly are the treatment of choice in this age group.

Table 62.3—Chemotherapy Issues in Geriatric Oncology

Issue	Comments
General	Comorbidities and multiple medications add complexity.
Pharmacokinetic changes	A progressive delay with age in the elimination of renally excreted medications, due to a reduction in glomerular filtration rate, can account in part for more severe toxicity.
Pharmacodynamic changes	Possible enhanced resistance with age to antitumor agents. Increased expression of the multidrug resistance gene has been reported in some older adults. Other proteins that result in drug efflux have been shown to have prognostic importance, but age-associated changes have not been described. Increased tumor hypoxia with age has been observed in a murine model.
Toxicity	Mucositis, cardiotoxicity, and peripheral and central neurotoxicity become more common and more severe with aging (SOE=B). Cardiotoxicity is a complication of anthracyclines and anthraquinones, mitomycin C, and high-dose cyclophosphamide; incidence of cardiotoxicity increases with age. Peripheral neurotoxicity with vincristine is more common and more severe in older adults. The incidence of cerebellar toxicity from high-dose cytosine arabinoside increases with age.
Myelotoxicity	Chemotherapy-related myelotoxicity can become more severe and more prolonged with aging, but moderately toxic treatment regimens, such as CMF (cyclophosphamide, methotrexate, fluorouracil), cisplatin and fluorouracil, and cisplatin and etoposide are tolerated by many patients ≥70 yr old without life-threatening neutropenia or thrombocytopenia (SOE=A). However, infections are markedly increased among older acute leukemia patients undergoing intensive induction treatment; in these cases, it is possible that the disease itself, rather than an age-associated change in "marrow reserve," is responsible for the depletion of hemopoietic stem cells.
Recent advances	Granulocyte colony-stimulating factor and granulocyte-macrophage colony-stimulating factor have reduced the incidence of neutropenic infections in patients receiving intensive treatment, and their effectiveness does not appear to be diminished with advancing patient age. Certain new medications or new formulations may be particularly suitable to older patients, eg, oral etoposide and fludarabine, gemcitabine, vinorelbine, capecitabine, paclitaxel protein-bound particles, and liposomal doxorubicin.

Table 62.4—Hormonal Agents Commonly Used in Treating Cancer

Site	Hormonal Agents
Breast	*Antiestrogens*: tamoxifen, toremifene *Progestational agents*: medroxyprogesterone acetate *Aromatase inhibitors*: aminoglutethimide, letrozole, anastrozole, exemestane
Prostate	*Luteinizing hormone-releasing hormone analogs*: goserelin, leuprolide *Estrogens*: diethylstilbestrol *Antiandrogens*: flutamide, bicalutamide
Endometrium	Progestational agents Antiestrogens

Diethylstilbestrol is an estrogenic compound with serious cardiovascular risks (eg, stroke, heart attack, thromboembolism) when used to treat prostate cancer in older men.

Biologic Therapy

Modulation of immune response is a particularly attractive option in treating older adults, whose natural defenses against cancer can be impaired by immune senescence. Only a limited number of options are clinically available, and these are clearly inadequate to restore a normal immune response in older adults.

Recombinant α-interferon at moderate dosages (eg, 3 million units, three times weekly) is reasonably well tolerated by patients of all ages. At higher dosages, α-interferon causes myelodepression, severe fatigue, flu-like illness, malaise, fever, neuropathy, and abnormalities of liver enzymes. Delirium, depression, and dementia after α-interferon use have been reported in patients ≥65 yr old. More information on the safety of α-interferon in older patients would be desirable. This is particularly important because interferon has been shown to be effective therapy for chronic myeloid leukemia, hairy cell leukemia, and multiple myeloma, hematologic malignancies that are more common among older adults (SOE=A). It may also prolong survival after chemotherapy for follicular lymphoma. It is being tested at higher, more toxic dosages in patients with Stage II melanoma after surgical resection of the primary lesion. About 15% of patients with metastatic melanoma can experience a partial response from α-interferon.

Interleukin-2 is used to treat metastatic melanoma and renal cancer. When administered daily at 3 million units/m^2, it may produce partial responses in about 15% of patients and complete remissions in about 5% of patients, many of which are long lasting. Interleukin-2 can produce severe dose-related toxicity, including capillary leak syndrome, hypotension, adult respiratory distress syndrome, cardiac arrhythmias, peripheral edema, renal failure (prerenal), cholestatic liver dysfunction, skin rashes, and thrombocytopenia. These complications tend to appear gradually in less severe form; generally, patients do not suddenly deteriorate. The toxicities reverse completely within a few days of stopping the drug. It is a strong clinical impression that interleukin-2 toxicities are less severe and develop later in older patients.

Monoclonal antibodies directed against CD20 (rituximab) expressed on B-cell lymphomas and against HER-2/*neu* (trastuzumab) expressed on breast cancer and other epithelial malignancies are effective treatments. In most patients, the antibodies are given just before combination chemotherapy; the antibodies appear to augment the response to the drugs. These humanized antibodies generally have mild toxicities. Patients can develop hypotension or shortness of breath with the first infusion because of complement fixation. Symptoms clear when the infusion rate is slowed down, and such symptoms rarely recur. Other antibodies against cancers are in development.

Radiation Therapy

Radiation therapy provides palliation for virtually all cancers, and it may be part of a treatment plan for lymphomas and cancers of the prostate, bladder, cervix, esophagus, breast, and head and neck area. In combination with cytotoxic chemotherapy, radiation therapy has allowed organ preservation in cancers of the anus, bladder, and larynx, and in extremity sarcomas. A central issue for radiation therapy in older adults is safety. There has been a trend for almost five decades to use radiation therapy as an alternative to surgery in poor surgical candidates, mainly patients ≥65 yr old, with the implied expectation that such an approach is less toxic. In fact, published reports have indicated that radiation therapy is both safe and effective in older patients (SOE=A). However, concern remains when treatment involves irradiation of the whole brain (fear of neurologic sequelae, including dementia) or pelvis (fear of marrow aplasia or myelodysplasia or radiation enteritis), but no systematic investigation has categorically substantiated these concerns.

Advances in radiation therapy include techniques that allow a more restricted radiation field (especially partial brain irradiation), new applications of brachytherapy (insertion of radiation sources into the tumor bed), the development of radiosurgery (gamma ray knife, a precisely focused external beam of radiation) that allows destruction of small lesions (diameter ≤4 cm) of the CNS without craniotomy, and the development of new radiosensitizers.

Surgery

Concerns related to cancer surgery in older adults are safety and rehabilitative potential. Several reports indicate that age itself is not a risk factor for elective cancer surgery, but the length of hospital stay and the time to full recovery become longer with advancing age. Similar results have been reported both from referral centers and community hospitals.

Advances in anesthesia and surgery have benefited older patients. Included among these are endoscopic procedures that provide valuable palliation for the many tumors of the GI tract, and the more widespread use of spinal anesthesia for major abdominal interventions, with a substantial decline in perioperative complications and mortality. More widespread use of laparoscopic surgical techniques and application of laser and photodynamic therapy is also broadening the surgical armamentarium and providing more older patients with potential palliation and cure.

The trend to manage cancer without deforming surgery can preclude the need for complex rehabilitation and can be of special value for older adults. Organ preservation without compromise of treatment outcome is obtainable for cancer of the anus and larynx, and is being studied for cancers of the oropharynx, esophagus, bladder, and vulva. Also, the use of initial (neoadjuvant) chemotherapy before primary surgery has been effective in patients with large primary breast and lung cancers. Such an approach results in less extensive and potentially more curative surgical procedures.

See also "Perioperative Care," p 92.

Quality-of-Life Issues

Several studies have determined that the perception of quality of life is highly subjective and poorly reproduced by external observers, even by those who have close relationships with the patient or by healthcare providers who are very familiar with the patient's physical condition. Furthermore, there is considerable discrepancy between the clinician's determination of the patient's quality of life and the patient's own assessment, with clinicians tending to underestimate the patient's quality of life (SOE=B).

Early assessments of quality of life focused on functional status and freedom from pain, but these factors, although important, are inadequate for evaluating far-reaching consequences of serious diseases on all domains of life. In the past decade, several instruments for measuring quality of life have been validated and used successfully to study specific problems, such as the effects on quality of life of intensive care, the consequences of limb amputation or of partial and total mastectomy, and iatrogenic impotence. These instruments are questionnaires querying an individual to rate his or her own well-being in several dimensions with a categorical or a visual analog scale. Unfortunately, these instruments have not been adjusted to the special needs of older adults. While it is reasonable to assume that the importance of some factors, such as professional or job satisfaction, may decline with age, the importance of others, including social support and the perception of family burden, can become more prominent.

Other problems related to assessing quality of life include the complexity of some questionnaires, which can overwhelm some older adults. In addition, little progress has been made in the assessment of quality of life in cognitively impaired individuals. Studies of pain in demented individuals have demonstrated the reliability of repetitive behavioral testing in assessing discomfort, even in patients with cognitive impairment. Perhaps the same principles can be applied to assessing quality of life in demented patients.

At present, the main application of quality-of-life assessment in clinical decision making concerns the choice between interventions yielding comparable survival. An area of potential use is in medical decisions involving limited survival benefits at the price of a decline in quality of life. At present, the value of this trade-off is evaluated with measures known as "quality of life adjusted survival" or "quality-adjusted time without symptoms or toxicity," both of which include complex interviews of limited application to adults ≥70 yr old.

SPECIFIC CANCERS

Breast Cancer

Controversy surrounds several critical issues in the management of this most common malignancy in older women. These issues include the following.

Postoperative Irradiation After Lumpectomy

Although irradiation after lumpectomy is safe in women ≥65 yr old, it may be a source of significant inconvenience and cost. The value of postoperative irradiation has been questioned because the local recurrence rate of breast cancer may decrease with age, and the inconvenience of daily radiation treatment protocols may outweigh the limited benefits for some.

Need for Axillary Lymphadenectomy

Given the benefits of adjunct tamoxifen in all postmenopausal women with estrogen receptor–positive breast cancer (regardless of nodal status), axillary dissection when the axilla is clinically nega-

tive can add unnecessary morbidity. This is particularly true if the procedure requires general anesthesia. However, proponents of lymphadenectomy claim that the procedure not only has a staging function but also may improve the curability of breast cancer or reduce the duration of adjuvant tamoxifen treatment. In some centers, axillary dissection is being replaced by biopsy of the sentinel node, the first lymph node draining the area of the breast that harbors the cancer. This is determined at surgery by injecting a dye into the site of the resected lump and removing the first node that turns blue. Data suggest that sentinel node sampling is just as accurate as axillary dissection but considerably less toxic (SOE=A).

Adjunct Hormonal Treatment

Adjunct treatment with tamoxifen for at least 2 yr prolongs both the disease-free survival and the overall survival of postmenopausal women (SOE=A). The benefits and risks of more prolonged treatment, especially for women >70 yr old, remain controversial. Aromatase inhibitors are currently licensed as second-line hormonal treatment for those on tamoxifen whose cancer has progressed. Aromatase inhibitors are used as first-line treatment in women with estrogen receptor–positive tumors, and the medication is given for at least 5 yr. Aromatase inhibitors are both more effective and less toxic than tamoxifen (SOE=A). In women currently on tamoxifen, it is recommended that tamoxifen treatment be continued for a 5-yr duration, followed by 5 yr of an aromatase inhibitor.

Initial Management of Metastatic Breast Cancer

Women ≥65 yr old with metastatic, hormone receptor–positive breast cancer are likely to have effective palliation with hormonal therapy, such as tamoxifen. Hormonal treatment has been shown to benefit older women with hormone receptor–poor tumors, but chemotherapy has also been shown to be safe and effective in this group of patients. Generally, single agents are used and treatment is begun at full dosage with modifications based on any toxicities that develop. In frail older adults, treatment can usually begin safely at 75% of the recommended dosage.

Lung Cancer

Lung cancer is becoming increasingly common in older women for reasons that are not completely understood. The increase may possibly be due to higher smoking rates among women. In addition, some data suggest that women are at greater risk (than men) of developing lung cancer per unit of tobacco exposure. Lung cancer currently is the leading cause of cancer death in both men and women.

Early recognition and surgical resection remain the best chance for cure. For patients with lesions in a location that precludes surgery, occasionally localized radiation produces long-term survival. Over the past decade, chemotherapy has produced clinical responses and provided effective palliation for a portion of patients with metastatic disease. Survival has been prolonged, but the added increment is measured in weeks to months. New chemotherapeutic agents, such as vinorelbine and gemcitabine, and more established agents such as paclitaxel or docetaxel used in lower-dose weekly schedules, have proved to produce responses, improve quality of life, and prolong overall survival by a few months for older patients with lung cancer (SOE=A).

Colon Cancer

Two-thirds of colon cancer cases are seen in adults ≥65 yr old. With advancing age, there is a greater likelihood of right-sided lesions and presentations with anemia rather than pain. Colonoscopy has become the mainstay of diagnosis, primarily because it enables direct visualization of the entire colon and biopsy. Surgical excision may be adequate for lesions confined to the colon, but if regional nodes are involved, postoperative adjuvant chemotherapy (usually 5-fluorouracil plus leucovorin) has reduced recurrence by 40%–50%. Survival of patients with metastatic disease in the liver or other organs remains disappointing, despite the appearance of new medications, such as irinotecan, that can induce partial remissions in a subset of patients. New medications that target a tyrosine kinase (an integral enzyme for cellular proliferation) within tumor cells and neutralize vascular endothelial growth factor (thought to promote angiogenesis) are currently in development and offer great promise. Surgical excision of solitary hepatic lesions has offered a survival advantage for selected patients, primarily those with smaller lesions, five or fewer lesions confined to a single hepatic lobe, and a longer interval from original tumor resection until the diagnosis of hepatic metastasis. See also Colonic Polyps and Colon Cancer in "Gastrointestinal Diseases and Disorders," p 402.

Prostate Cancer

See "Prostate Disease," p 423.

Hematologic Malignancies, Lymphomas, and Multiple Myeloma

Leukemias

Acute myeloid leukemia (AML) after myelodysplastic syndromes, as is seen more commonly among older adults, is more likely to be refractory to treatment and to have a smoldering course, requiring only supportive care. What is not clear is whether the prevalence of unfavorable cytogenetic abnormalities and of multilineage neoplastic involvement increases with age in de novo AML. The subset of patients with myelodysplasia who do not have excess blasts or overt leukemia but are neutropenic and have recurrent infections may benefit from intermittent treatment with granulocyte colony-stimulating factor.

In a trial with older patients with AML, delayed treatment was much less effective than immediate treatment. Although this study established the value of timely chemotherapy, the choice of treatment (whether full-dose induction or low-dose cytarabine) remains controversial. In one study, the survival of older patients with leukemia treated with low-dose cytarabine was superior to the survival of those receiving standard induction, because of lower treatment-related mortality. However, others have obtained different results and claimed the superiority of standard treatment.

Chronic lymphocytic leukemia is the most common form of leukemia in the Western world; about 12,500 cases are diagnosed each year in the United States. The incidence is declining for unknown reasons. The median age at diagnosis is 61 yr. The diagnosis is most often made incidentally when a peripheral WBC count reveals leukocytosis with a small-lymphocyte count >4,000/μL. Treatment is generally instituted only to control a life-threatening or symptomatic complication. The major complications are infection and marrow failure. Because about 25% of patients develop autoimmune anemia or thrombocytopenia sometime in the course of the disease, it is important to investigate the mechanism of any decline in peripheral blood cell counts. Autoimmune mechanisms can be treated with glucocorticoids or splenectomy, whereas marrow infiltration by tumor cells requires antitumor therapy. Chlorambucil and fludarabine are the two most active agents. Median survival varies with the stage of disease. Once anemia or thrombocytopenia develops as a consequence of marrow failure, median survival is about 18 mo.

Non-Hodgkin's Lymphoma

Although there are about 38 named varieties of lymphoma, the two most common forms (diffuse large B-cell lymphoma and follicular lymphoma) account for about 75% of cases. The prognosis of non-Hodgkin's lymphoma worsens with age, but the explanation remains unclear. It is likely that older adults are more susceptible to the complications of intensive treatment.

The treatment of older adults with diffuse large B-cell lymphoma has improved in recent years. In this group, 60%–70% of patients obtain a durable complete remission with combination chemotherapy

(CHOP, ie, cyclophosphamide, doxorubicin, vincristine, prednisone) plus rituximab (a monoclonal antibody against CD20 on B cells). Administration of lower-than-normal dosages results in a poorer outcome. Hematopoietic growth factors can lessen the hematopoietic toxicity of treatment.

The treatment of follicular lymphoma is more controversial. Localized forms of the disease (seen in 15% of patients) are curable with radiation therapy. In the 85% of patients with more advanced disease, single agent and combination chemotherapy can sometimes induce long, complete remissions (median duration 6–7 yr). However, in patients with other serious morbidities and a remaining life expectancy of 5 yr, treatment may not be needed because of the indolent nature of the disease progression.

Hodgkin's Disease

Hodgkin's disease exhibits a curious bimodal age-incidence curve, with a second peak late in life. Compared with younger patients, older patients with advanced disease may respond less well to therapy and have poorer survival rates (SOE=C). Several factors can contribute to this poorer prognosis: more extensive disease at presentation, biologic variations from true Hodgkin's disease, greater toxicity with standard treatment regimens, and less aggressive treatment. Older adults can usually tolerate full doses of ABVD (ie, doxorubicin, bleomycin, vinblastine, dacarbazine) without life-threatening bone marrow toxicity.

Multiple Myeloma and Monoclonal Gammopathy of Uncertain Significance (MGUS)

Multiple myeloma is diagnosed in about 19,900 people each year in the United States. The median age at diagnosis is 68 yr; it is rare in people <40 yr old. The incidence in black Americans is twice that in white Americans. The classic triad of myeloma is marrow plasmacytosis (>10%), lytic bone lesions, and a serum or urine (or both) monoclonal gammopathy. Monoclonal gammopathy is common in older adults, estimated at 6% of those ≥70 yr old. When an abnormal paraprotein is discovered on serum immunoelectrophoresis, the best diagnostic test to distinguish myeloma from MGUS is a skeletal survey. If the skeletal survey is normal, a bone marrow biopsy is still indicated to determine the presence of marrow plasmacytosis. Patients with MGUS have marrow plasma cells constituting <10% of the total cell number, do not have lytic bone lesions, and usually do not have other features of myeloma, including hypercalcemia, renal failure, anemia, or susceptibility to infection. MGUS progresses to multiple myeloma or a related malignancy at a rate of 1% per year (SOE=B).

Patients with myeloma require treatment when the lytic bone lesions become symptomatic or progressive, infections are recurrent, or the serum paraprotein increases. Standard treatment consists of lenalidomide plus dexamethasone for those who will go on to receive high-dose therapy plus an autologous stem cell transplant. For those who are not transplant candidates, intermittent pulses of an oral alkylating agent (eg, melphalan), prednisone, and lenalidomide are given for 4–7 days every 4–6 weeks. Supportive care includes bisphosphonates to decrease bone turnover, erythropoietin and other hematinics for the anemia, intravenous immunoglobulin for recurrent infections, radiation for specific symptomatic bone lesions, maintenance of hydration to preserve renal function, and adequate analgesia.

PRINCIPLES OF MANAGEMENT

Both the incidence and prevalence of cancer increase with age, and older adults more often present with advanced-stage disease. Screening older populations for colon and breast cancer can lead to early detection of more curable lesions. Older patients can have less physiologic reserve than younger patients, but unless a specific comorbid illness is influencing baseline organ function, cancer treatments with curative or palliative potential should be offered to most patients in most settings, regardless of age. Curative surgical procedures may require more prolonged convalescence, but recovery from most procedures is expected. Radiation therapy is safe and effective in the same settings in which it is used in younger patients. Chemotherapy may need to be adjusted to the individual patient's level of tolerance of the adverse events, but usually the changes should be made in the face of toxicities that actually develop rather than on toxicities anticipated to develop. Biologic therapies are usually safe; some are less toxic in older than in younger patients.

See also "Dermatologic Diseases and Disorders," p 333, for the diagnosis and treatment of skin cancers; and "Persistent Pain," p 109; and "Palliative Care," p 114, for the management of pain and end-of-life care.

ACOVE-3* Quality Indicators Pertaining to Oncology

BREAST CANCER

Mammogram

- If a female vulnerable older adult is <70 yr old, then she should be offered mammographic screening for breast cancer every 2 yr.

History

- If a female vulnerable older adult is diagnosed with breast cancer, then physical and psychosocial performance status should be evaluated.
- If a female vulnerable older adult is diagnosed with breast cancer, then comorbid illnesses should be evaluated.

Discussion of options

- If a female vulnerable older adult has a new diagnosis of breast cancer, then there should be documentation of a discussion regarding:
  - Surgical options and goals of therapy
  - Posttreatment quality of life
  - Functional outcomes
  - Risk and benefits of adjuvant therapy

Surgical documentation

- If a female vulnerable older adult is diagnosed with locally invasive breast cancer, then tumor size, grade, and margins should be recorded after surgery.

Estrogen receptor status

- If a female vulnerable older adult is diagnosed with locally invasive breast cancer, then the estrogen and progesterone receptor status of the tumor should be documented.

HER-2/neu receptor status

- If a female vulnerable older adult is diagnosed with locally invasive breast cancer and chemotherapy is planned, then at the time of diagnosis, HER-2/neu receptor status should be evaluated.
- If a female vulnerable older adult is diagnosed with locally invasive breast cancer, chemotherapy is planned, and she has a score of 2+ for HER-2/neu overexpression according to immunohistochemistry testing, then HER-2/neu receptor status should be confirmed using fluorescence in situ hybridization.

Bone evaluation

- If a female vulnerable older adult with locally invasive breast cancer has symptoms of bone pain, increased serum alkaline phosphatase, tumor size >5 cm, or positive lymph nodes, then radiographic bone imaging should be performed during the staging examination.

Surgical care

- If a female vulnerable older adult is diagnosed with early-stage locally invasive breast cancer (Stage I–III) and chemotherapy is planned, then she should undergo axillary staging with a sentinel lymph node biopsy or a complete axillary lymph node dissection at the time of surgery.
- If a female vulnerable older adult is diagnosed with only lobular carcinoma in situ, then further surgical resection should not be performed.
- If a female vulnerable older adult is diagnosed with ductal carcinoma in situ or early-stage invasive breast cancer, then breast-conserving surgery should be offered.
- If a female vulnerable older adult with locally invasive breast cancer is treated with a mastectomy, then she should be offered breast reconstruction.

Radiation therapy

- If a female vulnerable older adult is diagnosed with early-stage invasive breast cancer and undergoes a lumpectomy, then breast radiation therapy should be discussed.
- If a female vulnerable older adult is diagnosed with invasive breast cancer with a tumor >5 cm or four or more positive lymph nodes and undergoes mastectomy, then postoperative radiation therapy should be discussed within 2 mo after surgery or after chemotherapy.

Hormonal therapy

- If a female vulnerable older adult is diagnosed with estrogen receptor–positive locally invasive breast cancer >1 cm, then adjuvant hormonal therapy should be offered.

Adjuvant chemotherapy

- If a female vulnerable older adult with a life expectancy of >5 yr is diagnosed with locally invasive breast cancer with four or more positive lymph nodes, then adjuvant chemotherapy should be offered.
- If a female vulnerable older adult with normal cardiac function and a life expectancy >5 yr is diagnosed with locally invasive breast cancer with positive lymph nodes and HER-2/neu receptor overexpression, then adjuvant chemotherapy with trastuzumab should be offered.

Limiting surveillance

- If a female vulnerable older adult is diagnosed with nonmetastatic breast cancer and receives primary treatment, then she should not receive follow-up surveillance with imaging (eg, CT scan) or laboratory studies (eg, CA 15–3, CA 27.29, carcinoembryonic antigen).

Metastatic disease

- If a female vulnerable older adult is diagnosed with advanced breast cancer with symptomatic or osteolytic bone metastasis, then bisphosphonate treatment should be offered.

- If a female vulnerable older adult is diagnosed with advanced estrogen receptor–positive breast cancer with bone metastasis and without extensive visceral involvement, then endocrine therapy should be offered.

- If a female vulnerable older adult has symptomatic multifocal metastatic hormone-refractory breast cancer or symptomatic hormone receptor–negative breast cancer with extensive visceral metastasis, then treatment with systemic chemotherapy should be offered.

- If a female vulnerable older adult with normal cardiac function with HER-2/neu-positive metastatic breast cancer is treated with systemic chemotherapy, then trastuzumab should be offered.

COLORECTAL CANCER

Screening

- If a vulnerable older adult is <70 yr old, then there should be documentation that the option of colorectal cancer screening was discussed.

History

- If a vulnerable older adult is diagnosed with colorectal cancer, then physical and psychosocial performance status should be evaluated.

- If a vulnerable older adult is diagnosed with colorectal cancer, then comorbid illnesses should be evaluated.

Staging evaluation

- If a vulnerable older adult has a new diagnosis of colorectal cancer and is a candidate for therapy, then he or she should have a pretreatment carcinoembryonic antigen (CEA) level.

- If a vulnerable older adult with a new diagnosis of colon or rectal cancer is a candidate for elective resection of the primary tumor and has an increased (or unknown) CEA, then pretreatment imaging with a CT scan (or similar imaging) of the abdomen and pelvis should be done.

- If a vulnerable older adult has a new diagnosis of rectal cancer with a normal CEA and is a candidate for elective resection of the primary tumor, then pelvic imaging should be performed using ultrasound (endoscopic ultrasound or transrectal ultrasound), MRI, or CT.

Colon examination

- If a vulnerable older adult has a new diagnosis of colorectal cancer and is a candidate for potential cure, then he or she should have a total colonic examination before surgery.

- If a vulnerable older adult underwent colorectal cancer resection for cure and total colonic examination was not performed preoperatively (eg, because of an obstructing lesion), then total colonic examination should be performed within 6 mo after surgery.

Discussion of options

- If a vulnerable older adult has a new diagnosis of colorectal cancer, then there should be documentation of a discussion regarding:
  ○ Surgical options and goals of surgery
  ○ Posttreatment quality of life
  ○ Functional outcomes
  ○ Risks and benefits of adjuvant therapy (if colon cancer) or neoadjuvant therapy (if rectal cancer)

Discussion of surgical findings

- If a vulnerable older adult undergoes surgery for colorectal cancer, then a qualified physician (eg, surgeon, oncologist, radiation oncologist) should discuss with the patient or caregiver final pathology (eg, stage, status of lymph nodes, margins) and indications for further treatment (eg, chemotherapy, radiation therapy).

Nonsurgical treatment plan

- If a vulnerable older adult has a new diagnosis of colorectal cancer and is not a candidate for surgical therapy, then this should be noted, as well as an alternative treatment plan.

- If a vulnerable older adult is diagnosed with incurable, metastatic colorectal cancer, then prognosis and end-of-life discussions should be documented.

Preoperative examination

- If a vulnerable older adult with a new diagnosis of rectal cancer is to be treated surgically, then the surgeon should preoperatively (or pre-neoadjuvant therapy) assess the mass (eg, digital rectal examination or flexible sigmoidoscopy).

Preoperative ostomy siting

■ If a vulnerable older adult with a new diagnosis of colorectal cancer is to have elective abdominal perineal resection or other procedure with planned creation of an ostomy, then the ostomy should be sited preoperatively and documented in the medical record (eg, enterostomal therapy note or operative note).

Adjuvant therapy

■ If a vulnerable older adult has Stage III colon cancer, then adjuvant chemotherapy should be given within 4 mo of surgery.

■ If a vulnerable older adult is thought to have Stage II or III mid-low rectal cancer and is a candidate for surgery, then preoperative neoadjuvant chemotherapy and radiation therapy should be given.

■ If a vulnerable older adult had surgical resection for Stage II or III rectal cancer and did not receive neoadjuvant radiation or chemotherapy, then postoperative adjuvant chemotherapy, radiation therapy, or both should be provided within 4 mo of surgery.

Postoperative surveillance

■ If a vulnerable older adult with greater than Stage I colorectal cancer underwent resection for cure, then a history and physical examination should be performed every 6 mo for the first 2 yr after surgery and annually during years 3 to 5.

■ If a vulnerable older adult with greater than Stage I colorectal cancer underwent resection for cure, then a CEA level should be performed every 6 mo for the first 2 yr after surgery and annually during years 3 to 5.

■ If a vulnerable older adult underwent colorectal cancer resection for cure, then a colonoscopy should be performed within 3 yr after surgery.

Evaluate rising CEA

■ If a vulnerable older adult had prior colorectal cancer resection for cure and has a CEA >7.5 (confirmed by retesting if <10), then further examination should be initiated (eg, colonoscopy, radiologic imaging).

Related quality indicators for Oncology

■ Goals of care surrogate discussion (see "Legal and Ethical Issues," p 23)

■ End-of-Life care preferences and management (see "Palliative Care," p 102)

■ Pain management (see "Persistent Pain," p 109)

*Assessing Care of Vulnerable Elders – 3rd Set. See inside front cover for explanation.

REFERENCES

■ Albrand G, Terret C. Early breast cancer in the elderly: assessment and management considerations. *Drugs Aging.* 2008;25(1):35–45.

■ Mitry E, Rougier P. Review article: benefits and risks of chemotherapy in elderly patients with metastatic colorectal cancer. *Aliment Pharmacol Ther.* 2009;29(2):161–171.

■ Monfardini S, Gridelli C, Pasetto LM, et al. Vulnerable and frail elderly: an approach to the management of the main tumour types. *Eur J Cancer.* 2008;44:488–493.

Normal Laboratory Values*
Referenced in the Questions and Critiques

BLOOD, PLASMA, SERUM CHEMISTRIES

Alanine aminotransferase (ALT)   0–35 U/L

Aspartate aminotransferase (AST)   0–35 U/L

Bicarbonate (CO_2)   21–30 mEq/L

Blood gas studies:

   PO_2 83–108 mmHg

   PCO_2 Women: 32–45 mmHg; Men: 35–48 mmHg

   pH   7.35–7.45

   Oxygen saturation   95%–98%

Blood urea nitrogen (BUN)   8–20 mg/dL

Calcium   8.8–10.3 mg/dL

Calcium, ionized   4.5–5.6 mEq/L

Carcinoembryonic antigen   <2.5 ng/mL

Chloride   98–106 mEq/L

Cholesterol:

   Total   Desirable: <200 mg/dL

   High-density lipoprotein (HDL)   Desirable: >39 mg/dL

   Low-density lipoprotein (LDL)   Recommended: <130 mg/dL, lower for those with CHD risk factors or vascular disease; evidence limited for adults ≥85 yr old

      Moderate risk: 130–159 mg/dL

      High risk: ≥160 mg/dL

Creatinine   0.7–1.5 mg/dL

Creatine kinase   Women: 26–140 U/L; Men: 38–174 U/L

Digoxin (therapeutic level)   0.8–2.0 ng/mL for rate control; 0.6–0.8 for heart failure

Ferritin   20–250 ng/mL

Folate   2.2–17.3 ng/mL

Glucose   Fasting: 70–105 mg/dL
         2-hour postprandial: <140 mg/dL

Hemoglobin A_{1c} 5.3%–7.5%

Homocysteine   5–15 μmol/L

Iron   50–150 mcg/dL; iron saturation ([iron/iron-binding capacity] × 100) ≤10% abnormal

Iron-binding capacity, total   250–450 mcg/dL

Lactate dehydrogenase   60–100 U/L

Methylmalonic acid (MMA)   0.08–0.56 μmol/L

Magnesium   1.8–3.0 mg/dL

Parathyroid hormone   10–65 pg/mL

Phosphatase, acid   0.5–5.5 U/L

Phosphatase, alkaline   20–135 U/L

Phosphorus (≥60 yr old)   Women: 2.8–4.1 mg/dL
                        Men: 2.3–3.7 mg/dL

Potassium   3.5–5 mEq/L

Prostate-specific antigen (PSA)   <4 ng/mL

Protein, total   6.4–8.3 g/dL

   Albumin   3.5–5.5 g/dL

   Globulin   2.0–3.5 g/dL

Rheumatoid factor, latest test   >1:80 is abnormal

Sodium   136–145 mEq/L

Testosterone:

   Women   <3.5 nmol/L (<100 ng.dL)

   Men   10–35 nmol/L (300–1,000 ng/dL)

Thyrotropin (TSH)   0.5–5.0 μU/mL

Thyroxine (T_4)   Total: 5–12 mcg/dL; Free: 0.9–2.4 ng/dL

Triglycerides   Recommended: <150 mg/dL

Uric acid   2.5–8.0 mg/dL

Vitamin B_{12} 200–950 pg/mL

25(OH) vitamin D (total)   30–75 mcg/L

HEMATOLOGY

RBC count   Women: 4.2–5.4 × 10^6/μL; Men: 4.7–6.1 × 10^6/μL

Erythrocyte sedimentation rate (Westergren)   0–35 mm/h

Hematocrit   Women: 33%–43%; Men: 39%–49%

Hemoglobin   Women: 11.5–15.5 g/dL; Men: 14–18 g/dL

WBC count and differential   4,800–10,800/μL
   Segmented neutrophils 54%–62%
   Band forms 3%–5%
   Lymphocytes 23%–33%
   Monocytes 3%–7%
   Eosinophils 1%–3%
   Basophils <1%

Mean corpuscular hemoglobin   28–32 pg

Mean corpuscular volume   86–98 fL (86–98 mm³)

Platelet count   150,000–450,000/μL

URINE

Creatinine clearance   90–140 mL/min

Creatinine, urine   Women: 11–20 mg/kg/24 h
                  Men: 14–26 mg/kg/24 h

Urine, postvoid residual volume   <50 mL, normal; >200 mL, abnormal; 50–200 mL, equivocal

---

* Note: Because normal ranges vary among laboratories, data in this table may not conform with that of all laboratories.

QUESTIONS

Directions: Each of the questions or incomplete statements below is followed by four or five suggested answers or completions. Select the ONE answer or completion that is BEST in each case and circle or place an "X" through the letter you have selected for each answer on the answer sheet. Answer sheets for self-assessment are available to download at: http://www.americangeriatrics.org/publications/gnrs3. The repeated questions with answers and supporting critiques are located on p 565. The table of Normal Laboratory Values on the previous page may be consulted for any of the questions in this book.

1. An 84-yr-old nursing home resident is evaluated because she has been sleeping more over the last few days. At the beginning of the visit, the patient is still sleeping in bed in her nightgown; this is unusual for her. Staff reports that she recently seems less likely to recognize familiar people. The patient has no complaints and is distracted by the birds chirping outside her window. History includes stroke with persistent left hemiplegia, hypertension, dyslipidemia, diabetes, and mild dementia. Her hypertensive medications were recently adjusted by her cardiologist to improve blood pressure control. On examination, vital signs are unremarkable. She is disoriented to place and time. Her neurologic examination is otherwise unchanged from previous evaluations.

   Which of the following is the most likely cause of her cognitive and behavioral changes?

   (A) Progressive dementia
   (B) Major depressive disorder
   (C) Delirium
   (D) New stroke

2. A 92-yr-old man who resides in an assisted-living facility has increasing shortness of breath with activity and increasing frequency of chest pain. The chest pain responds promptly to sublingual nitroglycerin. He walks daily, reads, and plays the piano. History includes severe aortic valve stenosis with preserved ejection fraction confirmed by echocardiography, paroxysmal atrial fibrillation accompanied by shortness of breath, hypertension, dyslipidemia, osteoarthritis, lumbar spine disease, gastroesophageal reflux, benign prostatic hyperplasia, and depression. Medications include furosemide, losartin, warfarin, atorvasatin, mirtazepine, tamulosin, finasteride, acetaminophen, calcium, and vitamin D.

On examination, the patient is pale and appears younger than his stated age. Weight is 84 kg (185 lb), blood pressure is 120/70 mmHg, heart rate is 76 beats per minute and regular. There is a 3/6 harsh late-peaking systolic murmur audible at the apex and left sternal edge. There are no bruits, and his lungs are clear. His score on the Mini–Mental State Exam is 29/30. The Charlson Comorbidity Index = 6.

Laboratory results
Creatinine   1.1 mg/dL with an estimated
                 GFR >60 mL/min
Electrolytes   normal
CBC   normal

Which of the following is the best diagnostic test to further evaluate this patient's cardiac status?

   (A) Transthoracic echocardiogram
   (B) Treadmill stress test
   (C) Coronary angiography
   (D) Persantine thallium stress test
   (E) Cardiac MRI

3. Which of the following assistive devices is most appropriate for a 72-yr-old man with Parkinson's disease who has postural instability and festination?

   (A) Cane
   (B) Front-wheeled walker
   (C) Hemi-walker
   (D) Pick-up walker
   (E) 4-Wheeled walker

4. A 76-yr-old man is brought to the office by his older sister to establish care. The patient has significant autism. He lives with his sister, who reports that over the past 3 mo he has been rocking, pacing, and yelling more often, and has hit himself twice. The behaviors have slowly increased in frequency and intensity

to a degree that she has not seen for several years. His sleep is disrupted and he often paces during the night. His sister is his guardian; she reports that his care is increasingly difficult for her. She recently moved them from their family home to an apartment, and they are getting out less frequently for walks and shopping. He has no history of significant illnesses and is on no routine medications.

On examination, the patient is slightly underweight. He rocks and hums nearly constantly during the office visit. His skin is intact, and there are no bruises. The examination is essentially normal other than his repetitive behaviors.

Which of the following is the most appropriate initial step in managing the patient's behaviors?

(A) Begin quetiapine 25 mg.
(B) Begin zolpidem 5 mg at bedtime.
(C) Begin mirtazapine 15 mg.
(D) Reevaluate in 2 wk if the behavior persists.
(E) Begin methylphenidate 5 mg.

5. A 75-yr-old woman comes to the office because she has had repeated episodes of profound dizziness and syncope, along with at least 2 episodes in which she found herself on the floor but was unaware of how she fell. Each episode has been preceded by a prodrome during which she feels warm and is diaphoretic and progressively lightheaded. The episodes are most likely to occur when she has been standing for a long time, such as during church services. History includes hypertension, for which she takes hydrochlorothiazide daily.

On physical examination, blood pressure is 142/84 mmHg while supine and 110/70 mmHg while upright; heart rate is 76 beats per minute while supine and 80 beats per minute while upright. There is no jugular venous distension or carotid bruit. Lungs are clear. Carotid upstroke is slightly delayed, with a II/VI systolic murmur at the base; the second heart sound is intact, and there is no gallop.

Which of the following is the most appropriate next step?

(A) Stop hydrochlorothiazide.
(B) Begin oral midodrine 5 mg three times daily (about 4 h apart, not too close to bedtime).
(C) Begin fludrocortisone 0.1 mg q12h.
(D) Obtain tilt-table test.

6. Which one of the following statements about smoking and older adults is true?

(A) Older smokers who quit gain substantial health benefits.
(B) Most smokers will attempt to quit only if they are supported by counseling or pharmacologic treatments.
(C) Older hospitalized patients are as likely as younger inpatients to receive smoking cessation interventions.
(D) Medicare does not cover tobacco cessation counseling for beneficiaries who have smoking-related illnesses.
(E) Brief interventions delivered by health care professionals do not affect rates of smoking cessation.

7. A 65-yr-old recently retired man comes to the office because he has recurring episodes of urinary frequency associated with perineal discomfort. He reports that he has had a "nervous bladder" for much of his life but had never seen a clinician for this. Over the last year, however, he has had a mild to moderately uncomfortable sensation that initially seemed to come and go but now is present most days and uncomfortable enough to cause him distress. He has been married for 35 yr and has been sexually active and monogamous for that time. He reports no problems associated with sexual activity, and has no chills, fever, incontinence, or difficulty starting or stopping urinary stream. He has never sought counseling or medical care for anxiety. He has no chronic disorders and takes no medications.

On examination, blood pressure is 140/80 mmHg and pulse is 80 beats per minute. His prostate is estimated at 15 mL, with no asymmetry, nodule, or induration. He notes mild tenderness during palpation. Urinalysis done after digital rectal examination reveals 3 or 4 WBCs per high-power field and is otherwise unremarkable. Cultures from that urine sample (including for *Mycobacterium tuberculosis*) are unremarkable. Prostate-specific antigen level is 3.2 ng/mL, and urine cytologies are negative.

Which of the following is the most appropriate next step?

(A) Finasteride therapy
(B) α-Agonist therapy
(C) Transrectal ultrasonography
(D) CT of the pelvis
(E) Psychiatric evaluation

8. Which of the following is meant by culturally competent care?

(A) Allocation of resources in proportion to the cultural composition of the community.
(B) Delivery of health services according to the cultural practices of the caregiver.
(C) Delivery of health services that acknowledge cultural diversity in the clinical setting.
(D) Characterizing patients based on their cultural backgrounds rather than their individual preferences.

9. An 81-yr-old man comes to the office for follow-up after myocardial infarction 5 wk earlier. He has not needed nitroglycerin for angina since 4 days after the infarct. He would like to resume sexual relations with the woman he has dated since his wife died 2 yr ago. In the past year, before the infarct, he was able to maintain an erection sufficient for intercourse about half of the time. He is anxious because he is now unable to achieve erections sufficient for intercourse. History includes well-controlled hypertension with left ventricular hypertrophy, and transurethral resection of the prostate 15 yr ago for benign prostatic hyperplasia. Medications include atenolol 50 mg/d, simvastatin 40 mg/d, aspirin 81 mg/d, and nitroglycerin as needed.

On examination, peripheral pulses are diminished. His score on the Geriatric Depression Scale is 3, and he denies symptoms of depression.

Which of the following is the most appropriate next step in assessing this patient?

(A) Refer to cardiologist.
(B) Measure serum testosterone and bioavailable testosterone.
(C) Measure nocturnal penile tumescence.
(D) Refer to psychiatrist.

10. Which of the following statements is true?

(A) Aged skeletal muscle cells are more likely than younger skeletal muscle cells to undergo apoptosis (cell death) as a result of physical inactivity.
(B) The reductions in skeletal muscle tone and contractility that occur with aging are due primarily to changes in muscle mass.
(C) Muscles do not lose any tone with aging if they are exercised regularly.
(D) The rate and extent of muscle changes is determined almost entirely by exercise and does not have a genetic component.

11. A 79-yr-old woman comes to the office to establish care. She reports that she often feels sleepy. History includes osteoporosis, hip fracture, systolic heart failure, hypertension, frequent falls, chronic kidney disease, and post-herpetic neuralgia. Medications include extended-release metoprolol 100 mg/d, gabapentin 600 mg q8h, alendronate 35 mg/wk, vitamin D 800 IU/d, calcium carbonate 500 mg q8h, and aspirin 81 mg/d. Serum creatinine is 1.5 mg/dL, with estimated creatinine clearance of 30 mL/min.

Which of the following would be most likely to relieve this patient's sleepiness?

(A) Reduce gabapentin dosage to 600 mg q12h.
(B) Start lisinopril 2.5 mg/d.
(C) Discontinue alendronate.
(D) Increase vitamin D to 1200 IU/d.
(E) Switch extended-release metoprolol to metoprolol 50 mg q12h.

12. A 90-yr-old woman comes to the office because, over the past year, she has had increasing difficulty walking. Her gait is slower, and she feels as if she might fall backward at times. She has hypertension, hypothyroidism, and osteoarthritis, and she had coronary artery

bypass surgery 10 yr ago, with no recurrence of angina.

On examination, she has moderate dorsal kyphosis and arthritic changes in her fingers and knees. Strength and reflexes are symmetric. She has some increased muscle tone. She uses her arms to push up from the chair; once standing, she has difficulty starting to walk. Her gait is symmetric, with a normal base, but her foot clearance and stride length are both decreased. She turns slowly and carefully, with an increased number of steps.

Which of the following is the most likely cause of her gait abnormality?

(A) Osteoarthritis
(B) Proprioceptive deficits
(C) Cerebrovascular disease
(D) Parkinson's disease
(E) Cautious gait

13. A 69-yr-old black man comes to the office for evaluation because routine laboratory tests showed an increased total calcium concentration (10.8 mg/dL). Three years ago, the concentration was 10.6 mg/dL. He has no symptoms of hypercalcemia, such as nausea, constipation, personality changes, or renal stones. There is a family history of hypertension; he is unaware of any family history of calcium disorders. The patient has an enlarged prostate and hypertension. Medications include amlodipine, hydrochlorothiazide, and saw palmetto. He does not take any vitamin supplements.

On physical examination, blood pressure is 140/80 mmHg, and he has mild prostatic hyperplasia. The remainder of the physical examination is normal. Levels of creatinine and $1,25(OH)_2D$ are normal. Parathyroid hormone concentration is 78 pg/mL and thyrotropin concentration is 2.1 mU/L.

Which of the following tests should be ordered next?

(A) Genetic testing for familial benign hypercalciuria hypocalciuria mutation
(B) 25(OH)D
(C) Parathyroid sestamibi (nuclear scan)
(D) A 24-hour urine collection for calcium and creatinine
(E) DEXA scan of the spine, hip, and forearm

14. Which of the following is true regarding how the nursing-home population has changed since 1985?

(A) The number of residents has increased.
(B) Among adults ≥85 yr old, men now outnumber women.
(C) The level of disability has declined.
(D) The number of admissions has increased.

15. A 79-yr-old woman was discharged from the hospital yesterday after a 2-wk stay for diverticular bleeding. She underwent transfusion with 8 units of RBCs and declined surgery. She has diabetes and osteoarthritis and was in bed for most of the past 2 wk. Her husband calls to report that she is very weak. She needs follow-up laboratory tests in 2 days in compliance with hospital discharge instructions, but he does not think he can transport her to the office. He wants to know if she can receive home health care to address her needs.

Which of the following is an allowable indication for home health care in this patient?

(A) Follow-up laboratory testing
(B) Physical therapy
(C) Home aide services
(D) Monitoring of glycemic control
(E) Durable medical equipment

16. A 76-yr-old woman is transferred from a rehabilitation facility to the hospital after she falls and fractures her right hip. She was recovering from a recent hospitalization for pneumonia and exacerbation of COPD that left her profoundly deconditioned. She uses a combined steroid and long-acting β-agonist inhaler and takes oral steroids for exacerbations. She is not oxygen dependent. She has no history of dementia but believes she has been more forgetful over the past year.

She is hydrated, her pain is controlled with narcotics, and surgery is planned for the next morning under general anesthesia.

Which of the following would be most likely to reduce her risk of postoperative delirium?

(A) Start low-dose intravenous haloperidol and continue for 48 h after surgery.
(B) Start oral donepezil and continue indefinitely.
(C) Obtain a preoperative comprehensive geriatric evaluation to develop a multifactorial risk-reduction strategy.
(D) Provide stress doses of intravenous steroids perioperatively.
(E) Avoid opioid analgesia after surgery.

17. Which of the following is the most reliable screen for hearing impairment?

(A) Screening version of the Hearing Handicap Inventory for the Elderly (HHIE-S)
(B) Abbreviated Profile of Hearing Aid Benefit
(C) Tinnitus Handicap Questionnaire
(D) Whisper test

18. A 72-yr-old man comes to the office because he has increased difficulty with urination, including poor stream, straining to void, and occasional urinary incontinence. History includes benign prostatic hyperplasia, dyslipidemia, type 2 diabetes mellitus, and painful peripheral neuropathy; past medical history is significant for transient ischemic attack. Medications include clopidogrel 75 mg/d, doxazosin 2 mg at bedtime, glipizide 10 mg/d, atorvastatin 20 mg/d, and gabapentin 400 mg q8h. The patient's peripheral neuropathy has been difficult to manage. Further increase of gabapentin is not possible because it causes him dizziness. Nortriptyline 25 mg at bedtime was started 2 wk ago, and the patient reports decreased pain.

On examination, the patient's prostate is not enlarged, nor is his bladder palpable. Urinalysis is normal.

Which of the following should be done next to manage this patient's voiding difficulties?

(A) Increase doxazosin.
(B) Discontinue nortriptyline.
(C) Begin tolterodine.
(D) Obtain postvoid residual level.
(E) Obtain prostate-specific antigen level.

19. A 69-yr-old woman with a history of deep venous thrombosis of right leg presents after diagnosis and surgical resection of estrogen and progesterone receptor-positive early stage breast cancer. She has been offered a balanced discussion of the risks and benefits of adjuvant therapy in the setting of early stage breast cancer. Her most recent dual x-ray absorptiometry (DEXA) results revealed no evidence of osteopenia.

Which of the following therapies is the best option for adjuvant therapy to reduce risk of recurrence and increase survival?

(A) Chemotherapy
(B) Tamoxifen
(C) Raloxifene
(D) Aromatase inhibitor therapy

20. An 86-yr-old man comes to the office to establish care. His wife died 10 yr ago; he recently moved to the area to be closer to his children and grandchildren. History includes visual impairment secondary to macular degeneration, osteoarthritis of the hip and knee, insomnia, benign prostatic hyperplasia, and mild nocturia. Medications include aspirin and tamsulosin daily, and meloxicam and temazepam, each 3 or 4 times weekly. His alcohol history comprises 1 highball each night before dinner and 1 glass of wine with dinner. At least once a week, the patient has a second glass of wine during dinner. The patient reports that his current pattern of drinking has remained the same for the past 40 yr. His CAGE (**C**ut down, **A**nnoyed, **G**uilty, **E**ye opener) score is 0 of 4.

On examination, he has decreased visual acuity, an enlarged prostate, and an antalgic gait.

Which one of the following is the most appropriate intervention?

(A) Recommend continuing alcohol intake at this level.
(B) Recommend restricting alcohol intake to no more than 1 drink per day.
(C) Measure liver enzyme levels to assess for alcohol-related liver impairment.
(D) Defer discussion of alcohol consumption until relationship with patient is more established.
(E) Defer renewing prescriptions for meloxicam and temazepam until he agrees to abstain from alcohol.

21. A 67-yr-old man comes to the office with his family to obtain a second medical opinion. He has lost 18 kg (40 lb) in the past 6 mo, is weak, spends most of his time in bed, no longer participates in family activities, and is no longer interested in watching sporting events on television. He tends to sit quietly and let his family answer questions, but when questioned directly, he indicates that he cannot swallow solids or liquids because his throat is blocked. His family reports that he eats and drinks small amounts. He believes he has undiagnosed cancer that the doctors have yet to find.

Physical examination and cognitive assessment reveal some mild difficulties in recall. According to the medical records he provides, radiography and CT of the chest are normal, and upper endoscopy is unremarkable. Physical examination and several sets of blood work have been obtained, none of which indicate dehydration, anemia, or hepatic or renal dysfunction.

Which of the following is the most likely explanation for these findings?

(A) Occult lung cancer
(B) Vascular dementia
(C) Alzheimer's disease
(D) Major depressive disorder with psychotic features
(E) Parkinson's disease with psychotic symptoms

22. An 84-yr-old man comes to the office because he has pain in his lower back and right buttock. The pain has progressively worsened over the past year. It is most pronounced when he stands or walks for a prolonged period, and is often relieved when he sits. The pain is most severe when he first stands after sitting and when he tries to get in or out of an automobile. He has difficulty climbing stairs.

On examination, there is mild symmetric immobility of the lumbar spine. The straight-leg raise test is normal bilaterally. He has full strength of the proximal and distal muscles of both lower legs. There is 30° abduction, 45° external rotation, and 10° internal rotation of the left hip; and 10° abduction, 20° external rotation, and no internal rotation of the right hip. When the patient walks, he limps favoring his right leg.

Which of the following is the most appropriate next step?

(A) Radiography of the lumbar spine
(B) MRI of the lumbar spine
(C) Nerve conduction studies of the right lower leg
(D) Radiography of the right hip
(E) Bone scan

23. A 70-yr-old woman comes to the office for a routine examination. She is cognitively intact and has a history of hypertension, macular degeneration, and osteoarthritis, mainly in her knees. She takes a multivitamin, lisinopril, and extra-strength acetaminophen as needed for pain.

Physical examination is normal, except that she wears pads. She reluctantly admits to having "accidents." She is embarrassed and worried, and has given up weekly bridge sessions. Lately she has been rushing to the bathroom frequently to prevent accidents. Which of the following is the most appropriate next step?

(A) Start an oxybutynin trial and schedule follow-up in 2 wk.
(B) Ask patient to keep a voiding diary and schedule follow-up in 2 wk.
(C) Start bladder retraining program and schedule follow-up in 2 wk.
(D) Obtain urology consultation.
(E) No further intervention is necessary.

24. A 79-yr-old man is discharged from the hospital after treatment for acute cholecystitis. History includes insulin-dependent diabetes mellitus, mild dementia, major depressive disorder, and recurrent falls (two in the past 6 mo). He has been hospitalized twice in the past year. He was delirious during the current hospitalization but is less confused at discharge. He lives with his daughter, who assists him with bathing and dressing. Arrangements are in place for a visiting nurse during the period immediately after discharge.

Medications during hospitalization included NPH and regular insulin, donepezil, acetaminophen, and a third-generation cephalosporin with metronidazole.

Which of the following is most likely to reduce this patient's risk of falls immediately after discharge?

(A) Supplemental vitamin D
(B) In-home occupational therapy
(C) Consultation with a podiatrist
(D) Consultation with an optometrist

25. A 73-yr-old woman comes to the office for follow-up and medication refills. Her examination is unchanged since her last visit 3 mo ago, except that her weight has decreased from 99.8 kg (220 lb) to 92.5 kg (204 lb). She expresses surprise about the weight loss: "It's a miracle I didn't gain a ton. Since my daughter and grandchildren moved out, all I do is watch TV!"

Which one of the following is most appropriate?

(A) Set exercise and diet goals, and schedule follow-up in 2 mo.
(B) Discuss the weight loss and evaluate her for causes.
(C) Administer the Simplified Nutritional Assessment Questionnaire.
(D) Encourage her to continue to lose weight.
(E) Suggest a nutritional supplement to help her regain the lost weight.

26. A 65-yr-old woman comes to the office to request advice about quitting smoking. She has a 40-pack-year smoking history. She wants to know whether she is too old to benefit from quitting.

Which of the following is a benefit of smoking cessation as an older adult?

(A) Circulation improves 5 yr after cessation.
(B) Lung function improves 5 yr after cessation.
(C) She would live longer.
(D) The risk of dying from heart disease decreases to 5 times that of a nonsmoker.

27. A 79-yr-old man comes to the office because he has increasing difficulty understanding conversations with his grandchildren.

Which of the following is the most likely diagnosis?

(A) Presbycusis
(B) Sociocusis
(C) Ototoxicity
(D) Acoustic neuroma

28. A 70-yr-old retired mailman comes to the office because he now has difficulty climbing 1 flight of stairs. He has dyspnea on exertion that has progressed slowly over 5 yr. He wheezes occasionally. He has had a minimally productive morning cough for many years but no chest pain or discomfort. He has a 50-pack-year cigarette smoking history and still smokes.

On examination, temperature is 36° C (96.8° F), blood pressure is 115/75 mmHg, heart rate is 98 beats per minute, and respiratory rate is 22 breaths per minute. There is no accessory muscle use. Bibasilar crackles are audible. Cardiac and abdominal examinations are normal. There is trace peripheral edema but no cyanosis or clubbing. Chest radiography is normal.

Pulmonary function tests:

FVC	65% of predicted
FEV_1	70% of predicted
FEV_1/FVC ratio	75%

After bronchodilation, FEV_1 increases by 9% and FVC increases by 8%.

Which of the following is the most likely cause of this patient's dyspnea?

(A) Asthma
(B) COPD
(C) Idiopathic pulmonary fibrosis
(D) Pleural effusion
(E) Pulmonary embolism

29. An 80-yr-old woman comes to the office because she has lost 4.5 kg (10 lb) in the preceding year, feels that everything she does is an "effort," and has begun using her arms to lift herself from her chair. She states that she is not depressed. She is accompanied by her daughter, with whom she lives.

Physical examination is normal except that she appears tired and has a slow, steady gait. She scores one positive response on the Geriatric Depression Scale. Results of a CBC, BUN, creatinine, electrolytes, and thyroid and liver function tests are normal. Frailty is diagnosed.

Which of the following is the most appropriate next step?

(A) Begin a trial of methylphenidate.
(B) Begin protein supplements.
(C) Begin a resistance-training exercise program.
(D) Encourage increased social interaction.
(E) Initiate a palliative care approach.

30. A 78-yr-old woman comes to the office because she has pain when she urinates. She has been seen three times for this problem in the last 3 mo. Each time she was told she had a urinary tract infection and was given a course of antibiotics. She has carefully followed the instructions for the antibiotics but has had no relief of symptoms.

Results of her last urinalysis:

WBCs	2 to 3/high-power field
RBCs	0 to 2/high-power field
Epithelial cells	Few
Nitrite	Negative
Leukocyte esterase	Negative

Which of the following should be done next?

(A) Send a clean-catch urine specimen for urinalysis and culture.
(B) Perform pelvic examination.
(C) Reassure the patient that she has asymptomatic bacteruria and that antibiotics are unlikely to help.
(D) Refer for cystoscopy.
(E) Order pelvic ultrasonography.

31. An 82-yr-old man comes to the office for preoperative evaluation before elective hip replacement. He cannot walk 2 blocks without incapacitating hip pain. He has no chest pain or dyspnea, and there is no history of myocardial infarction, stroke, or diabetes mellitus. He has hypertension and dyslipidemia. Medications are atenolol 50 mg/d and lovastatin 20 mg/d.

On physical examination, blood pressure is 140/70 mmHg and heart rate is 76 beats per minute and regular. On auscultation, chest and lungs are clear; there is a 2/6 systolic ejection murmur, and there is no third or fourth heart sound. There is no edema, and pulses are intact. ECG shows normal sinus rhythm with left-ventricle hypertrophy.

Which of the following is indicated as part of his preoperative evaluation?

(A) Stress echocardiography
(B) Nuclear stress test
(C) Coronary angiography
(D) Measurement of creatinine
(E) Measurement of brain natriuretic peptide

32. An active 75-yr-old man with no significant medical history has a chief complaint of dry scaling feet and thickened nails. The patient indicates that, for >20 yr, he has had thick nails starting in the great toes. Over the last few years, this has spread to his lesser digits. His main complaint is chronic itching and scaling feet. Self-care has included nail trimming and OTC hand cream, which he applies a few times a week. Physical examination shows dry erythematous scaling in a moccasin distribution bilaterally, web-space scaling, and thickened yellow nails. Neurovascular examination is within normal limits.

What is the most likely causative organism?

(A) *Candia albicans*
(B) *Microsporum canis*
(C) *Trichophyton rubrum*
(D) *Corneum bacterium*

33. An 85-yr-old woman is brought to the emergency department after she is found on the bathroom floor at home. She has retrograde amnesia for the circumstances surrounding the episode, and denies any confusion after the episode. There were no witnesses. History includes hypertension, for which she takes atenolol 25 mg/d and hydrochlorothiazide 25 mg/d.

On physical examination, she has a right periorbital ecchymosis. Blood pressure is 152/84 mmHg while supine and 146/86 mmHg while upright, and heart rate is 76 beats per minute while supine and 86 beats per minute while upright. There is no jugular venous distension or carotid bruit. Lungs are clear. Carotid upstroke is delayed, with a II/VI midpeaking systolic murmur at the base; the second heart sound is not audible.

CT of the head and facial bones shows a large, right periorbital contusion and no fractures.

Which of the following is the most appropriate next step in the evaluation of this patient?

(A) Blood tests
(B) Echocardiography
(C) Holter monitoring
(D) Event monitor
(E) Tilt-table test

34. A 92-yr-old man with Alzheimer's disease is brought to the office by his daughter because over the past several months he has become increasingly aggressive toward his wife and home health aide. His daughter is worried about their safety and asks that he be given medication to control his aggression. Discussion ensues regarding different psychotropic options.

Which of the following is associated with increased mortality?

(A) Antipsychotic agents
(B) Antidepressant agents
(C) Mood stabilizers
(D) Anticholinesterase agents

35. An 88-yr-old man comes to the clinic for the first time in 18 mo, accompanied by his son. The patient states that he has no active medical problems. He has lived alone since his wife's death 10 yr ago. He is not sexually active and does not smoke or drink alcohol. The son states that his father has lost weight, is less active socially than he used to be, has little energy or endurance, and spends most of his time reading or watching television. On detailed questioning, the patient indicates that he often skips meals but otherwise feels his appetite is unchanged. He does all his own cooking. His son notes that when his dad comes to his house on weekends,

he eats well. The patient indicates that he does not have problems sleeping, swallowing, or voiding. He has had no change in bowel habits, no incontinence, and no depressive symptoms. History includes early-stage prostate cancer, for which he had a prostatectomy 8 yr ago; at follow-up 1 yr ago, his urologist told him there was no evidence of recurrence. Screening colonoscopy done 2 yr ago was normal. The patient takes a daily multivitamin.

On examination, the patient weighs 62.6 kg (138 lb; body mass index, 22 kg/m²), which, according to medical records, is 13% less than he weighed 18 mo ago. The rest of his physical examination is normal. His score on the Mini–Mental State Examination is 29/30; his score on the Yesavage Geriatric Depression Scale–Short Form is 2/15. Fecal guaiac is negative. Urinalysis, CBC, electrolytes, vitamin B_{12}, and liver, renal, and thyroid function tests are normal, and prostate-specific antigen is undetectable. ECG reveals normal sinus rhythm, and chest radiography is normal.

Which of the following is the most appropriate next step?

(A) CT of the chest, abdomen, and pelvis
(B) Upper and lower endoscopy
(C) Upper GI series with small-bowel follow-through
(D) Complete radiographic bone survey
(E) No further diagnostic testing

36. A 70-yr-old woman comes to the office because she has had a malodorous vaginal discharge for 1 wk. She has vulvovaginal burning, itching, and soreness that have intensified over the past few months. At menopause 15 yr ago, she had similar symptoms, minus the discharge, and hot flashes. She was treated with cyclic oral estrogen and progesterone, but she stopped hormone replacement therapy after several years because she was concerned about adverse events. After the hot flashes abated, she had increasing vaginal soreness, pain, and burning after intercourse. In the past 10 yr, she has had 2 urinary tract infections, the most recent >1 yr ago. She recently tried application of aloe vera gel in an effort to relieve the itching, without effect. She does not wish to go back on hormone therapy.

On examination, there is redness and erythema in the vulvovaginal area, sparse pubic hair, and decreased vaginal moisture. Insertion of an adult speculum is moderately difficult and results in slight bleeding. Mucosa appears inflamed. Occasional vaginal petechiae are evident, and there are some fissures on the vaginal walls. There are no vaginal folds. No growths, plaques, or suspicious structures are seen or palpated. Serosanguineous discharge is present, with a pH of 6.8. A vaginal smear taken from the upper lateral third of the vagina reveals increased parabasal cells, an inflammatory exudate, and classic "blue blobs" (basophilic structures).

Which of the following is the most likely explanation for these findings?

(A) Candidiasis
(B) Atrophic vaginitis
(C) Psoriasis
(D) Vaginal cancer

37. A 72-yr-old retired bookkeeper is brought to the office by her husband because she has had gradually increasing problems with her memory over the past year. At first he noticed that his wife had trouble remembering the names of new acquaintances. This progressed to difficulty recalling details of books they read together, and more recently she had to telephone him for help because she could not recall where she had parked her car. Last month the husband had to take control of managing the household finances, a job she had performed competently throughout their marriage. Alzheimer's disease is diagnosed after physical examination and evaluation including laboratory tests and structural neuroimaging. The couple asks you about cholinesterase inhibitor treatment.

Which of the following statements is the most appropriate response?

(A) The most common adverse events are headache and somnolence.
(B) Liver function must be monitored for the first 6 mo of treatment.
(C) Improvement of cognitive symptoms is sustained during the first 5 yr of treatment.
(D) Benefits are likely to be clinically subtle.
(E) Cholinesterase inhibitors differ significantly from one another in their effectiveness.

38. A 67-yr-old woman comes to the office for advice regarding diet. She recently had a modified radical mastectomy for stage I breast cancer. She chose this approach because she wanted to avoid radiation and chemotherapy. She has always had a healthy lifestyle. She asks whether there are any dietary changes she could make to avoid recurrence of breast cancer.

Which of the following is most likely to reduce breast cancer recurrence?

(A) Increase soy foods.
(B) Drink 4 cups of green tea daily.
(C) Restrict fats to <10% of diet.
(D) Follow a strict vegetarian diet.

39. An 89-yr-old man presents to you complaining of generalized weakness. General physical examination and neurologic examination are normal. He lives with his wife in a rural community, is independent in ADLs and IADLs, and rarely drives. He has avoided medical care for most of his life. He is on no medications other than calcium, vitamin D, and aspirin 81 mg/d.

Laboratory tests:

Hgb	11.9 g/dL
Hematocrit	35%
Mean corpuscular volume	102 mm^3
Serum B$_{12}$	200 pg/mL (low normal)
Methylmalonic acid	300 nmol/L (increased)
Homocysteine	18 μmol/L (increased)
RBC folate	normal
Ferritin	250 ng/mL

What is the best next step?

(A) Prescribe oral vitamin B$_{12}$ 1000 mcg/d
(B) Administer vitamin B$_{12}$ 1000 mcg IM weekly for 8 wk, followed by 1000 mcg IM monthly
(C) Administer a 3-part Schilling test.
(D) Recommend upper and lower endoscopy to exclude pernicious anemia and bacterial overgrowth syndrome.

40. A 70-yr-old man comes to the office because he has diarrhea with associated crampy abdominal pain and low-grade fever. The diarrhea began 3 days earlier; he is passing up to 5 watery, nonbloody bowel movements daily.

History includes venous insufficiency, and he was recently treated with a 7-day course of cephalexin for lower-extremity cellulitis.

On examination, he does not look ill, and vital signs are normal. Abdominal examination demonstrates mild, nonspecific diffuse tenderness without guarding or rebound. Bowel sounds are present. Laboratory results are normal except for a WBC count of 11,000/μL. Abdominal radiography demonstrates a nonspecific gas pattern. Enzyme immunoassay detects the presence of *Clostridium difficile* toxin A. His symptoms improve with a 10-day course of oral metronidazole, but diarrhea recurs within 1 week, and enzyme immunoassay again detects *C difficile* toxin A.

Which of the following should be prescribed next?

(A) Rifampin and metronidazole
(B) Metronidazole
(C) Vancomycin
(D) Cholestyramine
(E) *Saccharomyces boulardii*

41. A 78-yr-old man comes to the office because he volunteers at the local hospital and is required to get a tuberculin skin test annually. A tuberculosis skin test (PPD) using 5 tuberculin units was done a year ago when he first started. At that time, the test was read as 4 mm of induration and interpreted as negative. On retesting now a year later, there is 16 mm of induration. He has no symptoms, and chest radiograph is negative. He is on coumadin for atrial fibrillation but has no other problems and no other medications.

What is the most appropriate next step in management?

(A) Observation only
(B) Annual chest radiography
(C) Repeat PPD testing in 6 mo
(D) Treatment with pyrazinamide plus rifampin for 2 mo
(E) Treatment with isoniazid for 9 mo

42. A 70-yr-old male smoker has a history of hypertension, dyslipidemia, diabetes mellitus, and nonvalvular atrial fibrillation.

Which of the following most increases his risk of stroke?

(A) Cigarette smoking
(B) Hypertension
(C) Dyslipidemia
(D) Atrial fibrillation

43. The Seventh Report of the *Joint National Committee on Prevention, Detection, Evaluation, and Treatment of High Blood Pressure (JNC7)* recommends which of the following for the initial treatment for hypertension in older adults?

(A) ACE inhibitor
(B) Thiazide diuretic
(C) Calcium channel blocker
(D) β-Blocker
(E) Angiotensin-receptor blocker

44. A 69-yr-old woman comes to the office because she has had anorexia, nausea, and vague lower abdominal pain associated with the onset of constipation 1 wk earlier. She also believes she has had a low-grade fever.

On examination, she appears uncomfortable. Temperature is 37.2° C (99.0° F), blood pressure is 130/80 mmHg, pulse is 90 beats per minute, and respiratory rate is 14 breaths per minute. She has suprapubic fullness and abdominal tenderness with localized guarding but no rebound. Bowel sounds are decreased. Laboratory results are normal except for mild anemia and a WBC count of 12,000/μL with a left shift. Radiography demonstrates a nonspecific ileus pattern.

Which of the following studies should be performed next?

(A) Barium enema
(B) Ultrasonography of pelvis
(C) CT of abdomen and pelvis
(D) Small-bowel series
(E) Colonoscopy

45. A 79-yr-old woman comes to the office because she has knee discomfort that is exacerbated by walking, and as a consequence, she undertakes little or no physical activity. She has moderate osteoarthritis of both knees and takes acetaminophen irregularly for pain.

On examination, the patient is 1.6 m (64 in) and weighs 65 kg (144 lb). She has bilateral synovial swelling and mild varus deformity of the left knee. There is no significant ligament laxity, and no joint effusions, warmth, or tenderness on palpation. She has full range of motion (extension and flexion) of both knees, but crepitus is present on the left side. Quadriceps strength is 4+/5 bilaterally. She walks slowly but with good balance.

Which of the following is the most appropriate recommendation for physical activity?

(A) Flexibility stretching exercises 1 day/wk
(B) Aquatic exercises 1 day/wk
(C) Isotonic quadriceps exercises 5 days/wk
(D) Isotonic quadriceps exercises 2 days/wk
(E) Moderate-intensity aerobic exercise, 5 days/wk

46. A 72-yr-old man with mild dementia returns to the office because he has had difficulty both falling and staying asleep for the past 4 mo. In addition, he has had vivid dreams a few times per month. His sleep disturbance emerged shortly after a clinician prescribed a new medication.

Which of the following is most likely to cause these symptoms?

(A) Buspirone
(B) Trazodone
(C) Donepezil
(D) Melatonin
(E) Ramelteon

47. A 75-yr-old woman calls the office to discuss a church-based screening program in which carotid arteries, abdominal aorta, and heel-bone density are evaluated using ultrasonography. She wonders whether it is worth the $85 charge.

Which of the following is the most appropriate response?

(A) The screening is a bargain, because each of these tests usually cost >$85 at the local hospital.
(B) The screening may result in expensive or potentially risky procedures.
(C) If the sensitivity is high, the screening would be valuable.
(D) The screening should be done at the local hospital.

48. A 94-yr-old nursing home resident with Alzheimer's disease is evaluated because she has been disturbing other patients by screaming for help and banging on her recliner throughout the day for the past 4 wk.

Which of the following is most likely to reduce the patient's agitation?

(A) Nonpharmacologic intervention
(B) Second-generation antidepressant
(C) Second-generation antipsychotic agent
(D) Cholinergic agent

49. An 80-yr-old man with diabetes and osteoporosis comes to the office for consultation regarding his pain regimen. He has severe pain related to diabetic neuropathy and back pain related to multiple compression fractures. He takes hydrocodone/acetaminophen 2 tablets q6h, which helps the back pain but does little for the neuropathic pain.

Which of the following medications is an appropriate alternative to hydrocodone/acetaminophen for control of this patient's pain?

(A) Meperidine
(B) Butorphanol
(C) Nalbuphine
(D) Methadone

50. An 82-yr-old man comes to the office because he has had excessive daytime sleepiness for about 6 mo. He falls asleep during the day, particularly in the late morning. He falls asleep easily around 8 PM, but wakes up every 2–3 hours throughout the night. His wife's sleep is often disturbed by his awakenings, and they have not been able to participate in social activities because of his intermittent daytime napping. History includes

stroke (with residual mild leg weakness), hypertension, and mild cognitive impairment.

The patient is referred for actigraphy, a 24-hour graphing of sleep and wake intervals that uses a unit (actigraph) worn on the nondominant wrist. Results show 3 sleep intervals during the 24-hour test, with no single, clearly defined major nocturnal sleep period.

Which of the following is the most likely diagnosis?

(A) Idiopathic hypersomnia
(B) Advanced sleep phase disorder
(C) Irregular sleep/wake rhythm disorder
(D) Sundowning
(E) REM sleep behavior disorder

51. A 79-yr-old woman presents with a lump on right upper quadrant of her left breast. Mammography reveals a 1.3-cm spiculated lesion. Biopsy reveals a high-grade, poorly differentiated, infiltrating ductal carcinoma of the breast, with negative margins and no evidence of lymphovascular invasion. She is concerned that breast conservation treatment (ie, lumpectomy or partial mastectomy) and postoperative radiotherapy would not be "as good as" a full mastectomy.

Which of the following statements is true?

(A) Breast conservation treatment is the standard of care for all patients with early disease.
(B) Breast conservation treatment is associated with the same quality of life as mastectomy.
(C) Overall survival and disease-free survival are worse for breast conservation treatment than mastectomy.
(D) Older patients are more likely to be offered breast conservation therapy than younger patients.

52. An 84-yr-old woman undergoes total hip replacement after falling and fracturing her hip. She lives at home with her 82-yr-old husband, who is confined to a wheelchair because of severe rheumatoid arthritis. The patient has diabetes mellitus, osteoporosis, and mild dementia. She has insurance coverage through standard fee-for-service Medicare Parts A and B.

On the third hospital day, she has no fever and her lungs are clear. She is taking adequate nourishment, and her weight is stable. Warfarin was begun after surgery; INR is 1.5. She requires a maximal assist of 1 to transfer and ambulate, and she has normal functioning of her arms. She tolerates physical therapy for 20 min before she is too fatigued to continue. Hospital discharge for the next day is discussed.

Which of the following is the most appropriate setting for now?

(A) Inpatient rehabilitation facility
(B) Nursing home with rehabilitation services
(C) Nursing home with dementia unit
(D) Her own home with home physical therapy
(E) She is not ready for discharge and should stay in the hospital.

53. An active, 70-yr-old moderately obese woman presents with a chief complaint of a painful left heel over the last few months. She has pain on first getting out of bed and after periods of rest. She denies any previous treatments. Past medical history is unremarkable. Physical examination of the left heel reveals pain at the medial tuberosity of the calcaneus. Dorsiflexion at the ankle joint is decreased but pain free, and foot structure is normal. A radiograph of her left heel is unremarkable.

What is the most likely diagnosis?

(A) Heel spur
(B) Calcaneal stress fracture
(C) Partial tear of Achilles tendon
(D) Posterior tibial tendonitis
(E) Plantar fasciitis

54. An 82-yr-old nursing home resident is evaluated because she has increased pain in her knee. She has refused to walk for the past several days. History includes dementia, osteoporosis, atrial fibrillation, and renal insufficiency.

On physical examination, temperature is 37.4° C (99.3° F), blood pressure is 110/80 mmHg, and pulse is 78 beats per minute. The knee is warm and tender and causes pain with movement. An effusion is palpable. There is bony enlargement of the first carpal-metacarpal and distal interphalangeal joints. Radiography of the knee demonstrates joint space narrowing, chondrocalcinosis, and osteophytes of the medial compartment.

Which of the following diagnostic tests should be obtained next?

(A) Westergren sedimentation rate
(B) Arthrocentesis and synovial fluid analysis
(C) Radiography of knee while bearing weight
(D) MRI of the knee

55. A 79-yr-old widower is seen in the office for self-reported anhedonia and depression. He has a history of affective disorder, lives alone, and has no nearby relatives. Recently his best friend died, and his social network has been getting smaller because of disabilities and deaths of associates. Three of his aquarium fish died this week, and he has not attended church for several months. He indicates that, increasingly, ADLs have become burdensome and problematic. There is no evidence of cognitive impairment on the Mini–Mental State Examination.

Which of the following is the next best step?

(A) Refer to grief counseling group.
(B) Evaluate suicide risk.
(C) Evaluate for alcohol abuse.
(D) Refer to a psychotherapist.

56. An 86-yr-old female resident of an assisted-living facility has urinary frequency, urgency, urge incontinence, leakage of urine when bending over and walking up or down stairs, and a sensation of incomplete bladder emptying. History includes hypertension, mild Alzheimer's disease, and lumbosacral degenerative joint disease, for which she uses a walker. Medications include a cholinesterase inhibitor, a thiazide diuretic, and an angiotensin-receptor blocker.

On physical examination, there is mild atrophic vaginitis, a moderate cystocele, normal rectal sphincter tone, and no fecal impaction. While the patient is standing, a cough test for stress incontinence is positive. She voids 100 mL; post-void residual volume is 225 mL. Urinalysis is positive for trace of protein.

Which of the following is the most likely diagnosis?

(A) Stress incontinence
(B) Diuretic-induced incontinence
(C) Cholinesterase inhibitor–induced incontinence
(D) Detrusor hyperactivity with impaired bladder contractility
(E) Urinary retention and incontinence due to cystocele

57. A 79-yr-old woman comes to the office because she has a fever and a cough. History includes hypertension, dyslipidemia, stable coronary disease, and osteoarthritis. She is enrolled in traditional Medicare Parts A and B; clinicians in the office are participating Medicare providers. On physical examination, it is evident that a CBC is needed to exclude bacterial infection. The patient explains that she is financially strapped and needs to know what her out-of-pocket costs will be for the office visit and blood work. Today's visit is her fifth this year; the office visits have been her only medical encounters for the year.

How much is the patient's out-of-pocket cost for this visit?

(A) Nothing
(B) 20% of the office visit fee and 0% of the laboratory fee
(C) 20% of the office visit fee and 20% of the laboratory fee
(D) 20% of the office visit fee and 100% of the laboratory fee
(E) 100% of the office visit fee and 100% of the laboratory fee

58. A 72-yr-old woman comes to the office because of persistent pain in her left hip. History includes osteoarthritis, as well as a life-threatening episode of GI bleeding related to use of NSAIDs. Oral acetaminophen 1000 mg q6h decreases the pain for a short time. She follows her physical therapy regimen routinely.

Which of the following is the most appropriate intervention?

(A) Increase acetaminophen to 1000 mg q4h.
(B) Start ibuprofen 600 mg q6h.
(C) Start oxycodone 2.5 mg q4h as needed.
(D) Start long-acting morphine 15 mg q12h.

59. A 65-yr-old woman is brought to the office by her niece because she believes that a neighbor has been coming into her apartment to steal items such as paper towels and sponges. She has called the police several times to report these thefts, and she complains regularly to her niece. This behavior began about 6 mo ago. The niece reports that her aunt has always been a little suspicious of other people. There is no history of alcohol or substance abuse. She has no hallucinations or depressive symptoms, and she has no other medical disorders. She is able to conduct her normal daily activities. Physical examination is normal except that she displays some mild memory loss. MRI is unremarkable.

Which of the following is the most likely explanation for her symptoms?

(A) Late-onset schizophrenia
(B) Delusional disorder
(C) Alzheimer's disease
(D) Bipolar disease
(E) Paranoid personality disorder

60. Two residents of a for-profit nursing home want to share a bed but can do so only with the cooperation of the staff. One is a 90-yr-old man who is blind and a double-amputee with well-controlled heart failure. The other is an 86-yr-old woman with severe rheumatoid arthritis and a colostomy. Both have outlived spouses after long marriages and have been residents in the facility for some time; both have a normal mental status. The residents have had two falls when in her single room alone, and they have asked for staff assistance to undress and share a bed. Some staff members are uncomfortable and want the medical director to call the families to stop this behavior. Both residents say that they do not want their families informed. There is no relevant statement regarding the facility's protocols or limitations in the materials provided at admission.

Which of the following is the best course of action?

(A) Have a private conversation with the lead family member in each family.
(B) Research civil rights laws to determine the legality of the couple's request.
(C) Pursue a compromise, such as working only with volunteer staff or getting married, with the couple and the staff.
(D) Advise the couple that sexual activity is hazardous to their health and cannot be allowed.

61. An 83-yr-old otherwise healthy woman is brought to the office by her daughter because the mother has become confused and forgetful since beginning treatment with extended-release oxybutynin 10 mg for urge urinary incontinence 6 mo ago. The incontinence has improved, yet the daughter is unwilling to continue the oxybutynin because of the increased confusion. The mother, when asked, has no new complaints about memory or cognition.

Which of the following is the most appropriate next step?

(A) Discontinue extended-release oxybutynin 10 mg; begin immediate-release oxybutynin 2.5 mg q6h.
(B) Begin memantine, titrating over 3 wk from starting dose of 5 mg/d to 20 mg/d.
(C) Begin donepezil 5 mg/d, titrating to 10 mg/d if needed.
(D) Reassure the daughter that the medication is unlikely to produce cognitive adverse events.
(E) Discontinue extended-release oxybutynin 10 mg; implement behavioral therapy for incontinence.

62. An 83-yr-old nursing home resident with advanced Alzheimer's disease has steadily lost nearly 8.2 kg (18 lb), or 11% of his weight, over 11 mo. His current weight is 66.2 kg (146 lb; body mass index, 22 kg/m²). He gained about 8.2 kg (18 lb) 6 yr ago, after he entered the nursing home, and then maintained his weight until this year. He has not had any hospitalizations, acute infections, or other serious medical problems in the last 20 mo. Since his admission, he has had a slow,

steady decline in cognitive function. He is fully ambulatory and attends most meals in the residents' dining hall; he needs minimal feeding assistance (set-up only). He is on a 2,600-kcal regular diet that was modified to include finger foods and nightly snacks. According to chart documentation, he only rarely consumes <75% of the food served, but a 2-day calorie count indicates that his consumption is closer to 40% of what he is served.

Besides a comprehensive evaluation for potentially reversible causes of the resident's weight loss, which of the following should be done?

(A) Prescribe 1 can (240 mL) of a polymeric oral supplement with each meal.
(B) Refer the resident for placement of a percutaneous endoscopic gastrostomy tube.
(C) Change the diet from regular to puréed.
(D) Implement a program of individualized feeding assistance.
(E) Start mirtazapine.

63. A 73-yr-old man in a rehabilitation facility is evaluated for irritable mood, poor motivation for rehabilitation, and demanding and verbally abusive behavior toward staff. He entered rehabilitation after an above-knee amputation. He acknowledges having felt depressed and anxious for a long time, and he has taken a low dose of an antidepressant for several years. Family members report that he previously was extroverted and tended to be provocative and hot-tempered. In recent years, he has had increasing difficulty tolerating disability and reliance on others, prompting arguments that have frayed already estranged relations with his children. He admits to frequent verbal outbursts toward staff because "I need help and they just walk by!" Staff members believe he is just seeking attention. He has pervasive irritable mood, anhedonia, feelings of worthlessness, reduced appetite, poor sleep, and low energy. He inconsistently attends physical therapy sessions. Cognitive examination and thyroid function are normal, and his symptoms are not due to medication or substance abuse.

Which of the following is most likely to improve this patient's behavior?

(A) Increase dosage of antidepressant and refer for psychotherapy.
(B) Maintain and monitor on current dosage of antidepressant.
(C) Discontinue antidepressant treatment and screen for mania.
(D) Advise staff to ignore attention-seeking behavior.

64. An 89-yr-old man is admitted to a nursing home for rehabilitation after being hospitalized for pneumonia. He is anxious and fidgety. He is widowed and lives in the community. History includes hypertension, benign prostatic hyperplasia, major depressive disorder, and chronic back pain. Medications on transfer from the hospital to the nursing home include metoprolol, oxybutynin, paroxetine, acetaminophen with codeine, and amitriptyline.

Which of the following medications is *least* likely to contribute to delirium?

(A) Amitriptyline
(B) Acetaminophen with codeine
(C) Oxybutynin
(D) Paroxetine
(E) Metoprolol

65. Which of the following is the mostly likely cause of new onset vaginal bleeding in a 70-yr-old woman?

(A) Pyometra
(B) Endometrial cancer
(C) Endometrial hyperplasia
(D) Vaginal atrophy
(E) Hormonal effect

66. An 86-yr-old man who lives alone is prepared for discharge after hospitalization for an open leg wound and cellulitis that followed a fall at home. He is a retired professor; he reports no difficulty with ambulation, ADLs, or IADLs. Notes from the emergency medical services personnel indicate that they had difficulty gaining access to the patient's apartment because of clutter, and they noted the smell of urine and visible cockroaches. The patient reports no past medical history and takes no prescription medications.

On initial examination, the patient's temperature was 38.3°C (101°F), blood pressure was 180/90 mmHg, and heart rate was 110 beats per minute; body mass index was 18. Blood glucose level by fingerstick was 350 mg/dL. He was disheveled and wore stained and malodorous clothing. He had several bags of papers with him. On his right medial mallelolus there was a 4-cm, round, clean-based open ulcer with surrounding erythema and warmth. He had erythematous patches in his intertriginous areas and long dystrophic nails. Score on the Mini–Mental State Examination was 27 (he recalled only 1 of 3 words and was unable to draw intersecting pentagons). WBC count was 13,000/μL with 90% neutrophils, BUN was 30 mg/dL, creatinine was 1.6 mg/dL, and hemoglobin A_{1C} was 9%.

He was treated with intravenous antibiotics, an antihypertensive agent, and long-acting insulin. On discharge, he refuses home care services, home-delivered meals, and all prescription medications, insisting that he can take care of himself.

Which of the following is the most likely explanation for these findings?

(A) Dementia
(B) Delirium
(C) Depression
(D) Self-neglect
(E) Delusional disorder

67. An 86-yr-old woman with dementia and heart failure has difficulty getting to the bathroom and is increasingly incontinent. She can no longer prepare food for herself or take medications reliably. She lives in the city with her son, who is away from home during the day. He is no longer comfortable leaving his mother alone, but neither he nor his mother wants her to move to a nursing home. The patient qualifies for Medicare and Medicaid.

If available, which of the following is the most appropriate recommendation?

(A) Enrollment in a social health maintenance organization (HMO)
(B) Admission to a nearby nursing home
(C) Referral to Program of All-inclusive Care of the Elderly (PACE)
(D) Hiring a full-time nurse to care for the patient at home
(E) Referral to state Department of Aging for assessment

68. A 55-yr-old man with Down syndrome is brought to the office by his caregivers because over the past year he has become confused and forgetful and has needed increasingly more frequent prompts for his assigned tasks. Although they do not have specific written records, the caregivers think that his speech and movement have slowed, that he is more socially withdrawn, and that he is having more outbursts with peers and staff. In the last 4 mo, he has twice lost his balance and fallen. He has been physically healthy overall and is on no medications. His last routine physical examination was 8 mo ago, at which time there were no indications of any problem.

During the visit, the patient seems shy and anxious and has a congruent affect. He has no complaints. His expressive abilities are limited and consistent with his low-moderate level of mental retardation.

Which of the following options is the most appropriate next step?

(A) Order head CT.
(B) Perform office-based, appropriate cognitive testing.
(C) Begin fluoxetine.
(D) Begin donepezil and, if well-tolerated, add memantine.
(E) Refer patient to a psychiatrist who specializes in neurodevelopmental disabilities.

69. A 72-yr-old man with chronic emphysema is being discharged home after spending 3 wk on a ventilator after a probable viral infection. The patient receives oxygen at home. Several months ago, he was on a ventilator for a few days. During preparations for discharge, the

patient emphatically states that he does not want ventilator care ever again. His wife died a year ago and he lives alone, with no friendly contacts. He cannot smoke because of the oxygen, and he cannot go fishing or leave his apartment to play poker any more. He asks that arrangements be made so that he is not readmitted and placed on the ventilator again.

Which of the following strategies is most likely to reassure the patient?

(A) Refer patient to a hospice with an inpatient unit.
(B) Order continuous positive airway pressure for home.
(C) Legally document a "do not resuscitate" directive.
(D) Refer patient to a hospice that can provide sedation at home.
(E) Evaluate patient for major depressive disorder.

70. An 80-yr-old woman comes to the office because she has been dizzy. When asked for specifics, she is vague, but states that she often feels unsteady when walking. She has also felt lightheaded a few times when getting up in the morning. She has had no falls. History includes hypertension, type 2 diabetes mellitus, dyslipidemia, and anxiety. Medications are hydrochlorothiazide, lisinopril, aspirin, metformin, simvastatin, and trazodone.

On examination, blood pressure is 125/82 mmHg and pulse is 80 beats per minute with no orthostatic changes. Her gait is slightly wide but otherwise normal. There is evidence of mild peripheral neuropathy. Her score on the Geriatric Depression Scale is 3/15.

Which of the following is the most likely cause of her dizziness?

(A) Anxiety
(B) Somatization disorder
(C) Medication adverse event
(D) Multifactorial triggers

71. A 72-yr-old man comes to the office for evaluation because he has impaired fasting glucose levels. Fasting levels were between 110 and 120 mg/dL on 3 occasions. He has well-controlled hypertension. His body mass index is 29.5.

Which of the following is most likely to prevent development of type 2 diabetes mellitus in this patient?

(A) Reduce caloric intake and increase physical activity to 150 min/week.
(B) Increase physical activity and begin metformin.
(C) Begin metformin.
(D) Reduce caloric intake.

72. A 77-yr-old woman comes to the office because she has frequent falls. She has difficulty walking unassisted and frequently feels that her feet get tangled together. She is also urinating more frequently. She has no burning on urination, fever, chills, or flank pain.

On examination, there are no significant abnormalities of joints in the limbs. There is good mobility of the lumbar spine and mild immobility of the cervical spine, with 45-degree rotation to the right and left and limited extension. Arm reflexes are 2+, with occasional fasciculations in the biceps and triceps muscles. Hoffmann's sign is present in both hands. There is increased tone in the lower extremities. Reflexes are 3+ at the knees and ankles. Both toes are upgoing.

Which of the following is the most appropriate next step?

(A) Bone scan
(B) MRI of the lumbar spine
(C) MRI of the cervical spine
(D) Radiography of the cervical spine
(E) Radiography of the thoracic spine

73. An 80-yr-old man comes to the office for a routine visit. He is enrolled in traditional fee-for-service Medicare Parts A and B and has a Part D policy. He has seen advertisements for an insurance plan called SeniorGold, which is described as a Medicare Advantage organization with a Medicare contract. He wishes to discuss advantages and disadvantages of switching his insurance coverage to this plan.

Which of the following is most likely to occur if he switches insurance coverage to SeniorGold?

(A) He would lose some Part A benefits.
(B) He would lose some Part B benefits.
(C) He would have to drop Part D prescription drug coverage.
(D) He would not get coverage for vision examination and eyeglasses.
(E) He would not get to choose his providers.

74. A 75-yr-old man comes to the office with several vague complaints and concerns. He is retired and has been married for 50 yr. Over the past 6 mo, he has come to the office repeatedly and has become increasingly homebound. He describes leg weakness, fatigue, and overall malaise that prevent him from engaging in once-pleasurable activities, such as playing cards at the senior center. He has become fearful of driving and of being alone, and his sleep and appetite are poor. He has lost approximately 4.5 kg (10 lb). History includes hypertension and spinal stenosis. Major depressive disorder is diagnosed, and a trial of an antidepressant is begun.

Which of the following is characteristic of late-life major depressive disorder?

(A) Strong family history of mood disorder
(B) Sudden onset of symptoms
(C) Preferential response to treatment with first-generation antidepressants
(D) Higher prevalence of somatic symptoms

75. A 66-yr-old man comes to the office because his family has noticed increasing apathy, forgetfulness, and confusion over the past few months. For example, he now gets lost on his way home from familiar places. He and his wife lived in England for 20 yr before her death 10 yr ago. He then moved to the United States and has dated occasionally. He has no significant comorbidities and is on no medications. There is no history of sexually transmitted disease. His family is concerned that he may have early Alzheimer's disease.

Physical examination is normal except for the neurologic exam, which reveals slowing of rapid finger and toe tapping, increased reflexes, short-term memory deficits, and an inability to do relatively simple calculations. He scores

22/30 on the Mini–Mental State Examination. His affect is normal. A cranial CT scan reveals mild to moderate atrophy, but no other changes. There are no metabolic or endocrine abnormalities on laboratory testing.

What is the most likely cause of this patient's dementia?

(A) Syphilis
(B) Creutzfeldt-Jakob disease
(C) Human immunodeficiency virus (HIV) antibody
(D) Lyme disease

76. An 85-yr-old man comes to the office to discuss the recurrence of anxiety attacks, of which he has a chronic history. He describes periods of intense fear and anxiety that last from 30 min to several hours and that are accompanied by physical and autonomic symptoms. He does not drink, has no history of alcohol or drug abuse, and has no other psychiatric issues. History includes hypertension, osteoarthritis, and urinary retention related to prostatic hyperplasia. He was diagnosed with panic disorder as an adult and took diazepam for the panic attacks, although not for the past 20 yr. He is interested in restarting treatment with diazepam.

Physical examination and laboratory evaluation (thyrotropin, CBC, metabolic profile) indicate nothing likely to cause new-onset panic attacks.

Which of the following is the most appropriate treatment?

(A) Benzodiazepines plus an SSRI
(B) Benzodiazepines plus cognitive-behavioral therapy
(C) An SSRI plus cognitive-behavioral therapy
(D) Benzodiazepines plus nortriptyline
(E) Mirtazapine plus an SSRI

77. A 76-yr-old woman with end-stage heart failure (New York Heart Association class IV) has worsening dyspnea at rest and has become dependent in all ADLs except feeding. She sometimes feels as though she is suffocating and becomes very anxious. She began home hospice care 4 mo ago. She had been feeling relatively well since an increase in her furosemide dosage and the addition of supplemental oxygen last month. The cardiologist believes that she would

not benefit from increasing her current dosages of carvedilol, enalapril, and spironolactone, and she has been compliant with her medication regimen and diet.

On a home visit by the hospice nurse, the patient is alert, oriented, and in mild distress. Temperature is 36.5° C (97.7° F), blood pressure is 126/64 mmHg, heart rate is 105 beats per minute, respiratory rate is 24 breaths per minute, and O_2 saturation is 97% on 4 L/min oxygen by nasal cannula. She has decreased breath sounds at the right base with dullness on percussion approximately one-fourth of the way up; a few crackles are heard at the left base. Jugular venous pressure is 12 mmHg. Hepatojugular reflex is positive, and leg edema is minimal.

The hospice nurse calls to discuss the care plan and recommends increasing the dosage of furosemide.

Which of the following is the most appropriate next step for this patient?

(A) Admit to the hospital for inpatient diuresis.
(B) Increase dosage of furosemide and arrange for outpatient, ultrasound-guided pleurocentesis.
(C) Increase dosage of furosemide and increase oxygen to 6 L/min by nasal cannula.
(D) Increase dosage of furosemide and add nebulized albuterol 2.5 mL q4h as needed for dyspnea.
(E) Increase dosage of furosemide and start morphine 5 mg po q3h as needed for dyspnea.

78. A 90-yr-old woman comes to the office to establish care. She has difficulty breathing with exertion and awakens several times each night to urinate. These symptoms began a year ago. She has a history of chronic poorly controlled hypertension, diabetes mellitus controlled by diet, and rheumatoid arthritis. On examination, jugular venous pressure is 9 cm H_2O. Lungs are clear. The abdomen is mildly distended with no tenderness, and there is 1+ edema in her legs. Brain natriuretic peptide (BNP) concentration is 76 pg/mL.

Which of the following is the most likely diagnosis?

(A) Deconditioning
(B) Heart failure with diastolic dysfunction
(C) Interstitial lung disease
(D) Pulmonary embolism
(E) Cirrhosis of the liver

79. Which of the following is true regarding health literacy?

(A) Health literacy is the degree to which a person can obtain, process, and understand information to make appropriate health decisions.
(B) People with limited health literacy are more likely to ask questions about care during clinician visits.
(C) Health status, rate of hospitalization, and health care costs of people with limited health literacy are similar to those of persons with adequate literacy.
(D) In the United States, 12% of the population lacks health literacy.

80. Which of the following has been shown to be of benefit in reducing pressure ulcers in acute-care settings?

(A) Standard nutritional supplements for older patients
(B) Specialized foam mattress hospital bed
(C) Patient rotation q4h on regular hospital mattress
(D) Specialized foam-mattress overlay on operating table
(E) Standard sheepskin overlay on hospital bed

81. A 75-yr-old man is evaluated because he has sudden onset of shortness of breath; sharp, pleuritic left-sided chest pain; and cough productive of blood-tinged sputum. He had elective hip replacement surgery 6 days ago. He has been (and is) wearing pneumatic compression devices on both legs. He has a 20-yr history of COPD. He is taking a proton-pump inhibitor for a duodenal ulcer diagnosed 2 wk ago and albuterol as needed.

On examination, temperature is 38.0° C (100.4° F), blood pressure is 165/90 mmHg, heart rate is 110 breaths per minute, and respiratory rate is 26 breaths per minute.

There is no accessory muscle use. He has slight expiratory wheezing. There is no jugular venous distension. A left-sided S4 gallop is audible. The abdomen is soft without masses or hepatosplenomegaly. There is no cyanosis, clubbing, edema, or thigh or calf pain.

WBC count is 13,800/μL, with 85% polymorphonuclear cells and 6% bands. Enzyme-linked immunosorbent assay reports D-dimer <500 ng/mL.

Arterial blood gas on room air:

pH	7.48
PaO_2	70 mmHg
$PaCO_2$	30 mmHg

An ECG reveals sinus tachycardia. Chest radiography reveals left lower-lobe atelectasis or infiltrate. Ventilation-perfusion (V/Q) scan indicates a low probability for pulmonary embolism. Bilateral lower-extremity Doppler ultrasonography demonstrates no evidence of deep vein thrombosis (DVT).

Which of the following is the most appropriate next step?

(A) Treat with heparin.
(B) Place an inferior vena cava filter.
(C) Treat with antibiotics and steroids.
(D) Obtain CT of chest.
(E) Obtain CT angiography of chest.

82. A 92-yr-old woman is brought to the office by her daughter because she is moving more slowly and unsteadily. She has not had any falls. She lives with her family and she is independent in ADLs. Until 2 yr ago, she took walks 3 times a week. Now her aerobic activity is limited to climbing 7 household steps about twice daily. She has a distant history of breast cancer and mild osteoarthritis. Medications include acetaminophen, vitamin D, and calcium.

On examination, vital signs are normal. There is no tremor or rigidity, and motor strength is symmetric and only slightly reduced. She stands unassisted but sways on standing and reaches out for contact assistance. She walks across the examination room without assistance but reaches out to touch the examination table. Her Mini–Mental State Examination score is normal.

Which of the following is the most appropriate next step?

(A) Establish a graduated balance-training program.
(B) Establish a high-intensity quadriceps strengthening program with 10 to 15 repetitions per session.
(C) Establish a moderate-intensity walking program of ≥1000 steps per day.
(D) Establish a high-intensity walking program of ≥5000 steps per day.
(E) Prescribe pain medication to be taken immediately before exercise.

83. A 75-yr-old man comes to the office for a routine physical examination. He feels well. He has a known history of chronic kidney disease; history also includes long-term type 2 diabetes mellitus, peripheral vascular disease, and coronary artery disease. Medications include insulin, metoprolol, sevelamer, and calcitriol. Examination is unremarkable.

Laboratory results (blood sample drawn at dialysis):

BUN	20 mg/dL
Creatinine	2.0 mg/dL
Sodium	140 mEq/L
Potassium	4.4 mEq/L
Hemoglobin	10 g/dL
Iron	within normal limits

Which of the following is the most appropriate next step?

(A) Begin epoetin-α with a target hemoglobin concentration of 13–14 mg/dL.
(B) Begin epoetin-α with a target hemoglobin concentration of 11–12 mg/dL.
(C) Begin epoetin-α if hemoglobin concentration falls to <9 mg/dL.
(D) Begin epoetin-α if symptoms develop.

84. A 78-yr-old widowed woman is in a nursing facility after hemicolectomy for metastatic cancer. She is dependent in ADLs, and her medical prognosis is poor. She presents herself as a woman who had unparalleled success in her career and numerous offers of marriage. Her brother reports that her lifelong tendency to become enraged after perceived slights has alienated her from her children and other relatives. Although at times she is tearful, she

enjoys making herself the focus of unit activities. She has not had changes in sleep or appetite. As her medical problems worsen, she is increasingly demanding and verbally abusive of nursing staff.

Mental status examination reveals normal rate of speech and psychomotor activity, and cognitive examination is normal.

Which of the following is the most likely diagnosis?

(A) Bipolar disorder, manic type
(B) Histrionic personality disorder
(C) Major depressive disorder
(D) Narcissistic personality disorder

85. A 75-yr-old man comes to the office for his annual visit. He has a family history of heart disease and wonders whether he would benefit from taking aspirin. He exercises frequently. History includes borderline dyslipidemia. On examination, blood pressure is 130/70 mmHg.

Which of the following is true about the role of aspirin in primary prevention?

(A) Enteric coating decreases the risk of aspirin-related GI bleeding.
(B) The recommended dose for primary prevention is 325 mg/d.
(C) Aspirin reduces the number of cardiovascular events in men.
(D) Aspirin reduces the risk of ischemic stroke in men.

86. A 76-yr-old man comes to the office because he recently read about the new "shingles shot" and wants to know if he should have it. He had an isolated case of herpes zoster in the past and does not want a recurrence.

Which of the following is true regarding the herpes zoster vaccine Zostavax?

(A) It is recommended for people with acute zoster or ongoing post-herpetic neuralgia.
(B) It is less effective in preventing post-herpetic neuralgia in adults ≥70 yr old than in younger adults.
(C) People with a history of herpes zoster infection were excluded from the stage 3 trial.
(D) Before administration of the vaccine, the patient's history of varicella exposure should be confirmed.

87. A 78-yr-old man comes to the office because he recently fell for no apparent reason. He has had cognitive problems for 5 yr. At first, friends noticed that he often seemed inattentive and was easily distractible. He began having trouble navigating to the location of his poker game, held at a different person's house each month. His family noticed that he was intermittently confused and often talked of seeing different friends (deceased) at his house. He is no longer able to organize his social calendar or prepare a tax return, which he previously did with ease. The family believes that recently his memory has begun "failing" as well. The history suggests dementia with Lewy bodies.

Which of the following statements is most accurate about dementia with Lewy bodies?

(A) Clinical suspicion is increased if parkinsonism was present ≥2 yr before the dementia.
(B) A history of exposure to neuroleptic agents with no adverse event excludes the diagnosis.
(C) Occipital lobe hypermetabolism is seen on positron emission tomography (PET).
(D) Associated visual hallucinations are usually complex and vivid.

88. A 68-yr-old woman is brought to the emergency department because she woke up from an afternoon nap with a sudden onset of rotational vertigo and clumsiness of the right arm. She feels as though the world is tilting toward the right. She is unable to walk even with assistance, and she has a headache. History includes hypertension and type II insulin-dependent

diabetes. Her medications include lisinopril, metformin, and aspirin.

On examination, temperature is 37.5°C (99.5°F). Blood pressure is 180/95 mmHg, pulse is 80 beats per minute, and respiratory rate is 16 breaths per minute. She has horizontal nystagmus and a negative head thrust test. She has difficulty both with making rapid alternating movements with the right arm and with toe-tapping or heel-to-shin movements on the right leg.

Which of the following is the most likely diagnosis?

(A) Cerebellar infarct
(B) Dorsolateral medullary stroke
(C) Meniere disease
(D) Herpes zoster infection of the inner ear (Ramsay Hunt syndrome)
(E) Benign paroxysmal positional vertigo

89. A 72-yr-old woman comes to the office for preoperative evaluation before left total-knee replacement. Despite the worsening pain in her left knee, she remains active, and gardens and plays golf 4 days a week. She has no known allergies and has never smoked. Both her parents lived into their nineties. History includes mild hypertension, for which she takes atenolol 25 mg/d.

On physical examination, blood pressure is 121/82 mmHg and resting heart rate is 70 beats per minute. Other than osteoarthritic changes in both knees, left worse than right, her examination is unremarkable. Serum chemistries and CBC are within normal limits. ECG shows no conduction delays and no ischemic changes.

Which of the following is most appropriate for perioperative management of this patient?

(A) Increase atenolol dosage to 50 mg/d; continue perioperatively.
(B) Discontinue atenolol immediately before surgery; restart 48 h after surgery.
(C) Continue atenolol at the current dosage.
(D) Discontinue atenolol; begin an ACE inhibitor plus a statin.

90. An 80-yr-old patient comes to the office for a routine physical examination. She has mild hearing loss and is otherwise healthy. She takes

a multivitamin and calcium citrate with vitamin D, and walks 1 mile daily. She states that she wishes to live to be 100 yr old and asks for advice about following the Mediterranean diet.

Which of the following is consistent with following the Mediterranean diet?

(A) Reduce fat intake.
(B) Reduce consumption of fish.
(C) Increase consumption of poultry.
(D) Increase consumption of legumes and whole grains.
(E) Increase consumption of bread and rice.

91. An 82-yr-old woman comes to the office because she has urine leakage when she coughs or sneezes, as well as urinary frequency and urgency. History includes COPD, hypertension, and aortic stenosis.

On pelvic examination, there is grade III pelvic prolapse. Postvoid residual volume is 200 mL.

Which of the following is most likely to be effective for this patient?

(A) Vaginal pessary
(B) Burch colposuspension
(C) Kegel exercises
(D) Oxybutynin

92. Which of the following statements regarding treatment for major depressive disorder is true?

(A) Most older adults with the diagnosis are treated by a psychiatrist.
(B) In older adults on an effective dosage of antidepressants, the response rate is close to 80% after 8 wk.
(C) Risk of recurrence or relapse is higher in patients who did not reach full remission.
(D) Augmentation with a second agent is not appropriate after a partial response to one antidepressant.
(E) Psychosocial interventions have little impact on rate of remission or risk of recurrence.

93. A 75-yr-old woman with established osteoporosis wishes to discuss advertisements she has seen for ibandronate and risedronate. She currently takes alendronate and wonders whether she would benefit more from a different agent. She has not had a fracture.

Which of the following is the best agent for preventing fracture?

(A) Alendronate
(B) Ibandronate
(C) Pamidronate
(D) Risedronate
(E) Data are not available to answer her question.

94. An 84-yr-old-man comes to the office to get information on minimizing muscle loss. He is vigorous and healthy, with no chronic diseases. He has heard that muscle loss is a serious problem with aging and may contribute to frailty. He would like to take medication to delay or minimize muscle loss associated with aging.

Which of the following is most likely to minimize the patient's muscle loss?

(A) Testosterone
(B) Dehydroepiandrosterone
(C) Growth hormone
(D) Vitamin D
(E) No medication

95. Which of the following statements is true of older versus younger adults with anxiety disorders?

(A) Older adults are less likely to respond to medication for anxiety disorders.
(B) Older adults are less likely to respond to psychotherapy for anxiety disorders.
(C) Older adults are less likely to cite anxiety as a primary complaint.
(D) Older adults are less likely to have an anxiety disorder.

96. An 82-yr-old man who lives in a nursing facility is evaluated because he has a facial rash. He has been taking ciprofloxacin therapy for 5 days for a urinary tract infection. History includes Parkinson's disease and dementia.

On examination, the rash comprises mild erythematous plaques with fine scales along the frontal hairline of the scalp as well as moderate erythema with increased scales along the nasolabial folds bilaterally.

Which of the following would be effective as an initial step in managing this patient's rash?

(A) Discontinue ciprofloxacin
(B) Open wet dressings
(C) 5% Fluorouracil ointment
(D) Ketoconazole cream and topical low-potency steroid
(E) Skin biopsy

97. A 79-yr-old man is brought to the office by his daughter; both are concerned about his recent deterioration and want to know his prognosis. The patient has hypertension, peripheral vascular disease, and stage IV colon cancer. Poorly differentiated adenocarcinoma of the colon, metastatic to liver and peritoneum, was diagnosed 2 yr ago. He did well after surgical resection of his tumor and treatment with bevacizumab. However, now there is increased involvement of his liver and peritoneum along with new pulmonary nodules. He has constant abdominal pain that is well controlled with a fentanyl patch and oxycodone as needed for breakthrough pain. He has become increasingly debilitated over the last 6 mo. Because of fatigue and pain, he is unable to do most IADLs, and in the last 4 wk he has become dependent in all ADLs except feeding.

Which of the following patient characteristics is most predictive of a poor prognosis?

(A) Low performance status
(B) Advanced tumor stage
(C) Multiple comorbidities
(D) Advanced age
(E) Opioid use

98. An 80-yr-old man comes to the office because he has had a left frontal headache and blurry vision for 2 wk. In addition, he has been feeling more tired, and his jaw aches when he eats. He denies nausea, vomiting, neck stiffness or visual loss. On examination, there is no nuchal rigidity or temporal tenderness. His pupils are round, equal in size, and reactive to light. Visual acuity, visual fields, fundoscopic examination, and extraocular movements are normal.

Which of the following is most likely to confirm the diagnosis?

(A) CT of the head
(B) Temporal artery biopsy
(C) Slit-lamp examination
(D) Tonometry
(E) Cerebral angiography

99. A 68-yr-old resident of a nursing facility is admitted to the hospital because he has increasing pain and erythema related to a sacral pressure ulcer for which he had been receiving treatment. He has a history of stroke and right-sided hemiparesis.

On examination, vital signs are stable. There is a 3 cm × 6 cm midline sacral ulcer with a dry, black eschar covering the entire wound, surrounding warmth, and erythema. It is tender to touch, and when pressed, it exudes moderate amounts of pus.

Which of the following is the most appropriate treatment for the pressure ulcer?

(A) Hydrocolloid dressings applied every 3 to 5 days
(B) Sharp debridement of eschar
(C) Papain-urea cream applied to eschar twice daily
(D) Wet-to-dry dressings applied twice daily
(E) Hydrogel dressings applied twice daily

100. An 85-yr-old woman is brought to the emergency department by her family because of increasingly erratic behavior. Normally, she functions independently, but over the past few days she has been forgetful, confused, and disoriented. History includes pneumonia 6 mo ago, hypertension, and gastroesophageal reflux. Medications include hydrochlorothiazide, omeprazole, lisinopril, and a multivitamin.

On examination, her vital signs are within normal limits. She is inattentive and scores 16/30 on the Mini–Mental State Examination.

Laboratory results:
Sodium   128 mmol/L
Potassium   3.2 mmol/L
BUN   10 mg/dL
Creatinine   0.8 mg/dL
Urine sodium   80 mmol/L
Urine osmolality   450 mOsm/kg

Which of the following is the most likely cause of this patient's hyponatremia?

(A) Syndrome of inappropriate arginine vasopressin secretion
(B) Water intoxication
(C) Hydrochlorothiazide
(D) Omeprazole
(E) Volume depletion and poor oral intake

101. An 82-yr-old man, previously independent, comes to the emergency department with 2 days of difficulty swallowing, productive cough, and dyspnea. History includes hypertension and controlled type 2 diabetes mellitus. On examination, he has a low-grade fever and increased blood pressure. Physical examination and chest radiography are consistent with consolidation in the left lower lobe. On bedside testing, he immediately sputters and coughs after drinking a small amount of water from a cup. There are no other neurologic findings. Laboratory testing suggests mild dehydration, and WBC count is slightly increased. MRI reveals a new, small brain-stem infarction and mild generalized cerebral atrophy.

Treatment for aspiration pneumonia is instituted. Seven days after onset of symptoms, swallowing has not improved, and formal evaluation shows aspiration with most consistencies.

Which of the following is the best recommendation?

(A) Careful oral feeding
(B) Gastrostomy feeding
(C) Hospice
(D) Nasogastric feeding
(E) Total parenteral nutrition

102. An 84-yr-old woman had a total thyroidectomy 3 mo ago because of gradually worsening compression symptoms. The symptoms were due to a benign multinodular goiter. Since thyroidectomy, the patient has taken levothyroxine 88 mcg/d. She also takes calcium and vitamin D for osteopenia.

After thyroidectomy, the patient's thyrotropin and free T_4 levels increased and total T_3 level decreased.

Thyroid function tests	Before thyroidectomy	After thyroidectomy
Thyrotropin	1.2 mIU/L	1.6 mIU/L
Free T$_4$	1.1 ng/dL	1.4 ng/dL
Total T$_3$	140 ng/dL	119 ng/dL

Which of the following is the best management option?

(A) Continue levothyroxine 88 mcg/d.
(B) Increase levothyroxine to 100 mcg/d.
(C) Add liothyronine 25 mcg/d.
(D) Switch to Armour desiccated thyroid 60 mg/d.

103. Which of the following is the most common nonpharmacologic intervention for urinary incontinence in nursing-home residents?

(A) Briefs or pads
(B) Toileting program
(C) Indwelling catheter
(D) External catheter

104. An 82-yr-old man living in a nursing facility is evaluated because of gradual functional decline. He has lost 4.5 kg (7% of body weight) since he entered the nursing facility 6 mo ago after hospitalization for acute myocardial infarction. During that hospitalization, type 2 diabetes was diagnosed. In the nursing home he has remained hyperglycemic, with periodic blood glucose concentrations spiking to 300 mg/dL and a recent hemoglobin A$_{1c}$ level of 7.9 g/dL. He is on an American Diabetic Association low-fat diet. He takes several medications, including glipizide, pravastatin, hydrochlorothiazide, metoprolol, lisinopril, and aspirin.

Laboratory results:
Creatinine	1.4 mg/dL
Low-density lipoprotein	100 mg/dL
High-density lipoprotein	34 mg/dL
Triglycerides	170 mg/dL

Which of the following is the most appropriate next step in management of this patient?

(A) Increase glipizide dosage.
(B) Add metformin.
(C) Add acarbose.
(D) Add niacin.
(E) Liberalize his diet.

105. An 80-yr-old man uses a handheld magnifier to read medication labels and the newspaper. He has never been prescribed eyeglasses. History includes successful cataract surgery 8 yr ago. At a routine ophthalmology examination 6 mo ago, his vision was recorded as 20/40 in his right eye and 20/50 in his left eye for distance with no correction. Near vision was not recorded. He was told he had the "eyes of a 30-yr-old" and was scheduled to return in 1 yr.

Which of the following is the most likely cause of his inability to read without a magnifier?

(A) Early exudative (wet) macular degeneration
(B) Early nonexudative (dry) macular degeneration
(C) Glaucoma
(D) Opacification of the posterior capsule of his lens after cataract surgery
(E) Lack of eyeglasses

106. An 88-yr-old man comes to you for evaluation after having two previous systolic blood pressure readings >160 mmHg. He is remarkably healthy, with a history only of osteoarthritis, macular degeneration, and multiple basal cell cancers that have been treated successfully. He takes calcium, vitamin D, and acetaminophen as needed.

On examination, blood pressure is 170/88 mmHg and pulse is 70 beats per minute, without postural changes. His physical examination is otherwise unremarkable. His ECG is normal, as are all laboratory tests except for a low-density lipoprotein cholesterol of 128 mg/dL. He eats a healthy diet, exercises regularly, and is not interested in further lifestyle changes.

What is the best approach to treating his blood pressure at this point?

(A) Measure home blood pressure on at least 3 separate occasions.
(B) Begin a thiazide diuretic.
(C) Begin a β-blocker.
(D) Begin an α-blocker.

107. An 88-yr-old black woman with peripheral arterial disease is admitted to the hospital because she has gangrene in 2 toes and soft-tissue infection of her distal foot. She is a widow

and lives alone; her daughter visits at least weekly.

On admission, her blood pressure is 140/80 mmHg, respiratory rate is 16 breaths per minute, pulse is 90, and temperature is 38° C (100.4° F). She is acutely confused and inattentive. Her speech is rambling.

Which of the following factors is most likely to increase her risk of in-hospital functional decline and nursing home placement?

(A) Marital status
(B) Race
(C) Gender
(D) Delirium

108. A 76-yr-old woman comes to the office because over the past day she has had progressive painful swelling of the wrist, such that she is now unable to use her left hand. She has had similar episodes involving her knee and ankle over the past year. History includes hypertension, coronary artery disease, and osteoarthritis of the hands. Medications include aspirin 81 mg/d, hydrochlorothiazide 12.5 mg/d, and acetaminophen 1 g q8h.

On examination, the patient has no fever. Her left hand is diffusely swollen, with wrist pain and tenderness; her right hand is tender over the second and third metacarpophalangeal joints. Her knees are warm to touch and hurt with movement. Uric acid level is 10.2 mg/dL, BUN is 30 mg/dL, and creatinine is 2.5 mg/dL.

In addition to discontinuing her hydrochlorothiazide, which of the following treatments is most appropriate?

(A) Intra-articular corticosteroid injection
(B) Oral corticosteroids and attention to adequate oral fluid intake
(C) Oral colchicine
(D) Oral probenecid
(E) Oral allopurinol

109. An 82-yr-old woman is brought to the office to establish care. She requires complete assistance with ADLs. History includes moderate vascular dementia, atrial fibrillation, and systolic heart failure; medications include warfarin, atenolol, simvastatin, and lisinopril.

On physical examination, she has a 6-cm rectangular yellow bruise on her right buttock, a 3-cm circular purple bruise on her left forearm, and a 4-cm oval red bruise on her posterior neck.

Which of the following bruise characteristics raises suspicion of physical abuse?

(A) Size
(B) Shape
(C) Number
(D) Location
(E) Color variation

110. A 74-yr-old woman comes to the office because she has a rash on her neck. It has been present for a few months and is getting thicker and redder. The area is itchy, and sometimes she finds herself scratching without realizing she is doing so; it is difficult for her to stop scratching, especially when she is worried and tired. She has been under stress recently because she is in the process of selling her house, to move in with her daughter. She does not use make-up or jewelry and has not changed detergent. Her usual emollient cream has not helped the rash.

On examination, she is afebrile and appears well. She has a 9-cm lichenified plaque on her neck that is erythematous, with areas of more intense erythema where it was recently scratched. The plaque feels thick and leathery to touch and is not warmer than the surrounding skin.

Which of the following is the most likely diagnosis?

(A) Nodular prurigo
(B) Xerosis
(C) Lichen simplex chronicus
(D) Asteatotic dermatitis
(E) Dyshidrotic eczematous dermatitis

111. A 69-yr-old man comes to the office to establish care. His wife is being treated for osteoporosis and she wants know whether her husband should also undergo a screening assessment.

Which of the following is the strongest risk factor for osteoporosis in men?

(A) Androgen deprivation therapy
(B) Low dietary intake of vitamin D
(C) Respiratory disease
(D) Thyroid replacement therapy
(E) Type 2 diabetes mellitus

112. An 85-yr-old man with macular degeneration is evaluated because of a sudden change in behavior and weight loss. He is recently widowed and has moved into an assisted-living facility. When his family visits, they are stunned to find him withdrawn, quiet, and losing weight. Previously, he had lived in his home for 50 yr and had managed ADLs and IADLs with assistance from his wife. Several years ago, he received services from a local agency for the blind and visually impaired.

Physical examination is normal except for low vision. Results of the Mini–Mental State Examination and Geriatric Depression Scale are normal. Examination by his ophthalmologist shows no change in the macular degeneration.

Which of the following is the most appropriate next step?

(A) Start antidepressant medications.
(B) Encourage participation in group activities.
(C) Obtain a complete medical evaluation to assess the weight loss.
(D) Refer to a vision rehabilitation specialist.
(E) Refer to a geriatric psychiatrist.

113. An 80-yr-old woman comes to the office because she recently has had difficulty eating and swallowing solid food. She notes that when she prepares to swallow, the food scrapes her cheeks and the roof of her mouth. History includes hypertension, diabetes mellitus, kidney stones, and major depressive disorder. Medications include hydrochlorothiazide, metformin, and fluoxetine. For the first time in many years, a recent dental examination revealed several cavities, which were located at the roots of the teeth.

Which of the following is the most likely explanation for these oral problems?

(A) Usual aging
(B) Salivary ductal stones
(C) Adverse effect of metformin
(D) Adverse effect of hydrochlorothiazide and fluoxetine
(E) Immune dysfunction

114. A 79-yr-old Asian-American woman is brought to the office because she has increasing forgetfulness; apathy; and behavioral changes of irritability, agitation, and aggression. Her primary caregiver reports that she is disruptive, occasionally screaming at imaginary people, and is frequently becoming combative. The patient has Alzheimer's disease but no history of psychosis or major depressive disorder. Physical examination, CBC, and serum chemistries are normal.

Which of the following is the next best step?

(A) Treat with a first-generation antipsychotic agent.
(B) Treat with a second-generation antipsychotic agent.
(C) Admit to a psychiatric unit for further evaluation.
(D) Review behavioral interventions with the caregiver.

115. A 75-yr-old man comes to the office because he has an ulcer on his tongue that is not painful except when he eats acidic or spicy foods. He does not remember when he first noticed it. His last dental examination was 2 yr ago. He smoked 2 packs daily for 30 yr, but stopped smoking 20 yr ago. He has hypertension controlled with medication.

On examination, there is a 2 × 2-cm nonhealing, indurated ulcer on the left lateroventral border of the tongue next to a broken filling.

Which of the following is the next best step?

(A) Refer patient to dentist to have filling restored.
(B) Refer for immediate biopsy of the lesion.
(C) Instruct patient to use an OTC local anesthetic gel to relieve the pain.
(D) Explain to patient that this is a canker sore that will resolve on its own in 7–10 days.
(E) Recommend that the patient avoid acidic or spicy foods until the sore heals.

116. An 80-yr-old woman is admitted to the hospital with urosepsis. On examination, she weighs 60 kg (132 lb) and has a low-grade fever and increased respiratory rate. There is a consolidation in the right lower lobe. Laboratory results show normal electrolyte concentrations and a serum creatinine concentration of 1.8 mg/dL, which is her recent baseline value. She responds well to 2 days of intravenous antibiotics, and cultures reveal *Escherichia coli* sensitive to trimethoprim/sulfamethoxazole. Your pharmacist reminds you that this medication requires adjustment for patients with renal impairment.

Based on published equations, what is her estimated glomerular filtration rate (GFR)?

(A) >90 mL/min
(B) 60–90 mL/min
(C) 30–60 mL/min
(D) 10–30mL/min
(E) <10 mL/min

117. An 88-yr-old man comes to the office because he has been feeling more tired than usual, and yesterday he fell in his bedroom. He was hospitalized with pneumonia 2 mo ago; he received daily physical and occupational therapy in a nursing facility for 4 wk and was then discharged home at maximal function. He has a history of Parkinson's disease, hypertension, and osteoarthritis. Medications include carbidopa/levodopa, hydrochlorothiazide, metoprolol, and acetaminophen.

Which of the following is most likely to yield additional information useful for reducing his risk of falling?

(A) Serum electrolytes
(B) Vitamin D level
(C) Postural blood pressure
(D) Timed Up and Go test

118. Which of the following statements describing response to common homeostatic challenges is true?

(A) Aging is associated with increased complexity of responses to auditory frequencies.
(B) Aging is associated with a decreased ability to respond to glucose challenges.
(C) Hypothermia in older adults exposed to cold temperatures is caused primarily by decreased thermogenesis.
(D) When exposed to stress, older adults have a shorter period of activation of the sympathetic nervous system than younger adults.

119. A 72-yr-old man comes to the office because he has anejaculatory orgasms. Over the last 3 yr, he has not consistently ejaculated with orgasm, and he has had no ejaculations for 3 mo. For the past 5 yr, he has taken tamsulosin 0.4 mg/d for lower urinary tract symptoms associated with benign prostatic hyperplasia. He has had no pelvic trauma, pain, or change in his lower urinary tract symptoms. He is monogamous and has intercourse once or twice a week with his wife of 40 yr.

Digital rectal examination reveals an asymmetric prostate of approximately 25 mL, with a hard nodule in the left lower lobe. The remainder of the examination is normal. Urinalysis is normal. His prostate-specific antigen (PSA) level is 9.5 ng/mL.

Which of the following is the most appropriate next step?

(A) Referral to a urologist
(B) Bone scan
(C) CT of the pelvis
(D) MRI of the pelvis
(E) Measurement of free PSA

120. A 75-yr-old woman with Alzheimer's disease is admitted to the hospital with a femoral neck fracture of the left hip and undergoes successful cemented hip arthroplasty within 24 h of admission. She resides in an assisted-living facility and walked independently before the fracture. Two weeks before the fracture, her score on the Mini–Mental State Examination was 15/30. Her daughter asks about rehabilitation options for her mother.

Which of the following is most appropriate for this patient?

(A) Arrange for immediate trial of rehabilitation.

(B) Do not recommend rehabilitation because of patient's dementia.

(C) Postpone rehabilitation because of patient's dementia.

(D) Postpone rehabilitation because of cemented prosthesis.

QUESTIONS, ANSWERS, AND CRITIQUES

1. An 84-yr-old nursing home resident is evaluated because she has been sleeping more over the last few days. At the beginning of the visit, the patient is still sleeping in bed in her nightgown; this is unusual for her. Staff reports that she recently seems less likely to recognize familiar people. The patient has no complaints and is distracted by the birds chirping outside her window. History includes stroke with persistent left hemiplegia, hypertension, dyslipidemia, diabetes, and mild dementia. Her hypertensive medications were recently adjusted by her cardiologist to improve blood pressure control. On examination, vital signs are unremarkable. She is disoriented to place and time. Her neurologic examination is otherwise unchanged from previous evaluations.

Which of the following is the most likely cause of her cognitive and behavioral changes?

(A) Progressive dementia
(B) Major depressive disorder
(C) Delirium
(D) New stroke

ANSWER: C

The key element in this patient's presentation is the acute change in her cognition and behavior. The most plausible explanation for her group of symptoms is delirium: an acute change in mental status (behavior and cognition), altered level of consciousness, and inattention. Delirium is often under-recognized in community-living, cognitively intact adults (SOE=B); it is even more difficult to detect in nursing-home residents with preexisting cognitive deficits. Nurses who interact with patients on a regular basis are most likely to identify cognitive and behavioral changes in their patients quickly. Recognition of delirium is essential—it is often the only symptom of an occult acute medical problem. Any suspicion of delirium must be followed with complete history and physical examination and targeted laboratory and radiologic tests.

The changes in the patient's behavior and cognition are too pronounced and acute to be due to progression of dementia, unless the patient has had a stroke or trauma that is not apparent in the neurologic examination. Dementia is most often slowly progressive, without sudden changes. Inattention is usually seen in advanced dementia or in dementias with Lewy bodies, neither of which is present in this case. Major depressive disorder can cause behavior changes but does not usually cause the degree of lethargy or inattention seen in this patient. Depression also would present more gradually.

Given the lack of additional changes in this patient's neurologic examination, it is premature to assume that her delirium is due to stroke or trauma. Although stroke or trauma can present with delirium, more likely causes are acute medical illness, medication toxicity, and metabolic disturbances.

2. A 92-yr-old man who resides in an assisted-living facility has increasing shortness of breath with activity and increasing frequency of chest pain. The chest pain responds promptly to sublingual nitroglycerin. He walks daily, reads, and plays the piano. History includes severe aortic valve stenosis with preserved ejection fraction confirmed by echocardiography, paroxysmal atrial fibrillation accompanied by shortness of breath, hypertension, dyslipidemia, osteoarthritis, lumbar spine disease, gastroesophageal reflux, benign prostatic hyperplasia, and depression. Medications include furosemide, losartan, warfarin, atorvasatin, mirtazepine, tamulosin, finasteride, acetaminophen, calcium, and vitamin D.

On examination, the patient is pale and appears younger than his stated age. Weight is 84 kg (185 lb), blood pressure is 120/70 mmHg, heart rate is 76 beats per minute and regular. There is a 3/6 harsh late-peaking systolic murmur audible at the apex and left sternal edge. There are no bruits, and his lungs are clear. His score on the Mini–Mental State Exam is 29/30. The Charlson Comorbidity Index = 6.

Laboratory results

Creatinine	1.1 mg/dL with an estimated GFR >60 mL/min
Electrolytes	normal
CBC	normal

Which of the following is the best diagnostic test to further evaluate this patient's cardiac status?

(A) Transthoracic echocardiogram
(B) Treadmill stress test
(C) Coronary angiography
(D) Persantine thallium stress test
(E) Cardiac MRI

ANSWER: C

This patient with previously diagnosed aortic stenosis presents with worsening symptoms. The only definitive therapy is valve replacement, and the information needed to guide the procedural approach is the presence or absence of concomitant coronary artery disease or mitral valve disease. The gold standard for acquiring information on coronary artery anatomy is coronary angiography (SOE=A).

Echocardiography has been performed in this patient and suggests severe aortic stenosis. Repeat transthoracic echocardiography is unlikely to contribute additional information to guide therapy because it is not highly accurate in precisely quantifying the degree of aortic stenosis, which depends on both the gradient across the valve and the flow, and because it cannot define the coronary anatomy (SOE=B). MRI can provide anatomic information on the valves and function, and limited information on very proximal coronary anatomy. However, it is expensive and does not fully delineate the coronary artery anatomy in most, if not all, cases. Both treadmill stress tests and dobutamine echocardiograms are used to determine the likelihood and area of coronary artery disease but do not define the anatomy. There tests are

accompanied by increases in blood pressure and heart rate that can precipitate symptoms and heart failure. These symptoms can be catastrophic in patients with aortic stenosis, because cardiopulmonary resuscitation is unlikely to be successful in severe aortic stenosis. External cardiac compression cannot generate the very high ventricular pressures necessary to open the stenotic aortic valve. Persantine thallium testing and imaging can provide only the likelihood and area of coronary artery disease. It also carries increased risk in patients with aortic stenosis. This is due to their limited ability to further increase contractility, as well as the decrease in diastolic filling and wall tension development that accompanies reflex tachycardia precipitated by the persantine-induced drop in blood pressure. CT with calcium scoring was not offered as a choice. However, it is not very specific in older adults: vascular calcifications are common but do not correlate with the presence or absence of obstructive coronary artery disease and cannot define the coronary anatomy (SOE=D).

3. Which of the following assistive devices is most appropriate for a 72-yr-old man with Parkinson's disease who has postural instability and festination?

(A) Cane
(B) Front-wheeled walker
(C) Hemi-walker
(D) Pick-up walker
(E) 4-Wheeled walker

ANSWER: B

Walking devices are extremely helpful for people with gait disorders. They increase mobility, reduce risk of falls, and facilitate independence. The walking device must be targeted to the patient's functional deficits to avoid increasing risk, and the patient must be trained, preferably by a physical therapist, to use the device safely. The patient described has the classic mobility problems of Parkinson's disease—postural instability (often associated with backward falls) and festination (gradual increasing of forward speed while walking). The device chosen should facilitate maintenance of forward center of gravity (to limit backward falls), yet not be so mobile that it could facilitate festination. A front-wheeled walker best meets these requirements.

Standard pick-up walkers and front-wheeled walkers both decrease a patient's gait speed. However, patients using the standard walker have increased freezing and slow gait speed. Front-wheeled walkers do not increase freezing and are associated with a gait speed intermediate between no walker and a standard walker (SOE=B).

A cane is not the best choice for this patient because the posturing of arms (internal rotation) could lead to tripping. A hemi-walker is used by patients with a hemiparesis. A pick-up walker promotes a very slow gait and can accentuate backward movement when lifting, thereby increasing the risk of a fall. The four-wheeled walker rolls very easily but could promote festination. For patients (with or without Parkinson's disease) who do not have festination and can use them safely, 4-wheeled walkers are preferred because they promote a more normal gait pattern (SOE=D).

4. A 76-yr-old man is brought to the office by his older sister to establish care. The patient has significant autism. He lives with his sister, who reports that over the past 3 mo he has been rocking, pacing, and yelling more often, and has hit himself twice. The behaviors have slowly increased in frequency and intensity to a degree that she has not seen for several years. His sleep is disrupted and he often paces during the night. His sister is his guardian; she reports that his care is increasingly difficult for her. She recently moved them from their family home to an apartment, and they are getting out less frequently for walks and shopping. He has no history of significant illnesses and is on no routine medications.

On examination, the patient is slightly underweight. He rocks and hums nearly constantly during the office visit. His skin is intact, and there are no bruises. The examination is essentially normal other than his repetitive behaviors.

Which of the following is the most appropriate initial step in managing the patient's behaviors?

(A) Begin quetiapine 25 mg.
(B) Begin zolpidem 5 mg at bedtime.
(C) Begin mirtazapine 15 mg.
(D) Reevaluate in 2 wk if the behavior persists.
(E) Begin methylphenidate 5 mg.

ANSWER: C

Adults with autism or autism-spectrum disorders characteristically have diminished social interaction; diminished expressive communication; repetitive and obsessive, ritualistic, or compulsive behaviors; a narrow range of interests or activities; and intolerance to change of routine or circumstances. Despite their diminished expressive ability, adults with autism can have good receptive ability and perception of the environment. Anxiety in response to change is common and can cause increased repetitive or stereotypic behaviors. Self-injurious behaviors, ranging from mild scratching to severe, potentially life-threatening injury, can begin or increase. A significant amount of clinical experience supports off-label use of second-generation antidepressants to decrease the intensity and frequency of self-injury (SOE=D).

This patient's changes in residence and familiar activities are the likely causes of his increased anxiety. The best choice among the options in this case would be to initiate a second-generation antidepressant at an appropriate dosage and carefully monitor the results.

Off-label use of the agents naltrexone and risperidone has been investigated for challenging behaviors in adults with autism, and risperidone has been approved for use in children with autism. In the choice between a relatively safe, well-studied, second-generation antidepressant, such as mirtazapine, with anxiolytic effects and a second-generation antipsychotic agent, such as quetiapine, the antidepressant offers better risk/benefit potential. If the patient's behaviors were markedly more dangerous to himself or to others, urgency may make the antipsychotic agent the wiser option.

A sedative is unlikely to produce much benefit in this case. The patient's sleep is probably disturbed by anxiety related to changes or frustrated compulsive needs. It is better to treat the anxiety that causes the behavior than to sedate an older patient.

Waiting to reevaluate the patient while someone is at risk of injury is not a good option. Although some challenging behaviors resolve with time or change in the environment, both the patient and his sister are currently at risk.

Because this patient has no evidence of attention deficit/hyperactivity disorder, methylphenidate is not an appropriate option.

Finally, the healthcare provider should ask the patient's sister about the extent of formal and informal social support available.

5. A 75-yr-old woman comes to the office because she has had repeated episodes of profound dizziness and syncope, along with at least 2 episodes in which she found herself on the floor but was unaware of how she fell. Each episode has been preceded by a prodrome during which she feels warm and is diaphoretic and progressively lightheaded. The episodes are most likely to occur when she has been standing for a long time, such as during church services. History includes hypertension, for which she takes hydrochlorothiazide daily.

On physical examination, blood pressure is 142/84 mmHg while supine and 110/70 mmHg while upright; heart rate is 76 beats per minute while supine and 80 beats per minute while upright. There is no jugular venous distension or carotid bruit. Lungs are clear. Carotid upstroke is slightly delayed, with a II/VI systolic murmur at the base; the second heart sound is intact, and there is no gallop.

Which of the following is the most appropriate next step?

(A) Stop hydrochlorothiazide.
(B) Begin oral midodrine 5 mg three times daily (about 4 h apart, not too close to bedtime).
(C) Begin fludrocortisone 0.1 mg q12h.
(D) Obtain tilt-table test.

ANSWER: A

Physical examination of this patient reveals orthostatic hypotension, an important cause of syncope in older adults. When a standing position is assumed, gravity induces pooling of blood in the lower extremities. Blood pressure

is normally maintained by vasoconstriction and increased heart rate when circulatory volume is decreased. The incidence and prevalence of orthostatic hypotension in older adults are affected by numerous age-related changes in cardiovascular structure and function, such as impaired baroreflex function, diastolic dysfunction, higher prevalence of disorders that directly or indirectly impair autonomic function, common use of vasoactive medications, and impaired salt and water balance.

The most commonly accepted definition of orthostatic hypotension is a decrease of >20 mmHg in systolic blood pressure or >10 mmHg in diastolic blood pressure on standing. In most patients with orthostatic hypotension, the drop in blood pressure is detected within 2 min of assuming an upright posture. Some patients, however, have delayed orthostatic intolerance, and blood pressure falls progressively over 15–45 min. This dysautonomic response to upright posture can be detected during a tilt-table test. In this particular patient, the diagnosis of orthostatic hypotension is apparent on physical examination, which eliminates the need for the tilt-table test.

Initial treatments for orthostatic hypotension include withdrawal of potentially exacerbating medications; accordingly, stopping hydrochlorothiazide is the best option in this patient (SOE=B). If necessary, physiologic interventions should be introduced next (eg, compressive devices such as stockings or abdominal bands, counterpressure maneuvers like squatting or leg crossing). Pharmacologic therapy (eg, fludrocortisone and midodrine) should be used only if other measures fail. Patients should be 1) reassured that the problem can be controlled; 2) taught to avoid predisposing factors and triggering events, such as volume depletion and prolonged upright posture; and 3) taught maneuvers to abort an episode of orthostasis. In older adults, supine hypertension can coexist with and be exacerbated by treatment of orthostatic hypotension. Some degree of supine hypertension may have to be tolerated to minimize the short-term risk of orthostasis and associated falls.

6. Which one of the following statements about smoking and older adults is true?

(A) Older smokers who quit gain substantial health benefits.
(B) Most smokers will attempt to quit only if they are supported by counseling or pharmacologic treatments.
(C) Older hospitalized patients are as likely as younger inpatients to receive smoking cessation interventions.
(D) Medicare does not cover tobacco cessation counseling for beneficiaries who have smoking-related illnesses.
(E) Brief interventions delivered by health care professionals do not affect rates of smoking cessation.

ANSWER: A

Approximately 1 in 10 older adults currently smokes. Quitting at an older age can yield substantial health benefits: compared with adults who continue smoking, men ≥65 yr old who quit gain 1.4–2 yr in longevity, and women ≥65 yr old who quit gain 2.7–3.7 yr. Improvements are observed in comorbid conditions as well (SOE=B).

The vast majority of smokers who attempt to quit each year do so without benefit of either behavioral or pharmacologic treatments. Among adults hospitalized for acute myocardial infarction, older adults who smoke are significantly less likely to receive interventions for smoking cessation than younger patients who smoke. Clinicians are less aggressive when counseling older adults about smoking cessation.

In 2005, the Centers for Medicaid and Medicare Services (CMS) estimated that 10% of its total annual budget is spent on smoking-related illnesses. As a result of the analysis, CMS now covers cessation counseling for Medicare beneficiaries who have smoking-related illnesses or who are taking medications that are affected by tobacco use. Medicare's prescription drug benefit now covers clinician-prescribed smoking cessation treatments.

There is substantial evidence that brief interventions by healthcare providers can affect smoking cessation rates. The 5-step intervention is one such evidence-based approach: 1) **ask** about smoking at every visit; 2) **advise** every smoker to stop; 3) **assess** the patient's readiness to quit; 4) **assist** patients, whether they are ready to quit or not; and 5) **arrange** for a follow-up visit to readdress smoking cessation.

7. A 65-yr-old recently retired man comes to the office because he has recurring episodes of urinary frequency associated with perineal discomfort. He reports that he has had a "nervous bladder" for much of his life but had never seen a clinician for this. Over the last year, however, he has had a mild to moderately uncomfortable sensation that initially seemed to come and go but now is present most days and uncomfortable enough to cause him distress. He has been married for 35 yr and has been sexually active and monogamous for that time. He reports no problems associated with sexual activity, and has no chills, fever, incontinence, or difficulty starting or stopping urinary stream. He has never sought counseling or medical care for anxiety. He has no chronic disorders and takes no medications.

On examination, blood pressure is 140/80 mmHg and pulse is 80 beats per minute. His prostate is estimated at 15 mL, with no asymmetry, nodule, or induration. He notes mild tenderness during palpation. Urinalysis done after digital rectal examination reveals 3 or 4 WBCs per high-power field and is otherwise unremarkable. Cultures from that urine sample (including for *Mycobacterium tuberculosis*) are unremarkable. Prostate-specific antigen level is 3.2 ng/mL, and urine cytologies are negative.

Which of the following is the most appropriate next step?

(A) Finasteride therapy
(B) α-Agonist therapy
(C) Transrectal ultrasonography
(D) CT of the pelvis
(E) Psychiatric evaluation

ANSWER: B

This patient has chronic pelvic pain syndrome. While this syndrome can present at any age, the risk increases with age; it has been reported in up to 13% of men ≥65 yr old. Chronic pelvic pain syndrome is a clinical diagnosis based on history of chronic pelvic pain and symptoms associated with voiding in the absence of inflammatory processes in the urinary tract.

Urinary tract cancer and recurrent infection—including tuberculosis—must be excluded. There is no specific test for this syndrome. Administration of α-blockers for 3–6 mo had a beneficial effect in most published trials, although differences in study design and outcome measures limit the strength of the evidence.

Measurement of prostate-specific antigen is not helpful, and increased levels in the absence of active infection would warrant an evaluation independent of pelvic pain. Imaging of any kind is not useful unless other diagnoses are suspected. Finasteride has not been shown to be helpful in the treatment of chronic pelvic pain syndrome. While anxiety and psychologic diagnoses must be considered, this patient has no overt evidence of significant psychopathology; thus, psychiatric evaluation is not indicated at this time.

8. Which of the following is meant by culturally competent care?

   (A) Allocation of resources in proportion to the cultural composition of the community.
   (B) Delivery of health services according to the cultural practices of the caregiver.
   (C) Delivery of health services that acknowledge cultural diversity in the clinical setting.
   (D) Characterizing patients based on their cultural backgrounds rather than their individual preferences.

ANSWER: C

Over the last few decades, globalization and changing geopolitics have caused major changes in immigration trends in the United States. In contrast to the predominantly European immigration during the earlier part of the 20th century, large numbers of people are migrating from other regions, especially Asia and Africa, thereby increasing the ethnic and cultural diversity of older Americans. Cultural diversity of older Americans poses significant challenges for optimal delivery of health care: clinical encounters should be characterized by a patient-centered approach to and respect for cultural, social, and ethnic differences—ie, cultural competency.

Culturally competent care involves delivery of health services in a manner consonant with customs, beliefs, values, behaviors, and norms of an individual patient. It involves aspects that directly or indirectly affect delivery of health care, including language, communication style, attire, food, reaction to pain, and participation in decision-making. All of these components influence patients' decisions regarding acceptance of and adherence to treatment plans.

Allocation of resources according to the cultural composition of the community is not consistent with equitable, nondiscriminatory, need-based distribution that would ensure health care for all segments of the community.

The beliefs and cultural practices of the patient, not of the care provider, should influence care. Attempts should be made to identify and incorporate a patient's health beliefs, social values, family dynamics, dietary practices, and privacy issues, and to overcome language barriers.

Beliefs and attitudes vary greatly even among specific cultural groups. Hence, to provide culturally competent care, it is essential to treat each patient as an individual rather than as a cultural, religious, socioeconomic, or ethnic stereotype. The nurse as advocate is ideally positioned to promote addressing the unique needs and preferences of the individual patient.

9. An 81-yr-old man comes to the office for follow-up after myocardial infarction 5 wk earlier. He has not needed nitroglycerin for angina since 4 days after the infarct. He would like to resume sexual relations with the woman he has dated since his wife died 2 yr ago. In the past year, before the infarct, he was able to maintain an erection sufficient for intercourse about half of the time. He is anxious because he is now unable to achieve erections sufficient for intercourse. History includes well-controlled hypertension with left ventricular hypertrophy, and transurethral resection of the prostate 15 yr ago for benign prostatic hyperplasia. Medications include atenolol 50 mg/d, simvastatin 40 mg/d, aspirin 81 mg/d, and nitroglycerin as needed.

On examination, peripheral pulses are diminished. His score on the Geriatric Depression Scale is 3, and he denies symptoms of depression.

Which of the following is the most appropriate next step in assessing this patient?

(A) Refer to cardiologist.
(B) Measure serum testosterone and bioavailable testosterone.
(C) Measure nocturnal penile tumescence.
(D) Refer to psychiatrist.

ANSWER: A

The probability of erectile dysfunction increases from 40% to 70% between ages 40 and 70. Dyslipidemia, hypertension, coronary artery disease, neurologic disorders (eg, stroke), use of certain medications, psychologic factors (eg, fear of failure, anxiety, unresolved grief, depression), hormonal changes, and hypogonadism can all be associated with erectile dysfunction. This patient has coronary artery disease as well as evidence of peripheral vascular disease, and thus has a significant vascular component to his erectile dysfunction. Consensus guidelines (SOE=C) have been developed for men with coronary artery disease to assess risk of sexual intercourse. Patients at low risk have asymptomatic coronary artery disease and no more than 2 of the following: controlled hypertension, mild stable angina, successful revascularization, previous uncomplicated revascularization, mild valvular disease, and heart failure with left ventricular dysfunction. This patient has more than 2 of the criteria. He is at intermediate risk and should be evaluated by a cardiologist. An exercise stress test should be ordered, because intercourse requires the ability to perform moderate metabolic equivalents of activity. Results of the test can also be used to evaluate whether the patient would benefit from treatment with phosphodiesterase inhibitors.

Generally, testosterone and bioavailable testosterone levels would not be measured immediately, unless libido is low, there is other evidence of hypogonadism, or the patient does not respond to treatment for erectile dysfunction (SOE=B). While hypogonadism increases in prevalence with age, this patient's erectile dysfunction is most likely related to vascular disease, which is the most common cause of erectile dysfunction (SOE=B).

The patient's score on the Geriatric Depression Scale does not increase his likelihood of having major depression and h denies depressive symptoms. Because he ha erections before the infarct, it is unlikely that unresolved grief related to being widowed is the cause of his erectile dysfunction. Sudden death due to intercourse is rare, and results of a stress test should reassure him. Thus, psychiatric evaluation is not warranted.

10. Which of the following statements is true?

(A) Aged skeletal muscle cells are more likely than younger skeletal muscle cells to undergo apoptosis (cell death) as a result of physical inactivity.
(B) The reductions in skeletal muscle tone and contractility that occur with aging are due primarily to changes in muscle mass.
(C) Muscles do not lose any tone with aging if they are exercised regularly.
(D) The rate and extent of muscle changes is determined almost entirely by exercise and does not have a genetic component.

ANSWER: A

Loss of muscle mass and declines in muscle function with aging are the major clinical features of sarcopenia. The pathophysiology of this highly prevalent condition remains unknown.

Older animals are more likely to develop apoptosis of skeletal muscle cells in response to physical inactivity. Declines in muscle quality with aging include decreased regenerative potential and increased tissue fibrosis. Muscle stem cells (satellite cells) from aged mice have a greater tendency to convert from a myogenic to a fibrogenic lineage as they begin to proliferate. Moreover, this conversion appears to be mediated by circulating factors present in serum from aged mice that induce Wnt signaling. Age-related reductions in muscle tone and contractility result from both aging changes in the nervous system as well as changes involving the quality of the muscle tissue. The rate and extent of muscle changes seems to be, at least in part, genetically determined and is also influenced by physical activity.

11. A 79-yr-old woman comes to the office to establish care. She reports that she often feels sleepy. History includes osteoporosis, hip

fracture, systolic heart failure, hypertension, frequent falls, chronic kidney disease, and post-herpetic neuralgia. Medications include extended-release metoprolol 100 mg/d, gabapentin 600 mg q8h, alendronate 35 mg/wk, vitamin D 800 IU/d, calcium carbonate 500 mg q8h, and aspirin 81 mg/d. Serum creatinine is 1.5 mg/dL, with estimated creatinine clearance of 30 mL/min.

Which of the following would be most likely to relieve this patient's sleepiness?

(A) Reduce gabapentin dosage to 600 mg q12h.
(B) Start lisinopril 2.5 mg/d.
(C) Discontinue alendronate.
(D) Increase vitamin D to 1200 IU/d.
(E) Switch extended-release metoprolol to metoprolol 50 mg q12h.

ANSWER: A

In patients with chronic kidney disease who take medications that are primarily eliminated by the kidneys, dosage adjustments are often needed to avoid adverse drug events. This patient's lethargy may be related to the excessive gabapentin dosage, particularly in light of her renal impairment. Gabapentin is eliminated by the kidneys unchanged. In patients with creatinine clearance between 30 and 59 mL/min, the total dosage recommendation for gabapentin is 400–1400 mg.

Because this patient has systolic heart failure, an ACE inhibitor may improve survival and reduce morbidity (SOE=A). It may also slow progression of her kidney disease. However, it is unlikely to cause her sleepiness.

Discontinuing alendronate will not reduce the patient's sleepiness. According to the manufacturer, alendronate (and other bisphosphonates) are not recommended for patients with severe renal impairment (creatinine clearance <35 mL/min), because experience in this population is limited. Available evidence suggests that bisphosphonates can be used safely in women with stage 3 chronic kidney disease, such as this patient (SOE=A). There are no comparable data for patients with stage 4 or 5 renal disease.

The recommended vitamin D dosage is 800–1000 IU/d (SOE=A). Increasing the patient's dosage to 1200 IU/d will not improve her lethargy. Likewise, changing from extended-

release to regular metoprolol will not affect the lethargy.

12. A 90-yr-old woman comes to the office because, over the past year, she has had increasing difficulty walking. Her gait is slower, and she feels as if she might fall backward at times. She has hypertension, hypothyroidism, and osteoarthritis, and she had coronary artery bypass surgery 10 yr ago, with no recurrence of angina.

On examination, she has moderate dorsal kyphosis and arthritic changes in her fingers and knees. Strength and reflexes are symmetric. She has some increased muscle tone. She uses her arms to push up from the chair; once standing, she has difficulty starting to walk. Her gait is symmetric, with a normal base, but her foot clearance and stride length are both decreased. She turns slowly and carefully, with an increased number of steps.

Which of the following is the most likely cause of her gait abnormality?

(A) Osteoarthritis
(B) Proprioceptive deficits
(C) Cerebrovascular disease
(D) Parkinson's disease
(E) Cautious gait

ANSWER: C

This older patient has known vascular disease. The difficulty starting to walk, the slow gait with decreased foot clearance, and the tendency to fall backward suggest subclinical cerebrovascular disease (SOE=A). Her advanced age and history of hypertension place her at risk of microvascular disease affecting cerebral white matter and of lacunar infarcts. More advanced cerebrovascular disease can result in vascular parkinsonism, with poor standing balance, rigidity, masked face, parkinsonian gait, and cognitive impairment.

The patient has osteoarthritis, yet she does not have evidence of pain on walking and does not complain of her legs "giving way." Her gait is symmetric; with painful osteoarthritis, there is usually some gait asymmetry. Proprioceptive deficits, with loss of position sense, lead to a wide-based, steppage gait, which she does not have. The typical gait of Parkinson's disease involves initial hesitation, then small, shuffling steps with no arm swing and difficulty with balance. Associated findings would include tremor, masked face, and cogwheel rigidity. Fear of falling can lead to a slow, cautious gait, with decreased step length. Although this patient is probably being cautious because she fears falling, she has objective abnormalities, including difficulty rising from a chair, difficulty with starting to walk, and decreased foot clearance.

13. A 69-yr-old black man comes to the office for evaluation because routine laboratory tests showed an increased total calcium concentration (10.8 mg/dL). Three years ago, the concentration was 10.6 mg/dL. He has no symptoms of hypercalcemia, such as nausea, constipation, personality changes, or renal stones. There is a family history of hypertension; he is unaware of any family history of calcium disorders. The patient has an enlarged prostate and hypertension. Medications include amlodipine, hydrochlorothiazide, and saw palmetto. He does not take any vitamin supplements.

On physical examination, blood pressure is 140/80 mmHg, and he has mild prostatic hyperplasia. The remainder of the physical examination is normal. Levels of creatinine and $1,25(OH)_2D$ are normal. Parathyroid hormone concentration is 78 pg/mL and thyrotropin concentration is 2.1 mU/L.

Which of the following tests should be ordered next?

(A) Genetic testing for familial benign hypercalcemia hypocalciuria mutation
(B) 25(OH)D
(C) Parathyroid sestamibi (nuclear scan)
(D) A 24-hour urine collection for calcium and creatinine
(E) DEXA scan of the spine, hip, and forearm

ANSWER: B

Although this patient's increased calcium and parathyroid hormone levels suggest primary hyperparathyroidism, it is also possible that the hypercalcemia is due to the thiazide he takes, and that the increased parathyroid hormone is secondary to vitamin D deficiency. An appropriate approach would be to switch to a

different class of antihypertensive medi[cation] and to check the level of 25(OH)D, whic[h is] the best measure of the body's vitamin D[.] The $1,25(OH)_2D$ level is often not helpful ... diagnosing vitamin D deficiency because its production is tightly regulated by the kidney, and the serum concentration is often normal (SOE=C).

Vitamin D deficiency is found in up to 50% of older adults. Darker-skinned people have reduced synthesis of vitamin D because of decreased absorption of ultraviolet B radiation. Epidemiologic studies have shown that low levels of vitamin D are linked not only to decreased calcium absorption and bone mineralization, but also to poorer physical performance (SOE=B), frailty, falls (SOE=A), risk of cardiovascular disease (SOE=B), and increased incidence of cancers (SOE=B).

Genetic testing for familial benign hypercalciuria hypocalciuria is not indicated until the previous steps are taken, and then only if hypocalciuria is confirmed on a 24-hour urine collection for calcium and creatinine. Familial benign hypercalcemia hypocalciuria is usually asymptomatic. Previously increased calcium concentrations are an important diagnostic clue (SOE=C).

Parathyroid sestamibi (nuclear scan) and DEXA scans of the forearm would be appropriate if primary hyperparathyroidism turns out to be the diagnosis. Localization of an adenoma via nuclear scan would allow a surgeon to remove a gland through minimally invasive surgery. The DEXA scan, together with other laboratory findings and patient symptoms, would help in determining whether the primary hyperparathyroidism should be managed medically or surgically (SOE=C). No randomized trials demonstrate a reduction in fractures in patients undergoing surgery rather than medical treatment.

14. Which of the following is true regarding how the nursing-home population has changed since 1985?

(A) The number of residents has increased.
(B) Among adults ≥85 yr old, men now outnumber women.
(C) The level of disability has declined.
(D) The number of admissions has increased.

ANSWER: D

The number of nursing home admissions has increased since 1994, because more facilities now offer short-term medical services and rehabilitation care after a hospitalization. The number of nursing-home residents has remained approximately constant since 1985; overall, the percentage of older people living in nursing homes has actually declined. In the United States, about 2% of adults 65–84 yr old, and about 14% of adults ≥85 yr old, live in nursing homes. Nationally, the occupancy rates in nursing homes have declined from about 92% to about 88% in the last 20 yr.

The level of disability among nursing-home residents has increased over the past decade. Dementia remains the most prevalent condition, affecting an estimated 50%–70% of residents. Between 48% and 65% of residents have urinary or fecal incontinence, and more than half are confined to a wheelchair or bed. About 25% require assistance with 1 or 2 ADLs, and about 75% require assistance with 3 or more.

According to the National Nursing Home Survey, 674,000 adults ≥85 yr old lived in nursing homes in 2004; of those, 18% were men and 82% were women.

15. A 79-yr-old woman was discharged from the hospital yesterday after a 2-wk stay for diverticular bleeding. She underwent transfusion with 8 units of RBCs and declined surgery. She has diabetes and osteoarthritis and was in bed for most of the past 2 wk. Her husband calls to report that she is very weak. She needs follow-up laboratory tests in 2 days in compliance with hospital discharge instructions, but he does not think he can transport her to the office. He wants to know if she can receive home health care to address her needs.

Which of the following is an allowable indication for home health care in this patient?

(A) Follow-up laboratory testing
(B) Physical therapy
(C) Home aide services
(D) Monitoring of glycemic control
(E) Durable medical equipment

ANSWER: B

This patient qualifies for Medicare Part A home health agency care, both for nursing assessment and teaching, and for rehabilitative physical and occupational therapy. Physical therapy to help a homebound patient recover functionally from deconditioning that resulted from a recent illness is a qualifying service; the patient does not need to have nursing care to begin Part A home health services.

Drawing blood for laboratory testing was removed as an independent qualifying service need, effective February 1998 as part of the Balanced Budget Act of 1997. Drawing blood as part of a care plan to actively manage a recently unstable medical condition is permitted.

Although home health agencies must provide home health aide care as part of their service portfolio, agencies are not required to provide home health aide services to each patient, and the amount of service to be provided is under the agency's control. Requiring only a home health aide is not sufficient to qualify for home health services under Medicare Part A.

Teaching related to diabetes care can be the primary indication for home health care in a homebound patient if the diabetes has been newly diagnosed or is newly unstable, or if the patient lacks knowledge and ability in self-care of this condition. However, overseeing glycemic control is not an indication for home health care, and there is no suggestion that this patient's diabetes has recently been uncontrolled.

Unlike hospice, in which some home medical equipment is arranged or paid for by the hospice, in Medicare Part A home health care, the agency's responsibility is limited to providing services (eg, nursing, physical therapy) plus some related supplies (eg, wound care). In general, durable medical equipment is covered by Medicare Part B, and medications are covered by Medicare Part D (for those who are enrolled in Part D). Home health services are not required to provide durable medical equipment covered by Part B.

16. A 76-yr-old woman is transferred from a rehabilitation facility to the hospital after she falls and fractures her right hip. She was recovering from a recent hospitalization for pneumonia and exacerbation of COPD that left her profoundly deconditioned. She uses a combined steroid and long-acting β-agonist

inhaler and takes oral steroids for exacerbations. She is not oxygen dependent. She has no history of dementia but believes she has been more forgetful over the past year.

She is hydrated, her pain is controlled with narcotics, and surgery is planned for the next morning under general anesthesia.

Which of the following would be most likely to reduce her risk of postoperative delirium?

(A) Start low-dose intravenous haloperidol and continue for 48 h after surgery.
(B) Start oral donepezil and continue indefinitely.
(C) Obtain a preoperative comprehensive geriatric evaluation to develop a multifactorial risk-reduction strategy.
(D) Provide stress doses of intravenous steroids perioperatively.
(E) Avoid opioid analgesia after surgery.

ANSWER: C

The prevalence of delirium in older hospitalized adults is as high as 60%. In-hospital development of delirium is associated with increased mortality, functional decline, longer hospital stay, and discharge to a long-term–care facility. Risk factors associated with development of in-hospital delirium are older age, chronic cognitive impairment, immobility, sleep deprivation, compromised hearing or vision, dehydration or volume overload, malnutrition, polypharmacy, bladder catheterization, anemia, pain, electrolyte disturbances, hypoxemia, and infection. Proactive geriatrics consultation to address common risk factors reduced the occurrence of delirium by one-third in patients undergoing hip surgery (SOE=B). In addition to addressing the aforementioned complications, it is critical to collaborate with the nursing staff to develop and implement a plan for mobilization, physical activity, and comfort.

The use of prophylactic haloperidol does not prevent delirium but can decrease the severity of the delirium and reduce the length of stay (SOE=B). However, in some studies, use of antipsychotics in patients with dementia has resulted in increased mortality; until there is further data about the safety of antipsychotics in patients with delirium, they should be used

cautiously (SOE=D). The use of prophylactic noncompetitive cholinesterase inhibitors, such as donepezil, offers no benefit over placebo (SOE=B). Stress doses of intravenous steroids may have been necessary if this patient had used systemic steroids chronically before surgery. Because this patient uses oral steroids only for exacerbations, stress doses may add to the patient's confusion through adverse events affecting the CNS.

Withholding analgesics would not decrease the risk of delirium. In fact, poorly controlled pain is a risk factor for delirium (SOE=B).

17. Which of the following is the most reliable screen for hearing impairment?

(A) Screening version of the Hearing Handicap Inventory for the Elderly (HHIE-S)
(B) Abbreviated Profile of Hearing Aid Benefit
(C) Tinnitus Handicap Questionnaire
(D) Whisper test

ANSWER: A

Medicare offers a one-time preventive examination. Two self-report measures, the screening version of the HHIE-S and the Dizziness Handicap Inventory, are recommended for use by clinicians. The HHIE-S is widely used to assess hearing handicap, ie, hearing loss that interferes with performing ADLs. The HHIE-S consists of 10 questions regarding hearing difficulty in various situations: half of the questions cover self-reported emotional consequences of hearing loss, and half cover self-reported activity limitations and restrictions. The screen is quick and easy to administer and inexpensive. It has high reliability and validity, as well as adequate sensitivity and specificity. Patients who score >8 should be referred to an audiologist to evaluate hearing and to determine the need for medical or nonmedical interventions.

An alternative screening tool is a hand-held otoscope (AudioScope), which generates pure tones at 500, 1000, 2000, and 4000 Hz and at two intensity levels, 25 or 40 dB. Outcome on the HHIE–S predicts need for hearing aids, whereas the AudioScope screen predicts level of hearing impairment.

The Tinnitus Handicap Questionnaire assesses self-reported handicapping effects of tinnitus. It can be used before and after treatment to measure effectiveness of therapy for tinnitus. The Abbreviated Profile of Hearing Aid Benefit is often used to assess outcomes with hearing aids. It quantifies the self-reported disabling effects of hearing impairment and assesses ease of communication, reverberation, speech understanding in the presence of background noise, and aversiveness to sound.

The whisper test, in which the tester whispers words at a measured distance from the patient's ear, is not as accurate a screen for hearing loss as the HHIE-S.

18. A 72-yr-old man comes to the office because he has increased difficulty with urination, including poor stream, straining to void, and occasional urinary incontinence. History includes benign prostatic hyperplasia, dyslipidemia, type 2 diabetes mellitus, and painful peripheral neuropathy; past medical history is significant for transient ischemic attack. Medications include clopidogrel 75 mg/d, doxazosin 2 mg at bedtime, glipizide 10 mg/d, atorvastatin 20 mg/d, and gabapentin 400 mg q8h. The patient's peripheral neuropathy has been difficult to manage. Further increase of gabapentin is not possible because it causes him dizziness. Nortriptyline 25 mg at bedtime was started 2 wk ago, and the patient reports decreased pain.

On examination, the patient's prostate is not enlarged, nor is his bladder palpable. Urinalysis is normal.

Which of the following should be done next to manage this patient's voiding difficulties?

(A) Increase doxazosin.
(B) Discontinue nortriptyline.
(C) Begin tolterodine.
(D) Obtain postvoid residual level.
(E) Obtain prostate-specific antigen level.

ANSWER: D

Although this patient's benign prostatic hyperplasia may be progressing, the recent addition of nortriptyline warrants excluding urinary retention due to introduction of a new medication. This is best accomplished through ultrasonography or straight catheterization assessment of postvoid residual. Medications with anticholinergic effects, such as

nortriptyline, can cause urinary retention by inhibiting contraction of bladder smooth muscle. Although nortriptyline has less anticholinergic activity than amitriptyline, it can cause urinary retention in susceptible individuals. Because nortriptyline[OL] has provided some pain relief in this patient, it should not be discontinued until the postvoid residual is accurately measured. If the residual is normal, it is unlikely that nortriptyline is contributing to his urinary symptoms.

The patient is on a low dosage of doxazosin for benign prostatic hyperplasia; increasing the dosage is a reasonable option to manage his symptoms after drug-induced urinary retention is excluded (SOE=A).

Tolterodine has anticholinergic activity and is used to treat symptoms of overactive bladder (eg, urinary frequency, urgency, urge incontinence). If this patient has urinary retention, tolterodine-related urinary retention could worsen incontinence. Adding anticholinergic bladder medication (eg, tolterodine) to α-adrenergic blocker therapy can improve symptoms in men with benign prostatic hyperplasia and symptoms of overactive bladder (SOE=A). Tolterodine could be considered after both α-blocker therapy has been maximized and postvoid residual has been excluded. Measuring the level of prostate-specific antigen is unlikely to assist in management of this patient's voiding symptoms.

19. A 69-yr-old woman with a history of deep venous thrombosis of right leg presents after diagnosis and surgical resection of estrogen and progesterone receptor-positive early stage breast cancer. She has been offered a balanced discussion of the risks and benefits of adjuvant therapy in the setting of early stage breast cancer. Her most recent dual x-ray absorptiometry (DEXA) results revealed no evidence of osteopenia.

Which of the following therapies is the best option for adjuvant therapy to reduce risk of recurrence and increase survival?

(A) Chemotherapy
(B) Tamoxifen
(C) Raloxifene
(D) Aromatase inhibitor therapy

ANSWER: D

While the use of 5 yr of adjuvant tamoxifen is well known to significantly decrease tumor recurrence and mortality in women with hormone-receptor–positive breast cancer, both with or without chemotherapy, the prevalence of breast cancer recurrence at 15 yr remains high at 30% with tamoxifen. Furthermore, tamoxifen is associated with significant adverse events, including thromboembolism and cerebrovascular events. A randomized trial of letrozole versus placebo in a group of 5,187 postmenopausal women after 5 yr of tamoxifen therapy for early stage breast cancer revealed significantly improved disease-free survival with 5 yr of letrozole therapy after completion of standard tamoxifen regimen. Results of this trial led to the direct comparison of aromatase inhibitor therapy to tamoxifen versus the combination of aromatase inhibitor and tamoxifen.

Based on results of the Arimidex, Tamoxifen, Alone or in Combination (ATAC) trial, aromatase inhibitors are now recommended as adjuvant treatment for postmenopausal women with hormone-receptor–positive early stage breast cancer. This trial showed significant efficacy and tolerability advantages over tamoxifen during the treatment phase, including a significantly prolonged disease-free survival and time to recurrence, and fewer occurrences of thromboembolism, ischemic cerebrovascular events and endometrial cancer. Based on the 100-mo follow-up analysis, lower recurrence rates are maintained with anastrazole, even after treatment has been completed. However, anastrazole was associated with an increase in fracture episodes as well as arthralgias.

Currently, most experts recommend that baseline bone mineral density examinations should be performed before aromatase inhibitor therapy is started in those suspected clinically to be at risk of osteopenia or osteoporosis.

Even though adjuvant chemotherapy is effective in treating breast cancer, by itself it is not as effective as either adjuvant tamoxifen or aromatase inhibitors in an older patient with estrogen- and progesterone-receptor–positive disease

 20. An 86-yr-old man comes to the office to establish care. His wife died 10 yr ago; he recently moved to the area to be closer to his children and grandchildren. History includes visual impairment secondary to macular degeneration, osteoarthritis of the hip and knee, insomnia, benign prostatic hyperplasia, and mild nocturia. Medications include aspirin and tamsulosin daily, and meloxicam and temazepam, each 3 or 4 times weekly. His alcohol history comprises 1 highball each night before dinner and 1 glass of wine with dinner. At least once a week, the patient has a second glass of wine during dinner. The patient reports that his current pattern of drinking has remained the same for the past 40 yr. His CAGE (**C**ut down, **A**nnoyed, **G**uilty, **E**ye opener) score is 0 of 4.

On examination, he has decreased visual acuity, an enlarged prostate, and an antalgic gait.

Which one of the following is the most appropriate intervention?

(A) Recommend continuing alcohol intake at this level.
(B) Recommend restricting alcohol intake to no more than 1 drink per day.
(C) Measure liver enzyme levels to assess for alcohol-related liver impairment.
(D) Defer discussion of alcohol consumption until relationship with patient is more established.
(E) Defer renewing prescriptions for meloxicam and temazepam until he agrees to abstain from alcohol.

ANSWER: B

Although light to moderate alcohol consumption has been associated with cardioprotective benefits in both middle-aged and older adults, it also poses substantial risk (SOE=A). Alcohol-related risk increases with age, due in part to age-related physiologic changes (decreased volume of distribution and gastric alcohol dehydrogenase levels) that result in higher blood alcohol levels in older adults than in younger adults. Thus, current guidelines recommend no more than 1 drink per day for people ≥65 yr old. This patient meets criteria for at-risk drinking: he has an average of 15 drinks per week, and regularly uses medications (a benzodiazepine and an NSAID) that may interact negatively with alcohol and increase his risk of alcohol-related morbidity.

Liver function tests have limited sensitivity as markers of alcohol-related liver injury in older adults and would not help to establish a diagnosis in this particular case. Failing to address the patient's alcohol consumption at the initial visit would be inappropriate, particularly given his comorbidity and medication list. Furthermore, his insomnia may be exacerbated by his alcohol intake. Substantial research has demonstrated that brief interventions can lead to substantial and sustained reductions in alcohol consumption, and should be instituted at the time of screening if at all possible (SOE=A).

Although elimination of either alcohol or benzodiazepines would be optimal, a stepwise approach to reducing both is more realistic than immediate abstinence.

21. A 67-yr-old man comes to the office with his family to obtain a second medical opinion. He has lost 18 kg (40 lb) in the past 6 mo, is weak, spends most of his time in bed, no longer participates in family activities, and is no longer interested in watching sporting events on television. He tends to sit quietly and let his family answer questions, but when questioned directly, he indicates that he cannot swallow solids or liquids because his throat is blocked. His family reports that he eats and drinks small amounts. He believes he has undiagnosed cancer that the doctors have yet to find.

Physical examination and cognitive assessment reveal some mild difficulties in recall. According to the medical records he provides, radiography and CT of the chest are normal, and upper endoscopy is unremarkable. Physical examination and several sets of blood work have been obtained, none of which indicate dehydration, anemia, or hepatic or renal dysfunction.

Which of the following is the most likely explanation for these findings?

(A) Occult lung cancer
(B) Vascular dementia
(C) Alzheimer's disease
(D) Major depressive disorder with psychotic features
(E) Parkinson's disease with psychotic symptoms

ANSWER: D

In older adults, the presentation of major depressive disorder with psychotic features is often masked by concomitant physical symptoms. This patient has a sustained belief of a physical abnormality not supported by medical evidence. The belief alone, however, is not sufficient for diagnosis of major depressive disorder with psychotic features. The patient has other suggestive signs and symptoms: psychomotor retardation, loss of interest, loss of energy, social withdrawal, and increased time in bed. These symptoms likely reflect depressive disorder rather than physical impairment, with the normal test results. Patients with occult malignancy can present with weight loss and poorly articulated physical complaints. However, the preponderance of depressive symptoms and his loss of interest in activities (eg, watching sports on television) that are unaffected by his physical limitations make occult malignancy unlikely. A primary psychiatric concern is also suggested by his delusional belief that he cannot swallow. This is contradicted by his family, as well as by his previous examinations.

Diagnosis of dementia requires the presence of memory impairment and at least one other deficit in another cognitive area such as language, executive function, or fine-motor coordination. Consequently, vascular dementia and Alzheimer's disease are unlikely. However, in a subgroup of older depressed adults with memory problems, dementia developed in subsequent years. The absence of symptoms of a movement disorder tends to exclude Parkinson's disease, although major depressive disorder can precede the onset of movement disorder in a subgroup of patients.

22. An 84-yr-old man comes to the office because he has pain in his lower back and right buttock. The pain has progressively worsened over the past year. It is most pronounced when he stands or walks for a prolonged period, and is often relieved when he sits. The pain is most severe when he first stands after sitting and when he tries to get in or out of an automobile. He has difficulty climbing stairs.

On examination, there is mild symmetric immobility of the lumbar spine. The straight-leg raise test is normal bilaterally. He has full strength of the proximal and distal muscles of both lower legs. There is 30° abduction, 45° external rotation, and 10° internal rotation of the left hip; and 10° abduction, 20° external rotation, and no internal rotation of the right hip. When the patient walks, he limps favoring his right leg.

Which of the following is the most appropriate next step?

(A) Radiography of the lumbar spine
(B) MRI of the lumbar spine
(C) Nerve conduction studies of the right lower leg
(D) Radiography of the right hip
(E) Bone scan

ANSWER: D

Hip disease is the great masquerader in musculoskeletal conditions. It classically causes pain in the groin, but it can present with pain in the thigh, lateral hip, buttock, and knee. Differentiation of hip from back disease is often difficult in patients with buttock and lateral hip pain. Pain when changing from supine to sitting position and with bending or stooping suggests the back as the cause of buttock pain. Hip disease is suggested if there is significant pain when a patient first gets out of a chair or bed or when there is difficulty ascending stairs, because hip flexion is the most important action when climbing. The patient should be assessed while he or she is walking. A limp is characteristic of hip disease and is rarely seen in back disease in the absence of sciatica.

For this patient, the most appropriate next step in the evaluation would be plain radiography of the right hip (SOE=D). The normal straight-leg raise test and absence of weakness of the proximal and distal leg muscles make back disease less likely. The presence of a limp especially suggests the hip as the cause of the pain, as do decreased range of motion of the right hip and relatively normal range of the left. In a study that compared hip with spine disease as a cause of back and leg pain, features that best predicted hip disease were groin pain, limp, and limited internal rotation of the hip. Therefore, radiography and MRI of the lumbar spine are not indicated.

The absence of sciatica makes lumbosacral radiculopathy less likely as the cause of this patient's pain, making nerve conduction studies

of the right lower leg a less useful diagnostic study in this patient. A bone scan in this patient would probably show increased uptake at the hips and other joints, consistent with degenerative joint disease. However, this finding is nonspecific and would be of little use in the evaluation of this patient.

23. A 70-yr-old woman comes to the office for a routine examination. She is cognitively intact and has a history of hypertension, macular degeneration, and osteoarthritis, mainly in her knees. She takes a multivitamin, lisinopril, and extra-strength acetaminophen as needed for pain.

Physical examination is normal, except that she wears pads. She reluctantly admits to having "accidents." She is embarrassed and worried, and has given up weekly bridge sessions. Lately she has been rushing to the bathroom frequently to prevent accidents. Which of the following is the most appropriate next step?

(A) Start an oxybutynin trial and schedule follow-up in 2 wk.
(B) Ask patient to keep a voiding diary and schedule follow-up in 2 wk.
(C) Start bladder retraining program and schedule follow-up in 2 wk.
(D) Obtain urology consultation.
(E) No further intervention is necessary.

ANSWER: B

This patient has involuntary loss of urine severe enough to affect her quality of life. From the history, it is not clear what type of incontinence she has. A voiding diary can help identify her exact symptoms and the severity of the problem. In addition, a medication review is indicated. Urinary incontinence is not a part of normal aging, although prevalence of the syndrome increases with age. Prevalence is higher in women than in men up to age 80, after which the prevalence is equal.

Conservative measures are highly effective for urinary incontinence in women. Kegel exercises significantly reduce symptoms of stress incontinence, although the cure rate is low (SOE=A). Bladder training should be first-line treatment for overactive bladder, because it is as effective as medication (SOE=A). Because the type of incontinence and its possible precipitants are unknown at this point, a trial of oxybutynin is premature and could be harmful. Clinical practice guidelines for urinary incontinence in adults recommend referral to specialists when there is no clear diagnosis, poor correlation between symptoms and clinical findings, inadequate response to therapy, hematuria without infection, comorbid conditions, or when surgery is a consideration (SOE=C).

24. A 79-yr-old man is discharged from the hospital after treatment for acute cholecystitis. History includes insulin-dependent diabetes mellitus, mild dementia, major depressive disorder, and recurrent falls (two in the past 6 mo). He has been hospitalized twice in the past year. He was delirious during the current hospitalization but is less confused at discharge. He lives with his daughter, who assists him with bathing and dressing. Arrangements are in place for a visiting nurse during the period immediately after discharge.

Medications during hospitalization included NPH and regular insulin, donepezil, acetaminophen, and a third-generation cephalosporin with metronidazole.

Which of the following is most likely to reduce this patient's risk of falls immediately after discharge?

(A) Supplemental vitamin D
(B) In-home occupational therapy
(C) Consultation with a podiatrist
(D) Consultation with an optometrist

ANSWER: B

The risk of a fall at home is greatest in the 2-wk period immediately after hospital discharge. Risk factors for falls during this period include impaired balance, new confusion or delirium, use of first-generation antidepressants, history of ≥2 falls in the past year, previous use of an assistive device for ambulation, prehospitalization dependency for ADLs, and greater number of hospitalizations in the prior year. This patient is at substantial risk.

Two studies on interventions designed to decrease falls in the period immediately after discharge both examined the value of home visits by an occupational therapist. In each study, the intervention included modification of environmental hazards, training in safe behaviors, and inclusion of mobility or functional aids. In both studies, patients who had home visits by an occupational therapist had fewer falls than patients who did not have occupational therapy at home (SOE=B).

A meta-analysis suggested that vitamin D supplements may reduce fall risk by about 20%, but a more recent study found that supplementation with cholecalciferol and calcium had a neutral effect on fall risk in men. There are no data on the use of vitamin D supplements to specifically reduce the risk of falls immediately after hospital discharge.

Podiatric or optometric consultation may theoretically reduce the risk of falls early after discharge, but these interventions in this setting have not been studied. However, in one randomized study of frail older outpatients, comprehensive vision and eye assessment with appropriate treatment did not reduce fall risk.

25. A 73-yr-old woman comes to the office for follow-up and medication refills. Her examination is unchanged since her last visit 3 mo ago, except that her weight has decreased from 99.8 kg (220 lb) to 92.5 kg (204 lb). She expresses surprise about the weight loss: "It's a miracle I didn't gain a ton. Since my daughter and grandchildren moved out, all I do is watch TV!"

Which one of the following is most appropriate?

(A) Set exercise and diet goals, and schedule follow-up in 2 mo.
(B) Discuss the weight loss and evaluate her for causes.
(C) Administer the Simplified Nutritional Assessment Questionnaire.
(D) Encourage her to continue to lose weight.
(E) Suggest a nutritional supplement to help her regain the lost weight.

ANSWER: B

This patient's unintentional weight loss is clinically significant (>5% in 3 mo) and requires attention even though she is overweight (SOE=A). Discussion of weight loss and evaluation for reversible causes are appropriate. Laboratory evaluation is part of a thorough evaluation for unintentional weight loss (SOE=C), as is age-appropriate screening for cancer. This patient may have provided an important clue to the cause of her weight loss: she may feel isolated (watching television most of the time and her family relocating to a different area). Screening for major depressive disorder may be warranted, because it is a common cause of weight loss and anorexia in older adults (SOE=B). If evaluation confirms that the patient is healthy, her goals for weight management (healthy, nonrestrictive diet and exercise) should be discussed.

Offering nutritional supplements to a patient with clinically significant unintentional weight loss without understanding the causes of the weight loss is inappropriate. Increasing caloric intake can lead to increased body fat and obese sarcopenia, because the patient is sedentary. This in turn can lead to functional decline (SOE=B).

The Simplified Nutritional Assessment Questionnaire is a validated risk-assessment instrument for community-dwelling and institutionalized adults. It is highly predictive for weight loss (SOE=B). In this case, however, significant weight loss is already present, and the questionnaire alone will not provide an evaluation of the causes of weight loss.

26. A 65-yr-old woman comes to the office to request advice about quitting smoking. She has a 40-pack-year smoking history. She wants to know whether she is too old to benefit from quitting.

Which of the following is a benefit of smoking cessation as an older adult?

(A) Circulation improves 5 yr after cessation.
(B) Lung function improves 5 yr after cessation.
(C) She would live longer.
(D) The risk of dying from heart disease decreases to 5 times that of a nonsmoker.

ANSWER: C

Current data suggest that 9% of people >65 yr old smoke, despite increased risk of death, lung cancer, dementia, stroke, and heart attack. Of the approximately 440,000 deaths each year from smoking-related diseases, 300,000 occur in adults ≥65 yr old. Advocating for smoking cessation is an important role for clinicians, and older adults are encouraged to quit when their clinicians discuss the benefits with them.

Lung function and circulation begin to improve immediately after smoking cessation. Irrespective of age or length of time since quitting, former smokers have cardiovascular mortality rates similar to those of nonsmokers. Longevity studies show that among smokers who quit at age 65, men gain 1.4–12 yr of life and women gain 2.7–3.4 yr (SOE=A).

Clinicians who use the 5-step approach—**ask** about smoking, **advise** to quit, **assess** a patient's willingness, **assist** the patient in developing a quitting plan, and **arrange** for follow-up—can significantly improve the health of older patients who smoke (SOE=A).

27. A 79-yr-old man comes to the office because he has increasing difficulty understanding conversations with his grandchildren.

Which of the following is the most likely diagnosis?

(A) Presbycusis
(B) Sociocusis
(C) Ototoxicity
(D) Acoustic neuroma

ANSWER: A

Approximately 40%–50% of adults ≥75 yr old have age-related hearing loss (presbycusis); it is the fourth most common chronic condition and contributes to cognitive and physical decline. Characteristic pathologic changes in the temporal bone correlate with six types of presbycusis, each having a distinctive pattern of hearing loss. The hearing loss is sensorineural, bilateral, symmetric, and gradual in onset. Manifestations include difficulty understanding speech, especially in noisy situations. Older adults with presbycusis report that they can hear people speaking but cannot make out the words.

Sociocusis refers to non-workplace-related hearing loss due to exposure to noise. Ototoxicity refers to the toxic effects of medications on the sensory and balance structures of the inner ear. Aminoglycosides, salicylates, and cisplatin are toxic to the hearing mechanism and can cause hearing or balance problems. Older adults are often susceptible to ototoxicity, especially when kidney function is compromised. Hearing testing and laboratory tests can be used to monitor the early onset of ototoxic effects. Presbycusis is more common than ototoxicity.

Acoustic neuroma usually causes unilateral hearing loss.

It is often difficult for audiologists to determine from the audiogram whether hearing loss is due solely to the effects of aging, because environmental factors and ototoxicity are also associated with loss that is sensorineural and affects primarily high-frequency hearing.

28. A 70-yr-old retired mailman comes to the office because he now has difficulty climbing 1 flight of stairs. He has dyspnea on exertion that has progressed slowly over 5 yr. He wheezes occasionally. He has had a minimally productive morning cough for many years but no chest pain or discomfort. He has a 50-pack-year cigarette smoking history and still smokes.

On examination, temperature is 36° C (96.8° F), blood pressure is 115/75 mmHg, heart rate is 98 beats per minute, and respiratory rate is 22 breaths per minute. There is no accessory muscle use. Bibasilar crackles are audible. Cardiac and abdominal examinations are normal. There is trace peripheral edema but no cyanosis or clubbing. Chest radiography is normal.

Pulmonary function tests:

FVC	65% of predicted
FEV_1	70% of predicted
FEV_1/FVC ratio	75%

After bronchodilation, FEV_1 increases by 9% and FVC increases by 8%.

Which of the following is the most likely cause of this patient's dyspnea?

(A) Asthma
(B) COPD
(C) Idiopathic pulmonary fibrosis
(D) Pleural effusion
(E) Pulmonary embolism

ANSWER: C

This patient's FEV_1/FVC ratio is ≥70%, which is consistent with either normal spirometry or restrictive disease. Because the FVC is <70% of predicted, the patient's spirometry is consistent with restrictive disease. Spirometry measures the rate of airflow out of the lungs during rapid, forceful, and complete expiration from total lung capacity to residual volume (forced vital capacity maneuver). This test provides an indirect measure of the flow-resistive properties of the lungs. The critical values to interpret are the FEV_1, the FVC, and the FEV_1/FVC ratio. FEV_1 is a measure of airflow, and FVC a measure of volume. The "reversibility" of airflow obstruction is evaluated by repeating spirometry 15 min after administration of a bronchodilator, usually a β_2-agonist such as albuterol. While the presence of "reversibility" indicates that asthma is a component of the disease, it is not pathognomonic for asthma. A reasonable normal range for FEV_1 and FVC is between 80% and 100% of predicted, and ≥70% (actual number, not percent predicted) for the FEV_1/FVC ratio. However, because structural changes occur in the airways with age, some experts recommend using an FEV_1/FVC ratio of ≥65% for adults ≥70 yr old. Significant reversibility is defined as ≥12% increase in either FEV_1 or FVC.

Asthma and COPD cause obstructive, not restrictive, disease. Pulmonary embolism is a pulmonary vascular disease and usually causes neither obstruction nor restriction. Although both pleural effusion and idiopathic pulmonary fibrosis can cause restriction, the absence of pleural disease on chest radiography makes effusion unlikely. Between 10% and 15% of cases of interstitial lung disease are associated with normal chest radiography. This patient's normal chest radiograph is consistent with idiopathic pulmonary fibrosis (SOE=A).

29. An 80-yr-old woman comes to the office because she has lost 4.5 kg (10 lb) in the preceding year, feels that everything she does is an "effort," and has begun using her arms to lift herself from her chair. She states that she is not depressed. She is accompanied by her daughter, with whom she lives.

Physical examination is normal except that she appears tired and has a slow, steady gait. She scores one positive response on the Geriatric Depression Scale. Results of a CBC, BUN, creatinine, electrolytes, and thyroid and liver function tests are normal. Frailty is diagnosed.

Which of the following is the most appropriate next step?

(A) Begin a trial of methylphenidate.
(B) Begin protein supplements.
(C) Begin a resistance-training exercise program.
(D) Encourage increased social interaction.
(E) Initiate a palliative care approach.

ANSWER: C

The clinical syndrome of frailty presents with multiple areas of decline: weakness, low energy or exhaustion, slowed walking speed, low physical activity, and weight loss. Many studies, each using different definitions of the syndrome, have found frailty to be associated with poor clinical outcomes, such as falls, functional decline, and mortality. A few studies have addressed interventions. Resistance training increases strength and function in frail nursing-home residents (SOE=A) and in patients recovering from hip fracture (SOE=A). Ongoing evaluation of the patient response including tolerance of the program is essential.

Methylphenidate has been studied in small trials of medically ill adults, but results have been inconsistent. Protein supplements also have not consistently improved clinical outcomes. Social isolation appears to contribute to functional decline, but interventions to enhance social interactions have not yet been shown to improve frailty. There is emerging evidence that severe frailty may not be reversible and that palliative care may be warranted. However, palliative care is premature in this patient, because treatment has not yet been attempted.

30. A 78-yr-old woman comes to the office because she has pain when she urinates. She has been seen three times for this problem in the last 3 mo. Each time she was told she had a urinary tract infection and was given a course of antibiotics. She has carefully followed the instructions for the antibiotics but has had no relief of symptoms.

Results of her last urinalysis:

WBCs	2 to 3/high-power field
RBCs	0 to 2/high-power field
Epithelial cells	Few
Nitrite	Negative
Leukocyte esterase	Negative

Which of the following should be done next?

(A) Send a clean-catch urine specimen for urinalysis and culture.
(B) Perform pelvic examination.
(C) Reassure the patient that she has asymptomatic bacteruria and that antibiotics are unlikely to help.
(D) Refer for cystoscopy.
(E) Order pelvic ultrasonography.

ANSWER: B

In this patient's previous visits, the urine specimen may not have been a clean catch, and positive cultures may represent contamination. After several rounds of antibiotics with no improvement in symptoms, the diagnosis of urinary tract infection should be suspect. Pelvic examination should be performed before additional laboratory work, ultrasonography, or referral for cystoscopy (SOE=D).

Urinary tract structures, deriving from the same embryologic origin as the genital tract, contain estrogen receptors and are estrogen dependent. The bladder, urethra, pelvic floor musculature, and endopelvic fascia are affected by a hypoestrogenic state, as is the vaginal epithelium with menopause. Possible consequences of urinary tract atrophy include urethral discomfort, frequency, hematuria, dysuria, and increased likelihood of urinary tract infection. Pelvic laxity and stress incontinence can also occur.

Diagnosis of vaginal atrophy is based on characteristic symptoms in the history and on findings of the physical examination. Classic findings include pale, dry vaginal epithelium that is smooth and shiny, with loss of most rugae. Laboratory tests are unnecessary and not diagnostic.

Unless contraindicated, systemic or local estrogen is the most effective treatment (SOE=A). Vaginal administration minimizes the degree of systemic absorption, although it can increase plasma levels of estrogen.

Local estrogen applications include low-dose creams, rings, and tablets. One strategy is low-dose vaginal estrogen cream 0.5 g/d for 3 wk, with twice-weekly administration thereafter. The estradiol ring (Estring®) delivers 6–9 mcg of estradiol to the vagina daily for 3 mo. The vaginal estrogen tablet (Vagifem®) is usually recommended every day for 2 wk, then twice weekly. Progestins are not prescribed routinely for women treated with low-dose vaginal estrogen. In women with breast cancer, vaginal estrogen is not used for symptoms of urogenital atrophy unless recommended by the woman's oncologist.

Although asymptomatic bacteruria should not be treated with antibiotics, reassuring the patient will not address her urogenital symptoms.

31. An 82-yr-old man comes to the office for preoperative evaluation before elective hip replacement. He cannot walk 2 blocks without incapacitating hip pain. He has no chest pain or dyspnea, and there is no history of myocardial infarction, stroke, or diabetes mellitus. He has hypertension and dyslipidemia. Medications are atenolol 50 mg/d and lovastatin 20 mg/d.

On physical examination, blood pressure is 140/70 mmHg and heart rate is 76 beats per minute and regular. On auscultation, chest and lungs are clear; there is a 2/6 systolic ejection murmur, and there is no third or fourth heart sound. There is no edema, and pulses are intact. ECG shows normal sinus rhythm with left-ventricle hypertrophy.

Which of the following is indicated as part of his preoperative evaluation?

(A) Stress echocardiography
(B) Nuclear stress test
(C) Coronary angiography
(D) Measurement of creatinine
(E) Measurement of brain natriuretic peptide

ANSWER: D

This patient has poor functional capacity (<4 metabolic equivalents) and is scheduled for elective noncardiac surgery. The need for additional preoperative testing is based on the number of clinical risk factors and the type of surgery planned. In patients with no clinical risk factors, no additional testing is required. In patients with 1 or 2 clinical risk factors and controlled heart rate, cardiac stress testing is at the discretion of the clinician. In patients with ≥3 clinical risk factors, stress testing is recommended before vascular surgery and is optional before intermediate-risk surgery (SOE=B).

According to the Revised Cardiac Risk Index, clinical risk factors include a history of ischemic heart disease, heart failure, cerebrovascular disease (ie, history of transient ischemic attack or stroke), diabetes mellitus, and renal insufficiency (preoperative serum creatinine >2 mg/dL). This patient's creatinine concentration must be obtained to calculate his risk factor score. If the concentration is <2 mg/dL, his score would be 0 because he has no other clinical risk factors. Therefore, no cardiac evaluation would be indicated. If his creatinine concentration is >2 mg/dL, his score would be 1 and further cardiac noninvasive evaluation would be optional. He is on a β-blocker and his heart rate is controlled. His β-blocker should be continued perioperatively. Any patient on a β-blocker preoperatively should be continued on β-blockers in the perioperative period (SOE=A).

Measurement of brain natriuretic peptide would not useful in this patient with no signs or symptoms of heart failure.

32. An active 75-yr-old man with no significant medical history has a chief complaint of dry scaling feet and thickened nails. The patient indicates that, for >20 yr, he has had thick nails starting in the great toes. Over the last few years, this has spread to his lesser digits. His main complaint is chronic itching and scaling feet. Self-care has included nail trimming and OTC hand cream, which he applies a few times a week. Physical examination shows dry erythematous scaling in a moccasin distribution bilaterally, web-space scaling, and thickened yellow nails. Neurovascular examination is within normal limits.

What is the most likely causative organism?

(A) *Candia albicans*
(B) *Microsporum canis*
(C) *Trichophyton rubrum*
(D) *Corneum bacterium*

ANSWER: C

The incidence of onychomycosis rises with age and often leads to chronic athlete's feet. It is usually caused by a dermatophyte infection. *Trichophyton rubrum* has been reported to be the infecting organism in up to 90% of cases (SOE=A). *Microsporum canis*, another dermatophyte, has been demonstrated to cause onychomycosis, although this type of infection is rare. Yeast infections do not usually involve the toenails, and more commonly cause fingernail infections in patients chronically exposed to water. Bacterial infections do affect the feet but do not present with chronic scaling. *Corneum bacterium* is associated with pitted keratolysis and presents with moisture and odor limited to web spaces and weight-bearing plantar skin.

33. An 85-yr-old woman is brought to the emergency department after she is found on the bathroom floor at home. She has retrograde amnesia for the circumstances surrounding the episode, and denies any confusion after the episode. There were no witnesses. History includes hypertension, for which she takes atenolol 25 mg/d and hydrochlorothiazide 25 mg/d.

On physical examination, she has a right periorbital ecchymosis. Blood pressure is 152/84 mmHg while supine and 146/86 mmHg while upright, and heart rate is 76 beats per minute while supine and 86 beats per minute while upright. There is no jugular venous distension or carotid bruit. Lungs are clear. Carotid upstroke is delayed, with a II/VI midpeaking systolic murmur at the base; the second heart sound is not audible.

CT of the head and facial bones shows a large, right periorbital contusion and no fractures.

Which of the following is the most appropriate next step in the evaluation of this patient?

(A) Blood tests
(B) Echocardiography
(C) Holter monitoring
(D) Event monitor
(E) Tilt-table test

ANSWER: B

This patient's clinical history suggests syncope, although in the absence of a definitive history, an unexplained fall is also possible. In older adults, syncope and unexplained falls can be indistinguishable clinical manifestations of the same pathophysiologic process, and for this reason many clinicians treat them as the same. This patient's physical examination suggests significant aortic stenosis. While the murmur is not loud and is midpeaking, the absence of a second heart sound indicates potentially severe aortic stenosis. Echocardiography can characterize the degree of aortic stenosis noninvasively. Because structural heart disease is the most important risk factor in unexplained syncope, echocardiography should be the next test ordered.

Echocardiographic findings of severe valvular abnormalities, ventricular hypertrophy with outflow obstruction, severe pulmonary hypertension, and atrial myxoma or thrombus are rare in the absence of a suggestive initial evaluation. In a study of 650 consecutive patients with syncope (average age 60 yr, with 44% of patients ≥75 yr old), echocardiography was useful mainly in confirming suspected severe aortic stenosis and for using ejection fraction to stratify patients with known cardiac disease. Echocardiography was normal or irrelevant in all patients who had no history, physical examination, or electrocardiography suggesting cardiac disease (SOE=A).

Blood tests have an extremely low diagnostic yield for patients with unexplained syncope. For example, hypoglycemia does not result in a transient loss of consciousness but rather requires intervention to reverse the metabolic derangement that could be contributing to symptoms. Unless it uncovers frequent ventricular ectopy or nonsustained ventricular tachycardia, short-term continuous electrocardiographic monitoring, such as telemetry, Holter monitor, or an event monitor, is not useful for identifying the cause of syncope because weeks, months, or even years can pass before the next arrhythmia-related event. Also, most arrhythmias detected in patients with syncope are brief and result in no symptoms.

Triage decisions and management should be based on preexisting cardiac disease or echocardiographic abnormalities, which are important predictors of arrhythmic syncope and mortality, rather than on symptoms. A tilt-table test would be appropriate only after structural heart disease has been excluded.

34. A 92-yr-old man with Alzheimer's disease is brought to the office by his daughter because over the past several months he has become increasingly aggressive toward his wife and home health aide. His daughter is worried about their safety and asks that he be given medication to control his aggression. Discussion ensues regarding different psychotropic options.

Which of the following is associated with increased mortality?

(A) Antipsychotic agents
(B) Antidepressant agents
(C) Mood stabilizers
(D) Anticholinesterase agents

ANSWER: A

The FDA mandates that second-generation antipsychotic agents carry a black-box warning of increased risk of mortality when taken by patients with dementia. Most placebo-controlled studies of dementia patients treated with second-generation antipsychotic agents (eg, olanzapine, aripiprazole, quetiapine, risperidone) report greater mortality (SOE=A), primarily from cardiac effect or infection. It is not clear what mechanism underlies this risk. In one meta-analysis, the absolute risk of death for dementia patients exposed to antipsychotic agents was 3.5%, while the absolute risk in patients given a placebo was 2.3%, yielding an NNH (number needed to harm) of 83 for that outcome.

Several studies suggest that the risk of death in patients with dementia is higher with first-generation than with second-generation antipsychotics. A recent meta-analysis comparing second-generation agents with haloperidol identified a relatively higher

mortality risk with haloperidol. In a 12-mo study comparing first- or second-generation antipsychotics with nonantipsychotic psychotropic medications in outpatients with dementia, antipsychotic agents were associated with significantly higher mortality rates (23%–29%) than nonantipsychotic psychotropics (15%) (SOE=B). The study did not differentiate among cerebrovascular, cardiovascular, or infection-related deaths in patients taking antipsychotics versus other psychotropic drugs. However, not all studies have replicated this finding, and no pathophysiologic mechanism has been clearly identified. It is not known whether the association between higher mortality and antipsychotic use reflects a direct medication effect or the pathophysiologic process associated with the symptoms that necessitated their use.

35. An 88-yr-old man comes to the clinic for the first time in 18 mo, accompanied by his son. The patient states that he has no active medical problems. He has lived alone since his wife's death 10 yr ago. He is not sexually active and does not smoke or drink alcohol. The son states that his father has lost weight, is less active socially than he used to be, has little energy or endurance, and spends most of his time reading or watching television. On detailed questioning, the patient indicates that he often skips meals but otherwise feels his appetite is unchanged. He does all his own cooking. His son notes that when his dad comes to his house on weekends, he eats well. The patient indicates that he does not have problems sleeping, swallowing, or voiding. He has had no change in bowel habits, no incontinence, and no depressive symptoms. History includes early-stage prostate cancer, for which he had a prostatectomy 8 yr ago; at follow-up 1 yr ago, his urologist told him there was no evidence of recurrence. Screening colonoscopy done 2 yr ago was normal. The patient takes a daily multivitamin.

On examination, the patient weighs 62.6 kg (138 lb; body mass index, 22 kg/m²), which, according to medical records, is 13% less than he weighed 18 mo ago. The rest of his physical examination is normal. His score on the Mini–Mental State Examination is 29/30; his score on the Yesavage Geriatric Depression Scale–Short Form is 2/15. Fecal guaiac is negative. Urinalysis, CBC, electrolytes, vitamin B_{12}, and liver, renal, and thyroid function tests are normal, and prostate-specific antigen is undetectable. ECG reveals normal sinus rhythm, and chest radiography is normal.

Which of the following is the most appropriate next step?

(A) CT of the chest, abdomen, and pelvis
(B) Upper and lower endoscopy
(C) Upper GI series with small-bowel follow-through
(D) Complete radiographic bone survey
(E) No further diagnostic testing

ANSWER: E

Involuntary weight loss in older adults is always cause for concern. It is often a harbinger of subsequent adverse clinical events, including death. The risk of death increases in direct proportion to the amount and rate of the weight loss. As a general rule, loss of >5% body weight within 1 mo or >10% in 6 mo should prompt a careful evaluation. However, even lesser amounts of weight loss can be clinically significant. Among community-dwelling older adults, weight loss of 5% over 3 yr is associated with increased mortality.

In older patients, potential causes of involuntary weight loss are often readily identifiable by history and physical examination alone. When this is not the case, more thorough diagnostic evaluation is warranted, using the same basic, focused panel of tests as was obtained for this patient. Additional tests are ordered only as required to investigate abnormalities identified in the initial screen. If the initial screen is unrevealing, a period of "watchful waiting" is appropriate, rather than more extensive undirected testing (SOE=B). In the case presented, the initial evaluation did not identify any abnormalities that would warrant further diagnostic testing. Addressing the patient's known risk factors for weight loss, such as social isolation and low level of physical activity, would probably benefit him more than additional tests.

Use of CT of the chest, abdomen, and pelvis is controversial when the initial diagnostic evaluation is normal in older adults with weight loss (SOE=D). Although several studies have demonstrated that such an approach will

sometimes identify unrecognized malignancy or other serious disease, there is no evidence that this information results in improved patient outcome. Such testing is also associated with a high probability of false-positive results that can lead to further, potentially harmful diagnostic testing. Substituting MRI for CT can decrease the risk of contrast-induced pathology but does not improve diagnostic accuracy. Similar concerns pertain to the use of endoscopy or barium studies. Because this patient has no evidence of metastatic cancer, a bone survey is not warranted.

36. A 70-yr-old woman comes to the office because she has had a malodorous vaginal discharge for 1 wk. She has vulvovaginal burning, itching, and soreness that have intensified over the past few months. At menopause 15 yr ago, she had similar symptoms, minus the discharge, and hot flashes. She was treated with cyclic oral estrogen and progesterone, but she stopped hormone replacement therapy after several years because she was concerned about adverse events. After the hot flashes abated, she had increasing vaginal soreness, pain, and burning after intercourse. In the past 10 yr, she has had 2 urinary tract infections, the most recent >1 yr ago. She recently tried application of aloe vera gel in an effort to relieve the itching, without effect. She does not wish to go back on hormone therapy.

On examination, there is redness and erythema in the vulvovaginal area, sparse pubic hair, and decreased vaginal moisture. Insertion of an adult speculum is moderately difficult and results in slight bleeding. Mucosa appears inflamed. Occasional vaginal petechiae are evident, and there are some fissures on the vaginal walls. There are no vaginal folds. No growths, plaques, or suspicious structures are seen or palpated. Serosanguineous discharge is present, with a pH of 6.8. A vaginal smear taken from the upper lateral third of the vagina reveals increased parabasal cells, an inflammatory exudate, and classic "blue blobs" (basophilic structures).

Which of the following is the most likely explanation for these findings?

(A) Candidiasis
(B) Atrophic vaginitis
(C) Psoriasis
(D) Vaginal cancer

ANSWER: B

With menopause, loss of estrogen results in atrophy of vulvar and vaginal epithelium. In vaginal atrophy, the number of superficial mature cells of the vagina are reduced, with a shift in cell structure to parabasal cells with a high nuclear/cytoplasmic ratio. These cells do not produce much glycogen, on which lactobacilli depend. Vaginal pH becomes higher than 4.5 because of decreased lactic acid production, and lactobacilli become fewer or disappear. There may be a shift toward coliform organisms. Vaginal rugae smooth out, the mucosa thins, and fissures may develop. Vaginal smears show WBCs and decreased or no lactobacilli (SOE=A).

   Candidiasis usually causes a cheesy discharge with hyphae, not a serosanguineous discharge. It is usually seen at a younger age, or in the setting of diabetes or recent antibiotic use (SOE=B). This patient has no history of psoriasis. When psoriasis is present, its spread is symmetric, it does not involve the vagina, and it causes scaly red lesions. Cervical or vaginal cancer, although uncommon in this age group, can also be associated with a serosanguineous discharge. Usually, there is evidence of suspicious lesions, new growths, or areas of induration, any of which should be biopsied. Because no suspicious lesions were seen or palpated, vaginal cancer is unlikely. The 2003 guidelines from the U.S. Preventive Services Task Force recommend discontinuing screening for cervical cancer after age 65 if previous results were consistently normal (SOE=B). However, Pap smear would be prudent in the presence of a serosanguineous discharge (SOE=B).

 37. A 72-yr-old retired bookkeeper is brought to the office by her husband because she has had gradually increasing problems with her memory over the past year. At first he noticed that his wife had trouble remembering the names of new acquaintances. This progressed to difficulty recalling details of books they read together, and more recently she had to telephone him for help because she could not recall where she had parked her car. Last month the husband had to take control of managing the household finances, a job she had performed competently throughout their marriage. Alzheimer's disease is diagnosed after physical examination and evaluation including laboratory tests and structural neuroimaging. The couple asks you about cholinesterase inhibitor treatment.

Which of the following statements is the most appropriate response?

(A) The most common adverse events are headache and somnolence.
(B) Liver function must be monitored for the first 6 mo of treatment.
(C) Improvement of cognitive symptoms is sustained during the first 5 yr of treatment.
(D) Benefits are likely to be clinically subtle.
(E) Cholinesterase inhibitors differ significantly from one another in their effectiveness.

ANSWER: D

Since their introduction in 1997, cholinesterase inhibitors (eg, donepezil, galantamine, and rivastigmine) have become first-line treatment for Alzheimer's disease. Although their pharmacologic properties differ slightly, they all work by inhibiting acetylcholine esterase, the primary enzyme involved in breaking down the neurotransmitter acetylcholine. A 2006 Cochrane review concluded that all three medications are efficacious for mild to moderate Alzheimer's disease (SOE=B).

   The most common adverse events reported with cholinesterase inhibitors are nausea, vomiting, and diarrhea. Because the adverse events are cholinergic and tend to be dose-related, cholinesterase inhibitors require low starting dosages with gradual upward titration. No laboratory monitoring is routinely required.

   Most studies have examined treatment response for 1–2 yr, so there is little evidence on duration of effectiveness. Cumulative results to date indicate that use of a cholinesterase inhibitor has a statistically significant positive effect on tests of cognition for 6–12 mo, although effect is generally modest. Benefits include improved performance on the ADAS-Cog Scale (a global scale of cognition), better ratings of global clinical state by clinicians blinded to other measures, and better ratings on scales of behavior and ADLs. Few studies have reported results in terms of improvements that are likely to be evident to patients and caregivers. Clinically apparent benefits can be subtle or can occur primarily via slowed progression. Patients and caregivers are at risk of therapeutic nihilism in the absence of counseling about treatment expectations.

There have been few comparative trials of different cholinesterase inhibitors. Most have been supported at least in part by pharmaceutical companies and have methodologic weaknesses, such as inadequate study duration. In a 2-yr, double-blind, randomized, multicenter trial from the United Kingdom in which rivastigmine and donepezil were compared, more frequent adverse events were reported for rivastigmine during the titration phase (SOE=A). Although some statistically significant differences between the two medications were reported in subgroup analyses, overall efficacy on cognition and behavior was similar.

38. A 67-yr-old woman comes to the office for advice regarding diet. She recently had a modified radical mastectomy for stage I breast cancer. She chose this approach because she wanted to avoid radiation and chemotherapy. She has always had a healthy lifestyle. She asks whether there are any dietary changes she could make to avoid recurrence of breast cancer.

Which of the following is most likely to reduce breast cancer recurrence?

(A) Increase soy foods.
(B) Drink 4 cups of green tea daily.
(C) Restrict fats to <10% of diet.
(D) Follow a strict vegetarian diet.

ANSWER: B

Green tea has been shown to reduce the recurrence of stages I and II breast cancer. A meta-analysis of 13 studies indicated a lower risk of breast cancer with green (but not black) tea consumption. There are multiple mechanisms for the role of tea in cancer prevention: tea has antioxidant and antiangiogenic properties, and it suppresses proliferation of neoplastic cells,

inhibits formation of N-nitroso compounds, inhibits cell division by telomerase inhibition, upregulates intracellular gap junction communication, interferes with estrogen metabolism, and increases apoptosis in cancer cells. The recommended amount for cancer prevention is 4 to 5 cups daily (SOE=B).

The recommendation to eat soy foods is controversial for women who have had breast cancer. Epidemiologic data support soy food as preventive of breast cancer only if it is consumed during adolescence. In vitro data show both tumor growth and suppression with exposure to soy (SOE=C).

The Women's Health Initiative did not show a statistically significant reduction in recurrence of breast cancer with a low-fat diet. In this 8-yr study, women were asked to reduce fat to 20% of total calories. Only 31% of the women were able to meet the goal at year 1, and only 14% at year 6; the result was an underpowered study (SOE=A).

A strict vegetarian diet has not been assessed for prevention of breast cancer. There is epidemiologic evidence of increased risk with beef and with any burnt animal flesh (SOE=D).

39. An 89-yr-old man presents to you complaining of generalized weakness. General physical examination and neurologic examination are normal. He lives with his wife in a rural community, is independent in ADLs and IADLs, and rarely drives. He has avoided medical care for most of his life. He is on no medications other than calcium, vitamin D, and aspirin 81 mg/d.

Laboratory tests:

Hgb	11.9 g/dL
Hematocrit	35%
Mean corpuscular volume	102 mm^3
Serum B$_{12}$	200 pg/mL (low normal)
Methylmalonic acid	300 nmol/L (increased)
Homocysteine	18 μmol/L (increased)
RBC folate	normal
Ferritin	250 ng/mL

What is the best next step?

(A) Prescribe oral vitamin B$_{12}$ 1000 mcg/d
(B) Administer vitamin B$_{12}$ 1000 mcg IM weekly for 8 wk, followed by 1000 mcg IM monthly
(C) Administer a 3-part Schilling test.
(D) Recommend upper and lower endoscopy to exclude pernicious anemia and bacterial overgrowth syndrome.

ANSWER: A

Many patients with B$_{12}$ deficiency have no or mild hematologic or neurologic symptoms. In one study, less than one-third of patients with documented B$_{12}$ deficiency had anemia or macrocytosis (SOE=B). The diagnosis of vitamin B$_{12}$ deficiency can be made with relative certainty (specificity of ≥95%) when the serum concentration is <200 pg/mL (<148 pmol/L) (SOE=B). For indeterminate result (200–300 pg/mL (148–241 pmol/L), increased methylmalonic acid and homocysteine concentrations can help establish the diagnosis with a sensitivity of 94% and specificity of 99% (SOE=A).

Causes of B$_{12}$ deficiency include pernicious anemia, history of gastrectomy, malapsorption syndromes, ileal resection or bypass, pancreatic insufficiency, diet, and a number of medications (eg, proton pump inhibitors). While many authors argue that a cause for B$_{12}$ deficiency must be found, it has never been demonstrated that identifying a cause for B$_{12}$ deficiency improves clinical outcomes (SOE=B). The clinician needs to think carefully about whether finding the cause of B$_{12}$ deficiency will be helpful in managing a particular patient. Anti-intrinsic factor antibodies are highly specific for pernicious anemia and can help establish the diagnosis. Schilling tests are rarely necessary (SOE=C).

Recommended options for vitamin B$_{12}$ replacement include oral or sublingual delivery of 500–2000 mcg/d, intranasal administration of 500 mcg/wk in one nostril, and intramuscular or deep subcutaneous delivery of 30 mcg/day for 5 to 10 days, followed by a maintenance dose of 100–200 mcg/mo; parenteral and oral options have equivalent efficacy in most patients, even in the absence of intrinsic factor (SOE=B). A response to therapy should be documented, and in the rare patient in whom oral therapy is not effective, the dosage should be increased or parenteral therapy should be substituted (SOE=C).

In this patient, who lives in a rural area, does not drive, and is not an enthusiastic consumer of medical care, a trial of oral B$_{12}$ therapy should be initiated. Parenteral therapy would be a reasonable alternative if the patient were able to get into the clinic or receive injections at home, or if he did not respond to oral therapy. A Schilling test would be unlikely to influence therapy in this patient who is otherwise asymptomatic. Endoscopy and colonoscopy are not indicated in an 89-yr-old man with no evidence of iron deficiency anemia (SOE=B).

40. A 70-yr-old man comes to the office because he has diarrhea with associated crampy abdominal pain and low-grade fever. The diarrhea began 3 days earlier; he is passing up to 5 watery, nonbloody bowel movements daily. History includes venous insufficiency, and he was recently treated with a 7-day course of cephalexin for lower-extremity cellulitis.

On examination, he does not look ill, and vital signs are normal. Abdominal examination demonstrates mild, nonspecific diffuse tenderness without guarding or rebound. Bowel sounds are present. Laboratory results are normal except for a WBC count of 11,000/μL. Abdominal radiography demonstrates a nonspecific gas pattern. Enzyme immunoassay detects the presence of *Clostridium difficile* toxin A. His symptoms improve with a 10-day course of oral metronidazole, but diarrhea recurs within 1 week, and enzyme immunoassay again detects *C difficile* toxin A.

Which of the following should be prescribed next?

(A) Rifampin and metronidazole
(B) Metronidazole
(C) Vancomycin
(D) Cholestyramine
(E) *Saccharomyces boulardii*

ANSWER: B

Clostridium difficile, the most common enteric pathogen, can colonize the large intestine of patients taking antibiotics. Infection can be asymptomatic, or symptoms can range from mild diarrhea to fulminant pseudomembranous colitis. Recent outbreaks of *C difficile* infection in North America have been due to a more virulent and possibly more resistant strain (BI/NAP1) that causes more severe disease.

The offending antibiotic must be stopped immediately, and medications with antiperistaltic activity avoided unless absolutely necessary. The CDC recommends that oral metronidazole be used as first-line therapy rather than vancomycin for all but seriously ill patients and those with complicated or fulminant infections or multiple recurrences. Most sources suggest stopping treatment after 10 days if symptoms have resolved (SOE=C); complicated cases may require longer or individualized treatment regimens (SOE=D). Metronidazole is less expensive than vancomycin, and its use avoids the risk of colonization with vancomycin-resistant organisms. Metronidazole and vancomycin are equally effective for treatment of mild *C difficile*–associated disease; vancomycin is superior for treating severe *C difficile*–associated disease (SOE=A). A trial of combination rifampin and metronidazole therapy for first-episode cases found the combination to be no better than therapy with metronidazole alone.

Despite successful initial therapy, *C. difficile* infection recurs in >20% of patients. Typically, relapse does not result in progression of disease or symptom severity. First relapses should be treated with the original medical regimen: up to 90% of cases can be treated successfully on first recurrence with the agent that was initially used (SOE=C).

Different regimens are used for patients with multiple relapses. These include continuous or pulsed dosing of oral vancomycin, anion exchange resins such as cholestyramine or colestipol that bind to *C difficile* toxins in the colon, probiotics (ie, *Saccharomyces boulardii*, *Lactobacillus rhamnosus* strain GG, and *Lactobacillus acidophilus*), intravenous immunoglobulin, and feces transplant. All of these measures are successful some of the time, but none is successful all of the time.

44. A 78-yr-old man comes to the office because he volunteers at the local hospital and is required to get a tuberculin skin test annually. A tuberculosis skin test (PPD) using 5 tuberculin units was done a year ago when he first started. At that time, the test was read as 4 mm of induration and interpreted as negative. On retesting now a year later, there is 16 mm of induration. He has no symptoms, and chest radiograph is negative. He is on coumadin for atrial fibrillation but has no other problems and no other medications.

What is the most appropriate next step in management?

(A) Observation only
(B) Annual chest radiography
(C) Repeat PPD testing in 6 mo
(D) Treatment with pyrazinamide plus rifampin for 2 mo
(E) Treatment with isoniazid for 9 mo

ANSWER: E

The proper interpretation of this PPD is that the patient is a recent converter (ie, induration enlarged from <10 mm to ≥15 mm within 2 yr). However, it is possible he has undergone a "booster" response in which the first PPD done a year ago "boosted" his T-cell memory so that a second PPD resulted in a greater reaction. This is why two-step testing is recommended for new long-term–care residents and staff and for all healthcare personnel. In either case, a positive test warrants therapy. All patients with a positive PPD should have active disease excluded by a thorough examination and chest radiograph; if this evaluation is negative, 9 mo of INH is the appropriate treatment. This is true despite the drug interaction with warfarin; this patient will simply need his INR monitored closely. In this case, he also would qualify for INH therapy based only on the size of the PPD reaction (≥15 mm) which is always considered positive regardless of other factors, including age, underlying illness, prior administration of BCG vaccine, etc. In those with specific risk factors, which are quite common in older adults (eg, diabetes, gastrectomy/achlorhydria, excessive weight loss, chronic renal disease, etc), a PPD ≥10 mm of induration is considered positive. In immunocompromised patients, in those with changes on chest radiographs typical of prior tuberculosis, and in those recently exposed to someone with active disease, a PPD ≥5 mm of induration is considered positive.

This patient has a 10% risk of developing active tuberculosis within 2 yr and works in a healthcare setting; thus, observation and annual chest radiography are not indicated. Repeat PPD testing will not change management options and is not needed. Treatment with pyrazinamide and rifampin has been shown effective in treating latent tuberculosis in patients with human immunodeficiency virus infection but is considered a second-line therapy to 9 mo of isoniazid treatment (SOE=A).

42. A 70-yr-old male smoker has a history of hypertension, dyslipidemia, diabetes mellitus, and nonvalvular atrial fibrillation.

Which of the following most increases his risk of stroke?

(A) Cigarette smoking
(B) Hypertension
(C) Dyslipidemia
(D) Atrial fibrillation

ANSWER: D

Among men, the incidence of stroke is 4.5 per 1,000 between the ages of 65 and 74 yr, and 9.3 per 1,000 between 75 and 84 yr. The contribution of factors to a person's stroke risk varies by age. For a 70-yr-old man, the relative risk from nonvalvular atrial fibrillation is 3.3; the relative risk from hypertension is 2; from cigarette smoking, 1.8; and from dyslipidemia, 2 (SOE=B).

The high prevalence of hypertension makes it the largest overall contributor to stroke risk in the population, with a population-attributable risk of 30%. This relationship is true in all age groups, except in adults >80 yr old, in whom the increased prevalence of nonvalvular atrial fibrillation results in a population-attributable risk of 23%, while that of hypertension is 20%.

43. The Seventh Report of the *Joint National Committee on Prevention, Detection, Evaluation, and Treatment of High Blood Pressure (JNC7)* recommends which of the following for the initial treatment for hypertension in older adults?

(A) ACE inhibitor
(B) Thiazide diuretic
(C) Calcium channel blocker
(D) β-Blocker
(E) Angiotensin-receptor blocker

ANSWER: B

JNC7 guidelines state that thiazide diuretics, either in combination or alone, should be the initial treatment for hypertension in most patients (SOE=A). However, thiazide diuretics are not necessarily the first choice for patients with other conditions. *JNC7* identifies compelling indications for the use of medications other than hydrochlorothiazide for initial management of hypertension. ACE inhibitors and β-blockers are recommended for initial treatment of hypertension in asymptomatic patients with impaired left ventricular systolic function. ACE inhibitors or angiotensin-receptor blockers are recommended for patients with hypertension and early chronic kidney disease. Calcium channel blockers are recommended in patients with diabetes or a high risk of coronary disease (SOE=A). In each of these diseases, clinical trials have demonstrated benefit of specific classes of antihypertensive agents.

44. A 69-yr-old woman comes to the office because she has had anorexia, nausea, and vague lower abdominal pain associated with the onset of constipation 1 wk earlier. She also believes she has had a low-grade fever.

On examination, she appears uncomfortable. Temperature is 37.2° C (99.0° F), blood pressure is 130/80 mmHg, pulse is 90 beats per minute, and respiratory rate is 14 breaths per minute. She has suprapubic fullness and abdominal tenderness with localized guarding but no rebound. Bowel sounds are decreased. Laboratory results are normal except for mild anemia and a WBC count of 12,000/μL with a left shift. Radiography demonstrates a nonspecific ileus pattern.

Which of the following studies should be performed next?

(A) Barium enema
(B) Ultrasonography of pelvis
(C) CT of abdomen and pelvis
(D) Small-bowel series
(E) Colonoscopy

ANSWER: C

The prevalence of diverticulosis increases with age and is estimated to be 70% among adults ≥80 yr older. Diverticulitis (inflammation of a diverticulum) is the most common clinical complication of diverticular disease, affecting 10%–25% of patients with diverticula. Most diverticula (80%) are located in the sigmoid and descending colon regions of the large intestine. Diverticulitis is commonly accompanied by gross or microscopic perforation and usually involves the sigmoid or descending colon.

Contained perforation can result in abscess formation, fistulization, small-bowel obstruction from adhesions, and after repeated episodes, large-bowel obstruction from fibrotic narrowing of the colon lumen. Free perforation will likely lead to frank peritonitis.

Diverticulitis typically causes left lower-quadrant abdominal pain, although the location of the pain can be variable because of the redundancy of the sigmoid colon. Leukocytosis is generally present, and low-grade fever and obstipation are common. Urinary symptoms may occur with adjacent bladder irritation.

CT is recommended as the initial radiologic examination (SOE=C). It has high sensitivity (approximately 93%–97%) and specificity approaching 100% for the diagnosis. It also allows the extent of disease to be delineated. CT can also reveal other disease processes that cause lower abdominal pain, such as appendicitis or carcinoma, and may be of value in predicting the need for surgery. In patients with evidence of abscess on CT, conservative therapy often fails; CT findings can be used to stratify cases that should be referred for early surgical intervention.

Because of the risk of perforation or other exacerbation, colonoscopy and sigmoidoscopy are contraindicated. While limited-contrast studies of the descending colon and rectum with water-soluble contrast media can help distinguish between diverticulitis and carcinoma, barium enema should be avoided during the acute attack because of possible leakage of barium into the peritoneal cavity. Ultrasonography can be used to diagnose acute colonic diverticulitis, but its use is limited by what has been described as "the unhappy triad" of too much pain, too much gas, and too much fat.

45. A 79-yr-old woman comes to the office because she has knee discomfort that is exacerbated by walking, and as a consequence, she undertakes little or no physical activity. She has moderate osteoarthritis of both knees and takes acetaminophen irregularly for pain.

On examination, the patient is 1.6 m (64 in) and weighs 65 kg (144 lb). She has bilateral synovial swelling and mild varus deformity of the left knee. There is no significant ligament laxity, and no joint effusions, warmth, or tenderness on palpation. She has full range of motion (extension and flexion) of both knees, but crepitus is present on the left side. Quadriceps strength is 4+/5 bilaterally. She walks slowly but with good balance.

Which of the following is the most appropriate recommendation for physical activity?

(A) Flexibility stretching exercises 1 day/wk
(B) Aquatic exercises 1 day/wk
(C) Isotonic quadriceps exercises 5 days/wk
(D) Isotonic quadriceps exercises 2 days/wk
(E) Moderate-intensity aerobic exercise, 5 days/wk

ANSWER: D

Light to moderate exercise has a preventive and perhaps restorative role in people with osteoarthritis and should be started immediately along with the pharmacologic regimen. An appropriate program includes flexibility, strengthening, and aerobic components. For this patient, stretching once per week is insufficient; she should stretch at least 3 times per week, preferably before strengthening sessions for quadriceps muscle (SOE=D). Because quadriceps muscle weakness is a risk factor in osteoarthritis, strengthening the muscle is a critical component of the physical activity program (SOE=A). Pain control with a fixed dose of acetaminophen or NSAID is likely to be necessary, as will a graded approach to exercise. Isotonic or isometric exercises should begin at a low intensity (<50% of the person's one repetition maximum of 6 to 8 repetitions, working up to 10 to 15 repetitions daily (SOE=C). Although weight lifting can generally be conducted at 48-hr intervals, a maximum of 2 days/wk is recommended for people who have osteoarthritis (SOE=C). An aerobic exercise program will improve bone strength and contribute to weight loss, but it is highly unlikely that this patient can engage at a moderate-intensity level; she should instead start at a low-intensity level. Aquatic exercises once a week are insufficient to provide the necessary strength or endurance to meet this patient's needs (SOE=C).

46. A 72-yr-old man with mild dementia returns to the office because he has had difficulty both falling and staying asleep for the past 4 mo. In addition, he has had vivid dreams a few times per month. His sleep disturbance emerged shortly after a clinician prescribed a new medication.

Which of the following is most likely to cause these symptoms?

(A) Buspirone
(B) Trazodone
(C) Donepezil
(D) Melatonin
(E) Ramelteon

ANSWER: C

In older adults, medications are a common cause of insomnia or they can exacerbate preexisting insomnia. Donepezil, an acetylcholinesterase inhibitor commonly used for treatment of cognitive function in patients with Alzheimer's disease, has been shown to disturb sleep, as well as increase rapid eye movement (REM) sleep. REM sleep is the stage most commonly associated with dreaming; vivid dreams have been reported by patients when they have taken donepezil in the evening.

Activation of cholinergic systems increases wakefulness and alertness, as well as REM sleep, and can contribute to sleep disturbances. In clinical trials, insomnia and vivid dreams have been identified as potential adverse events

of donepezil (SOE=A). In a study examining the use of donepezil and hypnotic agents in older adults with Alzheimer's disease living in the community, use of hypnotic agents was higher among patients prescribed donepezil.

Buspirone, an anxiolytic medication, and trazodone, a sedating antidepressant, are unlikely to cause insomnia (SOE=B); indeed, trazodone is often used off-label for treatment of insomnia (SOE=B). Melatonin is a nutritional supplement with sleep-promoting properties (SOE=B), and ramelteon is a melatonin-receptor agonist hypnotic medication that does not promote insomnia (SOE=A).

47. A 75-yr-old woman calls the office to discuss a church-based screening program in which carotid arteries, abdominal aorta, and heel-bone density are evaluated using ultrasonography. She wonders whether it is worth the $85 charge.

Which of the following is the most appropriate response?

(A) The screening is a bargain, because each of these tests usually cost >$85 at the local hospital.
(B) The screening may result in expensive or potentially risky procedures.
(C) If the sensitivity is high, the screening would be valuable.
(D) The screening should be done at the local hospital.

ANSWER: B

The United States Preventive Services Task Force (USPSTF) publishes screening recommendations based on a comprehensive literature review. The USPSTF recommends screening of the abdominal aorta by ultrasonography in men 65–75 yr old who have ever smoked, because surgical repair of abdominal aortic aneurysms >5.5 cm decreases mortality (SOE=B). However, the USPSTF recommends against screening of the abdominal aorta in women, because the prevalence of abdominal aneurysm in women is low (approximately one-sixth the prevalence in men). In fact, evidence suggests that screening and early treatment in asymptomatic women results in an increased incidence of unnecessary surgery, with an increase in associated morbidity and mortality.

The USPSTF recommends screening all women ≥65 yr old for osteoporosis with dual x-ray absorptiometry (DEXA) scanning, preferably of the hip. There is substantial discordance in results between ultrasonography of the heel and central DEXA scanning, such that the former is not a useful test. The USPSTF recommends against screening for asymptomatic carotid artery stenosis in the general adult population.

While each of these tests would cost >$85 at the local hospital, it is not a good deal if the tests are unnecessary. Although undergoing unnecessary tests at the local hospital may improve the quality of the study, it does not make the tests more appropriate.

48. A 94-yr-old nursing home resident with Alzheimer's disease is evaluated because she has been disturbing other patients by screaming for help and banging on her recliner throughout the day for the past 4 wk.

Which of the following is most likely to reduce the patient's agitation?

(A) Nonpharmacologic intervention
(B) Second-generation antidepressant
(C) Second-generation antipsychotic agent
(D) Cholinergic agent

ANSWER: A

Nonpharmacologic interventions are first-line treatment in management of agitated behavior in patients with dementia (SOE=B). Analysis of the behavioral pattern can help identify stimuli or unmet needs that can trigger agitation. For example, specific environmental triggers, such as bathing, dressing, and under- or over-stimulation can cause increased agitation, as can reversible precipitants, such as pain and medical illness. Treating the pain or reconfiguring the environment may reverse or reduce agitation.

Once offending stimuli and unmet needs have been addressed, use of a second-generation antipsychotic agent is a second-line strategy for managing agitation. Use of second-generation antidepressants is another approach to managing agitation. Citalopram is somewhat effective in reducing irritability and disruptive vocalizations over 4–6 wk. In placebo-controlled studies in patients treated with fluvoxamine, no significant improvement was seen in irritability, anxiety, panic, restlessness, and mood. Reports have been mixed for other antidepressants, such as trazodone (SOE=C).

First-generation antipsychotic agents are somewhat effective for agitation but poorly tolerated (SOE=B). Their use is associated with high risk of extrapyramidal symptoms, tardive dyskinesia, hypotension, sedation, anticholinergic adverse events, and cognitive and functional impairment. Second-generation antipsychotics, such as risperidone, aripiprazole, and olanzapine, can also help reduce agitation and are associated with a lower incidence of extrapyramidal symptoms but high incidence of other adverse events (SOE=B). Safety concerns for these agents include metabolic syndrome, stroke risk, and increased mortality.

A review of the effect of cholinesterase inhibitors and memantine on cognition in patients with dementia incidentally found that several studies noted positive outcomes on a variety of behavioral measures (SOE=B). Mood symptoms appeared most responsive to cholinesterase inhibitors; improvements in aggression and agitation were observed most with memantine. There was great variability between studies. In general, trials with negative behavioral outcomes primarily involved institutionalized patients. As a whole, cholinesterase inhibitors and memantine appear to have a greater role in prevention, rather than treatment, of behavioral disturbance.

49. An 80-yr-old man with diabetes and osteoporosis comes to the office for consultation regarding his pain regimen. He has severe pain related to diabetic neuropathy and back pain related to multiple compression fractures. He takes hydrocodone/acetaminophen 2 tablets q6h, which helps the back pain but does little for the neuropathic pain.

Which of the following medications is an appropriate alternative to hydrocodone/acetaminophen for control of this patient's pain?

(A) Meperidine
(B) Butorphanol
(C) Nalbuphine
(D) Methadone

ANSWER: D

Using a single agent for this patient's two different types of pain—nociceptive and neuropathic—would be ideal. Opioids have some efficacy in treating neuropathic pain, although tricyclic antidepressants and anticonvulsants are more effective (SOE=A).

Of the medications listed, methadone is the most appropriate. In addition to having mu-opioid receptor activity, methadone has antagonist activity at the NMDA receptor, making it useful in cases of opioid tolerance and neurotoxicity. Methadone inhibits reuptake of both norepinephrine and serotonin, making it potentially more effective than other opioids in the treatment of neuropathic pain, although this claim is debated (SOE=C). Methadone should be used cautiously because it has complicated pharmacokinetics and can cause prolongation of the QT_c interval (SOE=C).

Meperidine is not recommended for use in older adults (SOE=B). Meperidine is metabolized to normeperidine, which has no analgesic properties but can accumulate in patients with decreased kidney function, causing tremulousness, myoclonus, and seizures. Mixed agonist-antagonist agents such as nalbuphine and butorphanol can cause restlessness and tremulousness, and therefore should be avoided in older adults (SOE=C).

50. An 82-yr-old man comes to the office because he has had excessive daytime sleepiness for about 6 mo. He falls asleep during the day, particularly in the late morning. He falls asleep easily around 8 PM, but wakes up every 2–3 hours throughout the night. His wife's sleep is often disturbed by his awakenings, and they have not been able to participate in social activities because of his intermittent daytime napping. History includes stroke (with residual mild leg weakness), hypertension, and mild cognitive impairment.

The patient is referred for actigraphy, a 24-hour graphing of sleep and wake intervals that uses a unit (actigraph) worn on the nondominant wrist. Results show 3 sleep intervals during the 24-hour test, with no single, clearly defined major nocturnal sleep period.

Which of the following is the most likely diagnosis?

(A) Idiopathic hypersomnia
(B) Advanced sleep phase disorder
(C) Irregular sleep/wake rhythm disorder
(D) Sundowning
(E) REM sleep behavior disorder

ANSWER: C

The patient's sleep pattern is consistent with circadian rhythm sleep disorder, irregular sleep/wake rhythm type. This condition is characterized by fragmented nocturnal sleep and daytime napping (SOE=B): there are at least 3 sleep periods throughout the 24-hour cycle, with no clearly defined, single, major nocturnal sleep period. The disorder is common in older adults with dementia; lack of structured exposure to light and to social and physical activities can precipitate or perpetuate the problem. A combination of increased light exposure and increased social and physical activity during the day is often recommended (SOE=B). Education of the patient and family about these interventions and the use of a sleep diary to monitor their effectiveness is warranted.

Although the patient complains of daytime sleepiness, the history indicates daytime napping and lack of consolidation of nocturnal sleep. The frequent daytime napping is most likely due to a decrease in the amplitude of the circadian rhythm, rather than to idiopathic hypersomnia. Advanced sleep phase disorder is characterized by one major nocturnal sleep period that is advanced relative to conventional sleep-wake times. This patient does not have one major sleep period, but rather several irregular periods of sleep and wake during the 24-hour cycle. The history does not indicate abnormal behavior during sleep (REM sleep behavior disorder) or agitation in the evening (sundowning).

51. A 79-yr-old woman presents with a lump on right upper quadrant of her left breast. Mammography reveals a 1.3-cm spiculated lesion. Biopsy reveals a high-grade, poorly differentiated, infiltrating ductal carcinoma of the breast, with negative margins and no evidence of lymphovascular invasion. She is concerned that breast conservation treatment (ie, lumpectomy or partial mastectomy) and postoperative

radiotherapy would not be "as good as" a full mastectomy.

Which of the following statements is true?

(A) Breast conservation treatment is the standard of care for all patients with early disease.
(B) Breast conservation treatment is associated with the same quality of life as mastectomy.
(C) Overall survival and disease-free survival are worse for breast conservation treatment than mastectomy.
(D) Older patients are more likely to be offered breast conservation therapy than younger patients.

ANSWER: A

Breast conservation treatment consists of breast-conserving surgery (ie, lumpectomy or partial mastectomy) and postoperative radiotherapy. It is recommended as the standard of care for patients of all ages with early stage breast cancer and has been shown in large randomized trials to have efficacy similar to that of mastectomy (SOE=A). It has also been shown to be associated with a better quality of life than mastectomy in patients ≥70 yr old (SOE=A). Furthermore, most older women prefer breast conservation to mastectomy but are less likely to receive such treatment.

Many factors must be considered when deciding the optimal treatment regimen for older women, including estimated life expectancy, medical comorbidites, functional status, goals of care, and ability to travel to a radiation oncology facility.

52. An 84-yr-old woman undergoes total hip replacement after falling and fracturing her hip. She lives at home with her 82-yr-old husband, who is confined to a wheelchair because of severe rheumatoid arthritis. The patient has diabetes mellitus, osteoporosis, and mild dementia. She has insurance coverage through standard fee-for-service Medicare Parts A and B.

On the third hospital day, she has no fever and her lungs are clear. She is taking adequate nourishment, and her weight is stable. Warfarin was begun after surgery; INR is 1.5. She requires a maximal assist of 1 to transfer and ambulate, and she has normal functioning of her arms. She tolerates physical therapy for 20 min before she

is too fatigued to continue. Hospital discharge for the next day is discussed.

Which of the following is the most appropriate setting for now?

(A) Inpatient rehabilitation facility
(B) Nursing home with rehabilitation services
(C) Nursing home with dementia unit
(D) Her own home with home physical therapy
(E) She is not ready for discharge and should stay in the hospital.

ANSWER: B

This patient is medically stable and requires rehabilitation after hip replacement. Because she needs nursing services (eg, medication monitoring) and rehabilitation (ie, physical therapy and other rehabilitation services <3 h/day), discharge to a nursing home with rehabilitation services is the most suitable option. The first 20 days of nursing-home care after hospitalization is fully covered through Medicare Part A.

The patient no longer requires hospitalization; she can continue to receive anticoagulation adjustments outside the hospital. According to Medicare rules, a patient must require hospital-level care—ie, a relatively intense, multidisciplinary team approach to rehabilitative care—to qualify for coverage in an inpatient rehabilitation facility. Because this patient is medically stable, requires only physical therapy without other types of rehabilitation, and can tolerate only 20 min of physical therapy at a time, she is not a candidate for admission to an inpatient rehabilitation facility. Her dementia is mild and not the chief cause of her current disability, making admission to a nursing-home dementia unit less appropriate. Discharge to home is also inappropriate, because her husband is unable to assist her with transfers and other ADLs.

53. An active, 70-yr-old moderately obese woman presents with a chief complaint of a painful left heel over the last few months. She has pain on first getting out of bed and after periods of rest. She denies any previous treatments. Past medical history is unremarkable. Physical examination of the left heel reveals pain at the medial tuberosity of the calcaneus. Dorsiflexion at the ankle joint is decreased but pain free, and

foot structure is normal. A radiograph of her left heel is unremarkable.

What is the most likely diagnosis?

(A) Heel spur
(B) Calcaneal stress fracture
(C) Partial tear of Achilles tendon
(D) Posterior tibial tendonitis
(E) Plantar fasciitis

ANSWER: E

Plantar fasciitis is a common condition seen after age 40 and is usually diagnosed through symptoms and physical examination findings. Patients typically have pain on rising in the morning and after periods of rest. During periods of nonactivity, the plantar ligament shortens; subsequently, the first few steps cause a sudden stretch, resulting in significant pain that usually decreases as the ligament is lengthened. An associated factor is ankle equinus or reduction in dorsiflexion of the ankle joint demonstrated on physical examination. This leads to increased stress on the plantar fascia during walking. Pain is usually maximal at the insertion of the plantar fascia on the medial tuberosity of the calcaneus. A pain-free range of motion in the ankle excludes a partial Achilles tear, because this tear is associated with end-range pain. Normal radiographs exclude heel spur and most calcaneal stress fractures; although stress fractures can be missed on plain radiographs, pain due to a stress fracture would not improve with ambulation. A normal foot structure and symptoms not worsening during ambulation (as the medial arch is stressed) exclude tendonitis.

54. An 82-yr-old nursing home resident is evaluated because she has increased pain in her knee. She has refused to walk for the past several days. History includes dementia, osteoporosis, atrial fibrillation, and renal insufficiency.

On physical examination, temperature is 37.4° C (99.3° F), blood pressure is 110/80 mmHg, and pulse is 78 beats per minute. The knee is warm and tender and causes pain with movement. An effusion is palpable. There is bony enlargement of the first carpal-metacarpal and distal interphalangeal joints. Radiography of the knee demonstrates joint space narrowing,

chondrocalcinosis, and osteophytes of the medial compartment.

Which of the following diagnostic tests should be obtained next?

(A) Westergren sedimentation rate
(B) Arthrocentesis and synovial fluid analysis
(C) Radiography of knee while bearing weight
(D) MRI of the knee

ANSWER: B

This patient has acute monoarthritis; direct evaluation of the synovial fluid is required to ascertain its cause. The presence of chondrocalcinosis suggests crystalline arthritis (calcium pyrophosphate deposition disease). Although her low-grade fever and inability or unwillingness to walk can be manifestations of this painful arthritis, an infectious cause must be excluded by arthrocentesis. Given her history of atrial fibrillation, she may be on anticoagulant therapy. Anticoagulant therapy is not a contraindication for arthrocentesis and has not been demonstrated to increase risk. Fluid samples should be immediately viewed with a polarizing microscope for crystals, and sent for cell count, Gram stain, and culture (SOE=B).

Arthrocentesis may yield a bloody effusion that, together with the history of osteoporosis, raises the possibility of a tibial plateau fracture. MRI is the best diagnostic test for detection of tibial plateau fracture and is useful in elucidating the integrity of ligaments and structures around and within the knee, including periarticular bone. MRI would not be helpful in distinguishing infectious from other inflammatory causes of monoarthritis. Although radiographs of the knee bearing weight are required to assess the joint space more accurately, they will not distinguish infectious from crystalline arthritis and may be difficult to obtain in a patient who is unable or unwilling to bear weight. The Westergren sedimentation rate increases with age and anemia and will not distinguish infectious from other inflammatory etiologies.

55. A 79-yr-old widower is seen in the office for self-reported anhedonia and depression. He has a history of affective disorder, lives alone, and has no nearby relatives. Recently his best friend died, and his social network has been getting

smaller because of disabilities and deaths of associates. Three of his aquarium fish died this week, and he has not attended church for several months. He indicates that, increasingly, ADLs have become burdensome and problematic. There is no evidence of cognitive impairment on the Mini–Mental State Examination.

Which of the following is the next best step?

(A) Refer to grief counseling group.
(B) Evaluate suicide risk.
(C) Evaluate for alcohol abuse.
(D) Refer to a psychotherapist.

ANSWER: B

This patient is at high risk of suicide because of his anhedonia, past affective disorder, diminishing social network, recent losses, and increasing difficulties with ADLs. The suicide risk should be addressed immediately before other courses of treatment are considered.

In the United States, suicide rates for men increase notably into old age (SOE=A). Psychologic autopsy studies identify five factors that contribute to risk: history of affective disorder, blunted hedonic response, medical illness, stressful life events, and diminished functional status. The risk increases substantially in individuals who are without an active social network.

56. An 86-yr-old female resident of an assisted-living facility has urinary frequency, urgency, urge incontinence, leakage of urine when bending over and walking up or down stairs, and a sensation of incomplete bladder emptying. History includes hypertension, mild Alzheimer's disease, and lumbosacral degenerative joint disease, for which she uses a walker. Medications include a cholinesterase inhibitor, a thiazide diuretic, and an angiotensin-receptor blocker.

On physical examination, there is mild atrophic vaginitis, a moderate cystocele, normal rectal sphincter tone, and no fecal impaction. While the patient is standing, a cough test for stress incontinence is positive. She voids 100 mL; post-void residual volume is 225 mL. Urinalysis is positive for trace of protein.

Which of the following is the most likely diagnosis?

(A) Stress incontinence
(B) Diuretic-induced incontinence
(C) Cholinesterase inhibitor–induced incontinence
(D) Detrusor hyperactivity with impaired bladder contractility
(E) Urinary retention and incontinence due to cystocele

ANSWER: D

This patient's symptoms and findings on examination are typical of detrusor hyperactivity with impaired bladder contractility. Affected patients have two simultaneous abnormalities of bladder function: involuntary bladder contractions, and weakness of the detrusor muscle resulting in incomplete bladder emptying with involuntary (and voluntary) bladder contractions (SOE=A). Detrusor hyperactivity with impaired bladder contractility can cause several different symptoms, as in this patient, and can mimic stress incontinence.

Diuretics can exacerbate symptoms of detrusor hyperactivity, but a thiazide diuretic is unlikely to be the primary cause of symptoms in this patient. Cholinesterase inhibitors can increase bladder contractility and possibly contribute to symptoms of overactive bladder (SOE=B). In older women with severe pelvic prolapse, urethral obstruction can develop, causing difficulty with bladder emptying (SOE=C). This patient, however, does not have severe pelvic prolapse. Even some obstruction of her urethra due to the cystocele would not account for all of her symptoms.

57. A 79-yr-old woman comes to the office because she has a fever and a cough. History includes hypertension, dyslipidemia, stable coronary disease, and osteoarthritis. She is enrolled in traditional Medicare Parts A and B; clinicians in the office are participating Medicare providers. On physical examination, it is evident that a CBC is needed to exclude bacterial infection. The patient explains that she is financially strapped and needs to know what her out-of-pocket costs will be for the office visit and blood work. Today's visit is her fifth this year; the office

visits have been her only medical encounters for the year.

How much is the patient's out-of-pocket cost for this visit?

(A) Nothing
(B) 20% of the office visit fee and 0% of the laboratory fee
(C) 20% of the office visit fee and 20% of the laboratory fee
(D) 20% of the office visit fee and 100% of the laboratory fee
(E) 100% of the office visit fee and 100% of the laboratory fee

ANSWER: B

Outpatient services for this patient are covered through Medicare Part B. Because this is her fifth office visit this year, by this time she likely has paid all of her Part B deductible. After the deductible is paid, Medicare Part B covers 80% of office visits and 100% of diagnostic laboratory fees. The patient would be responsible for the other 20% of the office visit. In this case, CMS would reimburse the participating Medicare provider directly for 80% of the office visit and 100% of the laboratory fees, and the patient would then be billed for the remaining 20% of the office fee.

58. A 72-yr-old woman comes to the office because of persistent pain in her left hip. History includes osteoarthritis, as well as a life-threatening episode of GI bleeding related to use of NSAIDs. Oral acetaminophen 1000 mg q6h decreases the pain for a short time. She follows her physical therapy regimen routinely.

Which of the following is the most appropriate intervention?

(A) Increase acetaminophen to 1000 mg q4h.
(B) Start ibuprofen 600 mg q6h.
(C) Start oxycodone 2.5 mg q4h as needed.
(D) Start long-acting morphine 15 mg q12h.

ANSWER: C

Following the dosage dictum to "start low and go slow" for older adults, the most appropriate next step is to prescribe oral oxycodone 2.5 mg q4h as needed (SOE=B). If the pain relief remains inadequate, then the dosage can be increased

to 5 mg q4h. If the pain relief is adequate and adverse events are tolerable, a long-acting regimen can be introduced. All patients beginning opioid therapy should also be started on a scheduled bowel regimen of an osmotic laxative (eg, lactulose) and a stimulant laxative (eg, senna), with a rescue regimen (eg, bisacodyl suppository or enema).

Increasing the acetaminophen dosage to q4h would be incorrect because the total daily dose would be above the limit for liver toxicity of 4000 mg/d. Starting ibuprofen is inappropriate given this patient's history of life-threatening GI bleeding with NSAIDs. In an opioid-naive patient, starting long-acting morphine is unsafe before completing a dose-finding trial with a short-acting opioid. If long-acting morphine is started, the patient may have excessive drowsiness or respiratory depression. Once an effective opioid dose is found, changing the patient to a long-acting opioid would be appropriate.

 59. A 65-yr-old woman is brought to the office by her niece because she believes that a neighbor has been coming into her apartment to steal items such as paper towels and sponges. She has called the police several times to report these thefts, and she complains regularly to her niece. This behavior began about 6 mo ago. The niece reports that her aunt has always been a little suspicious of other people. There is no history of alcohol or substance abuse. She has no hallucinations or depressive symptoms, and she has no other medical disorders. She is able to conduct her normal daily activities. Physical examination is normal except that she displays some mild memory loss. MRI is unremarkable.

Which of the following is the most likely explanation for her symptoms?

(A) Late-onset schizophrenia
(B) Delusional disorder
(C) Alzheimer's disease
(D) Bipolar disease
(E) Paranoid personality disorder

ANSWER: B

Delusional disorder is characterized by nonbizarre delusions involving situations that can occur in real life, such as theft, suffering from a disease, spousal infidelity, or being followed. According to the *DSM-IV-TR* it is rare; its precise prevalence is unknown, but it is estimated to be 0.03% in the general population, typically beginning in middle to late adulthood. Findings are mixed regarding the association of delusional disorder with hearing loss. Antipsychotic agents often are effective, especially in agitated delusional patients (SOE=C), but patients with delusions typically deny their illness. Consequently, they commonly do not adhere to medication regimens. Cognitive-behavioral therapy may also be effective. Modified electroconvulsive therapy has been reported as successful for refractory cases.

Delusional disorder is differentiated from schizophrenia by a lack of prominent auditory or visual hallucinations and by the absence of deterioration in areas of functioning outside the delusional scope. It can be distinguished from dementia by absence of cognitive and functional impairment, and from mood disorders by delusions preceding any mood disturbances. Although a history of schizotypal or paranoid personality disorders is more common in delusional disorder, the latter can be distinguished from personality disorders by the presence of delusions.

Delusional disorders can be difficult to differentiate from paranoid schizophrenia, but the latter has more bizarre delusions and auditory hallucinations. Poor psychosocial functioning in delusional disorder is directly related to the delusional beliefs.

60. Two residents of a for-profit nursing home want to share a bed but can do so only with the cooperation of the staff. One is a 90-yr-old man who is blind and a double-amputee with well-controlled heart failure. The other is an 86-yr-old woman with severe rheumatoid arthritis and a colostomy. Both have outlived spouses after long marriages and have been residents in the facility for some time; both have a normal mental status. The residents have had two falls when in her single room alone, and they have asked for staff assistance to undress and share a bed. Some staff members are uncomfortable and want the medical director to call the families to stop this behavior. Both residents say that they do not want their families informed. There is no relevant statement regarding the facility's protocols or limitations in the materials provided at admission.

Which of the following is the best course of action?

(A) Have a private conversation with the lead family member in each family.
(B) Research civil rights laws to determine the legality of the couple's request.
(C) Pursue a compromise, such as working only with volunteer staff or getting married, with the couple and the staff.
(D) Advise the couple that sexual activity is hazardous to their health and cannot be allowed.

ANSWER: C

Sexual activity among residents in nursing homes usually raises questions of competence, exploitation, harassment of staff, or other adverse behaviors that can justify efforts to eliminate the behavior. However, disabled adults generally have the right to create and follow relationships on the same grounds as nondisabled adults. They do not have to notify children or justify their choices. Yet the facility has to respect the sentiments of staff members and cannot dictate that staff members cooperate, especially if there is strong support in the community for limiting sexual activity to marriage. A reasonable compromise may be possible. Very likely, some staff members are not personally troubled and are willing to assist the couple. Senior leaders (the nursing director, medical director, and social work director) will need to take a strong stand of being willing to be among those helping out. Local advocates for people living with disabilities could be of help, or some volunteers at the nursing home may be supportive.

Informing the families over the explicit objections of competent adults is contrary to medical ethical principles and probably illegal. Legal advice from responsible public agencies is unlikely to help the situation or to be authoritative. Advising the couple that sexual activity would be hazardous to their health is generally not true, because people with well-controlled heart failure, stable arthritis, and colostomies can enjoy sex without harm. Furthermore, even if there is some risk, the nursing home cannot require that the couple make their decisions in accordance with the nursing home's view of risk.

61. An 83-yr-old otherwise healthy woman is brought to the office by her daughter because the mother has become confused and forgetful since beginning treatment with extended-release oxybutynin 10 mg for urge urinary incontinence 6 mo ago. The incontinence has improved, yet the daughter is unwilling to continue the oxybutynin because of the increased confusion. The mother, when asked, has no new complaints about memory or cognition.

Which of the following is the most appropriate next step?

(A) Discontinue extended-release oxybutynin 10 mg; begin immediate-release oxybutynin 2.5 mg q6h.
(B) Begin memantine, titrating over 3 wk from starting dose of 5 mg/d to 20 mg/d.
(C) Begin donepezil 5 mg/d, titrating to 10 mg/d if needed.
(D) Reassure the daughter that the medication is unlikely to produce cognitive adverse events.
(E) Discontinue extended-release oxybutynin 10 mg; implement behavioral therapy for incontinence.

ANSWER: E

While most patients receiving anticholinergic bladder-relaxant therapy have no discernable cognitive decline, some will have cognitive adverse events (SOE=C). Because the symptoms may be a adverse event of medication, the agent should be discontinued (SOE=C). Adding memantine or donepezil would not be appropriate because cholinesterase inhibitors can worsen symptoms of overactive bladder in some patients.

Cognitive adverse events of oxybutynin are related to peak medication concentration (SOE=A). Immediate-release medication with the same total dosage could potentially worsen this effect.

Behavioral therapy is an effective therapy for urge incontinence (SOE=A). If this patient is not cognitively intact enough to fully participate in behavioral therapy, she might benefit from the use of toileting assistance protocols such as prompted voiding (SOE=A).

62. An 83-yr-old nursing home resident with advanced Alzheimer's disease has steadily lost nearly 8.2 kg (18 lb), or 11% of his weight, over 11 mo. His current weight is 66.2 kg (146 lb; body mass index, 22 kg/m²). He gained about 8.2 kg (18 lb) 6 yr ago, after he entered the nursing home, and then maintained his weight until this year. He has not had any hospitalizations, acute infections, or other serious medical problems in the last 20 mo. Since his admission, he has had a slow, steady decline in cognitive function. He is fully ambulatory and attends most meals in the residents' dining hall; he needs minimal feeding assistance (set-up only). He is on a 2,600-kcal regular diet that was modified to include finger foods and nightly snacks. According to chart documentation, he only rarely consumes <75% of the food served, but a 2-day calorie count indicates that his consumption is closer to 40% of what he is served.

Besides a comprehensive evaluation for potentially reversible causes of the resident's weight loss, which of the following should be done?

(A) Prescribe 1 can (240 mL) of a polymeric oral supplement with each meal.
(B) Refer the resident for placement of a percutaneous endoscopic gastrostomy tube.
(C) Change the diet from regular to puréed.
(D) Implement a program of individualized feeding assistance.
(E) Start mirtazapine.

ANSWER: D

Of the choices provided, the best option is to work with the nursing staff to implement a program of individualized feeding assistance (SOE=B). Several recent controlled-intervention trials demonstrate that 90% of residents with inadequate nutrient intake increase food consumption by at least 15% in response to feeding assistance provided by appropriately trained staff. As part of this program, residents with low nutrient intake are monitored more closely and provided social stimulation, encouragement to eat, verbal cueing, and help in choosing menu items. Physical assistance is provided only as needed. Studies indicate that a 2-day trial of feeding assistance is a valid method of determining whether a given resident would respond. The intervention is offered both during and between meals.

The resident in this case is probably an ideal candidate for individualized feeding assistance. His progressive decline in cognitive function places him at increased risk of a continued decline in nutrient intake, as confirmed by the 2-day calorie counts. Nursing staff consider him a self-feeder; self-feeders often respond better than others to individualized feeding assistance.

One drawback of individualized feeding assistance is that it requires significantly more time than nursing home staff usually spend on feeding care. To address this issue, nursing homes can adopt alternative staffing models such as the "paid feeding assistant" program. A second issue is identifying residents in need of assistance. Chart documentation may not be accurate, and nursing staff tend to overestimate how much food residents consume, particularly when the resident is considered to be a self-feeder. A decline in a nursing home resident's intake can initially go unnoticed. For this reason, the nutrient intake of residents who are losing weight should be carefully assessed.

Although each of the other options has merit, none is optimal for the patient at this time. If nutrient intake remains low after implementing the feeding assistance program, a polymeric oral supplement can be added. However, supplements are generally most effective when offered between, rather than with, meals. Because there is no specific indication for a puréed diet, this option is not appropriate at this time. If the assessment provides evidence that the patient is depressed, a trial of an antidepressant would be appropriate. However, there is little evidence that mirtazapine is more effective than other types of antidepressants in improving nutrient intake (SOE=B).

63. A 73-yr-old man in a rehabilitation facility is evaluated for irritable mood, poor motivation for rehabilitation, and demanding and verbally abusive behavior toward staff. He entered rehabilitation after an above-knee amputation. He acknowledges having felt depressed and anxious for a long time, and he has taken a low dose of an antidepressant for several years. Family members report that he previously was extroverted and tended to be provocative and hot-tempered. In recent years, he has had increasing difficulty tolerating disability and reliance on others, prompting arguments that have frayed already estranged relations with his children. He admits to frequent verbal outbursts toward staff because "I need help and they just walk by!" Staff members believe he is just seeking attention. He has pervasive irritable mood, anhedonia, feelings of worthlessness, reduced appetite, poor sleep, and low energy. He inconsistently attends physical therapy sessions. Cognitive examination and thyroid function are normal, and his symptoms are not due to medication or substance abuse.

Which of the following is most likely to improve this patient's behavior?

(A) Increase dosage of antidepressant and refer for psychotherapy.
(B) Maintain and monitor on current dosage of antidepressant.
(C) Discontinue antidepressant treatment and screen for mania.
(D) Advise staff to ignore attention-seeking behavior.

ANSWER: A

Some older adults have chronic, unremitting major depressive disorder. If the behavior is of long duration and characterized by irritable mood and an abrasive interpersonal style, a mood disorder may be mistaken for an Axis II personality disorder. Although major depressive and personality disorders can coexist, features of personality disorder can overshadow depressive symptoms. Distinguishing a personality disorder from persisting mood disorder is challenging and may be possible only after adequate treatment for depressive disorder (SOE=C).

This patient may have major depressive disorder superimposed on medical illness and an underlying personality disorder. The continuation of his symptoms despite long-term, low-dose treatment with an antidepressant suggests that the dosage is inadequate and should be reevaluated. In contrast to the goal of major depression, the goal of treating personality disorders in older adults is not remission but reduction in frequency and intensity of symptoms.

It is unlikely that this patient's behavior would disappear if ignored by staff. Although irritability can be a symptom of mania, it is also common in older depressed adults. In patients with depressive symptoms, irritability does not suggest mania if symptoms of mania (eg, inflated self-esteem, decreased need for sleep, increased involvement in pleasurable activity) are absent.

64. An 89-yr-old man is admitted to a nursing home for rehabilitation after being hospitalized for pneumonia. He is anxious and fidgety. He is widowed and lives in the community. History includes hypertension, benign prostatic hyperplasia, major depressive disorder, and chronic back pain. Medications on transfer from the hospital to the nursing home include metoprolol, oxybutynin, paroxetine, acetaminophen with codeine, and amitriptyline.

Which of the following medications is *least* likely to contribute to delirium?

(A) Amitriptyline
(B) Acetaminophen with codeine
(C) Oxybutynin
(D) Paroxetine
(E) Metoprolol

ANSWER: E

All of these medications have some anticholinergic properties, but the metoprolol has the least potential impact on mental status (SOE=B). Amitriptyline, codeine, and oxybutynin have strong anticholinergic properties, are associated with delirium, and should be avoided. Both amitriptyline and codeine also have active metabolites, which can result in accumulation of drug and metabolite in the system, especially during times of stress and illness. Similarly, paroxetine has significant anticholinergic effects in older adults.

Although the pathophysiology of delirium is unknown and may be multifactorial, there is consensus that suppression of cholinergic neurons contributes to delirium (SOE=C). Older adults with impaired cholinergic systems, such as those with Alzheimer's dementia, are more susceptible to delirium. Thus, anticholinergic medications should be avoided in older adults, especially when they are most susceptible to delirium, such as while hospitalized.

In some studies, delirium symptoms and severity have been associated with serum anticholinergic activity level; other studies have not shown a clear association. Adjustments to

medications with anticholinergic properties can reduce the serum anticholinergic activity level and improve delirium symptoms (SOE=B). If delirium develops, the medication regimen should be reviewed to eliminate or reduce agents with anticholinergic properties.

65. Which of the following is the mostly likely cause of new onset vaginal bleeding in a 70-yr-old woman?

(A) Pyometra
(B) Endometrial cancer
(C) Endometrial hyperplasia
(D) Vaginal atrophy
(E) Hormonal effect

ANSWER: D

Vaginal atrophy is the most common cause of postmenopausal bleeding (SOE=A). In a series of 1,138 postmenopausal women (49–91 yr old) who had bleeding, atrophy was the histopathologic diagnosis in 59% of cases. Polyp was the next most frequent cause (12% of cases). Endometrial cancer and hyperplasia caused about 10% of cases, and hormonal effect caused 7%. Cervical cancer accounted for <1% of postmenopausal bleeding. Other causes (eg, hydrometra, pyometra, and hematometra), combined accounted for 2%. Even though 95% of postmenopausal bleeding is due to benign causes, all postmenopausal women with unexpected vaginal bleeding should be evaluated for endometrial cancer, because it is highly treatable.

Vaginal and endometrial atrophy is caused by hypoestrogenism. Classic findings include a pale, dry vaginal epithelium that is smooth and shiny, is easily friable, and has decreased rugae. Atrophic endometrial surfaces in the uterus contain little or no fluid to prevent intracavitary friction. This results in microerosions of the surface epithelium and subsequent chronic inflammatory reaction. The inflammatory reaction produces a chronic endometritis, which is prone to light bleeding or spotting.

The main objective in evaluating postmenopausal bleeding is to exclude cancer. Endometrial biopsy is the initial diagnostic test. If the patient cannot tolerate biopsy in the office, then transvaginal ultrasonography is an alternative. A biopsy is not required if the endometrial lining is <4–5 mm thick and appears homogeneous, without increased echogenicity (SOE=A).

Unless contraindicated, systemic or local estrogen is the most effective treatment for vaginal atrophy. Vaginal administration minimizes systemic absorption, although it can increase plasma levels of estrogen. Local estrogen applications include low-dose creams, rings, and tablets. One strategy is low-dose vaginal estrogen cream 0.5 g/d for 3 wk, with twice-weekly administration thereafter. The estradiol ring (Estring®) delivers 6-9 mcg of estradiol to the vagina daily for 3 mo. The vaginal estrogen tablet (Vagifem®) is usually recommended every day for 2 wk, then twice weekly. Progestins are not prescribed routinely for women treated with low-dose vaginal estrogen. In women with breast cancer, vaginal estrogen is not used for symptoms of urogenital atrophy unless recommended by the woman's oncologist.

66. An 86-yr-old man who lives alone is prepared for discharge after hospitalization for an open leg wound and cellulitis that followed a fall at home. He is a retired professor; he reports no difficulty with ambulation, ADLs, or IADLs. Notes from the emergency medical services personnel indicate that they had difficulty gaining access to the patient's apartment because of clutter, and they noted the smell of urine and visible cockroaches. The patient reports no past medical history and takes no prescription medications.

On initial examination, the patient's temperature was 38.3°C (101°F), blood pressure was 180/90 mmHg, and heart rate was 110 beats per minute; body mass index was 18. Blood glucose level by fingerstick was 350 mg/dL. He was disheveled and wore stained and malodorous clothing. He had several bags of papers with him. On his right medial mallelolus there was a 4-cm, round, clean-based open ulcer with surrounding erythema and warmth. He had erythematous patches in his intertriginous areas and long dystrophic nails. Score on the Mini–Mental State Examination was 27 (he recalled only 1 of 3 words and was unable to draw intersecting pentagons). WBC count was 13,000/μL with 90% neutrophils, BUN was 30 mg/dL,

creatinine was 1.6 mg/dL, and hemoglobin A_{1C} was 9%.

He was treated with intravenous antibiotics, an antihypertensive agent, and long-acting insulin. On discharge, he refuses home care services, home-delivered meals, and all prescription medications, insisting that he can take care of himself.

Which of the following is the most likely explanation for these findings?

(A) Dementia
(B) Delirium
(C) Depression
(D) Self-neglect
(E) Delusional disorder

ANSWER: D

This patient exhibits several cardinal features of self-neglect. Although there is no uniform, validated definition, expert consensus characterizes self-neglect as the presence of at least one of the following: 1) persistent inattention to personal hygiene or environment, 2) repeated refusal of services that can reasonably be expected to improve quality of life, and 3) self-endangerment through unsafe behaviors (SOE=C). Self-neglect can also be associated with disorders of aging that lead to executive dysfunction, which in turn leads to functional impairment in the setting of absent but needed medical or social services. When the individual loses the ability to recognize potentially unsafe living conditions, self-neglect ensues. According to prevalence estimates derived from Adult Protective Services data, self-neglect constitutes the most common category of investigated reports. In 2004, over 46,000 reports of self-neglect were made to Adult Protective Services, but this likely underestimates the true prevalence.

Dementia has been associated with self-neglect in longitudinal studies of cases identified by Adult Protective Services. Memory loss, especially executive dysfunction, plus impaired judgment can inhibit self-care. Dementia can also be associated with clutter if executive dysfunction impairs the individual's ability to sort and discard unnecessary items. Although this patient has a normal score on the Mini–Mental State Examination, it may actually reflect a decrease from his baseline, given his former occupation. However, the diagnosis of dementia alone does not adequately explain his refusal of medically indicated services. Self-neglect is also seen in the absence of cognitive impairment.

The hallmarks of delirium are an acute change in mental status, symptoms that fluctuate over minutes or hours, and inattention, in addition to altered level of consciousness or disorganized thinking. Although this patient was at risk of delirium because of his age, infection, and hospitalization, he does not exhibit features of acute delirium.

Depression has also been associated with self-neglect, possibly because it can increase the risk of nonadherence to medication, or because it can result in executive dysfunction. The patient in this case, however, has no other features of depression (eg, anhedonia, difficulty concentrating, sleep or appetite disturbance, fatigue, psychomotor changes, or suicidal ideation).

Delusional disorder most often develops in mid to late life and can manifest as poor insight and judgment and disorganized thinking. If this is seen concurrently with self-neglect, it can preclude the individual from seeking help. While this patient may misperceive his own environment—leading to apathy about the state of his apartment—he does not have any evidence of paranoia or any firmly held belief in something that is not true.

67. An 86-yr-old woman with dementia and heart failure has difficulty getting to the bathroom and is increasingly incontinent. She can no longer prepare food for herself or take medications reliably. She lives in the city with her son, who is away from home during the day. He is no longer comfortable leaving his mother alone, but neither he nor his mother wants her to move to a nursing home. The patient qualifies for Medicare and Medicaid.

If available, which of the following is the most appropriate recommendation?

(A) Enrollment in a social health maintenance organization (HMO)
(B) Admission to a nearby nursing home
(C) Referral to Program of All-inclusive Care of the Elderly (PACE)
(D) Hiring a full-time nurse to care for the patient at home
(E) Referral to state Department of Aging for assessment

ANSWER: C

PACE is a managed-care program developed to address the needs of older adults who have a level of disability that makes them eligible for nursing-home care. It was modeled after the innovative program in San Francisco, On Lok, which focused on caring for Asian Americans in their home community. PACE services are provided by an interdisciplinary team comprising primary care physicians; nurse practitioners; nurses; social workers; physical, occupational, and recreational therapists; pharmacists; dieticians; home care coordinators; PACE center managers; personal care attendants; and drivers. Daily services are commonly provided at an adult day healthcare center, and multidisciplinary care is highly coordinated. Enrollment in PACE is associated with higher patient satisfaction, improved health status and function, fewer nursing-home admissions, improved quality of life, and lower mortality than usual care (SOE=B). PACE is a comprehensive managed-care program that is paid for through Medicare and Medicaid funds and by the participant's own contributions. Unfortunately, the program is available only in selected, primarily urban environments.

The social HMO was also developed with the intent of keeping older adults in the community. It is a capitated program for frail Medicare recipients with complex medical needs. A social HMO provides the full range of Medicare benefits offered by standard HMOs plus additional services that include care coordination, chronic care benefits covering short-term nursing-home care, and home- and community-based services. Evaluations indicate mixed results regarding cost and effectiveness of social HMOs in caring for frail older adults (SOE=C).

The patient and her son do not want her to be admitted to a nursing home, although Medicaid would cover the costs of this long-term care. Hiring a full-time nurse to care for the patient at home would not be covered by either Medicare or Medicaid and would be very expensive. Referral to the state Department of Aging for assessment may result in more home support than is usually available from the Medicaid program, but full-day care by any type of care provider would not likely be covered. Of the options, only PACE would provide the comprehensive care coordination best suited for this patient.

68. A 55-yr-old man with Down syndrome is brought to the office by his caregivers because over the past year he has become confused and forgetful and has needed increasingly more frequent prompts for his assigned tasks. Although they do not have specific written records, the caregivers think that his speech and movement have slowed, that he is more socially withdrawn, and that he is having more outbursts with peers and staff. In the last 4 mo, he has twice lost his balance and fallen. He has been physically healthy overall and is on no medications. His last routine physical examination was 8 mo ago, at which time there were no indications of any problem.

During the visit, the patient seems shy and anxious and has a congruent affect. He has no complaints. His expressive abilities are limited and consistent with his low-moderate level of mental retardation.

Which of the following options is the most appropriate next step?

(A) Order head CT.
(B) Perform office-based, appropriate cognitive testing.
(C) Begin fluoxetine.
(D) Begin donepezil and, if well-tolerated, add memantine.
(E) Refer patient to a psychiatrist who specializes in neurodevelopmental disabilities.

ANSWER: B

Patients with developmental disabilities are now surviving to middle age and presenting with geriatric conditions, such as dementia and osteoporosis. This patient has symptoms consistent with dementia in Down syndrome. Early symptoms in patients both with and without Down syndrome include more short-term than distant memory loss, forgetfulness, and confusion. Patients with Down syndrome also have earlier frontal lobe symptoms, such as slowing of speech, language, and motor activities; social withdrawal; and problems with sleep, balance, and emotional regulation (SOE=B). This patient displays many of the symptoms of dementia, but diagnostic tests and additional history are needed before determining an appropriate treatment strategy. The cognitive testing necessary in this situation is available through psychology and psychiatry services and does not require consultation with a specialist in neurodevelopmental disabilities.

Despite the caregivers' report of falls, brain imaging is not likely to yield additional clinically useful information. Although some of the patient's symptoms suggest depression, more information would be needed before making a diagnosis of depression.

The degree of severity and patient values should guide treatment for dementia. The patient's presentation suggests mild rather than moderate or severe dementia. A medication regimen that combines two agents is not an appropriate first choice. In addition, cognitive assessment must be performed first.

69. A 72-yr-old man with chronic emphysema is being discharged home after spending 3 wk on a ventilator after a probable viral infection. The patient receives oxygen at home. Several months ago, he was on a ventilator for a few days. During preparations for discharge, the patient emphatically states that he does not want ventilator care ever again. His wife died a year ago and he lives alone, with no friendly contacts. He cannot smoke because of the oxygen, and he cannot go fishing or leave his apartment to play poker any more. He asks that arrangements be made so that he is not readmitted and placed on the ventilator again.

Which of the following strategies is most likely to reassure the patient?

(A) Refer patient to a hospice with an inpatient unit.
(B) Order continuous positive airway pressure for home.
(C) Legally document a "do not resuscitate" directive.
(D) Refer patient to a hospice that can provide sedation at home.
(E) Evaluate patient for major depressive disorder.

ANSWER: D

A patient who faces dyspnea and suffocation cannot be served humanely without a ventilator unless the care team can provide sedation. A hospice that can provide home sedation would allow the patient to be confident that he will be comfortable at home until there is a final exacerbation. It would be wise to document the care plan and his role in shaping it; that documentation is usually sufficient without such legal requirements as a second witness or a notary. The patient could be evaluated for major depressive disorder, but his response to his situation is reasonable, and he is not so much withdrawn as isolated by illness. He might benefit from interventions to decrease his isolation, such as visits from hospice volunteers, nearby church or veterans organizations, and meals programs. Any consideration of more treatment, such as continuous positive airway pressure, should have been part of his ongoing evaluation; it should not be likely that additional treatment could offer major gains now. All hospice programs are required to have inpatient care available, which may be useful for him at a later point.

70. An 80-yr-old woman comes to the office because she has been dizzy. When asked for specifics, she is vague, but states that she often feels unsteady when walking. She has also felt lightheaded a few times when getting up in the morning. She has had no falls. History includes hypertension, type 2 diabetes mellitus, dyslipidemia, and anxiety. Medications are hydrochlorothiazide, lisinopril, aspirin, metformin, simvastatin, and trazodone.

On examination, blood pressure is 125/82 mmHg and pulse is 80 beats per minute with no orthostatic changes. Her gait is slightly wide but otherwise normal. There is evidence of mild peripheral neuropathy. Her score on the Geriatric Depression Scale is 3/15.

Which of the following is the most likely cause of her dizziness?

(A) Anxiety
(B) Somatization disorder
(C) Medication adverse event
(D) Multifactorial triggers

ANSWER: D

Complaints of dizziness are often vague, and its diagnosis and treatment can be frustrating for both patients and practitioners. Dizziness in older adults may be thought of as a geriatric syndrome that is often caused by several underlying risk factors. In one study, 56% of older adults who described dizziness had multiple different sensations, and 74% had multiple different triggers. In many of these adults, no obvious, single diagnosis could be made. Characteristics associated with "dizziness syndrome" included anxiety, depressive symptoms, impaired hearing, use of 5 or more medications, postural hypotension, impaired balance, and past myocardial infarction. Authors of the study suggested that a strategy to reduce several factors might be an effective approach for many older adults with dizziness.

A multifactorial origin of dizziness is most likely in this patient, because her sensations of dizziness vary and have no obvious cause on physical examination. Although it would be reasonable to look at different interventions to address her dizziness, including adjusting antihypertensive medications and initiating physical therapy, there is no proof that such an approach improves outcome (SOE=C).

71. A 72-yr-old man comes to the office for evaluation because he has impaired fasting glucose levels. Fasting levels were between 110 and 120 mg/dL on 3 occasions. He has well-controlled hypertension. His body mass index is 29.5.

Which of the following is most likely to prevent development of type 2 diabetes mellitus in this patient?

(A) Reduce caloric intake and increase physical activity to 150 min/week.
(B) Increase physical activity and begin metformin.
(C) Begin metformin.
(D) Reduce caloric intake.

ANSWER: A

The landmark trial from the Diabetes Prevention Program Research Group evaluated patients at risk of new-onset diabetes who were randomly assigned to 1) lifestyle intervention (goal of 7% weight loss through reducing caloric intake and increasing physical activity by 150 min/wk), 2) educational materials plus metformin 850 mg q12h, or 3) educational materials only (control). Participants were overweight and had both fasting and post-load hyperglycemia at levels not yet diagnostic of diabetes. Lifestyle intervention was the most effective approach to diabetes prevention: the incidence of diabetes in this group was reduced by >50% versus in patients who received only educational materials. The incidence of diabetes was also reduced in the group that received metformin plus educational materials versus in patients who received only educational materials, but to a lesser extent (by 25%). Intensive lifestyle intervention worked especially well for older participants. Metformin was most effective in participants with a lower body mass index and in participants with lower fasting glucose concentrations (SOE=A).

72. A 77-yr-old woman comes to the office because she has frequent falls. She has difficulty walking unassisted and frequently feels that her feet get tangled together. She is also urinating more frequently. She has no burning on urination, fever, chills, or flank pain.

On examination, there are no significant abnormalities of joints in the limbs. There is good mobility of the lumbar spine and mild immobility of the cervical spine, with 45-degree rotation to the right and left and limited extension. Arm reflexes are 2+, with occasional fasciculations in the biceps and triceps muscles. Hoffmann's sign is present in both hands. There is increased tone in the lower extremities.

Reflexes are 3+ at the knees and ankles. Both toes are upgoing.

Which of the following is the most appropriate next step?

(A) Bone scan
(B) MRI of the lumbar spine
(C) MRI of the cervical spine
(D) Radiography of the cervical spine
(E) Radiography of the thoracic spine

ANSWER: C

This patient has symptoms and signs of cervical spinal stenosis (ie, cervical myelopathy). The most significant physical findings are upper motor neuron signs in the legs (increased muscle tone, increased reflexes, and upgoing toes) with both lower (fasciculations) and upper motor neuron signs (Hoffmann's signs) in the hands. Hoffmann's test involves flicking the terminal phalanx of the third finger; if the terminal phalanx of the thumb flexes into the palm, the test is positive. (This is analogous to Babinski's sign for the lower extremities.) The presence of Hoffmann's sign indicates interruption of the corticospinal tract, usually in the cervical spine.

Any patient with gait disorders and increased frequency of urination should be evaluated for cervical myelopathy. MRI of the cervical spine is the most appropriate study (SOE=D).

MRI of the lumbar spine would not be helpful, because this patient has upper motor neuron signs indicating disease above L1 (SOE=D). Tumor of the cervical spine rarely causes cervical myelopathy. A much more common cause is cervical spinal stenosis. Plain radiography of the cervical spine is not likely to be helpful, because 80% of radiographs are abnormal in adults ≥55 yr old (SOE=D).

Radiography of the thoracic spine would not be helpful, because the presence of Hoffmann's sign in both hands indicates stenosis of the cervical spine, not the thoracic spine (SOE=D). A bone scan cannot demonstrate compression of the spinal cord and is not indicated in this patient.

73. An 80-yr-old man comes to the office for a routine visit. He is enrolled in traditional fee-for-service Medicare Parts A and B and has a Part D policy. He has seen advertisements for

an insurance plan called SeniorGold, which is described as a Medicare Advantage organization with a Medicare contract. He wishes to discuss advantages and disadvantages of switching his insurance coverage to this plan.

Which of the following is most likely to occur if he switches insurance coverage to SeniorGold?

(A) He would lose some Part A benefits.
(B) He would lose some Part B benefits.
(C) He would have to drop Part D prescription drug coverage.
(D) He would not get coverage for vision examination and eyeglasses.
(E) He would not get to choose his providers.

ANSWER: E

A potential disadvantage of a Medicare Advantage plan is that the provider network may be restricted, because this is a key strategy for controlling costs in managed-care systems. Medicare Advantage plans are required by law to provide all services covered in traditional Medicare Parts A and B. Participants may enroll in a Medicare Advantage plan and have a separate, stand-alone Part D policy, or attach a Part D policy to the Medicare Advantage plan. Traditional Medicare does not cover vision examination and eyeglasses; many Medicare Advantage plans cover such services as an enticement to get patients to enroll.

74. A 75-yr-old man comes to the office with several vague complaints and concerns. He is retired and has been married for 50 yr. Over the past 6 mo, he has come to the office repeatedly and has become increasingly homebound. He describes leg weakness, fatigue, and overall malaise that prevent him from engaging in once-pleasurable activities, such as playing cards at the senior center. He has become fearful of driving and of being alone, and his sleep and appetite are poor. He has lost approximately 4.5 kg (10 lb). History includes hypertension and spinal stenosis. Major depressive disorder is diagnosed, and a trial of an antidepressant is begun.

Which of the following is characteristic of late-life major depressive disorder?

(A) Strong family history of mood disorder
(B) Sudden onset of symptoms
(C) Preferential response to treatment with first-generation antidepressants
(D) Higher prevalence of somatic symptoms

ANSWER: D

In general, major depressive disorder presents with sad mood and a variety of symptoms affecting energy level, sleep, appetite, cognitive skills, and overall ability to derive enjoyment from activities. It can be complicated by psychotic symptoms (eg, delusions or hallucinations) and suicidal ideation. It is a recurring illness, and it is more prevalent in family members of patients.

When major depressive disorder is first seen after age 65, the presentation is distinctive. Dementia is described in up to one-third of patients within 5 yr of the depression. The family history of mood disorder is weaker than in younger patients. The onset of symptoms is slow, subtle, and insidious. Psychotic symptoms and somatic complaints are more prevalent. Nonetheless, recommendations for treatment are similar in those for major depressive disorder with onset before age 65: because of their more favorable adverse event profile and low rates of death in overdose, second-generation antidepressants are first-line treatment for major depressive disorder in adults, regardless of age at onset. There is no evidence that any class of antidepressants is superior to another for treatment of late-life depressive disorder. Tolerability and potential drug-drug interactions in patients on several medications should guide the choice of treatment.

75. A 66-yr-old man comes to the office because his family has noticed increasing apathy, forgetfulness, and confusion over the past few months. For example, he now gets lost on his way home from familiar places. He and his wife lived in England for 20 yr before her death 10 yr ago. He then moved to the United States and has dated occasionally. He has no significant comorbidities and is on no medications. There is no history of sexually transmitted disease.

His family is concerned that he may have early Alzheimer's disease.

Physical examination is normal except for the neurologic exam, which reveals slowing of rapid finger and toe tapping, increased reflexes, short-term memory deficits, and an inability to do relatively simple calculations. He scores 22/30 on the Mini–Mental State Examination. His affect is normal. A cranial CT scan reveals mild to moderate atrophy, but no other changes. There are no metabolic or endocrine abnormalities on laboratory testing.

What is the most likely cause of this patient's dementia?

(A) Syphilis
(B) Creutzfeldt-Jakob disease
(C) Human immunodeficiency virus (HIV) antibody
(D) Lyme disease

ANSWER: C

One of every 11 new diagnoses of HIV is in an adult >50 yr old. In the United States, older adults are the cohort least likely to practice safe sex; most cases of HIV infection in older adults are acquired through sexual activity. Older adults are more likely than young adults to meet criteria for acquired immune deficiency syndrome (AIDS) at the time of HIV diagnosis, perhaps because nonspecific symptoms such as weight loss, dementia, and failure to thrive are more common in older adults and because, untreated, AIDS progresses faster in older adults. However, once diagnosed, older adults with HIV are as likely to benefit from anti-HIV therapy as young adults, with regard to both survival and immunologic recovery.

HIV-associated dementia can present with many different clinical syndromes. The most common characteristics include fairly rapid decline in memory and concentration, emotional disturbances, and psychomotor slowing. Spasticity, tremor, and ataxia can also be present. This patient's presentation is consistent with HIV-associated dementia, and epidemiologically this is the most prevalent infectious dementia in this age group. Arrest and even reversal of HIV-associated dementia are widely described and expected with combinations of antiretroviral drugs that penetrate the CNS. Although hyperlipidemia, accelerated atherosclerosis, and other metabolic complications are seen in patients on antiretroviral therapies, these effects do not offset the marked benefit of therapy. If treated, this patient can expect marked improvement in his memory and his chance of surviving at least 3 yr is >80%. He should be counseled regarding safe sex and routes of transmission. All his sexual partners within the last 5 yr should be tested for HIV.

Neurosyphilis is a late manifestation of infection with *Treponema pallidum*. Findings include neurocognitive decline and prominent frontal lobe signs. Creutzfeldt-Jakob disease is a rapidly progressive dementia associated with myoclonus, and pyramidal and extrapyramidal signs, which this patient does not exhibit. *Borrelia burgdorferi* is an unusual cause of infectious dementia. Patients can have a history of tick bite, as well as the typical rash of *erythema chronicum migrans*, transient arthritis, cranial nerve palsies, and cardiac conduction disturbances that would precede dementia caused by *B burgdorferi*.

76. An 85-yr-old man comes to the office to discuss the recurrence of anxiety attacks, of which he has a chronic history. He describes periods of intense fear and anxiety that last from 30 min to several hours and that are accompanied by physical and autonomic symptoms. He does not drink, has no history of alcohol or drug abuse, and has no other psychiatric issues. History includes hypertension, osteoarthritis, and urinary retention related to prostatic hyperplasia. He was diagnosed with panic disorder as an adult and took diazepam for the panic attacks, although not for the past 20 yr. He is interested in restarting treatment with diazepam.

Physical examination and laboratory evaluation (thyrotropin, CBC, metabolic profile) indicate nothing likely to cause new-onset panic attacks.

Which of the following is the most appropriate treatment?

(A) Benzodiazepines plus an SSRI
(B) Benzodiazepines plus cognitive-behavioral therapy
(C) An SSRI plus cognitive-behavioral therapy
(D) Benzodiazepines plus nortriptyline
(E) Mirtazapine plus an SSRI

ANSWER: C

In at least one large-scale epidemiologic study, panic disorder was identified in about 1% of community-dwelling older adults. Classic panic disorder (ie, frequent, unexplained panic attacks with marked fear and autonomic symptoms) with first onset in late life appears to be rare. However, panic-like symptoms are common in late life, particularly in the context of cardiac or respiratory illness or Parkinson's disease. In addition, because panic disorder, like other anxiety disorders, tends to be chronic and relapsing, its recurrence or persistence in old age is unsurprising (SOE=B).

Benzodiazepines are among the most commonly prescribed medications in older adults. They are effective for anxiety symptoms, including panic attacks. The risk of dependence with these medications tends to be low in older adults, particularly if there is no history of alcohol or drug dependence. However, older adults are more likely to suffer falls, fall-related injury, delirium, and cognitive impairment when taking benzodiazepines, and chronic use can accelerate cognitive decline (SOE=B). Thus, benzodiazepines are not first-line treatment in anxiety disorders in older adults. Better options for this patient include a third-generation antidepressant (eg, SSRI or serotonin-norepinephrine–reuptake inhibitor) and cognitive-behavioral therapy. When beginning treatment with antidepressants, adjunctive treatment with benzodiazepines may be considered until therapeutic levels of the antidepressant are reached, as long as the trial is brief and the patient is aware of the risks (SOE=C).

77. A 76-yr-old woman with end-stage heart failure (New York Heart Association class IV) has worsening dyspnea at rest and has become dependent in all ADLs except feeding. She sometimes feels as though she is suffocating and becomes very anxious. She began home hospice care 4 mo ago. She had been feeling relatively well since an increase in her furosemide dosage and the addition of supplemental oxygen last month. The cardiologist believes that she would not benefit from increasing her current dosages of carvedilol, enalapril, and spironolactone, and she has been compliant with her medication regimen and diet.

On a home visit by the hospice nurse, the patient is alert, oriented, and in mild distress. Temperature is 36.5° C (97.7° F), blood pressure is 126/64 mmHg, heart rate is 105 beats per minute, respiratory rate is 24 breaths per minute, and O$_2$ saturation is 97% on 4 L/min oxygen by nasal cannula. She has decreased breath sounds at the right base with dullness on percussion approximately one-fourth of the way up; a few crackles are heard at the left base. Jugular venous pressure is 12 mmHg. Hepatojugular reflex is positive, and leg edema is minimal.

The hospice nurse calls to discuss the care plan and recommends increasing the dosage of furosemide.

Which of the following is the most appropriate next step for this patient?

(A) Admit to the hospital for inpatient diuresis.
(B) Increase dosage of furosemide and arrange for outpatient, ultrasound-guided pleurocentesis.
(C) Increase dosage of furosemide and increase oxygen to 6 L/min by nasal cannula.
(D) Increase dosage of furosemide and add nebulized albuterol 2.5 mL q4h as needed for dyspnea.
(E) Increase dosage of furosemide and start morphine 5 mg po q3h as needed for dyspnea.

ANSWER: E

Dyspnea is common in many patients with advanced heart failure, even in those who are not in overt fluid overload. This patient shows evidence of mild fluid overload, and her furosemide dosage should be adjusted as recommended by the home hospice nurse. Because the cardiologist does not think her symptoms would improve by adjusting her other current medications, the addition of opioids should be considered (SOE=C). In patients who are not already taking an opioid, morphine, 5 mg po q3–6h as needed, can offer significant relief. Given this patient's persistent and distressing dyspnea, the morphine should be started at a low dosage as needed and adjusted for symptom relief.

Admission for inpatient diuresis is not indicated. If this patient's dyspnea was moderate or severe, and the hospice nurse and clinician did not believe that her symptoms could be managed effectively at home, then admission to the hospital for general inpatient care under the Medicare Hospice Benefit would be recommended. Although she likely has a right-sided pleural effusion, pleurocentesis is not likely to relieve her dyspnea and may cause significant complications, eg, pneumothorax. In addition, the effusion may improve with an increase in the furosemide dosage.

Supplemental oxygen can improve dyspnea in patients with heart failure, including those who are not hypoxemic. However, this patient is already on a moderate amount of supplemental oxygen, with normal O_2 saturation. Increasing supplemental oxygen to 6 L/min is unlikely to provide additional benefit. Nonpharmacologic methods that may be effective in the treatment of dyspnea include breathing training, walking aids, neuroelectrical muscle stimulation, and chest wall vibration (SOE=B). The use of fans and fresh air can also provide relief in patients with dyspnea (SOE=D).

There is no evidence to suggest that addition of nebulized albuterol relieves dyspnea in patients with heart failure without bronchospasm. This patient does not have evidence of reactive airway disease, she has no history of asthma or COPD, and she has no wheezing or other signs of obstruction. The addition of nebulized albuterol could exacerbate her tachycardia and dyspnea.

78. A 90-yr-old woman comes to the office to establish care. She has difficulty breathing with exertion and awakens several times each night to urinate. These symptoms began a year ago. She has a history of chronic poorly controlled hypertension, diabetes mellitus controlled by diet, and rheumatoid arthritis. On examination, jugular venous pressure is 9 cm H_2O. Lungs are clear. The abdomen is mildly distended with no tenderness, and there is 1+ edema in her legs. Brain natriuretic peptide (BNP) concentration is 76 pg/mL.

Which of the following is the most likely diagnosis?

(A) Deconditioning
(B) Heart failure with diastolic dysfunction
(C) Interstitial lung disease
(D) Pulmonary embolism
(E) Cirrhosis of the liver

ANSWER: B

Heart failure with diastolic dysfunction is common in patients with chronic hypertension, particularly women. Findings include dyspnea, edema, and increased jugular venous pressure. However, it is difficult on physical examination to differentiate systolic from diastolic heart failure. Lung examination is often normal in patients with chronic heart failure, despite evidence on physical examination of volume overload such as increased jugular venous pressure and edema. BNP is secreted by the myocardium as a result of increased stretch of the ventricular myocytes. BNP levels can be normal in patients with heart failure. Diagnosis of heart failure should therefore be based on physical signs and symptoms of heart failure, not on serum testing of BNP alone.

Deconditioning does not lead to increased jugular venous pressure. Interstitial lung disease due to rheumatoid arthritis is usually associated with an abnormal respiratory examination. While chronic pulmonary embolism could cause this patient's symptoms, diastolic dysfunction is more likely, given her chronic hypertension. Cirrhosis of the liver is unlikely to cause shortness of breath in the absence of significant ascites.

79. Which of the following is true regarding health literacy?

    (A) Health literacy is the degree to which a person can obtain, process, and understand information to make appropriate health decisions.

    (B) People with limited health literacy are more likely to ask questions about care during clinician visits.

    (C) Health status, rate of hospitalization, and health care costs of people with limited health literacy are similar to those of persons with adequate literacy.

    (D) In the United States, 12% of the population lacks health literacy.

ANSWER: A

Health literacy is the degree to which a person can obtain, process, and understand health information to make appropriate health decisions. Literacy level appears to be an important determinant of a patient's participation in medical encounters: people with limited health literacy are less likely to ask questions about care during clinician visits and more likely to make medication errors. Limited health literacy can affect a person's ability to learn about his or her medical conditions and treatments.

People with limited health literacy have less health knowledge, worse health status, more hospitalizations, higher healthcare costs, and poorer outcomes than people with adequate literacy (SOE=A). They are less likely to use preventive services and more likely to use hospitals and emergency departments. Inadequate knowledge about health, incorrect use of medication, poorer health status, and higher hospitalization rates related to limited health literacy increase healthcare costs by almost $100 billion each year.

According to the National Assessment of Adult Literacy survey conducted in 2003 by the U.S. Department of Education, only 12% of the adult population has sufficient skills to allow them to deal with complex and challenging tasks requiring health literacy. An additional 53% has intermediate skills, meaning they can deal with most tasks they encounter that require health literacy. The remainder of the population—36%, or nearly 90 million adults—has inadequate health literacy skills.

80. Which of the following has been shown to be of benefit in reducing pressure ulcers in acute-care settings?

    (A) Standard nutritional supplements for older patients

    (B) Specialized foam mattress hospital bed

    (C) Patient rotation q4h on regular hospital mattress

    (D) Specialized foam-mattress overlay on operating table

    (E) Standard sheepskin overlay on hospital bed

ANSWER: D

The prevalence of pressure ulcers in acute-care settings ranges from 0.4% to 38% based on observational studies. Patients with pressure ulcers have a mortality risk 2–6 times greater than patients with intact skin. In 2000 and 2001, pressure ulcers were cited as 1 of the top 3 in-hospital errors that lead to patient deaths; in an effort to improve care, as of October 2008 CMS no longer reimburses hospitals for costs due to pressure ulcers that develop during hospitalization.

In 2006, in a systematic review of trials of different interventions, evidence was sufficient to support use of specialized foam-mattress overlays on operating tables to reduce pressure ulcers (SOE=B). There was no difference in prevention of pressure ulcers between specialized foam mattresses and regular hospital beds (SOE=B). Special support surfaces may allow patients to be turned less frequently than q2h, but turning q4h has not been shown to reduce pressure ulcers. Specialized sheepskin overlays, which are thicker and denser than standard sheepskin overlays, help prevent pressure ulcers; standard sheepskin overlays do not (SOE=B).

The relationship between nutritional intake and prevention of pressure ulcers is based on limited evidence. Which specific nutrients offer the best protection is unclear. Evidence is mounting that nutritional supplementation for malnourished patients prevents wounds and helps healing (SOE=C), but there is no strong evidence that it benefits healthy older adults.

81. A 75-yr-old man is evaluated because he has sudden onset of shortness of breath; sharp, pleuritic left-sided chest pain; and cough productive of blood-tinged sputum. He had elective hip replacement surgery 6 days ago. He has been (and is) wearing pneumatic compression devices on both legs. He has a 20-yr history of COPD. He is taking a proton-pump inhibitor for a duodenal ulcer diagnosed 2 wk ago and albuterol as needed.

On examination, temperature is 38.0°C (100.4°F), blood pressure is 165/90 mmHg, heart rate is 110 breaths per minute, and respiratory rate is 26 breaths per minute. There is no accessory muscle use. He has slight expiratory wheezing. There is no jugular venous distension. A left-sided S4 gallop is audible. The abdomen is soft without masses or hepatosplenomegaly. There is no cyanosis, clubbing, edema, or thigh or calf pain.

WBC count is 13,800/µL, with 85% polymorphonuclear cells and 6% bands. Enzyme-linked immunosorbent assay reports D-dimer <500 ng/mL.

Arterial blood gas on room air:

pH	7.48
PaO_2	70 mmHg
$PaCO_2$	30 mmHg

An ECG reveals sinus tachycardia. Chest radiography reveals left lower-lobe atelectasis or infiltrate. Ventilation-perfusion (V/Q) scan indicates a low probability for pulmonary embolism. Bilateral lower-extremity Doppler ultrasonography demonstrates no evidence of deep vein thrombosis (DVT).

Which of the following is the most appropriate next step?

(A) Treat with heparin.
(B) Place an inferior vena cava filter.
(C) Treat with antibiotics and steroids.
(D) Obtain CT of chest.
(E) Obtain CT angiography of chest.

ANSWER: E

The individual symptoms, signs, laboratory data, and predisposing factors for pulmonary thromboembolism (PTE) are neither sensitive nor specific (SOE=A). When the clinical presentation suggests the possibility of PTE, pretest probability must be determined. In a validated clinical decision rule (Wells score), points are assigned based on history and clinical signs and symptoms. Pretest probability is based on total points (SOE=A). This patient's total Wells score is 6.5 (heart rate >100 beats per minute = 1, immobilization = 1.5, hemoptysis = 1, PTE more likely than alternative diagnosis = 3), indicating a high probability for PTE.

The results of all investigations must be interpreted in light of this high pretest probability. D-dimer is highly sensitive for DVT and PTE. Because several conditions (eg, sepsis, recent surgery, liver disease, malignancy) can increase D-dimer, the test is not specific for DVT or PTE. Consequently, a negative D-dimer (<500 ng/mL) by enzyme-linked immunosorbent assay, in the setting of low or intermediate probability of DVT or PTE, makes DVT and PTE unlikely (SOE=A). In this case, however, with the high pretest probability of PTE, the normal D-dimer does not result in a post-test probability low enough to preclude further evaluation, so the test result is not useful (SOE=A).

The only clinically useful results of a V/Q scan are normal and high probability. Because a V/Q scan is highly sensitive, a normal scan provides compelling evidence against PTE (SOE=A). In patients with a high pretest probability for PTE, a high probability V/Q scan confirms the diagnosis (SOE=A). V/Q scans other than normal or high probability require additional diagnostic evaluation (SOE=A). In this patient, the low-probability V/Q scan does not exclude PTE. In the Prospective Investigation of Pulmonary Embolism Diagnosis (PIOPED), 40% of patients with a low-probability V/Q scan in whom the clinical suspicion of PTE was high had angiographically confirmed PTE.

The sensitivity and specificity for diagnosing *symptomatic* proximal DVT by Doppler ultrasonography is ≥95% (SOE=A). However, its sensitivity and specificity in the setting of *asymptomatic* proximal DVT ranges from 47% to 62%. Again, a negative result cannot exclude PTE in this patient.

In almost all circumstances, prolonged treatment of PTE (eg, with inferior vena cava filter or heparin) requires objective documentation. Although treatment with heparin is recommended during evaluation for suspected PTE, in this case heparin is contraindicated because of the patient's recent history of a duodenal ulcer. CT of the chest could be useful for diagnosing pulmonary causes of this patient's presentation other than PTE, ie, pulmonary infiltrate consistent with pneumonia. However, given the high pretest probability of PTE, CT angiography is required to exclude PTE.

82. A 92-yr-old woman is brought to the office by her daughter because she is moving more slowly and unsteadily. She has not had any falls. She lives with her family and she is independent in ADLs. Until 2 yr ago, she took walks 3 times a week. Now her aerobic activity is limited to climbing 7 household steps about twice daily. She has a distant history of breast cancer and mild osteoarthritis. Medications include acetaminophen, vitamin D, and calcium.

On examination, vital signs are normal. There is no tremor or rigidity, and motor strength is symmetric and only slightly reduced. She stands unassisted but sways on standing and reaches out for contact assistance. She walks across the examination room without assistance but reaches out to touch the examination table. Her Mini–Mental State Examination score is normal.

Which of the following is the most appropriate next step?

(A) Establish a graduated balance-training program.
(B) Establish a high-intensity quadriceps strengthening program with 10 to 15 repetitions per session.
(C) Establish a moderate-intensity walking program of ≥1000 steps per day.
(D) Establish a high-intensity walking program of ≥5000 steps per day.
(E) Prescribe pain medication to be taken immediately before exercise.

ANSWER: A

This patient is at risk of falls and loss of function. She has not engaged in exercise over the past 2 yr, and her balance has deteriorated significantly. She requires a comprehensive physical activity program. However, the program should be initiated slowly to reduce

the risk of injury and to improve the likelihood of adherence. Graduated balance-training exercises should begin immediately, with static exercises such as single-leg stands and side-to-side weight shifts, and dynamic exercises such as tandem walk and heel walk (SOE=C). Strengthening exercises of the quadriceps and hip flexors would be beneficial but should not be high intensity (ie, maximum that can be lifted). The aerobic component of the program should start at low intensity. Setting a goal based on number of steps per day is not useful, even with a pedometer, because it is difficult to translate number of steps into minutes of continuous exercise (SOE=C). Pain medication can be used if needed, but there is no indication that pain is limiting her activity.

83. A 75-yr-old man comes to the office for a routine physical examination. He feels well. He has a known history of chronic kidney disease; history also includes long-term type 2 diabetes mellitus, peripheral vascular disease, and coronary artery disease. Medications include insulin, metoprolol, sevelamer, and calcitriol. Examination is unremarkable.

Laboratory results (blood sample drawn at dialysis):

BUN	20 mg/dL
Creatinine	2.0 mg/dL
Sodium	140 mEq/L
Potassium	4.4 mEq/L
Hemoglobin	10 g/dL
Iron	within normal limits

Which of the following is the most appropriate next step?

(A) Begin epoetin-α with a target hemoglobin concentration of 13–14 mg/dL.
(B) Begin epoetin-α with a target hemoglobin concentration of 11–12 mg/dL.
(C) Begin epoetin-α if hemoglobin concentration falls to <9 mg/dL.
(D) Begin epoetin-α if symptoms develop.

ANSWER: B

Erythropoietin has become a standard part of therapy for patients with chronic or end-stage renal disease, because it improves both physiologic and clinical parameters and quality of life (SOE=A). Recommendations are to treat patients with anemia of chronic renal disease when the hemoglobin concentration falls to <9 g/dL (SOE=C). However, better outcomes have been most consistently associated with hemoglobin concentrations of 11–12 g/dL (hematocrit 33%–36%) (SOE=B). Evidence is increasing for worse clinical outcomes when hemoglobin concentration ≥13 g/dL (hematocrit ≥39%) is targeted and maintained in dialysis and predialysis patients (SOE=B). The U.S. Normal Hematocrit Study was terminated prematurely because patients in the group targeted to normal hematocrit values had a higher mortality that approached statistical significance. Other possible adverse consequences associated with normal or near-normal hemoglobin concentrations include stroke, arteriovenous access thrombosis, and hypertension. The updated 2007 guidelines from the National Kidney Foundation Dialysis Outcomes Quality Initiative (DOQI) recommend target hemoglobin concentrations of 11–12 g/d, not to exceed 13 g/dL (SOE=B). Similar target levels are recommended in Canadian, European, and Japanese guidelines.

84. A 78-yr-old widowed woman is in a nursing facility after hemicolectomy for metastatic cancer. She is dependent in ADLs, and her medical prognosis is poor. She presents herself as a woman who had unparalleled success in her career and numerous offers of marriage. Her brother reports that her lifelong tendency to become enraged after perceived slights has alienated her from her children and other relatives. Although at times she is tearful, she enjoys making herself the focus of unit activities. She has not had changes in sleep or appetite. As her medical problems worsen, she is increasingly demanding and verbally abusive of nursing staff.

Mental status examination reveals normal rate of speech and psychomotor activity, and cognitive examination is normal.

Which of the following is the most likely diagnosis?

(A) Bipolar disorder, manic type
(B) Histrionic personality disorder
(C) Major depressive disorder
(D) Narcissistic personality disorder

ANSWER: D

This patient has personality disorder, which is characterized by a long-standing, pervasive pattern of disturbances in emotionality, cognition, interpersonal functioning, and impulse control that cause significant distress or impaired functioning. Patients with narcissistic personality disorder tend to exaggerate achievements, seek admiration, and exhibit arrogant behavior and limited empathy toward others. In late life, such behaviors and traits become particularly troublesome when interpersonal environmental demands change. Unavoidable dependency, transition to institutional living, and the need to rely on others to meet one's daily needs always require time to achieve a new equilibrium. But when the need to adjust is compounded by chronic interpersonal vulnerabilities, persistent dysequilibrium can be the result. When a "situational adjustment reaction" seems extreme or overlong, a personality disorder should be considered.

Patients with histrionic personality disorder display excessive emotionality and seek attention but do not have the inflated sense of self-importance or entitlement seen with narcissistic personality disorder.

Patients with bipolar disorder, manic type, can demonstrate persistently elevated or irritable mood during an episode, which can manifest as inflated self-esteem, as well as excessive engagement in pleasurable activities, decreased need for sleep, and increased rate of speech.

Because the patient is not pervasively dysphoric, enjoys daily activities, and does not report changes in sleep or appetite, major depressive disorder is unlikely.

85. A 75-yr-old man comes to the office for his annual visit. He has a family history of heart disease and wonders whether he would benefit from taking aspirin. He exercises frequently. History includes borderline dyslipidemia. On examination, blood pressure is 130/70 mmHg.

Which of the following is true about the role of aspirin in primary prevention?

(A) Enteric coating decreases the risk of aspirin-related GI bleeding.
(B) The recommended dose for primary prevention is 325 mg/d.
(C) Aspirin reduces the number of cardiovascular events in men.
(D) Aspirin reduces the risk of ischemic stroke in men.

ANSWER: C

The role of aspirin in primary prevention of ischemic stroke and cardiovascular events has been studied with varying results for years. Several randomized, controlled trials demonstrate that aspirin reduces the risk of myocardial infarction in men (SOE=A). Depending on the study and the risk factors of the cohort, the number needed to treat to prevent one myocardial infarction over 5 yr ranges from 65 to 667. The randomized trials did not show a reduction in death or ischemic stroke, but they were underpowered to assess these outcomes.

Study results have been mixed regarding the role of aspirin in primary prevention of heart disease in women. In the Nurses' Health Study, fewer cardiovascular events were observed in women ≥55 yr old who used aspirin, but aspirin did not prevent stroke or death from any cause. In contrast, the Women's Health Study showed a decrease in stroke but not in cardiovascular events for women taking aspirin 100 mg every other day.

The current consensus is to consider the individual patient's risk of coronary artery disease, including sex, age, diabetes, cholesterol level, blood pressure, and smoking and family history. Organizations such as the U.S. Preventive Services Task Force recommend aspirin for patients in whom the risk of coronary artery disease in 5 yr is ≥3%.

The optimal dose of aspirin for men appears to be between 75 mg and 160 mg daily or every other day. Enteric-coated preparations do not decrease the risk of GI bleeding. Over a 5-yr period, aspirin causes GI bleeding in 4 to 12 per 1,000 older adults, and hemorrhagic stroke in 0 to 2 per 1,000 adults. These risks are likely higher in patients who have uncontrolled hypertension, use NSAIDs, or are >75 yr old, and in patients taking higher dosages of aspirin.

86. A 76-yr-old man comes to the office because he recently read about the new "shingles shot" and wants to know if he should have it. He had an isolated case of herpes zoster in the past and does not want a recurrence.

Which of the following is true regarding the herpes zoster vaccine Zostavax?

(A) It is recommended for people with acute zoster or ongoing post-herpetic neuralgia.
(B) It is less effective in preventing post-herpetic neuralgia in adults ≥70 yr old than in younger adults.
(C) People with a history of herpes zoster infection were excluded from the stage 3 trial.
(D) Before administration of the vaccine, the patient's history of varicella exposure should be confirmed.

ANSWER: C

Herpes zoster develops in approximately 30% of adults over a lifetime. The risk of herpes zoster increases with age: by age 85, 50% of adults have had herpes zoster. The incidence of post-herpetic neuralgia increases with age. Approximately 40% of adults ≥60 yr older are likely to have neuralgia after an episode of herpes zoster.

The zoster vaccine (Zostavax) was licensed for prevention of herpes zoster after being studied in a large (38,546 participants), double-blind, placebo-controlled trial of adults ≥59 yr old; 90% of participants had more than one underlying chronic medical illness. The average duration of follow-up was 3 yr, and 95% of participants completed the study. The vaccine was more effective in preventing zoster in adults between the ages of 60 and 69 than for those >70 yr old. However, the incidence of post-herpetic neuralgia was lower in the group ≥70 yr old than in adults 60–69 yr old. From this study, 17 persons would need to be vaccinated to prevent 1 case of herpes zoster, and approximately 31 would need to be vaccinated to prevent 1 case of post-herpetic neuralgia (SOE=A).

Adults with a history of zoster were excluded from the trial, possibly because of the risk of recurrent zoster. However, use of the vaccine does not appear to present safety concerns for this group, and patients do not need to be asked about varicella exposure or have a varicella titer determined before receiving the vaccine.

The vaccine is not used to treat people with acute zoster or to treat ongoing post-herpetic neuralgia. It is contraindicated for patients who are immunosuppressed, have a history of tuberculosis, or have recently taken either steroids or chemotherapy for cancer. Typical adverse events of the vaccine are local, varicella-like rash, erythema, pain, swelling, and pruritus at the site of injection.

87. A 78-yr-old man comes to the office because he recently fell for no apparent reason. He has had cognitive problems for 5 yr. At first, friends noticed that he often seemed inattentive and was easily distractible. He began having trouble navigating to the location of his poker game, held at a different person's house each month. His family noticed that he was intermittently confused and often talked of seeing different friends (deceased) at his house. He is no longer able to organize his social calendar or prepare a tax return, which he previously did with ease. The family believes that recently his memory has begun "failing" as well. The history suggests dementia with Lewy bodies.

Which of the following statements is most accurate about dementia with Lewy bodies?

(A) Clinical suspicion is increased if parkinsonism was present ≥2 yr before the dementia.
(B) A history of exposure to neuroleptic agents with no adverse event excludes the diagnosis.
(C) Occipital lobe hypermetabolism is seen on positron emission tomography (PET).
(D) Associated visual hallucinations are usually complex and vivid.

ANSWER: D

Diagnostic criteria for dementia with Lewy bodies are subdivided into central, core, suggestive, and supportive features. The central feature, dementia, is required, although memory impairment is often less conspicuous than deficits in attention, executive function, and visuospatial ability, especially early in

the disease course. Core features consist of fluctuating cognition, recurrent visual hallucinations, and spontaneous parkinsonism. Suggestive features consist of rapid-eye movement (REM) sleep behavior disorder, severe neuroleptic sensitivity, and low dopamine-transporter uptake in the basal ganglia observed on single-proton emission CT or PET. Supportive features, such as syncope, delusions, or autonomic dysfunction, are common but do not have diagnostic specificity. Diagnosis usually specifies degree of certainty by denoting "probable" or "possible" dementia with Lewy bodies. The central feature (dementia) must always be present.

The criteria make formal note of the temporal sequence of symptoms, specifying that parkinsonism should occur after or concurrent with the onset of dementia to warrant the diagnosis of dementia with Lewy bodies. If parkinsonism is well established by the time dementia occurs, then the diagnosis is Parkinson's disease dementia. A gap of at least 1 yr between onset of dementia and parkinsonism is recommended to facilitate distinction between dementia with Lewy bodies and Parkinson's disease dementia.

Visual hallucinations in dementia with Lewy bodies are often complex, detailed, and vivid. The hallucinations tend to be recurrent, and patients often retain a degree of insight into their unreality. The degree of insight can be helpful in deciding whether to initiate antipsychotic therapy, which can cause clinical deterioration in a patient with Lewy body dementia.

Neuroleptic sensitivity is suggestive of dementia with Lewy bodies. Because 50% of patients with dementia with Lewy bodies do not react adversely, past neuroleptic use without adverse event does not exclude the diagnosis. Sensitivity reactions are characterized by acute onset or exacerbation of parkinsonism and impaired consciousness.

88. A 68-yr-old woman is brought to the emergency department because she woke up from an afternoon nap with a sudden onset of rotational vertigo and clumsiness of the right arm. She feels as though the world is tilting toward the right. She is unable to walk even with assistance, and she has a headache. History includes hypertension and type II insulin-dependent

diabetes. Her medications include lisinopril, metformin, and aspirin.

On examination, temperature is 37.5°C (99.5°F). Blood pressure is 180/95 mmHg, pulse is 80 beats per minute, and respiratory rate is 16 breaths per minute. She has horizontal nystagmus and a negative head thrust test. She has difficulty both with making rapid alternating movements with the right arm and with toe-tapping or heel-to-shin movements on the right leg.

Which of the following is the most likely diagnosis?

(A) Cerebellar infarct
(B) Dorsolateral medullary stroke
(C) Meniere disease
(D) Herpes zoster infection of the inner ear (Ramsay Hunt syndrome)
(E) Benign paroxysmal positional vertigo

ANSWER: A

The sudden onset of vertigo with other focal neurologic symptoms makes a stroke most likely. A diagnosis of cerebellar or posterior fossa infarction should be considered in any patient with acute onset of vertigo. The patient should undergo immediate imaging, especially given her history of headache (SOE=C). In the event of posterior fossa hemorrhage, surgical evaluation may be lifesaving (SOE=D). The nystagmus in a cerebellar infarct may look similar to a peripheral nystagmus (horizontal torsional).

A head thrust test (or head impulse test) can help distinguish vestibular neuritis from stroke (SOE=C). With rapid, passive head rotation as the patient fixes on a central target, the normal response (ie, a negative test) is an equal and opposite eye movement that keeps the eyes stationary in space. The inability to maintain fixation after head rotation that requires a corrective gaze shift is abnormal (ie, a positive test). Vertigo with a negative head thrust test suggests central stroke. A positive head thrust test suggests a peripheral cause but does not absolutely exclude a stroke.

Patients can also present with an ocular tilt reaction that can be on the same side or on the opposite side of the cerebellar infarct. Dorsolateral medullary stroke (Wallenberg's syndrome) is usually accompanied by other

focal neurologic signs and symptoms, including ipsilateral Horner's pupil, ipsilateral facial pain and loss of temperature sensation, ipsilateral central facial (lower face only) weakness, and contralateral pain and loss of temperature sensation in the arms and legs. It is often associated with artery-to-artery emboli from vertebral artery atherosclerosis to the posterior inferior cerebellar artery. Meniere disease, Ramsay Hunt syndrome, and benign paroxysmal positional vertigo do not present with clumsiness of the extremities.

89. A 72-yr-old woman comes to the office for preoperative evaluation before left total-knee replacement. Despite the worsening pain in her left knee, she remains active, and gardens and plays golf 4 days a week. She has no known allergies and has never smoked. Both her parents lived into their nineties. History includes mild hypertension, for which she takes atenolol 25 mg/d.

On physical examination, blood pressure is 121/82 mmHg and resting heart rate is 70 beats per minute. Other than osteoarthritic changes in both knees, left worse than right, her examination is unremarkable. Serum chemistries and CBC are within normal limits. ECG shows no conduction delays and no ischemic changes.

Which of the following is most appropriate for perioperative management of this patient?

(A) Increase atenolol dosage to 50 mg/d; continue perioperatively.
(B) Discontinue atenolol immediately before surgery; restart 48 h after surgery.
(C) Continue atenolol at the current dosage.
(D) Discontinue atenolol; begin an ACE inhibitor plus a statin.

ANSWER: C

This patient has a Revised Cardiac Risk Index of 0 (normal creatinine level; no heart failure, ischemic heart disease, or diabetes; and no history of cerebrovascular disease). For patients at low cardiac risk (index of 0 or 1) who are already on a β-blocker for hypertension, angina, arrhythmias, or other cardiac problems, β-blocker treatment should be continued perioperatively (SOE=C).

Perioperative β-blockers should not be started in patients at low cardiac risk (index of 0 or 1) who do not already take a β-blocker; in these patients, β-blockers offer no benefit and may be harmful (SOE=B). The available evidence suggests that benefit from β-blockers is primarily limited to patients with a Revised Cardiac Risk Index >2 who are undergoing major noncardiac surgery.

Increasing the dosage of β-blocker in a low-risk patient affords no benefit and may precipitate perioperative hypotension or bradycardia. Abrupt discontinuation of the β-blocker could result in rebound hypertension and tachycardia. In this patient, there is no indication for starting an ACE inhibitor.

90. An 80-yr-old patient comes to the office for a routine physical examination. She has mild hearing loss and is otherwise healthy. She takes a multivitamin and calcium citrate with vitamin D, and walks 1 mile daily. She states that she wishes to live to be 100 yr old and asks for advice about following the Mediterranean diet.

Which of the following is consistent with following the Mediterranean diet?

(A) Reduce fat intake.
(B) Reduce consumption of fish.
(C) Increase consumption of poultry.
(D) Increase consumption of legumes and whole grains.
(E) Increase consumption of bread and rice.

ANSWER: D

Mediterranean diets are characterized by high intake of vegetables, legumes, fruits, and unrefined cereals; moderate to high intake of fish; low to moderate intake of dairy, mostly as cheese and yogurt; low intake of meat; and modest intake of alcohol, mostly as wine. Mediterranean diets have up to 40% fat. What makes them healthy is the balance of fats: low intake of saturated fats; high intake of monounsaturated fats, especially olive oil; and intake of polyunsaturated fats to provide sufficient omega-3 fatty acid.

The Mediterranean diet has been associated with longevity in several studies. In a recent large-scale, prospective trial conducted by the National Institutes of Health and the American Association for Retired Persons, the Mediterranean diet was associated with reduced all-cause and cause-specific mortality. In men, the multivariate hazard ratios comparing high to low conformity to diet for all-cause, cardiovascular disease, and cancer mortality were 0.79 (95% CI, 0.76–0.83), 0.78 (95% CI, 0.69–0.87), and 0.83 (95% CI, 0.76–0.91), respectively. In women with high conformity to diet, this study found decreased risks that ranged from 12% for cancer mortality to 20% for all-cause mortality (P = .04 and P <.001, respectively).

Possible mechanisms of action for the Mediterranean diet include a high antioxidant capacity and low concentrations of oxidized low-density lipoprotein; high fiber and a low omega-6 to omega-3 fatty acid ratio, which potentially prevent cancer initiation and progression; and less chronic inflammation as evidenced by lower levels of C-reactive protein, interleukin-6, homocysteine, and fibrinogen, and by lower WBC counts (SOE=B).

91. An 82-yr-old woman comes to the office because she has urine leakage when she coughs or sneezes, as well as urinary frequency and urgency. History includes COPD, hypertension, and aortic stenosis.

On pelvic examination, there is grade III pelvic prolapse. Postvoid residual volume is 200 mL.

Which of the following is most likely to be effective for this patient?

(A) Vaginal pessary
(B) Burch colposuspension
(C) Kegel exercises
(D) Oxybutynin

ANSWER: A

Support and space-filling pessaries are used to treat pelvic organ prolapse. A support pessary can be used to treat all stages of pelvic organ prolapse and stress urinary incontinence, whereas a space-filling pessary is mostly used for severe prolapse. Use of a vaginal pessary for pelvic organ prolapse is appropriate if a patient does not want surgery, if there is a need to delay surgery, or if the patient is a poor surgical candidate (SOE=C).

Most pessaries are made of silicone, which is nonallergenic and durable, and does not retain odors. They are fit by trial and error. A ring pessary, which provides support, is the most commonly used and is likely to be successful for stage II or III prolapse. A Gellhorn pessary is more likely to be successful with stage III prolapse. After a pessary is fitted, a follow-up visit is scheduled for 1–2 wk later. The pessary is removed and cleaned, and the vagina is examined for erosions. If the patient is unable to remove and reinsert the pessary, follow-up is again scheduled in 1–2 wk, and then every 3–4 mo thereafter. Common adverse events include vaginal erosion, bleeding, and discharge. They usually occur in the setting of vaginal atrophy and can be treated or prevented by use of low-dose vaginal estrogen cream. Serious complications from vaginal pessaries are rare. For women with urinary incontinence, 1-mo efficacy is approximately 60%. In about 60% of cases, there is long-term (6–12 mo) satisfaction and continued use.

This patient's COPD and aortic stenosis make surgery, such as colposuspension, less attractive and perhaps not feasible. Kegel exercises are not indicated for the treatment of incontinence due to prolapse. Oxybutynin, which is useful in the treatment of urge incontinence, is contraindicated in the presence of a larger postvoid residual volume.

92. Which of the following statements regarding treatment for major depressive disorder is true?

(A) Most older adults with the diagnosis are treated by a psychiatrist.
(B) In older adults on an effective dosage of antidepressants, the response rate is close to 80% after 8 wk.
(C) Risk of recurrence or relapse is higher in patients who did not reach full remission.
(D) Augmentation with a second agent is not appropriate after a partial response to one antidepressant.
(E) Psychosocial interventions have little impact on rate of remission or risk of recurrence.

ANSWER: C

Most older adults with major depressive disorder present to their primary care clinician with multiple somatic symptoms, anxiety, poor sleep, or concerns about decline in cognitive performance. Because of the nonspecific nature of the symptoms, the inability of many patients to voice sadness, and the limited time available to primary care clinicians to address multiple medical problems and medications, major depressive disorder is often overlooked. Patients are often treated with anxiolytic or sleep agents, and symptoms are likely to worsen. Even with correct diagnosis, patients are rarely referred to a psychiatrist. For patients without suicidal thoughts or psychosis, referral to a psychiatrist is often unnecessary; second-generation antidepressant medications and nonpharmacologic interventions can be effectively prescribed by primary care clinicians.

Often these medications are prescribed at inappropriately low dosages, or for too short a time. All antidepressant medications require a trial of 8 wk at full therapeutic dosage before their efficacy in a particular patient can be evaluated; the best evidence indicates that a significant percentage of nonresponders or partial responders will achieve remission if the trial is continued until week 12. However, even under the best conditions, the response rate is unlikely to exceed 60% (in many trials it can be as low as 40%, barely reaching statistical significance), particularly at 8 wk. In some trials, it approached 80% after ≥12 wk.

In many trials, a significant reduction in symptoms is considered as a response to treatment. However, partial response is associated with a high risk of relapse and recurrence (SOE=A). Full remission is a return to a fully euthymic mood with no residual symptoms. Remission is associated with a higher level of psychosocial function, significantly lower risk of relapse or recurrence, and overall improvement in quality of life indicators. Remission is rarely achieved with a single medication. Results of the STAR-D trial support the practice of switching interventions for patients in whom the initial agent failed, or dosage augmentation for patients who have a partial response to treatment (SOE=A). The morbidity and mortality associated with untreated major depressive disorder are significant, and most of the medications currently used as first- and second-line treatment are well tolerated, even in combination. Several studies provide evidence in support of psychosocial interventions to improve response to medications, improve functioning, and decrease risk of relapse or recurrence.

93. A 75-yr-old woman with established osteoporosis wishes to discuss advertisements she has seen for ibandronate and risedronate. She currently takes alendronate and wonders whether she would benefit more from a different agent. She has not had a fracture.

Which of the following is the best agent for preventing fracture?

(A) Alendronate
(B) Ibandronate
(C) Pamidronate
(D) Risedronate
(E) Data are not available to answer her question.

ANSWER: E

Bisphosphonates are effective in reducing fracture risk among postmenopausal women with osteoporosis. When compared with placebo, these agents prevent vertebral, nonvertebral, and hip fractures (SOE=A). Patients are exposed to considerable advertising about the benefits of these agents, different dosing regimens, and convenience. Studies have not been identified that demonstrate the superiority of one agent over another in preventing fractures (SOE=A). A systematic review of studies of agents used to treat osteoporosis identified the following design issues: 1) few studies compared different agents within the same class; 2) most head-to-head comparisons of agents from different classes reported intermediate outcomes (eg, changes in bone mineral density or in markers of bone turnover) rather than differences in fracture incidence; and 3) no trial with head-to-head comparisons of ≥2 agents had a sufficient sample size to detect even large differences in fracture risk.

Only 2 head-to-head trials were designed to compare fracture outcomes. In one, no difference was found between risedronate and etidronate for the prevention of vertebral fractures. In the other, which compared raloxifene and alendronate, not enough participants were recruited to test differences in fracture outcomes. The authors of the above-mentioned systematic review

concluded that "1) within the bisphosphonate class, superiority for prevention of fractures has not been shown for any agent; 2) superiority for the prevention of vertebral fractures has not been demonstrated for bisphosphonates compared with calcitonin, calcium, or raloxifene; and 3) on the basis of 6 inadequately powered randomized trials, fracture prevention did not differ between bisphosphonates and estrogen."

94. An 84-yr-old-man comes to the office to get information on minimizing muscle loss. He is vigorous and healthy, with no chronic diseases. He has heard that muscle loss is a serious problem with aging and may contribute to frailty. He would like to take medication to delay or minimize muscle loss associated with aging.

Which of the following is most likely to minimize the patient's muscle loss?

(A) Testosterone
(B) Dehydroepiandrosterone
(C) Growth hormone
(D) Vitamin D
(E) No medication

ANSWER: E

No supplement or medication has been proved to increase function in older men with sarcopenia without significant adverse events. Studies of testosterone replacement have been inconclusive, although one trial showed improvement in function.

Dehydroepiandrosterone has not been shown to consistently improve strength or function in older men. Growth hormone can improve muscle strength, but the adverse events and cost prohibit its use. Vitamin D supplements are associated with fewer falls in frail older adults with vitamin D insufficiency, but its role in preventing sarcopenia is unknown. The therapy consistently shown to prevent sarcopenia is resistance training and exercise (SOE=A).

95. Which of the following statements is true of older versus younger adults with anxiety disorders?

    (A) Older adults are less likely to respond to medication for anxiety disorders.

    (B) Older adults are less likely to respond to psychotherapy for anxiety disorders.

    (C) Older adults are less likely to cite anxiety as a primary complaint.

    (D) Older adults are less likely to have an anxiety disorder.

ANSWER: C

Older adults are less likely than younger adults to cite emotional distress as a chief complaint; this may be a cohort effect specific to the current generation of patients. Thus, clinicians need to be vigilant for anxiety disorders and their associated somatic presentations.

Anxiety disorders are seen in older adults, although phobias and panic disorder are unlikely to have first onset in old age. Because they are common in young adults as well as highly chronic and relapsing in nature, anxiety disorders are present in many older adults (SOE=C).

Age is not a determinant of responsiveness to medication or psychotherapy in anxiety disorders.

96. An 82-yr-old man who lives in a nursing facility is evaluated because he has a facial rash. He has been taking ciprofloxacin therapy for 5 days for a urinary tract infection. History includes Parkinson's disease and dementia.

On examination, the rash comprises mild erythematous plaques with fine scales along the frontal hairline of the scalp as well as moderate erythema with increased scales along the nasolabial folds bilaterally.

Which of the following would be effective as an initial step in managing this patient's rash?

    (A) Discontinue ciprofloxacin
    (B) Open wet dressings
    (C) 5% Fluorouracil ointment
    (D) Ketoconazole cream and topical low-potency steroid
    (E) Skin biopsy

ANSWER: D

This patient has an exacerbation of seborrheic dermatitis, which is common in men and in patients with Parkinson's disease. Exacerbations of dermatitis can be triggered by stress and illness (eg, urinary tract infection). Seborrheic dermatitis is diagnosed based on its appearance. The findings on examination in this case are typical: inflammatory changes with erythematous scaling, and pruritic plaques in the affected sites of the scalp and nasolabial folds. Treatment of seborrheic dermatitis includes an antifungal preparation, such as ketoconazole (SOE= A), to decrease colonization by yeast, and topical steroids to address the inflammatory and erythematous eruption. The need for combination therapy is based on the severity of symptoms and the degree of pruritus or erythema involved. A mild steroid (class IV-VI) should be used first, for a limited period of therapy. Although topical steroids are associated with several adverse events, including skin atrophy, discoloration, and telangiectasia, appropriate use of the least-potent steroid can minimize these outcomes. If response to the low-potency steroid is inadequate, a higher potency, class III steroid can be used. If response is still inadequate, a class II or I steroid may be considered, or a referral to a dermatologist.

The characteristics and location of the patient's lesions are not consistent with drug allergy reactions or actinic keratosis. Drug eruption can present with a fine erythematous maculopapular rash, hives, or scale, but the distribution should include the trunk and often the extremities. Open wet dressings can be useful for any inflammatory or pruritic eruption but would not specifically treat seborrheic dermatitis. Skin biopsy would be useful for diagnosing actinic keratosis or squamous cell carcinoma. Typically, actinic keratoses are slightly pink and rough to touch, but they may be skin colored or pigmented. Although lesions can be as large as several centimeters in diameter, more typically they average 5 mm. Actinic keratoses can be treated with 5% fluorouracil ointment.

97. A 79-yr-old man is brought to the office by his daughter; both are concerned about his recent deterioration and want to know his prognosis. The patient has hypertension, peripheral vascular disease, and stage IV colon cancer.

Poorly differentiated adenocarcinoma of the colon, metastatic to liver and peritoneum, was diagnosed 2 yr ago. He did well after surgical resection of his tumor and treatment with bevacizumab. However, now there is increased involvement of his liver and peritoneum along with new pulmonary nodules. He has constant abdominal pain that is well controlled with a fentanyl patch and oxycodone as needed for breakthrough pain. He has become increasingly debilitated over the last 6 mo. Because of fatigue and pain, he is unable to do most IADLs, and in the last 4 wk he has become dependent in all ADLs except feeding.

Which of the following patient characteristics is most predictive of a poor prognosis?

(A) Low performance status
(B) Advanced tumor stage
(C) Multiple comorbidities
(D) Advanced age
(E) Opioid use

ANSWER: A

Performance status is the best predictor of prognosis in patients with advanced cancer (SOE=A). It is a global measure of a patient's functional capacity, or ability to maintain independence in daily life. A number of different tools are available to assess performance status, including the Karnofsky Performance Score and the Palliative Performance Scale, Version 2.

In some studies, tumor stage, comorbidity, advanced age, and opioid dependence have been shown to influence prognosis, but the findings are not consistent. These factors are usually most prognostic in less advanced disease.

98. An 80-yr-old man comes to the office because he has had a left frontal headache and blurry vision for 2 wk. In addition, he has been feeling more tired, and his jaw aches when he eats. He denies nausea, vomiting, neck stiffness or visual loss. On examination, there is no nuchal rigidity or temporal tenderness. His pupils are round, equal in size, and reactive to light. Visual acuity, visual fields, fundoscopic examination, and extraocular movements are normal.

Which of the following is most likely to confirm the diagnosis?

(A) CT of the head
(B) Temporal artery biopsy
(C) Slit-lamp examination
(D) Tonometry
(E) Cerebral angiography

ANSWER: B

Temporal (giant cell) arteritis is a vasculitis that affects the large- and medium-size blood vessels. Criteria that distinguish giant cell arteritis from other types of vasculitis include age >50 yr old, localized headache, tenderness or decreased pulse of the temporal artery, RBC sedimentation rate >50 mm/h, and a biopsy positive for necrotizing arteritis. The presence of 3 criteria has a sensitivity of 93% and specificity of 91.2%. Other common symptoms include fever, fatigue, weight loss, jaw claudication, and visual loss.

If temporal arteritis is suspected, temporal artery biopsy is indicated. In a meta-analysis of 21 studies, biopsy was positive in 39% of patients with suspected temporal arteritis. In this meta-analysis, the features associated with an increased likelihood of temporal arteritis were jaw claudication (positive likelihood ratio 4.2) and diplopia (positive likelihood ratio 3.4). Normal sedimentation rate was associated with a decreased likelihood of temporal arteritis (negative likelihood ratio 0.2) (SOE=A).

99. A 68-yr-old resident of a nursing facility is admitted to the hospital because he has increasing pain and erythema related to a sacral pressure ulcer for which he had been receiving treatment. He has a history of stroke and right-sided hemiparesis.

On examination, vital signs are stable. There is a 3 cm × 6 cm midline sacral ulcer with a dry, black eschar covering the entire wound, surrounding warmth, and erythema. It is tender to touch, and when pressed, it exudes moderate amounts of pus.

Which of the following is the most appropriate treatment for the pressure ulcer?

(A)   Hydrocolloid dressings applied every 3 to 5 days
(B)   Sharp debridement of eschar
(C)   Papain-urea cream applied to eschar twice daily
(D)   Wet-to-dry dressings applied twice daily
(E)   Hydrogel dressings applied twice daily

ANSWER: B

This patient has an unstageable pressure ulcer with a black eschar and signs of infection. He has no contraindications to local excision. The wound needs to be opened and cleansed to promote healing. The eschar requires sharp debridement with a scalpel, scissors, or forceps (SOE=C). Antibiotic therapy is required as well.

Hydrocolloid dressings are appropriate for stage II and III ulcers and provide a good environment for autolytic debridement but are contraindicated in infected ulcers (SOE=C). Papain-urea cream is a form of enzymatic debridement that dissolves devitalized tissue and is helpful with patients who cannot tolerate surgery or procedures (SOE=C), but it is also contraindicated in infected ulcers.

Wet-to-dry dressings promote mechanical debridement; they are inappropriate in the setting of an infected, unstageable ulcer. Wet-to-dry dressings can also cause damage to healing granulated tissue (SOE=B).

Hydrogel dressings are cross-linked polymer gels that are often shaped into sheets to provide and maintain a moist wound environment; they need to be combined with gauze dressings. They are appropriate for stage II, III, and IV ulcers (SOE=B). By increasing moisture content, hydrogel dressings help clean and debride necrotic tissue. They may be appropriate for treatment of this patient's ulcer, but only after the eschar has been removed, the wound cleansed, and the stage of the ulcer identified.

100.   An 85-yr-old woman is brought to the emergency department by her family because of increasingly erratic behavior. Normally, she functions independently, but over the past few days she has been forgetful, confused, and disoriented. History includes pneumonia 6 mo ago, hypertension, and gastroesophageal reflux.

Medications include hydrochlorothiazide, omeprazole, lisinopril, and a multivitamin.

On examination, her vital signs are within normal limits. She is inattentive and scores 16/30 on the Mini–Mental State Examination.

Laboratory results:
Sodium   128 mmol/L
Potassium   3.2 mmol/L
BUN   10 mg/dL
Creatinine   0.8 mg/dL
Urine sodium   80 mmol/L
Urine osmolality   450 mOsm/kg

Which of the following is the most likely cause of this patient's hyponatremia?

(A)   Syndrome of inappropriate arginine vasopressin secretion
(B)   Water intoxication
(C)   Hydrochlorothiazide
(D)   Omeprazole
(E)   Volume depletion and poor oral intake

ANSWER: C

Hyponatremia—an excess of total body water relative to sodium—is the most common electrolyte problem in older adults, with a prevalence as high as 14%. Symptoms of hyponatremia are generally manifested in the CNS and can include somnolence, cognitive impairment, seizures, and possibly coma. The symptoms are due to swelling of neurons caused by the change in osmotic gradient between the cells and the extracellular fluid. Most patients, however, exhibit no or few symptoms.

Thiazide diuretics are among the most common antihypertensive medications prescribed, and their use has increased since studies have found them highly effective in preventing serious cardiovascular outcomes in hypertensive patients. They are clearly implicated in causing many electrolyte abnormalities, including hyponatremia (SOE=B). Older adults seem particularly vulnerable: in one study, 26% of cases of hyponatremia in patients ≥65 yr old were attributable to thiazide diuretics. Older women are especially susceptible; the reason is unclear but may be related to the low-calorie, low-protein diet ("tea and toast") common in this population. The "tea and toast" diet leads to a lower urinary osmolar clearance and impaired free-water clearance. The exact pathogenesis of the condition is unknown. It may be caused by a combination of impaired urinary diluting ability, sodium loss, intracellular potassium depletion, and increases in arginine vasopressin (AVP) from mild volume depletion. The effects are often compounded by the concomitant sodium restriction that is prescribed for treatment of hypertension. More severe hyponatremia can be seen in patients who are ingesting large quantities of water. Thiazide diuretics must be discontinued in any patient presenting with hyponatremia.

The syndrome of inappropriate arginine vasopressin secretion (SIADH) is the causative factor in up to 26% of cases of hyponatremia. In the absence of thiazide diuretic use, SIADH is the likely diagnosis if renal function, adrenal function (ie, cortisol levels), pituitary and thyroid function, cardiac function, and hepatic function are all normal. Patients with SIADH have urine osmolality >100 mOsm/kg and urine sodium >20 mmol/L in the setting of euvolemia. In addition, the serum sodium concentration improves with restriction of water alone. SIADH is not diagnosed in patients on long-term diuretic therapy, because the volume depletion induced by the diuretic leads to secondary AVP secretion.

Water intoxication can lead to hyponatremia by overwhelming the capacity of the kidney to excrete water. Generally, renal excretory capacity is >8–12 L/d, so the water intake has to be excessive. Water intoxication is generally seen in patients with severe psychiatric disorders (psychogenic polydipsia).

Numerous medications are associated with development of hyponatremia through SIADH. The most common of these are third-generation antidepressants, anticonvulsants, and some antidiabetes agents. Case reports have associated many other medications with SIADH, but the instances are too anecdotal to attribute causation. For example, while omeprazole has been associated in case reports with SIADH, the incidence is likely extremely low, given the large number of patients who take omeprazole long-term. In the current case, thiazide use is a far more likely cause of the hyponatremia.

Hyponatremia can develop in patients with poor oral intake and volume depletion through activation of AVP. Generally, these patients appear clinically volume depleted and have very low levels of urine sodium.

101. An 82-yr-old man, previously independent, comes to the emergency department with 2 days of difficulty swallowing, productive cough, and dyspnea. History includes hypertension and controlled type 2 diabetes mellitus. On examination, he has a low-grade fever and increased blood pressure. Physical examination and chest radiography are consistent with consolidation in the left lower lobe. On bedside testing, he immediately sputters and coughs after drinking a small amount of water from a cup. There are no other neurologic findings. Laboratory testing suggests mild dehydration, and WBC count is slightly increased. MRI reveals a new, small brain-stem infarction and mild generalized cerebral atrophy.

Treatment for aspiration pneumonia is instituted. Seven days after onset of symptoms, swallowing has not improved, and formal evaluation shows aspiration with most consistencies.

Which of the following is the best recommendation?

(A) Careful oral feeding
(B) Gastrostomy feeding
(C) Hospice
(D) Nasogastric feeding
(E) Total parenteral nutrition

ANSWER: B

This patient most likely has pharyngeal-phase dysphagia resulting from brain-stem infarction. He will not be able to obtain adequate nutrition via an oral route at this time. The safest oral feeding may require pureed solids and honey-thick liquids; most people cannot obtain adequate intake with this restrictive diet. Nearly half of patients with dysphagia due to stroke recover effective swallowing within 7 days (SOE=B). Many patients with this type of injury will have significant, if not complete, recovery within 1 yr with rehabilitation (SOE=C). Hospice is not appropriate at this time: given the patient's relatively good premorbid functional status and lack of serious comorbidities, substantial recovery is likely, and he should be encouraged to undergo optimal treatment. Early placement of a gastrostomy tube with appropriate nutritional support and judicious rehabilitation gives this patient the best opportunity to return to his premorbid condition. Many patients can manage their own feeding tube and return to their prior residence (SOE=C).

Nasogastric feeding is a short-term treatment associated with greater need for tube replacement. Nasogastric feeding might be appropriate temporarily if placement of a gastrostomy tube is delayed. Total parenteral nutrition is associated with bacterial and fungal sepsis and makes fluid management more difficult; it also requires central venous access with its associated risks, and thus is not appropriate.

102. An 84-yr-old woman had a total thyroidectomy 3 mo ago because of gradually worsening compression symptoms. The symptoms were due to a benign multinodular goiter. Since thyroidectomy, the patient has taken levothyroxine 88 mcg/d. She also takes calcium and vitamin D for osteopenia.

After thyroidectomy, the patient's thyrotropin and free T_4 levels increased and total T_3 level decreased.

Thyroid function tests	Before thyroidectomy	After thyroidectomy
Thyrotropin	1.2 mIU/L	1.6 mIU/L
Free T_4	1.1 ng/dL	1.4 ng/dL
Total T_3	140 ng/dL	119 ng/dL

Which of the following is the best management option?

(A) Continue levothyroxine 88 mcg/d.
(B) Increase levothyroxine to 100 mcg/d.
(C) Add liothyronine 25 mcg/d.
(D) Switch to Armour desiccated thyroid 60 mg/d.

ANSWER: A

The thyrotropin concentration is the best monitor during treatment for hypothyroidism. Because this patient's thyrotropin concentration remains normal, no changes to therapy are needed. The thyroid gland makes T_4 and to a lesser extent T_3, most of which is derived through peripheral conversion of T_4. After thyroidectomy, the peripheral conversion of levothyroxine to T_3 maintains the concentration of total

T_3 similar to that before thyroidectomy (SOE=C). Often, however, the free T_4 concentration on levothyroxine therapy is significantly higher than the free T_4 concentration before thyroidectomy.

Increasing the levothyroxine dosage can lower the thyrotropin concentration below the lower limit of normal, and can increase bone turnover and the incidence of atrial fibrillation (SOE=B).

There is no proven benefit to combination therapy of levothyroxine and T_3 (liothyronine) versus levothyroxine alone (SOE=B). Many studies of combination therapy are limited by small sample size, iatrogenic hyperthyroidism, and different thyrotropin levels between treatment groups. The serum concentration of T_3 can fluctuate widely depending on the time of ingestion of T_3.

Most endocrinologists do not recommend therapy with Armour thyroid because the amount of desiccated animal T_4 and T_3 is not consistent (SOE=D).

Many substances, such as calcium, iron, and multivitamins, interfere with absorption of thyroid medications. Because this patient takes medication for both hypothyroidism and osteopenia, the schedule for medication administration should be structured and followed carefully.

103. Which of the following is the most common nonpharmacologic intervention for urinary incontinence in nursing-home residents?

(A) Briefs or pads
(B) Toileting program
(C) Indwelling catheter
(D) External catheter

ANSWER: A

In the United States, from 48% to 65% of nursing-home residents have urinary incontinence. Urinary incontinence is associated with poor health status, urinary tract infections, skin breakdown, falls and fall-related injury, decreased quality of life, poor self-rated health, and psychologic distress. The cost of care for an incontinent resident is 2.5 times that of a continent resident, including extra nursing time, cleaning supplies, and laundry. The predominant nonpharmacologic intervention for urinary incontinence in long-term settings is use of briefs or pads (84%). Less frequently used are toileting programs (39%), indwelling catheters (3.5%), and external catheters (1.2%). Despite strong evidence that toileting programs are effective, most incontinent residents do not receive the scheduled interventions documented in the care plan.

Maintaining an effective continence program in nursing homes requires system-wide involvement of nursing-home administration and staff. Overcoming barriers in management of urinary incontinence requires better recognition of the correlation between incontinence and poor quality of life.

104. An 82-yr-old man living in a nursing facility is evaluated because of gradual functional decline. He has lost 4.5 kg (7% of body weight) since he entered the nursing facility 6 mo ago after hospitalization for acute myocardial infarction. During that hospitalization, type 2 diabetes was diagnosed. In the nursing home he has remained hyperglycemic, with periodic blood glucose concentrations spiking to 300 mg/dL and a recent hemoglobin A_{1c} level of 7.9 g/dL. He is on an American Diabetic Association low-fat diet. He takes several medications, including glipizide, pravastatin, hydrochlorothiazide, metoprolol, lisinopril, and aspirin.

Laboratory results:

Creatinine	1.4 mg/dL
Low-density lipoprotein	100 mg/dL
High-density lipoprotein	34 mg/dL
Triglycerides	170 mg/dL

Which of the following is the most appropriate next step in management of this patient?

(A) Increase glipizide dosage.
(B) Add metformin.
(C) Add acarbose.
(D) Add niacin.
(E) Liberalize his diet.

ANSWER: E

Older adults with recently diagnosed diabetes, other chronic disease, and functional impairment are at high risk of micro- and especially macrovascular complications of diabetes. This patient is at especially grave risk of medical complications and death because of his weight loss and functional decline. Moreover, changes

in his medication regimen carry added risk for him. The most rational approach in this exceptionally vulnerable patient is also the most conservative: make no change in his (already complex) regimen of multiple medications and increase his caloric intake (SOE=D).

Increasing the dose of glipizide to lower this patient's hemoglobin A_{1c} level (to below <7 g/dL) might increase his risk of hypoglycemia and death (SOE=A). Marginal renal function is likely, given his creatinine level of 1.4 mg/dL and probable low muscle mass. Adding metformin to glipizide might increase anorexia and the risk of lactic acidosis. When this approach was tried in the United Kingdom Prospective Diabetes Study (albeit in individuals who were overweight and diabetic), the death rate was unexpectedly increased (SOE=A).

Adding acarbose to his current dose of glipizide might reduce his hyperglycemia and possibly moderate postprandial glycemic excursions. However, acarbose has common and predictable GI adverse events (eg, flatulence, diarrhea) that often limit compliance in patients with diabetes. In this patient with progressive weight loss and functional decline, acarbose is inappropriate and perhaps unsafe (SOE =D). Also, addition of acarbose would complicate an already complex regimen. The first priority is to stop his weight loss.

Niacin is associated with increased levels of high-density lipoprotein and reduced triglyceride levels. It would be unlikely to lower this patient's low-density lipoprotein level (the additional benefit of which would be controversial in any event); moreover, his high-density lipoprotein and triglyceride levels are as likely attributable to his frailty and marginal nutritional status as to his diabetes (SOE=D). Niacin also might exacerbate his hyperglycemia.

105. An 80-yr-old man uses a handheld magnifier to read medication labels and the newspaper. He has never been prescribed eyeglasses. History includes successful cataract surgery 8 yr ago. At a routine ophthalmology examination 6 mo ago, his vision was recorded as 20/40 in his right eye and 20/50 in his left eye for distance with no correction. Near vision was not recorded. He was told he had the "eyes of a 30-yr-old" and was scheduled to return in 1 yr.

Which of the following is the most likely cause of his inability to read without a magnifier?

(A) Early exudative (wet) macular degeneration
(B) Early nonexudative (dry) macular degeneration
(C) Glaucoma
(D) Opacification of the posterior capsule of his lens after cataract surgery
(E) Lack of eyeglasses

ANSWER: E

One of the most common causes of decreased vision in the United States is uncorrected refractive error (SOE=A). The patient had an excellent response to cataract surgery and can see at a distance. However, the ophthalmologist did not perform a refraction to determine if eyeglasses would improve his vision. Although there are intraocular lens implants that can provide for near and distant vision, they are not the lens of choice for all patients. This patient has good distant vision but did not receive eyeglasses to improve his near vision. He has "solved" the problem himself by using magnifiers. By providing him with a prescription for eyeglasses, he will likely be more independent, able to read more comfortably, and drive with better acuity.

Exudative and nonexudative macular degeneration affects near acuity and distant vision. An early sign of macular degeneration is central visual distortion or scotoma, which would also be apparent with distance. Some patients with early macular changes report that the door frame appears distorted or wavy. This patient was recently seen by his ophthalmologist, who gave the patient a good report.

Vision loss from glaucoma presents with peripheral field constriction. Near vision is not affected until the disease has progressed (SOE=A). Opacification of the posterior capsule develops after intraocular lens implantation; it affects distant as well as near vision.

106. An 88-yr-old man comes to you for evaluation after having two previous systolic blood pressure readings >160 mmHg. He is remarkably healthy, with a history only of osteoarthritis, macular degeneration, and multiple basal cell cancers that have been treated successfully. He takes

calcium, vitamin D, and acetaminophen as needed.

On examination, blood pressure is 170/88 mmHg and pulse is 70 beats per minute, without postural changes. His physical examination is otherwise unremarkable. His ECG is normal, as are all laboratory tests except for a low-density lipoprotein cholesterol of 128 mg/dL. He eats a healthy diet, exercises regularly, and is not interested in further lifestyle changes.

What is the best approach to treating his blood pressure at this point?

(A) Measure home blood pressure on at least 3 separate occasions.
(B) Begin a thiazide diuretic.
(C) Begin a β-blocker.
(D) Begin an α-blocker.

ANSWER: B

Systolic hypertension in older adults is common and associated with poor outcomes. In several clinical trials (SHEP, Syst-Eur), treatment of systolic hypertension reduced the incidence of stroke, coronary heart disease, and heart failure (versus placebo) (SOE=A). A meta-analysis of eight trials of treatment of systolic hypertension also showed a mortality benefit (SOE= B). Most experts recommend that thiazide diuretics should be the initial agent in the absence of comorbidities that would make other agents preferable (eg, coronary artery disease—β-blockers; diabetes—ACE inhibitors) (SOE=C). However, all four major classes of antihypertensive drugs (diuretics, β-blockers, ACE inhibitors/angiotensin-receptor blockers, and calcium channel blockers) have been shown to reduce cardiovascular events (SOE=A). α-Agonists were found to be inferior to other classes of blood pressure agents in improving clinical outcomes (SOE=A). Recently, some analyses have suggested that β-blockers may be inferior to other agents in older adults (SOE=B). In many cases, combination medication therapy is necessary.

Treatment of systolic hypertension in adults >80–85 yr old has benefits, but optimal agents and the goals of treatment are a topic of continued interest. The recent Hypertension in the Very Elderly Trial (HYVET) showed that treatment of hypertension in patients ≥80 yr old with indapamise with or without perindopril with a target blood pressure of <150/80 mmHg was associated with reduced all-cause mortality, cardiovascular events, stroke-related death, and heart failure. In other studies, hypertensive patients >80 yr old who achieved systolic blood pressures of <140 mmHg appeared to have increased mortality rates, so the ideal blood pressure target in adults >80 yr old is still being debated. Because this patient's systolic blood pressure has been >160 mmHg on three separate occasions, additional home blood pressure recordings before treatment are not indicated. Home blood pressure measurements are most useful when office readings are inconsistent, the diagnosis of hypertension is in question, or when the diagnosis of "white coat" hypertension is being considered (SOE=C).

107. An 88-yr-old black woman with peripheral arterial disease is admitted to the hospital because she has gangrene in 2 toes and soft-tissue infection of her distal foot. She is a widow and lives alone; her daughter visits at least weekly.

On admission, her blood pressure is 140/80 mmHg, respiratory rate is 16 breaths per minute, pulse is 90, and temperature is 38°C (100.4°F). She is acutely confused and inattentive. Her speech is rambling.

Which of the following factors is most likely to increase her risk of in-hospital functional decline and nursing home placement?

(A) Marital status
(B) Race
(C) Gender
(D) Delirium

ANSWER: D

Factors that predict both in-hospital functional decline (as measured by ability to perform ADLs) and nursing-home placement include older age, dependence in IADLs, delirium, and other cognitive impairment, such as dementia (SOE=B). Factors more predictive of nursing-home admission than of functional decline include living alone and patient and family preference for institutional care. Gender, race, and marital status have less influence as predictors of either outcome.

The effect of race on in-hospital functional decline has been examined. There was no difference between older black and older white patients in improvement in ADLs by the time of hospital discharge or by 90 days after discharge. At the same time points, however, improvement in IADLs was significantly less likely among black patients than among white patients. The geriatric clinician is critical in supporting in-hospital function-focused care; educating the staff, patient, and family about its importance; and collaborating with the interdisciplinary team to develop individualized plans to prevent functional decline.

108. A 76-yr-old woman comes to the office because over the past day she has had progressive painful swelling of the wrist, such that she is now unable to use her left hand. She has had similar episodes involving her knee and ankle over the past year. History includes hypertension, coronary artery disease, and osteoarthritis of the hands. Medications include aspirin 81 mg/d, hydrochlorothiazide 12.5 mg/d, and acetaminophen 1 g q8h.

On examination, the patient has no fever. Her left hand is diffusely swollen, with wrist pain and tenderness; her right hand is tender over the second and third metacarpophalangeal joints. Her knees are warm to touch and hurt with movement. Uric acid level is 10.2 mg/dL, BUN is 30 mg/dL, and creatinine is 2.5 mg/dL.

In addition to discontinuing her hydrochlorothiazide, which of the following treatments is most appropriate?

(A) Intra-articular corticosteroid injection
(B) Oral corticosteroids and attention to adequate oral fluid intake
(C) Oral colchicine
(D) Oral probenecid
(E) Oral allopurinol

ANSWER: B

This patient has polyarticular gout. Flares are best managed with intramuscular or short-term oral corticosteroid therapy (prednisone 30 mg/d for 5 days). Joint aspiration and intra-articular corticosteroid therapy are appropriate for gout attacks of 1 or 2 accessible joints (knee, wrist, elbow, ankle) but not if there is concurrent involvement of small hand joints (SOE=C).

If corticosteroids and NSAIDs are contraindicated, analgesics alone are an acceptable alternative. Colchicine can alleviate an acute attack, but at dosages associated with significant nausea, vomiting, and diarrhea. Urate-lowering therapy should not be started during an acute gouty attack.

The patient will continue to be susceptible to flares once this episode resolves. It is reasonable to consider urate-lowering therapy weeks after the current attack resolves. Initial intervention may include discontinuing diuretic therapy: 90% of cases of chronic hyperuricemia in older adults result from reduced renal excretion that is due to renal disease or medications, especially diuretics. Although aspirin at low dosages reduces uric acid clearance, it may be required for cardiovascular prophylaxis. Probenecid, a uricosuric agent, is less effective in patients with renal insufficiency (creatinine clearance <40 mm/h). Allopurinol lowers serum urate concentration by blocking uric acid formation but should not be used during an acute flare.

109. An 82-yr-old woman is brought to the office to establish care. She requires complete assistance with ADLs. History includes moderate vascular dementia, atrial fibrillation, and systolic heart failure; medications include warfarin, atenolol, simvastatin, and lisinopril.

On physical examination, she has a 6-cm rectangular yellow bruise on her right buttock, a 3-cm circular purple bruise on her left forearm, and a 4-cm oval red bruise on her posterior neck.

Which of the following bruise characteristics raises suspicion of physical abuse?

(A) Size
(B) Shape
(C) Number
(D) Location
(E) Color variation

ANSWER: D

Among older adults, the risk of accidental bruising is increased by gait instability, medications, thinning of the epidermis, reduced subcutaneous fat, and increased capillary

fragility. Older adults are more likely to take warfarin or NSAIDs, which add to ease of bruising. However, the location of this patient's bruises on her buttocks and neck raise suspicion of mistreatment rather than accidental trauma. In one study comprising 101 people (average age, 78 yr) from the community and nursing homes who were examined daily, 108 bruises were identified during the study period. Of these, 89% were on the extremities. No bruises were seen on the ears, neck, genitalia, buttocks, or soles of the feet. On the first day of observation, 16% of bruises were predominantly yellow. Reddish coloration was observed throughout the course of the bruises.

Although the size of a bruise does not necessarily suggest mistreatment, patients are more likely to recall the circumstance surrounding a large bruise (5–20 cm) on the trunk. It is cause for concern if an older adult has a large bruise on the trunk but cannot recall how it happened or gives an explanation inconsistent with the physical examination.

The shape of the bruise can be important if it suggests a pattern or method of injury, eg, a circular cigarette burn, or circumferential abrasions around the wrists suggesting restraint. In the absence of any suspicious pattern, the shape of the bruises on this patient does not suggest mistreatment.

The number of bruises would not trigger further assessment for abuse. However, multiple bruises clustered in a pattern inconsistent with the history should raise suspicion and prompt further assessment and documentation (SOE=C).

110. A 74-yr-old woman comes to the office because she has a rash on her neck. It has been present for a few months and is getting thicker and redder. The area is itchy, and sometimes she finds herself scratching without realizing she is doing so; it is difficult for her to stop scratching, especially when she is worried and tired. She has been under stress recently because she is in the process of selling her house, to move in with her daughter. She does not use make-up or jewelry and has not changed detergent. Her usual emollient cream has not helped the rash.

On examination, she is afebrile and appears well. She has a 9-cm lichenified plaque on her neck that is erythematous, with areas of more intense erythema where it was recently scratched. The plaque feels thick and leathery to touch and is not warmer than the surrounding skin.

Which of the following is the most likely diagnosis?

(A) Nodular prurigo
(B) Xerosis
(C) Lichen simplex chronicus
(D) Asteatotic dermatitis
(E) Dyshidrotic eczematous dermatitis

ANSWER: C

The location of this patient's lesion is consistent with psoriasis, but the clinical description is more consistent with lichen simplex chronicus (neurodermatitis). Lichen simplex chronicus is a localized area of lichenification caused by repetitive rubbing and scratching. It involves areas that are easily reached by the dominant hand: legs, ankles, arms, scrotal skin, neck, and upper trunk. Many patients have a history of atopic dermatitis and have anxiety disorders or emotional stresses. It is difficult to treat unless the patient stops scratching. Treatment includes education on the importance of breaking the itch-scratch-itch cycle, addressing psychologic factors, and application of topical steroids with occlusive dressing.

Psychogenic factors also play a role in nodular prurigo, in which emotional tensions induce a self-perpetuating pruritic sensation, but patients scratch in multiple locations and develop dome-shaped nodules rather than plaques. The nodules can be several millimeters to 2 cm in diameter; they can be excoriated and ulcerated when the patient picks at them with fingernails.

Dyshidrotic eczematous dermatitis is a vesicular dermatitis that involves palms, fingers, and soles. It starts with pruritic vesicles that can progress to scaling fissures and lichenification.

Xerosis, or dry skin, is a common cause of generalized itching in older adults. It gets worse in winter with low humidity and frequent bathing. Clinically, the skin is dry and scaly; in more severe cases, the skin becomes inflamed, with fissuring or cracking of the stratum corneum that resembles "cracked porcelain" (erythema craquelé or asteatotic dermatitis). Xerosis

usually involves legs, arms, and hands, rather than the neck.

111. A 69-yr-old man comes to the office to establish care. His wife is being treated for osteoporosis and she wants know whether her husband should also undergo a screening assessment.

Which of the following is the strongest risk factor for osteoporosis in men?

(A) Androgen deprivation therapy
(B) Low dietary intake of vitamin D
(C) Respiratory disease
(D) Thyroid replacement therapy
(E) Type 2 diabetes mellitus

ANSWER: A

Osteoporosis is a problem in older men, but data on screening guidelines are still being accrued. Literature review indicates that the most important risk factors for osteoporotic fractures in men are age ≥70 yr old and low body weight (body mass index <25 kg/m^2 or weight <70 kg [154 lb]) (SOE=A). Other risk factors include weight loss, physical inactivity, corticosteroid use, previous osteoporotic fracture, and androgen deprivation therapy (SOE=A). Androgen deprivation therapy (pharmacologic or by orchiectomy) is a strong predictor of both osteoporosis and fracture.

Multiple other risk factors for osteoporosis in men have been reported, but the strength of the association is inconclusive in most cases. Some of the other reported risk factors include cigarette smoking, alcohol use, vitamin D and calcium intake, respiratory disease, thyroid replacement therapy, and type 2 diabetes mellitus. These possible risk factors have plausible physiologic rationales, and some are supported by data on osteoporosis and fractures in women or inconsistent data in men.

112. An 85-yr-old man with macular degeneration is evaluated because of a sudden change in behavior and weight loss. He is recently widowed and has moved into an assisted-living facility. When his family visits, they are stunned to find him withdrawn, quiet, and losing weight. Previously, he had lived in his home for 50 yr and had managed ADLs and IADLs with assistance from his wife. Several years ago, he

received services from a local agency for the blind and visually impaired.

Physical examination is normal except for low vision. Results of the Mini–Mental State Examination and Geriatric Depression Scale are normal. Examination by his ophthalmologist shows no change in the macular degeneration.

Which of the following is the most appropriate next step?

(A) Start antidepressant medications.
(B) Encourage participation in group activities.
(C) Obtain a complete medical evaluation to assess the weight loss.
(D) Refer to a vision rehabilitation specialist.
(E) Refer to a geriatric psychiatrist.

ANSWER: D

The patient functioned well in his home. He knew where everything was located. He was able to get a cup of tea, dial the phone, go for a walk, and visit friends. Although he and his wife depended on each other for support, they could function independently at home. Thinking he could no longer live alone, his family did not take into account the benefits of a known home layout. In the new facility, his room layouts are unfamiliar. It is likely that he has difficulty accessing the dining room without assistance. A vision rehabilitation specialist can assess the new environment and ensure that the patient receives additional instruction in orientation and mobility so that he can navigate independently and safely. He may benefit from a talking watch to assist him to be on time for meals. The rehabilitation specialist can provide information on lighting to the staff, so that the patient can have sufficient light to eat his meals, and can instruct staff in creating plates that accentuate the color contrast of the food. With this assistance, he may obtain independence (and gain weight) in the new setting.

Loss of vision is associated with major depressive disorder in older adults. The prevalence of depression among patients with age-related macular degeneration is approximately 30%; depression is a major cause of excess disability (SOE=A). A return to independence may prevent major depressive disorder in this patient.

Encouraging participation in group activities may be beneficial but will be more successful once the patient has the tools for more independence. A complete medical evaluation is indicated if weight loss persists after the patient is oriented to the dining hall and his own room, and it is clear that he has access to meals.

113. An 80-yr-old woman comes to the office because she recently has had difficulty eating and swallowing solid food. She notes that when she prepares to swallow, the food scrapes her cheeks and the roof of her mouth. History includes hypertension, diabetes mellitus, kidney stones, and major depressive disorder. Medications include hydrochlorothiazide, metformin, and fluoxetine. For the first time in many years, a recent dental examination revealed several cavities, which were located at the roots of the teeth.

Which of the following is the most likely explanation for these oral problems?

(A) Usual aging
(B) Salivary ductal stones
(C) Adverse effect of metformin
(D) Adverse effect of hydrochlorothiazide and fluoxetine
(E) Immune dysfunction

ANSWER: D

This patient's difficulty eating and swallowing solid foods in the context of new dental cavities is most consistent with xerostomia, or decreased saliva. Saliva has several functions: it is a protective cleanser with antibacterial activity, a buffer that inhibits demineralization, a lubricant, and a transport medium to taste sensors. These functions are seriously altered in xerostomia. Signs and symptoms of xerostomia include oral dryness or burning, changes in tongue surface or taste, dysphasia, cheilosis, difficulty with speech, and development of root caries. Many conditions and treatments contribute to xerostomia, such as radiation or chemotherapy; psychologic, endocrine, and nutritional disorders; and adverse effect of medication (>200 commonly used medications can cause xerostomia). Antihypertensive medications (especially diuretics) and antidepressants (especially first-generation SSRIs) reduce saliva flow. Metformin is not known to decrease salivary flow. Immune diseases, such as Sjögren syndrome, and diabetes can increase cavities but are not likely to produce xerostomia.

While older adults are likely to have a decreased amount of active glandular tissue, salivary flow does not decrease significantly with age. The causes of salivary stones (sialoliths) are largely unknown; theories include autoimmune and inflammatory causes. Kidney stones are unrelated to salivary stones. Salivary stones do not usually cause xerostomia; they usually affect only one gland (commonly the submandibular gland) on only one side, so saliva is still present in the other major and minor salivary glands.

Treatment for patients with xerostomia includes scrupulous oral hygiene with a soft toothbrush, fluoride rinses, reduced alcohol consumption, frequent intake of water, saliva substitutes, and avoidance of highly acidic foods (SOE=B).

114. A 79-yr-old Asian-American woman is brought to the office because she has increasing forgetfulness; apathy; and behavioral changes of irritability, agitation, and aggression. Her primary caregiver reports that she is disruptive, occasionally screaming at imaginary people, and is frequently becoming combative. The patient has Alzheimer's disease but no history of psychosis or major depressive disorder. Physical examination, CBC, and serum chemistries are normal.

Which of the following is the next best step?

(A) Treat with a first-generation antipsychotic agent.
(B) Treat with a second-generation antipsychotic agent.
(C) Admit to a psychiatric unit for further evaluation.
(D) Review behavioral interventions with the caregiver.

ANSWER: D

The behavior reported by the caregiver could lead to nursing-home admission and requires rapid intervention. However, treatment with either a first- (SOE=B) or second-generation antipsychotic (SOE=A) is more often associated with adverse events necessitating discontinuation than with meaningful benefit. As a result, antipsychotics are not considered first-

line treatment for agitation among individuals with dementia and should not be started until behavioral interventions have proved inadequate. Admission to a psychiatric unit before exhausting behavioral and pharmacologic interventions is premature. It may be necessary ultimately but will initially exacerbate disorientation and combativeness. Consensus suggests that a cholinesterase inhibitor is the first-line pharmacologic treatment combined with behavioral interventions when objectionable behaviors either are not the expressions of the patient's unmet needs or exceed the caregiver's tolerance.

115. A 75-yr-old man comes to the office because he has an ulcer on his tongue that is not painful except when he eats acidic or spicy foods. He does not remember when he first noticed it. His last dental examination was 2 yr ago. He smoked 2 packs daily for 30 yr, but stopped smoking 20 yr ago. He has hypertension controlled with medication.

On examination, there is a 2 × 2-cm nonhealing, indurated ulcer on the left lateroventral border of the tongue next to a broken filling.

Which of the following is the next best step?

(A) Refer patient to dentist to have filling restored.
(B) Refer for immediate biopsy of the lesion.
(C) Instruct patient to use an OTC local anesthetic gel to relieve the pain.
(D) Explain to patient that this is a canker sore that will resolve on its own in 7–10 days.
(E) Recommend that the patient avoid acidic or spicy foods until the sore heals.

ANSWER: B

The clinical appearance of the ulcer—large and indurated, with rolled, firm edges—and its unknown duration make biopsy essential. Oral cancer claims approximately 8,000 lives in the United States each year. It is most common in people ≥40 yr old, especially in those with a history of smoking. Although head and neck cancer accounts for only 3% of all new cancer cases and 2% of all cancer deaths in the United States annually, it is the fifth most common malignancy worldwide. Tobacco and alcohol are the primary etiologic agents.

Squamous cell carcinoma, which accounts for 96% of all oral cancers, is usually preceded by dysplasia presenting as white epithelial lesions on the oral mucosa (leukoplakia), red and white lesions (erythroplakia), or a nonhealing ulcer. Early diagnosis and treatment markedly improve outcome and survival.

Although the defective tooth filling could have precipitated the ulcer, the duration and clinical appearance of the ulcer indicate a precancerous or cancerous lesion. An OTC local anesthetic gel may provide temporary pain relief, but it does not treat precancerous, cancerous, or any other oral lesions. Canker sore is unlikely: a canker sore has a short duration and is a shallow ulcer covered by a yellowish white, removable, fibrinous membrane and surrounded by an erythematous halo.

Avoiding spicy or acidic foods is not indicated; the patient needs immediate biopsy of the lesion (SOE=C).

116. An 80-yr-old woman is admitted to the hospital with urosepsis. On examination, she weighs 60 kg (132 lb) and has a low-grade fever and increased respiratory rate. There is a consolidation in the right lower lobe. Laboratory results show normal electrolyte concentrations and a serum creatinine concentration of 1.8 mg/dL, which is her recent baseline value. She responds well to 2 days of intravenous antibiotics, and cultures reveal *Escherichia coli* sensitive to trimethoprim/sulfamethoxazole. Your pharmacist reminds you that this medication requires adjustment for patients with renal impairment.

Based on published equations, what is her estimated glomerular filtration rate (GFR)?

(A) >90 mL/min
(B) 60–90 mL/min
(C) 30–60 mL/min
(D) 10–30mL/min
(E) <10 mL/min

ANSWER: D

The most useful measure of kidney function is GFR (SOE=A). Other measures of kidney function, such as tubular function, acid-base and electrolyte excretion, and hormonal production, tend to run in parallel with GFR and are harder to measure. Serum creatinine

alone may not give an accurate estimate of GFR in older adults. This is partly because of the decrease in lean muscle mass with aging and the concomitant decrease in creatinine production. The most common and clinically useful way to determine GFR in older adults is to use the serum creatinine concentration in one of several regression formulas. Currently, the Modification of Diet in Renal Disease (MDRD) formula for determining GFR is best validated in middle-aged people and is recommended by the National Kidney Foundation (SOE=A). This complex equation can be obtained by using an on-line calculator such as that found on www.nephron.com. Most laboratories also report this value with routine serum chemistries. This equation has not been validated in patients >70 yr old. An alternative equation is the Cockcroft-Gault formula, which also has not been validated in adults >80 yr old. The Cockcroft-Gault formula is:

GFR = (140 − age) × weight / 72 × serum creatinine (multiply by 0.85 for women).

Despite these shortfalls, these equations provide a prompt and reasonable estimate of GFR for clinical decision-making. The formulas assume that the patient is in a steady state without a rapidly changing serum creatinine concentration.

For this patient with a serum creatinine concentration of 1.8 mg/dL, the Cockcroft-Gault estimated GFR is 23.6 mL/min. The MDRD is not validated in a person her age but would yield an estimated GFR of 29 mL/min. With either estimate, despite an only moderately increased serum creatinine, the GFR is extremely depressed and requires dosing adjustments to avoid complications. Thus, with older adults, normal kidney function cannot be assumed in the setting of apparently normal serum creatinine concentration. In situations in which a very accurate GFR determination is needed (eg, chemotherapy), a 24-h creatinine clearance should be measured.

117. An 88-yr-old man comes to the office because he has been feeling more tired than usual, and yesterday he fell in his bedroom. He was hospitalized with pneumonia 2 mo ago; he received daily physical and occupational therapy in a nursing facility for 4 wk and was then

discharged home at maximal function. He has a history of Parkinson's disease, hypertension, and osteoarthritis. Medications include carbidopa/levodopa, hydrochlorothiazide, metoprolol, and acetaminophen.

Which of the following is most likely to yield additional information useful for reducing his risk of falling?

(A) Serum electrolytes
(B) Vitamin D level
(C) Postural blood pressure
(D) Timed Up and Go test

ANSWER: C

Up to 70% of patients with Parkinson's disease fall in a given year. This patient's recent fall and his fatigue may be related to the orthostasis associated both with Parkinson's disease and with carbidopa/levodopa (SOE=A). He should be evaluated for postural hypotension. Furthermore, he has had several recent transitions—from the hospital to a nursing facility to home. Changes in medication regimen are a common cause of complications in transition of care, raising the possibility that the patient's hypertension is being overtreated. Both hydrochlorothiazide and metoprolol may be lowering his blood pressure excessively.

Serum electrolytes should be checked because of the patient's fatigue and because he takes hydrochlorothiazide. Low sodium or potassium concentrations could cause the patient's symptoms, but orthostasis remains the primary consideration in this case. Inadequate levels of vitamin D are common in older adults, and supplementation with vitamin D_3 can decrease fall risk. Checking the vitamin D level is appropriate in the overall management of fall risk but is a secondary consideration in this situation. The Timed Up and Go test is a good screen for functional balance, strength, and gait but would not yield specific useful information in this situation. Because the patient has recently undergone intensive rehabilitation, results of the Timed Up and Go test are not likely to lead to further interventions to improve his physical function.

118. Which of the following statements describing response to common homeostatic challenges is true?

(A) Aging is associated with increased complexity of responses to auditory frequencies.
(B) Aging is associated with a decreased ability to respond to glucose challenges.
(C) Hypothermia in older adults exposed to cold temperatures is caused primarily by decreased thermogenesis.
(D) When exposed to stress, older adults have a shorter period of activation of the sympathetic nervous system than younger adults.

ANSWER: B

Aging is associated with a variety of well-described deficits in the ability of cells, tissues, and organisms to respond to common homeostatic challenges. For example, older adults are less able to maintain normal glucose levels in response to oral or intravenous glucose challenges. While both insulin secretion and tissue sensitivity to insulin decline in old age, tissue insulin responsiveness is heavily influenced by changes in body composition and physical activity.

Although many physiologic parameters remain relatively unchanged with age when measured at a single point in time, the complexity of their behavior often declines with aging when more extensive measurements and analyses are conducted. Examples of physiologic variables that decline in terms of complexity with age include narrowing of auditory frequency responsiveness, decreased long-range correlations in time-series data such as blood pressure measurements, and increased randomness or stochastic activity in terms of cardiac intervals. Together with declines in structural complexity of bone microarchitecture and brain connectivity, these changes increase the vulnerability of older adults when confronting common homeostatic challenges.

Older adults are less able to maintain a normal body temperature when exposed to low environmental temperatures. Multiple relevant mechanisms include decreased sensation of cold, declines in shivering intensity, inadequate thermogenesis, and poor vasoconstriction;

inadequate thermogenesis is not the primary cause.

When exposed to physical or emotional stress, older adults demonstrate greater and more prolonged activation of both sympathetic (eg, norepinephrine levels) and hypothalamic-pituitary-adrenal (eg, cortisol levels) systems than younger adults.

A key impact of aging on homeostatic mechanisms is also reflected in the observation that older adults are often able to respond adequately to individual homeostatic challenges, yet become vulnerable when exposed to more than one concurrent challenge. For example, many healthy older adults who maintain normal blood pressure in response to orthostasis or mild diuretic-induced sodium depletion are unable to do so in the face of both challenges.

119. A 72-yr-old man comes to the office because he has anejaculatory orgasms. Over the last 3 yr, he has not consistently ejaculated with orgasm, and he has had no ejaculations for 3 mo. For the past 5 yr, he has taken tamsulosin 0.4 mg/d for lower urinary tract symptoms associated with benign prostatic hyperplasia. He has had no pelvic trauma, pain, or change in his lower urinary tract symptoms. He is monogamous and has intercourse once or twice a week with his wife of 40 yr.

Digital rectal examination reveals an asymmetric prostate of approximately 25 mL, with a hard nodule in the left lower lobe. The remainder of the examination is normal. Urinalysis is normal. His prostate-specific antigen (PSA) level is 9.5 ng/mL.

Which of the following is the most appropriate next step?

(A) Referral to a urologist
(B) Bone scan
(C) CT of the pelvis
(D) MRI of the pelvis
(E) Measurement of free PSA

ANSWER: A

Based on his physical examination and PSA level, this patient most likely has prostate cancer. In a patient with a remaining life expectancy of >5 yr, the next step is transrectal ultrasound-guided biopsy (SOE=C). The

optimal treatment for prostate cancer in men of this age has not yet been determined, so treatment decisions are usually based on patient preference and estimated remaining life expectancy.

The patient's anejaculatory orgasms most likely represent retrograde ejaculation due to either benign prostatic hyperplasia or tamsulosin therapy and are not directly related to the current findings. A bone scan is reserved for detecting metastasis in the presence of known disease and is unlikely to be informative in patients with a PSA level <10 ng/mL. CT or MRI of the pelvis is reserved for identifying local spread or evaluating patients in whom the suspicion of cancer is high despite negative biopsy findings. A high proportional free PSA level will not exclude prostate cancer with a high enough level of certainty given this patient's symptoms and physical findings.

120. A 75-yr-old woman with Alzheimer's disease is admitted to the hospital with a femoral neck fracture of the left hip and undergoes successful cemented hip arthroplasty within 24 h of admission. She resides in an assisted-living facility and walked independently before the fracture. Two weeks before the fracture, her score on the Mini–Mental State Examination was 15/30. Her daughter asks about rehabilitation options for her mother.

Which of the following is most appropriate for this patient?

(A) Arrange for immediate trial of rehabilitation.
(B) Do not recommend rehabilitation because of patient's dementia.
(C) Postpone rehabilitation because of patient's dementia.
(D) Postpone rehabilitation because of cemented prosthesis.

ANSWER: A

According to results of a randomized, controlled trial, patients with mild to moderate dementia who fracture a hip are likely to have better outcomes with rehabilitation than without. Patients with mild dementia are as successful as patients with normal cognitive function in returning to independent living. Further, after 1 yr, significantly fewer patients with moderate dementia who received rehabilitation are in institutional care (SOE=A).

There is no evidence that waiting to start rehabilitation is beneficial, and any delay in mobilization can lead to serious adverse outcomes, such as deconditioning, pressure sores, and pneumonia (SOE=A).

Mobilization is allowed on the second or third postoperative day with compression screws and uncemented or cemented prostheses. Adequate pain control is essential to promote full participation in rehabilitation (SOE=D).

In older adults with hip fracture, surgery within 24 hours is associated with reduced pain and length of hospital stay. Cemented prostheses are associated with less pain at 1 yr and later, and may be associated with better mobility. Rehabilitation after hip fracture improves outcome in terms of functional status. Home-based care can be as effective as care provided in a rehabilitation facility for patients with dementia.

GRS7 CONTRIBUTING CHAPTER AUTHORS

Sumaira Z. Aasi, MD
Associate Professor
Department of Dermatology
Yale University School of Medicine
New Haven, CT

Harold P. Adams, Jr., MD
Professor and Director
Division of Cerebrovascular Diseases
Department of Neurology
Iowa City, IA

Reva N. Adler, MD, MPH, FRCPC
Medical Director
STAT Centre & At Home Supports
Vancouver General Hospital
Vancouver Community Services
Clinical Professor
Division of Geriatric Medicine
Associate, Centre for International Health
University of British Columbia
Vancouver, BC

Marc E. Agronin, MD
Associate Professor of Psychiatry
University of Miami Miller School of Medicine
Medical Director for Mental Health and Clinical Research
Miami Jewish Health Systems
Miami, FL

Douglas A. Albreski, DPM
Assistant Professor, Department of Dermatology
University of Connecticut School of Medicine
Director of the Podiatric Dermatology Clinic
Farmington, CT

Cathy A. Alessi, MD, AGSF
Deputy Director and Associate Director
Clinical/Health Services Research
Geriatric Research, Education and Clinical Center
Veterans Administration Greater Los Angeles Healthcare
  System
Professor, David Geffen School of Medicine at UCLA
Los Angeles, CA

Neil B. Alexander, MD
Director, Mobility Research Center
Professor, Department of Internal Medicine
Division of Geriatric Medicine; Research Professor
Institute of Gerontology
University of Michigan
Director, VA Ann Arbor Health Care System GRECC
Ann Arbor, MI

Priscilla F. Bade, MD, FACP, CMD
Associate Professor of Internal Medicine
Sanford School of Medicine at the University of South
  Dakota
Rapid City, SD

Leen Bakkali, MD
Yale New Haven Geriatric Services, PC
New Haven, CT

Cynthia Barton, RN, MSN
Geriatric Nurse Practitioner
Memory and Aging Center
Assistant Clinical Professor, School of Nursing
University of California, San Francisco
San Francisco, CA

Sarah D. Berry, MD, MPH
Instructor in Medicine
Hebrew SeniorLife
Institute for Aging Research
Boston, MA

Marc R. Blackman, MD
Associate Chief of Staff for Research & Development
Veterans Affairs Medical Center
Professor of Medicine
George Washington University
Department of Medicine
Washington, DC
Professor of Medicine
Johns Hopkins University School of Medicine
Professor of Medicine
University of Maryland
Baltimore, MD

Caroline S. Blaum, MD, MS
Professor of Internal Medicine
Division of Geriatric Medicine
University of Michigan
Research Scientist, Ann Arbor DVAMC GRECC
Ann Arbor, MI

Chad Boult, MD, MPH, MBA
Professor of Public Health
Director of the Lipitz Center for Integrated Health Care
Johns Hopkins Bloomberg School of Public Health
Baltimore, MD

Cynthia J. Brown, MD, MSPH
Associate Professor of Medicine
University of Alabama at Birmingham
Birmingham, AL

David M. Buchner, MD, MPH
Shahid and Ann Carlson Khan Professor in Applied
  Health Sciences
Department of Kinesiology and Community Health
University of Illinois at Urbana-Champaign
Champaign, IL

David Bush, MD
Director, Cardiac CT
Associate Director, Cardiac Catheterization Laboratory
Johns Hopkins Bayview Medical Center
Associate Professor of Medicine
Johns Hopkins University School of Medicine
Baltimore, MD

R. Charles Callison, MD
Associate
University of Iowa Hospitals and Clinics
Department of Radiology and Neurology
Interventional Neuroradiology and Cerebrovascular
    Divisions
Iowa City, IA

Julie C. Chapman, PsyD
Neuroscientist
War Related Illness and Injury Study Center
Veterans Affairs Medical Center
Instructor of Neurology
Georgetown University School of Medicine
Washington, DC

Gurkamal S. Chatta, MD
Associate Professor of Medicine
Division of Hematology-Oncology
University of Pittsburgh
Pittsburgh, PA

Jaehyuk Choi, MD, PhD
Department of Dermatology
Yale University School of Medicine
New Haven, CT

Colleen Christmas, MD
Program Director, Internal Medicine
Johns Hopkins Bayview Medical Center
Assistant Professor of Medicine
Division of Geriatric Medicine and Gerontology
Johns Hopkins University
Baltimore, MD

Anne L. Coleman, MD, PhD
The Fran and Ray Stark Professor of Ophthalmology
Professor of Epidemiology
Jules Stein Eye Institute
UCLA David Geffen School of Medicine
Los Angeles, CA

Leo M. Cooney, Jr., MD
Professor of Medicine
Yale University School of Medicine
New Haven, CT

Steven R. Counsell, MD, AGSF
Mary Elizabeth Mitchell Professor
Director, IU Geriatrics
Scientist, IU Center for Aging Research
Indiana University School of Medicine
Indianapolis, IN

G. Willy Davila, MD
Chairman, Department of Gynecology
Head, Section of Urogynecology and Reconstructive Pelvic
    Surgery
Cleveland Clinic Florida
Weston, FL

Maria L. Diaz, MD
Head, Section of Ambulatory Gynecology
Department of Gynecology
Cleveland Clinic Florida
Weston, FL

Margaret A. Drickamer, MD
Associate Professor
Yale University School of Medicine
New Haven, CT

Catherine E. DuBeau, MD
Professor of Medicine
Clinical Chief of Geriatrics
Departments of Medicine, Family Medicine and
    Community Health, and Obstetrics and Gynecology
University of Massachusetts Medical School
UMass Memorial Medical Center
Worcester, MA

G. Paul Eleazer, MD, FACP, AGSF
Director, Division of Geriatrics
University of South Carolina School of Medicine
Columbia, SC

E. Wesley Ely, MD, MPH
Associate Professor of Medicine
Allergy, Pulmonary and Critical Care
Vanderbilt University School of Medicine
Nashville, TN

William B. Ershler, MD
Deputy Clinical Director
Intramural Research Program
National Institute on Aging
National Institutes of Health
Baltimore, MD

Neal S. Fedarko, PhD
Associate Professor
Division of Geriatrics
Department of Medicine
Director, Institute for Clinical and Translation Research
    Clinical Core Laboratory
Director, Translational Research Training Program in
    Gerontology & Geriatrics
Johns Hopkins University
Baltimore, MD

Mark H. Fleisher, MD, FAPA
Associate Professor of Psychiatry
Director, Division of Public and Community Psychiatry
Director, Neurodevelopmental Psychiatry
Medical Director, Public and Community Psychiatry
    Clinics
University of Nebraska College of Medicine
Associate Clinical Professor of Psychiatry
Creighton University School of Medicine
Omaha, NE

Linda P. Fried, MD, MPH, AGSF
Dean and DeLamar Professor of Public Health
Columbia University Mailman School of Public Health
Professor of Epidemiology and Medicine
Senior Vice President, Columbia University Medical
    Center
New York, NY

Terry Fulmer, PhD, RN, FAAN, AGSF
The Erline Perkins McGriff Professor &
Dean, College of Nursing
New York University
New York, NY

Angela Gentili, MD
Associate Professor of Internal Medicine
Director, Geriatrics Fellowship Training Program
VAMC/Virginia Commonwealth University
Richmond, VA

JoAnn A. Giaconi, MD
Assistant Clinical Professor of Ophthalmology
Jules Stein Eye Institute
UCLA David Geffen School of Medicine
Greater Los Angeles VA Healthcare Center
Los Angeles, CA

Thomas M. Gill, MD
Humana Foundation Professor of Geriatric Medicine
Professor of Medicine, Epidemiology & Investigative
    Medicine
Yale University School of Medicine
New Haven, CT

Suzanne M. Gillespie, MD, RD
Assistant Professor of Medicine
Division of Geriatrics/Aging
University of Rochester School of Medicine and Dentistry
Rochester, NY

Lisa J. Granville, MD, AGSF
Professor and Associate Chair,
Department of Geriatrics,
Florida State University College of Medicine
Tallahassee, FL

David A. Gruenewald, MD
Associate Professor of Medicine
Division of Gerontology and Geriatric Medicine
Department of Medicine
University of Washington School of Medicine
Staff Physician, Geriatric Research, Education, and
    Clinical Center
Seattle, WA

Kenneth Hepburn, PhD
Professor and Associate Dean for Research
Director of Graduate Studies
Nell Hodgson Woodruff School of Nursing
Emory University
Atlanta, GA

Kevin P. High, MD, MS, FACP
Chief, Section on Infectious Diseases
Professor of Medicine, Sections on Infectious Diseases
Hematology/Oncology and Molecular Medicine
Co-Director, Molecular Medicine Graduate Program
Wake Forest University Health Sciences
Winston Salem, NC

Amanda Itzkoff, MD
Assistant Professor
Department of Psychiatry
Mount Sinai School of Medicine
New York, NY

Gordon L. Jensen, MD, PhD
Professor and Head, Department of Nutritional Sciences
Professor of Medicine
Pennsylvania State University
University Park, PA

Jennifer M. Kapo, MD
Assistant Professor of Clinical Medicine
Division of Geriatric Medicine
Department of Medicine
University of Pennsylvania
Medical Director, Palliative Care Services
Philadelphia Veteran's Medical Center
Philadelphia, PA

Paul R. Katz, MD, AGSF
Professor of Medicine
Chief of Geriatrics/Aging
University of Rochester School of Medicine and Dentistry
Rochester, NY

Gary J. Kennedy, MD
Professor and Director, Division of Geriatric Psychiatry
Albert Einstein College of Medicine
Montefiore Medical Center
Bronx, NY

Anne M. Kenny, MD
Associate Professor of Medicine
Traveler's Center on Aging
University of Connecticut Health Center
Farmington, CT

Ali Khanmohamadi, MD
Staff Psychiatrist
Bellevue Hospital Center
New York, NY

Douglas P. Kiel, MD, MPH
Associate Professor of Medicine
Harvard Medical School
Director Medical Research
Hebrew SeniorLife
Institute for Aging Research
Boston, MA

C. Seth Landefeld, MD
Professor of Medicine
Chief, Division of Geriatrics and Director, Center on
    Aging,
University of California, San Francisco
Associate Chief of Staff, Geriatrics and Extended Care,
    San Francisco
VA Medical Center
San Francisco, CA

Melinda S. Lantz, MD
Chief of Geriatric Psychiatry
Beth Israel Medical Center
New York, NY

Susan W. Lehmann, MD
Assistant Professor
Department of Psychiatry and Behavioral Sciences
The Johns Hopkins School of Medicine
Baltimore, MD

Shari M. Ling, MD
Assistant Professor
Division of Geriatric Medicine & Gerontology
Johns Hopkins University School of Medicine
Assistant Clinical Professor
Division of Rheumatology and Clinical Immunology
University of Maryland School of Medicine
Baltimore, MD

Dan L. Longo, MD
Scientific Director
National Institute on Aging
Baltimore, MD

Courtney H. Lyder, ND, GNP, FAAN
Dean and Professor, School of Nursing
Assistant Director for Academic Nursing,
Ronald Reagan UCLA Medical Center
University of California, Los Angeles
Los Angeles, CA

William L. Lyons, MD
Associate Professor
Section of Geriatrics and Gerontology
Department of Internal Medicine
University of Nebraska Medical Center
Omaha, NE

Edward R. Marcantonio, MD, SM
Director of Research
    Division of General Medicine and Primary Care
    Beth Israel Deaconess Medical Center
    Associate Professor of Medicine
    Harvard Medical School
    Boston, MA

Alvin M. Matsumoto, MD
Professor of Medicine
Geriatric Research, Education, and Clinical Center
VA Puget Sound Health Care System
Division of Gerontology and Geriatric Medicine
Department of Medicine and Population Center for
    Research in Reproduction
University of Washington School of Medicine
Seattle, WA

Robert McCann, MD, AGSF
Professor of Medicine
University of Rochester School of Medicine and Dentistry
Highland Hospital Department of Medicine
Rochester, NY

Paige E. Miller, MS
Department of Nutritional Sciences
Pennsylvania State University
University Park, PA

R. Sean Morrison, MD
Director, National Palliative Care Research Center
Hermann Merkin Professor of Palliative Care
Professor of Geriatrics and Medicine
Vice-Chair for Research
Brookdale Department of Geriatrics
Mount Sinai School of Medicine
New York, NY

Thomas Mulligan, MD, AGSF
Director, Center on Aging and
Medical Director, Senior Services
St. Bernards Healthcare
Jonesboro, AR

Aman Nanda, MD
Assistant Professor of Medicine
Program Director
Geriatric Medicine Fellowship Program
The Warren Alpert Medical School of Brown University
Providence, RI

Judith Neugroschl, MD
Alzheimer's Disease Research Center
Division of Geriatric Psychiatry
Department of Psychiatry
Mount Sinai School of Medicine
New York, NY

David W. Oslin, MD
Assistant Professor
University of Pennsylvania
Geriatric and Addiction Psychiatry
Philadelphia, PA

James T. Pacala, MD, MS, AGSF
Associate Professor
Distinguished University Teaching Professor
Department of Family Medicine and Community Health
University of Minnesota Medical School
Minneapolis, MN

Sanjeevkumar R. Patel, MD, MS
Assistant Professor,
Division of Nephrology
University of Michigan Medical School
Ann Arbor, MID

Alfred J. Phillips, DPM, FACFAS
Chief of Podiatry
Cambridge Health Alliance, Cambridge MA
Cambridge, MA

Stacie T. Pinderhughes, MD
Associate Medical Director
North General Hospital
Chief, Division of Hospice & Palliative Medicine
Assistant Professor Geriatrics
Albert Einstein College of Medicine
New York, NY

Margaret Pisani, MD
Yale University School of Medicine
Pulmonary & Critical Care Medicine
New Haven, CT

James S. Powers, MD. AGSF
Associate Professor of Medicine
Vanderbilt University Medical Center
Associate Clinical Director, TVHS GRECC
Nashville, TN

Michael W. Rich, MD, AGSF
Professor of Medicine
Washington University School of Medicine
Cardiovascular Division, Washington University
St. Louis, MO

David Sarraf, MD
Associate Clinical Professor of Ophthalmology
Retinal Disorders and Ophthalmic Genetics Division
Jules Stein Eye Institute
UCLA David Geffen School of Medicine
Greater Los Angeles VA Healthcare Center
Los Angeles, CA

Mara A. Schonberg, MD
Instructor in Medicine
Beth Israel Deaconess Medical Center
Brookline, MA

Todd P. Semla, MS, PharmD, BCPS, FCCP, AGSF
Clinical Pharmacy Specialist
Pharmacy Benefits Management Services
Department of Veterans Affairs
Associate Professor
Departments of Medicine, and Psychiatry and Behavioral Sciences
The Feinberg School of Medicine
Northwestern University
Evanston, IL

Kenneth Shay, DDS, MS
Director of Geriatrics Programs
VA Office of Geriatrics and Extended Care
Ann Arbor VA Medical Center
Ann Arbor, MI

Richard Sims, MD
Professor of Medicine
Director, the UAB Geriatric Medicine Fellowship Program
Chief, Geriatrics Section
Birmingham VA Medical Center
Birmingham, AL

Richard G. Stefanacci, DO, MGH, MBA, AGSF, CMD
CMS Health Policy Scholar 2003-04
The Institute for Geriatric Studies
Center for Medicare Medication Management (cm^3)
Mayes College of Healthcare Business & Policy
University of the Sciences in Philadelphia
Philadelphia, PA

Mark A. Supiano, MD, AGSF
Professor and Chief, Division of Geriatrics
University of Utah Health System
Director, VA Salt Lake City Geriatric Research, Education and Clinical Center
Executive Director, University of Utah Center on Aging
Salt Lake City, UT

Pamela Taxel, MD
Associate Professor of Medicine
Department of Medicine
Center on Aging and
Division of Endocrinology and Metabolism
University of Connecticut Health Center
Farmington, CT

George Triadafilopoulos, MD
Clinical Professor of Medicine
Division of Gastroenterology and Hepatology
Stanford University School of Medicine
Stanford, CA

Jocelyn E. Wiggins, MA, BM, BCh, MRCP
Assistant Professor
Division of Geriatrics
University of Michigan Medical School
Ann Arbor, MI

Jennifer L. Wolff, PhD
Associate Professor
Department of Health Policy and Management
Johns Hopkins Bloomberg School of Public Health
Baltimore, MD

Pui Yin Wong, MD
Staff Psychiatrist
Maimonides Medical Center
Brooklyn, NY

Kristine Yaffe, MD
Associate Professor
Departments of Psychiatry, Neurology, Biostatistics and Epidemiology
University of California, San Francisco
Chief, Geriatric Psychiatry
San Francisco Veterans Administration Medical Center
San Francisco, CA

GRS7 CONTRIBUTING QUESTION WRITERS

Tara Aghaloo, DDS, MD, PhD
Associate Professor
Oral and Maxillofacial Surgery
UCLA School of Dentistry
Los Angeles, CA

Douglas A. Albreski, DPM
Assistant Professor, Department of Dermatology
University of Connecticut School of Medicine
Director of the Podiatric Dermatology Clinic
Farmington, CT

Kathryn A. Atchison, DDS, MPH
Interim Vice-Provost Intellectual Property and
Industry Relations Associate
Vice Chancellor for Research
UCLA Office of Intellectual Property Administration
Los Angeles, CA

R. Morgan Bain, MD
Medical Director, Palliative Care Program
Section on General Internal Medicine
Section on Gerontology and Geriatric Medicine
Wake Forest University School of Medicine
Winston-Salem, NC

Rachelle Bernacki, MD, MS
Director of Quality Initiatives
Pain and Palliative Care Program
Dana Farber Cancer Institute
Harvard Medical School
Boston, MA

Peter A. Boling, MD, AGSF
Professor of Internal Medicine
Virginia Commonwealth University
Richmond, VA

Rebecca Boxer, MD
Assistant Professor of Medicine
Department of Medicine
Case Western Reserve University
Cleveland, OH

Kenneth Brummel-Smith, MD, AGSF
Charlotte Edwards Maguire Professor and Chair,
Department of Geriatrics
Florida State University College of Medicine
Tallahassee, FL

Susan Charette, MD
Associate Clinical Professor
Division of Geriatrics
Department of Medicine
University of California, Los Angeles
Los Angeles, CA

Carl I. Cohen, MD
Professor and Director
Division of Geriatric Psychiatry
SUNY Downstate Medical Center
Brooklyn, NY

Leo M. Cooney, Jr., MD
Professor of Medicine
Yale University School of Medicine
New Haven, CT

Ann R. Datunashvili, MD
Yale School of Medicine
Clinical Instructor in Medicine (Geriatrics)
New Haven, CT

Michelle Eslami, MD
Professor of Medicine
Division of Geriatrics
David Geffen School of Medicine at UCLA
Los Angeles, CA

Helen M. Fernandez, MD
Associate Professor
Geriatrics Fellowship Program Director
Brookdale Department of Geriatric and Palliative Medicine
Mount Sinai School of Medicine
New York, NY

Mark H. Fleisher, MD
Associate Professor of Psychiatry
Director, Division of Public and Community Psychiatry
Director, Neurodevelopmental Psychiatry
University of Nebraska College of Medicine
Omaha, NE

Gordana Gataric, MD
Assistant Professor
Department of Geriatrics
Wright State University-Boonshoft School of Medicine
Dayton, OH

Angela Gentili, MD
Associate Professor of Internal Medicine
Director, Geriatrics Fellowship Training Program
VAMC/Virginia Commonwealth University
Richmond, VA

Shelly L. Gray, PharmD, MS
Professor
School of Pharmacy
University of Washington
Seattle, WA

Blaine S. Greenwald, MD
Vice Chairman, Combined Department of Psychiatry
Long Island Jewish Medical Center/North Shore University
    Hospital
Director, Geriatric Psychiatry Division
The Zucker Hillside Hospital
Glen Oaks, NY

William R. Hazzard, MD, AGSF
Chief, VA Section
Division of Gerontology & Geriatric Medicine
Professor of Medicine
University of Washington
Seattle, WA

Kevin P. High, MD, MS, FACP
Chief, Section on Infectious Diseases
Professor of Medicine, Sections on Infectious Diseases
Hematology/Oncology and Molecular Medicine
Co-Director, Molecular Medicine Graduate Program
Wake Forest University Health Sciences
Winston Salem, NC

Lyn M. Holley, PhD
Assistant Professor
Department of Gerontology
University of Nebraska at Omaha
Omaha, NE

Sam J. Holley, PhD
Professor and Director of Academics,
Offutt Campus
Embry-Riddle Aeronautical University Worldwide
Offutt AFB, NE

Michael S. Irwig, MD, FACE
Assistant Professor of Medicine
George Washington University School of Medicine
Division of Endocrinology, Medical Faculty Associates
Director, Center for Andrology
Washington, DC

Gail Ishiyama, MD
Associate Professor
UCLA David Geffen School of Medicine
Department of Neurology
Division of Neurotology
Reed Neurological Research Center
Los Angeles, CA

Jerry C. Johnson, MD, AGSF
Chief of the Division of Geriatric Medicine
Professor of Medicine
Senior Fellow of the Institute on Aging
University of Pennsylvania
Ralston-Penn Center
Philadelphia, PA

Theodore M. Johnson II, MD, MPH
Associate Professor of Medicine
Emory School of Medicine
Director, Division of Geriatric Medicine and Gerontology
Interim Director, Woodruff Health Sciences Center for
    Health in Aging
Atlanta Site Director, Birmingham/Atlanta VA GRECC
Atlanta, GA

C. Bree Johnston, MD, MPH
Professor of Clinical Medicine
Associate Chief for Geriatrics Education
Division of Geriatrics
University of California, San Francisco
San Francisco, CA

Fran E. Kaiser, MD, AGSF, FGSA
Adjunct Professor of Medicine
St. Louis University School of Medicine
St Louis, MO
Executive Medical Director
Region Medical Director Program
Merck and Co., Inc
Upper Gwynedd, PA

Catherine McVearry Kelso, MD
Medical Director, Hospice and Palliative Care Service
Site Director, Hospice and Palliative Medicine Fellowship
Ethics Consultation Coordinator
McGuire VA Medical Center
Academic Affiliate Virginia Commonwealth University
Richmond, VA

Anne Kenny, MD
Associate Professor of Medicine
Traveler's Center on Aging
University of Connecticut Health Center
Farmington, CT

Mary B. King, MD
Geriatrician
Williamstown Medical Associates
Williamstown, MA

Steve Koenig, MD
Medical Director
Keswick Sleep Institute
Charlottesville, VA

George A. Kuchel, MD, FRCP, AGSF
Professor of Medicine
Citicorp Chair in Geriatrics & Gerontology
Director, UConn Center on Aging
Chief, Division of Geriatric Medicine
University of Connecticut Health Center
Farmington, CT

Larry W. Lawhorne, MD
Chair, Department of Geriatrics
Boonshoft School of Medicine
Wright State University
Elizabeth Place, East Medical Building
Dayton, OH

Eric Lenze, MD
Associate Professor
Department of Psychiatry
Washington University School of Medicine
St. Louis, MO

Michael C. Lindberg, MD, FACP
Director, Department of Medicine
Hartford Hospital
Hartford, CT
Clinical Associate Professor,
University of Connecticut School of Medicine
Farmington, CT

Shari M. Ling, MD
Assistant Professor
Division of Geriatric Medicine & Gerontology
Johns Hopkins University School of Medicine
Assistant Clinical Professor
Division of Rheumatology and Clinical Immunology
University of Maryland School of Medicine
Baltimore, MD

Joanne Lynn, MD, MA, MS, AGSF
Bureau Chief, Cancer and Chronic Disease
Community Health Administration
Department of Health
Government of the District of Columbia
Washington, DC

Bill Lyons, MD
Associate Professor
Section of Geriatrics and Gerontology
Department of Internal Medicine
University of Nebraska Medical Center
Omaha, NE

Victoria Maizes, MD
Executive Director
Arizona Center for Integrative Medicine
Associate Professor
Medicine, Family Medicine and Public Health
University of Arizona
Tucson, AZ

Mathew S. Maurer, MD
Associate Professor of Clinical Medicine
Director, Clinical Cardiovascular Research Laboratory for
    the Elderly
Columbia University Medical Center, College of Physicians
    and Surgeons
New York, NY

Ellen M. McMahon, MD
Clinical Preceptor
Department of Family Practice and Community Health
University of Massachusetts
Worcester, MA
Martha's Vineyard Hospital
Oak Bluffs, MA

Lynn McNicoll, MD
Assistant Professor of Medicine
Warren Alpert School of Medicine
Brown University
Rhode Island Hospital
The Miriam Hospital
Providence, RI

Daniel Ari Mendelson, MS, MD, FACP
Associate Professor of Medicine, Division of Geriatrics
University of Rochester School of Medicine & Dentistry
Highland Hospital, Department of Medicine
Rochester, NY

Diana V. Messadi, DDS, MMSc, DMSc
Professor and Chair
Section of Oral Medicine and Orofacial Pain
Division of Oral Biology & Medicine
UCLA School of Dentistry
Los Angeles, CA

Karin Ouchida, MD
Assistant Professor of Medicine
Montefiore Medical Center
Albert Einstein College of Medicine
Medical Director
Montefiore Medical Center Home Health Agency
Bronx NY

Joseph G. Ouslander, MD, AGSF
Professor of Clinical Biomedical Science and Associate
    Dean for Geriatric Programs
Charles E. Schmidt College of Biomedical Science
Professor (Courtesy), Christine E. Lynn College of Nursing
Florida Atlantic University
Boca Raton, FL
Professor of Medicine (Voluntary),
University of Miami Miller School of Medicine
Miami, FL

Arash Naeim, MD, PhD
Assistant Professor of Medicine
University of California, Los Angeles
Los Angeles, CA

James T. Pacala, MD, MS, AGSF
Associate Professor
Distinguished University Teaching Professor
Department of Family Practice and Community Health
University of Minnesota Medical School
Minneapolis, MN

Joe W. Ramsdell, MD
Professor and Head,
Division of General Internal Medicine
University of California, San Diego
UCSD Medical Center
San Diego, CA

M. Carrington Reid, MD, PhD
Associate Professor of Medicine
Division of Geriatrics and Gerontology
Weill Cornell Medical College
New York, NY

Julie Robison, PhD
Associate Professor of Medicine
Center on Aging
University of Connecticut Health Center
Farmington, CT

Mitchell H. Rosner, MD
Associate Professor
Vice Chairman, Department of Medicine
Director, Nephrology Fellowship Training Program
Division of Nephrology
University of Virginia Health System
Charlottesville, VA

Amy E. Sanders, MD
Assistant Professor of Neurology
Albert Einstein College of Medicine
Bronx, NY

Alessandra Scalmati, MD
Director, Montefiore Aging and Memory Center
Assistant Professor of Psychiatry and Behavioral Sciences
Albert Einstein College of Medicine
Associate Director Fellowship in Geriatric Psychiatry
Montefiore Medical Center
Bronx, NY

Gary J. Schiller, MD
Professor, Department of Medicine
Director, Hematological Malignancy/Stem Cell Transplant
    Program
David Geffen School of Medicine at UCLA
Los Angeles, CA

Janice B. Schwartz, MD
Clinical Professor of Medicine and Biopharmaceutical
    Sciences
University of California, San Francisco
Director of Research, Jewish Home of San Francisco
San Francisco, CA

Pushpendra Sharma, MD
Attending Geriatrician,
Jewish Home Lifecare
Site Medical Director,
Prison Health Services
Manhattan Detention Complex
New York, NY

David H. Stern, MD
Associate Medical Director
S+AGE (Specialized Ambulatory Geriatric Evaluation
    Clinic)
Sherman Oaks, CA

Gwen K. Sterns, MD
Chief, Department of Ophthalmology
Rochester General Hospital
Clinical Professor of Ophthalmology
University of Rochester School of Medicine and Dentistry
Chief, Department of Ophthalmology
Rochester General Hospital
Rochester, NY

Dennis H. Sullivan, MD, AGSF
Director, Geriatric Research, Education, and Clinical
  Center
Central Arkansas Veterans Healthcare System (3J/NLR)
Professor, Geriatrics and Internal Medicine
Donald W. Reynolds Department of Geriatrics
University of Arkansas for Medical Sciences
Little Rock, AR

Joe Verghese, MD, MS
Associate Professor of Neurology
Director, Division of Cognitive & Motor Aging
Albert Einstein College of Medicine
Bronx, NY

Katie Ward, MD
Assistant Clinical Professor
Division of Geriatrics
David Geffen School of Medicine at UCLA
Los Angeles, CA

Barbara E. Weinstein, PhD
Professor and Executive Officer
Health Sciences Doctoral Programs
The Graduate Center
The City University of New York
New York, NY

Phyllis C. Zee, MD, PhD
Professor of Neurology, Neurobiology and Physiology
Director Sleep Disorders Center
Chicago, IL

Richard A. Zweig, PhD
Director, Ferkauf Older Adult Program
Associate Professor of Psychology
Ferkauf Graduate School-Yeshiva University
Assistant Professor of Psychiatry
Albert Einstein College of Medicine
Bronx, NY

Steven Zweig, MD, MSPH
Paul Revare Family Professor and Chairman
Family and Community Medicine
Director, Interdisciplinary Center on Aging
University of Missouri Columbia, MO

DISCLOSURE OF FINANCIAL INTERESTS

As an accredited provider of Continuing Medical Education, the American Geriatrics Society continuously strives to ensure that the education activities planned and conducted by our faculty meet generally accepted ethical standards as codified by the ACCME, the Food and Drug Administration, and the American Medical Association's Guide for Gifts to Physicians. To this end, we have implemented a process wherein everyone who is in a position to control the content of an education activity has disclosed to us all relevant financial relationships with any commercial interests within the past 12 months as related to the content of their presentations and under which we work to resolve any real or apparent conflicts of interest. In order to help ensure content objectivity, independence, and fair balance, conflicts of interest in this particular educational activity have been resolved by having the content independently peer reviewed before publication by the Editorial Board.

The following authors (and/or their spouses/partners) have reported real or apparent conflicts of interest that have been resolved through a peer review content validation process.

Harold P. Adams, Jr., MD
Dr. Adams receives grant support from NMT Medical, Merck, and Schering Plough.

Marc Agronin, MD
Dr. Agronin receives grant support from Janssen, Medivation, Eli Lilly, Cardiokine, and Merck and is a member of the Speaker's Bureau for Astra-Zeneca, Merck, and Novartis.

Cathy A. Alessi, MD, AGSF
Dr. Alessi serves as a paid consultant for Prescription Solutions Inc.

Priscilla Faith Bade, MD
Dr. Bade serves as a paid consultant (as Medical Director) for Golden Living Bella Vista and Hospice of the Hills.

Peter A. Boling, MD, AGSF
Dr. Boling serves as a paid consultnat for Home Instead Senior Care and Amedisys

Chad Boult, MD, MPH, MBA
Dr. Boult serves as a paid consultant for Zist Services and Sacred Independence.

Cynthia J. Brown, MD, MSPH
Dr. Brown receives grant support from NIH SBIR in conjunction with AugmenTech, Inc.

Kenneth Brummel-Smith, MD, AGSF
Dr. Brummel-Smith serves as a paid consultant for Scan Health Plan and receives grant support from University of California, Irvine.

Julie C. Chapman, PsyD
Dr. Chapman receives grant support from Dept. of Veterans Affairs and the Institute for Clinical Research.

Gurkamal S. Chatta, MD
Dr. Chatta receives grant support from Novartis and Sanofi Aventis and is a member of the Speaker's Bureau for Sarnoff Aventis.

Anne L. Coleman, MD, PhD
Dr. Coleman receives grant support from Aleon, Allergan, and Pfizer.

G. Willy Davila, MD
Dr. Davila serves as a paid consultant and is a member of the Speaker's Bureau for Astellas, Watson Pharma and American Medical Systems. He also receives grant support from Astella, American Medical Systems and CL Medical.

Maria L. Diaz, MD
Dr. Diaz serves as a paid consultant for Ethican Women's Health.

Catherine E. DuBeau, MD
Dr. DuBeau serves as a paid consultant for Pfizer, Astellas, Novartis, and Watson and receives grant support from Pfizer.

E. Wesley Ely, MD, MPH
Dr. Ely is a member of the Speaker's Bureau, serves as a paid consultant and receives grant support from Lilly, Pfizer, Hospira, GlaxoSmithKline, and Aspect.

Elizabeth Galik, PhD, CRNP
Dr. Galik serves as a paid consultant for Novartis.

John D. Gazewood, MD, MSPH
Dr. Gazewood serves as a paid consultant for Elsevier Publishing.

Thomas M. Gill, MD
Dr. Gill serves as a paid consultant for Asobio Pharmaceuticals.

Kevin P. High, MD, MS, FACP
Dr. High receives grant support from Pfizer, Optimer, Chimerix and is a member of the advisory board of Optimer.

Gordon L. Jensen, MD, PhD
Dr. Jensen serves as a paid consultant for Baster Healthcare, Nestle, and Abbott. He is a member of the Speaker's Bureau and receives grant support from Abbott and Baster.

Theodore M. Johnson, MD, MPH
Dr. Johnson serves as a paid consultant for Pfizer, Johnson & Johnson, and Ferring. He receives grant support in the form of Federal Funds from Aventis.

Fran E. Kaiser, MD, AGSF
Dr. Kaiser holds significant shares and is an employee of Merck & Co., Inc.

Paul R. Katz, MD, AGSF
Dr. Katz serves as a paid consultant for Omnicare.

Catherine McVearry Kelso, MD
Dr. Kelso receives grants support from Virginia Commonwealth University, Center on Aging.

Gary J. Kennedy, MD
Dr. Kennedy receives grant support from Forest Laboratories and speaker honoraria from Pfizer, Inc. Myriad Pharmaceuticals.

Eric Lenze, MD
Dr. Lenze serves as a paid consultant for Fox Learning Systems and receives grant support from Forest.

Courtney H. Lyder, RN, ND
Mr. Lyder serves as a paid consultant and is a member of the Speaker's Bureau for ConvaTec and Kenetic Concepts Inc. He receives grant support from ConvaTec.

Alvin M. Matsumoto, MD
Dr. Matsumoto serves as a paid consultant for GlaxoSmithKline, Solvay, GTL, Amgen, and Quatrx. He receives grant support from GSK, Solvay, Ascend, Auxilium, and Ardana.

Mathew S. Maurer, MD
Dr. Maurer serves as a paid consultant from Bio. Reference Labs, Inc. and St. Jude Medical. He receives grant support from Fold RX, Inc. and Novartis, Inc.

Daniel Ari Mendelson, MS, MD
Dr. Mendelson serves as a paid consultant for and receives grant support from Synthes.

Arash Naeim, MD, PhD
Dr. Naeim serves as a paid consultant for Amgen, receives grant support from Genetech and Pfizer, and is a member of the Speaker's Bureau for Amgen and Pfizer.

David W. Oslin, MD
Dr. Oslin receives grant support from the NIH, VA, commonwealth of Pennsylvania, and Hazelden Foundation.

Joseph G. Ouslander, MD, AGSF
Dr. Ouslander serves as an advisory board member for Pfizer and is a paid consultant for Pfizer and Amgen.

Stacie T. Pinderhughes, MD
Dr. Pinderhughes is a member of the Speaker's Bureau for Wyeth.

James Powers, MD
Mr. Powers serves as a paid consultant for Healthways and Healthspring.

Joe W. Ramsdell, MD
Dr. Ramsdell serves as the principal investigator through the University California, San Diego for Clinical Trials for Astra Zeneca, Boehringer Ingelheim, Centecor Research & Development Inc., Chiesi Inc., DeepBreeze LTC, Forest Research Institute, GlaxoSmithKline.

Michael W. Rich, MD, AGSF
Dr. Rich receives grant support from Astellas Pharma US and serves as a paid consultant from Medco PBM.

Gary Schiller, MD
Dr. Schiller serves as a paid consultant for Vion Pharmaceuticals, receives grant support from Novartis, Johnson & Johnson, Wollennium, Celzine, Genzyme, and is a member of the Speaker's Bureau for Novartis.

Todd P. Semla, MS, PharmD, BCPS, FCCP, AGSF
Dr. Semla serves as a paid consultant for Omnicare Pharmacy and Therapeutic Committee, Ovations and Evercare. He also has a significant financial relationship with Lexi Corp, Inc. Publishing.

Richard Sims, MD
Dr. Sims is a member of the Speaker's Bureau for Merck & Co. Inc.

Richard G. Stefanacci, DO, MGH, MBA, AGSF, CMD
Dr. Stefanacci is a member of the Speaker's Bureau for Pfizer, Forest Laboratories, Amgen, Merck, BMS, and Eisai. He serves as a paid consultant for NewCourtland Elder Services, and has served as a member of an advisory board for Novartis.

Gail M. Sullivan, MD, MPH, AGSF
Dr. Sullivan serves as a paid consultant for Medicare Advocacy, Inc.

Pam Taxel, MD
Dr. Taxel is a member of the Speaker's Bureau for Novartis and Amgen.

Joe Verghese, MD, MS
Dr. Verghese is a member of the Speaker's Bureau for Pfizer.

Jennifer L. Wolff, PhD
Dr. Wolff receives grant support from NIMH, Center for Healthcare Strategies.

Kristine Yaffe, MD
Dr. Yaffe serves as a paid consultant and is a member of the Speaker's Bureau for Novartis.

Phyllis C. Zee, MD, PhD
Dr. Zee serves as a paid consultant for Takeda, Sanofi-Aventis, Cephalon, Zeo, and Philips and receives grant support from Takeda.

The following authors have returned disclosure forms indicating that they (and/or their spouses/partners) have no affiliation with, or financial interest in, any commercial interest that may have direct interest in the subject matter of their chapters/questions:

Sumaira Z. Aasi, MD
Reva N. Adler, MD, MPH, FRCPC
Tara Aghaloo, DDS, MD, PhD
Susan E. Aiello, DVM, ELS
Douglas Albreski, MD
Neil Alexander, MD
Kathryn A. Atchison, DDS, MPH
Carolyn Auerhahn, EdD, ANP, GNP-BC, FAANP
R. Morgan Bain, MD
Leen Bakkali, MD
Cynthia Barton, RN, MSN
Judith L. Beizer, PharmD, CGP, FASCP
Rachelle Bernacki, MD, MS
Sarah D. Berry, MD MPH
Marc R. Blackman, MD
Caroline S. Blaum, MD, MS
Marie Boltz, PhD, RN, GNP-BC
Rebecca Boxer, MD
David M. Buchner, MD, MPH
David Bush, MD
R. Charles Callison, MD
Elizabeth Capezuti, PhD, RN, FAAN
Susan Charette, MD
Jaehyuk Choi, MD, PhD
Colleen Christmas, MD
Carl I. Cohen, MD
Leo M. Cooney, Jr., MD
Steven R. Counsell, MD, AGSF
Ann R. Datunashvili, MD
Margaret A. Drickamer, MD
Carmel Bitondo Dyer, MD, AGSF
G. Paul Eleazer, MD
William B. Ershler, MD
Anne Fabiny, MD
Neal S. Fedarko, PhD
Helen M. Fernandez, MD
Ellen Flaherty, PhD, RN, GNP-BC
Mark H. Fleisher, MD
Linda P. Fried, MD, MPH, AGSF
Terry Fulmer, PhD, RN, FAAN, AGSF
Gordana Gataric, MD
Angela Gentili, MD
JoAnn Giaconi, MD
Suzanne M. Gillespie, MD, RD
Lisa J. Granville, MD, AGSF
Shelly L. Gray, PharmD, MS
Blaine S. Greenwald, MD
David A. Gruenewald, MD
William R. Hazzard, MD, AGSF
Kenneth Hepburn, PhD
Lyn M. Holley, PhD
Sam J. Holley, PhD
Michael S. Irwig, MD

Gail Ishiyama, MD
Amanda Itzkoff, MD
Jerry C. Johnson, MD, AGSF
C. Bree Johnston, MD, MPH
Jennifer M. Kapo, MD
Anne Kenny, MD
Douglas P. Kiel, MD, MPH
Mary B. King, MD
Steve Koenig, MD
George A. Kuchel, MD, AGSF
C. Seth Landefeld, MD
Melinda S. Lantz, MD
Larry W. Lawhorne, MD
Susan Lehmann, MD
Michael C. Lindberg, MD
Shari M. Ling, MD
Dan L. Longo, MD
Joanne Lynn, MD, MA, MS, AGSF
Bill Lyons, MD
Victoria Maizes, MD
Edward R. Marcantonio, MD, SM
Robert McCann, MD, AGSF
Ellen McMahon, MD
Lynn McNicoll, MD
Annette Medina-Walpole, MD, AGSF
Diana V. Messadi, DDS, MMSc, DMSc
Paige E. Miller, MS
R. Sean Morrison, MD
Thomas Mulligan, MD, AGSF
Aman Nanda, MD
Judith Neugroschl, MD
Karin Ouchida, MD
James T. Pacala, MD, MS
Sanjeevkumar R. Patel, MD, MS
Alfred Jordan Phillips, DPM, FACFAS
Margaret Pisani, MD
M. Carrington Reid, MD
Barbara Resnick, PhD, CRNP, FAANP, FAAN
Julie Robison, PhD
Dalia Ritter Rosenberg
Mitchell H. Rosner, MD
Amy E. Sanders, MD
David Sarraf, MD
Alessandra Scalmati, MD
Mara A. Schonberg, MD
Janice B. Schwartz, MD
Pushpendra Sharma, MD
Kenneth Shay, DDS, MS
Andrea Sherman, MS
David H. Stern, MD
Gwen K. Sterns, MD
Dennis H. Sullivan, MD, AGSF
Mark A. Supiano, MD, AGSF
George Triadafilopoulos, MD
Katie Ward, MD
Barbara E. Weinstein, PhD
Jocelyn E. Wiggins, MA, BM, BCh, MRCP
Richard A. Zweig, PhD
Steven Zweig, MD, MSPH

INDEX

Page references followed by *t* and *f* indicate tables and figures, respectively. Numbers preceded by "q" indicate question numbers (not page numbers) and critiques.

Androgens, adrenal, 500
Anemia, 514–519
  of chronic disease, 516–517
  diagnostic criteria for, 514
  evaluation of, 515
  hemolytic, 515, 515t, 518–519
  hypoproliferative, 515–518, 515t, 516f
  ineffective, 515, 515t
  of inflammation, 516–517
  iron dosing for, 521
  laboratory evaluation of, 515, 516f, 517f
  management of, 412
  physiologic classification of, 515, 515t
  and rehabilitation, 134
  sideroblastic, 518
  valve-associated, 519
Aneurysms, abdominal aortic (AAA), 372
  indications for repair, 373
  screening for, 62t, 66
Angina, unstable, 362
Angiodysplasia, 401
  colonic, 401–402
Angiography, coronary, q2
Angiotensin-converting enzyme (ACE) inhibitors
  for acute coronary syndrome, 362
  adverse drug events, 76–77, 77t
  for chronic CAD, 364
  for comorbid vascular disease, 391
  drug interactions, 77, 78t
  early, 374
  for heart failure, 378t, 379, 380
  for hypertension, 387
  and incontinence, 208t
  for MI and heart failure, 374
  quality indicators for, 375, 382
Angiotensin-receptor blockers (ARBs)
  for acute coronary syndrome, 362
  adverse drug events, 76–77, 77t
  for heart failure, 378, 378t, 379, 380
  for hypertension, 387–388
Angular cheilitis, 350–351, 350f
Anhedonia, q55
Ankle, 462–464
Ankle-brachial index (ABI), 340, 372
Anorexia, 105
Antacids
  adverse drug events, 76–77, 77t
  nutrient interactions, 197–198, 198t
Antagonistic pleiotropy theory, 9
Antalgic gait, 219t
Anterior ischemic optic neuropathy, 175, 175f
Anthropometrics, 196
Antiandrogens, 427t
Antianxiety agents, 319
Antiarrhythmics
  for acute coronary syndrome, 363
  adverse drug events, 76–77, 77t
  drug interactions, 77, 78t
  quality indicators for, 383
Antibiotics
  minimum criteria for initiation in long-term
    care settings, 481–482, 482t

nutrient interactions, 197–198, 198t
  perioperative, 93–95, 95t
  for prostatitis, 428–429
Anticholinergics
  adverse drug events, 76–77, 77t
  for COPD, 356, 357t
  and delirium, 268, 270t, q64
  and incontinence, 208t
  quality indicators for, 80
Anticoagulation
  for atrial fibrillation, 375, 477
  cessation before surgery, 95, 96t
  for hip fracture, 101
  for hip replacement, 101
  perioperative, 93–95, 95t
Anticonvulsant therapy
  adverse drug events, 76–77, 77t
  and delirium, 270t
  for persistent pain, 112t, 117
  for seizures, 474, 475t
  to stabilize mood in mania and bipolar
    disorder, 301, 302t
Antidepressants
  adverse drug events, 76–77, 77t
  for anxiety disorders, 310
  for anxiety with autism, q4
  choice of, 305
  and delirium, 270t
  for dementia, 254
  for depression, 298–301, 299t–300t
  for depressive features of behavioral
    disturbances in dementia, 259, 260t
  drug interactions, 77, 78t
  indications for, 296, 296t
  interventions for preventing falls with, 231t
  for major depressive disorder with personality
    disorder, q63
  for persistent pain, 112t–113t, 117
  for personality disorders, 320
  second-generation, q48
  sedating, 281, 281t
  tricyclic, 112t, 208t, 259, 260t, 270t, 299t,
    305
Antidiuretic hormone, inappropriate secretion of,
  405, 406, 407, 499
Antihistamines
  adverse drug events, 76–77, 77t
  for anxiety disorders, 310
  and delirium, 270t
  quality indicators for sleep problems, 282
  sedating, 277
Antihypertensives, 76–77, 77t
Antimicrobial management, 481–482
Antimuscarinics, 212–214, 213t, 215
Antinuclear antibodies (ANAs), 438
Antioxidants, 253
Antiparkinsonian agents
  adverse drug events, 76–77, 77t
  and delirium, 270t
Antiplatelet therapy
  adverse drug events, 76–77, 77t
  quality indicators for cardiovascular diseases
    and disorders, 375

Antipsychotics
  adverse drug events, 76–77, 77t
  atypical, 270t
  and delirium, 268, 270t, q16
  dosing and adverse events of, 313, 314t
  drug interactions, 77, 78t
  and incontinence, 208t
  interventions for preventing falls with, 231t
  for personality disorders, 319
  for psychosis in dementia, 261–262, 261t
  quality indicators for, 80
  second-generation, 270t, q34, q48
  sedating, 281
  to stabilize mood in mania and bipolar
    disorder, 301, 302t
Antiretroviral therapy, highly active, 488
Antisocial personality disorder
  features of, 316, 317t
  therapeutic strategies for, 318–319, 319t
Antithrombotic therapy, 362–363
Anxiety
  with autism, q4
  with depression, 309
  features of anxious or fearful behaviors, 316,
    317t
  marked anxiety, 309
Anxiety attacks, q76
Anxiety disorders, 307–311, q95
  classes of, 307–309
  comorbidity, 309
  generalized anxiety disorder, 309, 310t
  and incontinence, 209t
  and medical disorders, 309, 310t
  pharmacologic management of, 309–310
  psychologic management of, 311
  treatment strategies for, 310t
Aortic regurgitation (AR), 366
  clinical features and treatment of, 367t
  diagnosis of, 366
  epidemiology of, 366
Aortic stenosis (AS), 366, q2, q33
  clinical features and treatment of, 367t
  diagnosis of, 366
  prevalence of, 366
Apathetic thyrotoxicosis, 494
Apathy, q114
Aphthous ulcers, 351, 351f
Apidra (insulin glulisine), 511t
Apolipoprotein E gene (APOE), 246
Appetite stimulants, 200
APS. See Adult Protective Services
Aqueous outflow facilitators, 175t
Aqueous suppressants, 175t
AR. See Aortic regurgitation
ARBs. See Angiotensin-receptor blockers
Area Agencies on Aging, 254
ARF (acute renal failure), 409–411
Arformoterol, 357t
Aripiprazole
  dosing and adverse events of, 313, 314t
  for psychosis in dementia, 261–262, 261t

Aripiprazole *(continued)*
　to stabilize mood in mania and bipolar
　　disorder, 301, 302*t*
Armour thyroid, q102
Aromatase inhibitor therapy, q19
Aromatherapy, 311
Arrhythmias
　bradyarrhythmias, 370–371
　cardiac, 188, 368–371
　cardiac syncope due to, 191, 192*t*
　indications for permanent pacemaker
　　implantation, 371, 371*t*
　supraventricular, 370
　ventricular, 370
Arterial ulcers, 339–340, 339*t*
Arteriosclerotic parkinsonism, 220
Arteriovascular disease, 209*t*
Arteriovenous malformation, 401
Arthritis, 437
　crystalline, q54
　differential diagnosis of, 437, 438*t*
　of elbow, 439
　exercise for, 441
　of foot, 463–464
　general management of, 441, 442
　of knee, 440
　monoarthritis, q54
　osteoarthritis, 442–443, 444*f*, q58
　prevalence of symptoms, 3, 4*f*
　rheumatoid arthritis, 443–444, 445*t*
　of wrist, 439
Arthritis Foundation, 112
Arthrocentesis, 438, 446, q54
Arthroplasty, total hip and knee, 123–124
Arthroscopic debridement, 443
Artificial feeding, 201
Artificial sphincter, 213*t*, 215
AS. *See* Aortic stenosis
ASA (American Society of Anesthesiologists), 93,
　93*t*
Asian Americans
　burning mouth syndrome in, 351
　cancer incidence, 523, 523*t*
　end-of-life care, 103
　nursing-home population, 142
　older population, 1
　urinary incontinence, 207
Aspiration, 204
Aspiration pneumonia, 128, 134, 204
Aspirin therapy
　for acute coronary syndrome, 362
　adverse drug events, 76–77, 77*t*
　for atrial fibrillation, 369
　for chronic CAD, 364
　early, 374, 478
　perioperative, 93–95, 95*t*
　for peripheral arterial disease, 372
　for persistent pain, 118
　for prevention of cardiovascular events, q85
　preventive, 63*t*, 69
　quality indicators for, 374
　quality indicators for diabetes mellitus, 513

quality indicators for GI diseases and
　disorders, 403
quality indicators for neurologic diseases and
　disorders, 478
for stroke prevention, 466
Assessment, 43–48. *See also* Screening
　of amputation, 139
　of behavioral problems in dementia, 257–258
　Berg Balance Test, 227
　cardiac risk assessment for noncardiac
　　surgery, 93, 94*f*
　cognitive, 45–46
　comprehensive geriatric assessment (CGA),
　　48, 67, 135–136, 157–158
　Confusion Assessment Method (CAM), 122,
　　264–265, 266*t*
　Confusion Assessment Method for the
　　Intensive Care Unit (CAM-ICU),
　　264–265, 266*t*, 267*t*
　continuity of tests, 160
　of decisional capacity, 24–25
　discharge, 128
　falls risk assessment, 62*t*
　of frailty, 164–165
　of hearing loss, 178
　in home care, 152
　at hospital admission, 120, 121*t*
　of hospitalized older patients, 120–124
　MacArthur Competency Assessment Tool for
　　Treatment, 26
　Mini-Cog Assessment Instrument for
　　Dementia, 46, 68, 123, 247
　Mini–Mental State Examination (MMSE), 25,
　　44*t*, 46, 68, 123, 247, 265, 267*t*
　of nutrition, 196–198, q25
　of older drivers, 47
　Outcome and Assessment Information Set
　　(OASIS), 132, 151
　of pain management, 118
　performance-based functional assessment, 221
　Performance-Oriented Mobility Assessment
　　(POMA), 45, 227–229
　of persistent pain, 109–111
　physical, 44–45
　of physical activity, 58–59
　preoperative, 92–97
　of pressure ulcers, 288, 294
　psychologic, 46
　quality indicators for, 48
　rapid screening followed by, 43, 44*t*
　related quality indicators for, 48
　rolling, 43
　social, 46
　of suicide risk, q55
　systematic, 120, 121*t*
　Timed Up and Go (TUG) test, 44*t*, 221, 227
　of total hip and knee arthroplasty, 138
　Try This, 43
　of urinary incontinence, 216
　vertebral fracture assessment (VFA), 239
Assessment instruments, 132*t*
Assisted-living facilities, 6, 155–156
Assistive devices, 5–6, 139
　ambulatory, 449

for balance disorders, 223
hearing aids, 179–182
listening devices, 179, 181*t*, 183
nonambulatory, 449
for postural instability and festination, q3
review of, 233
Asthma, 355
At-risk substance use, 322
Atenolol, q89
Atherosclerosis
　in diabetes mellitus, 507–508
　prevention and management of, 507–508
Athlete's foot, q32
ATN (acute tubular necrosis), 409–410
Atorvastatin, 362
Atrial fibrillation, 368–370, q42
　anticoagulation for, 375, 477
　clinical features, 368
　diagnosis of, 368–369
　epidemiology of, 368
　in hospitalized patients, 121*t*
　interventions for, 121*t*
　management of, 369
Atrial natriuretic hormone, 499
Atrioventricular block, 371, 371*t*
Atrophic vaginitis, q30, q36, q65
Atrophy
　multiple system, 471
　urogenital, 416–417
　vaginal, 431, q30, q36, q65
　vulvovaginal, 416, 417*f*
Attention
　inattention, 264–265, 266*t*
　tests of, 265, 267*t*
Attention Screening Examination, 265
Attitudes
　regarding disclosure and consent, 52
　toward advance directives, 53
　toward North American health services, 51
Atypical antipsychotics, 270*t*
Audiologic evaluation, 232*t*
Audiometry screening, 64*t*, 68, 182
AudioScope test, q17
AUDIT-C Questionnaire, 325, 326*t*
Auditory system changes, 176–177
Autism, q4
Autoimmune skin conditions, 334–339
Autonomy, 19
　in dementia, 29–30
　respect for, 23
Avandamet (rosiglitazone and metformin), 510*t*
Avandaryl (rosiglitazone and glimepiride), 510*t*
Avandia (rosiglitazone), 510*t*, 511
Aventyl (nortriptyline), 112*t*
Avoidant personality disorder
　features of, 316, 317*t*
　therapeutic strategies for, 318–319, 319*t*
Axillary lymphadenectomy, 527
Azithromycin, 486, 488*t*
Azotemia, prerenal, 409

Blindness
    causes of, 167, 168t
    definition of, 167
    irreversible, 168t
    reversible, 168t
Blood glucose screening, 62t
Blood pressure. *See also* Hypertension;
    Hypotension
    classification of, 384, 384t
    orthostatic hypotension, q5
    postural, q117
    screening, 62t
    transient decreases in, 188
Blood pressure control, 513
Blood pressure goals, 390, 391
Blood pressure monitoring
    ambulatory, 385
    indirect or cuff, 385
    quality indicators for diabetes mellitus, 513
    quality indicators for hypertension, 390
Blood testing, q33
BMI. *See* Body mass index
Body composition changes, 195
Body dysmorphic disorder, 320
Body language, 50
Body mass index (BMI), 45, 68, 196
    body size classification based on, 196, 196t
    quality indicators for, 70
    risk threshold for, 196
Body size classification, 196, 197t
Body weight, 57–58
Bone
    age-related changes in, 12t, 13
    formation changes, 236
    musculoskeletal complaints, 437
Bone densitometry, 64t
Bone disease
    calcium, phosphorus, and renal bone disease,
        412
    Paget's disease of bone, 498–499
Bone evaluation, 530
Bone infections, 487
Bone loss, 235. *See also* Osteomalacia;
    Osteoporosis
Bone mineral density testing, 238–239
    diagnostic criteria for osteoporosis, 234
    indications for, 238, 238t
    recommendations for, 238
Bone remodeling, 235
Bone-specific alkaline phosphatase, 237, 238t
Bone turnover, 235, 239
Boost Drink, 199t
Boost Glucose Control, 199t
Boost Plus, 199t
Borderline personality disorder
    features of, 316, 317t
    therapeutic strategies for, 318–319, 319t
Bordetella pertussis infection, 355
Botulinum toxin, 214
Bowel control difficulties, 142–143, 143t
BPH. *See* Benign prostatic hyperplasia

BPPV. *See* Benign paroxysmal positional vertigo
Brachytherapy, 426t, 427
Braden Scale, 286
Bradyarrhythmias, 370–371
Bradycardia, 371, 371t
Bradykinesia, 469
Brain imaging studies, 247
Breast cancer, 527
    adjunct hormonal treatment of, 527
    adjuvant therapy for, q19
    CAM for, 86
    characteristics of, 522
    discussion of options, 530
    early, q51
    ethnic and racial differences in incidence,
        523, 523t
    history, 530
    hormonal therapy for, 524–525, 525t
    metastatic, 527, 531
    prevention of recurrence, q38
    quality indicators for, 530–531
    racial differences in diagnosis and survival,
        523, 523t
    screening for, 63–65
    treatment of, q51
Breast conservation treatment, q51
Breast self-examination (BSE), 65
Breath, shortness of, q81
Breathing disorders, sleep-related, 275
Breathlessness, 106
Bright light, 279, 279t, 280
Brimonidine, 175t
British Geriatrics Society (BGS), 229–230, 232
Bronchodilators
    inhaled, 356, 357t
    long-acting, 359
    rapid-acting, 359
Brown-bag evaluation, 78–79
Bruises, q109
BSE (breast self-examination), 65
Bulk laxatives, 399t
Bullous pemphigoid, 337, 337f
Bunions, 457t, 458–459
Buprenorphine, 327
Bupropion, 259, 260t, 300t, 301
Burch operation (colposuspension), 214
Burning mouth syndrome, 351
Bursitis, 437
    olecranon, 439
    subacromial, 439
Buspirone, q46
    for anxiety disorders, 310, 310t
    for depression, 300t, 301
Butorphanol, 118, q49
Byetta (exenatide), 510t
Bypass surgery, 365–366

C

C-reactive protein, 361
Cachexia, 105, 457t
CAD. *See* Coronary artery disease

Caffeine, 231t
CAGE Questionnaire, 325, 326t
Calcaneal spur, 457t
Calcitonin, 241t, 242
Calcitriol, 236
Calcium
    coronary artery content, 361
    deficiency of, 236
    dietary intake, 240
    disorders of metabolism of, 495–499
    drug interactions, 197–198, 198t
    foods that contain, 240, 240t
    homeostasis changes, 495–496, 496t
    RDAs for adults ≥ 71 yr old, 196t
    and renal bone disease, 412
    screening for secondary osteoporosis, 237,
        238t
Calcium channel blockers
    adverse drug events, 76–77, 77t, 197–198
    for chronic CAD, 365
    drug interactions, 77, 78t
    for heart failure, 383
    for hypertension, 388
    and incontinence, 208t, 214
Calcium-containing antacids, 76–77, 77t
Calcium pyrophosphate dihydrate deposition
        disease, 445–446
Calcium supplements
    for osteoporosis prevention and treatment, 237,
        237t, 240, 245
    preventive, 63t, 69
    quality indicators for, 70
California Healthcare Foundation, 507
CAM. *See* Complementary and alternative
        medicine; Confusion Assessment Method
Canalith repositioning procedure, 187, 187f
Cancer, 521
    advanced, q97
    biologic therapy for, 525–526
    biology of, 522–523
    breast cancer, 527, 530–531, q19, q38, q51
    CAM for, 86
    cervical cancer, 65, q36
    characteristics of, 522–523
    chemotherapy for, 524, 525t
    colon cancer, 402–403, 528
    colorectal cancer, 402–403, 404, 531–532
    diagnosis of, 523, 523t
    esophageal cancer, 395
    ethnic differences in incidence, 523, 523t
    hormonal therapy for, 525–526, 525t
    incidence of, 523, 523t
    lip cancer, 349
    lung cancer, 527–528
    mortality of, 523
    oral cancer, 349–350, q115
    pain assessment and, 118
    physical activity recommendations for, 56t
    prevalence of, 3, 4f, 522
    principles of management of, 523–527, 529
    prostate cancer, 423–428, q119
    pseudodisease, 63
    quality-of-life issues, 526–527

Chondrocalcinosis, 445, 446f, q54

Choosing Long-Term Care: A Guide for People with Medicare (CMS Publication No. 02223), 40

Chorea, 472

Choroidal neovascularization, 172, 172f

Chronic athlete's foot, q32

Chronic benzodiazepine use, 278, 283

Chronic constipation, 397, 398t

Chronic coronary artery disease, 363–366
  medical therapy for, 364–365
  presentation and diagnosis of, 363–364

Chronic cough, 354–355

Chronic disease, anemia of, 516–517

Chronic dislocated metatarsal phalangeal joint, 459f, 460

Chronic hospitalization, 127

Chronic hypnotic use, 281–282

Chronic kidney disease, 411–413
  classification of, 411, 411t
  management of, 411–413, q83
  medication use in, 411
  stages of, 411, 411t

Chronic lower respiratory disease, 5, 5t

Chronic lymphocytic leukemia, 528

Chronic myeloproliferative disorders, 520

Chronic obstructive pulmonary disease, 39t, 355–356
  anxiety and, 309
  diagnostic criteria for, 355–356, 355t
  GOLD guidelines for, 355–356, 355t
  inhaled bronchodilators for, 356, 357t
  quality indicators for, 359
  therapy for, 356, 357t

Chronic pain syndromes with developmental disabilities, 332t

Chronic pelvic pain syndrome, q7

Chronic subdural hematoma, 467

Chronic urethral catheters, 217

Chronulac (lactulose), 399t

Cigarette smoking, q42

Cilostazol, 372

CIMT (constraint-induced movement therapy), 136–137

Ciprofloxacin, 400

Circadian rhythm sleep disorders, 276, q50

Circulatory system disorders
  with acute myocardial infarction, 39t
  amputation for, 39t

Circumduction, 219t

Citalopram, 259, 260t, 299t, 301, q48

Citroma (magnesium citrate), 399t

Citrucel (methylcellulose), 399t

Clarithromycin, 486, 488t

Clindamycin, 486, 488t

Clinical breast examination (CBE), 65

Clinical settings
  promoting physical activity in, 58
  rehabilitation services, 131t

Clock-drawing test, 46, 68

Clomipramine, 310t

Clonazepam (Klonopin)
  for persistent pain, 112t, 117
  for REM sleep behavior disorder, 277

Clonidine, 416

Clopidogrel
  for acute coronary syndrome, 363
  for atrial fibrillation, 369
  for peripheral arterial disease, 372
  quality indicators for, 374
  for stroke prevention, 466

Clostridium difficile infection, 402, q40

Clotting factor deficiencies, 520

Clozapine
  and delirium, 270t
  dosing and adverse events of, 313, 314t
  for Parkinson's disease and hallucinations, 315
  for psychosis in dementia, 261–262, 261t

CMS. *See* Centers for Medicare and Medicaid Services

Coagulation, 519–520. *See also* Anticoagulation

Cochlear implants, 182
  characteristics of older candidates for, 182, 182t
  quality indicators for, 183

Cockcroft-Gault equation, 74, 96, 405, q116

Code of Federal Regulations, 146

Codeine, q64

Coenzyme Q$_{10}$, 82–83, 83t, 84, 85

Cognitive assessment, 45–46, q68
  Confusion Assessment Method, 122
  for dementia, 254
  at discharge, 101
  for falls, 232
  Mini-Cog Assessment Instrument for Dementia, 46, 68, 123, 247
  Mini–Mental State Examination (MMSE), 25, 44t, 46, 68, 123, 247, 265, 267t
  quality indicators for, 48, 254
  rapid screening, 43, 44t

Cognitive-behavioral therapy
  for anxiety attacks, q76
  for anxiety disorders, 310t
  for depression, 303, 304t
  for pain, 111–112
  for sleep problems, 278–279, 279t

Cognitive bibliotherapy, 303, 304t

Cognitive enhancers, 253–254

Cognitive impairment
  AGS guidelines for research on cognitively impaired older adults, 27, 27t
  in dementia, 249, 250t
  in hospitalized patients, 121t, 122–123
  interventions for, 121t
  interventions for preventing falls, 231t
  mild, 248, 248t
  pain assessment and treatment in, 111
  pain behaviors in, 111, 111t
  postoperative decline, 100
  screening for, 62t, 68, 71, 254
  sexuality and, 30–31

Cognitive rehabilitation, 251

Cognitive restructuring, 311

Cognitive training, 251

Colace (docusate), 399t

Colchicine, 197–198, 198t, q108

Cold therapy, 441

Colitis, pseudomembranous, 402

Collaboration, 53

Collapsing pes plano valgus foot, 456–458

Colon, 397–403

Colon cancer, 402–403, 528
  CAM for, 86
  ethnic and racial differences in incidence, 523, 523t
  racial differences in diagnosis and survival, 523, 523t

Colon cancer screening, 65
  Medicare coverage and cost-effectiveness of, 64t
  recommendations for, 62t, 65

Colon examination, 531

Colonic angiodysplasia, 401–402

Colonic ischemia, 402

Colonic polyps, 402–403, 403t

Colonic pseudo-obstruction, acute, 402

Colonoscopy, q44
  Medicare coverage and cost-effectiveness of, 64t
  recommendations for, 62t, 65
  virtual, 65

Colorectal cancer, 402–403
  adjuvant therapy for, 532
  discussion of options, 531
  discussion of surgical findings, 531
  history, 404, 531
  nonsurgical treatment plan, 531
  postoperative surveillance, 532
  preoperative examination, 531
  preoperative ostomy siting, 532
  quality indicators for, 531–532
  screening for, 404
  staging evaluation, 531

Colposuspension (Burch operation), 214

Combunox (oxycodone, immediate release), 114t

Communication
  addressing the healthcare provider, 50
  addressing the patient, 50
  with continuity physician, 128
  discussion of death, 103
  discussion of goal blood pressure, 390
  discussion of options, 530, 531
  discussion of surgical findings, 531
  with hearing-impaired people, 178, 179t
  medication discussion, 255
  patient-clinician, 43–44
  preoperative discussion, 100
  quality indicators for dementia, 255
  quality indicators for hospital care, 128
  respectful nonverbal communication, 50
  strategies to enhance, 43, 44t, 178, 179t
  during transition from hospital care, 127
  unspoken challenging medical issues, 51–52

Community-acquired pneumonia, 482, 483
Community-based care, 150–156
  services not requiring change in residence, 154–155
  services requiring change of residence, 155–156
Community-dwelling older Americans
  marital status and living arrangements of, 3, 3*t*
  Medicare beneficiaries with ADL limitations, 5, 7*f*
  Medicare beneficiaries without ADL or IADL disability, 5, 6*f*
  prevention of falls in, 227, 228*f*
  self-reported functional limitations of Medicare beneficiaries, 3, 5*f*
Competence, 24
  cultural, 54, q8
  MacArthur Competency Assessment Tool for Treatment, 26
  testamentary, 24–25
Complementary and alternative medicine (CAM), 81–86
  definition of, 81
  diversity of modalities, 81
  efficacy of, 83–86
  for managing illness in older adults, 83–86
  safety of, 82–83
  usage patterns, 82, 82*t*
Complete blood count (CBC), 237, 238*t*
Complicated grief therapy, 303, 304*t*
Comprehensive eye examination, 167
Comprehensive geriatric assessment (CGA), 48, 67
  in primary care, 157–158
  quality indicators for outpatient care systems, 160
  in rehabilitation, 135–136
Compulsions, 308, 310*t*
Computed tomography, 439, q44
Conduction disturbances, 371, 371*t*
Conductive hearing loss, 177, 183
Confusion Assessment Method (CAM), 122, 264–265, 266*t*
Confusion Assessment Method for the Intensive Care Unit (CAM-ICU), 264–265, 266*t*, 267*t*
Conivaptan, 407
Conjunctivitis
  allergic, 169*t*, 170
  viral, 169*t*, 170
Connective tissue malignancy, 39*t*
Consciousness
  altered level of, 264–265, 266*t*
  sudden loss of, 191, 192*t*
  transient loss of, 189, 190*f*
Consent
  attitudes regarding, 52
  capacity for, 24–27, 100
  informed consent for research, 27
Conservatorships, 26
Constipation, 397
  management of chronic constipation, 397, 398*t*

medications that may relieve, 397, 399*t*
  opioid-induced, 116, 118
  postoperative, 99
  in terminal illness, 104
Constraint-induced movement therapy (CIMT), 136–137
Consultation, outpatient, 157–158, 160
Continuing-care retirement communities (CCRCs), 156
Continuity physicians, 128
Continuous passive-motion (CPM) machines, 138–139
Continuous performance task, 267*t*
Continuous positive airway pressure, 275, 358
Control-relevant intervention, 303, 304*t*
Conversion disorder, 320
Coombs' test, 518
Coordination of care, 160
COPD. *See* Chronic obstructive pulmonary disease
Coping strategies, 20–21
Copper, 197–198, 198*t*
Corneal ulcers, 169*t*
Coronary angiography, q2
Coronary artery calcium content, 361
Coronary artery disease, 362
  chronic, 363–366
  diagnosis of, 363
  epidemiology of, 362
  medical therapy for, 364–365
Corticosteroids
  for COPD, 356, 357*t*
  for CPPD, 446
  for idiopathic pulmonary fibrosis, 358
  inhaled, 359
  ophthalmic, 170
  osteoporosis prophylaxis with, 244
  perioperative, 99
  for persistent pain, 117
  for polyarticular gout, q108
  stress doses, 99
Costs
  of assistive listening devices, 181*t*
  of health care, 32–42
  of hearing aids, 181–182, 181*t*
  of preventive measures, 61, 64*t*
Cough
  chronic, 354–355
  in terminal illness, 107
Councils on Aging, 254
Counseling
  on cancer screening and preventive health, 69–70
  dementia caregiver counseling, 303, 304*t*
  estrogen and progesterone, 375
  healthy lifestyle counseling, 61, 62*t*, 67
  for increasing physical activity, 59
  smoking cessation counseling, 62*t*, 64*t*, 67
COX-2 inhibitors
  for musculoskeletal pain, 442
  for persistent pain, 115, 117

CPAP (continuous positive airway pressure), 275, 358
CPM machines. *See* Continuous passive-motion machines
CPM (continuous passive-motion) machines, 138–139
CPPD (calcium pyrophosphate dihydrate deposition disease), 445–446
Creatinine, serum, 405, 406*f*, q31
Creatinine clearance, 74, 405, 406*f*
Critical illness, 125–126
Cross-cultural health care, 49, 54
Cross-over toe deformity, 459*f*, 460
Cross-training, 60
CRT (cardiac resynchronization therapy), 380–381
Crutches, 140
Cruzan v. Director, Department of Health of Missouri, 27–28
Crystalline arthritis, q54
CSA (central sleep apnea), 275
Cultural aspects of care, 49–54, 103
  alcohol use, 324
  quality indicators for, 54
Cultural differences, 24
Cultural identity, 49
Culturally competent care, 54, q8
Culture, 52
Cushing's disease, 237, 238*t*
Custodial care, 34*t*
Cutaneous horn, 343
Cymbalta (duloxetine), 113*t*
Cyproheptadine, 200
Cystic erosion, 457*t*
Cystocele, q56
Cysts, epidermal inclusion, 461
Cytochrome P450, 77–78

D

25(OH)D, q13
Dabigatran, 370
Daily rounds, 124
Dance, 251
Darifenacin, 213*t*, 214
Darvocet (propoxyphene), 117
Darvon (propoxyphene), 117
Day care, 154
Day hospitals, 154
Daytime sleepiness, q11, q50
DDIs (drug-drug interactions), 77–78, 78*t*, 305
Death
  interventions that can hasten, 28
  leading causes and numbers of, 5, 5*t*
  overall care near, 102–103
Debridement, 288, 291*t*
  sharp, q99
Decision making
  about institutionalization, 154
  approaches to, 52
  cultural aspects, 49–54, 103

Decision making *(continued)*
  end-of-life, 27–29, 52
  in extended-care settings, 29
  family decisions, 103
  hierarchy of strategies, 25, 25*t*, 26
  life-sustaining treatment decisions, 31
  for patients who lack decisional capacity, 26–27
  role of incapacitated patient in, 26
  treatment decisions, 29, 31
Decisional capacity, 24–27
  assessment of, 24–25
  decision making for patients who lack, 26–27
  elements of, 25, 25*t*
  standardized tests of, 25
  temporary loss of, 26–27
Decubitus ulcers, 285
Deep brain stimulation, 470
Deep venous thrombosis, 373, q19, q81
  guidelines for prophylaxis, 98, 98*t*
Defecography, 397
Degenerative joint disease, 332*t*
Degenerative nervous system disorders, 39*t*
Dehydroepiandrosterone (DHEA), 84, q94
  safety issues, 82–83, 83*t*
  supplements, 500
Delirium, 264–272, q1, q107
  agitated, 270–271, 271*t*
  and dementia, 267
  diagnosis of, 264–265, 265*t*
  differential diagnosis of, 264–265
  drug-induced, q64
  drugs to reduce or eliminate in management of, 268, 270*t*
  evaluation of, 128, 268, 272
  features of, q66
  incidence of, 264
  and incontinence, 209*t*
  management of, 268–271, 269*t*
  pharmacologic therapy for, 270–271, 271*t*
  postoperative, 100, 101, 267–268, q16
  preoperative assessment and management of, 97, 101
  prognosis for, 264
  psychotic symptoms in, 314
  quality indicators for, 272
  quality indicators for hospital care, 128
  quiet, 265
  related quality indicators for, 272
  reversible causes of, 267, 267*t*
  risk factors for, 265–267
  spectrum of, 265
  in terminal illness, 105
Delusional disorder, q59, q66
Delusions, 311
  antipsychotic medications for, 261–262, 261*t*
  in dementia, 257, 261–262, 261*t*
  evaluation of patient with, 311–312, 312*f*
  mood-congruent, 314
Dementia, 245–255
  aggression or agitation with, 263, q48, q114
  alcohol-related, 325
  of Alzheimer's disease, 85, 253

assessment methods for, 247
behavioral interventions for, 258, 259*t*
behavioral problems in, 256–263
behavioral symptoms of, 255, 263
CAM for, 85
definition of, 248
delirium and, 267
delusions in, 261–262, 261*t*
depression in, 259, 260*t*
diagnosis of, q21
diagnostic features of, 248, 248*t*
differential diagnosis of, 248–249
in Down syndrome, q68
epidemiology of, 246
ethical issues in, 29–31
frontotemporal, 246, 248*t*, 249
general progression of, 249, 250*t*
hallucinations in, 261–262, 261*t*
hip fracture with, q120
HIV-associated, q75
and incontinence, 209*t*
Lewy body, 246, 248*t*, 249, 315, q87
management of, 249–254
manic-like behavioral syndromes in, 259–261
with mental retardation, 331
Mini-Cog Assessment Instrument for Dementia, 46, 68, 123, 247
mixed, 246
mood disturbances in, 259
pharmacologic treatment of, 252–254
prevention of, 246–247
psychologic symptoms of, 255, 263
psychosis in, 261–262, 261*t*
psychotic symptoms in, 314–315
pugilistic, 331
quality indicators for, 254–255, 263
resources for, 254
reversible, 264
risk factors for, 246–247
safety concerns, 252
screening for, 62*t*, 68
with self-neglect, q66
sleep disturbances in, 262–263, 277
societal impact of, 246
supportive therapy for, 251
treatment of, 248*t*, 249–254
and urinary incontinence, 208
vascular, 246, 248–249, 248*t*
Dementia caregiver counseling, 303, 304*t*
Demography
  of aging, 1–7
  of nursing-home population, 142–143, 143*t*
Denosumab, 241*t*, 243
Dental anatomy, 346, 346*f*
Dental caries, 346–347
Dental cavities, q113
Dental decay, 346–347
Dental/oral conditions with developmental disabilities, 332*t*
Dental pulp changes, 346, 346*t*
Dental treatment, 352–353
Denture stomatitis, 350–351, 350*f*
Dentures, 348

Dependence
  benzodiazepine, 326–327
  definition of, 322
  opioid, 327
  physical, 115–116
  psychologic, 116
  tobacco, 327–328
Dependent personality disorder
  features of, 316, 317*t*
  therapeutic strategies for, 318–319, 319*t*
Depression, 295–306
  activity recommendations for, 56*t*
  bipolar, 301–303
  CAM for, 84–85
  in chronic kidney disease, 412
  clinical presentation of, 295–298
  in dementia, 256, 259
  with developmental disabilities, 332*t*
  diagnosis of, 295–298
  documenting symptoms, 305
  electroconvulsive therapy for, 301, 303
  epidemiology of, 295
  evaluation for, 478
  evaluation for comorbid conditions, 305
  follow-up, 305–306
  Geriatric Depression Scale, 297, 297*t*
  in hospitalized patients, 121*t*, 122
  indications to start antidepressant therapy based on PHQ-9, 296, 296*t*
  interventions for, 121*t*, 122
  interventions for preventing falls, 231*t*
  late-life, geriatric syndrome of, 295–296
  with macular degeneration, q112
  maintenance therapy for, 306
  major depressive disorder, q74, q92, q112
  major depressive disorder with personality disorder, q63
  major depressive disorder with psychosis, q21
  major depressive disorder without mania but with hypomania, 297
  mania with or without, 297
  with marked anxiety, 309
  minor, 295, 298
  pharmacotherapy for, 259, 260*t*, 298–301
  psychosocial interventions for, 303
  psychotherapy for, 303, 304*t*
  psychotic, 305
  quality indicators for, 305–306
  rapid screening followed by assessment and management of, 43, 44*t*
  recognizing, 305
  recommended preventive measures for, 62*t*
  and rehabilitation, 134
  related quality indicators for, 306
  remission of, 297
  with self-neglect, q66
  subclinical, 298
  subsyndromal, 295, 298
  suicide risk assessment, q55
  in terminal illness, 105–106
  treatment of, 298–303, 305–306
Depression care management, 303, 304*t*

Depression screening, 62t, 68, 296–297, 305
  quality indicators for cardiovascular diseases and disorders, 374
  quality indicators for dementia, 255
Depressive personality disorder
  features of, 316, 317t
  therapeutic strategies for, 318–319, 319t
Dermatitis
  dyshidrotic eczematous, q110
  neurodermatitis, 336
  seborrheic, 334–335, q96
  stasis dermatitis, 339
Dermatofibromas, 461
Dermatologic diseases and disorders, 334–345
  skin and nail disorders of foot, 461–462
  skin cancer, 343–345
Dermatomyositis, 448
Dermatophyte infection, q32
Desipramine (Norpramin)
  for depression, 299t
  for depressive features of behavioral disturbances in dementia, 259, 260t
  for persistent pain, 112t
Desvenlafaxine, 260t, 299t
DETERMINE checklist, 198
Detoxification, 325–326, 327
Detrusor hyperactivity with impaired bladder contractility, q56
Detrusor overactivity, 209
Detrusor underactivity, 209–210
Developmental disabilities, 329–333
  and dementia, q68
  and health problems, 332t
Device therapy, 380–381
DEXA (dual x-ray absorptiometry) scan, q13, q47
DHEA. *See* Dehydroepiandrosterone
Diabeta (glyburide), 509t
Diabetes mellitus, 39t, 504–514
  activity recommendations for, 56t
  atherosclerotic complications of, 507–508
  CAM for, 85–86
  and cardiovascular risk, 360
  classification of, 504
  clinical evaluation of, 505–506
  deaths due to, 5, 5t
  diagnosis of, 505
  education and self-management support, 511–512
  evaluation of, 505
  and foot, 462–464
  guidelines for care of older adults with, 507
  hyperglycemia in, 508–511
  and incontinence, 209t
  lactose-free oral products for, 199t
  management of, 505–511
  microvascular complications of, 508
  non-insulin agents for, 508–511, 509t–510t
  pathophysiology of, 504–505
  postoperative management of, 99, 101
  prediabetes, 504–505
  preoperative evaluation, 101
  prevalence of, 3, 4f
  prevention of, q71
  quality indicators for, 512–513
  screening for, 64t, 66
  self-management support for, 511–512
  type 1, 504
  type 2, 504, 505, q71
Diabetic foot examination, 464
Diabetic neuropathy, q49
Diabetic retinopathy, 168t, 172–174, 174f
Diagnostic and Statistical Manual of Mental Disorders, 4th edition, Text Revision (DSM IV-TR), 307
  criteria for bipolar disorder type 1, 297
  diagnostic criteria for delirium, 264–265, 266t
Diagnostic imaging, 34t
Diagnostic laboratory tests
  in falls, 229
  health insurance coverage for, 34t
  in heart failure, 382
Diagnostic-related groups (DRGs), 150
Dialectical behavior therapy, 303, 304t
Dialysis, renal, 413–414, 414t
Diarrhea, q40
  infectious, 489–490
  postoperative, 99
  in terminal illness, 105
Diazepam, 270t
DIC (disseminated intravascular coagulation), 519
Diclofenac sodium, 113t
Dicyclomine, 214
Diet
  to avoid breast cancer recurrence, q38
  and cancer, 86
  for chronic kidney disease, 412–413
  for diabetes type 2, q104
  Mediterranean diet, q90
  Modified Diet in Renal Disease (MDRD) formula, 74, 96, 404
  for pressure ulcers, 289
  vegetarian diet, q38
2005 Dietary Guidelines for Americans, 57
Dietary products, 82
Dietary Supplement Health and Education Act (DSHEA), 83
Dietary supplements, 200
  quality indicators for, 202
  safety of, 82–83, 83t
Dieticians, 133–134, 133t
Diffuse large B-cell lymphoma, 528–529
Digestive problems. *See* Gastrointestinal diseases and disorders
Digestive system changes, 12t, 14–15
Digit flexus, 457t
Digit quinti varus, 457t
Digit span test, 267t
Digital rectal examination, 424
  Medicare coverage and cost-effectiveness of, 64t
  recommendations for, 65
Digitalis, 77, 78t
Digoxin
  adverse drug events, 76–77, 77t, 197–198
  for heart failure, 379, 380
  nutrient interactions, 197–198, 198t
  toxicity of, 383
Dilaudid (hydromorphone), 114t
Diltiazem, 76–77, 77t
Dilutional hyponatremia, 406–407
Diogenes syndrome, 308
Diphenhydramine
  adverse drug events, 76–77, 77t
  and delirium, 270t
Dipivefrin, 175t
Diplopia, 169t
Disability
  developmental disabilities, 329–333, 332t, q68
  excess, 324
  International Classification of Functioning, Disability, and Health (ICF) (WHO), 130–131
  trends in, 4–5
Disability accommodation, 5–6
Disalcid (salsalate), 113t
Discharge assessment, 128
Discharge planning, 127
  cognition and function at discharge, 101
  primary diagnoses for "early" discharges regarded as "transfers" 38–39, 39t
Discharge summary, 128
Disclosure, 52
Discontinuing interventions, 27–28
Disease management, 159
Disease-modifying anti-inflammatory drugs (DMARDs), 444
Disequilibrium, 184, 185t
Dislocation
  of lesser metatarsal phalangeal joint, 457t
  of metatarsal phalangeal joint, 459f, 460
Disorganized thinking, 264–265, 266t
Disposable soma theory of aging, 9
Disseminated intravascular coagulation, 519
Disulfiram, 327
Diuretics
  adverse drug events, 76–77, 77t
  drug interactions, 77, 78t
  for heart failure, 379, 380
  for hypertension, 387
  loop, 208t, 379, 383
  nutrient interactions, 197–198, 198t
  thiazide, 387, q43
Divalproex sodium
  for behavioral disturbances in dementia with manic-like features, 259–261, 260t
  for personality disorders, 319–320
  to stabilize mood in mania and bipolar disorder, 301, 302t
Diversity, cultural, q8
Diverticular disease, 398–400
Diverticulitis, q44

Glucocorticoids
  adverse drug events, 76–77, 77t
  and bone loss, 237
  for dermatomyositis, 448
  for giant cell arteritis, 447
  for knee pain, 443
  for musculoskeletal pain, 442
  for polymyositis, 448
Glucophage (metformin), 509t
Glucophage XR (metformin), 509t
Glucosamine, 82–83, 83t
Glucose, fasting, q71
Glucose challenges, q118
Glucose intolerance, 505
Glucose screening, 62t
α-Glucosidase inhibitors, 509t, 511
Glucotrol (glipizide), 509t
Glucotrol XL (glipizide), 509t
Glucovance (glyburide and metformin), 510t
Glyburide (Diabeta, Micronase)
  for diabetes mellitus, 509t
  micronized (Glynase), 509t
Glyburide and metformin (Glucovance), 510t
Glycated hemoglobin, 512
Glycemic control, 512
Glycoprotein IIb/IIIa inhibitors, 363
Glycopyrrolate, 107
Glynase (micronized glyburide), 509t
Glyset (miglitol), 509t
Goiter, q102
Gout, 445
  polyarticular, q108
GRACE (Geriatric Resources for Assessment and Care of Elders), 158–159
Grand mal seizures, 473
Granulocyte colony-stimulating factor, 525t
Granulocyte-macrophage colony-stimulating factor, 525t
Green Prescription, 58
Green tea, q38
Grief, 19
GRN (Geriatric Resource Nurse) Model, 125
Group exercise, 221–222
Group homes, 156
Growth factors, 283–284, 291
Growth hormone, 200, 503, q94
Growth hormone deficiency, 503
Growth retardation, 332t
Guardian, 26
Guided Care, 159
Gustatory dysfunction
  medications that cause, 352, 352t
  nonpharmacologic causes of, 351–352, 352t
Gynecologic diseases and disorders, 415–420, 468–474

H

H₂-receptor antagonists
  adverse drug events, 197–198
  and delirium, 268, 270t

HAART (highly active antiretroviral therapy), 488
Haemophilus influenzae, 483
Haglund's deformity, 457t
Half-life, 73
Hallucinations, 311
  antipsychotic medications for, 261–262, 261t
  in dementia, 261–262, 261t
  in dementia associated with Lewy bodies, 315
  evaluation of patient with, 311–312, 312f
  isolated, 315
  visual, q87
Hallux abducto valgus, 457t, 459f
Hallux limitus, 457t, 459
Hallux rigidus, 457t
Hallux valgus, 457t, 458–459
Haloperidol, q16
  for agitated delirium, 271, 271t
  dosing and adverse events of, 313, 314t
Hammertoe, 457t, 459–460
Hand osteoarthritis, 442–443, 444f
Harpagophytum procumbens (devil's claw), 84
Harris-Benedict equations, 195, 196t
Harris Hip Questionnaire, 132t, 136
Hartford Institute for Geriatric Nursing
  Nurses Improving Care for Health System Elders (NICHE), 124–125
  Try This, 43
Head and neck cancer, 523, 523t
Head-impulse test, q88
Head-thrust test, 186, q88
Headaches, 39t, 467–468
Healers, 53
Healing
  cascade of, 283–284
  monitoring, 291
  Pressure Ulcer Scale for Healing, 291
Health beliefs, 51
Health care
  attitudes toward North American health services, 51
  costs of, 32–42
  coverage of, 32–42
  federal financing of, 41–42
  financing of, 32–42
  flow of funds for, 32, 33f
  GRACE model, 158
  trends in, 3–4
Health-enhancing physical activity, 54–55
Health insurance coverage
  for older Americans, 32–42, 34t
  for preventive services, 33, 34t
  for rehabilitation, 131–132
Health literacy, 2–3, q79
Health maintenance organizations (HMOs), 35, q67
Healthcare agent or proxy, 26
Healthcare Employers' Data Information System (HEDIS), 41–42
Healthcare providers
  addressing, 50

Medicare Advantage plan payments, 37–38, 38t
Healthy behaviors, 22
Healthy lifestyle counseling, 61, 62t, 67
Hearing
  age-related changes in, 176–177
  health insurance coverage for services, 34t
  normal, 176–177
Hearing aids, 179–182
  caring for, 182
  costs and styles of, 180–182, 181t
Hearing examination
  Medicare coverage and cost-effectiveness of, 64t
  quality indicators for, 70
Hearing Handicap Inventory for the Elderly–Screening Version (HHIE-S), 178, q17
Hearing impairment, 176–183
  assessment of, 45
  conductive hearing loss, 177, 183
  diagnosis of, 178
  effects of, 179–180, 180t
  epidemiology of, 177
  interventions for preventing falls with, 232t
  presbycusis, q27
  quality indicators for, 182–183
  rapid screening followed by assessment and management of, 43, 44t
  recommended preventive measures for, 62t, 68
  rehabilitation of, 179–180, 180t, 183
  screening for, 62t, 68, 182, q17
  sensorineural hearing loss, 177
  strategies to improve communication, 178, 179t
  treatment of, 178–182
Heart, 12t, 13
Heart disease
  deaths due to, 5, 5t
  ischemic, 391
  prevalence of, 3, 4f
  valvular, 366
Heart failure, 39t, 376–383
  Cheynes-Stokes breathing pattern of, 275
  clinical features of, 376–377
  device therapy for, 380–381
  diagnosis of, 377, 382
  diastolic, 380, q78
  education about, 383
  end-of-life care for, 381
  end-stage, q77
  epidemiology of, 376
  etiology of, 376
  examination of, 382
  history, 382
  and incontinence, 209t
  management of, 377–381
  outpatient visits, 383
  pathophysiology of, 376
  prognosis, 381
  quality indicators for, 382–383
  recurrent hospitalization for, 381
  systolic, 378–380

Heart rate abnormalities, 230

Heat therapy, 441

Heavy drinking, 324

HEDIS (Healthcare Employers' Data Information System), 41–42

Heel pain, q53

Heel spur, 457t

Heel ultrasonography, q47

Height measurement, 62t, 70

Helicobacter pylori infection, 395, 396

HELP. *See* Hospital Elder Life Program; Hospitalized Elderly Longitudinal Project

HELP (Hospital Elder Life Program), 125

Hemangioma, 461

Hematologic diseases and disorders, 513–521
malignancies, 528–529
quality indicators for, 521

Hematoma, subdural, 467

Hematopoiesis, 513–514

Hematopoietic stem cells, 513–514

Hematuria, 429

Hemodialysis, 413–414, 414t

Hemoglobin
glycated, 512
replacement, 412

Hemolytic anemia, 515, 515t, 518–519

Hemorrhage
intracerebral, 467
subconjunctival, 169t, 170, 171

Hepatitis B vaccinations, 64t

HER-2/neu receptor status, 530

Herbal/dietary products, 82

Herpes simplex, 351, 351f

Herpes simplex keratitis, 169t

Herpes zoster ("shingles"), 340–341, 340f, 489

Herpes zoster ophthalmicus
signs and symptoms of, 169t
treatment of, 169t, 171

Herpes zoster vaccine (Zostavax), 62t, 69, q86

HF. *See* Heart failure

HHIE-S (Hearing Handicap Inventory for the Elderly–Screening Version), 178, q17

HHRGs (home-health–related groups), 151

HHS (U.S. Department of Health and Human Services), 56–57

High T$_4$ syndrome, 494

Highly active antiretroviral therapy (HAART), 488

Hip disease, q22

Hip fracture, 39t, 137–138
epidemiology of, 137
prevention of recurrence, 138
rehabilitation after, 137–138, q120
surgical care of, 101, 137

Hip joint, 132t, 136

Hip osteoarthritis, q58

Hip pain, 440, q58

Hip protectors, 230–232

Hip replacement, q31, q52

Hip surgery
anticoagulation for, 101
for hip fracture, 137
procedures, 39t
total hip and knee arthroplasty, 138–139

Hispanic Americans
alcohol use, 324
cancer incidence, 523, 523t
community-dwelling Medicare beneficiaries with ADL limitations, 5, 7f
community-dwelling Medicare beneficiaries without ADL or IADL disability, 5, 6f
diabetes mellitus, 504
leading causes of death, 5, 5t
nursing-home population, 142
older population, 1
perceived health, 3, 3t
poverty rates, 2
urinary incontinence, 207

History of immigration or migration, 51

History of traumatic experiences, 50

Histrionic personality disorder, q84
features of, 316, 317t
therapeutic strategies for, 318–319, 319t

HIV (human immunodeficiency virus) antibody, q75

HIV (human immunodeficiency virus) infection, 145, 487–488, q75

Hmong, 19

HMOs (health maintenance organizations), 35, q67

Hodgkin's disease, 522–523, 529

Hoffmann's signs, q72

Holter monitoring, q33

Home care, 127, 150–154
codes, reimbursement, and requirements for certification, 151, 151t
ethical issues in, 154
falls risk in, 226t, 227
fee for service, 40
financing, 40–41
health insurance coverage for, 34t
indications for, q15
liability and legal issues, 153
limitations of, 153
managed care, 40
occupational therapy, q24
patient assessment, 152
preventing falls, 230, 232t
primary provider's role in, 151–152
prospective payment system for, 150–151
rehabilitation services, 131, 131t, 132
sedation, q69

Home-delivered meals, 200

Home-health–related groups (HHRGs), 151

Home hospital, 126, 155

Home safety evaluation, 232, 232t

Homeostasis, 283–284

Homeostatic challenges, q118

Homocysteine, 519

Hormonal regulation
influences in men, 236

of water and electrolyte balance, 499

Hormone therapy
for breast cancer, 527, 530
for cancer, 524–525, 525t
for erectile dysfunction, 436
estrogen therapy, 501–503
for female sexual dysfunction, 431, 432, 500
for incontinence, 208t, 213t, 214
for menopausal symptoms, 416
for neurologic diseases and disorders, 478
for osteoporosis, 241t, 242–243
preventive, 63t, 69
quality indicators for, 70, 478, 530
testosterone replacement therapy, 500–501
testosterone supplementation, 501, 502t
for vulvovaginal atrophy, 416–417

Horner's syndrome, 466

Hospice, 103–104, q69
cultural aspects, 19, 103
for end-stage kidney disease, 414
financing, 41
health insurance coverage for, 34t
requirements for access to, 103
services, 103, 104t

Hospital-acquired pneumonia, 483

Hospital care, 119–129
alternatives to, 126
chronic, 127
day hospitals, 154
falls risk in, 226t, 227
geriatric evaluation and management (GEM) units, 125, 158
health insurance coverage for, 34t
home hospital, 155
inpatient fall evaluation, 128, 233
oral intake evaluation, 201
posthospitalization appointments, 129
posthospitalization follow-up, 128
posthospitalization medications, 128
posthospitalization tests, 129
primary diagnoses for "early" discharges regarded as "transfers" 38–39, 39t
quality indicators for, 128–129
recurrent, 381
rehabilitation hospitals, 131t
systematic assessment on admission, 120, 121t
systems of care, 124–125
transitions from, 126–127

Hospital Elder Life Program (HELP), 125

Hospitalized Elderly Longitudinal Project (HELP), 102–103

Hospitalized patients
assessment of, 120–124
care preference documentation of vulnerable older adults, 31
hazards and opportunities commonly overlooked in, 120, 121t
management of, 120–124
sleep disturbances in, 277–278
systems of care for, 124–125

Hot flushes, 416

House calls, 151–152
    billing codes and reimbursement for, 151, 151*t*
    choosing patients for, 152
    equipment for, 152, 153*t*
    financial considerations, 152–153
    office-based programs, 152–153
    supplies for, 152, 153*t*
Housing and Urban Development programs, 156
Humalog (insulin lispro), 511*t*
Human growth hormone, 200
Human immunodeficiency virus (HIV) antibody, q75
Human immunodeficiency virus (HIV) infection, 145, 487–488, q75
Humulin (insulin), 511*t*
Hurley Discomfort Scale, 111
Hydralazine, 379–380
Hydrocephalus, normal-pressure (NPH)
    and incontinence, 209*t*
    surgery for, 222
Hydrochlorothiazide, 387, q5, q100, q113
Hydrocodone (Lorcet, Lortab, Vicodin, Vicoprofen), 113*t*
Hydrocolloid dressings, q99
Hydrocortisone, 99
Hydrogel dressings, q99
Hydromorphone (Dilaudid, Hydrostat), 114*t*
Hydrophilic drugs, 73
Hydrostat (hydromorphone), 114*t*
Hydroxychloroquine, 447–448
Hyoscyamine, 107, 214
Hyperactivity, 257
Hyperadrenocorticoidism, 499
Hypercalcemia, 497–498, q13
    differential diagnosis of, 497, 498*t*
    and incontinence, 209*t*
Hyperglycemia, q104
    management of, 508–511
    perioperative, 99
Hypericum perforatum (St. John's wort), 84
    for depression, 300*t*
    safety issues, 82–83, 83*t*
Hyperkalemia, 408
Hyperlipidemia
    quality indicators for neurologic diseases and disorders, 477
    screening for, 66–67
Hypernatremia, 407
Hyperparathyroidism, 497–498
    screening for secondary osteoporosis in, 237, 238*t*
    secondary, 236
Hypersexuality, 263
Hypertension, 384–391
    and cardiovascular risk, 360
    classification of, 384, 384*t*
    clinical evaluation of, 385
    diagnosis of, 390
    emergencies and urgencies, 389, 391
    epidemiology and physiology of, 384–385

evaluation of, 390
    follow-up visits, 388–389, 388*t*
    in long-term care setting, 389–390
    management of, 388, 388*t*, q43, q106
    nonpharmacologic therapy for, 386, 386*t*, 390
    persistent, 390
    pharmacologic treatment of, 386–388
    prehypertension, 384, 384*t*
    prevalence of, 3, 4*f*
    quality indicators for, 390–391
    recommended preventive measures for, 62*t*
    recommended treatment of, 386–387, 387*t*
    refractory, 390–391
    screening for, 66
    special considerations for, 389–390
    stage 1, 384*t*, 386–387, 386*t*, 387*t*
    stage 2, 384*t*
    and stroke, q42
    systolic, q106
    treatment of, 385–389, 387*t*
    white-coat, 385
Hyperthyroidism, 494–495
    screening for secondary osteoporosis in, 237, 238*t*
    subclinical, 494–495
Hypertonic saline, 407
Hypnotics
    chronic use of, 281–282
    and delirium, 270*t*
    and incontinence, 208*t*
    interventions for preventing falls with, 231*t*
    for sleep problems, 278
Hypoadrenocorticoidism, 499–500
Hypoaldosteronism, hyporeninemic, 499
Hypochondriasis, 320
Hypogonadism, 236
    male, 501
    screening for secondary osteoporosis in, 237, 238*t*
    testosterone preparations available for, 501, 502*t*
Hypokalemia, 408
Hypomania, 297–298
Hyponatremia, 405–406, q100
    dilutional, 406–407
    hypotonic, 406, 407
    treatment of, 407
Hypoproliferative anemia, 515–518, 515*t*
    due to iron deficiency, 515, 516*f*
    due to vitamin B_{12} or folate deficiency, 515, 517*f*
Hyporeninemic hypoaldosteronism, age-related, 499
Hypotension
    orthostatic, 194, 391, q5
    postprandial, 194
    postural, 229–230, q117
Hypothyroidism, 492–494, q102
    secondary, 492–494
    subclinical, 492
Hypotonic hyponatremia, 406, 407
Hypoxemia, 359

I

IADLs. *See* Instrumental activities of daily living
Ibandronate, 240, 241*t*, q93
IBS (irritable bowel syndrome), 397, 400–401
Ibuprofen
    for musculoskeletal pain, 442
    for persistent pain, 113*t*, 115, q58
ICD-9 (International Classification of Diseases), 151
ICDs. *See* Implantable cardiac defibrillators
Identity, cultural, 49
Idiopathic myelofibrosis, 520
Idiopathic pulmonary fibrosis, 358, q28
Iliotibial band syndrome, 440
Imaging
    abdominal ultrasonography, 62*t*
    brain imaging studies, 247
    of gait impairment, 220–221
IMF (idiopathic myelofibrosis), 520
Imipramine, 214, 270*t*
Immigration status, 50–51
Immobility
    in hospitalized patients, 121–122, 121*t*
    interventions for, 121*t*, 122
Immune function changes, 479, 480*t*
Immune senescence, 479
Immune system changes, 12*t*, 15
Immune theory of aging, 11
Immune thrombocytopenia, 520
Immunizations, 61, 62*t*, 69
    for hospitalized patients, 121*t*, 124
    interventions for, 121*t*
    Medicare coverage and cost-effectiveness of, 64*t*
    quality indicators for, 70
    recommendations for, 69
IMPACT (Improving Mood—Promoting Access to Collaborative Treatment), 159
Implantable cardiac defibrillators (ICDs)
    for heart failure, 380–381
    for ventricular tachyarrhythmias, 194
Implantable loop recorders, 192–193
Implants, cochlear, 182
    characteristics of older candidates for, 182, 182*t*
    quality indicators for, 183
Improving Mood—Promoting Access to Collaborative Treatment (IMPACT), 159
Inattention, 264–265, 266*t*
Incompetence, 24
Incontinence
    with developmental disabilities, 332*t*
    and rehabilitation, 134
    urinary, 67–68, 207–217, q23, q56
Incontinence history, 216
Individualized feeding assistance, q62
Indwelling bladder catheter, 128
Ineffective anemia, 515, 515*t*
Ineffective erythropoiesis, 518

M

M2 inhibitors, 484

MA. *See* Medicare Advantage

MacArthur Competency Assessment Tool for
  Treatment, 25

Macronutrient guidelines, 195

Macronutrient needs, 195

Macular degeneration, q112
  age-related, 168*t*, 171–172, 175

Magnesium
  drug interactions, 197–198, 198*t*
  RDAs for adults ≥ 71 yr old, 196*t*

Magnesium citrate (Citroma), 399*t*

Magnesium-containing antacids, 76–77, 77*t*

Magnesium hydroxide (Milk of Magnesia), 399*t*

Magnetic resonance imaging, 438–439
  cardiac, q2
  of cervical spine, q72

Major depressive disorder, q25
  characteristics of, q74
  with loss of vision, q112
  with psychotic features, q21
  treatment of, q63, q92
  without mania but with hypomania, 297

Maladaptive behaviors, 331

Malassezia furfur, 335

Male hypogonadism, 501

Male sexuality, 432–436

Malignancy
  connective tissue, 39*t*
  deaths due to, 5, 5*t*
  hematologic malignancies, 528–529
  musculoskeletal, 39*t*
  skin neoplasms, 461

Malignant melanoma, 461*f*, 462

Malnutrition, 195–202
  comorbid conditions, 201–202
  legal and ethical issues, 201
  quality indicators for, 201–202

Mammography, 63–65
  Medicare coverage and cost-effectiveness of,
    64*t*
  quality indicators for, 530
  recommendations for, 62*t*, 63

Managed care
  home-health care, 40
  inpatient care, 38
  nursing-home care, 41
  outpatient care, 36–38
  postacute rehabilitation, 40

Mandibular torus, 350, 350*f*

Mania
  DSM IV-TR criteria for, 297
  hypomania, 297–298
  late-onset, 297–298
  medications to stabilize mood in mania and
    bipolar depression, 301, 302*t*
  pharmacotherapy for, 301, 302*t*

Manic-like behavioral syndromes
  in dementia, 257, 259–261
  mood stabilizers for, 259–261, 260*t*
  treatment of, 259–260

Marche a petits pas, 220

Marital status
  of community-dwelling older Americans, 3, 3*t*
  of nursing-home population, 142–143, 143*t*

Massage
  for lower back pain, 84, 84*t*
  for musculoskeletal pain, 441

Master athletes, 60

McGill Pain Questionnaire, 110

MDRD (Modified Diet in Renal Disease)
  formula, 74, 96, 405

MDS. *See* Minimum Data Set; Myelodysplastic
  syndromes

Mechanical loading, 287

Mechanical ventilation
  preference for, 31
  withdrawal of, 108, 126

Mediators, 20–21

Medicaid, 2, 34*t*, 36
  advantages and disadvantages of, 36, 37*t*
  assisted-living benefits, 156
  continuing-care retirement community benefits,
    156
  future of, 42–43
  hearing aid benefits, 181–182
  hospice benefits, 103
  Program of All-inclusive Care of the Elderly
    (PACE), q67
  requirements for long-term care facilities, 147,
    148*t*

Medical decisions, 25, 25*t*

Medical directors, 147, 148*t*

Medical ethics, 23–24

Medical-legal interface, 91

Medical records, 160

Medical savings accounts (MSAs), 35

Medicare, 2, 32–36
  assisted-living benefits, 156
  billing codes and reimbursement for home
    visits, 151, 151*t*
  biofeedback benefits, 212
  cochlear implant coverage, 182
  community-dwelling beneficiaries with ADL
    limitations, 5, 7*f*
  community-dwelling beneficiaries without ADL
    or IADL disability, 5, 6*f*
  continuing-care retirement community benefits,
    156
  coverage of preventive health services, 70
  definition of weight loss, 196
  evaluation and management (E&M) codes, 36,
    37*t*
  fee-for-service (FFS), 33, 34*t*, 36, 37*t*
  future of, 42–43
  guidelines for erythropoietin therapy, 412
  hearing aid benefits, 181–182
  home-care benefits, 151, 152
  home-health benefits, 131, 132, q15
  hospice benefits, 103
  house-call benefits, 151, 152
  nursing-home care benefits, 144–145
  out-of-pocket expenses, 33–34, q57

outpatient benefits, q57
  Part A, 32, 33–34, 34*t*, 131–132, 131*t*, q15,
    q73
  Part B, 32, 33–34, 34*t*, 42, 131*t*, q57, q73
  Part C (*See* Medicare Advantage)
  Part D, 34*t*, 35, 42, 64*t*, q73
  postacute care benefits, 132
  preventive health service benefits, 61, 64*t*
  private contracts, 33
  Program of All-inclusive Care of the Elderly
    (PACE), q67
  prospective payment system (PPS), 144–145,
    150–151
  prospective reimbursement, 132, 132*t*
  rehabilitation benefits, 131–132, 131*t*
  requirements for long-term care facilities, 147,
    148*t*
  requirements for rehabilitation sites, 131*t*
  self-reported functional limitations of
    beneficiaries, 3, 5*f*
  skilled-nursing-facility benefits, 131*t*, 144–145
  smoking cessation counseling benefits, q6
  "Welcome to Medicare" physical examination,
    70

Medicare Advantage (MA), 34–35, 34*t*, q73
  advantages and disadvantages of, 36, 37*t*
  healthcare provider payments, 37–38, 38*t*
  types of plans, 35

Medicare Health Maintenance Organizations
  (HMOs), 35

Medicare Health Outcomes Survey, 42

Medicare Modernization Act of 2003, 42

Medicare Personal Plan Finder, 36

Medicare Prescription Drug Improvement and
  Modernization Act of 2003, 42

Medicare Prescription Drug Plan Finder, 35

Medicated urethral system for erection (MUSE),
  435*t*, 436

Medication discussion, 255

Medication lists, 80, 127

Medication review
  annual drug regimen review, 80
  brown-bag evaluation, 78–79
  discharge medication list, 127
  at hospital admission, 120, 121*t*
  quality indicators for dementia, 254
  requirements for long-term care facilities, 147,
    148*t*

Medications. *See* Drugs; Pharmacotherapy;
  specific medications

Medigap, 34*t*, 35–36, 37*t*

Mediterranean diet, q90

Megestrol, 200

Meglitinides, 509*t*

Melanoma, 344–345, 344*f*
  acral lentiginous, 344, 345*f*
  malignant, 461*f*, 462
  superficial spreading, 344, 344*f*

Melatonin, 503, q46

Melatonin receptor agonists, 281, 281*t*

Memantine, 253, q48

Membranoproliferative glomerulonephritis, 408

Membranous nephropathy, 408
Memory problems, q37. *See also* Cognitive
    impairment; Dementia
  three-item recall test for, 68
Memory retraining, 251
Meniere disease, 184, q88
Meningitis, bacterial, 488
Meniscus, 445, 446f
Menopausal symptoms
  CAM for, 85
  treatment of, 416
Menopause, 416, q36
Men's health
  alcohol use among men, 324
  benign prostatic hyperplasia (BPH), 420–423,
      q119
  BMD testing in, 238–239
  cardiovascular disease in, 361f
  criteria that define frailty, 163t
  erectile dysfunction in, 433–434
  gall stones in, 396–397
  hormonal influences in, 236
  indications for bone mineral density testing in,
      238, 238t
  leading causes of death for, 5, 5t
  life expectancy of, 2, 2t
  marital status and living arrangements of, 3,
      3t
  in nursing-home population, 142–143, 143t
  pharmacologic treatment of osteoporosis in,
      245
  prevention of cardiovascular events, q85
  prostate disease, 420–430
  RDAs for micronutrients, 196, 196t
  risk factors for osteoporosis, q111
  sarcopenia, q94
  screening DEXA scan for, 244
  self-reported functional limitations of Medicare
      beneficiaries, 3, 5f
  sexual problems, 67
  stroke in, 464
  suicide rates, 4
  testosterone supplementation for, 501, 502t
  treatment of osteoporosis in, 245
  urinary incontinence in, 207
  urinary tract infections in, 485
Mental health
  acute mental status change, 264–265, 266t
  health insurance coverage for outpatient care,
      34t
  rehabilitation and, 134
  requirements for long-term care facilities, 147,
      148t
  self-efficacy beliefs and, 20, 20t
  social networks and, 21–22, 21t
Mental health problems, 324–325
  diagnosis and treatment of, 331–333
  mental retardation with, 329–330, 330–333
  preadmission screening for, 147, 148t
  requirements for long-term care facilities, 147,
      148t
Mental retardation, 39t, 329–333
  definition of, 329

with developmental disabilities, 332t
  diagnostic issues, 330
  medical disorders with, 333
  mental disorders with, 329–330, 330–333
  preadmission screening for, 147, 148t
  prevalence of, 329–330
  psychiatric disorders with, 330–333
  requirements for long-term care facilities, 147,
      148t
  social conditions with, 333
  treatment issues, 330
Meperidine, 117, 270t, q49
Mesangial glomerulonephritis, 408
Metabolic disorders, 39t, 209t, 491–503
Metabolic encephalopathy, 264
Metabolism
  age-associated changes in, 73
  of drugs, 73
  preoperative assessment and management of,
      96–97
METAGLIP (glipizide and metformin), 510t
Metamucil (psyllium), 399t
Metastatic breast cancer
  initial management of, 527
  quality indicators for, 531
Metatarsal phalangeal joint dislocation, 459f,
      460
Metatarsalgia, 457t
Metformin (Glucophage, Glucophage XR), q104
  for diabetes mellitus, 509t, 511
  glipizide and metformin (METAGLIP), 510t
  glyburide and metformin (Glucovance), 510t
  nutrient interactions, 197–198, 198t
  pioglitazone and metformin (ACTOplus met),
      510t
  repaglinide and metformin (PrandiMet), 510t
  rosiglitazone and metformin (Avandamet), 510t
  sitagliptin and metformin (Janumet), 510t
Methadone, 327, q49
Methicillin-resistant *Staphylococcus aureus*
      (MRSA), 483
Methylcellulose (Citrucel), 399t
Methyldopa, 416
Methylmalonic acid, 519
Methylphenidate, 106, 259, 300t, q4
Methylprednisolone
  for COPD, 357t
  for CPPD, 446
  for dermatomyositis, 448
  for giant cell arteritis, 447
  for polymyositis, 448
Metoclopramide, 76–77, 77t
Metolazone, 379
Metoprolol, 378t, q64
Metronidazole
  for *C difficile*–associated disease, 402, q40
  for diverticulitis, 400
Mexican Curanderos, 82
Mexiletine (Mexitil), 113t
MGUS (monoclonal gammopathy of uncertain
      significance), 529

Michigan Alcoholism Screening Test
      (MAST)—Geriatric Version, 325
Micrographia, 469
Micronase (glyburide), 509t
Micronutrient requirements
  age-related changes in, 196
  recommended dietary allowances, 196, 196t
Micronutrient supplements, 200
Microsporum canis, q32
Microvascular complications of diabetes mellitus,
      508
Midodrine, 231t
Miglitol (Glyset), 509t
Migration history, 51
Mild cognitive impairment
  diagnostic features and treatment of, 248t
  differential diagnosis of, 248
Milk of Magnesia (magnesium hydroxide), 399t
Milnacipran (Savella), 113t
Mind-body relaxation techniques, 85
Mineral oil, 197–198, 198t
Mini-Cog Assessment Instrument for Dementia,
      46, 68, 123, 247
Mini-Nutritional Assessment (MNA), 198
Mini-Nutritional Assessment, short form
      (MNA-SF), 198
Minimal change disease, 408
Mini–Mental State Examination (MMSE), 25,
      44t, 46, 68, 123, 247, 265
  tests of attention, 267t
Minimum Data Set (MDS), 146, 196, 215
  quality measures for nursing homes based on,
      146, 147t
Miotics, 175t
Miralax (polyethylene glycol), 399t
Mirtazapine, q4, q62
  for depression, 300t, 301
  for depressive features of behavioral
      disturbances in dementia, 259, 260t
  for insomnia, 281, 281t
  for sleep disturbances in dementia, 262
  for undernutrition, 200
Mistreatment, 87–91
  bruise characteristics that raise suspicion of,
      q109
  definition of, 87
  financial, 89
  history, 87–88
  of hospitalized patients, 121t, 123–124
  incidence of, 87
  institutional, 90
  interventions for, 90–91, 121t
  medical-legal interface, 91
  physical, 88, q109
  prevalence of, 87
  prevention of, 87
  psychological abuse, 89
  questions to guide intervention for, 90
  risk factors for, 87, 88t
  screening for, 68, 88, 89t

Index

Neuraminidase inhibitors, 484

Neurodermatitis, 336, q110

Neurologic changes, age-related, 11, 12t

Neurologic diseases and disorders, 464–479
  CAM for, 85
  degenerative disorders of, 39t
  and incontinence, 209t
  quality indicators for, 477–478

Neurologic testing, 193
  quality indicators for dementia, 254

Neuroma, 460, q27

Neuromuscular electrical stimulation, 441

Neurontin (gabapentin), 112t

Neuropathic pain, 110–111

Neuropsychiatric concerns, preoperative, 97

Neuroreflexotherapy, 84, 84t

Neurosyphilis, 488–489, q75

New York University College of Nursing
  (NYUCN), 124–125

NHTSA (National Highway Traffic Safety
  Administration), 47

Niacin, q104
  drug interactions, 197–198, 198t
  RDAs for adults ≥ 71 yr old, 196t

NICHE (Nurses Improving Care for Health
  System Elders), 124–125

Nicotine dependence, 327–328

Nicotine replacement, 327

NIH Stroke Scale, 136, 465, 467

Nitrates
  adverse drug events, 76–77, 77t
  for chronic CAD, 365
  drug interactions, 77, 78t

NMES (neuromuscular electrical stimulation),
  441

Nociceptive pain, 110

Nocturia, 210, 210t

Nocturnal limb movements, 282

Nodular basal cell carcinoma, 343

Nodular melanoma, 344

Nodular prurigo, q110

Nodular thyroid disease, 495

Non-Hodgkin's lymphoma, 528–529

Nonadherence to medication regimens, 79–80

Nonconvulsive status epilepticus, 474

Nonmaleficence, 23

Nonsteroidal anti-inflammatory drugs (NSAIDs)
  adverse drug events, 76–77, 77t, 197–198,
    395–396, 396t
  gastric complications, 395–396
  for GI diseases and disorders, 403
  and incontinence, 208t, 214
  for musculoskeletal pain, 442
  for persistent pain, 113t, 115, 117, 118
  for polymyalgia rheumatica, 446
  reduction of, 390
  risk factors for upper GI adverse events,
    395–396, 396t

Nonverbal communication, respectful, 50

Norpramin (desipramine), 112t

Norton Scale, 285–286

Nortriptyline (Aventyl, Pamelor), q18
  for depression, 299t, 301
  for depressive features of behavioral
    disturbances in dementia, 259, 260t
  for persistent pain management, 112t

Novolin (insulin), 511t

Novolin 70/30 (isophane insulin + regular
  insulin), 511t

NovoLog (insulin aspart), 511t

NPH insulin (Humulin, Novolin), 511t

NSAIDs. See Nonsteroidal anti-inflammatory
  drugs

Nucynta (tapentadol), 114t

Numeric Rating Scale, 109–110

Nurse practitioners, 34t
  rehabilitation team role, 133–134, 133t

Nurses Improving Care for Health System Elders
  (NICHE), 124–125

Nursing, 133–134, 133t

Nursing facilities, 6
  staffing patterns, 145

Nursing-home care, 142–150
  availability of, 143–144
  clinical practice guidelines for, 149
  clinical practice in, 149–150
  demographic characteristics of older adults in,
    142–143, 143t
  falls risk in, 226t, 227
  fee for service, 41
  fever in, 481
  financing, 41, 144–145, 144f
  functional characteristics of older adults in,
    142–143, 143t
  health insurance coverage for, 34t
  for hip replacement, q52
  legislation influencing, 146–147
  length of stay in, 144
  managed care, 41
  medical care issues, 148–149
  placement factors, 145
  population, 142–143, 143t
  postacute care, 144
  quality issues, 146–147
  quality measures for, 146, 147t
  sexual activity among residents in, q60
  sleep in, 278
  spending for, 144, 144f
  staffing patterns, 145
  standards of care, 201
  unacceptable weight loss, 201
  urinary incontinence in, 215

Nursing-home populations, q14

Nursing-home–acquired pneumonia, 483

Nutrition
  alternative alimentation, 202
  for chronic kidney disease, 412–413
  disorders, 39t
  drug-nutrient interactions, 197–198, 198t
  for hospitalized patients, 121t, 123
  intake, 196–197
  interventions, 121t, 200

malnutrition, 195–202
  oral, 200
  for prevention of pressure ulcers, 286–287
  to reduce risk of osteoporosis, 237, 237t
  requirements for, 195, 196t
  risk factors for poor status, 198, 198t
  syndromes, 198–199
  total parenteral nutrition, q101
  undernutrition, 198–199

Nutrition assessment, 45, 196–198
  multi-item tools for, 198
  rapid screening followed by assessment and
    management, 43, 44t
  screening evaluations, 68
  threshold to trigger, 201

Nutrition Screening Initiative, 198

Nutritional assessment, q25

Nutritional supplements, q25
  for pressure ulcers, 289
  quality indicators for, 202

NYUCN (New York University College of
  Nursing), 124–125

O

OASIS (Outcome and Assessment Information
  Set), 132, 151

Obesity, 199
  cardiovascular risk, 360–361
  classification of, 196, 197t
  prevalence of, 199
  screening for, 68

OBRA (Omnibus Budget Reconciliation Act), 90,
  146–147, 201

Obsessive-compulsive disorder, 308
  features of, 316, 317t
  treatment strategies for, 310t, 318–319, 319t

Obstruction
  acute colonic pseudo-obstruction, 402
  emergent, 108
  postrenal ARF, 410–411

Obstructive pulmonary disease, chronic, 39t,
  355–356
  anxiety and, 309
  quality indicators for, 359

Obstructive sleep apnea, 209t, 275, 357

Occupational therapy, q24

Occupational therapy (OT), 34t
  for dementia, 251
  for pain, 441–442
  rehabilitation team role, 133–134, 133t

Odd or eccentric behaviors, 316, 317t

Office-based house-call programs, 152–153

Office visits, 43, 251

25(OH)D, 237, 238t, 496, q13

Olanzapine
  for agitated delirium, 270–271, 271t
  for depression, 301
  dosing and adverse events of, 313, 314t
  for Parkinson's disease and hallucinations,
    315

Pain management, 111–112
  in diabetic neuropathy, q49
  nonpharmacologic therapy, 111–112, 441–442
  pharmacologic therapy, 112–115, 442
  postoperative, 100
  reassessment of, 118
  in vertebral compression fractures, 243–244
Paliperidone, 261–262, 261t
Palliative care, 102–108
  cultural aspects of, 103
  endoscopic palliation, 395
  ethnographic data, 103
  frailty and, 167
  hospice, 103–104
  overall care near death, 103
  quality indicators for, 104, 107–108
Palsy, progressive supranuclear, 471–472
Pamelor (nortriptyline), 112t
Panic attacks, 307–308, q76
Panic disorder, 307–308, 310t
Pantothenic acid, 196t
Pao₂, 354
Pap smear, q36
  Medicare coverage and cost-effectiveness of,
    64t
  recommendations for, 62t, 65
Papaverine, 435t, 436
Paranoia, 257
Paranoid personality disorder
  features of, 316, 317t
  therapeutic strategies for, 318–319, 319t
Parathyroid hormone (teriparatide)
  for osteoporosis prevention and treatment,
    241t, 243
  and renal bone disease, 412
  screening for secondary osteoporosis, 237,
    238t
  secondary hyperparathyroidism, 236
Parathyroid hormone-related peptide (PTHrp),
  498
Parathyroid metabolism disorders, 495–499
Parathyroid sestamibi (nuclear scan), q13
Parkinson's disease, 468–471
  assistive devices for, q3
  CAM for, 85
  clinical features of, 469
  falls with, q117
  gait of, q12
  and incontinence, 209t
  interventions for preventing falls, 231t
  psychosis in, 315
  seborrheic dermatitis in, q96
Parkinson's plus disease, 471
Paronychia, 462
Paroxetine, 259, 260t, 299t, q64
Passive-aggressive personality disorder
  features of, 316, 317t
  therapeutic strategies for, 318–319, 319t
Past medical history, 120, 121t
Patient education
  about diabetes, 511–512
  about stroke, 478

guidelines for prevention of falls, 230
  HF education, 383
  for persistent pain, 118
  for pharmacotherapy, 80
  sleep hygiene education, 282
Patient Health Questionnaire (PHQ), 44t, 46, 68
  indications to start antidepressant therapy
    based on, 296, 296t
  screening questions and complete assessment,
    296, 296t
Patient safety. See also Safety
  quality indicators for dementia, 255
Pay for performance, 42
PCI. See Percutaneous coronary intervention
PE. See Pulmonary embolism
Peak expiratory flow meters and inhalers, 356
Pediculosis capitis, 342
Pediculosis corporis, 342
Pediculosis pubis, 342
Pegaptanib sodium, 172
Pelvic examination, 415–416
  Medicare coverage and cost-effectiveness of,
    64t
Pelvic floor support disorders, 418–419
Pelvic muscle exercises, 212
  with bladder training, 212t
  for urinary incontinence, 211, 212t
Pelvic organ prolapse, 418, 419t, q91
Pelvic Organ Prolapse Quantification (POPQ),
  418
Pelvic pain, q7
Pelvis, fracture of, 39t
Penile prosthesis, 435t, 436
Peptic ulcer disease, 396
Percocet (oxycodone, immediate release), 114t
Percodan (oxycodone, immediate release), 114t
Percutaneous coronary intervention (PCI)
  for acute coronary syndrome, 363
  for chronic CAD, 365
Percutaneous endoscopic gastrostomy or
  jejunostomy, 205
Percutaneous endoscopic gastrostomy tubes, q62
Performance-based functional assessment, 221
Performance-Oriented Mobility Assessment
  (POMA), 45, 227–229
Performance status, q97
Perindopril, 378t, 380
Periodic limb movements during sleep, 276
Periodic retinal examination, 512
Periodontal anatomy, 346, 346f
Periodontal ligament, 347
Periodontitis, 347
Periodontium, 347
Perioperative care, 92–102
  quality indicators for, 101
Periostitis, 457t
Peripheral arterial disease, 371–373
  diagnosis of, 372
  and foot, 463
  treatment of, 372–373

Peripheral neuropathy, 476–477
Peripheral vascular disease, 39t
Peripheral vasculature, 188
Peripheral venous insufficiency, 209t
Periurethral bulking injections, 213t
Perphenazine, 313, 314t
Persantine thallium testing, q2
Persistent pain, 109–119
  assessment of, 109–111
  education for, 118
  nonopioid medications to treat, 117
  pharmacotherapy for, 112–115, 112t–114t
  quality indicators for, 118
  screening for, 118
  treatment of, 111–117
Personality disorders, 316–320
  diagnostic challenges, 317–318
  differential diagnosis of, 318
  epidemiology of, 316–317
  features of, 316, 317t
  long-term course, 318
  major depressive disorder with, q63
  narcissistic, q84
  not otherwise specified, 316
  provisional, 316, 317t
  therapeutic strategies for, 318–319, 318–320,
    319t
Personhood, 30
Pes cavus, 457t
Pes planus, 456–458, 457t
Pes valgo planus, 457t
Pessaries, 214, 418–419, q91
Phantom limb pain, 139
Pharmacodynamics
  age-associated changes in, 74–75
  chemotherapy issues, 524, 525t
Pharmacokinetics
  age-associated changes in, 72–74
  chemotherapy issues, 524, 525t
Pharmacotherapy, 72–81
  adverse drug events, 76–77, 76t, 77t
  for agitated delirium, 270–271, 271t
  anticonvulsant therapy, 475t
  for benign prostatic hyperplasia, 421, 422t
  for dementia, 252–254
  for depression, 298–301
  for diastolic HF, 380
  for GI diseases and disorders, 403–404
  for hypertension, 386–388
  inappropriate prescribing, 75–76, 75t, 76t
  investigational agents for osteoporosis, 243
  for mania, 301, 302t
  for musculoskeletal diseases and disorders,
    442, 449
  non-insulin agents for diabetes mellitus,
    509t–510t
  nonadherence to regimens, 79–80
  optimizing prescribing, 75–76
  for osteoporosis, 240–243, 241t, 245
  for pain, 112–115
  for persistent pain, 112–115, 112t–114t
  prescribing cascade, 77

Poverty rates, 2

PPD (tuberculin skin test), q41

PPOs (preferred provider organizations), 35

PPS (prospective payment system), 144–145, 150–151

PQRI (Physician Quality Reporting Initiative), 42

Pra (Probability of Repeated Admission) Questionnaire, 160

Pradaxa (dabigatran etexilate), 370

Pramipexole, 469

Pramlintide (Symlin), 510t

PrandiMet (repaglinide and metformin), 510t

Prandin (repaglinide), 509t

Prasugrel, 363, 374

Prealbumin, 197

Precose (acarbose), 509t

Prediabetes, 504–505

Prednisolone, 447

Prednisone, q108
 for dermatomyositis, 448
 for giant cell arteritis, 447
 for gout, 445
 for musculoskeletal pain, 442
 for polymyalgia rheumatica, 446
 for polymyositis, 448
 for rheumatoid arthritis, 444

Preferred provider organizations (PPOs), 35

Pregabalin (Lyrica)
 and incontinence, 208t
 for persistent pain, 112t, 117

Prehabilitative approach, 125

Prehypertension, 384, 384t

Preoperative assessment and management, 92–97
 preoperative discussion, 100
 quality indicators for care, 100–101
 quality indicators for evaluation, 100–101

Presbycusis, 177–178, q27

Presbyesophagus, 203

Prescribing. See also Medication review
 inappropriate prescribing, 75–76, 75t, 76t
 optimizing, 75–76
 principles of, 78–79, 79t

Prescribing cascade, 77

Prescription drugs. See Drugs; Pharmacotherapy

Presenilin 1 (PS1), 246

Presenilin 2 (PS2), 246

Pressure Sore Status Tool, 291

Pressure Ulcer Scale for Healing, 291

Pressure ulcers, 285–293
 assessment of, 288, 289t, 294
 Braden Scale, 286
 complications from, 293
 control of infections in, 291–293
 dressings for, 288–289, 292t
 epidemiology of, 285–286
 guidelines for management, 288
 guidelines for prevention, 286
 management of, 288, 289t, 294
 monitoring healing of, 291
 Norton Scale, 285–286

prevention of, 286–288, 288t
 quality indicators for, 293–294
 reducing, in acute-care settings, q80
 and rehabilitation, 134
 risk-assessment scales, 285–286
 risk factors for, 285–286
 sacral, q99
 staging system for, 288, 290t, 291
 support surfaces for older adults at risk of, 287, 288t
 surgical repair of, 289
 treatment of, 288–293, q99

Presyncope, 184, 185t

Prevention, 61–71
 aspirin therapy, 63t, 69
 of atherosclerotic complications of diabetes mellitus, 507–508
 available health measures for, 61, 62t–63t
 cost-effectiveness of, 61, 64t
 counseling on, 69–70
 of falls, 225, 227, 228f, 229–230, 231t–232t
 health insurance coverage for services, 33, 34t
 of hip fracture recurrence, 138
 Medicare coverage for services, 61, 64t, 70
 of microvascular complications of diabetes mellitus, 508
 of mistreatment, 87
 osteoporosis advice, 244
 physical activity benefits for, 55
 of pressure ulcers, 286–288, 294
 quality indicators for, 70–71, 294
 recommended measures for, 61, 62t–63t
 of stroke, 466, 477
 of surgical site infections, 101

Prevention reminders, 71, 160

Primary care
 comprehensive geriatric assessment (CGA) in, 157–158
 enhanced, 158–159
 geriatrics in, 157–159
 GRACE model of, 158–159

Primidone, 270t

Private contracts, 33

Private FFS plans, 35

Probability of Repeated Admission Questionnaire (Pra), 160

Probenecid, 445, q108

Problem-solving therapy, 303, 304t

Problem substance use, 322

Productivity, 21

Progesterone
 estrogen and progesterone counseling, 375
 for hypersexuality in dementia, 263

Program of All-inclusive Care of the Elderly (PACE), 40–41, 154–155, q67

Progressive supranuclear palsy, 471–472

Prolapse
 pelvic organ, 418, 419t
 surgery for, 419

Prometheus Prescribing Program, 400–401

Prompted voiding, 212, 212t

Propantheline, 214

Propoxyphene (Darvon, Darvocet), 117, q49

Propulsion, 219t

Prospective payment system (PPS), 144–145, 150–151

Prostaglandins, 174–175, 175t

Prostate cancer, 423–428
 advanced, 426t–427t, 428
 CAM for, 86
 diagnostic tests, 424
 ethnic and racial differences in incidence, 523, 523t
 expectant or conservative management of, 425
 grading, 424
 hormonal therapy for, 524–525, 525t
 incidence and epidemiology of, 423
 locally advanced, 426t, 428
 management of, 425–427, 426t–427t, 428
 staging, 424–425, 424t
 surveillance, 425
 symptoms of, 423
 treatment of, q119

Prostate cancer screening, 424
 controversy, 423
 Medicare coverage and cost-effectiveness of, 64t
 recommendations for, 65–66

Prostate disease, 420–430
 indications for referral, 429
 quality indicators for, 429–430

Prostate-specific antigen testing, 424
 Medicare coverage and cost-effectiveness of, 64t
 quality indicators for prostate disease, 429
 recommendations for, 62t, 65–66

Prostatectomy, radical, 425–427, 426t

Prostatic hyperplasia, benign, 420–423
 anejaculatory orgasms with, q119
 CAM for, 85

Prostatism, 421

Prostatitis, 428–429

Prostheses, penile, 435t, 436

Prosthetic device infections, 486–487

Prosthetic Profile of the Amputee, 139

Prosthetic rehabilitation, 139

Prosthetists, 133–134, 133t

Protein-energy undernutrition, 199

Protein error theory of aging, 9–10

Protein intake guidelines, 195

Protein modification theory of aging, 10

Protein requirements, 195, 196t

Protein supplements, 202

Proteinuria, 512

Proton-pump inhibitors
 adverse drug events, 197–198
 for GERD, 393–394

Provider-sponsored organizations (PSOs), 35

Proxy, 26

Pruritus, 337–338

Pseudo-obstruction, acute colonic, 402

Pseudoaddiction, 116

Pseudoclaudication, 451

Resistance training
    exercise programs, q29
    for preventing falls, 231t
    for preventing sarcopenia, q94
    recommendations for, 56t
Resource Benecalorie, 199t
Resource Breeze, 199t
Resource utilization groups (RUGS), 39
Respect for autonomy, 23
Respect for life, 103
Respectful nonverbal communication, 50
Respiration, loud, 107
Respiratory diseases and disorders, 353–359
    antibiotic therapy for infections, 481–482,
        482t
    chronic lower respiratory disease, 5, 5t
    evaluation of symptoms, 359
    preoperative assessment and management of,
        95–96
    pulmonary disease, 355–358
    quality indicators for, 359
    symptoms and complaints, 354–355
Restless legs syndrome, 276
Restraints, 30, 124
    quality indicators for behavioral problems in
        dementia, 263
    quality indicators for dementia, 255
Retinal detachment, 169, 169t
Retinal examination, periodic, 512
Retinopathy, diabetic, 168t, 172–174, 174f
Retropubic suspension, 213t
Retropulsion, 219t
Revascularization
    for chronic CAD, 365–366
    for peripheral arterial disease, 372–373
    quality indicators for, 374
Review of systems at hospital admission, 120,
        121t
Rheumatic mitral stenosis, 366
Rheumatoid arthritis, 443–444, 445t
Rheumatoid factor, 438
Rheumatologic diseases, 442–448
Rhinosinusitis, 354
Rhythm abnormalities, 230
Riboflavin, 196t
Rifampin, 486
Rimantadine, 484
Risedronate, 240, 241t, q93
Risperidone
    for agitated delirium, 270–271, 271t
    dosing and adverse events of, 313, 314t
    for psychosis in dementia, 261–262, 261t
    to stabilize mood in mania and bipolar
        disorder, 301, 302t
Rituximab, 526
Rivastigmine, 252, 253
RLS (restless legs syndrome), 276
Role loss and acquisition, 19
Rolling assessment, 43
Ropinirole, 469
Rosacea, 335, 335f

Rosiglitazone (Avandia), 510t, 511
Rosiglitazone and glimepiride (Avandaryl), 510t
Rosiglitazone and metformin (Avandamet), 510t
Roxanol (morphine, immediate release), 114t
RUGS (resource utilization groups), 39

S

S-adenosylmethionine (SAM-e), 82–83, 83t,
        84–85
Sacral fractures, osteoporotic, 452
Sacral nerve neuromodulation, 214
Sacral pressure ulcers, q99
Safe Return, 252
Safety, 68–69
    attention to, 252
    of CAM therapies, 82–83
    and dementia, 252
    home safety evaluation, 232, 232t
    preventing injury, 68–69
    quality indicators for dementia, 255
Salflex (salsalate), 113t
Salicylates, 197–198, 198t
Saline laxatives, 399t
Saliva, decreased, q113
Salivary function, 348–349
Salivary glands, 346, 346t
Salivary stones (sialoliths), q113
Salix alba (white willow bark), 84
Salmeterol, 356, 357t
Salsalate (Disalcid, Mono-Gesic, Salflex), 113t
Salt depletion, primary, 406
SAM-e (S-adenosylmethionine), 82–83, 83t,
        84–85
Sarcopenia, 203, q10, q94
Sarcoptes scabei var hominis, 341
Savella (milnacipran), 113t
Saw palmetto (Serenoa repens)
    for benign prostatic hyperplasia, 85, 422
    safety issues, 82–83, 83t
Saxagliptin (Onglyza), 509t
Scabies, 341–342
Schizoid personality disorder
    features of, 316, 317t
    therapeutic strategies for, 318–319, 319t
Schizophrenia and schizophrenia-like syndromes,
        312–314
    clinical characteristics of, 313
    epidemiology of, 313
    late-onset schizophrenia, 312, 313
    treatment and management of, 313–314
Schizophrenia-like psychosis
    late-onset, 313
    very-late-onset, 312
Schizotypal personality disorder
    features of, 316, 317t
    therapeutic strategies for, 318–319, 319t
Sciatica, 451
Scissoring, 219t
Scleritis, 169, 169t
Scooters, motorized, 140

Screening, 66–67
    abdominal aorta, q47
    for cancer, 61–66, 524
    cognitive, 254
    for colorectal cancer, 404, 531
    criteria for recommending, 61
    for depression, 255, 296–297, 305, 374
    DEXA, 244
    for falls, 232
    functional, 254
    for hearing loss, 178, 182, q17
    for hypoxemia, 359
    for mistreatment, 88, 89t
    nutrition, 196–198
    for osteoporosis, q47
    for persistent pain, 118
    PHQ-9 questions, 296, 296t
    physical activity, 58
    for postoperative delirium, 101
    for prostate cancer, 423, 424
    quality indicators for, 48, 71
    rapid, 43, 44t
    recommendations for, 61, 62t
    for secondary osteoporosis, 237, 238t
    for sleep problems, 282
    for urinary incontinence, 210, 216
    USPSTF Screening Guidelines, 524
Seborrheic dermatitis, 334–335, q96
Seborrheic keratoses, 342, 342f
Section 8, Housing and Urban Development
        programs, 156
Sedating antidepressants, 281, 281t
Sedating antihistamines, 277
Sedating antipsychotics, 281
Sedation, home, q69
Sedative/hypnotics
    adverse drug events, 76–77, 77t
    chronic use, 281–282
    and incontinence, 208t
    interventions for preventing falls with, 231t
    for sleep problems, 278
Seizures, 39t, 473
    anticonvulsant therapy for, 474, 475t
    with developmental disabilities, 332t
    signs and symptoms of, 192t
Selective estrogen-receptor modulators, 241t, 242
Selective norepinephrine-reuptake inhibitors
        (SNRIs)
    for anxiety disorders, 310t
    for depression, 299t
    for depressive features of behavioral
        disturbances in dementia, 260t
Selective serotonin-reuptake inhibitors (SSRIs)
    adverse drug events, 76–77, 77t, 197–198
    for anxiety attacks, q76
    for anxiety disorders, 310t
    for dementia, 254
    for depression, 298–301, 299t
    for depressive features of behavioral
        disturbances in dementia, 259, 260t
    nutrient interactions, 197–198, 198t
    for vasomotor symptoms or hot flushes, 416

Somatoform disorders, 320–321
  clinical characteristics and causes of, 320
  not otherwise specified, 320
  treatment of, 321
  undifferentiated, 320
Somatoform pain disorders, 110
Sorbitol 70%, 399*t*
Soy foods, q38
Spasticity, 134
Special needs, 42
Special needs plans, 35
Specialty care, geriatric, 157
Speech, 177
Speech therapy, 34*t*
  quality indicators for neurologic diseases and
    disorders, 478
  rehabilitation team role, 133–134, 133*t*
Spinal cord dysfunction, 475
Spinal cord injury, 209*t*
Spinal deformities, 332*t*
Spinal manipulation, 84, 84*t*
Spinal stenosis, 209*t*
Spirituality, 22, 53–54
Spironolactone, 379
Squamous cell carcinoma, 344
  oral, 349
  oropharyngeal, 349
Squamous hyperplasia, 418
SSI (Supplemental Security Income), 156
SSRIs. *See* Selective serotonin-reuptake
    inhibitors
ST. *See* Speech therapy
St. John's wort *(Hypericum perforatum)*, 84
  for depression, 300*t*
  safety issues, 82–83, 83*t*
Stabilization, 325–326
Staffing patterns, 145
Staphylococcus aureus, 483
Starlix (nateglinide), 509*t*
Stasis dermatitis, 339
Statins
  for acute coronary syndrome, 362
  for atherosclerotic complications of diabetes
    mellitus, 508
  for chronic CAD, 364
  perioperative, 93–95, 95*t*
Stem cell/progenitor cell theory of aging, 11
Stem cells, hematopoietic, 513–514
Steppage gait, 219*t*
Stimulant laxatives, 399*t*
Stimulants, 300*t*
Stimulation-oriented treatment, 251
Stimulus control, 279*t*
STIs (sexually transmitted infections), 67
Stomach disorders, 395–397
Stomatitis, denture, 350–351, 350*f*
Strength training, q45
Streptococcus pneumoniae, 483
Stress
  caregiver, 108

mediators, 20–21
moderators, 21–22
posttraumatic stress disorder, 308–309, 310*t*
Stress incontinence, 207, q23
  and impaired urethral sphincter support, 209
  minimally invasive procedures for, 214
  surgery for, 214–215, 217
  treatment of, 212*t*–213*t*, 214
Stress management, 84
Stress testing
  noninvasive, 374
  preoperative, 93
Stress theory model, 17, 18*f*
Stressors, 17–19
Stroke
  acute ischemic, 466–467
  approach to management of, 136–137
  goals of rehabilitation after, 136
  guidelines for rehabilitation after, 136
  incidence of, 464
  and incontinence, 209*t*
  ischemic, 477
  NIH Stroke Scale, 136, 465, 467
  patient education about, 478
  prevalence of, 3, 4*f*
  prevention of, 255, 370, 466, 477
  quality indicators for, 477
  rehabilitation after, 136–137
  risk factors for, 464–465, q42
Stroke Impact Scale, 132*t*, 136
Strontium ranelate, 243
Subclinical hypothyroidism, 492
Subconjunctival hemorrhage, 169*t*, 170, 171
Subdural hematoma, 467
Subluxation, foot, 457*t*
Substance abuse
  at-risk use, 322
  counseling interventions for, 64*t*
  definition of, 322–323
  identifying substance-use disorders, 325
  Medicare coverage for treatment of, 64*t*
  outpatient management of, 327–328
  pharmacotherapy for, 327
  risks and benefits of, 324–325
  treatment of, 325–328
Substance Abuse and Mental Health Services
    Administration, 327
Substance dependence, 322
Substituted judgment, 25*t*, 26
Suicidality, 305
Suicide, 4
  physician-assisted, 28
Suicide risk assessment, q55
Sulfonylureas, 2nd-generation, 508, 509*t*
Superficial basal cell carcinoma, 343
Superficial spreading melanoma, 344, 344*f*
Supplemental Security Income (SSI), 156
Supplements, 200
Supplies for house calls, 152, 153*t*
Support groups, 251
Support surfaces, 287–288, 288*t*

Supraventricular arrhythmias, 370
Supraventricular tachycardia, 370
Surfactant laxatives, 399*t*
Surgical care
  for benign prostatic hyperplasia, 421,
    422–423, 422*t*
  for breast cancer, 530, q51
  breast conservation treatment, q51
  bypass surgery, 365–366
  for cancer, 526
  cardiac risk assessment for, 93, 94*f*
  discussion of surgical findings, 531
  for epilepsy, 474
  extensive operating room procedures unrelated
    to principal diagnosis, 39*t*
  for foot deformities, 461
  for gait disorders, 222
  for hip fracture, 137
  hip replacement, q31, q52
  iatrogenic complications, 97
  for incontinence, 214–215
  incontinence after, 212*t*, 213*t*
  knee replacement, q89
  noncardiac, 93, 94*f*
  for osteoarthritis, 443
  overview of operative therapy, 92
  for pelvic organ prolapse, q91
  perioperative care, 92–102
  postoperative delirium, 267–268, q16
  postoperative management of, 97–100
  postoperative surveillance, 532
  preoperative assessment and management of,
    92–97
  preoperative evaluation before hip
    replacement, q31
  preoperative examination, 531
  preoperative ostomy siting, 532
  for pressure ulcers, 289
  for prolapse, 419
  for prostate cancer, 425–427
  for stress incontinence, 213*t*, 217
  total hip and knee arthroplasty, 138–139
  for vertebral compression fractures, 244
Surgical documentation, 530
Surgical site infections, 101
Surveillance
  limiting, 531
  postoperative, 532
  for prostate cancer, 425
Suspiciousness, isolated, 313
Swallowing, 203–205
Swallowing difficulties, q101, q113
Swallowing training, 206
Swinging flashlight test, 168
Symlin (pramlintide), 510*t*
Syncope, 188–194
  causes of, 188, 189*t*
  classes of, 191, 192*t*
  evaluation of, 189–193, 190*f*
  history in, 189–191
  indications for permanent pacemaker
    implantation, 371, 371*t*
  natural history of, 188–189

Syncope *(continued)*
  with orthostatic hypotension, q5
  physical examination of, 191–192
  prognosis for, 189
  recurrent, 194, q5
  signs and symptoms of, 191, 192*t*
  treatment of, 193–194
  unexplained, q33
  vasovagal, 189, 192*t*, 194
Syndrome of inappropriate antidiuretic hormone
    (SIADH), 405, 406, 407, 499, q100
Syndromes, 161–293
Synovial fluid analysis, q54
Syphilis, 488–489, q75
Systematic assessment, 120, 121*t*
Systemic lupus erythematosus, 447–448
Systems biology
  and aging, 16
  of frailty, 166, 166*f*
Systems of care, 119–161
Systems review, 120, 121*t*
Systolic hypertension, q106

T

T$_3$ (L-triiodothyronine), 300*t*, 301
T$_3$ (triiodothyronine) thyrotoxicosis, 494
T$_4$. *See* Thyroxine
Tachy-brady syndrome, 371–372
Tachykinesia, 469
Tachyphemia, 469
Tacrine, 252
Tadalafil, 435–436, 435*t*
Tai Chi
  for preventing falls, 57, 229, 231*t*
  recommendations for, 56*t*, 67
  for sleep problems, 279–280
Tailor's bunion, 457*t*
Talk test, 56–57
Tamsulosin, q119
Tapentadol (Nucynta), 114*t*
Tardive dyskinesia, 313–314
Target theory of genetic damage, 9
Tarsal tunnel syndrome, 457*t*
Taste dysfunction
  age-related changes, 351–352
  medications that cause, 352, 352*t*
  nonpharmacologic causes of, 352, 352*t*
Teams, rehabilitation, 133–134, 133*t*
Technetium bone scan, 453–454
Teeth
  age-related changes in, 346, 346*t*
  anatomy of, 346, 346*f*
Tegretol (carbamazepine), 112*t*
Telecoil, 181
Telephone quit lines, 64*t*
Telmisartan, 378*t*
Temazepam, 280, 281*t*
Temporal (giant cell) arteritis, 446–447, q98
  headache due to, 468
  signs and symptoms of, 169
Temporal artery biopsy, q98

Tendinitis, 437
Tenosynovitis, 457*t*
TENS (transcutaneous electrical nerve
    stimulation), 441
Teriparatide (parathyroid hormone), 241*t*, 243
Terminal illness
  anorexia in, 105
  cachexia in, 105
  constipation in, 104
  cough in, 107
  delirium in, 105
  depression in, 105–106
  diarrhea in, 105
  dyspnea in, 106–107
  nause and vomiting in, 104–105
  palliative care, 104–107
Terminology
  glossary of gait abnormalities, 218, 219*t*
  preferred terms for cultural or religious
      identity, 49
  shoe terms, 460*t*
Testamentary competence, 24–25
Testosterone, 500–501
  screening for secondary osteoporosis, 237,
      238*t*
  for undernutrition, 200
Testosterone replacement therapy, 500–501
Testosterone supplementation
  available preparations, 501, 502*t*
  benefits and risks for men, 501, 502*t*
  for erectile dysfunction, 436
  for female sexual dysfunction, 432, 500
Tests
  continuity of, 160
  quality indicators for outpatient care systems,
      160
Tetanus booster, 62*t*, 69
Theophylline
  adverse drug events, 197–198
  nutrient interactions, 197–198, 198*t*
Theories of aging, 8–11
Thiamine, 196*t*
Thiazide diuretics, 387, q43
  for hypertension, q106
  side effects of, q100
Thiazolidinediones
  for diabetes mellitus, 509*t*–510*t*, 511
  and incontinence, 208*t*
Thinking problems. *See* Cognitive impairment
Thrombocythemia, essential, 520
Thrombocytopenia, 520
Thromboembolism
  pulmonary, 358
  venous, 98, 98*t*, 373–374
Thrombolytic therapy, 478
Thrombopathy, 520
Thrombosis, venous, 101, 128
Thrombotic thrombocytopenic purpura, 519
Thrush, 350–351, 350*f*
Thyroid disorders, 491–496
  cancer, 495

  with developmental disabilities, 332*t*
  nodular, 495
  screening for, 66
Thyroid hormone replacement, 492
Thyroid hormone requirements, 494
Thyroid medications, q102
Thyroid-stimulating hormone (thyrotropin), 237,
    238*t*
  low thyrotropin, 493*f*, 494
  screening test, 62*t*, 491
Thyroid ultrasonography, 495, 495*t*
Thyroidectomy, q102
Thyrotoxicosis
  apathetic, 494
  triiodothyronine (T$_3$), 494
Thyrotropin (thyroid-stimulating hormone)
  low thyrotropin, 493*f*, 494
  screening test, 62*t*, 491
Thyroxine (T$_4$)
  high T$_4$ syndrome, 494
  low T$_4$ syndrome, 492–494
  replacement therapy, 494
Tiagabine, 475*t*
Tibialis posterior dysfunction, 457*t*, 458, 458*f*
Ticlopidine, 375
Tilt-table testing, 193, q33
Timed Up and Go (TUG) test, 44*t*, 221, 227
Timolol, 175*t*
Tinnitus, 178
Tinnitus Handicap Questionnaire, q17
Tiotropium bromide, 357*t*
Tissue plasminogen activator
  inclusion and exclusion criteria for, 478
  recombinant tPA (alteplase), 466–467
TMP (trimethoprim), 197–198, 198*t*
TMP-SMX (trimethoprim-sulfamethoxazole),
    484–485, q116
Tobacco dependence, 70, 327–328
α-Tocopherol (vitamin E)
  for dementia, 253
  RDAs for adults $\geq$ 71 yr old, 196*t*
Tolcapone, 470
Tolerance, 116
Tolterodine, 213*t*, 214, q18
Tongue, black hairy, 351, 351*f*
Tongue ulcers, q115
Toothlessness, 347–348
Topiramate, 475*t*
Total hip and knee arthroplasty, 138–139
  assessment of, 138
  management of, 138–139
  natural history of, 138
  quality indicators for, 449
Total joint replacement
  hip replacement, q31, q52
  knee replacement, q89
  total hip and knee arthroplasty, 449
Total parenteral nutrition, q101
Toxic or metabolic encephalopathy, 264

Toxicity
  chemotherapy, 524, 525*t*
  digoxin, 383
  ototoxicity, q27
    water intoxication, q100
Tracheostomy, 39*t*
Tradition, 51
Tramadol (Ultram), 114*t*, 117
Trandolapril, 378*t*
Transcutaneous electrical nerve stimulation, 441
Transdermal fentanyl (Duragesic), 114*t*
Transesophageal echocardiography, 486
Transfer skills impairment, 231*t*
"Transfers" to postacute care, 39, 39*t*
Transient ischemic attack, 465
Transient loss of consciousness, 189, 190*f*
Transitions in care
  from hospital care, 126–127
  planning for, 100
Transplantation, kidney, 414
Tranylcypromine, 300*t*, 301
Trastuzumab, 526
Trauma
  history of traumatic experiences, 50
  posttraumatic stress disorder, 308–309, 310*t*
  urologic trauma, 429
Trazodone, q46
  adverse drug events, 76–77, 77*t*
  for depression, 300*t*
  for depressive features of behavioral
    disturbances in dementia, 260*t*
  for insomnia, 281, 281*t*
  for sleep disturbances in dementia, 262
Treadmill stress testing, q2
Treatment decisions
  ETHNICS mnemonic, 53–54
  in extended-care settings, 29
  following preferences, 31
  life-sustaining treatment decisions, 31
Treatment initiation programs, 303, 304*t*
Tremors
  essential tremor, 472–473
  "pill rolling" tremor, 249
Trendelenburg gait, 219*t*
Trends, 3–4
Triamcinolone acetonide, 446
Triazolam, 270*t*
Trichophyton rubrum, q32
Tricyclic antidepressants
  adverse drug events, 76–77, 77*t*
  and delirium, 270*t*
  for depression, 299*t*
  for depressive features of behavioral
    disturbances in dementia, 259, 260*t*
  ECG for use of, 305
  and incontinence, 208*t*
  for persistent pain, 112*t*, 117
L-Triiodothyronine (T₃), 300*t*, 301
Triiodothyronine (T₃) thyrotoxicosis, 494
Trimethoprim, 197–198, 198*t*

Trimethoprim-sulfamethoxazole (TMP-SMX),
  484–485, q116
Trospium, 213*t*, 214
Truth telling, 29
Try This, 43
TTP (thrombotic thrombocytopenic purpura), 519
Tube feeding, 204, 205
Tuberculin skin test (PPD), q41
Tuberculosis, 485–486, q41
Tubular necrosis, acute, 409–410
TUG (Timed Up and Go) test, 44*t*, 221, 227
Turn en bloc, 219*t*
Tylenol (acetaminophen), 112*t*
Tylox (oxycodone, immediate release), 114*t*

U

UI. *See* Urinary incontinence
Ulcers, 339–340
  aphthous ulcers, 351, 351*f*
  arterial ulcers, 339–340, 339*t*
  corneal, 169*t*
  decubitus ulcer, 285
  foot ulcers, 463
  NSAID-induced, 395–396
  peptic ulcer disease, 396
  pressure ulcers, 285–293, q80, q99
  tongue, q115
  venous ulcers, 339–340, 339*t*
Ultram (tramadol), 114*t*
Ultrasound
  abdominal, 62*t*, 66
  abdominal aorta, q47
  therapeutic, 441
  thyroid, 495, 495*t*
Undernutrition, 198–199, 200
Underprescribing, 75, 75*t*, 76
Unspoken challenging medical issues, 51–52
Unstable lumbar spine, 451
Urethral catheters, chronic, 217
Urethral sphincter support, impaired, 209
Urge incontinence, 207, q61
  minimally invasive procedures for, 214
  treatment of, 212*t*–213*t*
  and uninhibited bladder contractions, 209
Urgencies, hypertensive, 389, 391
Urinary frequency, q7
Urinary incontinence, 207–217, q23
  annual assessment of, 216
  behavioral therapies for, 211–212, 212*t*
  classification of, 217
  comorbid conditions that can cause or worsen,
    208, 209*t*
  discussion of treatment options, 217
  due to cystocele, q56
  evaluation of, 210–211
  functional, 207
  history in, 210
  with impaired bladder emptying, 209–210
  from incomplete emptying, 207
  incontinence examination, 216
  incontinence history, 216

lower urinary tract pathophysiology in,
    208–210
  management of, 211–215
  medications that can cause or worsen, 208,
    208*t*
  minimally invasive procedures for, 214
  mixed UI, 207, 209
  nonpharmacologic interventions for, q103
  in nursing-home residents, 215
  pathophysiology of, 208–210
  physical examination with, 210–211
  prevalence and impact of, 207–208
  prevention of, 67–68
  quality indicators for, 216–217
  response to treatment of, 217
  risk factors for, 208
  screening for, 62*t*, 210
  stress UI, 207, 209, q23
  supportive care for, 215
  surgery for, 214–215
  testing for, 211
  transient, 207
  treatment of, 211–215, 212*t*–213*t*
  types of, 207
  urge UI, 207, 209, q61
Urinary retention, q18, q56
Urinary system, 12*t*, 15
Urinary tract atrophy, q30
Urinary tract infections, 39*t*, 484–485
  antibiotic therapy for, 481–482, 482*t*
  in men, 485
  in women, 484–485
Urine evaluation, 216
  postvoid residual (PVR), 211, q18
  preoperative, 429
  quality indicators for prostate disease, 429
Urodynamic testing, 211, 217
Urogenital atrophy, 416–417
Urogenital symptoms, 416
Urogynecologic disorders, 85
Urologic trauma, 429
Urosepsis, q116
U.S. Department of Agriculture (USDA), 195
U.S. Department of Health and Human Services
  (HHS), 56–57
U.S. Preventive Services Task Force (USPSTF),
  61
  recommendations for BMD testing, 238
  recommendations for prostate cancer
    screening, 423
  Screening Guidelines, 524
Uveitis, 169, 169*t*

V

Vaccinations
  herpes zoster, 62*t*, 69, q86
  for hospitalized patients, 121*t*
  pneumococcal, 62*t*, 64*t*, 69, 121*t*, 483
Vacuum tumescence devices, 435*t*, 436
Vaginal atrophy, 431, q30, q36, q65
Vaginal bleeding, postmenopausal, 419–420,
  419*t*, q65